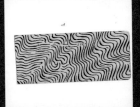

FUNDAMENTALS *of*
Sleep Medicine

FUNDAMENTALS *of*

Sleep Medicine

Richard B. Berry, MD
Professor of Medicine
University of Florida, Gainesville
Medical Director
University of Florida and Shands Sleep Disorder Center
Gainesville, Florida

1600 John F. Kennedy Blvd.
Ste 1800
Philadelphia, PA 19103-2899

FUNDAMENTALS OF SLEEP MEDICINE   ISBN: 978-1-4377-0326-9

Library of Congress Cataloging-in-Publication Data

Berry, Richard B., 1947–
    Fundamentals of sleep medicine / Richard B. Berry.
        p. ; cm.
    Includes bibliographical references and index.
    ISBN 978-1-4377-0326-9 (pbk. : alk. paper)   1. Sleep disorders.   2. Sleep–Physiological aspects.   I. Title.
    [DNLM: 1. Sleep–physiology.   2. Sleep Disorders. WL 108]
    RC547.B47 2012
    616.8′498—dc22   2011008073

Cover photograph copyright Calvin Hall, with permission

Acquisitions Editor: Julie Goolsby
Developmental Editor: Jessica Pritchard
Publishing Services Manager: Pat Joiner-Myers
Project Manager: Marlene Weeks
Design Manager: Louis Forgione
Marketing Manager: Carla Holloway

Printed in the United States of America

Last digit is the print number: 9   8   7   6   5   4   3   2

This book is dedicated to my wife Cathy, my son David,
and my daughter Sarah.
They are my greatest joy.

The goal of this book is to provide the reader with a core of fundamental knowledge about sleep medicine and polysomnography. I have tried to write the book so that a person without training in sleep medicine can start reading chapter one and progress until the end of the book. With the publication of the International Classification of Sleep Disorders, Second Edition, and the American Academy of Sleep Medicine scoring manual, there is a need for an up-to-date text using current terminology and diagnostic criteria. A single text cannot hope to cover all aspects of sleep medicine and sleep physiology. Therefore, I have tried to focus on information that I feel is the most clinically useful. The field of sleep medicine is changing so rapidly that any text is "out-of-date" before it is even published. To this end, there will be an associated website to allow for updates, corrections, review questions, illustrative case studies, and some video clips of parasomnias.

My inspiration for writing this book has come in part from the satisfaction and appreciation that I received from writing the text *Sleep Medicine Pearls*. *Sleep Medicine Pearls* had short fundamentals chapters mixed with cases and was heavy on graphics and illustrative sleep tracings. I have tried to amplify the fundamentals sections to provide what I hope is a concise and useful introduction to the entire spectrum of sleep disorders. In particular, I have tried to cover aspects of the technology of sleep monitoring and interpreting sleep studies that many new to the sleep field find difficult. The challenging but enjoyable experience of teaching sleep fellows and residents about sleep medicine has also prompted me to write a book covering the fundamentals both to serve as an introductory text and to assist those physicians actively taking care of sleep patients.

RICHARD B. BERRY, MD

Acknowledgments

I would like to express my gratitude for the support and encouragement of the University of Florida sleep physicians, including Dr. Abby Wagner, co-director of the University of Florida Sleep Medicine Fellowship, Dr. Stephan Eisenschenk, and Dr. Craig Foster. It is a pleasure to work with such a dedicated and talented group of individuals. I would also like to thank Dr. Klark Turpen for her assistance in editing the book chapters. The patience and assistance of the Elsevier editorial staff is also greatly appreciated. Jessica Pritchard helped assemble the chapters and many figures. Dolores Meloni, Senior Acquisitions Editor, was instrumental in developing the concept for the book and provided critical support in the planning stages. Julie Goolsby, Associate Acquisitions Editor, provided encouragement during the final stages of book preparation. I am also grateful for the patience and diligence of Berta Steiner of Bermedica Production, Ltd. during the production process.

Contents

Online Video Content

Chapter 1

Sleep Stages and Basic Sleep Monitoring

Chapter Points

- In the EEG or EOG derivation G_1-G_2, an upward deflection in the tracing is noted if input G_1 becomes negative with respect to input G_2 (negative upward polarity).
- To differentiate whether alpha waves or sleep spindles are present, change to a 10-second window and count the individual deflections in one second (see Fig. 1–3).
- K complexes and slow waves have the greatest amplitude in frontal derivations. Sleep spindles and saw-tooth waves have the greatest amplitude in central derivations.
- Alpha activity is any wave form with a frequency of 8 to 13 Hz. **Alpha rhythm** has a frequency of 8 to 13 Hz, is most prominent in the occipital derivations, and is enhanced by eye closure and attenuated by eye opening.
- The recommended EEG derivations are F_4-M_1, C_4-M_1, and O_2-M_1.
- The recommended EOG derivations are E_1-M_2 and E_2-M_2. Both eye electrodes are referred to a common mastoid electrode M_2.
- The front of the eye (cornea) is positive with respect to the back of the eye (retina). If the eyes move toward E_1-M_2 and away from E_2-M_2, this causes a downward deflection in E_1-M_2 and an upward deflection in E_2-M_2.
- In the recommended EOG derivations, eye movements result in out-of-phase deflections. K complexes result in in-phase deflections.
- In stage R, the chin EMG amplitude is equal to or lower than the lowest level in NREM sleep. The chin EMG activity can reach the REM level during NREM sleep. Transitions from NREM to stage R are not always associated with a drop in chin activity. Chin EMG activity is useful in differentiating stage R from stage W with the eyes open (REMs present).

Sleep is divided into non–rapid eye movement (NREM) and rapid eye movement (REM) sleep. Sleep staging is based on electroencephalographic (EEG), electro-oculographic (EOG), and submental (chin) electromyographic (EMG) criteria. EOG (eye movement recording) and chin EMG recordings are used to detect REM sleep, which is characterized by REMs and reduced muscle tone. Since 1968, sleep was usually staged according to *A Manual of Standardized Terminology, Techniques and Scoring System for Sleep Stages of Human Subjects,* edited by Rechtschaffen and Kales (R&K).[1] In the R&K scoring manual,[1] *NREM sleep* was divided into sleep stages 1, 2, 3, and 4. *REM sleep* was referred to as stage REM. Sleep stage nomenclature has changed following the publication of the *American Academy of Sleep Medicine (AASM) Manual for the Scoring of Sleep and Associated Events* (hereafter referred to as the AASM scoring manual).[2] The new nomenclature was introduced to denote sleep stages defined by new criteria. The old and new nomenclatures are shown in Table 1–1. Stages 3 and 4 are combined into stage N3.

Today, digital polysomnography (sleep recording) has virtually replaced recording on paper. However, previously sleep recording was performed with polygraphs using ink writing pens with a paper speed of 10 mm/sec. At this paper speed, a 30-cm page of paper contained 30 seconds of recording. A sleep stage was identfed for each page (30 sec) termed *an epoch.* The tradition of staging sleep in 30-second epochs has been retained in the recent AASM scoring manual. The sleep stage assigned to each epoch is the stage occupying the majority of time within that epoch. Digital recording allows display of data in one of several time windows (typically 5, 10, 30, 60, 90, 120, 240 sec). The 10-second window corresponds to a paper speed of 30 mm/sec and is used for clinical EEG monitoring. This time window also approximates electrocardiographic (ECG) recording that was typically performed using a paper speed of 25 mm/sec before the current use of digital ECG recording.

EEG ELECTRODE PLACEMENT

Monitoring to detect the presence and stage of sleep requires only a portion of the electrodes used in standard clinical EEG recording (Table 1–2). The nomenclature for the EEG electrodes follows the International 10–20 system.[3] The "10–20" refers to the fact that the electrodes are positioned at either 10% or 20% of the distance between landmarks. The major landmarks include the nasion (bridge of the nose),

TABLE 1–1

Sleep Stage Nomenclature

	R&K	AASM
Wake	Stage W	Stage W
NREM	Stage 1	Stage N1
	Stage 2	Stage N2
	Stage 3	Stage N3
	Stage 4	
REM	Stage REM	Stage R

AASM = American Academy of Sleep Medicine[2]; NREM = non–rapid eye movement; R&K = Rechtschaffen and Kales A[1]; REM = rapid eye movement; stages 3 and 4 are combined into stage N3.

TABLE 1–2

Electroencephalographic Electrode Nomenclature

	LEFT	RIGHT	MIDLINE
Frontopolar	F_{p1}	F_{p2}	F_{pz}
Frontal	F_3	F_4	F_z
Central	C_3	C_4	C_z
Occipital	O_1	O_2	O_z
Mastoid	M_1	M_2	

FIGURE 1–1 Electrode positions using the 10–20 system.

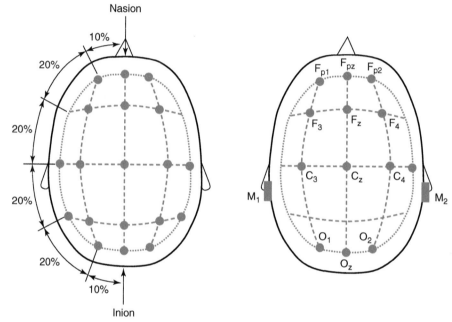

inion (prominence at base of the occiput), and preauricular points (Figs. 1–1 and 1–2). In the 10–20 system, even-numbered subscripts refer to the right side of the head and odd-numbered subscripts to the left. Electrodes are named for the part of the brain they are over. For example, F_{p1} and F_{p2} are the left and right **frontal pole** electrodes, F_3 and F_4 are the left and right **frontal** electrodes, C_3 and C_4 are the left and right **central** electrodes, and O_1 and O_2 are the left and right **occipital** electrodes. Electrodes in the midline in the frontopolar, frontal, central, and occipital regions are named F_{pz}, F_z, C_z, and O_z, respectively. The position of the electrode C_z is at the top of the head and is called the **vertex.** The left and right mastoid electrodes in the new AASM scoring manual nomenclature are named M_1 and M_2, respectively. They were previously named A_1 and A_2. The nomenclature of EEG electrodes used for sleep monitoring is listed in Table 1–2.

EEG Derivations

EEG signals are displayed as voltage differences between two electrodes. The term **derivation** refers to a set of two electrodes (and the voltage difference between the electrodes). The term **montage** refers to a particular set of derivations. In sleep monitoring, electrodes in the frontal, central, and occipital electrodes are referenced against the **opposite mastoid electrode.** The AASM scoring manual recommends that all of the following electrodes be placed (F_3, F_4, C_3, C_4, O_1, O_2, M_1, and M_2). The recommended derivations and the alternative derivations are listed in Table 1–3. The backup derivations are displayed if one of the electrodes in the recommended derivation fails. For example, if electrode F_4 fails, the derivation F_3–M_2 is used. In digital recording, one can easily display all six derivations if desired at the same time. In the original R&K scoring manual, only central derivations

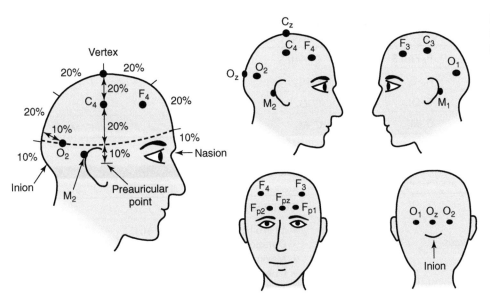

TABLE 1–3

Recommended Electroencephalographic Derivations with Backup Derivations

RECOMMENDED DERIVATIONS[2]	BACKUP DERIVATIONS
• F_4-M_1	• F_3-M_2
• C_4-M_1	• C_3-M_2
• O_2-M_1	• O_1-M_2

were utilized. However, additional derivations allow better visualization of the EEG patterns used to stage sleep.

Although the derivations cited previously are the most widely used, the AASM scoring manual lists alternative acceptable derivations (Table 1–4). The alternative derivations use the electrodes F_z, C_z, O_z, C_4, and M_1 with the backup electrodes F_{pz} (to replace F_z), C_3 (to replace C_z or C_4), O_1 (to replace O_z), and M_2 (to replace M_1).

It is common to place additional electrodes beyond those discussed in the AASM scoring manual to serve as a ground electrode and common reference. In sleep monitoring, a ground electrode is usually placed at or near F_{pz} and connected to the ground (or iso-ground) input on the electrode box. As discussed in Chapter 2, the ground is used to balance the individual AC differential amplifiers. One electrode (or two linked electrodes) is also placed to serve as a reference for referential recording (see Chapter 2). The reference electrode is commonly placed at or near C_z depending on which EEG electrodes are to be recorded for sleep monitoring.

EEG Patterns

Recognition of certain characteristic EEG patterns is essential for sleep staging.[1-6] EEG activity is recorded using a differential AC amplifier such that the signal recorded is the **difference in voltage** between two inputs (G1 and G2). By EEG convention, if input G1 is **negative** with respect to G2, this results in an **upward** deflection. As noted previously, the term *derivation* is used to describe the differential signal between two inputs. For example, in the derivation C_4-M_1, a change in the voltage between these electrodes results in an upward deflection if C_4 is negative with respect to M_1. EEG activity is described by frequency in cycles per second (hertz = Hz), amplitude (microvolts [μV]), and shape. The classically described EEG frequency ranges are delta (<4 Hz), theta (4–7 Hz), alpha (8–13 Hz), and beta (>13 Hz). Activity that is faster results in narrower deflections and slower frequency results in wider deflections. **Sharp waves** are narrow waves of 70 to 200 msec duration and **spikes** have a shorter duration of 20 to 70 msec.

Some of the characteristics of EEG patterns important for sleep staging are listed in Tables 1–5 through 1–9. In addition to frequency, the region of highest activity (amplitude) and the effects of maneuvers on the EEG activity are also important. For example, one could use the term "alpha activity" to describe any EEG activity with a frequency in the alpha range (8–13 Hz). However, **alpha rhythm** consists of activity most prominent in occipital derivations that is attenuated by eye opening and increased by eye closure (Fig. 1–3). An important part of biocalibrations (see Chapter 4) at the start of sleep recording is to ask patients to close and then open their eyes to document that they produce alpha rhythm. Bursts of alpha waves can also occur during stage R typically at a frequency 1 to 2 Hz slower than during wakefulness.

Sleep spindles[7-9] are bursts of activity with a frequency range of 11 to 16 Hz (usually 12–14) with a duration of 0.5 sec or greater (usually 0.5–1.5 sec). The term *spindle* is used because the shape of sleep spindle burst is often like that of a yarn spindle (see Fig. 1–3). If there is uncertainty about whether activity is a burst of alpha activity or a sleep spindle, one can display a 10-second window (see Fig. 1–3) and actually count the deflections (waves) per second. Sleep spindles arise from thalamocortical oscillations. The **reticular nucleus** of the thalamus is responsible for generating sleep spindles.

A **K complex**[1,2,8,9] is a high-amplitude biphasic wave composed of an initial negative sharp wave (deflection up)

TABLE 1–4

Alternative Electroencephalographic Derivations with Backup Derivations

ALTERNATIVE DERIVATIONS	F_z FAILS	C_z FAILS	O_z FAILS	C_4 OR M_1 FAILS
F_z-C_z	F_{pz}-C_z	F_{pz}-C_3	F_z-C_z	F_z-C_z
C_z-O_z	C_z-O_z	C_3-O_z	C_z-O_1	C_z-O_z
C_4-M_1	C_4-M_1	C_4-M_1	C_4-M_1	C_3-M_2

TABLE 1–5

Characteristics of Alpha Rhythm and Sleep Spindles

ALPHA RHYTHM	SLEEP SPINDLES
• 8–13 Hz. • Most prominent over the *occipital areas*. • Activity increased by eye closure. • Activity suppressed by eye opening. • Predominate EEG activity in drowsy, eyes closed stage W. • Common in REM sleep (1–2 Hz slower than during stage W or N1). • Can occur with arousals (brief awakenings). • 10% of persons do not produce alpha rhythm with eye closure.	• 11–16 Hz (classically 12–14 Hz). • Duration ≥ 0.5 sec (0.5–1.5 sec). • Maximal over *central areas*. • One of the defining characteristics of stage N2. • Thalamocortical oscillations (reticular thalamic nucleus). • Can be seen in stage N3 sleep. • Drug spindles (benzodiazepines) may be slightly faster.

EEG = electroencephalographic; REM = rapid eye movement.

TABLE 1–6

Characteristics of K Complex and Slow Wave Activity

K COMPLEX	SLOW WAVE ACTIVITY
• High amplitude–biphasic deflection. • A well-delineated negative sharp wave (upward) followed by a positive (downward) slow wave. • Stands out from the lower voltage background. • Duration ≥ 0.5 sec. • Characteristic of stage N2 sleep. • Maximal over *frontal areas* (frontal > central > occipital). • K complex–associated arousal requires arousal to start no more than 1 second after K complex termination.	• Frequency 0.5–2 Hz and > 75 µV peak to peak in the **frontal** derivations. • Used to define stage N3 sleep. • Stage N2 < 20% SWA (<6 sec). • Stage N3 ≥ 20% SWA (≥6 sec). • SWA is usually transmitted to eye derivations.

SWA = slow wave activity.

TABLE 1–7

Characteristics of Vertex Sharp and Saw-Tooth Waves

VERTEX SHARP WAVES	SAW-TOOTH WAVES
• Sharply contoured waves • Duration < 0.5 sec • Maximal over the central region (derivations containing C_3, C_4, C_z) and distinguishable from the background activity (higher amplitude). • Occurs in stage N1 often near transition to stage N2	• Trains of triangular waves, often serrated • 2–6 Hz waves • Maximal in amplitude in central derivations • Often, but not always, preceding a burst of REMs • Characteristic of stage R but not required for scoring stage R

REMs = rapid eye movements.

followed by a slow wave (Fig. 1–4). A burst of spindle activity is often superimposed on a K complex. A K complex stands out from the lower voltage background. K complex activity is greatest in frontal derivations (also central > occipital). A K complex is said to be associated with an arousal if the arousal commences no more than 1 second after the K complex. An arousal during sleep stages N1, N2, and N3 is scored if there is an abrupt shift of EEG frequency including alpha, theta, and/or frequencies greater than 16 Hz (but not spindles) that lasts *at least 3 seconds*, with at least 10 seconds of stable sleep preceding the change. Arousals are discussed in more detail in Chapter 3.

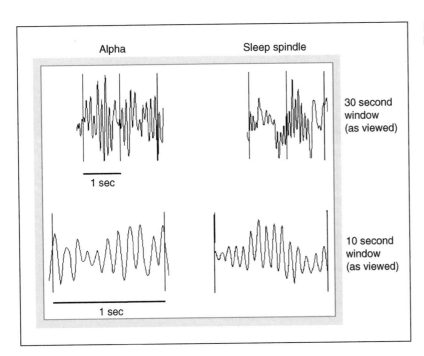

FIGURE 1–3 Alpha rhythm and sleep spindle activity as visualized in 30-second and 10-second windows.

TABLE 1–8
Summary of Important Wave Form Characteristics

	ALPHA RHYTHM	SLEEP SPINDLE	K COMPLEX	VERTEX SHARP WAVE	SLOW WAVE ACTIVITY	SAW-TOOTH WAVES
Frequency (Hz)	8–13	11–16	N/A	N/A	0.5–2	2–6
Amplitude/ shape	Oscillation	Spindle-shaped oscillation	High amplitude (usually > 100 µV) Stands out against EEG background Biphasic-negative sharp wave followed by positive component	Sharp wave	High-amplitude broad wave >75 µV peak to peak	Triangular, serrated
Duration	Variable	≥0.5	≥0.5 sec	<500 msec	0.5–2 sec	Variable
Location of highest amplitude	Occipital	Central	Frontal	Central (vertex)	Frontal	Central
Associated sleep stages/ events	Stage W Stage N1 Stage R Arousals	Stage N2 Stage N3	Stage N2 Stage N3	Stage N1	Stage N2 Stage N3	Stage R

EEG = electroencephalogram; N/A = not applicable.

TABLE 1–9
Electro-oculographic Derivations

RECOMMENDED	ALTERNATE
E_1-M_2	E_1-F_{pz}
E_2-M_2	E_2-F_{pz}

An example of a K complex associated with an arousal is shown in Figure 1–5. Also note that the K complex is seen in the EOG derivations E_1-M_1 and E_2-M_2 as an in-phase deflection.

As noted previously, the frequency of delta activity is less than 4 Hz. EEG activity in this range produces relatively wide duration deflections, often called *delta* or *slow waves* (see Fig. 1–4). However, for sleep staging, the designation **slow wave activity (SWA)**[2] specifically refers to waves with a frequency range of 0.5 to 2 Hz (2- to 0.5-sec duration) and

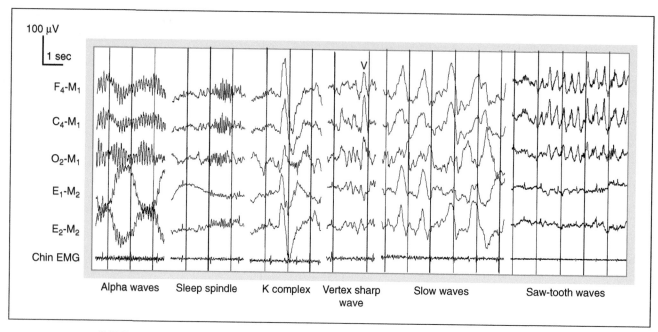

FIGURE 1–4 Important EEG patterns for sleep staging. The grid lines are 1 second apart. V = position of the vertex sharp wave.

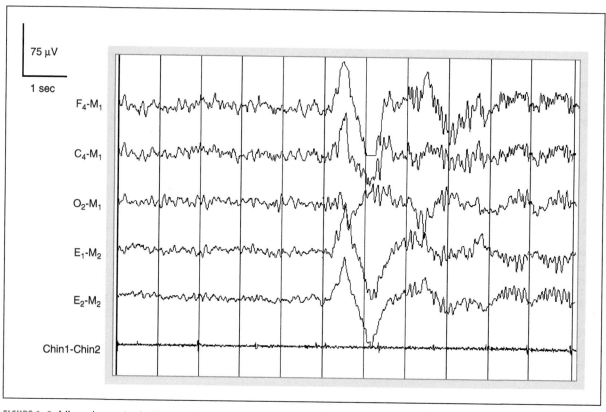

FIGURE 1–5 A K complex associated with an arousal. An abrupt shift in EEG frequency immediately follows the K complex that lasts greater than 3 seconds. To be considered associated with a K complex, an arousal must commence no later than 1 second after K complex termination.

a peak-to-peak amplitude of greater than 75 µV in the **frontal derivations** (see Fig. 1–4). SWA has the greatest amplitude over frontal areas. In the R&K definitions, only central derivations were utilized. Because slow wave amplitude is higher over the frontal areas, a given epoch of EEG activity would potentially have greater SWA (longer duration

meeting amplitude criteria) using the AASM scoring manual definition[2] (frontal derivations) compared with the R&K definition (using central derivations).

Vertex sharp waves (see Fig. 1–4) are narrow-duration waves (<500 msec according to the AASM scoring manual[2]) prominent in derivations containing electrodes near the

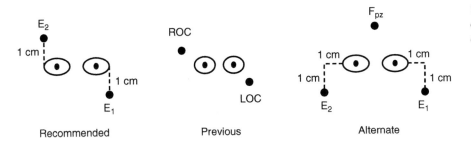

FIGURE 1–6 Recommended, previous, and alternate eye movement electrode positions. LOC = left outer canthus; ROC = right outer canthus.

vertex (C_z, C_3, C_4). They are often seen near the transition between stage N1 and stage N2 sleep. **Saw-tooth waves** (see Fig. 1–4) occur during REM sleep, although they are not always present during this sleep stage. They are triangular waves of 2 to 6 Hz of highest amplitude in the central derivations. The presence of saw-tooth waves is not required to score stage R. However, the presence of saw-tooth waves is very helpful when they occur.

EOG MONITORING FOR SLEEP

Recording of eye movements is possible because a potential difference exists across the eyeball with the front/cornea positive (+) and back/retina negative (–). Eye movements are detected by EOG recording of voltage changes associated with eye movement.

The recommended EOG electrodes in the AASM scoring manual[2] are illustrated in Figure 1–6. E_1 and E_2 refer to the left and right eye electrodes, respectively. Previously eye electrodes were named *right outer canthus (ROC)* and *left outer canthus (LOC)*. For comparison, the positions of the ROC and LOC electrodes are also shown. Please note that E_1 is placed below the LOC and E_2 is placed above the ROC, whereas LOC and ROC were placed lateral to the respective outer canthus. Because E_1 is below and E_2 above the eyes, vertical as well as horizontal movement can be detected. Alternate eye electrode positions were also recommended for use with alternate eye movement derivations (see Fig. 1–6). The AASM scoring manual recommends the EOG derivations E_1-M_2 and E_2-M_2 (see Table 1–9). Note that both eye derivations use the right mastoid (M_2) as the reference electrode. Previous ROC and LOC derivations varied between sleep centers, and these electrodes were referenced either to the same mastoid or to the opposite mastoid. The AASM scoring manual also specified the alternative eye movement derivations (E_1-F_{pz} and E_2-F_{pz}). If these eye movement derivations are used, **both** E_1 and E_2 are below and lateral to the LOC and ROC, respectively (see Fig. 1–6).

When the eyes move toward an electrode, a positive voltage is recorded (Fig. 1–7). Recall that in EEG recording, by polarity convention, if an eye electrode is negative compared with the reference electrode, the signal has an upward deflection. Thus, eye movement (cornea +) **toward an electrode** referenced to another electrode further away from the eyes results in a **downward** deflection.

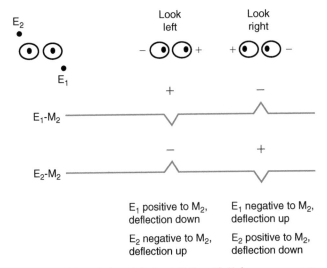

FIGURE 1–7 Schematic shows deflections in E_1-M_2 and E_2-M_2 from eye movements.

In the recommended EOG derivations, eye movements result in **out-of-phase deflections.** This is because eye movements are conjugate, and when both eyes move laterally or vertically, they both move toward one EOG electrode and away from the other EOG electrode. The polarity of the eye electrodes determines the net voltage difference of the EOG derivations because the electrodes are much closer to the eyes than M_2. The schematic in Figure 1–7 illustrates eye movements and the resulting deflections (this assumes that both eye derivation tracings have negative polarity upward which is standard).

Note that when the alternate EOG derivations E_1-F_{pz} and E_2-F_{pz} are used, both E_1 and E_2 are 1 cm *below* and 1 cm lateral to the LOC and ROC, respectively. In this scheme, **vertical** eye movements result in **in-phase deflections** and **lateral** eye movements result in **out-of-phase deflections** (Fig. 1–8). The advantages of the **alternative** EOG derivations are that vertical deflections tend to produce larger deflections (blinks are more prominent) and one can distinguish vertical (in-phase) from horizontal (out-of-phase) eye movements. In addition, it is easy to remember that downward eye movements result in downward deflections in the eye derivations and upward eye movements result in upward deflections. Alternatively, the **recommended** eye derivations make it easier to recognize artifacts or EEG activity transmitted to the eye derivations because these cause in-phase deflections while eye movements cause out-of-phase deflections (Fig. 1–9).

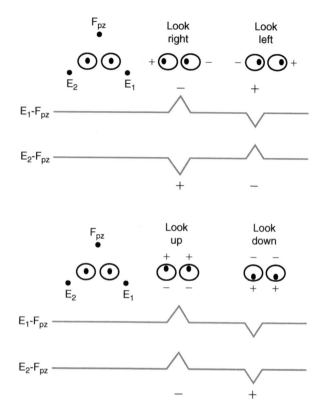

FIGURE 1–8 Schematic shows deflections in E_1-F_{pz} and E_2-F_{pz} due to horizontal and vertical eye movements. Note that, using these derivations, vertical eye movements result in in-phase deflections whereas lateral eye movements result in out-of-phase deflections. In addition, downward eye movements result in downward deflections.

Eye Movement Patterns

Typical eye movement patterns (Table 1–10) include blinks, slow eye movements (SEMs), REMs, and reading eye movements (Fig. 1–10). SEMs are typical of eyes closed drowsy, wakefulness, and stage N1 sleep. REMs are seen in eyes open wakefulness or stage R sleep. SEMs typically disappear with the onset of stage N2 sleep. However, patients on selective serotonin reuptake inhibitors (SSRIs) can have eye movements that are a mixture of slow and more rapid activity that persists into stage N2.[10,11] This pattern is called "Prozac eyes"

TABLE 1–10
Eye Movements Pattern Definitions
• **Eye blinks:** Conjugate vertical eye movements at a frequency of 0.5–2 Hz present in wakefulness with the eyes open or closed.
• **Reading eye movements:** Trains of conjugate eye movements consisting of a slow phase followed by a rapid phase in the opposite direction as the subject reads.
• **Slow eye movements:** Conjugate, fairly regular, sinusoidal eye movements with an initial deflection lasting > **500 msec.**
• **Rapid eye movements (REMs):** Conjugate, irregular, sharply peaked eye movements with an initial deflection usually lasting < 500 msec. Whereas rapid eye movements are characteristic of stage R sleep, *they may also be seen in wakefulness with eyes open* (as patients look around the room)

Adapted from Iber C, Ancoli-Israel S, Chesson A, Quan SF for the American Academy of Sleep Medicine: The AASM Manual for the Scoring of Sleep and Associated Events: Rules, Terminology and Technical Specifications, 1st ed. Westchester, IL: American Academy of Sleep Medicine, 2007.

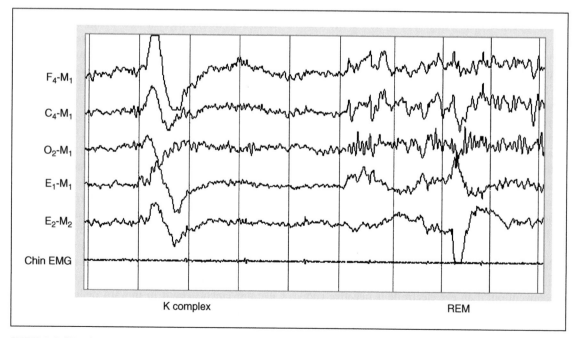

FIGURE 1–9 Using the recommended electro-oculographic (EOG) derivations, the K complex results in deflections that are in phase and the rapid eye movement (REM) results in out-of-phase deflections. The vertical lines are 1 second apart. EMG = electromyography.

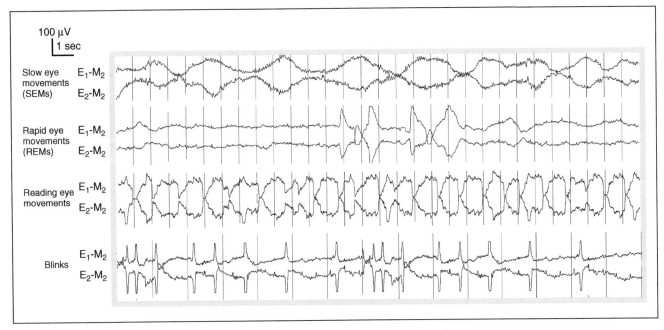

FIGURE 1–10　Eye movement patterns. The grid lines are 1 second apart.

but can occur with any of the SSRIs (see Chapter 4). Reading eye movements are due to a slow scan of the written page (left to right) followed by a rapid return to the left. This results in a slowly increasing downward deflection in E_2-M_2 followed by a rapid upward deflection. In E_1-M_2, there is a slow upward deflection followed by a rapid downward deflection (see Fig. 1–10).

Chin (Submental) EMG Monitoring

The monitoring of chin EMG activity is an essential element only for identifying stage R (REM sleep). In stage R, the chin EMG is relatively reduced: the amplitude is equal to or lower than the lowest EMG amplitude in NREM sleep.

The placement of EMG electrodes recommended by the AASM scoring manual is illustrated in Figure 1–11. The scoring manual defines the positions of the electrodes but does not assign them names.

For convenience, labels are assigned in Figure 1–11. The standard chin derivation consists of either of the electrodes below the mandible referred to the electrode above the mandible. That is chin2–chin1 or chin3–chin1. The electrode not used in the displayed derivation is placed as a backup.

If the EMG derivation sensitivity (gain) is adjusted high enough to show some activity in NREM sleep, a drop in activity **may** be seen on transition to REM sleep. However, the EMG can fall to the REM level before the onset of REM sleep. Depending on the gain, a reduction in the EMG amplitude from wakefulness to sleep and often a further reduction on transition from stage N1 to stage N3 may be seen. However, chin EMG activity is a requirement for

THREE ELECTRODES ARE RECOMMENDED
TO RECORD THE CHIN EMG

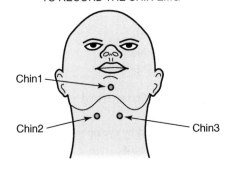

Electrode 1.　Midline 1 cm above interior edge of mandible

Electrode 2.　2 cm below inferior edge of mandible and 2 cm right of the midline

Electrode 3.　2 cm below inferior edge of mandible and 2 cm left of the midline

Standard chin EMG derivations Chin2 - Chin1 or Chin3 - Chin1

FIGURE 1–11　Submental (chin) EMG electrode positions. The terms Chin1, Chin2, and Chin3 are not specified in the American Academy of Sleep Medicine (AASM) scoring manual but are added for convenience. The standard derivation is either of the electrodes below the mandible referred to the electrode above the mandible.

identifying ONLY stage R. The reduction in the chin EMG amplitude during REM sleep is a reflection of the generalized skeletal-muscle hypotonia present in this sleep stage. In the tracings in Figure 1–12, there is a fall in chin EMG amplitude (A) just before saw-tooth waves (B) and the REMs (C) occur.

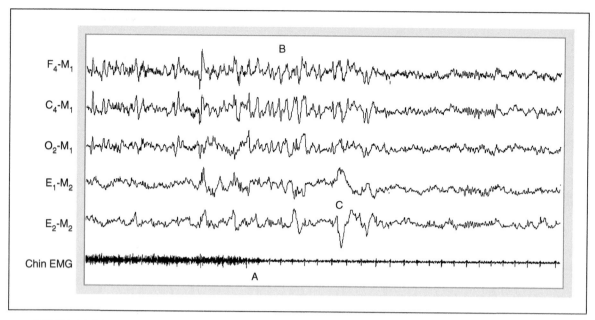

FIGURE 1–12 A 30-second tracing shows a reduction in the chin EMG on transition to stage R sleep (A). Note saw-tooth waves (B) and REMs (C).

CLINICAL REVIEW QUESTIONS:

1. The standard EEG montage for sleep recording is F_4-M_1, C_4-M_1, and O_2-M_1. If electrode C_4 fails, which of the following montages should be used?

   A. F_4-M_1, C_3-M_2, O_2-M_1

   B. F_4-M_1, C_3-M_1, O_2-M_1

   C. F_3-M_2, C_3-M_2, O_1-M_2

   D. F_4-M_2, C_3-M_2, O_2-M_2

2. Alpha rhythm is characterized by which of the following?

   A. 8–13 Hz, attenuated by eye opening, most prominent in occipital derivations

   B. 11–16 Hz, attenuated by eye closure, most prominent in occipital derivations

   C. 8–13 Hz, attenuated by eye opening, most prominent in frontal derivations

   D. 11–16 Hz, attenuated by eye opening, most prominent in central derivations

3. Sleep spindles are characterized by which of the following?

   A. 12–14 Hz activity, most prominent in the occipital areas

   B. 8–13 Hz, thalamocortical oscillations

   C. 11–16 Hz, most prominent in frontal derivations

   D. 11–16 Hz, generated by the reticular nucleus of the thalamus

4. SWA for sleep staging is characterized by which of the following?

   A. Minimum EEG amplitude peak to peak > 75 µV in central derivations, frequency 0.5–2 Hz

   B. Minimum EEG amplitude peak to peak > 75 µV in frontal derivations, frequency 0.5–2 Hz

   C. Minimum EEG amplitude peak to peak > 75 µV in frontal derivations, frequency < 4 Hz

   D. Minimum EEG amplitude peak to peak > 50 µV in frontal derivations, frequency < 4 Hz

5. On right lateral gaze, which of the following deflections are noted in the recommended EOG derivations?

   A. E_1-M_2 Deflection up E_2-M_2 Deflection down

   B. E_1-M_2 Deflection down E_2-M_2 Deflection up

   C. E_1-M_2 Deflection up E_2-M_2 Deflection up

   D. E_1-M_2 Deflection down E_2-M_2 Deflection down

6. Which of the following is true about SEMs (using the recommended eye derivations)?

   A. Can occur during stage W or N1, are sinusoidal out-of-phase eye movements.

   B. Can occur during stage W only, are sinusoidal out-of-phase eye movements.

   C. Can occur during stage W or N1, are sinusoidal in-phase movements.

   D. Can occur only during stage W only, are sinusoidal out-of-phase movements.

Answers

1. **A.** The alternate derivation for C_4-M_1 is C_3-M_2. It is not necessary to change the other derivations. (See FAQ for scoring manual V4. http://www.aasmnet.org/FAQs.aspx?cid=29)

2. **A.** Alpha rhythm is 8–13 Hz, attenuated by eye opening, most prominent in occipital derivations.

3. **D.** Sleep spindles have a frequency of 11–16 Hz and represent thalamocortical oscillations generated by the reticular nucleus of the thalamus. Sleep spindles are most prominent in central derivations.

4. **B.** SWA is characterized by a minimum amplitude peak to peak of > 75 μV in the frontal derivations with a frequency of 0.5 to 2 Hz.

5. **A.** In the recommended derivations, eye movements cause out-of-phase deflections. Because the cornea is positive with respect to the retina, a rightward gaze results in E_2 being positive with respect to M_2 (E_2 is closer to the cornea) and this results in a downward deflection. With a rightward gaze, E_1 is negative with respect to M_2 (upward deflection).

6. **A.** SEMs can occur during wake (eyes closed drowsy wake) or stage N1 and are sinusoidal out-of-phase movements.

REFERENCES

1. Rechtschaffen A, Kales A (eds): A Manual of Standardized Terminology, Techniques and Scoring System for Sleep Stages of Human Sleep. Los Angeles: Brain Information Service/Brain Research Institute, UCLA, 1968.
2. Iber C, Ancoli-Israel S, Chesson A, Quan SF for the American Academy of Sleep Medicine: The AASM Manual for the Scoring of Sleep and Associated Events: Rules, Terminology and Technical Specifications, 1st ed. Westchester, IL: American Academy of Sleep Medicine, 2007.
3. International Federation of Societies for Electroencephalography and Clinical Neurophysiology: Ten twenty electrode system. EEG Clin Neurophysiol 1958;10:371–375.
4. Williams RL, Karacan I, Hursch CJ: Electroencephalography of Human Sleep: Clinical Applications. New York: John Wiley & Sons, 1974.
5. West P, Kryger MH: Sleep and respiration: terminology and methodology. Clin Chest Med 1985;6:691–712.
6. Caraskadon MA, Rechschaffen A: Monitoring and staging human sleep. In Kryger MH, Roth T, Dement WC (eds): Principles and Practice of Sleep Medicine. Philadelphia: Elsevier Saunders, 2005, pp. 1359–1377.
7. DeGennaro L, Ferrara M: Sleep spindles: an overview. Sleep Med Rev 2003;7:423–440.
8. McCormick L, Nielsen T, Nicolas A, et al: Topographical distribution of spindles and K complexes in normal subjects. Sleep 1997;20:939–941.
9. Silber MH, Ancoli-Israel S, Bonnet MH, et al: The visual scoring of sleep in adults. J Clin Sleep Med 2007;15:121–131.
10. Schenck CH, Mahowlad MW, Kim SW, et al. Prominent eye movements during NREM sleep and REM sleep behavior disorder associated with fluoxetine treatment of obsessive-compulsive disorder. Sleep 1992;15:226–235.
11. Armitage R, Trivedi M, Rush AJ: Fluoxetine and oculomotor activity during sleep in depressed patients. Neuropsychopharmacology 1995;12:159–165.

The Technology of Sleep Monitoring: Differential Amplifiers, Digital Polysomnography, and Filters

Chapter Points

- Common mode rejection of unwanted signals by a differential AC amplifier depends on having low and fairly equal electrode impedances. An electrode impedance less than 5 KΩ is desirable (<10 KΩ acceptable).
- Digital PSG typically uses a combination of AC referential, AC true bipolar, and DC recording.
- In referential recording, each electrode is recorded in comparison with a common reference electrode. Any derivation (combination of differences between electrodes) can be displayed by digital subtraction $[(C_4\text{-Ref}) - (M_1\text{-Ref}) = C_4\text{-}M_1]$ during acquisition or later during review of the study. If the reference electrode is faulty, all channels will be affected.
- Most digital AC amplifiers record with a wide bandwidth ("wide open"), for example, a low-frequency filter of 0.03 and a high-frequency filter of 100 Hz. Each derivation is then displayed after processing with the desired low- and high-frequency digital filters. The recorded data are not changed by the display filters. This allows display with different filter settings if desired.
- Digital recording requires appropriate sampling rates by the A/D converter depending on the variable being recorded. A suitable high-frequency filter must be used to prevent aliasing distortion.
- The resolution of the monitor is usually what limits the possible resolution of the displayed data rather than the sampling rate.

In sleep monitoring (polysomnography [PSG]), electroencephalographic (EEG), electro-oculographic (EOG), and electromyographic (EMG) activity is recorded by differential AC amplifiers that amplify the difference in voltage between two inputs[1-3] (Fig. 2–1). Each differential amplifier has two inputs and a ground. By convention in EEG recording, if input 1 (G_1) is negative relative to input 2 (G_2), the deflection is upward (negative up polarity).

Signals common to both inputs are not amplified (common mode rejection) (Fig. 2–2). Actually, each of the inputs is recorded against the common ground and input 2 is inverted. This allows common signals to cancel each other but differences between input 1 and input 2 to be amplified. Use of differential amplifiers permits the recording of very low voltage EEG signals that are superimposed upon larger DC scalp voltage changes and 60-cycle interference from nearby AC power lines. Common mode rejection depends on the impedance at input 1 and 2 being relatively equal. Otherwise, common signals will produce unequal voltages at the two inputs. Making the intrinsic impedance of the inputs much higher than the impedance of the electrodes minimizes the effect of unequal electrode impedances. However, a poorly conducting electrode (high impedance) will typically result in a large amount of 60-Hz artifact (signal contamination). The ground of each differential AC amplifier is connected to the common patient ground (commonly, an electrode placed on the forehead). This common ground helps balance the inputs to all the differential amplifiers, thereby improving common mode rejection. The use of grounds in EEG recording is discussed at the end of the chapter.

It should be noted that a **localized** EEG transient (e.g., sharp wave) that is located midway between two electrodes will produce an equal signal in both sides of the differential AC amplifier that will cancel out (output approximately zero). This cancellation effect will alter the overall EEG signal amplitude less if electrodes are further apart. Thus, a greater distance between two electrode inputs will increase the amplitude of the recorded signal (less cancellation). This is one reason the recommended EEG derivations use contra-lateral mastoid references (C_4-M_1, not C_4-M_2).

REFERENTIAL AND BIPOLAR RECORDING

Most digital recording systems use a combination of referential, true bipolar, and DC recording (Table 2–1).[2] In true bipolar recording, each amplifier records the difference between two electrodes of interest (A–B, C–D). Before the digital era, paper recording was performed using a selector panel and dedicated individual differential amplifiers. Using this approach, it is possible to change the electrodes (derivation) that are recorded with a given amplifier (Fig. 2–3). However, changing the derivation once the signal is recorded (changing from A–B to A–D) is not possible. Today, selector panels are rarely used in digital sleep recording. However, true bipolar recording is still used for inputs that one would not desire to change in review—for example, the two inputs of the thermal flow sensor, respiratory effort bands (thorax

and abdomen), leg EMG inputs, and electrocardiographic (ECG) inputs.

In referential recording, multiple electrodes are recorded against a common electrical reference (often a single or two linked electrodes placed near the vertex). A **display** of any derivation using two referentially recorded electrodes is then obtained by digital subtraction [(electrode A − reference) − (electrode B − reference) = electrode A − electrode B] either during live recording or during review (see Fig. 2–3). The digital subtraction for display does NOT change the recorded data. For example, if the sleep technologist failed to observe that the electrode F_4 went bad during the recording, the reviewer can change the viewed frontal derivation to F_3-M_1 or F_3-M_2 (the recommended alternative) (Fig. 2–4). For this reason, both F_3 and F_4 are recorded (against the reference electrode) even though only F_4-M_1 may be displayed in the default montage. Of note, if the reference electrode is faulty, all referential signals are affected (Fig. 2–5). In Figure 2–5, note that the true bipolar channels are not affected by a faulty reference electrode. In most digital PSG systems, the EEG, EOG, mastoid, and chin EMG electrodes are recorded referentially (see Table 2–1). DC recording is used for nasal pressure, pulse oximetry, and other DC signals such as those

TABLE 2–1	
Types of Recording	
Referential recording	EEG: F_4, F_3, C_4, C_3, O_2, O_1, M_1, M_2 EOG: E_1, E_2, M_1, M_2 Chin1, Chin2, Chin3 Reference
True bipolar (two inputs each)	ECG, thermal flow, thorax and abdominal sensors, right and left anterior tibial EMG
DC	Nasal pressure, SpO_2, positive airway pressure device (flow, leak, pressure), end-tidal or transcutaneous PCO_2

ECG = electrocardiography; EEG = electroencephalography; EMG = electromyography; EOG = electro-oculography; PCO_2 = partial pressure of carbon dioxide; SpO_2 = pulse oximetry.

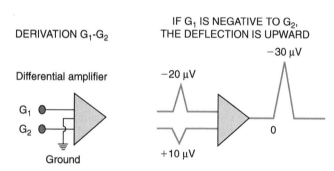

DERIVATION G_1-G_2

IF G_1 IS NEGATIVE TO G_2, THE DEFLECTION IS UPWARD

Differential amplifier

G_1
G_2

Ground

−30 µV
−20 µV
+10 µV
0

FIGURE 2–1 Differential amplifier. The difference between the two inputs is amplified (for simplicity, the amplification factor = 1).

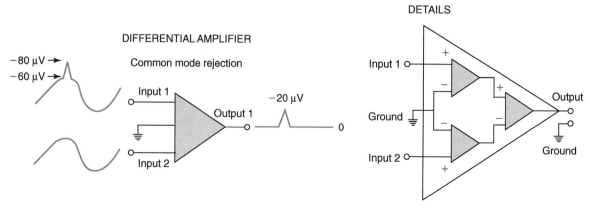

DIFFERENTIAL AMPLIFIER

Common mode rejection

−80 µV
−60 µV

Input 1
Output 1
Input 2

−20 µV
0

DETAILS

Input 1
Ground
Input 2

Output
Ground

FIGURE 2–2 Common mode rejection by a differential amplifier (for simplicity, the amplification factor = 1).

BIPOLAR RECORDING

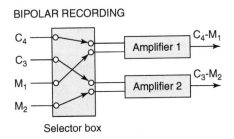

REFERENTIAL RECORDING

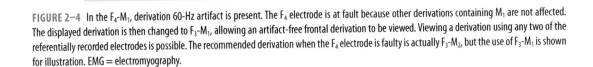

DISPLAY BIPOLAR VIEWS

$$C_4 - M_1 = (C_4 - Ref) - (M_1 - Ref)$$
$$C_3 - M_2 = (C_3 - Ref) - (M_2 - Ref)$$

FIGURE 2–3 The difference between true bipolar recording and referential recording. In referential recording, each electrode is recorded against a common reference. Specific derivations are then displayed by digital subtraction (during acquisition or review).

FIGURE 2–4 In the F_4-M_1, derivation 60-Hz artifact is present. The F_4 electrode is at fault because other derivations containing M_1 are not affected. The displayed derivation is then changed to F_3-M_1, allowing an artifact-free frontal derivation to be viewed. Viewing a derivation using any two of the referentially recorded electrodes is possible. The recommended derivation when the F_4 electrode is faulty is actually F_3-M_2, but the use of F_3-M_1 is shown for illustration. EMG = electromyography.

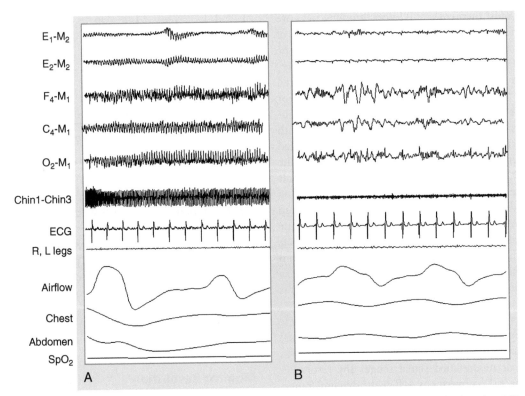

FIGURE 2–5 **A,** The reference electrode is faulty. All referentially recorded electrodes show artifact. The true bipolar channels and DC channels are not affected. In **B,** the reference electrode was repaired. SpO_2 = pulse oximetry.

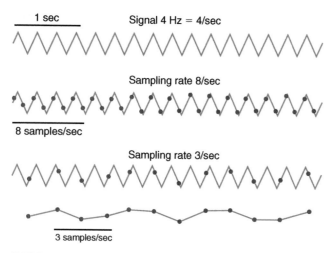

FIGURE 2–6 A signal at 4 Hz is sampled at 8/sec with fair reproduction. However, with sampling at 3/sec, the signal is distorted and a lower-frequency signal is introduced.

from the positive airway pressure device (flow, leak, tidal volume, delivered pressure), end-tidal, or partial pressure of carbon dioxide (PCO_2) device (end-tidal or transcutaneous).

Sampling Rate

Most digital recording systems use analog amplifiers that produce a continuous signal output. The signal is then sampled by an analog-to-digital (A/D) conversion board that converts the signal to a digital form that can be stored and manipulated by a computer. The sampling rate must be more than twice the frequencies being recorded to avoid signal distortion (Nyquist theorem).[1,2,4] If lower sampling rates are used, the signal can be very distorted and the addition of frequencies lower than the original signal sampled may be introduced (Fig. 2–6). For this reason, signals with a frequency higher than half the sampling rate must be filtered out because they can cause aliasing distortion.[2,4,5] For example, if the sampling rate is 200 samples/sec, the amplified signal must be processed by a high frequency filter with a cutoff frequency of 100 Hz or lower before being sampled (A/D converter). The required sampling rate depends on the frequency of the signal to be recorded. Slower varying signals require a lower sampling rate. In Table 2–2, the sampling rates recommended by the American Academy of Sleep Medicine (AASM) scoring manual[6] are illustrated. Some digital PSG systems have the ability to record different signals at different sampling rates. Ultimately, the computer program uses only a small portion of the data for the display because monitor resolution (in pixels per displayed time duration) is usually much less than the sampling rate.[5]

A/D conversion is also characterized by the dynamic range (the range of voltages accepted by the A/D converter) and the resolution. The dynamic range may be expressed as the amplified or unamplified signal range. The resolution depends on the A/D converter as well as the dynamic range. A 12-bit DC converter produces $2^{12} = 4096$ digital values (bits) or a 16-bit converter = 65,536 values across the dynamic

TABLE 2–2		
Recommended Sampling Rate for Various Polysomnographic Signals		
SAMPLING RATES	**DESIRABLE (HZ)**	**MINIMAL (HZ)**
EEG	500	200
EOG	500	200
EMG	500	200
ECG	500	200
Airflow	100	25
Oximetry	25	10
Nasal pressure	100	25
Esophageal pressure	100	25
Body position	1	1
Snoring	500	200
Rib cage/abdominal movements	100	25

ECG = electrocardiography; EEG = electroencephalography; EMG = electromyography; EOG = electro-oculography.
From Iber C, Ancoli-Israel S, Chesson A, Quan SF for the American Academy of Sleep Medicine: The AASM Manual for the Scoring of Sleep and Associated Events: Rules, Terminology and Technical Specifications, 1st ed. Westchester, IL: American Academy of Sleep Medicine, 2007.

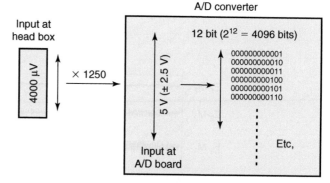

FIGURE 2–7 Dynamic range and resolution of an analog-to-digital (A/D) converter.

range. A typical A/D converter might have a dynamic range for the amplified signal of 5 V (±2.5 V). Commonly, a set amplification is applied to all AC signals before A/D conversion (e.g., a gain of 1250). If one assumes an amplification of 1250, then the dynamic range (peak to peak) of an A/D converter with an amplified voltage range of 5 V expressed as the unamplified signal would be approximately 4000 µV (4000 µV × 1250 = 5,000,000 µV = 5.0 V). If a 12-bit A/D converter is used, this would result in a resolution of 0.97 µV/bit (4000 µV/4096 digital values) (Fig. 2–7).

Monitor Resolution

An important limitation on the accuracy of signal recording and display is introduced by the fact that the monitor

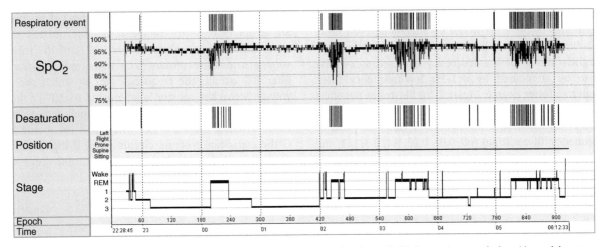

FIGURE 2–8 An overview of the entire night of the recording shows respiratory events, pulse oximetry (SpO₂), desaturation events, body position, and sleep stage (hypnogram). REM = rapid eye movement.

resolution is usually much lower than the data sampling rate. Because the sampling rate used for most digital systems is 200 samples/sec or higher, the resolution of the monitor is often the limiting factor in the accuracy of signal display. The minimum monitor resolution recommended by the AASM scoring manual is 1600×1200. Assuming 1600 pixels horizontally, the visual sampling rate for displays of a 30- or 10-second window of data corresponds to a sampling rate of approximately 50 and 150 samples/sec if the entire monitor display consists of waveforms. Then according to the Nyquist theorem, frequencies of 25 or 75 Hz or greater would be prone to aliasing. A monitor-induced aliasing distortion of data can sometimes be noted if switching from a 30-second to a 10-second view significantly changes the shape of the activity being visualized.[5]

Time Window for Display

During traditional paper-ink recording for sleep, the paper speed was 10 mm/sec, which produced 30-second pages (30-cm-wide paper). A faster speed was used for clinical EEG (30 mm/sec). However, such a fast paper speed would produce a very large amount of paper for each sleep study. In digital recording, one can choose various time windows during either acquisition or review. A 30-second window (equivalent to a paper speed of 10 mm/sec) is used for sleep staging and for scoring arousals. Time windows of 60 to 240 seconds may be used to view and score respiratory events and leg movements. Alternatively, viewing data in a 10-second window (equivalent to 30 mm/sec) is the usual method for clinical EEG recording. This allows better visualization of very brief events (sharp waves and spikes) and interictal or epileptiform activity. The 10-second window can also be useful for measuring the frequency of a group of oscillations or viewing the ECG result. The traditional ECG speed is 25 mm/sec, which is quite close to 30 mm/sec. Some systems allow split screens with different time windows in each screen. All digital sleep monitoring systems also provide

an all-night condensed view with graphs of the hypnogram (representation of sleep stages), arterial oxygen saturation (SpO₂ tracing), continuous positive airway pressure (CPAP) levels, respiratory events, and body position (Fig. 2–8). This allows a useful overview of the entire recording. One can usually select a time point (double click) on a given position in the summary view and be taken to that time point in the more detailed tracings.

FILTERS (LOW-FREQUENCY, HIGH-FREQUENCY, AND NOTCH FILTERS)

Any signal of interest can be contaminated by unwanted low- or high-frequency signals or 50- to 60-Hz artifact (from nearby AC power lines). Filters allow these components to be diminished. For example, a low-frequency filter (high-pass filter) attenuates the amplitude of low-frequency signals. A high-frequency filter (low-pass filter) attenuates the amplitude of high-frequency signals.[1] The amount of signal reduction due to a given analog or digital filter is given in decibels. The amount of signal reduction in decibels (dB) is given by the formula 20 log (voltage-out/voltage-in), where voltage-out and voltage-in are the amplitude of the signal entering and leaving the filter, respectively. A signal reduction of 30% and 50% (voltage-out/voltage-in ratios of ~ 0.7 and 0.5, respectively) corresponds to 3 dB and 6 dB reductions. Different filter settings (e.g., 0.3, 1) are named by the "cutoff frequency," which is the frequency of the signal that is reduced by 3 or 6 dB depending on the terminology and the type of filter the manufacturer uses. Therefore, a filter setting of "X Hz" means that the amplitude of a signal with a frequency of X is diminished by 30% or 50% depending on whether the 3 dB or 6 dB cutoff frequency is used to name the filter.

Low-Frequency Filter

A 1-Hz low-frequency filter (3 dB) attenuates a 1-Hz signal by 30% (or to 70% of the original signal). Similarly, a 6 dB filter would attenuate a 1-Hz signal by 50%. Signal strength of frequencies below 1 Hz would be attenuated even more (Figs. 2–9 and 2–10). It is important to realize that frequencies **slightly above** the low-frequency filter setting of 1 Hz will also be attenuated by a 1-Hz low-frequency filter, although to a lesser degree. Figure 2–10 illustrates the effect of various low-frequency filters (denoted by their 3 dB cutoff frequency) on low-frequency signals. A range of possible low-frequency filter settings (off, 0.01, 0.03, 0.1, 0.3, 1, 3, and 10) is commonly provided.

Sometimes low-frequency filter settings are specified as a time constant rather than as a cutoff frequency (Fig. 2–11). Traditional analog filters used resistance-capacitance (RC)

circuits. In RC circuits, an increase in step voltage produces an abrupt increase in voltage across the resistor, then an exponential fall in voltage to 1/e (0.37) of the maximum voltage in one time constant (TC). In a simple, low-frequency filter RC circuit, the frequency (fc) at which the output voltage across the resistor is attenuated to 0.37 of the input voltage is related to the TC by the formula fc = 1/(2π/TC). In RC circuits, the TC = RC, where R is the resistance and C the capacitance of the circuit. Even if digital filters are used, the relationship between the TC and the 3 dB frequency is given by Equation 2–1:

$$TC = 1/(2\pi \times \text{filter frequency}) \qquad \text{Equation 2–1}$$

FIGURE 2–9 A low-frequency filter setting of 1 Hz attenuates a signal of 1 Hz by 50% (6 dB filter). Signals with lower frequencies are attenuated more. Signals slightly above 1 Hz are also attenuated (but < 50%). Note that the horizontal axis uses a logarithmic scale and the vertical axis is linear.

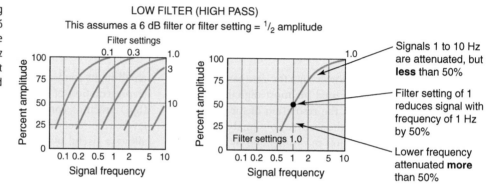

FIGURE 2–10 Effect of different low-frequency filter (LF) settings **(3 dB filter)** given in hertz on slow wave amplitude. Note that an LF 1 reduces a 1-Hz wave by about 30% (from 100 to 70 μV). An LF 0.3 Hz reduced the 1-Hz wave only slightly, whereas an LF 3 Hz essentially eliminated 1 Hz activity.

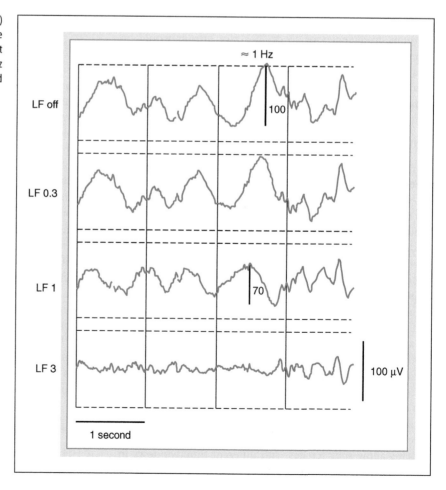

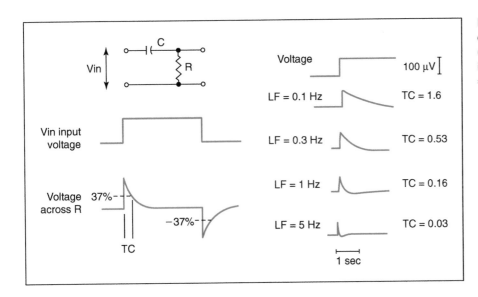

FIGURE 2-11 The lower the low-frequency filter cutoff frequency (LF), the longer the time constant (TC). Here, C is the capacitance and R is the resistance in a traditional resistance-capacitance (RC) filter. Vin = input voltage.

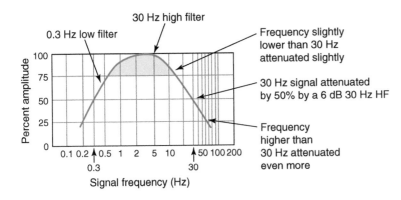

FIGURE 2-12 The effects of a high-frequency filter. A 6 dB 30-Hz filter attenuates a 30-Hz signal by 50%. Signals less than 30 Hz are attenuated less (low pass). Signals with a frequency higher than 30 Hz are attenuated much more. The *gray* shows a frequency range that is attenuated less than 0.70 by the combination of a 0.3-Hz low-frequency filter and a 30-Hz high-frequency filter (HF). This is often referred to as the *bandwidth* (or *bandpass* of the filters). Note that the horizontal axis of the plot uses a logarithmic scale and the vertical axis is linear.

For example, a 0.3-Hz low-frequency filter has a TC of approximately 0.53 second. Of note, the actual TC after a step increase in voltage may vary depending on the high-frequency filter setting as well. The lower the cutoff frequency, the longer the time constant (see Fig. 2–11). If amplifiers are calibrated by step (square wave) voltage change, the actual TC can be noted from the time it takes for the deflection to return to 0.37 of the maximum deflection.

High-Frequency Filters

A 35-Hz high-frequency filter attenuates a signal of 35 Hz by 50% (6 dB filter), and frequencies above 35 Hz would be attenuated more. In addition, frequencies **slightly below** the high-frequency filter setting will also be slightly attenuated. Figure 2–12 illustrates the effects of a 6 dB 30 Hz filter. A range of high-frequency filter settings is typically provided (off, 3, 15, 35, 70, and 100 Hz). Note that using a 30-Hz high-frequency filter (see Fig. 2–12) significantly attenuates 60-Hz signals. Therefore, the addition of a 60-Hz notch filter adds little if a 30- to 35-Hz filter is already being used.

Using the combination of a low-frequency and a high-frequency filter, a range of frequencies is amplified. Alternatively, if digital filters are applied to raw digital data, a range of frequencies is displayed. The range of signal displayed or amplified is called the *bandwidth*.

60-Hz or Notch Filters

Most amplifiers (digital PSG systems) provide optional notch filters to significantly attenuate a narrow range of frequency associated with power line signal contamination (e.g., 50 or 60 Hz). The notch filter can be added or removed. If the notch filter is turned on, it is applied to the signal in addition to the low-frequency and high-frequency filters. The routine use of a notch filter is usually not recommended. The sudden appearance of increased 60-Hz activity in a derivation is a clue that one or more electrodes is faulty. However, as previously mentioned, use of a high-frequency filter of 35 Hz (commonly used for EEG and EOG derivations) already substantially attenuates a 60-Hz signal (much the same as turning on the 60-Hz filter)

Turning on and off the 60-Hz (notch) filter can be useful in determining the degree of signal contamination by 60-Hz interference. If turning off the notch filter dramatically increases signal amplitude, this suggests considerable 60-Hz

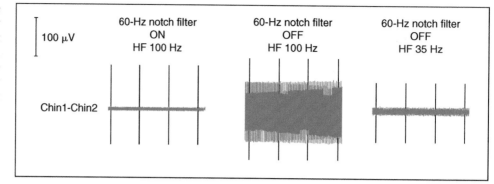

FIGURE 2–13 If signal amplitude increases significantly after the 60-Hz filter is turned off, this is evidence that significant 60-Hz activity is contaminating the signal. Turning on and off the 60-Hz filter will have less effect when the high-frequency filter setting is 35 Hz because much of the 60-Hz activity has already been filtered out.

signal contamination (Fig. 2–13). One would expect switching on and off the 60-Hz filter to have more effect if a high-frequency filter of 100 Hz was used (commonly used for EMG derivations) compared with a high-frequency filter of 35 Hz (EEG and EOG derivations). For this reason, 60-Hz contamination is most frequently visualized in the chin and leg EMG derivations even if the 60-Hz filter is turned on. Artifacts including 60-Hz artifact are discussed in more detail in Chapter 4.

AMPLIFIER FILTER SETTINGS FOR DIGITAL SLEEP RECORDING

Sleep recording with traditional dedicated bipolar AC amplifiers used RC circuits (RC filters) as filters and the recorded (on paper or computer) signal was filtered at the current amplifier settings. Today, most amplifiers used for digital recording (referential and true bipolar) record signals "wide open," that is, with default low-frequency filter (0.03–0.1) and a high-frequency filter setting usually at or less than half the sampling rate (e.g., 100-Hz for a sampling rate of 200/sec). Thus, "raw" signals are actually recorded over a wide frequency range or bandwidth (between default low and high frequencies) but are viewed (displayed) after application of selected digital low-frequency and high-frequency filters. The digital filters alter the displayed signal but NOT the recorded data. This allows multiple choices of filters if desired by the technologist or reviewer. The filter settings recommended by the AASM scoring manual[6,7] are shown in Table 2–3. The filter settings are selected to include the frequencies of interest in sleep monitoring. For example, to detect slow waves and eye movements but avoid the effect of scalp DC voltage changes (very low frequency), a low-frequency filter of 0.3 Hz is selected. Setting the low-frequency filter of the EEG or EOG channels higher would reduce slow wave and eye movement amplitude. For EMG and ECG channels, a low-frequency filter of 10-Hz is used, because the relevant activity is of a much higher frequency. For EEG and EOG monitoring, selection of a 35-Hz high-frequency filter removes unwanted higher frequencies but attenuates the characteristic EEG patterns such as sleep spindles (11–16 Hz) to a lesser degree. In contrast, the EMG frequences of interest are much higher and a high-frequency filter of 100 Hz is usually selected.

TABLE 2–3		
Recommended Filter Settings		
	LOW FREQUENCY	**HIGH FREQUENCY**
EEG	0.3 Hz	35 Hz
EOG	0.3 Hz	35 Hz
EMG	10 Hz	100 Hz
ECG	0.3 Hz	70 Hz
Respiration	0.1 Hz	15 Hz
Snoring	10 Hz	100 Hz

ECG = electrocardiography; EEG = electroencephalography; EMG = electromyography; EOG = electro-oculography.
From Iber C, Ancoli-Israel S, Chesson A, Quan SF for the American Academy of Sleep Medicine: The AASM Manual for the Scoring of Sleep and Associated Events: Rules, Terminology and Technical Specifications, 1st ed. Westchester, IL: American Academy of Sleep Medicine, 2007.

Clinical Example of the Effects of Filter Settings

As discussed in Chapter 7, monitoring nasal pressure provides a more accurate estimate of airflow than thermal sensors. During upper airway narrowing, the nasal pressure signal shows a flattening (flow plateau) during inspiration. Some sleep centers record nasal pressure with an AC amplifier instead of acquiring the signal in the DC mode. However, a low-frequency filter setting of 0.03 or less (or a long TC) is ideal to allow demonstration of a flow plateau in the nasal pressure signal (Fig. 2–14). To accurately record or display a very slowly varying signal, a sufficiently low cutoff frequency must be used for the low filter.

If the nasal pressure signal is unfiltered, vibration during snoring is often visible. However, the ability to see snoring (high-frequency vibration) depends on the high-frequency filter settings. Use of a fairly low high-frequency filter setting will reduce high-frequency signals such as noted in the nasal pressure tracing during snoring (Fig. 2–15). Ideally, one would use a high-frequency filter setting of 70 to 100 Hz.

DIGITIAL PSG SYSTEM OVERVIEW

The typical digital PSG system includes a headbox in which individual electrodes are attached to an amplifier. An

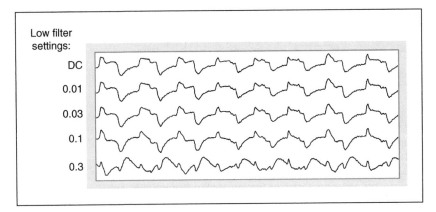

Low filter settings:

DC

0.01

0.03

0.1

0.3

FIGURE 2–14 Effects of different low-frequency filter settings on the nasal pressure signal. To visualize the plateau in the nasal pressure signal, either a DC recording or an AC recording with a very small low-frequency filter setting is needed (either 0.01 or 0.03 is ideal).

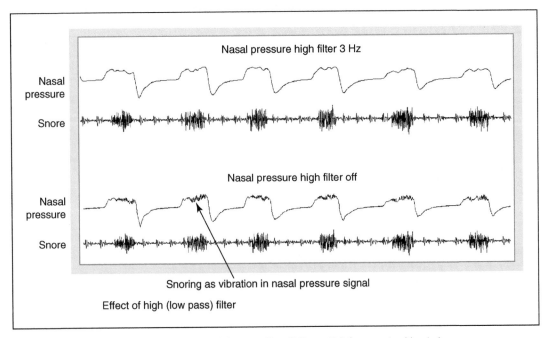

Nasal pressure high filter 3 Hz

Nasal pressure

Snore

Nasal pressure high filter off

Nasal pressure

Snore

Snoring as vibration in nasal pressure signal

Effect of high (low pass) filter

FIGURE 2–15 Effect of a high-frequency filter of 3 Hz on a high-frequency signal (snoring).

accessory box for DC channel inputs or dedicated input jacks on the amplifier are also usually available. The amplifier is then connected to the A/D converter. Today, the A/D converter is often contained within the amplifier that sits at the patient's bedside. The digitized signal can then be sent over ethernet cables to the computer or sent in the wireless mode to a computer, which then records the digital data. This arrangement avoids the difficulties that occur when an analog signal is sent over a long distance (60 Hz contamination or loss of signal strength). A schematic of a typical system is shown in Figure 2–16. A typical PSG amplifier often has a fixed gain and default low- and high-frequency filter settings (e.g., 0.1 and 100 Hz). AC signals are recorded over a wide frequency range (bandwidth). The A/D converter samples the signal and raw digital data are stored in the computer. After the raw data are digitized and stored, extensive manipulation is possible to produce the desired signal display. During acquisition and review, the computer program performs digital subtraction to display the desired

derivations and processes the data with the selected digital low-frequency and high-frequency filters. A display sensitivity is also chosen to determine the upper and lower limits of data to be displayed in the channel width (digital gain). The changes in the display (specific derivations, digital filters, digital gain) do not change the raw data that are recorded by the computer. The entire process is summarized in Figure 2–16.

Montages for Digital Recording

Digital systems allow the user to specify a number of user-defined display montages with the ability to select the number of channels (traces) to be displayed, the derivations for each channel, the order in which the desired derivations are displayed (the inputs for each channel), as well as the sensitivity (gain), low- and high-frequency filter settings, notch filter on or off, and the color of each tracing. A sample montage (Table 2–4) is displayed in Figure 2–17. Typically,

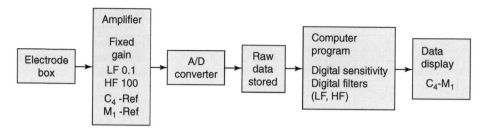

FIGURE 2–16 Schematic of a digital polysomnography (PSG) system. In many systems, the A/D converter is within the same unit housing the amplifier(s). Modern digital PSG systems usually perform a fixed amplification with default low (LF) and high (HF) filters permitting a wide frequency range to be amplified. The digitized data are stored on media (hard drive in the computer). The PSG software then scales the raw data, applies the selected low-frequency and high-frequency filters, and provides a display (either during acquisition or at review).

TABLE 2–4

Montage 1: Diagnostic Adult

CHANNEL (TRACING)	INPUT TYPE	INPUT 1	INPUT 2	SENSITIVITY (P-P) µV UNLESS DC	LF (HZ)	HF (HZ)	NOTCH FILTER
1	Ref	F_4	M_1	150	0.3	35	Off
2	Ref	C_4	M_1	150	0.3	35	Off
3	Ref	O_2	M_1	150	0.3	35	Off
4	Ref	F_3	M_2	150	0.3	35	Off
5	Ref	C_3	M_2	150	0.3	35	Off
6	Ref	O_1	M_2	150	0.3	35	Off
7	Ref	E_1	M_2	150	0.3	35	Off
8	Ref	E_2	M_2	150	0.3	35	Off
9	Ref	Chin1	Chin2	150	10	100	Off
10	BP	ECG1	ECG2	1500	0.3	70	Off
11	DC	Nasal pressure	N/A	−1 to +1 V†	DC	100	Off
12	BP	NOTF—input 1	Input 2	750*	0.1	15	Off
13	BP	Snore—input 1	Input 2	750*	10	100	Off
14	BP	Thorax—input 1	Input 2	1500*	0.1	15	Off
15	BP	Abdomen—input 1	Input 2	1500*	0.1	15	Off
16	DC	SpO$_2$	DC	0–1 V	DC	N/A	Off
17	BP	RAT—input 1	Input 2	150	10	100	Off
18	BP	LAT—input 1	Input 2	150	10	100	Off

*The sensitivity settings for bipolar channels depend on the output range for a particular device.
†Varies with transducer type.
BP = dedicated bipolar inputs (input-1, input-2); ECG = electrocardiography; HF = high frequency filter setting; LAT = left anterior tibial; LF = low frequency filter setting; N/A = not applicable; NOTF = nasal-oral thermal flow sensor; P-P = peak to peak; RAT = right anterior tibial; Ref = referential input; SpO$_2$ = pulse oximetry.

one montage is adapted for a diagnostic study and another for a positive-pressure titration. During review or acquisition, each individual channel may be altered if so desired or an entirely different montage may be displayed.

Channel Settings/Montages

Each channel (tracing) display can be changed by the viewer with respect to the inputs, sensitivity (sometimes called gain), low-frequency and high-frequency filters, channel width, and inversion of signal. Default settings for each channel can be specified, so they do not have to be individually set for each recording. Figure 2–17 illustrates typical channel controls. Recall that changes in channel settings do not change the recorded (and digitally stored) data.

In sleep recording using paper, the EEG was usually recorded at a sensitivity of 50 µV/cm in adults. In children, a lower sensitivity (100 µV/cm) was used because of the very high amplitude EEG activity. The term "gain" rather than sensitivity was also used. However, this implies an amplification of signal. In digital recording, amplification actually occurs before the signal is digitized. The size of the display of a given signal is varied by the computer program that scales the display based on the available channel width and the voltage limits or sensitivity. For example, if a channel width of 100 pixels represents 100 μV peak to peak, a signal of 50-μV peak to peak would vary between the 25th and the 75th pixel. The default digital displays for EEG often use 100 or 150 μV peak to peak per channel width (200 for children). Figure 2–18 shows two methods of adjusting the display (gain/voltage per division or peak-to-peak sensitivity). The

ultimate size of the channel width depends on the way the computer program scales the signal for display. Some programs have an option to allow signals either to overlap or to be cropped if they exceed the given channel width.

Impedance Checking and Referential Display View

Traditionally, after electrodes were applied to the patient's head, the impedance of each electrode was checked by plugging the electrodes into an impedance box that allowed comparison of any electrode referred to the ground electrode or a combination of all the other electrodes. Most digital systems can measure impedance on line using a signal from the amplifier. The values can then be stored with other digital data for later review. The AASM scoring manual recommends a maximum electrode impedance of 5 KΩ (<10 KΩ is acceptable). Another useful method of looking at the quality of each individual electrode is to display all of the unfiltered referentially recorded electrode against the common reference (rather than the digital subtraction of two referentially recorded electrodes). Figure 2–19 displays a referential view with all high-frequency filters set to 100 Hz. Electrode impedance is also displayed. One can tell that F$_4$, Chin2, and Chin3 electrodes are faulty and should be changed or fixed. As previously noted, if all tracings on the referential view are bad, this suggests a problem with the reference electrode. However, a faulty reference electrode does not affect the true bipolar channels (see Fig. 2–5).

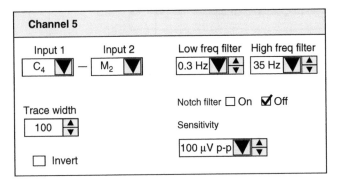

FIGURE 2–17 Example of typical controls for each display channel (tracing). Controls allow selection of the derivation, low-frequency and high-frequency filters, notch filter (on or off), and sensitivity. On most digital PSG systems, channel width and trace color can also be selected. p-p = peak to peak.

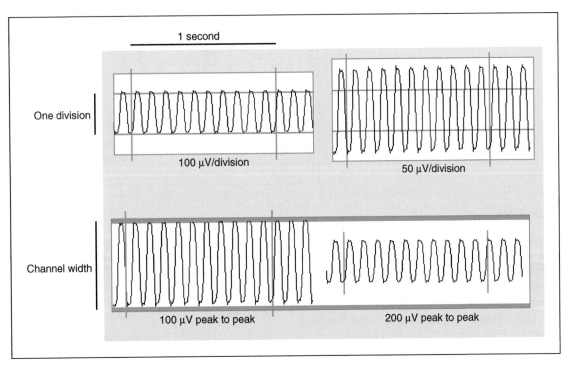

FIGURE 2–18 Two methods of adjusting the sensitivity (digital gain) are shown. A signal with a frequency of 10 Hz and amplitude of 100 uv is shown. The **top panels** specify a voltage per division value. A larger channel width is needed to display a given signal if the actual division size remains constant when voltage per division decreases. The **bottom panel** illustrates a method by which the peak-to-peak voltage of the entire channel width is specified. The actual channel width will depend on the way the computer program scales the display.

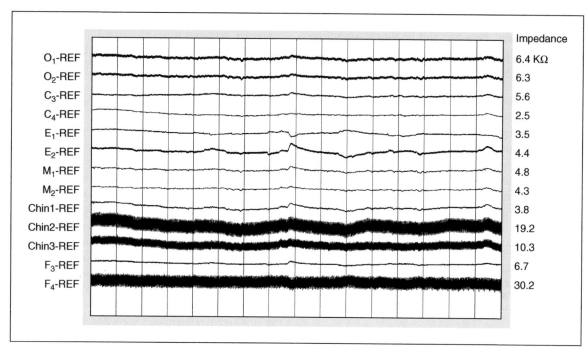

	Impedance
O$_1$-REF	6.4 KΩ
O$_2$-REF	6.3
C$_3$-REF	5.6
C$_4$-REF	2.5
E$_1$-REF	3.5
E$_2$-REF	4.4
M$_1$-REF	4.8
M$_2$-REF	4.3
Chin1-REF	3.8
Chin2-REF	19.2
Chin3-REF	10.3
F$_3$-REF	6.7
F$_4$-REF	30.2

FIGURE 2–19 A "referential display" with each electrode displayed against the common reference electrode. The electrode impedance is also displayed. One can see that the Chin2, Chin3, and F$_4$ electrodes should be replaced or repaired.

FIGURE 2–20 The three types of grounds used in a modern PSG amplifier are illustrated in a simplified schematic. The patient ground is separated from the earth ground by an isolation device or isolated section of the amplifier. (Courtesy of Marc Paliotta, Grass Technologies.) H = hot; N = neutral.

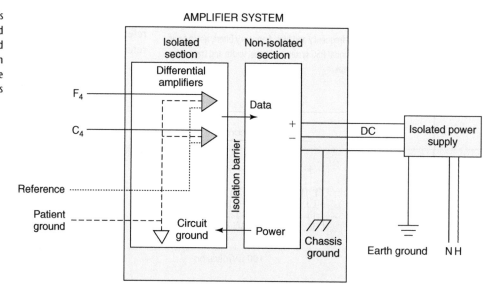

Video-Audio PSG

Today, most digital systems allow for the simultaneous recording of video and audio signals. Ideally, the video should be synchronized with the recorded EEG and other signals. This will allow the reviewer to see patient movement corresponding exactly to a given time point in the recorded PSG signals. For example, one could note facial twitching during a particular EEG pattern. Video PSG is an important development and allows the reviewer to confirm the patient position as well as document unusual behavior (e.g., parasomnias) during the night. Video files are often quite large and are usually compressed (e.g., MPEG4). The size of the file will depend on the quality of the video (10 or 25 frames/

sec). Simultaneous audio is also usually available and this is very useful for documenting teeth grinding (bruxism), talking during parasomnias, snoring, and other behaviors during the recording.

Grounds

The terminology is confusing with three different grounds being used in modern PSG recording (Fig. 2–20). These include

1. The patient ground (iso-ground input on the electrode box). This neutral electrode is usually connected to the

forehead. It is used to balance the inputs of all the differential amplifiers (essential for common mode rejection).

2. Chassis ground (container ground). Because a metal chassis is rarely used today, this would be the amplifier circuit ground (or the ground of the nonisolated portion of the amplifier).

3. Earth ground. In the three-wire power line (three-prong plug) AC input, the three wires are designated "hot (H)," "neutral (N)," and "earth" ground. Most amplifiers use an isolated medical-grade power supply that outputs low-level DC voltage to power the amplifiers.

In modern systems, the **patient ground is never directly connected to the earth ground.** A current-limiting device or isolation device is always placed between the patient ground and the earth ground. A common method is to use optical isolation in which the signal is transmitted by light within a small element of the circuit. Figure 2–20 illustrates one method in which part of the amplifier is isolated from the chassis and earth grounds.

CLINICAL REVIEW QUESTIONS

1. What (low, high) filter settings are recommended for PSG recording (display) of EEG and EOG derivations?
   A. 0.5, 70 Hz.
   B. 0.3, 35 Hz.
   C. 0.5, 70 Hz.
   D. 0.5, 35 Hz.

2. What are the recommended (low, high) filter settings for display of EMG?
   A. 1 Hz, 70 Hz.
   B. 0.3 Hz, 35 Hz.
   C. 10 Hz, 100 Hz.
   D. 10 Hz, 70 Hz.

3. What is the minimal recommended sampling rate for recording EEG, EOG, EMG, and ECG signals?
   A. 100 samples/sec.
   B. 200 samples/sec.
   C. 400 samples/sec.
   D. 500 samples/sec.

4. What is the minimal recommended sampling rate for airflow, rib cage and abdominal movements, and NP?
   A. 10 samples/sec.
   B. 25 samples/sec.
   C. 100 samples/sec.
   D. 200 samples/sec.

5. Which of the following is true about the effect of a low filter setting of 0.3 Hz?
   A. Has minimal effect on a 10-Hz signal.
   B. Does not affect the amplitude of slow wave activity (0.5–2 Hz).

C. Decreases the amplitude of a 0.1-Hz signal more than a 0.3-Hz signal.
   D. A and B.
   E. A and C.

6. If a sampling rate of 400 samples/sec is used, what is the highest frequency cutoff for the high filter that can be used and still avoid significant aliasing distortion?
   A. 400 Hz.
   B. 200 Hz.
   C. 100 Hz.
   D. 50 Hz.

7. Signals X, Y, and Z are recorded against a reference (referential) and W1 and W2 are acquired by bipolar recording (W1-W2) using digital PSG. Which of the following is **NOT** true?
   A. The derivation X-Y can be displayed.
   B. The derivation W1-X can be displayed.
   C. If all derivations containing X, Y, and Z show artifact, the reference electrode is probably faulty.
   D. The filter settings of the displayed derivation W1-W2 can be changed.

8. What is the minimum recommended sampling rate to record the oximetry signal?
   A. 50 samples/sec
   B. 25 samples/sec.
   C. 10 samples/sec.
   D. 100 samples/sec.

9. What is the recommended electrode impedance less than?
   A. 10 KΩ.
   B. 5 KΩ.
   C. 20 KΩ.
   D. 1 KΩ.

10. What are the recommended (low, high) filter settings for display of the ECG?
    A. 10, 100 Hz.
    B. 0.3, 35 Hz.
    C. 10, 70 Hz.
    D. 0.3, 70 Hz.

11. Using a high filter of 35 Hz for the EEG and EOG display (recording) reduces 60-Hz activity in the displayed signal.
    A. True
    B. False

12. What are the recommended (low, high) filter settings for display of the thermal airflow or chest and abdominal RIP signals?
    A. 0.3, 35 Hz.
    B. 0.1, 15 Hz.

C. 0.3, 15 Hz.

D. 0.1, 35 Hz.

Answers

1. **B.**

2. **C.**

3. **B.**

4. **B.**

5. **E.** A low filter of X Hz has some effect on signals with a slightly higher frequency than X. Therefore, a 0.3-Hz filter does have some effect on a frequency range of 0.5 to 2 Hz. The lower a frequency signal is compared with X Hz, the more the decrement in amplitude. A 0.3-Hz filter decreases the amplitude of a 0.1-Hz signal more than a 0.3-Hz signal.

6. **B. 200 Hz.** The Nyquist theorem states that the minimum sampling frequency to record a signal of X Hz is 2 X. Conversely, all frequencies greater than X are undersampled if a sampling rate of 2 X is used and if sampled can result in signal distortion. For this reason, a high filter of X must be applied to the signal to diminish those frequencies before the total signal reaches the A/D converter and is sampled.

7. **B.** True bipolar recording does not allow one part of the derivation (W1, W2) to be displayed against another electrode.

8. **C.** (10 samples/sec is the minimum recommended rate but 25 Hz is desirable).

9. **B.** 5 KΩ is recommended, <10 KΩ or less is acceptable.

10. **D.** Although a high filter of 70 Hz is the official recommendation, using a high filter setting of 100 Hz may allow better visualization of pacer spikes.

11. **True.** A high filter with a cutoff setting of X reduces the activity of frequency of signals higher than X. When using a high-frequency filter of 35 Hz, turning on and off the 60-Hz notch filter has less effect on the viewed signal.

12. **B.** Using a low filter of 0.1 instead of 0.3 allows more accurate visualization of a slowly varying signal.

REFERENCES

1. Tyner FS, Knott JR, Brem Mayer W: Fundamentals of EEG Technology. New York: Raven, 1983.
2. Fisch BJ: Spehlman's EEG Primer. New York: Elsevier, 1991, pp. 39–65.
3. Berry RB: Sleep Medicine Pearls, 2nd ed. Philadelphia: Hanley & Belfus, 2003, pp. 67–69.
4. Epstein C: Digital EEG. Trouble in paradise? J Clin Neurophysiol 2006;23:190–193.
5. Epstein CM: Aliasing in the visual EEG: a potential pitfall of video display technology. Clin Neurophysiol 2003;114:1974–1976.
6. Iber C, Ancoli-Israel S, Chesson A, Quan SF for the American Academy of Sleep Medicine: The AASM Manual for the Scoring of Sleep and Associated Events: Rules, Terminology and Technical Specifications, 1st ed. Westchester, IL: American Academy of Sleep Medicine, 2007.
7. Silber MH, Ancoli-Israel S, Bonnet MH, et al: The visual scoring of sleep in adults. J Clin Sleep Med 2007;15:121–131.

Sleep Staging in Adults

From 1968 to 2007, sleep was staged according to the manual by Rechtschaffen and Kales (R&K).[1,2] In the R&K manual, only central derivations were used to stage sleep, the term "movement time" was utilized to characterize epochs in which the electroencephalographic (EEG) and eye movement tracings are obscured by patient movement, and there was a 3-minute rule for the continuation of stage 2 (now known as *stage N2*). The *AASM Manual for the Scoring of Sleep and Associated Events*[3,4] was published in 2007 (subsequently referred to as the "AASM scoring manual"). This manual changed the rules of staging sleep and made recommendations about the methods used to monitor sleep.

The AASM scoring manual uses new nomenclature (Table 3–1) for the sleep stages, uses frontal and occipital as well as central EEG derivations, does not use the term "movement time," and has no 3-minute rule for stage N2 sleep. In addition, stages 3 and 4 are combined into stage N3. The succeeding discussion follows the new rules with some minor adaptations for brevity and clarity. Answers to questions posed to the AASM Scoring Manual Steering Committee and clarifications of the staging rules are posted in a frequently asked questions (FAQs) document on the internet (http://www.aasmnet.org/Resources/PDF/FAQsScoring Manual.pdf). The definitions of the EEG and eye movement patterns used for scoring are discussed in more detail in Chapter 1.

SCORING BY EPOCHS

The AASM scoring manual continues the convention of staging sleep in sequential 30-second epochs. Each epoch is assigned a sleep stage. If two or more stages coexist during a single epoch, the epoch is assigned the stage comprising the greatest portion of the epoch.

Stage W (Wake)

During wakefulness, patients make the transition from full alertness to the early stages of drowsiness. During **eyes open stage W** (Fig. 3–1), the EEG consists of low-amplitude activity (chiefly beta and alpha frequencies) without the rhythmicity of alpha rhythm (8–13 Hz most prominent over occipital derivations). Often, muscle artifact (high-frequency activity) is also present in the EEG. Rapid eye movements (REMs) and eye blinks (vertical movements 0.5–2 Hz) may occur. The submental (chin) electromyogram (EMG) is usually relatively increased compared with that during sleep. The majority of individuals with **eyes-closed stage W** will demonstrate alpha rhythm most prominent in the occipital area. Slow eye movements (SEMs) may also be present and the chin EMG activity is relatively high.

The rules for scoring stage W are listed in Table 3–2. In subjects who generate alpha rhythm, stage W is scored when more than 50% of the epoch contains alpha rhythm over the occipital region (see Table 3–2, rule A). SEMs may or may not be present during periods when alpha rhythm is present.

TABLE 3–1

Comparison of R&K and the American Academy of Sleep Manual

R&K*	AASM SCORING MANUAL†
Stage W	Stage W
Stages 1, 2, REM	Stages N1, N2, R
Stages 3, 4	Stage N3
Central EEG derivations	Frontal, central, and occipital derivations
3-minute rule for continuation of stage 2 after an epoch with K complexes or sleep spindles	No time limit on stage N2 continuation
Movement arousal based on EMG—an increase in the EMG of any channel accompanied by a change in pattern of any additional channel	Arousal based on EEG (and chin EMG for stage R)
Movement time when EEG and EOG obscured for more than half the epoch	No movement time Major body movement rules

*Rechtschaffen A, Kales A (eds): A Manual of Standardized Terminology Techniques and Scoring System for Sleep Stages of Human Sleep. Los Angeles: Brain Information Service/Brain Research Institute, UCLA, 1968.
†Iber C, Ancoli-Israel S, Chesson A, Quan SF for the American Academy of Sleep Medicine: The AASM Manual for the Scoring of Sleep and Associated Events: Rules, Terminology and Technical Specifications, 1st ed. Westchester, IL: American Academy of Sleep Medicine, 2007.
EEG = electroencephalography; EMG = electromyography; EOG = electro-oculography; REM = rapid eye movement.

TABLE 3–2

Stage W Rules

A. Score epochs as stage W when *more* than 50% of the epoch has alpha rhythm over the occipital region.
   1. EOG: Slow eye movements are characteristic of eyes-closed stage W but are not required criteria for scoring stage W.
   2. Chin EMG: The chin EMG amplitude is variable but is often higher than during sleep.

B. Score epochs **without visually discernible alpha rhythm (or portions of an epoch without alpha rhythm*)** as stage W if any of the following are present:
   1. Eye blinks are present at a frequency of 0.5–2 Hz.
   2. Reading eye movements are present.
   3. Irregular conjugate REMs are present associated with *normal or high chin muscle tone* (in contrast, stage R has low chin activity).

*Adaptation of AASM scoring manual stage W, rule B.
Notes:
1. Score stage W when the majority of an epoch has either alpha rhythm or eye movements consistent with wake as defined in B.
2. Eye movement patterns (see Chapter 1).
   A. Reading eye movements: trains of conjugate eye movements consisting of a slow phase followed by a rapid phase in the opposite direction as the subject reads.
   B. Blinks: conjugate vertical eye movements present in wakefulness with eyes open or closed.
   C. REMs: conjugate irregular, sharply peaked eye movements with an initial deflection lasting < 500 msec.
EMG = electromyogram; EOG = electro-oculogram; REMs = rapid eye movements.
Adapted from Iber C, Ancoli-Israel S, Chesson A, Quan SF for the American Academy of Sleep Medicine: The AASM Manual for the Scoring of Sleep and Associated Events: Rules, Terminology and Technical Specifications, 1st ed. Westchester, IL: American Academy of Sleep Medicine, 2007.

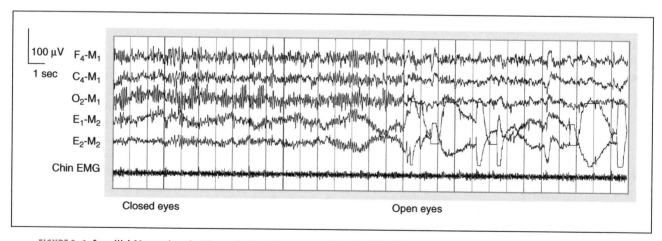

FIGURE 3–1 Stage W. A 30-second epoch with eyes closed and then eyes open. More than 50% of the epoch has occipital alpha activity. EMG = electromyogram.

Epochs without visually discernible alpha rhythm (see Table 3–2, rule B) are scored as stage W if any of the following are present: Eye blinks of a frequency of 0.5 to 2 Hz, reading eye movements, or irregular conjugate REMs with normal or high chin muscle tone. These eye movement patterns are characteristic of stage W. The requirement of normal or high chin EMG tone for REMs is because stage R (REM sleep) is characterized by REMs and low muscle tone.

How should one score epochs that contain both portions with alpha rhythm (but < 50% of the epoch) AND portions with eye movements consistent with wake? The AASM scoring manual did not specifically address this situation.

However, one can modify stage W rule B to apply to the **portions** of the epoch without alpha rhythm that contain eye movements consistent with wake (see Table 3–2, rule B). If the portions of the epoch containing alpha rhythm AND the portions of the epoch considered to be wake due to eye movements add up to more than 15 seconds (majority of the epoch), then the epoch is scored as stage W.

Of note, approximately 10% of subjects do not generate alpha rhythm on eye closure and a further 10% may generate limited alpha rhythm. In these subjects, the occipital EEG activity is similar during eye opening and eye closure. When alpha rhythm is not generated with eye closure, the rules for scoring stage W and stage N1 are somewhat different and sleep onset is more difficult to define (Tables 3–3 and 3–4). In patients who do not generate alpha rhythm, epochs satisfying rule B in Table 3–2 are scored as stage W. Otherwise, epochs are scored as stage W if they do NOT meet criteria for stages N1, N2, N3, or R. In contrast to patients generating alpha rhythm, the presence of SEMs is a criterion for scoring stage N1 in subjects who do not generate alpha rhythm (see Table 3–4).

In Figure 3–1, a 30-second tracing shows the transition from eyes-closed stage W to eyes-open stage W. Slightly more than 50% of the epoch contains alpha activity. Alpha activity is attenuated with eye opening and REMs are noted. In Figure 3–2, portions of the epoch contain alpha rhythm and other portions are considered stage W owing to the presence of eye movements consistent with wakefulness

---

TABLE 3–3

Stage N1 Rules

A. In subjects **who generate alpha rhythm with eye closure,** score stage N1 if
1. EEG: Alpha rhythm is attenuated and replaced by low-amplitude mixed-frequency (4–7 Hz) activity for **more than 50%** of the epoch (<50% of the epoch has alpha rhythm).
   a. EEG: Vertex sharp waves may be present but are *not required* for scoring stage N1.
2. EOG: Slow eye movements may be present in N1, but these are **not required** for scoring N1.
3. Chin EMG: Variable amplitude, often lower than wake.

B. In subjects *who do NOT generate alpha rhythm with eye closure,* score stage N1 commencing with the *earliest* of any of the following phenomena:
1. The EEG shows 4- to 7-Hz activity with slowing of background frequencies by 1 Hz or greater from those of stage W.
2. Vertex sharp waves.
3. Slow eye movements.

Note: Because slow eye movements often commence before attenuation of alpha rhythm, sleep latency may be slightly shorter for some individuals who do not generate alpha rhythm than for those who do.
EEG = electroencephalogram; EMG = electromyogram;
EOG = electro-oculogram.
Adapted from Iber C, Ancoli-Israel S, Chesson A, Quan SF for the American Academy of Sleep Medicine: The AASM Manual for the Scoring of Sleep and Associated Events: Rules, Terminology and Technical Specifications, 1st ed. Westchester, IL: American Academy of Sleep Medicine, 2007.

TABLE 3–4

Scoring Stage W and N1

		EEG*	EOG	CHIN EMG
Alpha rhythm on eye closure	Stage W Eyes closed	>50% of the epoch with alpha activity	SEMs may be present	Variable
	Stage W Eyes open	Low-amplitude beta and alpha frequencies	**REMs**	**Normal or high**
			Blinks	Variable
			Reading eye movements	
	Stage N1	>50% of epoch with alpha attenuation and replacement with low-amplitude mixed-frequency EEG	SEMs may be present	Variable
No alpha rhythm on eye closure	Stage W	Low-amplitude beta and alpha frequencies	**REMs**	**Normal or high**
			Eye blinks	Variable
			Reading eye movements **SEMs absent**	
	Stage N1	**Vertex sharp wave**	Variable	Variable
		Slowing of 4 to 7 Hz, slowing of frequency ≥ 1 Hz, compared to stage W	Variable	Variable
		Low-amplitude beta and alpha frequencies	**SEMs appear**	Variable

Note: **Bold text** denotes essential features.
*The EEG is assumed not to contain sleep spindles or K complexes not associated with arousal.
EEG = electroencephalogram; EMG = electromyogram; EOG = electro-oculogram; REMs = rapid eye movements; SEMs = slow eye movements.

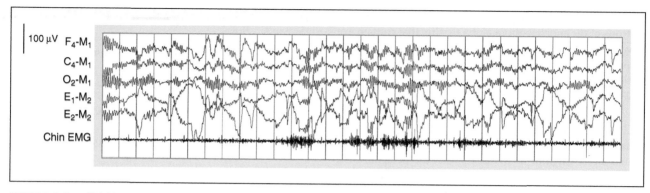

FIGURE 3–2 Stage W. A 30-second epoch containing rapid eye movements (REMs), high chin electromyographic (EMG) activity, and some alpha activity. The majority of the epoch contains either alpha activity or eye movements consistent with wakefulness.

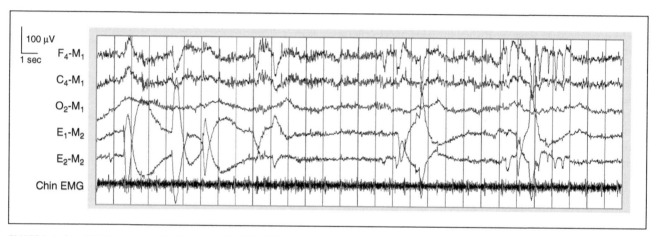

FIGURE 3–3 Stage W. A 30-second epoch is shown containing REMs, blinks, relatively high chin electromyographic (EMG) activity, and the absence of discernible alpha activity.

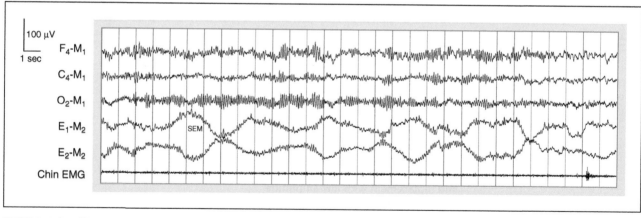

FIGURE 3–4 Stage W with the eyes closed. A 30-second epoch is shown. Note that alpha rhythm is more prominent in the occipital derivation and present for more than 50% of the epoch. Slow eye movements (SEMs) are present in this epoch. Although characteristic, they are not a criterion for scoring stage W or N1 in patients producing alpha rhythm with eye closure. The chin electromyography (EMG) has a low amplitude, but this is variable. In some patients, the chin EMG activity is higher in stage W than during sleep.

(see Table 3–2, stage W rule B). The majority of the epoch contains either alpha rhythm or eye movements consistent with wakefulness, and hence, the epoch is scored as stage W. In Figure 3–3, the chin EMG activity is relatively high, REMs and blinks are present, and there is no discernible alpha activity. The epoch is scored as stage W using stage W rule B (see Table 3–2). Figure 3–4 illustrates an example of eyes-closed stage W. Here, greater than 50% of the epoch has prominent alpha activity. SEMs are also present and the EMG activity is relatively decreased. It should be noted that SEMs can be seen during both eyes-closed stage W and stage N1. If patients produce alpha rhythm with eye closure, SEMs are not part of the criteria to score stage W (although they are characteristic during eyes-closed stage W).

Stage N1

Low-amplitude mixed-frequency (LAMF) activity is defined as a low-amplitude EEG pattern with predominantly 4- to 7-Hz activity. Stage N1 is characterized by LAMF activity and the **absence** of sleep spindles (SSs) and K complexes (KCs) not associated with arousal. SEMs may occur (see Table 3–3). At the transition from stage N1 to stage N2, vertex sharp waves may appear. In patients who produce alpha activity with eye closure (stage N1 rule A, see Table 3–3), the onset of stage N1 occurs when **more than 50% of the epoch is marked by alpha attenuation** (alpha activity in < 50% of the epoch) and replacement with LAMF EEG (Fig. 3–5). In individuals who do not produce alpha activity with eye closure (Fig. 3–6), the start of stage N1 occurs **at the earliest occurrence** of SEMs, a slowing of the EEG by 1 Hz or more from that in stage W, or the presence of vertex sharp waves (stage N1 rule B, see Table 3–3). Table 3–4 displays the characteristics of stage W and stage N1 for patients who do and do not produce alpha with eye closure. As noted in the AASM scoring manual, because SEMs may occur before alpha attenuation in subjects who have alpha activity with eye closure, the sleep onset may be scored somewhat earlier in patients who do not produce alpha activity with eye closure.

Stage N2

Stage N2 is characterized by the presence of one or more nonarousal KCs (i.e., KCs NOT associated with an arousal) or one or more trains of SSs (Fig. 3–7). Arousal rules are discussed later in this chapter. During epochs of stage N2, eye movements have usually ceased and the chin EMG is variable but usually at a level lower than that during wakefulness. Recall that a KC is said to be associated with an arousal (KC+Ar) if the arousal commences no more than 1 second after the termination of the KC. Also note that the KC activity is seen in the recommended electro-oculographic (EOG) derivations (E_1-M_2 and E_2-M_2) as in-phase deflections in contrast to REMs (out-of-phase deflections). The rules for scoring stage N2 are listed in Table 3–5 and summarized in Table 3–6.

Start and Continuation of Stage N2

According to the stage N2 rules (see Table 3–5, rule A), begin scoring stage N2 (see Fig. 3–7) when a KC (not associated with an arousal) or an SS occurs in the first half of the **current epoch** or the **last half of the previous epoch**. This assumes that the epoch does not meet criteria for stage N3 (slow wave activity [SWA] present in ≥ 20% of the epoch, i.e., ≥6 sec). Recall that SWA is defined as EEG activity of

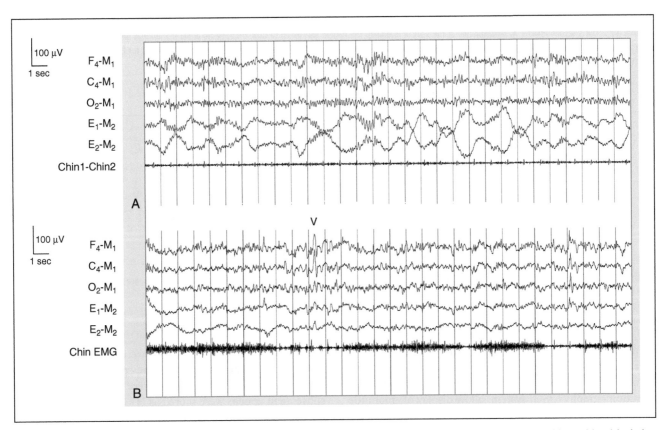

FIGURE 3–5   **A,** Stage N1. A 30-second epoch in which no sleep spindles or K complexes are noted in the electroencephalogram (EEG). Less than 50% of the epoch has alpha rhythm. The EEG shows alpha attenuation and low-amplitude mixed-frequency (4–7 Hz) activity for more than 50% of the epoch. Slow eye movements are present but not required. The chin electromyogram (EMG) is often lower than stage W. **B,** Stage N1. A vertex sharp wave (V) is noted. No sleep spindles or K complexes are seen in the EEG. The chin EMG is relatively high in this example.

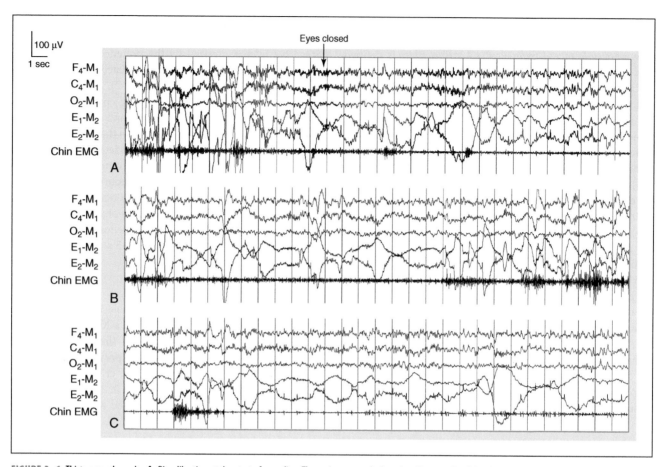

FIGURE 3–6 Thirty-second epochs. **A,** Biocalibration at the start of recording. The patient was asked to close his eyes. No alpha rhythm was generated. **B** and **C,** Consecutive 30-second epochs. **B,** An epoch of stage W with REMs and high chin electromyographic (EMG) activity. **C,** Slow eye movements are present and the EEG frequency slows. Therefore, epoch **C** is scored as an epoch of stage N1 sleep. The chin EMG also falls in **C,** but this is not a criterion used for scoring stage N1 sleep.

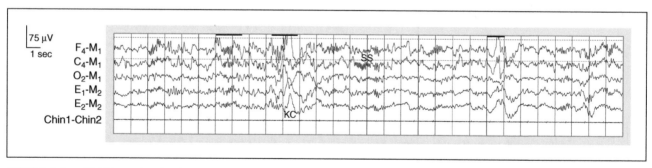

FIGURE 3–7 Stage N2: A 30-second epoch with sleep spindles (SS) and K complexes (KC). The *dark horizontal bars* at the top denote the presence of slow wave activity (>75 μV peak to peak, 0.5–2.0 Hz). The total duration of slow wave activity is less than 6 seconds. The *dotted lines* in F₄-M₁ are 75 μV apart.

0.5 to 2 Hz with greater than 75-μV peak-to-peak amplitude over the frontal areas. If the epoch in question contains 20% or more SWA, then stage N3 is scored (Fig. 3–8). Most digital polysomnography (PSG) systems allow display of amplitude grid lines, and placing lines at −37.5 μV + 37.5 μV in F_4-M_1 or F_3-M_2 allows one to easily note 75-μV peak-to-peak activity (see Figs. 3–7 and 3–8).

In the R&K scoring manual, stage 2 continued without additional SSs or KCs for a maximum of 3 minutes (the

3-min rule). If no new KCs or SSs were noted for more than 3 minutes, the epochs following the epoch with the last KC or SS (during the 3-min period) were scored as stage 1 and subsequent epochs were scored as N1 (unless there was new evidence for another sleep stage). In the AASM scoring manual, there is no such time limitation. Stage N2 continues until there is a reason to score an end of a period of stage N2 sleep (see Table 3–5, rule B). If an arousal occurs, a major body movement (MBM) followed by SEMs (signaling a

TABLE 3-5

Stage N2 Rules*

A. RULE DEFINING THE START OF N2 SLEEP

1. EEG: Begin scoring stage N2 (in the absence of evidence of N3, SWA < 6 sec) if one or both of the following occur during the ***first half of the current epoch*** or the ***last half of the previous epoch:***
   a. One or more K complexes *unassociated with arousals* or
   b. One or more trains of sleep spindles.
2. EEG: If the only K complexes present are associated with arousal, continue to score stage N1.
3. EOG: Usually no eye movements, slow eye movements have ended.
4. Chin EMG: Variable, usually less than wake.

Note: SWA = EEG activity 0.5–2 Hz with > 75 μV peak-to-peak amplitude in the frontal areas. If SWA ≥ 20% of the epoch (6 sec), score stage N3.

B. RULE DEFINING THE CONTINUATION OF STAGE N2 SLEEP

1. Continue to score epochs with low-amplitude mixed-frequency EEG activity without K complexes or sleep spindles as stage N2 if they are preceded by an epoch containing:
   a. K complexes unassociated with arousals or
   b. Sleep spindles.

C. RULE DEFINING THE END OF A PERIOD OF STAGE N2 SLEEP

1. End stage N2 sleep when one of the following events occurs:
   a. Transition to stage W, stage N3, or stage R.
   b. An **arousal** (change to stage N1 until a K complex unassociated with an arousal or a sleep spindle occurs).
   c. A **major body movement** followed by **slow eye movements** and low-amplitude mixed-frequency EEG without nonarousal associated K complexes or sleep spindles then score epochs after the major body movement as N1.
      i. If no slow eye movements follow the major body movement, score the epoch as stage N2.
      ii. The epoch containing the body movement is scored using criteria for major body movements.

*See later rules for arousal (see Table 3–15) and major body movements (see Table 3–14).
EEG = electroencephalography; EMG = electromyography; EOG = electro-oculography; SWA = slow wave activity.
Adapted from Iber C, Ancoli-Israel S, Chesson A, Quan SF for the American Academy of Sleep Medicine: The AASM Manual for the Scoring of Sleep and Associated Events: Rules, Terminology and Technical Specifications, 1st ed. Westchester, IL: American Academy of Sleep Medicine, 2007.

TABLE 3-6

Summary of Scoring Stage N2

START N2	CONTINUE N2	STOP N2
KC or SS in **first half** of current epoch or *last half* of the previous epoch.	• EEG with LAMF **without** KC or SS. • IF the epoch (or a group of epochs) is preceded by an epoch with a nonarousal KC or SS.	• Transition to stage W, N3, or R. • Arousal. • Major body movement followed by an SEM.

EEG = electroencephalogram; KC = K complex not associated with arousal; LAMF = low-amplitude mixed-frequency; SEM = slow eye movement; SS = sleep spindle.

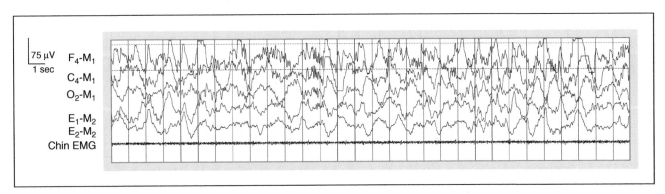

FIGURE 3–8 Stage N3 sleep (30-sec epoch). The *dotted lines* in F₄-M₁ are 75 μV apart. The grid lines are 1 second apart. Slow wave activity is present in all 30 seconds of the epoch (Table 3–7).

transition to stage N1), or the epoch meets criteria for stages W, N3, or R, then stage N2 ends (see Table 3–5, rule C.1.a).

Figure 3–9 is a schematic illustrating the start of stage N2 sleep. Epoch 101 has a KC not associated with an arousal in the first half of the epoch and is scored stage N2. In epoch 201, the KC begins in the second half of the epoch so stage N2 begins in epoch 202. Stage N2 continues in epochs 102 and 103 and 202 and 203 even though no SSs or KCs occur. Note that a KC+Ar is NOT evidence that stage N2 has begun (Fig. 3–10, epoch 101).

TABLE 3–7

Stage N3 Rules

A. Score stage N3 when **20% or more** of an epoch consists of SWA, irrespective of age (*20% of 30-sec epoch = 6 sec*).
 1. EEG: SWA ≥ 20% of the epoch (≥6 sec), sleep spindles may be present in stage N3.
 2. EOG: Eye movements are not typically seen during stage N3 sleep.
 3. EMG: In stage N3, the chin EMG is of variable amplitude, often lower than in stage N2 sleep and sometimes as low as in stage R sleep.

Definition: SWA = EEG activity 0.5–2 Hz with peak-to-peak amplitude > 75 µV measured over the frontal areas.
Note: SWA may be seen in the EOG derivations.
EEG = electroencephalogram; EMG = electromyogram;
EOG = electro-oculogram; SWA = slow wave activity.
Adapted from Iber C, Ancoli-Israel S, Chesson A, Quan SF for the American Academy of Sleep Medicine: The AASM Manual for the Scoring of Sleep and Associated Events: Rules, Terminology and Technical Specifications, 1st ed. Westchester, IL: American Academy of Sleep Medicine, 2007.

End of Stage N2: Effects of Arousals

Stage N2 ends following an arousal (see Table 3–5, rule C.1.b). Unless there is a transition to another sleep stage, stage N1 is scored until there is evidence for resumption of stage N2 (see Table 3–5, rule A). Note if an arousal interrupts stage N2 in the second half of the epoch, the epoch is still scored as stage N2 because the majority of the epoch is stage N2. The effects of an arousal are illustrated in Figure 3–10. An arousal occurs in epoch 201. Because the arousal occurs in the last half of the epoch, the current epoch remains as stage N2 but the next epoch is scored as stage N1. Stage N2 resumes only when there is evidence of a KC not associated with an arousal or SS (using rules for the start of stage N2).

End of Stage N2: Effect of MBM

A **major body movement** (MBM) is defined as movement and muscle artifact obscuring the EEG for more than half an epoch to the extent that the sleep stage cannot be determined. If stage N2 is interrupted by an MBM followed by an SEM and LAMF, stage N1 is scored until there is evidence to restart stage N2 (SS or KC not associated with an arousal) (see Table 3–5, rule C.1.c). If the MBM is NOT followed by an SEM, stage N2 does not end unless there is a transition to stage W, N3, or R (see Table 3–5, rule C.1.c). In Figure 3–11, an MBM interrupts stage N2 sleep. In Figure 3–11A, the MBM is not followed by SEMs and stage N2 continues. The epoch with the MBM is scored using rules discussed later. In Figure 3–11B, the MBM is followed by an SEM and LAMF EEG activity and the epoch after the MBM is scored as stage N1. Stage N2 resumes only when there is new

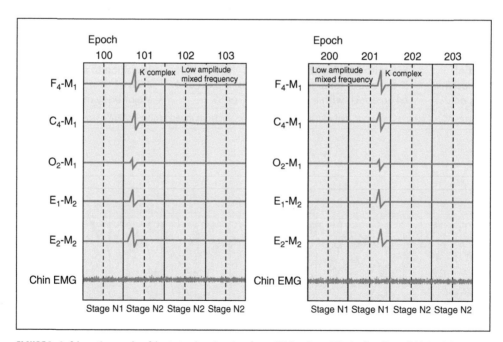

FIGURE 3–9 Schematic examples of the start and continuation of stage N2 sleep (stage N2 rules A and B; see Table 3–5). Score stage N2 in epoch 101 as a nonarousal—K complex is noted in the first half of the epoch. Stage N2 continues in epochs 102 and 103. In epoch 201, the K complex occurs in the last half of the epoch, so stage N2 begins in epoch 202. The schematics assume the EEG activity is low-voltage mixed-frequency unless otherwise depicted.

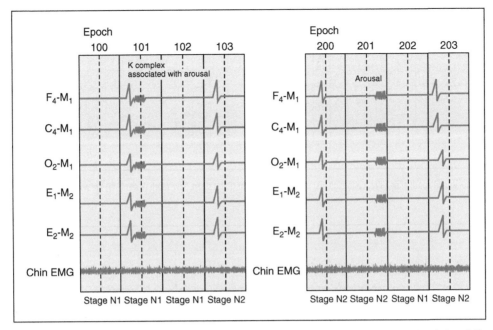

FIGURE 3–10 Schematics illustrating the effects of a K complex associated with an arousal (epoch 101) (stage N2 rule A; see Table 3–5) and an arousal interrupting stage N2 sleep (stage N2 rule C.1.b; see Table 3–5). Epoch 202 is scored as stage N1.

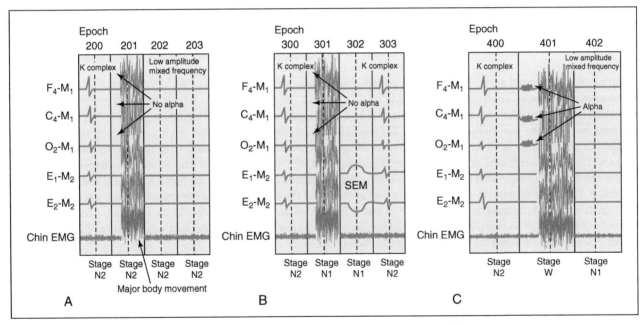

FIGURE 3–11 A major body movement (MBM) interrupts stage N2 (stage N2, rule C.1.c). **A,** If the epoch containing the MBM has no alpha and there are no slow eye movements (SEMs) in the subsequent epoch, stage N2 continues (epochs 202 and 203). **B,** If SEMs and low-amplitude mixed-frequency (LAMF) activity follow the MBM, a transition to stage N1 is scored (epoch 302). **C,** If the MBM epoch contains alpha, the epoch is scored as stage W (see MBM rules in Table 3–5, rule C.1.c). In this case, stage N2 ends. The next epoch of sleep without K complexes or sleep spindles is scored as stage N1.

evidence for this sleep stage (a KC not associated with an arousal or an SS).

As discussed in a subsequent section on MBM scoring, if any alpha is present in the epoch (even < 15 sec) containing the MBM, then the epoch is scored as stage W. In this case, the period of stage N2 ends (see Fig. 3–11C). If the epoch preceding or following an MBM is scored as stage W, the MBM epoch is scored as stage W. Otherwise, the MBM

epoch is scored based on the stage of the following epoch (see "Major Body Movements," later) (see Tables 3–13 and 3–14, later in this chapter).

Stage N3

In stage N3, the amount of SWA (SWA = EEG activity of 0.5–2 Hz and a peak-to-peak amplitude of > 75 µV

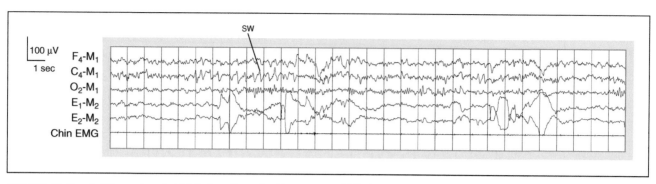

FIGURE 3–12 Stage R. A 30-second epoch of definite (unambiguous) rapid eye movement (REM) sleep. Saw-tooth waves (SW) are not required to score stage R but are helpful.

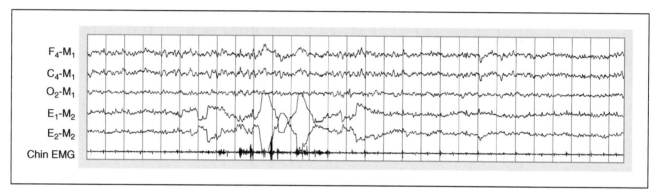

FIGURE 3–13 Stage R. A 30-second epoch containing transient muscle activity (TMA) in the chin EMG.

measured over the frontal areas) *is **equal to** or greater than* 20% of an epoch (≥6 sec). The SWA is also noted in the EOG derivations but SEM or REMs are not present. The chin EMG is variable but typically less than during wake. The amount of stage N3 decreases in adult men but not women as age increases. This is primarily due to a decrease in EEG amplitude (in the 0.2–2 Hz range) that occurs in men with aging. In Figure 3–7, SWA is denoted by dark horizontal bars at the top of the tracing and the total duration of SWA is less than 6 seconds. If SWA is ≥6 seconds, the epoch would be scored as stage N3. Figure 3–8 shows an epoch of stage N3. Nearly all of the epoch meets SWA amplitude criteria.

Stage R

The EEG activity in stage R resembles that of stage N1 and generally contains LAMF activity. However, alpha activity in stage R is usually more prominent than in stage N1 and usually has a frequency 1 to 2 Hz lower than during wakefulness. The three components of stage R are (1) a low-amplitude EEG without KCs or SSs, (2) REMs, and (3) low chin EMG tone (activity). In the AASM scoring manual, **low EMG tone** is defined as baseline EMG activity in the chin derivation no higher than in any other sleep stage and usually at the lowest level of the entire recording. These three components of stage R may not all start or stop at the same time. In addition, REMs are episodic and not all epochs of stage R have REMs. Therefore, special rules are needed for the start, continuation, and end of stage R as well as transitions from N2 to REM

sleep. Saw-tooth waves are often present in epochs of stage R. They are 2- to 6-Hz triangular waves maximal over central regions (Fig. 3–12). During burst of REMs, transient muscle activity (TMA) is also often seen during stage R. TMA is characterized by short irregular bursts of EMG activity (<0.25 sec) in the chin derivations superimposed on low chin activity (Fig. 3–13). Saw-tooth waves and TMA are NOT part of the criteria for scoring stage R but are strongly supportive that stage R is present. TMA may also occur in leg EMG derivations often associated with bursts of REMs.

Definite REM Sleep (REM Rule A)

When epochs have all three characteristics of REM sleep (Table 3–8, REM rule A), they are considered definite or unambiguous epochs of REM sleep (see Fig. 3–12). The EEG has low amplitude mixed frequency activity, REMs are present, and chin EMG tone is low. However, contiguous epochs (before or after definite epochs of REM sleep) that lack REMs but have a "REM-like EEG" with no sleep spindles or K complexes and low chin EMG activity are often scored as stage R, **if they meet criteria specified in the stage R rules.**

Stage REM typically follows epochs of stages N2 and, less commonly, stage W or stage N1. The AASM scoring manual lists rules for transition from stage N2 to stage R (see later). The manual does not address transitions from stage W or stage N1 to stage R. However, based on FAQ V7, stage R is not scored following stage W or N1 until an epoch of definite REM sleep is noted.

TABLE 3-8

Stage R Rule A (Definite REM Sleep)

A. Score stage R sleep in epochs with *all* the following phenomena (definite or unequivocal REM epochs):
   a. Low-amplitude mixed-frequency EEG.
   b. Low chin EMG tone (the baseline EMG activity in the chin derivation is no higher than in any other sleep stage and ***usually at the lowest level of the entire recording).***
   c. REMs.

Notes:
1. **Low chin EMG tone:** The baseline EMG activity in the chin derivation is no higher than in any other sleep stage and ***usually at the lowest level of the entire recording.***
2. **REMs:** Conjugate, irregular, sharply peaked eye movements with an initial deflection usually lasting < 500 msec.
3. **Definite stage R (unequivocal stage R)** = EEG without spindles or K complexes, REMs, low chin EMG activity (at REM level).

EEG = electroencephalogram; EMG = electromyogram; REM = rapid eye movement.

Adapted from Iber C, Ancoli-Israel S, Chesson A, Quan SF for the American Academy of Sleep Medicine: The AASM Manual for the Scoring of Sleep and Associated Events: Rules, Terminology and Technical Specifications, 1st ed. Westchester, IL: American Academy of Sleep Medicine, 2007.

TABLE 3-9

Continuation and End of Stage R (REM Rules B and C)

B. **Continuation of stage R:** Continue to score stage R sleep, *even in the absence of REMs,* for epochs **following** one or more epochs of stage R as defined above (unequivocal REM epochs), if
   a. EEG continues to show *low-amplitude mixed-frequency activity without K complexes or sleep spindles.*
   b. Chin EMG: Tone *remains low* (at REM level).

C. **End of stage R.**
   1. Stop scoring stage R sleep when one or more of the following occur:
      a. There is a transition to stage W or N3.
      b. An ***increase in chin EMG tone*** above the level of stage R is seen and criteria for stage N1 are met.
      c. An ***arousal*** occurs followed by low-amplitude mixed-frequency EEG and *slow eye movements* (score as stage N1; *if no slow eye movements and chin EMG tone remains low, continue to score as stage R*).
      d. **A major body movement followed by slow eye movements** and low-amplitude mixed-frequency EEG without nonarousal-associated K complexes or sleep spindles (score the epoch after the major body movement as stage N1; if **no slow eye movements** and the EMG tone remains low, continue to score as stage R; the epoch containing the body movement is scored using major body movement criteria).
      e. One or more nonarousal-associated K complexes or sleep spindles are present in the **first half** of the epoch in the **absence of REMs**, even if chin EMG tone remains low (score as stage N2).

EEG = electroencephalogram; EMG = electromyogram; REM = rapid eye movement.

Adapted from Iber C, Ancoli-Israel S, Chesson A, Quan SF for the American Academy of Sleep Medicine: The AASM Manual for the Scoring of Sleep and Associated Events: Rules, Terminology and Technical Specifications, 1st ed. Westchester, IL: American Academy of Sleep Medicine, 2007.

Continuation of REM Sleep (REM Rule B)

REM rule B (Table 3–9) is illustrated in the schematic in Figure 3–14. Epochs following epochs of definite stage R continue to be scored as stage R even if no REMs are present so long as the chin EMG stays at the REM level and there are no KCs or SSs in the EEG. If the EMG increases above the REM level for a majority of an epoch, stage R can no longer be scored (see Fig. 3–14, epoch 202).

End of REM Sleep

Stage R ends (see Table 3–9, REM rules C.l.a to C.1.e) when there is a transition to stage W or N3, the chin EMG increases above the REM level for the majority of the epoch, an arousal occurs followed by an SEM(s), an MBM occurs followed by SEMs, or there is a transition to stage N2 of sleep (appearance of KCs or SSs in the first half of the epoch).

End of REM Sleep: Transition to Stage W or N3

Stage R ends if there is a transition to stage W or stage N3 (stage R rule C.1.a). Transitions from stage R to stage N3 are very rare. However, awakenings out of REM sleep are common. Patients may often return to sleep and subsequently reenter stage R. The AASM scoring manual does not directly address transitions from stage W to stage R. However, based on FAQ V7 concerning transition from N1 to stage R (see later section), one would not resume scoring stage R unless an epoch of definite stage R was present (REM-like EEG, REMs, and low chin EMG tone) even if a preceding epoch had a chin EMG at the REM level. In Figure 3–15, stage R ends when there is a transition to stage W. Stage R begins when there is an epoch of definite stage R (epoch 204).

End of REM Sleep: Increase in Chin EMG Activity

Stage R ends if there is an ***increase in chin EMG tone*** above the level of stage R and criteria for stage N1 are met (see Table 3–9, rule C.1.b). In Figure 3–14, epoch 102 remains stage R because the chin EMG does not increase until the second half of the epoch. In epoch 202, the chin EMG increases above the REM level and criteria for stage N1 are met (see Table 3–9, stage R rule C.1.b).

End of REM Sleep: Arousal Followed by LAMF EEG and SEMs

Stage REM ends if there is an ***arousal*** followed by LAMF EEG and *SEMs* (score as stage N1). If the arousal is **not** followed by SEMs and the chin EMG remains low, stage R continues (see Table 3–9, REM rule C.1.c). In Figure 3–16A, an arousal interrupts stage R, but the epoch following the

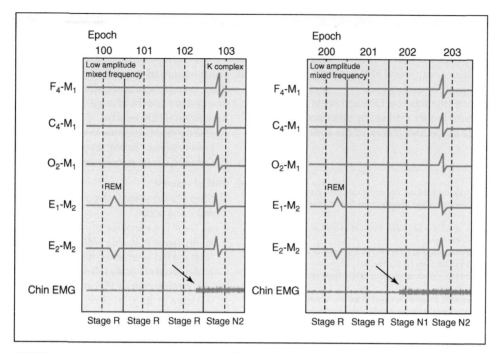

FIGURE 3–14 Schematics illustrate the continuation of REM sleep (stage R, rule B; see Table 3–9). Epochs 100 and 200 are definite (unequivocal) stage R. Subsequent epochs are scored as stage R even in the absence of REMs if the EEG does not have K complexes or sleep spindles and the chin EMG remains at the REM level. Epoch 102 is scored as stage R because the chin EMG activity remains low for the majority of the epoch. The *arrows* show the time when the chin EMG is no longer at the REM level.

FIGURE 3–15 An epoch of stage W interrupts stage R. Stage R starts again when a definite epoch of stage R is noted (epoch 204). EMG = electromyography; REM = rapid eye movement; SEM = slow eye movement. *(See frequently asked question [FAQ] V7 at http://www.aasmnet.org/Resources/PDF/FAQsScoringManual.pdf).*

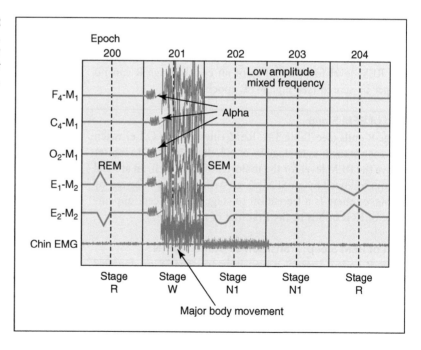

arousal continues to be scored as stage R (even in the absence of REMs) because the chin EMG remains at the REM level for the majority of the epoch and there is no evidence of stage N1 (no SEM following the arousal) or stage N2 (EEG with KCs or SSs). However, in Figure 3–16B, the arousal is followed by SEMs and stage N1 is scored.

End of REM Sleep: MBM Followed by LAMF EEG and SEMs

When REM sleep is interrupted by an **MBM followed by SEMs** and LAMF EEG without nonarousal-associated KCs or SSs, the epoch after the MBM is scored as stage N1 (see Table 3–9, REM rule C.1.d). If the MBM is not followed by

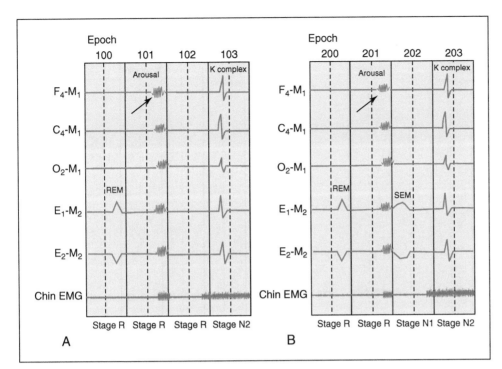

FIGURE 3–16 Stage R is interrupted by an arousal (stage R, rule C.1.c; see Table 3–9). The EEG in the following epoch has no sleep spindles or K complexes and the chin EMG returns quickly to the stage R level. **A,** No slow eye movement (SEM) follows the arousal, and because the chin EMG returns quickly to the REM level, stage R continues. **B,** An SEM follows the arousal and stage N1 is scored (epoch 202). REM = rapid eye movement.

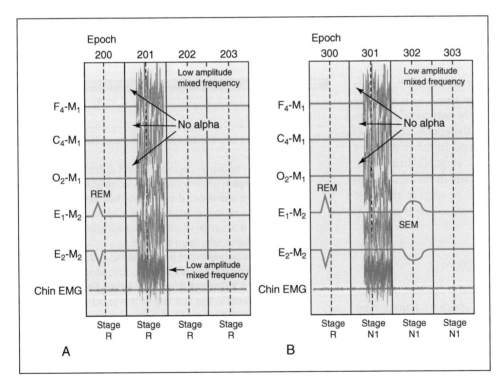

FIGURE 3–17 Rapid eye movement (REM) sleep interrupted by a major body movement (MBM) (stage R, rule C.1.d; see Table 3–9).

SEMs and the EMG tone remains low, stage R continues. The epoch containing the MBM is scored using MBM criteria (see Table 3–14). In Figure 3–17, stage R is interrupted by an MBM. In Figure 3–17A, the MBM epoch is not scored as wake owing to the absence of alpha activity (see MBM rules) and is not followed by an SEM. Therefore, stage R continues and the MBM epoch is scored based on the following epoch (stage R). In Figure 3–17B, an SEM follows the MBM,

signifying a change in sleep state. Stage R ends and the epoch is scored as stage N1. In this case, the MBM epoch (see MBM rules) is scored based on the following epoch (stage N1).

End of REM Sleep: Appearance of Nonarousal KCs or SSs in the EEG

If stage R is interrupted by one or more nonarousal-associated KCs or SSs that are present in the **first half** of the epoch in

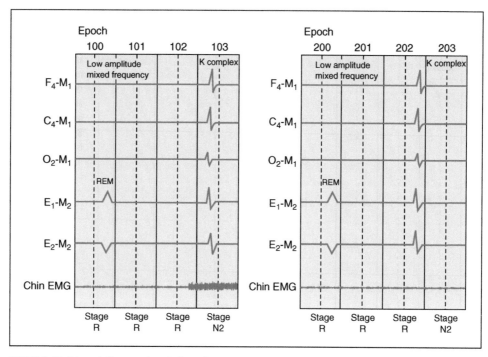

FIGURE 3–18 Schematic illustrates the end of stage R owing to transition to stage N2 (stage R, rule C.1.e; see Table 3–9). In epoch 202, the K complex appears only in the second half and the chin EMG is at the rapid eye movement (REM) level. Therefore, the next epoch is scored as stage N2.

the *absence of REMs is scored as stage N2* (even if chin EMG tone remains low) (see Table 3–9, REM rule C.1.e). In Figure 3–18A, stage R ends when a KC not associated with an arousal is present in **the first half of the epoch.** The start of N2 follows the N2 rule (KC/SS located in the first half of the epoch 103). Epoch 103 is scored as stage N2. In contrast, in Figure 3–18B, because the KC occurs in the second half of the epoch 202 and the chin EMG remains at the REM level, epoch 202 remains stage R but epoch 203 is scored as stage N2.

TRANSITIONS BETWEEN DEFINITE STAGE N2 AND STAGE R

Intervening epochs between that last epoch of definite stage N2 (KC or SS in the first half of the epoch or last half of the previous epoch) and definite stage R are scored according to REM rule D (Table 3–10).

If epoch(s) preceding and contiguous with an epoch of definite stage R has (have) a chin EMG at the REM level and no KCs or SSs in the EEG, such an epoch is (epochs are) scored as stage R even in the absence of REMs (Fig. 3–19) using stage R rule D1 (see Table 3–10). In Figure 3–19, epoch 101 is scored as stage R because the chin EMG is at the REM level for the majority of the epoch. Epoch 201 cannot be scored as stage R because the chin EMG is above the REM level for the majority of the epoch and is scored as N2.

If the chin EMG falls to the REM level in the first part of the epoch but a **KC or SS occurs in the epoch** contiguous

TABLE 3–10
Transitions between Stage N2 and Stage R (REM Rule D)

D. Score epochs of transition between stage N2 and stage R as follows:
1. In epochs between definite N2 and definite stage R, **score stage R** (even in the absence of REMs) if:
   a. There is a **distinct drop in the chin EMG to the REM level** in the first half of the epoch.
   b. There is absence of nonarousal-associated K complexes and sleep spindles.
2. In epochs between definite stage N2 and definite stage R, **score stage N2** if all the following are met:
   a. There is a **distinct drop in the chin EMG to the REM level** in the first half of the epoch.
   b. There is the presence of nonarousal-associated K complexes and sleep spindles.
   c. **Absence of REMs.**
3. In epochs between definite N2 and definite stage R, score stage R even in the absence of REMs if:
   a. There is a **low chin EMG activity (at the REM level)** for the entire epoch.
   b. There is absence of nonarousal-associated K complexes and sleep spindles.

EMG = electromyogram; REM = rapid eye movement.
Adapted from Iber C, Ancoli-Israel S, Chesson A, Quan SF for the American Academy of Sleep Medicine: The AASM Manual for the Scoring of Sleep and Associated Events: Rules, Terminology and Technical Specifications, 1st ed. Westchester, IL: American Academy of Sleep Medicine, 2007.

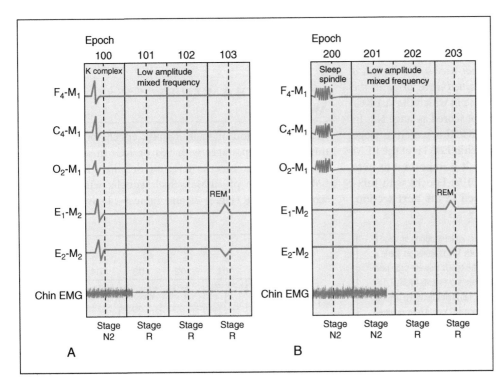

FIGURE 3–19 Transition from definite stage N2 to definite stage R. Epochs contiguous with definite stage R with the chin electromyogram (EMG) at the rapid eye movement (REM) level for the majority of the epoch and an EEG without sleep spindles or K complexes (not associated with an arousal) are scored as stage R even in the absence of REMs (stage R rule D1; see Table 3–10). **A,** Epochs 101, 102, and 103 are scored as stage R. **B,** Epoch 201 is scored as stage N2 by stage N2 continuation rules. The epoch is not stage R because the chin EMG remains above the REM level.

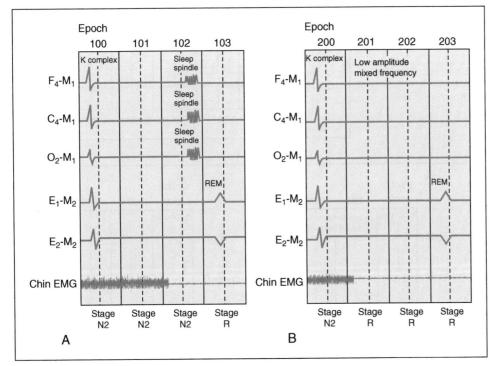

FIGURE 3–20 Schematics of 30-second epochs illustrate the transition from definite stage N2 to definite stage R. **A,** Epoch 102 is scored as stage N2 because the epoch contains a sleep spindle (stage R rule D2; see Table 3–10). **B,** Epochs 201 and 202 are scored as stage R even in the absence of rapid eye movements (REMs) because the chin electromyogram (EMG) is at the REM level, no nonarousal K complexes or sleep spindles are present in the EEG, and the epochs are contiguous with definite stage R (stage R rule D3; see Table 3–10).

with an epoch of definite stage R **and no REMs are present,** the epoch is scored as N2 (Fig. 3–20A) using REM rule D2 (see Table 3–10). There are two important points to note. First, the rule does not require that the SS or KC be in the first half of the epoch. The rationale is that without other evidence for a sleep stage transition, stage N2 sleep is present up until the last KC/SS in the epoch preceding definite stage R. Second, no REMs are present in the epoch containing the

KC or SS. Epochs with mixtures of KCs and REMs are discussed later. If the SS had been in the first half of epoch 202, the epoch would be scored as stage N2 by the stage N2 rules.

In transitions between epochs of definite N2 with chin EMG at the REM level and definite stage R the intervening epochs are scored as stage R in the absence of nonarousal-associated KCs or SSs in the EEG (see Fig. 3–20B) using

REM rule D3. This of course assumes that the chin EMG remains at the REM level.

During epochs in transition from stage N2 to stage R, the last epoch of definite stage N2 may not necessarily contain a KC or SS (if the previous epoch contained a KC or SS in the last half). Figure 3–21 illustrates a case in which the last KC/SS was in the last half of an epoch not scored as stage N2. In this case, epoch 102 following the KC/SS is scored as stage N2 based on the N2 rules even if the chin EMG is at the REM level and no KCs or SSs are present. It is important to note that no REMs are present in epoch 101. Epochs with mixtures of KCs and REMs are discussed in the next section.

After epoch 102, subsequent similar epochs are scored as stage R because the chin EMG is at the REM level and the EEG remains without KCs or SSs (FAQ V6).

EPOCHS WITH A MIXTURE OF SSs/KCs AND REMs

In the first period of stage R sleep, epochs often contain a mixture of sleep stages with SSs or KCs in an epoch that would otherwise meet criteria for definite REM (low chin EMG, presence of REMs). Such epochs **with REMs** are scored as stage R (Fig. 3–22 and Table 3–11). In Figure 3–22,

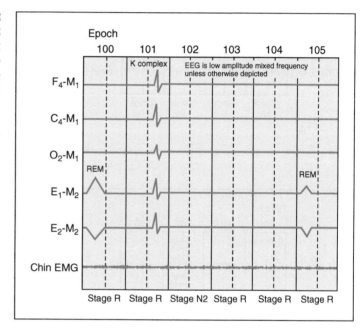

FIGURE 3–21 Schematic of 30-second epochs depict an interruption of stage R by a K complex not associated with an arousal. Epoch 101 is scored as stage R because the K complex occurs in the second half of the epoch. However, the next epoch is scored as stage N2 (in the absence of rapid eye movements [REMs]). The following epochs are scored stage R by the rules for transitions between definite stage N2 and definite stage R. If the K complex in epoch 101 would have occurred in the first half of epoch 101, the epoch would have been scored as stage N2 (in the absence of REMs). In this case, epoch 102 would have been scored as stage R using the rules for transition from definite stage N2 to definite stage R. EMG = electromyogram.

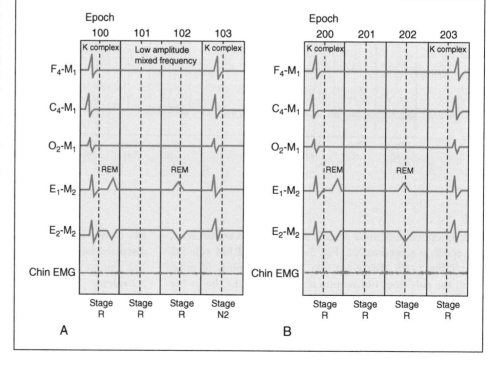

FIGURE 3–22 Schematics of 30-second epochs illustrate scoring when epochs meet criteria for definite rapid eye movement (REM) sleep except for the presence of K complexes or sleep spindles. **A,** Epoch 100 is scored as stage R because REMs are present and chin electromyographic (EMG) tone is low even if a K complex is present. Epoch 101 is scored using the continuation of stage R rules. Epoch 103 is scored as stage N2 because the K complex is in the first half of the epoch. **B,** Epoch 203 is scored as stage R because the K complex is in the second half of the epoch (stage R rule C.1.e; see Table 3–9).

TABLE 3-11

Epochs with a Mixture of Sleep Spindles/K Complexes and REMs

1. Epochs **with REMs** and low chin EMG tone (at the REM level) that would be scored as stage R except for the presence of either K complexes or sleep spindles are still scored as stage R.

2. Subsequent contiguous epochs **without REMs** but continued low chin EMG are scored by the REM continuation and end rules (REM rules B and C, Table 3-9) or stage N2 rules.

EMG = electromyogram; REM = rapid eye movement.
Adapted from Iber C, Ancoli-Israel S, Chesson A, Quan SF for the American Academy of Sleep Medicine: The AASM Manual for the Scoring of Sleep and Associated Events: Rules, Terminology and Technical Specifications, 1st ed. Westchester, IL: American Academy of Sleep Medicine, 2007.

TABLE 3-12

Major Points of Rapid Eye Movement Rules

CONTINUATION OF STAGE R	END OF REM
Following an epoch of definite stage R, continue scoring stage R in the absence of REMs. **IF** • Low chin EMG. • EEG **without** SS or nonarousal KC in the first half of the epoch.	• Transition to stage W or N3. • Arousal followed by SEM. • Body movement followed by SEM. • Nonarousal KC or SS in first half of epoch with no REMs (stage N2). • EMG above REM level for majority of epoch.

EEG = electroencephalogram; EMG = electromyogram; KC = K complex not associated with an arousal; REM = rapid eye movement; SEM = slow eye movement; SS = sleep spindle.

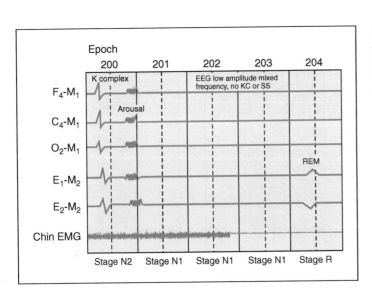

FIGURE 3-23 Schematic of 30-second epochs. Stage N1 is scored after an arousal during stage N2 sleep. Epoch 201 has an electromyogram (EMG) above the rapid eye movement (REM) level. Epoch 203 has a chin EMG at the stage R level and no K complexes (KCs) or sleep spindles (SSs). However, it is scored as stage N1 according to FAQ V7.

epochs 100 and 200 are scored as stage R. Epoch 101 is scored as stage R by the REM continuation rule because it contains no KC or SS. If epoch 100 had the KC in the second half of the epoch, it would still have been stage R. However, epoch 101 would be stage N2 by the stage N2 rules (KC or SS in last half of previous epoch). Note that epoch 203 is scored as stage R by the continuation of REM rule and the fact that the KC is in the second half of this epoch.

TRANSITIONS BETWEEN STAGE N1 AND STAGE R (FAQ V7 AASM SCORING RULES)

The AASM scoring manual did not provide rules for the transition from stage N1 to stage R.

One might assume that epochs intervening between definite stage N1 with low chin EMG and definite stage R would

be scored similarly to rules for stage N2 to stage R transitions. However, according to an FAQ V7, stage R would be scored only once REMs are present (definite stage R) (Fig. 3-23 and Table 3-12).

EFFECTS OF AROUSALS AND MBMS: STAGE N2 VERSUS STAGE R RULES

Given the complexity of sleep staging, it is helpful to note that arousals are treated slightly differently in scoring stage N2 and stage R. Stage N2 ends when an arousal occurs even in the absence of an SEM (see Fig. 3-10). Stage R ends following an arousal only if the arousal is followed by an SEM (see Fig. 3-16). In both stage N2 and stage R, the stage is assumed to end only if an intervening MBM is followed by an SEM. This assumes that the MBM epoch contains no

<table>
<tr><td colspan="2">

TABLE 3-13

When Arousals and Major Body Movements End Stage N2 and Stage R

</td></tr>
</table>

	YES
End of stage N2	Arousal MBM followed by SEM
End of stage R	Arousal followed by SEM MBM followed by SEM

MBM = major body movement; SEM = slow eye movement.

TABLE 3-14

Scoring Rules for Major Body Movements

A. Score stage W if alpha rhythm is present for part of the epoch (even if < 15 sec in duration).

B. Score stage W in the absence of alpha rhythm if an epoch scoreable as stage W either precedes or follows the epoch with the major body movement.

C. If neither A or B apply, score an epoch with a major body movement as the same stage as the epoch that follows it.

Adapted from Iber C, Ancoli-Israel S, Chesson A, Quan SF for the American Academy of Sleep Medicine: The AASM Manual for the Scoring of Sleep and Associated Events: Rules, Terminology and Technical Specifications, 1st ed. Westchester, IL: American Academy of Sleep Medicine, 2007.

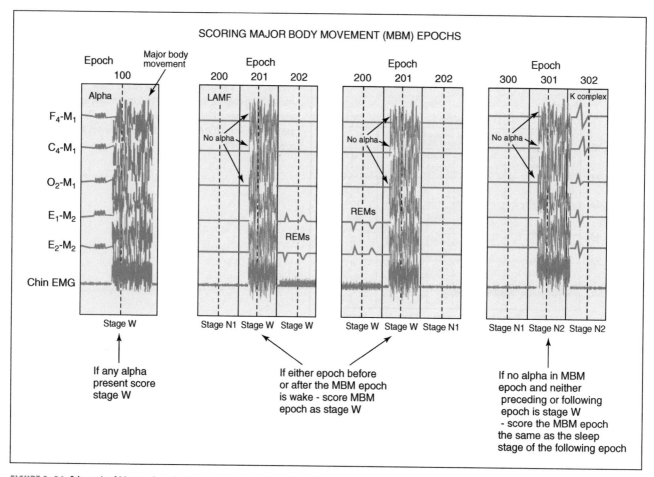

FIGURE 3-24 Schematic of 30-second epochs illustrate scoring rules for major body movements (MBMs). EMG = electromyogram; LAMF = low-amplitude mixed-frequency; REM = rapid eye movement.

alpha. If the epoch contains alpha, it is scored as stage W and either stage N2 or stage R end (transition to stage W) (Table 3–13).

MAJOR BODY MOVEMENTS

An MBM is defined as movement and muscle artifact obscuring the EEG for more than half an epoch to the extent that

the sleep stage cannot be determined (Table 3–14). The rules for scoring epochs containing MBM are illustrated in Figure 3–24. If any alpha is present in the MBM epoch, it is staged as stage W. The MBM epoch is also scored as stage W if either the epoch preceding or the one following the MBM epoch is scored as stage W. Finally, if the previous possibilities do not apply, the MBM epoch is scored the same as the following epoch.

TABLE 3–15

Arousal Rules

NREM AROUSAL CRITERIA

Score an arousal during sleep stages N1, N2, and N3 if there is an abrupt shift of EEG frequency including alpha, theta, and/or frequencies greater than 16 Hz (but not spindles) that lasts *at least 3 seconds*, with at least 10 seconds of stable sleep preceding the change.

REM AROUSAL CRITERIA

Score an arousal during sleep stage R if there is an abrupt shift of EEG frequency including alpha, theta, and/or frequencies greater than 16 Hz (but not spindles) that lasts *at least 3 seconds*, with at least 10 seconds of stable sleep preceding the change.
AND
There is a concurrent increase in submental EMG lasting at least *1 second in addition to the required EEG changes.*

EEG = electroencephalogram; EMG = electromyogram; NREM = non–rapid eye movement; REM = rapid eye movement.
Adapted from Iber C, Ancoli-Israel S, Chesson A, Quan SF for the American Academy of Sleep Medicine: The AASM Manual for Scoring of Sleep and Associated Events: Rules, Terminology and Technical Specifications, 1st ed. Westchester, IL: American Academy of Sleep Medicine, 2007.

TABLE 3–16

Summary of Arousal Rules

	EEG (NREM OR REM)	DURATION OF EEG CHANGE	INCREASE IN SUBMENTAL CHIN EMG
NREM	Abrupt shift in EEG frequency including alpha, theta, and frequencies greater than 16 but NO spindles	At least 3 sec	None required.
REM		At least 3 sec	At least 1 sec and concurrent with shift in EEG frequency.

EEG = electroencephalogram; EMG = electromyogram; NREM = non–rapid eye movement; REM = rapid eye movement.

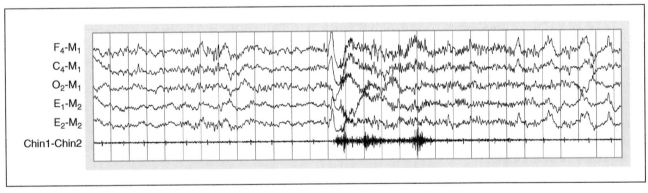

FIGURE 3–25 An arousal during non–rapid eye movement (NREM) sleep. A 30-second tracing is depicted. Note that the K complex was NOT included in criteria for the arousal. In addition, an increase in the chin electromyogram (EMG), although present, is NOT required.

Arousal Rules

Arousals are transient phenomenon that may lead to wakefulness or only briefly interrupt sleep. They are worth scoring because patients with frequent arousals may have daytime sleepiness even if the total sleep duration is normal. An arousal is scored during sleep stages N1, N2, and N3 (NREM sleep) if there is an abrupt shift of EEG frequency including alpha, theta, and/or frequencies greater than 16 Hz (but not spindles) that lasts *at least 3 seconds,* with at least 10 seconds of stable sleep preceding the change (Tables 3–15 and 3–16). An arousal is scored during REM sleep if there is a concurrent increase in submental EMG lasting at least 1 second in addition to the EEG changes required for NREM arousals. Because alpha bursts during stage R are common, the additional requirement of an increase in chin EMG was added.

Figure 3–25 illustrates an arousal during NREM sleep. In this example, the chin EMG also increases but this is not part of the criteria used to score an arousal. Note that there is a shift in EEG frequency greater than 3 seconds that does not include spindle activity. Also note that, although KCs may be associated with arousals, the presence of a KC alone (no 3-sec shift in EEG frequency) is not considered to indicate an arousal even if it is associated with an increase in the chin EMG. Figure 3–26 illustrates an arousal from stage R. Here both the EEG and the chin EMG changes meet arousal criteria. Figure 3–27 illustrates an epoch of stage R with a burst of alpha activity that is not concurrent with the brief increase in chin EMG activity and an arousal is not scored. Bursts of alpha are common during stage R. The alpha activity during REM sleep is often about 1 Hz slower than during non–rapid

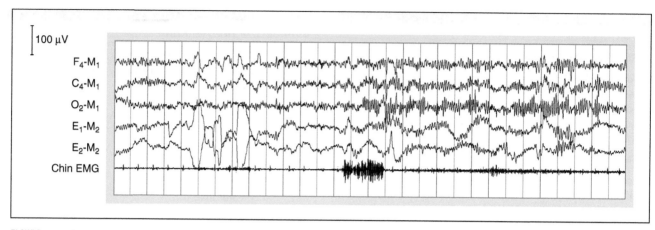

FIGURE 3–26 Stage R with an arousal. A 30-second epoch is depicted. Note that the increase in chin electromyogram (EMG) is greater than 1 second (the criteria for arousal in stage R is at least 1 sec).

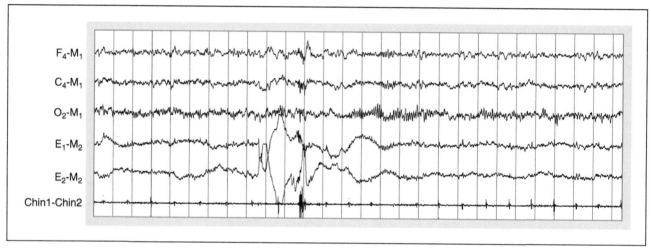

FIGURE 3–27 A 30-second epoch of Stage R is depicted. There is a burst of alpha activity after REMs. This is not an arousal. Note that the increase in EMG is less than 1 second and not concurrent with the burst of alpha.

eye movement (NREM) sleep. The burst of chin EMG activity in Figure 3–27 is less than 1 second in duration and there is no concurrent 3 seconds or longer abrupt shift in EEG frequency.

Although the choice of a 3-second EEG change appears arbitrary, studies have shown that reliability of scoring arousals is better with a 3-second EEG change than with shorter durations of required EEG change.[5] Although not specified in the recent AASM scoring manual, a previous American Sleep Disorders Association (ASDA) task force produced a number of additional recommendations for the scoring of arousals.[6] A summary of the most important points follows:

1. If one arousal is scored, at least 10 seconds of continuous intervening sleep must be present before a second arousal can be scored.
2. Arousals cannot be scored based on changes in submental EMG alone.
3. Artifacts, KCs, or delta waves are not scored as arousals unless accompanied by an EEG frequency shift, as defined previously.
4. Intrusions of alpha activity less than 3 seconds in duration into NREM sleep at a rate greater than one burst per 10 seconds is not scored as an EEG arousal. Three seconds of alpha sleep is not scored as an arousal unless a 10-second episode of alpha-free sleep precedes.
5. Transitions from one stage of sleep to another are not scored as arousals unless they meet the criteria indicated previously.

REFERENCES

1. Rechtschaffen A, Kales A (eds): A Manual of Standardized Terminology Techniques and Scoring System for Sleep Stages of Human Sleep. Los Angeles: Brain Information Service/Brain Research Institute, UCLA, 1968.

2. Caraskadon MA, Rechschaffen A: Monitoring and staging human sleep. In Kryger MH, Roth T, Dement WC (eds): Principles and Practice of Sleep Medicine, 2nd ed. Philadelphia: WB Saunders, 2005, pp. 1359–1377.

3. Iber C, Ancoli-Israel S, Chesson A, Quan SF for the American Academy of Sleep Medicine: The AASM Manual for the Scoring of Sleep and Associated Events: Rules, Terminology and Technical Specifications, 1st ed. Westchester, IL: American Academy of Sleep Medicine, 2007.

4. Silber MH, Ancoli-Israel S, Bonnet MH, et al: The visual scoring of sleep in adults. J Clin Sleep Med 2007;15:121–131.

5. Bonnet MH, Doghramji K, Roehrs T, et al: The scoring of arousals in sleep. Reliability, validity, and alternatives. J Clin Sleep Med 2007;3:133–145.

6. American Sleep Disorders Association—The Atlas Task Force: EEG arousals: scoring rules and examples. Sleep 1992;15: 174–184.

Chapter 4

Biocalibration, Artifacts, and Common Variants of Sleep

Chapter Points

- Recording a technically adequate biocalibration is an important part of every sleep study. Careful attention to the recorded biocalibration by the scorer or physician reviewing the study is essential for identifying the individual's pattern of eyes-open and eyes-closed wakefulness as well as the appearance of eye movements. The biocalibration may help the scorer differentiate stage W with REMs from stage R when the chin EMG is at a low level in both sleep stages.
- A 60-Hz artifact is recognized as a ropelike pattern. If there is a large increase in the signal amplitude when the 60-Hz notch filter is turned off (especially with a 100 Hz high filter setting), this implies significant 60-Hz contamination of the signal. High electrode impedance is a common cause of 60-Hz artifact.
- The ideal electrode impedance is less than 5 KΩ (acceptable <10 KΩ).
- ECG artifact can be minimized by correct mastoid electrode placement. During review, ECG artifact can be minimized by using an average of the mastoids (e.g., F₄-Avg) or linking the electrodes.
- Sweat artifact (sway) can be minimized by cooling the patient down or using different derivations if movement of one of the mastoid electrodes is causing the problem.
- Electrode popping is a serious artifact and requires replacement or fixing the faulty electrode (or preventing movement of the electrode with each breath) during recording.
- A large amount of sleep spindle activity may be a clue that the patient is taking a BZRA.
- Eye movements may persist in stage N2 sleep in patients taking SSRIs.
- Prominent alpha activity can be seen "riding" on top of SWA in alpha-delta sleep. Increasing the viewing window to 10 seconds and counting waveforms can help confirm that prominent alpha activity is present.

CALIBRATIONS AND BIOCALIBRATIONS

Calibrations

Calibration was especially critical during paper recording to document the individual amplifier sensitivity, polarity, and filter settings because these could not be changed once data were recorded. In the digital era, electroencephalographic (EEG), electro-oculographic (EOG), and electromyographic (EMG) data are acquired at a default gain and with a wide bandpass (e.g., 0.03 and 100 Hz, respectively). The desired channel sensitivity and filter settings for the display of individual channels (traces) can be changed during acquisition and review. In the paper era (Fig. 4–1), calibration was usually performed by sending a square wave voltage pulse (typically 50 µV). The sensitivity control was adjusted until a 50-µV signal produced a 10-mm pen deflection (others used 75 µV for 10 mm). Digital systems today often send a sine wave signal of standard frequency (5 or 10 Hz) and peak-to-peak voltage (100–500 µV) to the amplifier to document digital system accuracy (Fig. 4–2). Whereas the analog amplifier gain used in digital systems usually cannot be adjusted except by the manufacturer, the computer program can change calibration factors to more accurately display the recorded data. If large adjustments are necessary, the program will often provide notification that amplifier service is needed.

The output of each individual AC amplifier can be scaled by calibration factors so that they provide exactly equivalent outputs from the calibration signal. In Figure 4–2, a 500-µV calibration signal results in slightly different outputs from the amplifiers processing the C₄-Ref and M₁-Ref signals. Calibration factors are selected to scale the outputs to the input standard. After scaling, the digital values used for display match the input calibration voltage and, even more important, the two amplifiers deliver the same exact output from the calibration signal. This improves common mode rejection during referential recording. That is, the same signal applied to both amplifiers should result in zero output when the derivation using them is displayed (digital subtraction).

Of note, the display filter settings can change signal amplitude depending on the calibration signal frequency.

One advantage of a 5-Hz signal is that it is minimally changed by typical low- and high-frequency filter settings used in EEG derivations.

Calibration of DC signals (Fig. 4–3) is usually performed using a two-point calibration method. This is performed by sending a lower and higher signal (usually 0 and 1 V or –1 and 1 V) and specifying the parameter values corresponding to the two voltages. For example, a positive airway pressure device and analog module outputs 0 V for 0 cm H_2O pressure and 1 V for 30 cm H_2O. The device would be directed to send 0 V to the digital system and 0 cm H_2O pressure is specified using the polysomnography (PSG) software. Then 1 V is sent and 30 cm H_2O is specified. There is usually an option to type in the expected voltage or to actually measure

the voltage sent by the device at each of the two calibration points. For example, when the low calibration voltage is sent the set low button is pushed. This action displays the actual voltage in the voltage input 1 window (Fig. 4–3) and sends value to the computer for computation of the calibration factors. A similar procedure is performed when the high calibration voltage is sent. The computer then determines and stores the calibration factors.

Biocalibrations

Biocalibration (Table 4–1 and Fig. 4–4) is an important part of every PSG recording, but the value of the procedure is often unrecognized. During the biocalibration, signals are recorded while the patient performs maneuvers that verify that the monitoring equipment, electrodes, and sensors are working properly. The impedance of all EEG, EOG, and EMG electrodes should be checked. For the reviewer, noting the patient's EEG, EOG, and EMG pattern of eyes-open and

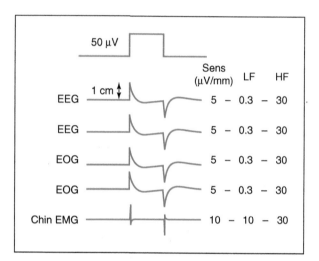

FIGURE 4–1 Example of calibration using analog amplifiers and paper recording. A square wave voltage signal of 50 μV is sent by pushing a button on the amplifier system and then releasing the button. The effects of the filters being used on the pen deflections can be seen (Chin EMG [electromyogram] channel). EEG = electroencephalogram; EMG = electromyogram; EOG = electro-oculogram; HF = high frequency; LF = low frequency.

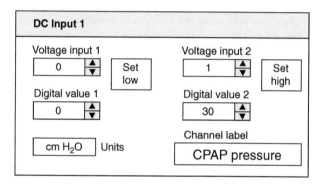

FIGURE 4–3 Schematic of computer screen used to calibrate DC signals. Most systems have an option to ask the system to measure the voltage input ("Get low value") rather than simply enter it. So voltage input 1 can be sent to the polysomnography (PSG) system and the actual voltage measured (acquired). CPAP = continuous positive airway pressure.

FIGURE 4–2 Schematic representation of scaling of amplifier outputs so that they both are accurate and provide the same output from the calibration signal. Here, Cal1 and Cal2 are the calibration factors and Ref is the reference electrode used for referential recording. A calibration signal of 500 μV is sent to all amplifier inputs.

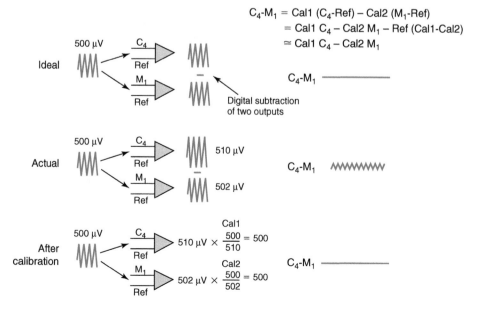

TABLE 4–1

Biocalibration Procedure

COMMAND	WHAT TO CHECK AND OBSERVE
While looking straight ahead, close your eyes	• Quality of alpha production. • Slow eye movements.
Open your eyes	• Attenuation of alpha. • EEG of wakefulness. • Pattern of eyes-open stage W. • REMs during wake.
Look right Look left Look up Look down Blink eyes	• Integrity of eye electrodes. • Pattern of the patient's REMs and blinks. • Ability to detect horizontal and vertical eye movements.
Grit teeth	• Function of chin EMG. • Sensitivity should be adjusted so that some activity is present during relaxed wake.
Breathe in, breathe out	• Airflow sensors show airflow working properly, adjust sensitivity. • Proper polarity for all respiratory sensors. That is, during inspiration, all deflections are upward or downward (depending on sleep center protocol). • Adjust sensitivity of chest and abdomen tracings.
Hold your breath	• Ability to detect apnea.
Wiggle your right toe Wiggle your left toe	• Ability to detect leg movements. • Adjust leg derivation sensitivity so movements can be easily seen in both legs.

EEG = electroencephalogram; EMG = electromyogram; REMs = rapid eye movements.

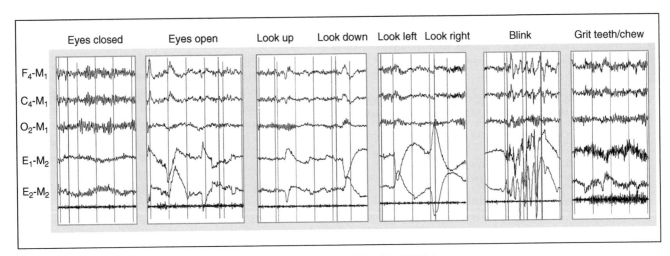

FIGURE 4–4 Biocalibration of EEG, EOG, and chin EMG derivations.

eyes-closed stage W can help with recognition of this sleep stage during the recording and during scoring of sleep. It is especially important to know whether the person being recorded generates alpha activity with eye closure because this affects the scoring criteria for stage W and stage N1 (see Chapter 3).

Figure 4–5 shows a portion of the biocalibration procedure in a patient with a prior left eye enucleation. Hopefully, technologist's notes and patient history would have alerted the reviewing physician to this situation. However, looking at the biocalibrations would also alert the physician that stage R sleep would have an unusual appearance.

ARTIFACTS

Artifacts in the EEG, EOG, and EMG derivations due to inadequate electrode application or the effects of patient movement and the environment are common in polysomnography.[1–4] It is essential that they be recognized during recording to allow for intervention by the sleep

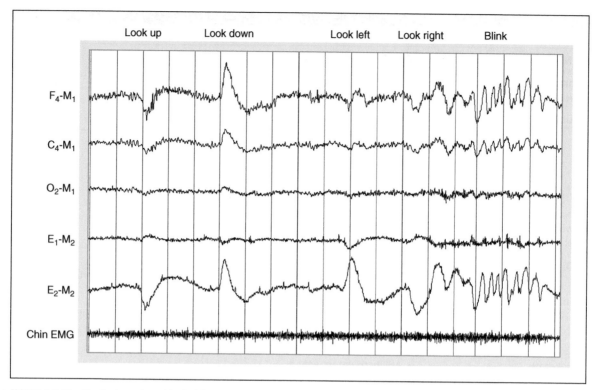

FIGURE 4–5 Biocalibration in a patient with prior left eye enucleation. The deflections in the frontal derivations are noted because these electrodes are relatively close to the eyes compared with other electrodes. The grid lines are 1 second apart. EMG = electromyogram.

TABLE 4-2
Electrode Popping Artifact
• Electrode popping artifact is a sudden, high-voltage deflection occurring at regular intervals, usually coincident with respiration.
• Electrode popping artifact is due to an electrode pulling away from the skin or the drying of electrode gel or paste.
• Noting the affected derivations can identify the problem electrode: • Several derivations with a common electrode. • One derivation with a unique electrode.
• Reapplication of the problem electrode, the addition of electrode paste, or change in the position of the electrode wire is indicated during recording.
• Review using a derivation not including the problem electrode will usually allow staging of sleep.

technologist. Postrecording maneuvers to minimize the effects of some artifacts on sleep staging are often possible.

Electrode Popping

Electrode popping is a common and severe artifact that makes the staging of sleep very difficult (Table 4–2). It is characterized by sudden, high-amplitude deflection (often with channel blocking) secondary to an electrode pulling

away from the skin (sudden loss of signal). The popping often tends to be regular and corresponds to body movement during breathing. Electrode popping may also be caused by the patient lying on one mastoid electrode or pulling on the wire connecting the electrode with the electrode box during respiration. For example, if the wire runs under the patient's body or through chest or abdominal bands, patient movement or respiration can pull on the electrode wire. Popping also can occur if the electrode gel dries out during the night. At the time of recording, adding electrode gel or reapplication of the problem electrode may eliminate the problem. Postrecording, the artifact can frequently be handled by switching to an alternative derivation that does not use the problem electrode. For example, if O_2 is the problem, the exploring occipital electrode is switched to O_1. This is one reason that redundant electrodes are routinely placed.

In Figure 4–6, regular high-voltage deflections are noted in all derivations containing M_1. Therefore, the problem is most likely in electrode M_1. Video monitoring confirmed that the patient was sleeping on the left side. After changing the reference electrode to M_2 (using derivations F_3-M_2, C_3-M_2, O_1-M_2, E_1-M_2, and E_2-M_2), the problem was eliminated. Displaying F_4-M_2, C_4-M_2, O_2-M_2 would also eliminate the artifact. However, using an exploring electrode opposite the reference is preferable because this produces a larger voltage signal. In fact, F_3-M_2, C_3-M_2, and O_1-M_2 are the alternate derivations recommended by the American Academy of Sleep Medicine (AASM) scoring manual. If an electrode in the standard derivation fails, use of corresponding

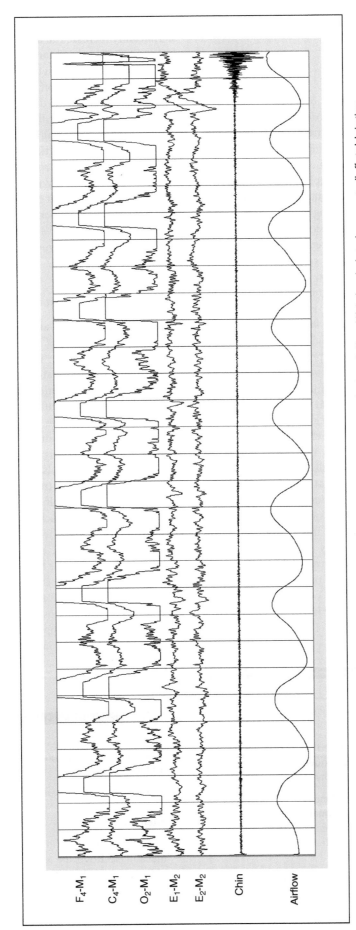

FIGURE 4–6 Electrode popping artifact. The problem electrode is M_1. The artifact is present only in derivations using the electrode M_1, and M_1 is the only electrode common to all affected derivations.

electrode in the alternate derivation set for sleep monitoring is recommended (see Chapter 1).

60-Cycle Artifact

A **60-cycle artifact** in EEG, EOG, or EMG tracings is a common problem in sleep study recording (Table 4–3). It is caused by 60-Hz electrical activity from power lines contaminating the recorded signal. A 60-Hz artifact can be minimized by correct application of electrodes and proper design of the sleep laboratory. EEG amplifiers are AC-coupled, which allows them to record low-voltage EEG activity while rejecting unwanted and sometimes higher-voltage AC or DC activity. Differential amplifiers can record low-voltage physiologic signals by amplifying the difference in voltage between two electrodes while rejecting the common-mode signal consisting of higher-voltage, 60-Hz, background activity. When recording the voltage difference between two electrodes, the background AC activity is rejected only if the electrode impedances are low and fairly equal. Although most AC amplifiers have notch filters to minimize 60-Hz activity, these filters may not prevent prominent 60-Hz activity when electrode impedances are very different (usually one defective electrode has very high impedance). The ideal impedance of electrodes is below 5 KΩ (acceptable <10 KΩ). Electrode impedance should be checked by the sleep technician after electrode application before recording starts. Routine use of 60-Hz notch filters makes recognition of 60-Hz contamination more difficult and is not recommended. It should be appreciated that use of a 35-Hz high-frequency filter for EEG and EOG derivations significantly attenuates 60-Hz activity. The effect of adding or removing the notch filter is more prominent in chin and leg EMG derivations that use a high-frequency filter of 100 Hz.

The sudden appearance of 60-Hz artifact usually means one electrode is faulty. In the days of paper PSG, the artifact caused a characteristic humming of the pens as they oscillated at 60 cycles/sec. If a 60-Hz contamination of a derivation is significant, turning off the 60-cycle filter will significantly increase the amplitude of the artifact (if a high filter of 100 Hz is used for the derivation). A 60-Hz artifact can also be recognized on the usual 30-second view by a very dense uniform squared off or "ropelike" tracing that does not vary. If 60-Hz artifact is due to a single electrode, it should be replaced during recording. Using a different display derivation after postrecording may solve the problem. In Figure 4–7, prominent 60-Hz artifact is noted in the chin derivation and produces a band or "ropelike" tracing. Application of the 60-Hz filter dramatically reduced the amplitude consistent with a significant amount of 60-Hz artifact. The problem was the chin2 electrode. When the derivation was changed, the artifact was eliminated even without the use of a 60-Hz filter. The ideal intervention would have been replacement of the chin2 electrode.

Slow-Frequency (Sweat) Artifact

Slow-frequency (sweat) artifact is characterized by a slowly undulating movement of the baseline of affected channels (Table 4–4 and Fig. 4–8). The movement may or may not be synchronous with the patient's respiration. When in-phase with the patient's respiration, the artifact also is called *respiratory artifact*. Sweat artifact is believed to be secondary to the effects of perspiration. Sweat alters the electrode potential, thereby producing an artifact that mimics delta waves and results in overscoring of stage N3. When the artifact is *not* present in all channels, the artifact may be secondary to pressure on an electrode (or pulling on the electrode). In this case, the artifact is usually coming from one or more electrodes on the side on which the patient is lying. For example, if the patient is sleeping with the left side down, derivations containing M_1 would be affected but not those containing M_2. If a single electrode is the problem, changing derivations to one that does not use the faulty electrode may be a solution. If this does not work or if the problem involves all derivations, other actions are necessary. Options include reducing the room temperature, uncovering the patient, and/or using a fan. As a last-ditch alternative, the setting of

TABLE 4–3
60-Hz Artifact
• 60-Hz artifact often produces a thick band or ropelike appearance in the tracing.
• 60-Hz contamination of the recorded signal may not be recognized if both a 35-Hz high-frequency filter and a 60-Hz notch filter are used for display.
• Recording with 60-Hz filter off will increase the ability to recognize the presence of 60-Hz signal contamination (usually a clue that an electrode needs replacement). 60-Hz artifact is more apparent with a high-frequency filter of 100 Hz.
• If turning on and off the 60-Hz notch filter significantly reduces (increases) signal amplitude, this is another clue that 60-Hz contamination is present in a given derivation.

TABLE 4–4
Slow-Frequency (Sweat) Artifact
• A slowly undulating signal (sway) is typical of sweat artifact.
• If sweat artifact is present in all derivations and the room or patient is warm, cooling of the patient should be attempted.
• If sway is present only in derivations utilizing a given mastoid electrode, the artifact may be due to movement of the mastoid electrode during respiration.
• Slow-frequency artifact may make scoring stage N3 very difficult.

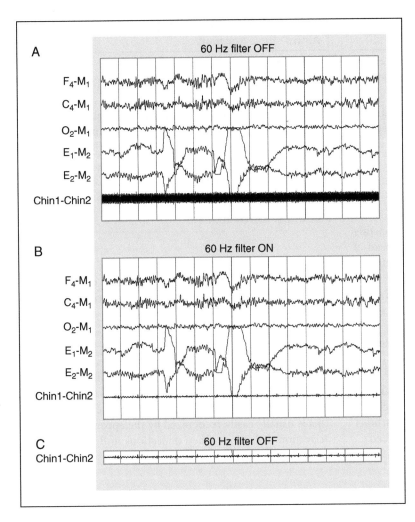

FIGURE 4–7 60-Hz artifact. **A,** The 60-Hz filter is off. Note the band or "ropelike" appearance of the chin EMG. **B,** Turning on the 60-Hz notch filter dramatically reduced the amplitude consistent with the presence of 60-Hz artifact. **C,** When chin2 was replaced with chin3, the EMG amplitude decreased dramatically and the epoch containing the 15-second fragment was scored as stage R (REM [rapid eye movement] sleep). The impedance of the faulty chin2 electrode was 55 KΩ (desired <5 KΩ).

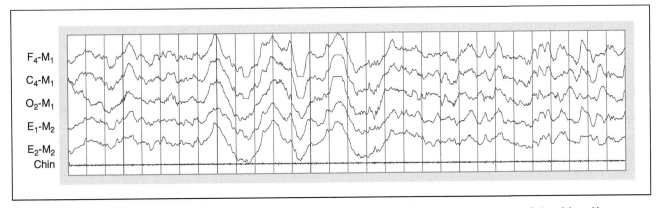

FIGURE 4–8 Slow-frequency (sweat) artifact is present in derivations containing both M$_1$ and M$_2$. Lowering the room temperature eliminated the problem.

the low-frequency filter may be increased (e.g., from 0.3 to 1). Unfortunately, this maneuver decreases the amount of slow wave activity (SWA) that is depicted, but still may be preferable to a totally unscorable record. Sweat artifact can be prevented by maintaining a low room temperature, especially when very obese or heavily perspiring patients are studied. One can quickly add a blanket, but cooling down a sleep room takes more time.

ECG Artifact

ECG artifact is one of the most common and easily recognizable recording artifacts (Table 4–5). It can be identified by sharp deflections in the signals of affected channels corresponding exactly in time to the QRS of the ECG tracing. Fortunately, this artifact does not usually interfere with visual sleep staging because the artifact does not mimic usual

TABLE 4-5
Electrocardiogram Artifact
• ECG artifact can be easily recognized as sharp deflections in the affected leads corresponding to the QRS complex in the ECG lead.
• Proper application of the mastoid electrodes and double referencing (using an average of M_1 and M_2) can prevent or minimize this artifact.
ECG = electrocardiogram.

TABLE 4-6
Alpha Sleep Anomaly
• Alpha sleep anomaly is characterized by the persistence of prominent alpha activity during NREM sleep (especially stage N3 sleep).
• The pattern has been associated with chronic pain syndromes or psychiatric disorders but can occur in normal individuals.
• Alpha anomaly makes scoring stage N1 and sometimes stage N2 sleep difficult.
Scoring stage N3 is less problematic.
NREM = non–rapid eye movement.

EEG patterns. It can mimic spike activity. The artifact can be minimized by placing the mastoid electrodes sufficiently high (behind the ear) so that they are over bone instead of neck tissue (fat). Either linking the two mastoid electrodes physically by a jumper cable at the electrode box or using derivations in which the reference electrode is an average of M_1 and M_2 can minimize ECG artifact. This is also sometimes called "double-referencing." These techniques work because, if the ECG voltage vector is toward one mastoid, it is away from the other. Hence, the ECG components of the two signals tend to cancel each other out. In Figure 4–9, ECG artifact is prominent in all derivations except one using an average of M_1 and M_2 (F_4-AVG). Two small dark circles in E_1-M_2 mark the artifact. In the tracing shown, ECG artifact is larger than desirable, but the record still can be scored.

Pulse Artifact

Pulse artifact is similar to ECG artifact except that, rather than electrical interference, the artifact is due to movement of an electrode caused by the pulsation of an underlying artery. Because the arterial pulse occurs after the QRS complex, the timing of the artifact is delayed after each QRS. Figure 4–10 shows the ECG (square) artifact and pulse artifact (circles).

Muscle Artifact

Muscle artifact in the EEG and EOG is due to increased muscle tone in the muscles underlying the EEG and EOG electrodes. Often, this will resolve as the patient relaxes and falls asleep (Fig. 4–11).

Snoring/Respiratory Chin EMG Artifact

An increase in chin EMG amplitude can sometimes be seen with each inspiration (Fig. 4–12). This is especially common when the upper airway resistance is high (e.g., during snoring). The genioglossus (tongue protruder) has inspiratory EMG activity that increases with more negative upper airway pressure.[5] The muscle attaches to the mandible in the midline. EMG electrodes below the mandible may pick up the increased inspiratory activity of the genioglossus or other nearby neck muscles associated with increased inspiratory effort induced by a high upper airway resistance. Another possible cause is simply movement of chin electrode wires with each inspiration. Nasal pressure monitoring is discussed in Chapter 7.

Eye Movement Artifact

Eye movements can be picked up in the frontal derivations because F_3 and F_4 are fairly close to the eyes. In Figure 4–5, note the deflections in F_4-M_1 associated with eye movements. This is usually easily recognized by the apperance of frontal derivation deflections when deflections in the EOG derivations are seen.

Ground Artifact

If one of the two inputs to a differential amplifier (say G_1 in Fig. 2–1) is disconnected (electrode unattached), the amplifier really records the difference between G_2 and the ground electrode. Because the ground electrode is typically attached to the forehead near the eyes, one can see deflections associated with eye movements in channels in which they are usually not visible (say, O_2-M_1). Usually, considerable 60-Hz artifact would also be seen. However, if the display of the derivation uses a 35-Hz high-frequency filter, which attenuates a great deal of the 60-Hz signal contamination, this might be missed. Therefore, the appearance of eye movements in unusual channels should trigger the technologist or reviewer to consider whether "ground artifact" is present.

COMMON VARIANTS SEEN DURING SLEEP MONITORING

Alpha Non–Rapid Eye Movement Sleep Anomaly

The finding of prominent alpha activity (8–13 Hz) during non–rapid eye movement (NREM) sleep is often called *alpha sleep, alpha intrusion,* or *alpha-delta* sleep (if noted in association with stage N3). It makes sleep staging more challenging (Table 4–6 and Fig. 4–13). The alpha activity may be more prominent in frontal than occipital regions in contrast to the typical alpha rhythm. When viewing a tracing of alpha-delta sleep in a 30-second window, there is the

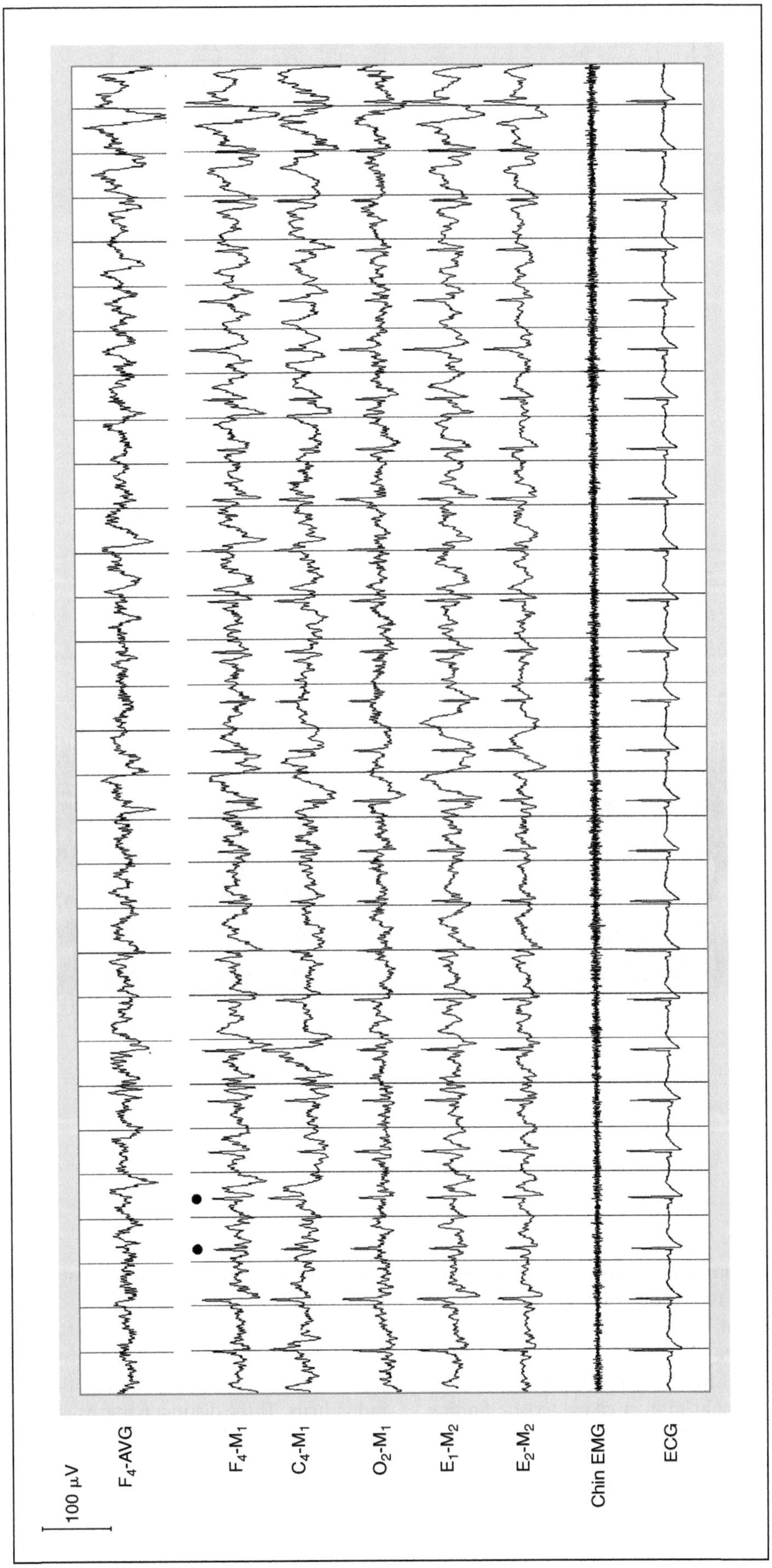

FIGURE 4–9 Electrocardiogram (ECG) artifact is present in all derivations except for the top one using an average of M_1 and M_2 as the reference (F_4-AVG). *Black dots* point out two deflections from the ECG artifact. EMG = electromyogram.

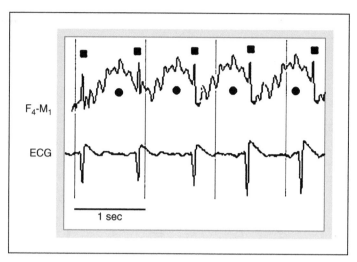

FIGURE 4–10 Pulse artifact *(circles)* follows the electrocardiogram (ECG) artifact in F_4-M_1 *(squares)* and the QRS in the ECG. The spike (narrow) deflection in the encephalogram (EEG) corresponds to the QRS in the ECG. This is followed by a "hump" in the EEG associated with the arterial pulse.

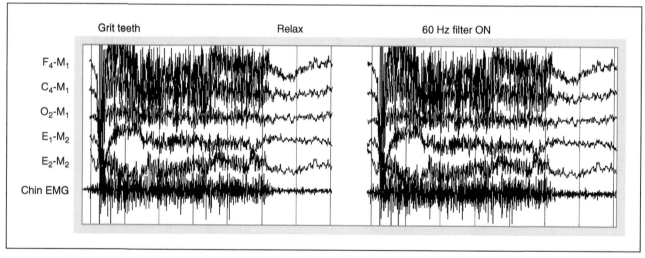

FIGURE 4–11 Muscle artifact. The patient was asked to grit his teeth then relax. Adding the 60-Hz filter makes little difference because the majority of signal activity is not due to 60-Hz signal contamination.

impression of a background of diffuse higher-frequency activity. By changing to a 10-second window, one can count the smaller wave forms in 1 second that are superimposed on slower activity (alpha 8–13 Hz).

First described in 1973 by Hauri and Hawkings,[6] alpha-delta sleep was once thought to be a characteristic finding associated with fibromyalgia (FM).[7] However, alpha sleep is not seen in all patients with FM and can occur in patients with other psychiatric and chronic pain disorders. Mahowald and Mahowald[8] concluded that alpha sleep was not specific for FM and was not necessarily associated with

symptoms of myalgia. It was present in 15% of normal subjects in undisturbed sleep.

Roizenblatt and coworkers[9] also studied patients with FM off medications and normal controls. Alpha rhythm was noted during sleep in 70% of FM patients and 16% of normal individuals. Three distinct patterns were noted: phasic alpha patterns—episodic alpha occurring simultaneously with delta activity (70% FM, 7% controls); tonic alpha continuously present throughout NREM sleep (20% of FM and 9% of controls); and low alpha pattern seen in 30% of FM patients and 84% of controls. The phasic pattern was

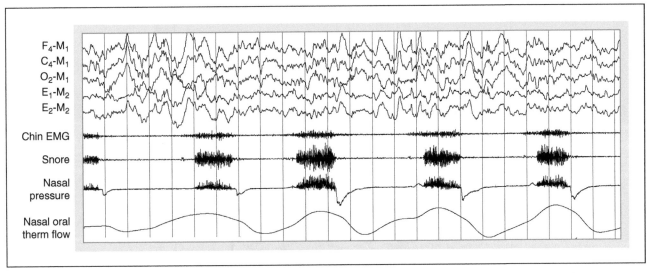

FIGURE 4–12 Snoring artifact is noted in the chin electromyogram (EMG). Note the evidence of snoring in the snore microphone and in the nasal pressure.

TABLE 4–7
Drug Spindles
• Frequent and prominent sleep spindle activity is often noted in patients taking benzodiazepine receptor agonists.
• Sleep spindle frequency is often at the higher end of the sleep spindle range.
• The pattern may be a useful clue that a hypnotic medication was taken before the sleep study.

TABLE 4–8
Eye Movements Associated with Selective Serotonin Reuptake Inhibitor Medications
• Prominent slow and rapid eye movement activity may be seen in stage N2 (and less commonly in stage N3) in patients taking SSRI antidepressants.
• The SSRI eye movements can be a mixture of slow and more rapid eye movements.
SSRI = selective serotonin reuptake inhibitor.

associated with lower sleep efficiency, decreased slow wave sleep, longer morning pain, and subjective feeling of superficial sleep. Further research is needed to confirm the findings.

Drug Spindles

Patients who are taking benzodiazepine receptor agonists (BZRAs) often have increased sleep spindle activity (Table 4–7 and Fig. 4–14).[10-12] Sleep spindle activity has a frequency of 11 to 16 Hz. Drug spindles often have a frequency in the higher end of the range. Benzodiazepines are associated with a decrease in slow wave amplitude (less stage N3 sleep) and an increase in higher EEG frequencies.[13] The nonbenzodiazepine BZRAs (zolpidem, zaleplon, eszopiclone) tend to have less effect on the amplitude of slow waves and, therefore, do not usually decrease the amount of stage N3 sleep. However, they do increase EEG frequencies during sleep, including sleep spindle activity.

Eye Movements Associated with Selective Serotonin Reuptake Inhibitor Medications

Slow eye movements are typically present during stage W with the eyes closed and during stage N1. They typically vanish with the onset of stage N2. However, in patients taking selective serotonin reuptake inhibitors (SSRIs), a mixture of slow and more rapid eye movements may persist into stage N2 or stage N3.[13,14] Because this phenomenon was first descibed with patients on fluoxetine, such eye movements are often called "Prozac eyes." Figure 4–15 shows a tracing from a patient on fluoxetine (Table 4–8).

Transient Muscle Activity during Rapid Eye Movement Sleep

Stage R (REM [rapid eye movement] sleep) is characterized by low chin EMG tone; that is, the baseline chin EMG activity in the chin derivation is no higher than in any other sleep stage and usually at the lowest level of the entire recording. However, transient bursts of EMG activity termed *transient muscle activity* (TMA; formerly called "phasic activity"), consisting of short irregular bursts of EMG activity (usually <0.25 sec), may be seen in the chin or anterior tibial EMG derivations during stage R[15,16] (Table 4–9). This activity is maximal in association with bursts of REMs (Fig. 4–16). In normal individuals, twitching in muscles may occur but usually no gross motor movements.

TMA is termed *excessive TMA* in REM sleep when more than 50% of 10 sequential 3-second miniepochs contain such

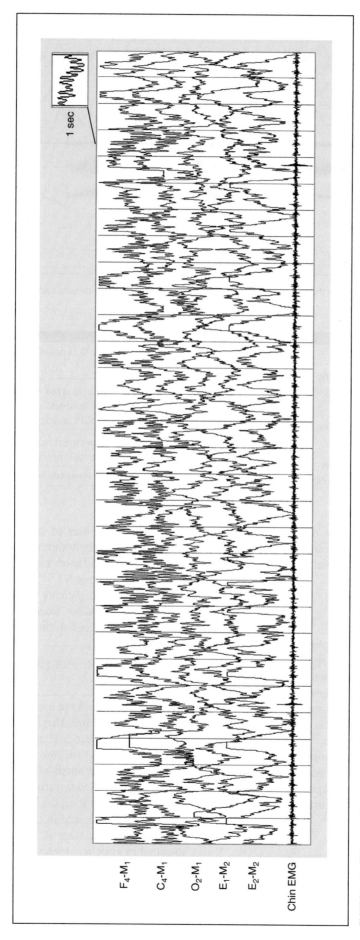

F₄-M₁
C₄-M₁
O₂-M₁
E₁-M₂
E₂-M₂
Chin EMG

1 sec

FIGURE 4–13 Alpha sleep. Prominent alpha activity is diffusely present in this 30-second epoch of stage N3 sleep. Note that the alpha activity is more prominent in the frontal and central derivations. A 1-second enlargement is shown. EMG = electromyogram.

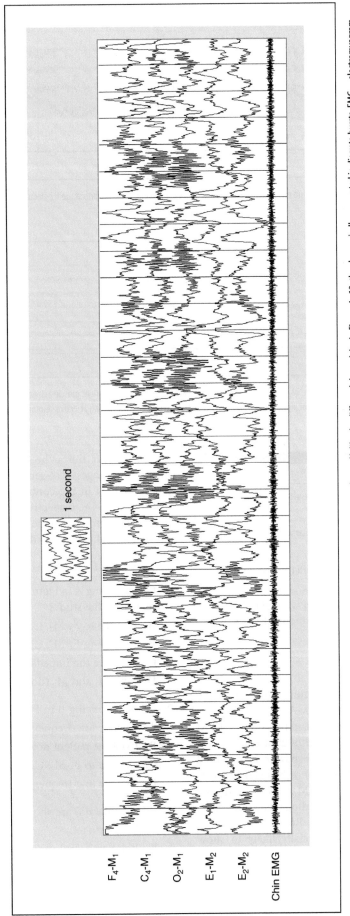

FIGURE 4–14 Prominent sleep spindle activity is noted in this 30-second tracing. A 1-second enlargement is shown. Unlike the diffuse alpha activity in Figure 4–13, the sleep spindles are noted in discrete bursts. EMG = electromyogram.

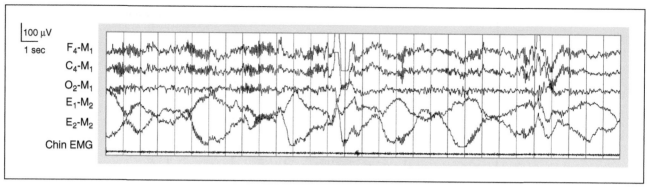

FIGURE 4–15 A 30-second tracing of a patient taking fluoxetine. Eye movements persist into stage N2 sleep. EMG = electromyogram.

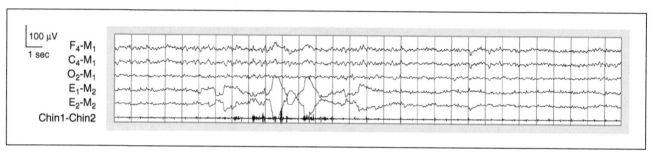

FIGURE 4–16 Bursts of EMG activity are noted on the background of reduced tonic chin EMG activity. The transient muscle activity often occurs in association with bursts of eye movements. Similar activity is not uncommon in normal individuals but is often more prominent in patients taking selective serotonin reuptake inhibitors.

TABLE 4–9
Transient Muscle Activity during Stage R
• Short irregular bursts of chin EMG activity (usually <0.25 sec).
• Most often seen in association with bursts of eye movements.
• Commonly seen in patients taking SSRI medications.
• Excessive TMA exists if >50% of 10 sequential 3-second miniepochs contain such activity with an amplitude at least four times greater than the background EMG activity.
EMG = electromyogram; SSRI = selective serotonin reuptake inhibitor; TMA = transient muscle activity.

activity with an amplitude at least four times greater than the background EMG activity. Excessive TMA (or an increase in tonic EMG activity during stage R) is said to represent REM sleep without atonia. If REM sleep without atonia is combined with abnormal dream-enacting behavior documented at the time of PSG (ideally video PSG) or by history, this is consistent with the presence of the REM sleep behavior disorder (see Chapter 28).[17] The EMG finding alone does NOT allow one to make the diagnosis of the REM sleep behavior disorder. Patients on SSRIs are especially likely to show TMA, although they usually do not meet criteria for excessive TMA. Winkelman and James[18] determined the number of 2-second bins during REM sleep that contained phasic chin (defined as EMG activity lasting 0.1–5 seconds with an amplitude four times the background EMG activity). The mean percentages of 2-second REM sleep bins containing phasic activity in the control group and SSRI groups were 2.36% and 9.54%, respectively ($P = .07$). See Chapter 12 for information on scoring the EMG activity associated with the REM sleep behavior disorder.

CLINICAL REVIEW QUESTIONS

1. Given tracing A in Figure 4–17, what should you do while reviewing the study?
   A. Change to F_3-M_2, C_3-M_2, O_1-M_2.
   B. Change to F_4-M_2, C_4-M_2, O_2-M_2.
   C. Measure the impedance of electrodes.
   D. Link M_1 and M_2 (double reference).

2. Based on tracing B in Figure 4–17, what should you do?
   A. Change low-frequency filter from 0.3 to 0.5 Hz.
   B. Cool the patient down.
   C. Change to F_3-M_2, C_3-M_2, O_1-M_2.
   D. Change low-frequency filter from 0.3 to 1.0 Hz.

3. What artifact(s) are shown in tracing C in Figure 4–17?
   A. ECG artifact.
   B. Pulse artifact.
   C. Sweat artifact.
   D. A and C.
   E. A and B.

FIGURE 4–17

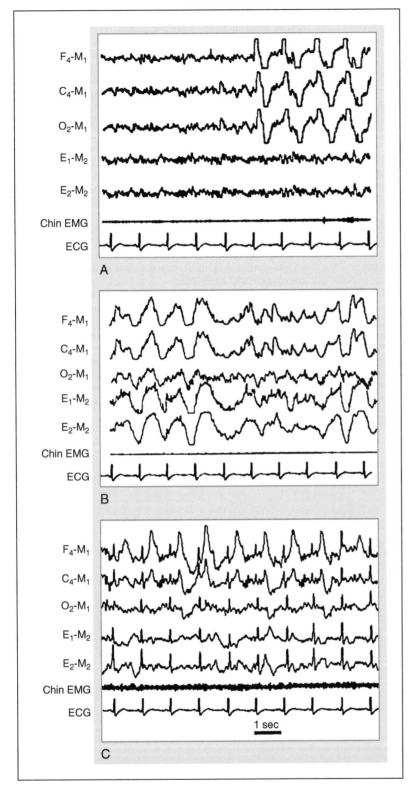

Answers

1. A. The electrode M_1 is faulty because only derivations containing M_1 have the artifact (electrode popping). The scoring rules state that if an electrode in the recommended derivations is faulty, then the alternative derivations (F_3-M_2, C_3-M_2, O_1-M_2) should be used (see Chapter 1).

2. B. Cool the patient down. Sweat artifact is shown. The first step is to cool the patient down with a fan, reducing the room temperature, or removing covers. Using a higher setting for the low-frequency filter (either 0.5 or 1 Hz) would remove much of the undulation but will also reduce the size of genuine slow waves, thus reducing the amount of activity in the 0.5- to 2-Hz range meeting the amplitude criteria for slow wave activity.

3. E. Both ECG and pulse artifact are noted. ECG artifact is visible in all of the derivations. Pulse artifact is best seen in F_4-M_1. Note the deflection follows the QRS and is usually broader than deflections due to ECG artifact.

REFERENCES

1. Caraskadon MA, Rechschaffen A: Monitoring and staging human sleep. In Kryger MH, Roth T, Dement WC (eds): Principles and Practice of Sleep Medicine, 4th ed. Philadelphia: WB Saunders, 2006, pp. 1359–1377.
2. Harris CD, Dexter D: Recording artifacts. In Shepard JW (ed): Atlas of Sleep Medicine. Mount Kisco, NY: Futura, 1991, pp. 50–51.
3. Butkov N. Clinical Polysomnography. Ashland, OR: Synapse Media, 1996, pp. 344–346.
4. Berry RB: Sleep Medicine Pearls, 2nd ed. Philadelphia: Hanley & Belfus, 2003, pp. 58–73.
5. White DP: Pathogenesis of obstructive and central sleep apnea. Am J Respir Crit Care Med 2005;172:1363–1370.
6. Hauri P, Hawkins DR: Alpha-delta sleep. Electroenceph Clin Neurophysiol 1973;34:233–237.
7. Moldofsky H, Scarisbrick P, England R, Smythe H: Musculoskeletal symptoms and non-REM sleep disturbance in patients with "fibrositis syndrome" and healthy subjects. Psychosom Med 1975;37:341–351.
8. Mahowald ML, Mahowald MW: Nighttime sleep and daytime functioning (sleepiness and fatigue) in less well defined chronic rheumatic disease with particular reference to "alpha-delta NREM sleep anomaly." Sleep Med 2000;1:195–207.
9. Roizenblatt S, Moldofsky H, Benedito-Silva AA, Tufik S: Alpha sleep characteristics in fibromyalgia. Arthritis Rheum 2001; 44:222–230.
10. Johnson LC, Hanson K, Bickford RG: Effect of flurazepam on sleep spindles and K complexes. Electroencephalogr Clin Neurophysiol 1976;40:67–77.
11. Johnson LC, Spinweber CL, Seidel WF, et al: Sleep spindle and delta changes during chronic use of a short acting and a long acting benzodiazepine hypnotic. Electroencephalogr Clin Neurophysiol 1983;55:662–667.
12. Obermeyer WH, Beneca RM: Effects of drugs on sleep. Neurol Clin 1996;14:827–840.
13. Schenck CH, Mahowald MW, Kim SW, et al: Prominent eye movements during NREM sleep and REM sleep behavior disorder associated with fluoxetine treatment of obsessive-compulsive disorder. Sleep 1992;15:226–235.
14. Armitage R, Trivedi M, Rush AJ: Fluoxetine and oculomotor activity during sleep in depressed patients. Neuropsychopharmacology 1995;12:159–165.
15. Iber C, Ancoli-Israel S, Chesson A, Quan SF for the American Academy of Sleep Medicine: The AASM Manual for the Scoring of Sleep and Associated Events: Rules, Terminology and Technical Specifications, 1st ed. Westchester, IL: American Academy of Sleep Medicine, 2007.
16. Silber MH, Ancoli-Israel S, Bonnet MH, et al: The visual scoring of sleep in adults. J Clin Sleep Med 2007;15:121–131.
17. American Academy of Sleep Medicine: International Classification of Sleep Disorders, 2nd ed. Westchester, IL: AASM, 2005, pp. 148–151.
18. Winkelman JW, James L: Serotonergic antidepressants are associated with REM sleep without atonia. Sleep 2004;15:317–321.

Sleep Staging in Infants and Children

The American Academy of Sleep Medicine (AASM) scoring manual[1,2] provides new scoring rules for infants older than 2 months and children. However, previously, the terminology for sleep staging for the newborn infant used different terminology, and sleep was staged according to the sleep scoring rules of Anders, Emde, and Parmelee.[3] These have been widely used for infants in the past and can still be used for scoring sleep in infants younger than 2 months

of age. The gestational age is the time from conception to birth (estimated from last menstrual period). The conceptional age (CA) is gestational age + time in weeks since birth. If one assumes term means 40 weeks, then the AASM rules would apply at 48 weeks' CA. For an infant born at 36 weeks, the AASM rules would apply at age 3 months (CA 48 wk).

BIPOLAR ELECTROENCEPHOGRAM RECORDING

In some of the tracings to follow, bipolar electroencephalogram (EEG) montages are illustrated using frontal (F_3, F_4, F_7, and F_8), central (C_3 and C_4), parietal (P_3, P_4, P_7, and P_8), and occipital (O_1 and O_2) electrodes (Fig. 5–1). Some of these electrodes are used in standard sleep recording and others are not. Clinical EEG is discussed in detail in Chapter 27. However, for reference, EEG electrode positions are illustrated in Figure 5–1.

SLEEP IN THE PREMATURE INFANT AND INFANTS YOUNGER THAN 48 WEEKS CA

Sleep Stages in the Newborn

Infant sleep is divided into **active sleep** (AS; corresponding to rapid eye movement [REM] sleep), **quiet sleep** (QS; corresponding to non–rapid eye movement [NREM] sleep) and **indeterminant sleep**, which is often a transitional sleep stage. Unlike adults, infants transition from wake to sleep via AS. The characteristics of each stage are listed in Table 5–1: The EEG patterns associated with wake, QS, and AS are discussed later.[1-6] The sleep of premature infants differs from that of term infants (CA 38–40 wks). The timing of the appearance of different EEG patterns characteristic of different sleep stages is illustrated in Figure 5–2. Behavioral observations are essential for sleep staging because EEG patterns may be associated with more than one state.

EEG Patterns

The EEG patterns of sleep in the pre-term and term infant are[3]

1. Tracé discontinue (TD): A discontinuous pattern consisting of high-voltage bursts with sharp features separated

by long, dramatically flat EEG periods of 10 to 20 seconds (Fig. 5–3). TD is seen at or before 30 weeks CA (see Fig. 5–2) and is the EEG pattern of QS in that age group.

2. Tracé alternant (TA): A discontinuous pattern (Figs. 5–4 and 5–5) that characterizes the QS of newborns after about 30 weeks CA (see Fig. 5–2). Bursts of mixed activity of 2 to 8 seconds are interspersed with periods of flatter EEG. The bursts are composed of high-voltage slow waves superimposed with rapid low-voltage sharp waves. There is a continuum between TD and TA, but in general, in TA, the high and low periods have fairly equal durations and the bursts do not have full bilateral synchrony. In TD, the flat is very flat and the bursts are very high voltage and have synchrony.

3. Low-voltage irregular (LVI): Continuous low-voltage mixed-frequency with prominent delta and theta rhythms and little variation. Voltage (14–35 μV), theta rhythm predominates (see Fig. 5–4).

4. High-voltage slow (HVS) pattern: Continuous, irregular mixed frequencies with higher voltages (50–100 μV) and more prominent delta frequencies (see Fig. 5–4).

5. Mixed pattern (M): Similar to LVI but with slightly higher voltages and more delta activity. Mixture of HVS and low-voltage polyrhythmic activity (see Fig. 5–4).

Premature Infants

In premature infants with a CA less than 30 weeks, QS usually shows a pattern of TD.[3,4] The pattern of TD is characterized by **electrical quiescence** between bursts of high-voltage activity. In contrast, TA is characterized by a lesser reduction in amplitude between periods of higher-amplitude activity. Another difference between TA and TD is that delta brushes (fast waves of 10–20 Hz) are superimposed on the delta waves in TD. As the infant matures, delta brushes disappear and the TA pattern replaces TD. Finally, at term, the EEG of QS is characterized by an HVS pattern. The EEG of AS in premature infants younger than 30 weeks may also show TD but later is typically LVI or M. The EEG pattern of wake and sleep is similar and states are distinguished by sustained eye closure (sleep) and open eyes (wake).

Term Infants

Wakefulness is characterized by crying, open eyes, and feeding. Non-nutritive sucking commonly continues during sleep. Sleep is often defined by sustained eye closure. The epochs during the transition from definite AS to QS are often scored as indeterminant sleep.

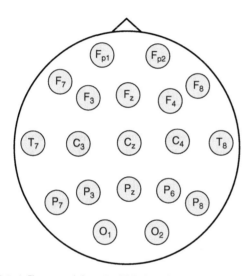

FIGURE 5–1 Electroencephalography (EEG) electrode positions. C = central; F = frontal; Fp = frontopolar; O = occipital; P = parietal; T = temporal.

TABLE 5–1					
Characteristics of Sleep Stages in Term Infants[3]					
	WAKE	**ACTIVE SLEEP**		**QUIET SLEEP**	**INDETERMINANT**
EEG	LVI or mixed	LVI M, HVS rarely		TA or HVS M rarely Premature: TD	Not meeting criteria for QS or AS
EOG	Eyes open	Eyes closed, horizontal REMs		Eyes closed Little or none	
Chin	Phasic	Low tonic between movements		High tonic	
Breathing	Irregular	Irregular, some postsigh pauses		Regular Deep and slow	
Body movements	Calm or active with eyes open	Squirming, sucking, grimacing Body: small digit or limb movements		Few, peaceful Sucking can occur	

AS = active sleep; EEG = electroencephalogram; EOG = electromyography; HVS = high-voltage slow; LVI = low-voltage irregular; M = mixed; QS = quiet sleep; REMs = rapid eye movements; TA = tracé alternant; TD = tracé discontinue.

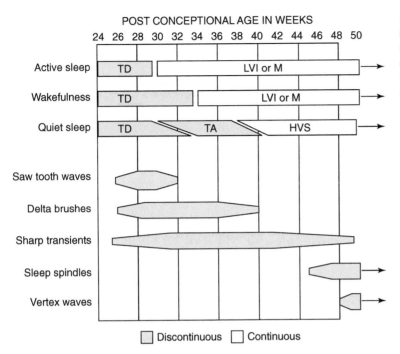

POST CONCEPTIONAL AGE IN WEEKS

FIGURE 5-2 Appearance of different EEG patterns by conceptional age in weeks. HVS = high-voltage slow; LVI = low-voltage irregular; M = mixed; TA tracé alternant; TD = tracé discontinue. The *dark bars* refer to discontinuous patterns. Examples of these patterns are illustrated in Figures 5–3 to 5–6. *From Libenson MH: Practical Approach to Electroencephalography. Philadelphia: Elsevier Saunders, 2010, p. 321.*

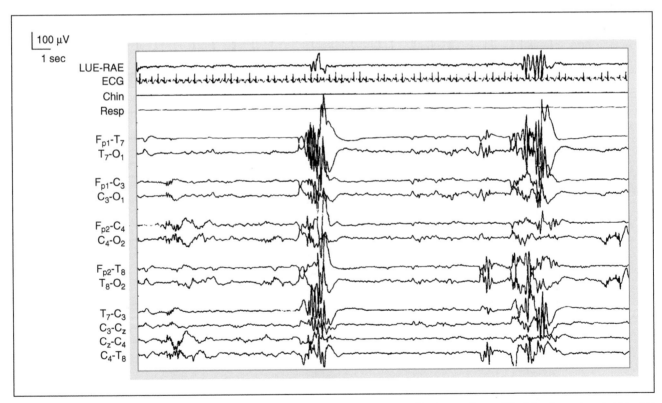

FIGURE 5-3 Tracé discontinue. Bursts of high-voltage activity alternate with long periods of flat EEG activity. ECG = electrocardiogram; LUE = left under eye electrode; RAE = right above eye electrode. *From Libenson MH: Practical Approach to Electroencephalography. Philadelphia: Elsevier Saunders, 2010, p. 307.*

AS is characterized by grimacing, sucking, an LVI EEG pattern, REMs, and low electromyogram (EMG) activity (Fig. 5–6; see also Table 5–1). Breathing is irregular in AS. QS (Fig. 5–7) is characterized by a peaceful infant with non-nutritive sucking and regular deep respiration. The EEG may show TA at early ages and HVS later. No or few eye movements are noted and the chin EMG is tonic and high.

Sleep Architecture

Newborn infants typically have periods of sleep lasting 3 to 4 hours interrupted by feeding, and the total sleep duration in 24 hours is usually 16 to 18 hours. They have cycles of sleep with a 45- to 60-minute periodicity with about 50% AS. In newborns, the presence of REM (AS) at sleep onset is the

FIGURE 5–4 EEG patterns of the newborn infant (30 sec tracings). HVS = high-voltage slow; LVI = low-voltage irregular; M = mixed. *Reproduced with permission from Anders T, Emde R, Parmelee A: A Manual of Standardized Terminology, Techniques and Criteria for Scoring of Stages of Sleep and Wakefulness in Newborn Infants. Los Angeles: Brain Information Service, UCLA, 1971.*

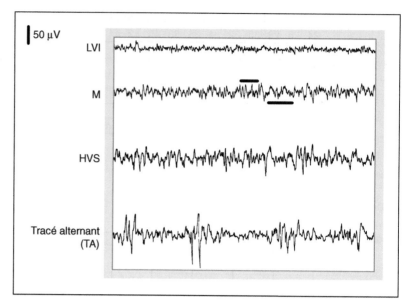

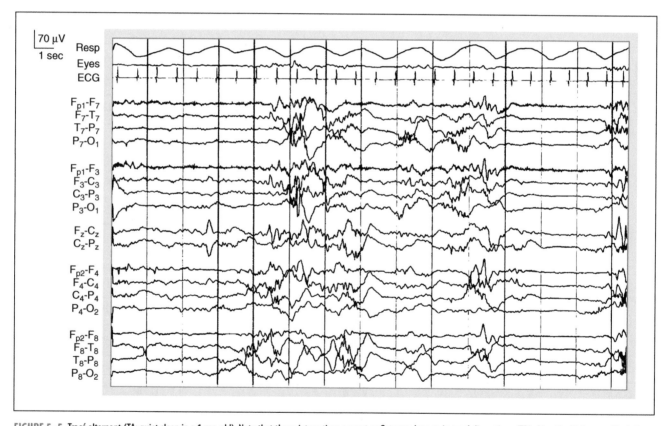

FIGURE 5–5 Tracé alternant (TA; quiet sleep in a 1-mo-old). Note that the quiet portions are not as flat or as long as in tracé discontinue (TD). Also, the higher-amplitude burst portions are longer and less synchronous. ECG = electrocardiogram. *From Libenson MH: Practical Approach to Electroencephalography. Philadelphia: Elsevier Saunders, 2010, p. 308.*

norm. In contrast, the adult sleep cycle is 90 to 100 minutes, REM occupies about 20% of sleep, and NREM sleep is noted at sleep onset.

After about 3 months, the percentage of REM sleep starts to diminish and the intensity of body movements during AS (REM) begin to decrease. The pattern of NREM at sleep onset begins to emerge. However, the sleep cycle period does not reach the adult value of 90 to 100 minutes until adolescence.[7-12]

As children mature, more typical adult EEG patterns begin to appear. The time of appearance is somewhat variable, but the values in Table 5–2 are typical. Sleep architecture in children is discussed in more detail in Chapter 6.

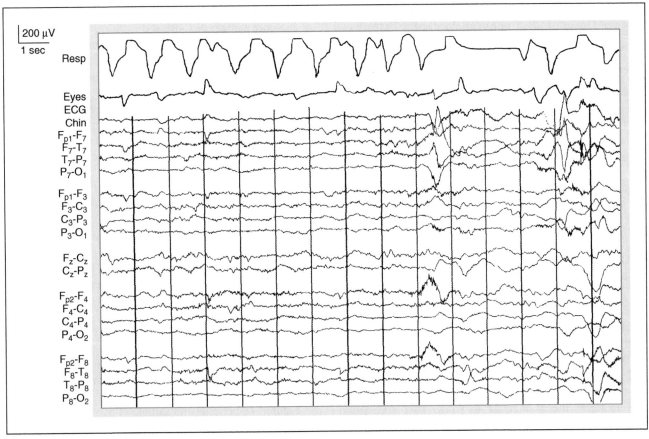

FIGURE 5–6 Active sleep. The EEG shows an LVI pattern. The respiration channel shows irregular respiration with a respiratory pause. The eye movement channel shows rapid eye movements. ECG = electrocardiogram. *Adapted from Libenson MH: Practical Approach to Electroencephalography. Philadelphia: Elsevier Saunders, 2010, p. 310.*

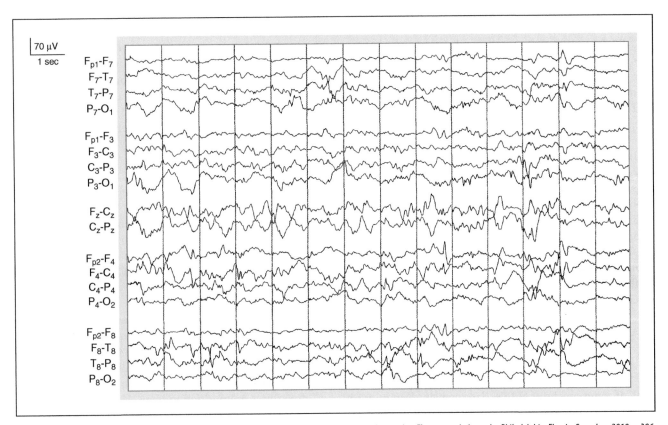

FIGURE 5–7 Quiet sleep showing an HVS EEG pattern in a term infant. *From Libenson MH: Practical Approach to Electroencephalography. Philadelphia: Elsevier Saunders, 2010, p. 306.*

TABLE 5-2

Age of Onset of Electroencephalographic Patterns

WAVE FORM	DESCRIPTION	AGE FIRST SEEN
Sleep spindles	12–16 Hz	2–3 mo
K complexes	Biphasic initial neg (up) Deflection	4–6 mo
Slow wave activity	>75 μV p-p in frontal derivation Frequency 0.5–2 Hz	4–5 mo postterm

p-p = peak-to-peak.

SCORING SLEEP IN INFANTS OLDER THAN 48 WEEKS CA AND CHILDREN

AASM Pediatric Rules for Scoring Sleep

Ages for which AASM Pediatric Sleep Scoring Rules Apply

A. Pediatric sleep scoring rules can be used to score sleep and wakefulness in children 2 months postterm or older.[2]

- *Postterm* means at least 40 weeks after conception (2 mo postterm = 48 wk CA). For example, for an infant born at 36 weeks postconception, the scoring rules apply 3 months after birth.
- For children younger than 2 months postterm, the AASM scoring manual refers the reader to the Pediatric Task Force review paper.[1] The scoring rules of Anders, Emde, and Parmelee can be used.
- There is no precise upper age limit for pediatric rules.

Terminology of Sleep Stages

A. The following terminology should be used when scoring sleep in children 2 months postterm or older:

1. Stage W (wakefulness)
2. Stage N1 (NREM 1)
3. Stage N2 (NREM 2)
4. Stage N3 (NREM 3)
5. Stage N (NREM)
6. Stage R (REM)

Scoring Sleep Stage

In the scoring of infant sleep, four possible scenarios are described:

A. If all epochs of NREM sleep contain no recognizable sleep spindles, K complexes, or high-amplitude 0.5- to 2-Hz slow wave activity (SWA), score all epochs of NREM sleep as **stage N (NREM)**.

B. If some epochs of NREM sleep contain sleep spindles or K complexes, score those as stage N2 (NREM 2). If the remaining NREM epoch contains no SWA comprising more than 20% of the duration of epochs, score as stage N (NREM).

C. If some epochs of NREM sleep contain greater than 20% SWA, score these as stage N3 (NREM 3). If the remaining NREM epochs contain no K complexes or spindles, score as stage N (NREM).

D. If NREM is sufficiently developed that some epochs contain sleep spindles and K complexes and other epochs contain sufficient amounts of SWA, score NREM sleep in the infant as either stage N1, N3, or N3 as in an older child or adult.

Notes:

1. Behavioral correlates are important in children 6 months postterm or younger.
2. NREM is characterized by regular respiration, no or rare vertical eye movements, and preserved EMG tone.
3. REM is characterized by irregular respiration, chin EMG atonia, and REMs.
4. Spontaneous eye closure in an infant indicates drowsiness.
5. **By age 6 months (and sometimes younger), stages N1, N2, and N3 can usually be scored.**

Figure 5–8 presents an example of a 3-month-old infant who had SWA but no definite sleep spindles or K complexes. NREM sleep was scored either stage N3 (epochs meeting criteria for stage N3) or stage N.

Dominant Posterior Rhythm

Dominant posterior rhythm (DPR) in both adults and children is defined as the predominant rhythm seen over **occipital derivations during eyes closed wakefulness that is reactive**. (Reactive = activity blocks or attenuates with eye opening and appears with passive eye closure.)

The DPR in **adults** is often called "alpha rhythm" and consists of activity most prominent over occipital derivations with an amplitude of less than 50 μV and a frequency of 8.5 to 13 Hz; it is reactive to eye opening (decreased amplitude).

Of note, 10% to 25% of adults have no or poorly defined alpha rhythm.

The DPR in **infants and children changes with age**. Table 5–3 shows the characteristic changes. A simple rule to remember is "greater than 8 by age 8," meaning that in normal awake children older than age 8, the DPR is greater than 8 Hz (8–13 Hz).

Additional Waveforms of Wakefulness

1. Posterior slow waves (PSWs) of youth: This waveform occurs in children between 8 and 14 years and has a frequency of 2.5 to 4.5 Hz. PSW usually occurs at the same time as DPR with eyes closed wake and disappears with drowsiness or transition to stage N1 sleep. Maximal incidence is 8 to 14 years of age, rare younger than 2 years or older than 21[1] (Fig. 5–9).

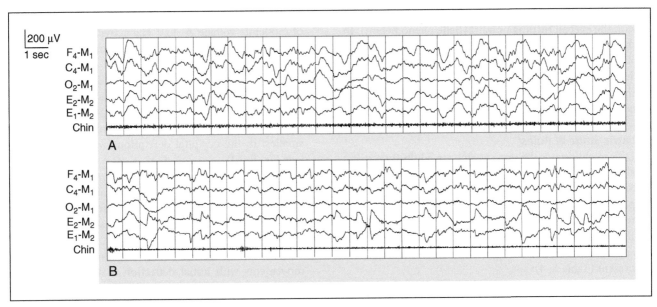

FIGURE 5–8 This 3-month-old infant had no sleep spindles or K complexes but had slow wave activity (non–rapid eye movement N3 [NREM 3]) and epochs of rapid eye movement (REM) sleep. This case shows stage N3 **(A)** and stage R **(B)**.

TABLE 5-3

Dominant Posterior Rhythm Characteristics by Age

	FREQUENCY (HZ)	% OF CHILDREN SHOWING THE PATTERN AT THIS AGE	AMPLITUDE (μV)	WAVEFORM	DISTRIBUTION
<3–4 mo	Slow	100	Not used	Irregular	Occipital
3–4 mo	3.5–4.5	75	50–100	Sinusoidal	Occipital
5–6 mo	5–6	70 by 12 mo	50–110	Sinusoidal	Occipital
3 yr	7.5–9.5	82		Sinusoidal	Occipital
6–9 yr	8–13	~88	Average 50–60	Sinusoidal	Occipital
>9 yr	8–13	90	Not used	Sinusoidal	Occipital

Memory tool: 4 Hz at 4 mo and 8 Hz at 8 yr.

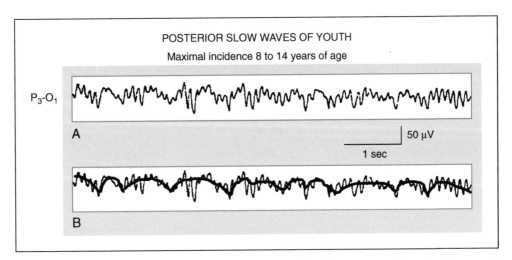

FIGURE 5–9 **A,** Posterior slow waves (PSWs) of youth in an occipital derivation. Alpha waves are superimposed on slow waves. **B,** Underlying slow wave activity. PSW is present only with eyes closed and disappears with drowsiness and sleep. PSW is a pattern of **relaxed wakefulness.**

2. Blinks: Eye blinks in children, as in adults, are associated with the eyeball turning upward (Bell's phenomenon). In children, they cause occipital sharp waves that are monophasic or biphasic (200–400 msec) and less than 200 μV that follow eye blinks.

3. Slow eye movements (SEMs) or REMs are defined the same as in adults.

Pediatric Stage W Rules[2]

A. DPR in children is the same as alpha in adults for scoring sleep and wake.

B. Score stage W when age-appropriate DPR or alpha occupies more than 50% of the epoch over the occipital region.

C. If there is no discernible reactive alpha or no age-appropriate DPR, score stage W when either of these is present (Table 5–4):

1. Eye blinks at a frequency of 0.5 to 2 Hz.
2. Reading eye movements.
3. Irregular conjugate REM associated with normal or high chin muscle tone.

Waveforms for Scoring Pediatric Stage N1[2]

In staging N1, the presence or absence of certain waveforms is important (Table 5–5).

TABLE 5-4

Pediatric Stage W Rules[1,2]

A. If there is alpha rhythm or age-appropriate DPR
1. Score wake if alpha/DPR is present for more than 50% of the epoch.

B. If there is no alpha or DPR, score wake when
1. Eye blinks are present.
2. Reading eye movements are present.
3. There are rapid eye movements with normal or high EMG tone.

DPR = dominant posterior rhythm; EMG = electromyography.

1. **Rhythmic anterior theta (RAT) activity** consists of runs of moderate voltage, 5- to 7-Hz, activity largest over the frontal regions. RAT activity is common in adolescents and young adults during drowsiness and first appears around 5 years of age[1,5] (Figs. 5–10 and 5–11).

2. **Hypnagogic hypersynchrony (HH)** is characterized by bursts of very high amplitude 3- to 4.5-Hz sinusoidal waves maximal in frontal and central derivations and smallest in the occipital derivation (widely distributed) (see Fig. 5–10).

3. **Low-amplitude mixed-frequency (LAMF):** Low-amplitude, predominantly 4- to 7-Hz activity.

4. **Vertex sharp waves** are sharply contoured waves with duration less than 0.5 second maximal over the central region and distinguishable from background activity.

5. **SEMs:** Conjugate, reasonably regular, sinusoidal eye movements with initial deflection that last longer than 500 msec.

Pediatric Stage N1 Rules[2]

A. If alpha/DPR is generated, score stage N1 if the posterior rhythm is **attenuated** or replaced by LAMF activity for more than 50% of the epoch (Fig. 5–12 and Table 5–6).

B. If alpha/DPR is not generated, score stage N1 commencing with the earliest of any of the following phenomena:

1. Activity in range 4 to 7 Hz **with** slowing of background frequencies by 1 to 2 Hz or higher from stage W (e.g., 5 Hz and stage W had 7 Hz).
2. SEMs.
3. Vertex sharp wave.
4. RAT activity.
5. HH.
6. Diffuse or occipital predominant high-amplitude rhythmic 3- to 5-Hz activity.

Pediatric Stage N2

Score as per adult rules:

Sleep spindles in children differ somewhat from those in adults. In infants, sleep spindles are often asynchronous until

TABLE 5-5

Waveforms Important for Scoring Pediatric Stage N1[1,2]

	FREQUENCY/DURATION	DISTRIBUTION	AMPLITUDE	AGE OF ONSET
LAMF	4–7 Hz	All regions	Low	
Vertex sharp waves	<0.5 sec (usually <200 msec)	Central, vertex	Stands out from background	2–3 mo (broad) 5 mo (adult-like)
RAT activity	5–7 Hz	Frontal regions	Not a criteria—generally low	Starts around age 5 yr Common in children and adolescents
Hypnagogic hypersynchrony	3–4.5 Hz	Frontal and central	Very large 75–350 μV	Appears around 3 mo Common 6–8 yr Rare > 12 yr

LAMF = low-amplitude mixed-frequency; RAT = rhythmic anterior theta.

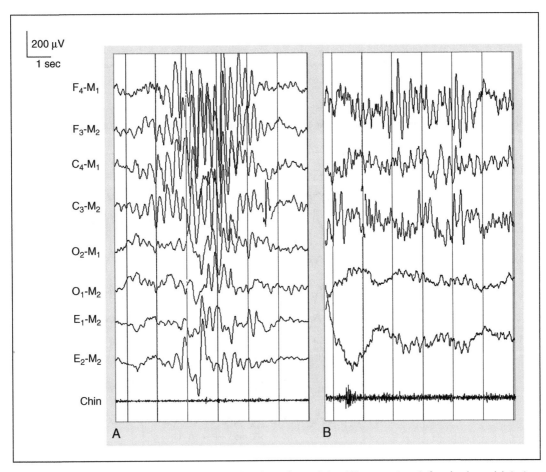

FIGURE 5–10 A, Hypnagogic hypersynchrony (HH). High-voltage bursts, frequently 3 to 4 Hz, are prominent in frontal and central derivations. **B,** Rhythmic anterior theta is faster than HH at 5 to 7 Hz and prominent in frontal derivations.

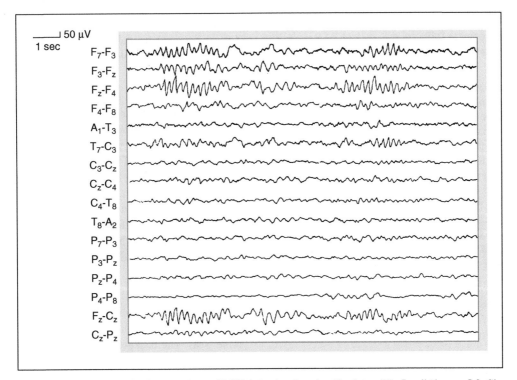

FIGURE 5–11 Rhythmic anterior theta in a 12-year-old child during drowsiness (considered stage N1). *From Neidermeyer E, Da Silva FL: Encephalography, Clinical Applications and Related Fields, 5th ed. Philadelphia: Lippincott Williams & Wilkins, 2005, p. 227.*

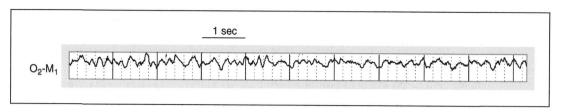

FIGURE 5–12 The dominant posterior rhythm slows from 4 to 4.5 Hz to 3 Hz in a 4-month-old during transition from stage W to stage N1.

FIGURE 5–13 Asynchronous sleep spindles in a 6-month-old girl. In the first part of the tracing, spindles are seen on the right (F₄-C₄) but not on the left. In the second part of the tracing, sleep spindles are seen on the left (F₃-C₃) but not on the right. *From Tyner FS, Knott JR, Mayer WB: Fundamentals of EEG Technology. New York: Raven, 1982, p. 243.*

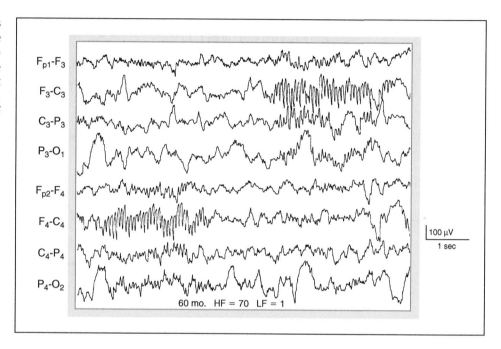

TABLE 5-6

Pediatric N1 Scoring Rules[2]

Score stage N1
In subjects who generate DPR
- DPR is **attenuated** or **replaced** by LAMF for > 50% of the epoch.

In subjects who do NOT generate DPR
- Score N1 beginning with the earliest of any of the following phenomenon:
  - Slowing of background frequencies > 1–2 Hz from those of stage W.
  - Slow eye movements.
  - Vertex sharp waves.
  - RAT activity.
  - Hypnagogic hypersynchrony.
  - Diffuse or occipital predominant **high-amplitude rhythmic 3- to 5-Hz activity.**

DPR = dominant posterior rhythm; LAMF = low-amplitude mixed-frequency; RAT = rhythmic anterior theta.

---

age 1 to 2 years. Figure 5–13 illustrates an example of asynchronous spindles.[1,6]

Sleep spindles in children:

- Sleep spindles occur independently at two different locations and frequencies in children and adolescents (Figs. 5–14 and 5–15; see also Fig. 5–13).

- Frontal spindles typically are 11 to 12.5 Hz compared with 12.5 to 14.5 Hz in centroparietal regions.

Centroparietal spindles show little change with age 4 to 24 years, whereas frontal spindles decreased dramatically in power and became stable about age 13.[1]

Pediatric Stage N3
Score as per adult rules (Table 5–7).

SWA for sleep staging is defined as greater than 75 μV peak to peak in the **frontal** derivation with a frequency of 0.5 to 2 Hz (2–0.5-sec width). Slow waves in children are often 100 to 400 μV (Fig. 5–16; see also Fig. 5–15). Slow waves appear as early as 3 months but more often about 3 to 4.5 months postterm. In scoring adult sleep, the major question for epochs containing low-frequency activity: "is the amplitude criteria met for at least 6 seconds?" In children, the major decision is what constitutes slow activity because nearly all activity exceeds 75 μV peak to peak.

Pediatric Stage R
Score as per adult rules.

The stage R of pediatric sleep differs from adults only in that the background activity may not look as familiar (Table 5–8). The background rhythm varies somewhat and can have some SWA (see Fig. 5–8B).

Pediatric Arousal Rules
Same as for adults.

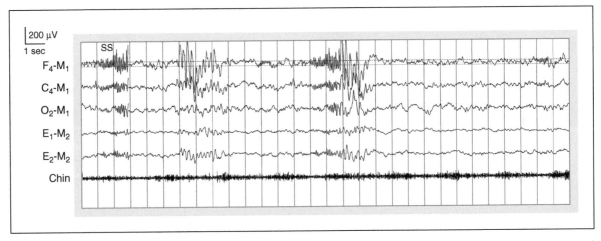

FIGURE 5–14 Stage N2 in a 5-year-old boy. Note the sleep spindle most prominent in the frontal derivation. In adults, sleep spindles are most prominent in central derivations. There are also bursts of theta activity (hypnagogic hypersynchrony).

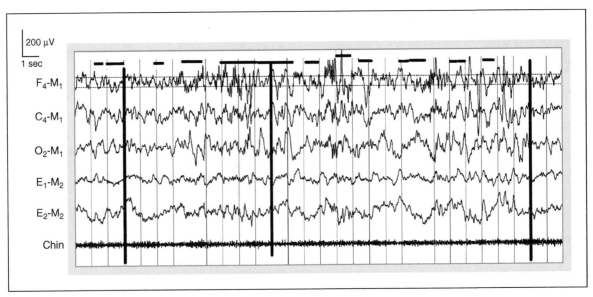

FIGURE 5–15 Stage N3 (30 second epoch). The patient is a 5-year-old boy. The horizontal amplitude lines in the derivation F_4-M_1 are 75 μV apart. The *dark bars* above F_4-M_1 show slow wave activity that exceeds 6 seconds in a 30-second epoch.

TABLE 5-7
Pediatric Stage N3 Scoring Rules[2]

Score stage N3
- Criteria: SWA (≥20% of epoch [6 sec]). SWA > 75 μV peak-to-peak in frontal derivation and frequency 0.5–2 Hz.
- Sleep spindles may or may not be present.
- Usually no eye movements in stage N3.
- Chin EMG is variable and not part of the scoring criteria.

EMG = electromyogram; SWA = slow wave activity.

TABLE 5–8	
REM Sleep in Children: Background Activity[1,2]	
AGE	BACKGROUND ACTIVITY DURING REM SLEEP
7 wk postterm	3 Hz
5 mo	4–5 Hz saw-tooth waves at 5 mo
9 mo	4–6 Hz
1–5 yr	5–7 Hz activity
5–10 yr	As adults

REM = rapid eye movement.

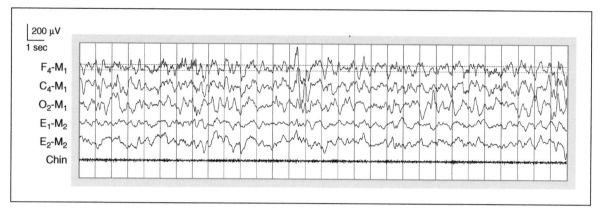

FIGURE 5–16 Stage N3 in a 5-month-old boy. The horizontal amplitude lines in F_4-M_1 are 75 µV apart.

CLINICAL REVIEW QUESTIONS

1. The sleep scoring rules of Anders, Emde, and Parmelee may be used for infants younger than what age?
   A. 3 months of age (term infant).
   B. 48 weeks conceptual age.
   C. 1 month post term.
   D. 6 months of age.

2. Which of the following is NOT true about the sleep of an infant 1 month post term?
   A. Usually enters sleep via AS.
   B. Active sleep accounts for 30% of the total sleep time.
   C. Grimacing and small digit and limb movements are normal in AS.
   D. Breathing is regular in QS.

3. What is the typical total sleep time and duration of the sleep cycle in term infants?
   A. 20 hours, 60 minutes.
   B. 16 hours, 90 minutes.
   C. 16 hours, 45 minutes.
   D. 20 hours, 30 minutes.

4. What is true about the DPR in young children?
   A. Increased with eye closure, attenuated with eye opening.
   B. Most prominent in central derivations.
   C. Score stage N1 if more than 50% of the epoch manifests the DPR.
   D. DPR reaches the 8-Hz range at about 12 years of age.

5. Posterior slow waves of youth occur in which sleep stage?
   A. Stage N3.
   B. Stage N1.
   C. Stage N2.
   D. Stage W.

6. Which of the following is true about HH?
   A. An important waveform for scoring stage N1.
   B. The frequent range is typically 4 to 7 Hz.
   C. Most prominent over occipital area.
   D. Moderate amplitude.

7. At what age do sleep spindles typically appear?
   A. 4 months.
   B. 2–3 months.
   C. 6 months.
   D. 8 months.

8. By what age can stage N1, N2, and N3 typically be scored?
   A. 2 months.
   B. 4 months.
   C. 6 months.
   D. 1 year.

Answers

1. **B.** 48 weeks conceptual age (equivalent to 2 mo post term).

2. **B.** AS accounts for around 50% of the total sleep time in a term infant.

3. **C.** Total sleep time is 16 to 18 hours and sleep cycle is about 45 minutes.

4. **A.** DPR reaches 8 Hz around 8 years of age and is most prominent in occipital derivations. Score stage W if more than 50% of the epoch manifests DPR.

5. **D.** Posterior slow waves of youth occur during eyes-closed wake and vanish with sleep onset.

6. **A.** HH is important for staging N1 in children. The frequency is usually 3 to 4.5 Hz and the waveform has a high amplitude most prominent in frontal and central areas and smallest in occipital regions.

7. B. Sleep spindles typically appear at 2 to 3 months of age.

8. C. Stage N1, N2, and N3 can typically be scored by 6 months of age (and sometimes sooner).

REFERENCES

1. Grigg-Damberger M, Gozal D, Marcus CL, et al: The visual scoring of sleep and arousal in infants and children. J Clin Sleep Med 2007;3:201–240.
2. Iber C, Ancoli-Israel S, Chesson A, Quan SF for the American Academy of Sleep Medicine: The AASM Manual for the Scoring of Sleep and Associated Events: Rules, Terminology and Technical Specifications, 1st ed. Westchester, IL: American Academy of Sleep Medicine, 2007.
3. Anders T, Emde R, Parmelee A: A Manual of Standardized Terminology, Techniques and Criteria for Scoring of Stages of Sleep and Wakefulness in Newborn Infants. Los Angeles: Brain Information Service, UCLA, 1971.
4. Libenson MH: Practical Approach to Electroencephalography. Philadelphia: Elsevier Saunders, 2010, p. 321.
5. Neidermeyer E, Da Silva FL: Encephalography, Clinical Applications and Related Fields, 5th ed. Philadelphia: Lippincott Williams & Wilkins, 2005, p. 227.
6. Tyner FS, Knott JR, Mayer WB: Fundamentals of EEG Technology. New York: Raven, 1982, p. 243.
7. Kahn A, Dan B, Grosswasser J, et al: Normal sleep architecture in infants and children. J Clin Neurophysiol 1996;13:184–297.
8. Seldon S: Polysomnography in infants and children. In Sheldon SH, Ferber R, Kryger MH (eds): Principles and Practice of Pediatric Sleep Medicine. Philadelphia: Elsevier Saunders, 2005, pp. 49–71.
9. Iglowstein I, Jenni OG, Molinari L, Largo RH: Sleep duration from infancy to adolescense: reference values and generational trends. Pediatrics 2003;111:302–307.
10. Montgomery-Downs HE, O'Brien LM, Gulliver TE, et al: Polysomnographic characteristics in normal preschool children. Pediatrics 2006;117:741–753.
11. Mason TB, Teoh L, Calabro K, et al: Rapid eye movement latency in children and adolescence. Pediatr Neurol 2008;39:162–169.
12. Beck SE, Marcus CL: Pediatric polysomnography. Sleep Med Clin 2009;4:393–406.

Chapter 6

Sleep Architecture Parameters, Normal Sleep, and Sleep Loss

Chapter Points

- Sleep in adults is characterized by 3 to 5 cycles of NREM/REM sleep, each lasting about 90 to 100 minutes.
- The duration of stage R in each cycle is typically longer in the second part of the night. The individual episodes of REM are also longer. The REM density (eye movements/time) is greater in the second part of the night.
- Most stage N3 occurs in the first part of the night.
- In adults, the TST and sleep efficiency decrease and the amount of wake increases with age. There is also a modest increase in the sleep latency and a decrease in the REM latency.
- In men, the amount of stage N3 decreases with age and the amount of stage N1 increases. In women, the amount of stage N3 does not decrease with age.
- In adults, the amount of stage R decreases slightly with age.
- The normal ArI increases with age.
- A number of medications increase the REM latency including selective serotonin reuptake inhibitors, tricyclic antidepressants, and lithium.
- Infants commonly enter sleep via stage R (or active sleep) and have a sleep cycle (45–60 min) that is much shorter than that of adults.
- After sleep deprivation, recovery sleep is usually characterized by an increase in stage N3 on the first recovery night with an increase in REM sleep on subsequent nights.
- Chronic sleep restriction can have a number of adverse health consequences. These include a reduction in leptin, an increase in ghrelin, and impaired glucose metabolism.

A number of parameters concerning the quantity and quality of sleep are usually included in polysomnography (PSG) reports[1,2] (Table 6–1). Typically, PSG data recording starts before lights out to verify that the electrodes and monitoring equipment are providing adequate signals. In addition, calibrations and biocalibrations are recorded as described in Chapter 4. **Lights out time** is the time at which the patient is allowed to fall asleep and marks the start of data that will be staged and analyzed. **Lights on** is the time that recording of sleep is terminated. **Total recording time** (TRT) is the time from lights out to lights on. Some sleep centers also record another set of biocalibrations after lights on. The **sleep latency** is the time from lights out to the start of the first epoch of sleep. **Wake after sleep onset (WASO)** as defined by the American Academy of Sleep Medicine (AASM) scoring manual includes all stage W after sleep onset (from the *start of the first epoch of sleep*) until lights on. It also includes out-of-bed wake time during the period from sleep onset until lights on. The total amount of stage W (during TRT) = sleep latency + WASO.

Previously, some clinicians used the term "sleep period time (SPT)," defined as the time from sleep onset to the final awakening. WASO was then defined as the duration of wake during the sleep period time ($WASO_{SPT}$). That is, $WASO_{SPT}$ = SPT − TST, where TST = total sleep time. The AASM scoring manual has standardized the definition of WASO and does not use the SPT as a standard parameter. However, a considerable number of publications[3] previously used SPT and $WASO_{SPT}$ (formerly identified as WASO), so the reader should be familiar with this terminology. The AASM scoring manual also recommends presentation of the durations of the sleep stages both as an absolute duration and as a percentage of TST. Some authors previously presented $WASO_{SPT}$ and the sleep stages as a percentage of SPT.

NORMAL SLEEP IN ADULTS

Sleep occurs in cycles, each usually composed of a period of non–rapid eye movement (NREM) sleep followed by stage R rapid eye movement (REM) sleep. There are usually three to five NREM/REM cycles per night (Table 6–2). A useful approach for presentation of sleep cycle data is the hypnogram. This is a plot of sleep stage versus time of night (Fig. 6–1). Although the sleep architecture parameters listed previously are useful, they obviously do not provide details about the pattern of sleep over the night. Hypnograms can be very informative, and many sleep centers include a hypnogram in their sleep report.

Sleep architecture is a term used to denote the structure of sleep. In young adults, stage N1 usually occupies approximately 5% to 10% of the TST.[3-5] It is a transitional state

TABLE 6-1

Sleep Architecture Parameters

TRT (min)	Time duration from lights out to lights on. TRT = SL + WASO + TST
Lights out time (hr:min)	Time of the start of the recording.
Lights on time (hr:min)	Time of the end of the recording.
TST (min)	Time spent in stages N1, N2, N3, and R.
SL (min)	Time from lights out until the start of the first epoch of sleep (stages N1, N2, N3, or R).
Stage R latency (min) (REM latency)	Time from start of first epoch of sleep until the start of the first epoch of stage R.
Sleep efficiency (%)	= TST × 100/TRT.
Stage W (min)	All minutes of stage W during TRT.
WASO	Stage W recorded after sleep onset until lights on time. = stage W − SL
Time in each sleep stage (min)	Minutes of stages N1, N2, N3, R.
Time in each sleep stage as a % of TST	Minutes of each sleep stage × 100/TST.
Arousal (number)	Total number of arousals.
ArI (#/hr)	Total number of arousals × 60/TST (min).

ArI = arousal index; REM = rapid eye movement; SL = sleep latency; TRT = total recording time; TST = total sleep time; WASO = wake after sleep onset.
After Iber C, Ancoli-Israel S, Chesson A, Quan SF for the American Academy of Sleep Medicine: The AASM Manual for the Scoring of Sleep and Associated Events: Rules, Terminology and Technical Specifications, 1st ed. Westchester, IL: American Academy of Sleep Medicine, 2007.

TABLE 6-2

Sleep Architecture Facts

- 3–5 sleep (NREM – REM) cycles during the night

- Stage N3
  - ⇒ Most stage N3 is during the first half of the night
  - ⇒ Delta power decreases with each NREM cycle

- Stage R
  - ⇒ Episodes of stage R are longer in the second part of the night
  - ⇒ REM density (number of eye movements per time during REM sleep) is higher in later episodes of REM sleep

NREM = non–rapid eye movement; REM = rapid eye movement.

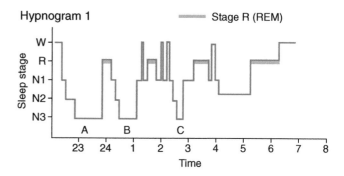

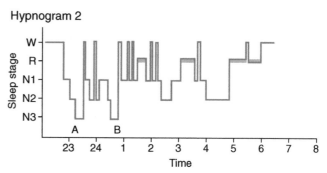

FIGURE 6–1 Hypnograms. Hypnogram 1 is from a normal individual. Hypnogram 2 is from a patient complaining of frequent nocturnal awakenings. The first rapid eye movement (REM) period is "missed" and there is a long REM latency. There are frequent awakenings during the night.

between wake and the other stages of sleep. Stage N2 occupies the greatest proportion of the TST and accounts for approximately 50% to 60% of sleep. Stage N3 occupies approximately 15% to 20% of the TST and stage R approximately 20% of the TST. The amplitude of the slow waves and amount of stage N3 is greatest in the first sleep cycle (see Fig. 6–1). Using spectral analysis, one can compute the delta power (the contribution of slow wave activity to the total electroencephalogram [EEG] activity) (Fig. 6–2). The delta power is highest during the initial cycle of NREM sleep. The episodes of stage R occur about every 90 to 120 minutes, and they are of longer duration as the night progresses. The REM

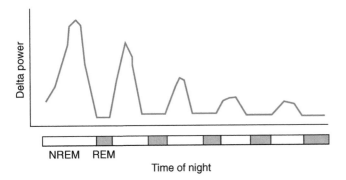

FIGURE 6–2 Schematic illustrating the fact that delta power (amount of slow wave activity) decreases with subsequent episodes of non–rapid eye movement (NREM) sleep. Note delta power is very low during episodes of rapid eye movement (REM) sleep.

TABLE 6–3
Stages in Sleep Architecture with Aging (20–60 yr)

	INCREASE WITH AGE	DECREASE WITH AGE
Changes with aging (20–60 yr)	Sleep latency WASO (most change after 40 yr) Stage N1 (%TST)[5] Stage N1 (%TST) men only[6] Stage N2 (%TST)[5] Stage N2 (%TST) men only[6]	Stage N3 (%TST)[5] Stage N3 (%TST) men only[6] Stage R (%TST)[5,6] REM latency TST Sleep efficiency

REM = rapid eye movement; TST = total sleep time; WASO = wake after sleep onset.

TABLE 6–4
Change in Sleep Architecture with Age (Sleep Heart Health Study)*

		AGE RANGE			
STAGE	SEX	QUARTILE 1 (37–54 YR)	QUARTILE 2 (55–60 YR)	QUARTILE 3 (61–70 YR)	QUARTILE 4 (>70 YR)
Stage N1	Men	5.8	6.3	7.1	7.6
	Women	4.6	5.0	5.0	4.9
Stage N2	Men	61.4	64.5	65.2	66.5
	Women	58.5	56.2	57.3	57.1
Stage N3	Men	11.2	8.2	6.7	5.5
	Women	14.2	17.0	16.7	17.2
Stage R	Men	19.5	19.1	18.4	17.8
	Women	20.9	20.2	19.3	18.8

*Stage as a % of TST in four age quartiles.
TST = total sleep time.
From Redline S, Kirchner L, Quan SF, et al: The effects of age, sex, ethnicity, and sleep-disordered breathing on sleep architecture. Arch Intern Med 2004;164:406–418.

density is the number of eye movements per time. The REM density tends to be the highest in the later REM periods. In fact, the initial REM period of the night is often difficult to score owing to infrequent REMs. The first REM period also may have K complexes or sleep spindles in epochs with **both** low chin electromyogram (EMG) and REMs. According to the AASM scoring manual, such epochs are scored as stage R[1] (see Chapter 3). During the last half of the night, most sleep is composed of stage N2 and stage R with intervening stage W and stage N1. In Figure 6–1, Hypnogram 1 presents a normal hypnogram. Hypnogram 2 shows a hypnogram with a longer sleep latency, a long REM latency, two episodes of stage N3 sleep, and more stage W.

CHANGES IN SLEEP ARCHITECTURE WITH AGING (ADULTS)

Sleep architecture changes as adults grow older (Table 6–3).[4–6] In general, sleep becomes lighter and more fragmented. There

is an increase in the sleep latency, WASO, and stages N1 and N2.[5] One study found an increase in stages N1 and N2 in men only.[6] There is a decrease in stage N3 (men only) and a small decrease in stage R. The REM latency decreases with age. Study of sleep architecture in older adults is complicated by inclusion of individuals with medical or mental disorders in some studies of the effect of aging on sleep architecture. Many early studies did not include a sufficient number of women. Ohayon and coworkers[5] performed a large meta-analysis of sleep architecture and attempted to specify normal values with and without exclusion of patients with mental diseases that could alter sleep architecture. Redline and colleagues[6] have published another analysis of the effect of age on sleep architecture (Sleep Heart Health Study). They studied a large group of patients using standardized recording and scoring techniques (Table 6–4). This study evaluated information from sleep studies of patients 37 years and older and divided the study group into four age quartiles. The sleep studies were performed at home. Van Cauter and associates[3] also published findings concerning the age-related changes in slow wave and REM sleep in healthy men.

Sleep Latency and REM Latency

In the meta-analysis by Ohayon and coworkers,[5] when studies that included individuals with sleep and mental disorders were excluded, sleep latency increased only minimally from ages 20 to 80 (~10 min) (Fig. 6-3). If patients with mental and medical disorders were included, there was not a significant increase in sleep latency with age. This is consistent with more reports of early morning awakening than sleep onset problems in the healthy elderly. In general, a sleep latency of 30 minutes or more is considered abnormal. In the same meta-analysis, the REM latency decreased with age.

TST and Sleep Efficiency

TST decreases with age as does the sleep efficiency (TST × 100/TRT) (Fig. 6-4). There tends to be a more rapid decrease

in TST from childhood to adolescence and then a slower decrease from age 20 to 80 years. Sleep efficiency decreases with age, especially after age 50.[5]

WASO and Stage N1 (as a Percentage of TST)

In the meta-analysis by Ohayon and coworkers,[5] WASO and stage N1 (as %TST) increased from age 20 to 60 years (Fig. 6-5). In the analysis of Redline and colleagues,[6] the amount of stage N1 increased over the four quartiles for men but not for women (Fig. 6-6).

Stage N2 (as a Percentage of TST)

In the meta-analysis of Ohayon and coworkers,[5] the amount of stage N2 increases with age (Fig. 6-7A). Redline and colleagues[6] found stage N2 to increase with age in men but not in women (see Fig. 6-7B). This is consistent with the findings of a decrease in stage N3 in men (see later). The amount of stage N2 was higher in men than in women when all age groups were considered.

Stage N3 (as a Percentage of TST)

In the large meta-analysis by Ohayon and coworkers,[5] the amount of stage N3 decreased with age (Fig. 6-8A). The

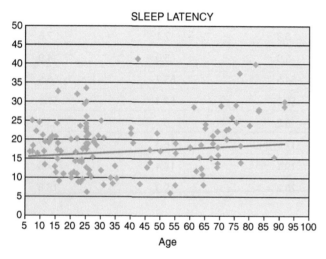

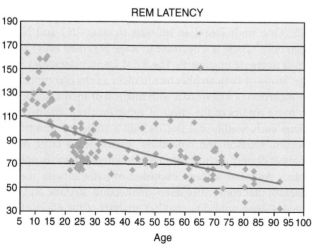

FIGURE 6-3 The sleep latency increases and rapid eye movement (REM) latency decreases with age. *From Ohayon MM, Carskadon MA, Guilleminault C, Viteiello MV: Meta-analysis of quantitative sleep parameters from childhood to old age in healthy individuals: developing normative sleep values across the human lifespan. Sleep 2004;27:1255–1273.*

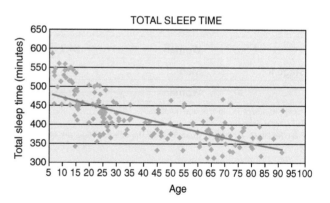

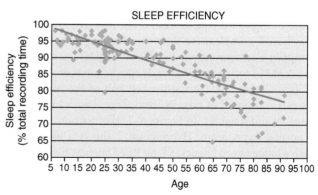

FIGURE 6-4 Changes in total sleep time and sleep efficiency with age. Both total sleep time and sleep efficiency decrease in older individuals. *From Ohayon MM, Carskadon MA, Guilleminault C, Viteiello MV: Meta-analysis of quantitative sleep parameters from childhood to old age in healthy individuals: developing normative sleep values across the human lifespan. Sleep 2004;27:1255–1273.*

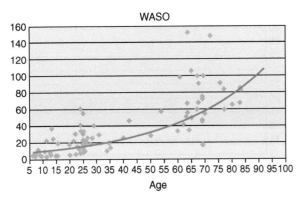

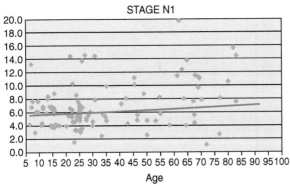

FIGURE 6-5 Wake after sleep onset (WASO) and stage N1 increase with age. *From Ohayon MM, Carskadon MA, Guilleminault C, Viteiello MV: Meta-analysis of quantitative sleep parameters from childhood to old age in healthy individuals: developing normative sleep values across the human lifespan. Sleep 2004;27:1255–1273.*

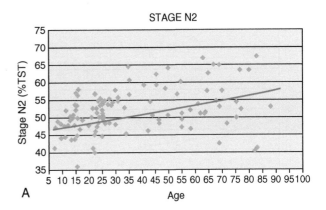

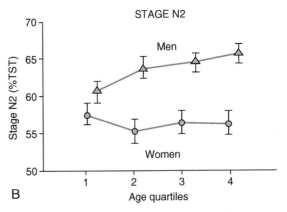

FIGURE 6-7 **A,** The relationship between the amount of stage N2 and age in the study of Ohayon and coworkers.[5] Stage N2 increased with age. **B,** Stage N2 increased with age only in men in the study of Redline and colleagues.[6] The age range for each quartile is defined in Table 6-4.

Stage R (as a Percentage of TST)

Ohayon and coworkers[5] found a decrease in stage R between 20 and 60 years of age (Fig. 6–9A). Most of the decrease in REM as a percentage of TST was noted between 10 and 35 years of age. In the data of Redline and colleagues[6] (see Table 6–4), there was a small but statistically significant decrease in stage R with age for both men and women (see Fig. 6–9B).

Sleep Architecture (as a Percentage of SPT)

Van Cauter and associates[3] also published information of sleep architecture in normal **men**. They found an increase in stage W but minimal change in combined stage N1 and N2 (Fig. 6–10). Their data were expressed as a percentage of sleep period time. They also found a decrease in stage N3 with age and a decrease in stage R most prominent after age 50 (Fig. 6–11).

ALTERNATIONS IN REM LATENCY

Various sleep disorders and medications[7] are associated with changes in the REM latency (Table 6–5). A short nocturnal REM latency can be seen in patients with narcolepsy, sleep apnea, and depression. Withdrawal from a REM-suppressing medication can also shorten the REM latency. A REM latency of 0 to 15 minutes is often referred to as *sleep-onset REM*. Sleep-onset REM is a defining characteristic of narcolepsy.

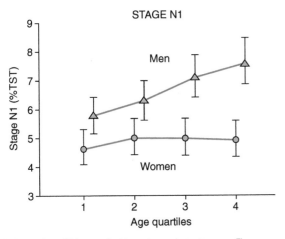

FIGURE 6-6 Stage N1 increased with age in men but not women. The age range of each quartile is defined in Table 6-4. TST = total sleep time. *Data from Redline S, Kirchner L, Quan SF, et al: The effects of age, sex, ethnicity, and sleep-disordered breathing on sleep architecture. Arch Intern Med 2004;164:406–418.*

effect size was greater in men than in women. In the study by Redline and colleagues,[6] the amount of stage N3 (%TST) decreased with age only in men (see Fig. 6–8B). The decrease in stage N3 was associated with increases in stages N1 and N2. Note that for the entire group of women (all ages), the amount of stage N3 was higher.

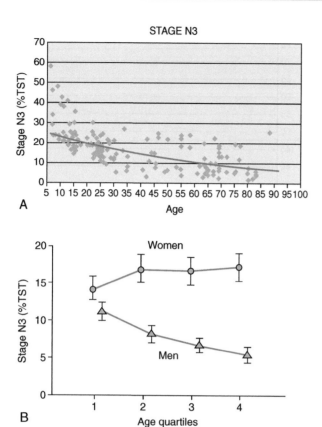

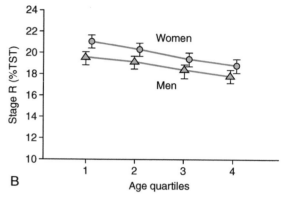

FIGURE 6–8 **A,** Stage N3 (%TST [total sleep time]) for men and women combined decreases in adults. **B,** Stage N3 (%TST) decreases with age only in men. The absolute amount of stage N3 for the study group as a whole was greater in women than in men. The age range for each quartile is defined in Table 6–4. **A,** From Ohayon MM, Carskadon MA, Guilleminault C, Viteiello MV: Meta-analysis of quantitative sleep parameters from childhood to old age in healthy individuals: developing normative sleep values across the human lifespan. Sleep 2004;27:1255–1273. **B,** Data from Redline S, Kirchner L, Quan SF, et al: The effects of age, sex, ethnicity, and sleep-disordered breathing on sleep architecture. Arch Intern Med 2004;164:406–418.

FIGURE 6–9 Stage R. **A,** The amount of stage R (%TST [total sleep time]) decreases with age. Most of the decrease comes between 20 and 30 years. **B,** There was a small decrease in rapid eye movement (REM) with age quartile. The age range for each quartile is defined in Table 6–4. In this study, only patients older than 37 years were included. **A,** From Ohayon MM, Carskadon MA, Guilleminault C, Viteiello MV: Meta-analysis of quantitative sleep parameters from childhood to old age in healthy individuals: developing normative sleep values across the human lifespan. Sleep 2004;27:1255–1273. **B,** Data from Redline S, Kirchner L, Quan SF, et al: The effects of age, sex, ethnicity, and sleep-disordered breathing on sleep architecture. Arch Intern Med 2004;164:406–418.

TABLE 6–5	
Short and Long REM Latency	
SHORT REM LATENCY	**LONG REM LATENCY**
Narcolepsy	Ethanol
Depression	SSRIs
Withdrawal of REM-suppressing medication	Tricyclic antidepressants Lithium
Sleep apnea	Sleep apnea
Previous REM deprivation	First-night effect
REM = rapid eye movement; SSRIs = selective serotonin reuptake inhibitors.	

In depression, REM latencies on the order of 40 minutes are typical but can be as short as those seen in patients with narcolepsy. In depression, the first episode of REM sleep is often prolonged with a higher REM density than usual. In contrast, a number of other sleep disorders that fragment sleep such as sleep apnea can prolong the REM latency. Medications known to prolong the REM latency include tricyclic antidepressants, selective serotonin reuptake inhibitors, monoamine oxidase inhibitors, and lithium. Some substances such as alcohol can also increase the REM latency.

Gender Differences

In adulthood, women of all ages tend to have more stage N3 than men at the expense of stages N1 and N2 (stage N1 and N2 are greater in men as %TST) (see Figs. 6–6 to 6–8). The amounts of stage R are similar in men and women.

First-Night Effect

The first-night effect was described by Agnew and coworkers[8] and Webb and Campbell[9] from analysis of individuals undergoing multiple sleep studies. The phenomenon consists of lower sleep efficiency, lower amount of REM sleep, and longer REM latency on the first night in the sleep center.

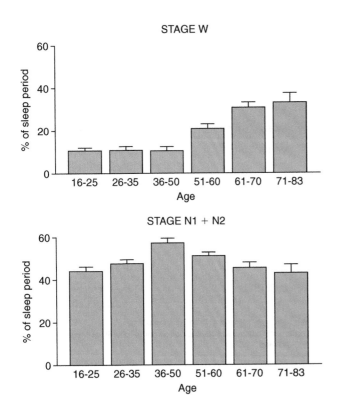

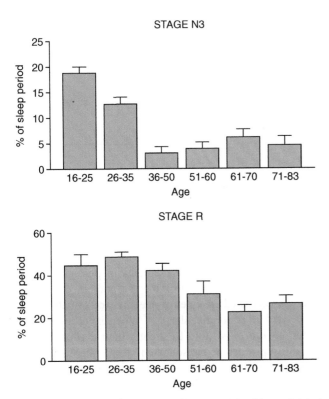

FIGURE 6–10 Changes in stage W and stage N1 + N2 expressed as a percentage of the sleep period time (time from first sleep until final awakening) in normal men. Stage W increased with age. There was minimal change in combined stage N1 + N2.

FIGURE 6–11 Change in stage N3 and stage R (as a percentage of sleep period time) with age in a group of normal men. Stage N3 decreased in the older age range as did stage R after age 50. *From Van Cauter E, Leprousl R, Plat L: Age-related changes in slow wave sleep and REM sleep and relationship with growth hormone and cortisol levels in healthy men. JAMA 2000;284:861–868.*

COMPARISON OF SLEEP STAGING BETWEEN THE AASM SCORING MANUAL AND RECHTSCHAFFEN AND KALES

Given that most previous work on sleep architecture was based on the scoring manual of Rechtschaffen and Kales (R&K),[10] normative values could be altered by the new AASM scoring manual. Therefore, studies comparing sleep architecture between R&K and the AASM scoring manual are needed. Moser and colleagues[11] found that the sleep latency, REM latency, TST, and sleep efficiency were not affected (similar in AASM and R&K). The absolute duration of sleep stage and the %TST in stage N1 increased and stage N2 decreased using AASM criteria compared with those of R&K. Stage R also differed but was age-dependent, being slightly higher using AASM criteria in older individuals. The amount of stage N3 was higher in AASM as expected with use of frontal derivations to assess slow wave activity (slow waves have the higher amplitude in frontal compared with central derivations). Danker-Hopfe and associates[12] compared interscorer reliability between the AASM and the R&K criteria and found slightly better agreement with the AASM criteria, although the difference was small. Novelli and coworkers[13] compared AASM (e.g., N1) and R&K (e.g., S1) for sleep scoring in children and adolescents. They found N1 > S1, N2 < S2, and R < stage REM. They found a low concordance between the systems. These studies are only the first of many to be expected in the future.

NORMAL SLEEP IN INFANTS AND CHILDREN

Sleep Architecture in Infants

As noted in Chapter 5, sleep stage scoring differs considerably between infants and adults. The sleep architecture in infants is also very different from that in adults (Table 6–6). Infants normally enter sleep via stage R (active sleep for age < 2 mo) and spend approximately 50% of the TST in this sleep stage. Infants have shorter sleep cycles of approximately 45 to 60 minutes (in contrast to adult cycles of 90–100 min).[14,15] By 3 months of age, the amount of REM sleep starts to decrease. Sleep begins to consolidate into longer nocturnal sleep periods with shorter naps during the day. Napping is rare after age 4 years.[16]

Children

The percentage of REM sleep decreases to approximately 30% at age 1 to 2 years and 20% to 25% at 3 to 5 years of age. As children move toward adolescence (Table 6–7), there tends to be a decrease in stage N3 sleep and stage R with an increase in stage N2. TST decreases from early childhood to adolescence from 14 hours at age 1 down to 9 hours in early adolescence.[16] Typical values for sleep parameters are listed in Tables 6–8 and 6–9.[17–19]

AROUSALS

Chapter 3 presents the scoring criteria for arousals.[2,20] Scoring of arousals is important because frequent arousals

TABLE 6-6
Normal Sleep Infants and Children

INFANTS < 3 mo

- Stage R (REM sleep, active sleep) at sleep onset.
- Total sleep time 16–18 hr.
- Sleep episodes of 3–4 hr duration interrupted by feeding.
- Sleep cycles 45- to 60-min periodicity (90–100 min in adults).
- Stage R about 50% of sleep.

INFANTS > 3 mo

- Percentage of REM sleep starts to decrease.
- Entering sleep through NREM sleep instead of stage R.
- Sleep consolidates into major episodes with daytime naps.

CHILDREN

- Sleep cycle period does not reach adult values until adolescence.

NREM = non–rapid eye movement; REM = rapid eye movement.
From Kahn A, Dan B, Grosswasser J, et al: Normal sleep architecture in infants and children. J Clin Neurophysiol 1996;13:184–197.

TABLE 6-7
Changes in Sleep Childhood to Adolescence

NO CHANGE	DECREASE	INCREASE
TST (recording nonschool days)	% Stage N3	Stage N2
Sleep efficiency	% REM sleep	
Sleep latency	TST (recording school days)	

REM = rapid eye movement; TST = total sleep time.
From Kahn A, Dan B, Grosswasser J, et al: Normal sleep architecture in infants and children. J Clin Neurophysiol 1996;13:184–197.

TABLE 6-8
Typical Sleep Architecture Values for Normal Children Aged 1–18

PARAMETER	USUAL VALUES
Sleep efficiency (%)	89%, large variability
Sleep latency (min)	23 min, large variability
REM latency (min)	87–155 (<10 yr) 136–156 (>10 yr)
Arousal index	9–16
Stage N1 (%TST)	4–5
Stage N2 (%TST)	44–56
Stage N3 (%TST)	29–32 (<10 yr) 20–32 (>10 yr)
Stage R (%TST)	17–21 (can be higher in younger children)

REM = rapid eye movement; TST = total sleep time.
From Beck SE, Marcus CL: Pediatric polysomnography. Sleep Med Clin 2009;4:393–406.

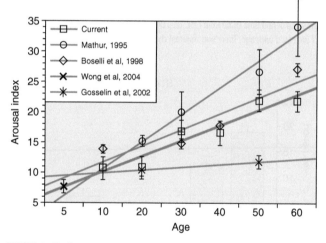

FIGURE 6–12 Change in arousal index with age. The data are from references 21–26. *Current* refers to data from reference 22. *From Bonnet M, Arand DL: EEG arousal norms by age. J Clin Sleep Med 2007;3:271–274.*

result in nonrestorative sleep even in the absence of a decrement in TST. The arousal index (ArI, number of arousals/hour of sleep) in normal individuals increases with age (Fig. 6–12).[21-25] Bonnet and Arand[21] found the ArI in 51- to 60-year-old individuals and 61- to 70-year-old individuals to be 21.9 ± 8.9/hr and 21.9 ± 6.8/hr, respectively (mean ± standard deviation [SD]). Therefore, the 95% confidence limits may approach 35/hr in older age groups. Conversely, an ArI of 25/hr would be high for a young adult. Figure 6–12 shows the data on the change in ArI with age from several studies.

SLEEP FRAGMENTATION

Although in clinical practice, sleep fragmentation and chronic partial sleep deprivation (chronic decreased TST) commonly occur together, studies have shown that frequent

arousals alone can cause decrements in performance and mood as well as increases in subjective and objective sleepiness. Consolidated episodes of sleep in excess of 10 minutes are needed for restorative sleep.[26,27] When experimental sleep disturbance occurs more frequently than every 3 minutes (<3-min episodes of consolidated sleep), there is a sharp decrease in the sleep latency by the multiple sleep latency test (MSLT)[27] (Fig. 6–13). This would correspond to an ArI greater than 20/hr. In sleep studies, some patients may have comparable ArIs but differ in the amount of preserved consolidated sleep. Table 6–10 lists the common clinical symptoms of sleep deprivation. Similar findings can occur with severe sleep fragmentation.

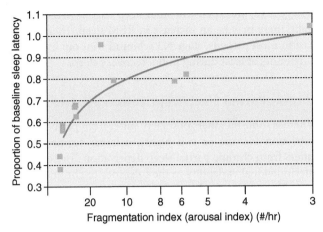

FIGURE 6–13 The sleep latency on the multiple sleep latency test (MSLT) decreases sharply when the frequency of sleep fragmentation (arousal index) during a preceding night of sleep is around 20/hr. The axis is logarithmic with larger numbers of the left. *From Bonnet MH, Arand DL: Clinical effects of sleep fragmentation versus sleep deprivation. Sleep Med Rev 2003;7:297–310.*

TABLE 6–9
Total Sleep Duration by Age in Normal Children

AGE	SLEEP DURATION (hr ± SD)
6 mo	14.2 ± 1.9
1 yr	13.9 ± 1.2
2 yr	13.2 ± 1.2
3 yr	12.5 ± 1.1
4 yr	11.8 ± 1.0
5 yr	11.4 ± 0.9
6 yr	11.0 ± 0.8
7 yr	10.8 ± 0.7
8 yr	10.4 ± 0.7
9 yr	10.1 ± 0.6
10 yr	9.8 ± 0.6
11 yr	9.6 ± 0.6
12 yr	9.3 ± 0.6
13 yr	9.0 ± 0.7
14 yr	8.7 ± 0.7
15 yr	8.4 ± 0.7
16 yr	8.1 ± 0.7

SD = standard deviation.
From Iglowstein I, Jenni OG, Molinari L, Largo RH: Sleep duration from infancy to adolescense: reference values and generational trends. Pediatrics 2003;111:302–307.

TABLE 6–10
Clinical Symptoms of Sleep Deprivation

- Longer reaction time
- Lapses in attention
- Lost information
- Poor short-term memory
- Poor mood
- Reduced motivation
- Sleepiness
- Poor performance
  ⇒ Worse at circadian low points
  ⇒ Worse when sedentary
  ⇒ Worse with no feedback
  ⇒ Worse with reduced light or sound
  ⇒ Worse with low motivation, interest or novelty

From Bonnet MH, Arand DL: Clinical effects of sleep fragmentation versus sleep deprivation. Sleep Med Rev 2003;7:297–310.

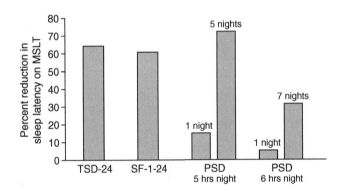

TSD-24 = 24 hours of total sleep deprivation

SF-1-24 = 24 hours of sleep fragmentation every 1 minute

PSD = partial sleep deprivation

FIGURE 6–14 Total sleep deprivation (TSD), frequent sleep fragmentation, and chronic sleep restriction all cause significant objective sleepiness. The effects of partial sleep deprivation (PSD) accumulate (5 nights have more effect than 1 night). MSLT = multiple sleep latency test. *Data redrawn from Bonnet MH, Arand DL: Clinical effects of sleep fragmentation versus sleep deprivation. Sleep Med Rev 2003;7:297–310.*

Total Sleep Deprivation

Some of the effects of total and partial sleep deprivation are listed in Table 6–10 and shown in Figure 6–14.[27] In general, the sleep latency (nocturnal and MSLT) decreases after both total and partial sleep deprivation as well as severe sleep fragmentation. In partial sleep deprivation, the effects will increase with repeated nights of partial sleep deprivations.

Selective Sleep Deprivation

If REM sleep is selectively impaired by induced arousals, the REM latency decreases and the amount of REM sleep increases on recovery nights.[27] In some patients with obstructive sleep apnea (OSA) on the first night of continuous positive airway pressure (CPAP), there may be a large increase in the amount of stage R (REM rebound). Withdrawal of REM-suppressant medications can also result in similar findings. Of note, other patients with OSA have a large increase in stage N3 on first CPAP night.

Recovery from Sleep Loss

The findings during recovery sleep after sleep deprivation are shown in Table 6–11.[27,28] On the first night, there is an increase

TABLE 6-11
Recovery from Acute Sleep Deprivation (Recovery Sleep)
FIRST RECOVERY NIGHT
• Shorter sleep latency
• Less stage W, stage N1, stage N2
• Longer TST (but ≤12–15 hr; if curtailed, longer TST on two or three recovery nights)
• Higher % stage N3
• Lower % stage R
• REM latency (unchanged younger, shorter in older adults)
SECOND RECOVERY NIGHT
• Increase stage R (REM rebound) most prominent in younger sleepers
• TST increased
• Stage N3 normal % TST
THIRD RECOVERY NIGHT
• Sleep variables approach normal
REM = rapid eye movement; TST = total sleep time. From Bonnet MH: Acute sleep deprivation. In Kryger MH, Roth T, Dement WC (eds): Principles and Practice of Sleep Medicine, 5th ed. St. Louis: Elsevier, 2011, pp 54–65.

in stage N3 at the expense of other sleep stages. On the second night, there may be an increase in REM sleep. Therefore, at least in most patients, stage N3 rebound wins out over stage R rebound, at least during initial recovery sleep.

Chronic Partial Sleep Deprivation (Restriction)

Whereas some members of society suffer from periodic sleep restriction for one or two nights, a larger segment likely suffers from chronic partial sleep deprivation. There is large interindividual variability in the tolerance to chronic partial sleep deprivation. Healthy humans appear to require 7 to 8 hours of sleep. A large-scale dose-response study on chronic sleep restriction estimated the daily sleep need to average 8.16 hours per night to avoid detrimental effects on waking functions. In one study of the psychomotor vigilance test (PVT), in which subjects respond to a randomly timed target, the frequency of lapses (missed target due to inattention) increased in proportion to total sleep debt or total accumulated excess time wake. The sleep deprivation and partial sleep loss conditions fit the same graph when expressed as PVT lapses versus total excess accumulated wake (Fig. 6–15). This study also found that the subjective feeling of sleepiness or impairment did not continue to worsen beyond a certain point. **Therefore, the chronically sleep-deprived individual does not recognize the degree of impairment.**[29] The results from this and other studies have demonstrated that chronic sleep restriction to less than 7 hours per night can have significant effects on cognitive functioning.[30]

Some of the many effects of chronic partial sleep loss are listed in Table 6–12. These include decreased performance, leptin, and response to immunization with increased cortisol, ghrelin (increased ghrelin causes hunger), and insulin resistance.[28,30–34] Some have hypothesized that the chronic partial sleep deprivation may contribute to the current obesity epidemic.

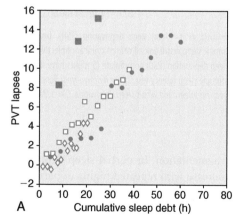
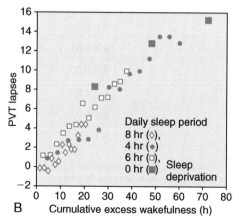

FIGURE 6–15 Progressive impairment with greater sleep debt or cumulative excess wakefulness. For example, if a person needs 8 hours of sleep (16 hr of wake tolerated), then after 2 nights of 6 hours of sleep, the cumulative sleep debt is 4 hours or the excess wake is 4 hours. In **A**, sleep deprivation causes much greater impairment expressed as sleep debt. **B**, When expressed as excess wake, the values are similar to those from chronic sleep loss of equal accumulated wake. PVT = psychomotor vigilance test. *From Van Dongen HPA, Maislin G, Mullington JM, et al: The cumulative cost of additional wakefulness: dose-response effects of neurobehavioral function and sleep physiology from chronic sleep restriction and total sleep deprivation. Sleep 2003;26:117–126.*

TABLE 6–12	
Effects of Chronic Partial Sleep Deprivation	
INCREASE WITH SD	**DECREASE WITH SD**
• Sleepiness (Subjective and objective) • Attention lapses • Norepinephrine • Cortisol and ACTH • Ghrelin (hunger) • Insulin resistance • Medical errors • Motor vehicle accidents	• Vigilance • Pain tolerance • Cognition and attention • Seizure threshold • Leptin • Acute antibody response to influenza and hepatitis A vaccination • Working memory • Cognitive processing (addition/subtraction)

ACTH = adrenocorticotropic hormone; SD = sleep deprivation.
Data from references 29–33.

CLINICAL REVIEW QUESTIONS

1. Which of the following does NOT decrease with age?
   A. TST.
   B. Sleep stage N1 (men).
   C. Stage N3 (men).
   D. Stage R.
   E. REM latency.

2. Which of the following decreases with age?
   A. Sleep latency.
   B. Sleep efficiency.
   C. ArI.
   D. WASO.

3. Which of the following is true about infant sleep?
   A. Enter sleep via stage R (active sleep).
   B. Active sleep about 50% of TST.
   C. Typical sleep cycle duration is 90 minutes.
   D. A and B.
   E. A and C.

4. Which of the following increase the REM latency?
   A. Depression.
   B. Lithium.
   C. Narcolepsy.
   D. Withdrawal of tricyclic antidepressants.

5. Sleep deprivation results in which of the following?
   A. Increased leptin.
   B. Increased ghrelin.
   C. Augmented response to immunization.
   D. Stage R rebound before stage N3 rebound in recovery sleep.

Answers

1. **B.** Stage N1 increases (men only in one study) or stays the same (women in one study).

2. **B.** Sleep efficiency decreases with age.

3. **D.** Infants enter sleep via active sleep, active sleep composes about 50% of TST, infant sleep cycle is about 45 to 60 minutes.

4. **B.** Lithium increases the REM latency.

5. **B.** Sleep deprivation increases ghrelin but decreases leptin and the response to immunization. In recovery, sleep increased stage N3 occurs on the initial recovery night. Increased stage R may occur on subsequent nights.

REFERENCES

1. Kushida CA, Littner MR, Morgenthaler T, et al: Practice parameters for the indications for polysomnography and related procedures: an update for 2005. Sleep 2005;28:499–521.
2. Iber C, Ancoli-Israel S, Chesson A, Quan SF for the American Academy of Sleep Medicine: The AASM Manual for the Scoring of Sleep and Associated Events: Rules, Terminology and Technical Specifications, 1st ed. Westchester, IL: American Academy of Sleep Medicine, 2007.
3. Van Cauter E, Leproult R, Plat L: Age-related changes in slow wave sleep and REM sleep and relationship with growth hormone and cortisol levels in healthy men. JAMA 2000;284:861–868.
4. Bliwise DL: Normal aging. In Kryger M, Roth T, Dement W (eds): Principles and Practice of Sleep Medicine. Philadelphia: Elsevier, 2005, pp. 24–38.
5. Ohayon MM, Carskadon MA, Guilleminault C, Viteiello MV: Meta-analysis of quantitative sleep parameters from childhood to old age in healthy individuals: developing normative sleep values across the human lifespan. Sleep 2004;27:1255–1273.
6. Redline S, Kirchner L, Quan SF, et al: The effects of age, sex, ethnicity, and sleep-disordered breathing on sleep architecture. Arch Intern Med 2004;164:406–418.
7. Harding SM, Hawkins JW: Sleep and internal medicine. In Carney P, Berry RB, Geyer J (eds): Clinical Sleep Medicine. Philadelphia: Lippincott Williams & Wilkins, 2005, pp. 456–470.
8. Agnew HW Jr, Webb WB, Williams RL: The first night effect: an EEG study of sleep. Psychophysiology 1966;2:263–266.
9. Webb WB, Campbell S: The first night effect revisited with age as a variable. Waking Sleeping 1979;3:319–324.
10. Rechtschaffen A, Kales A (eds): A Manual of Standardized Terminology Techniques and Scoring System for Sleep Stages of Human Subjects. Los Angeles: Brain Information Service/Brain Research Institute, UCLA, 1968.
11. Moser D, Anderer P, Gruber G, et al: Sleep classification according to AASM and Rechtschaffen & Kales: effects of sleep scoring parameters. Sleep 2009;32:139–149.
12. Danker-Hopfe H, Anderer P, Zeitlhofer J, et al: Interrater reliability for sleep scoring according to the Rechtschaffen & Kales and the new AASM standard. J Sleep Res 2009;18:74–84.
13. Novelli L, Ferri R, Bruni O: Sleep classification according to AASM and Rechtschaffen and Kales: effects on sleep scoring parameters of children and adolescents. J Sleep Res 2010;19:238–247.

14. Kahn A, Dan B, Grosswasser J, et al: Normal sleep architecture in infants and children. J Clin Neurophysiol 1996;13:184–197.

15. Seldon S: Polysomnography in infants and children: In Sheldon SH, Ferber R, Kryger MH (eds): Principles and Practice of Pediatric Sleep Medicine. Philadelphia: Elsevier Saunders, 2005, pp. 49–71.

16. Iglowstein I, Jenni OG, Molinari L, Largo RH: Sleep duration from infancy to adolescence: reference values and generational trends. Pediatrics 2003;111:302–307.

17. Montgomery-Downs HE, O'Brien LM, Gulliver TE, et al: Polysomnographic characteristics in normal preschool children. Pediatrics 2006;117:741–753.

18. Mason TB, Teoh L, Calabro K, et al: Rapid eye movement latency in children and adolescence. Pediatr Neurol 2008;39: 162–169.

19. Beck SE, Marcus CL: Pediatric polysomnography. Sleep Med Clin 2009;4:393–406.

20. Bonnet MH, Doghramji K, Roehrs T, et al: The scoring of arousal in sleep; reliability, validity, and alternatives. J Clin Sleep Med 2007;3:133–145.

21. Bonnet M, Arand DL: EEG arousal norms by age. J Clin Sleep Med 2007;3:271–274.

22. Wong TK, Galster P, Lau TS, et al: Reliability of scoring arousals in normal children and children with obstructive sleep apnea syndrome. Sleep 2004;27:1139–1145.

23. Mathur R, Douglas NJ: Frequency of EEG arousals from nocturnal sleep in normal subjects. Sleep 1995;18:330–333.

24. Gosselin N, Michaud M, Carrier J, et al: Age difference in heart rate changes associated with micro-arousals in humans. Clin Neurophysiol 2002;113:1517.

25. Boselli M, Parrino L, Smerieri A, et al: Effect of age on EEG arousals in normal sleep. Sleep 1998;21:351–357.

26. Bonnet MH. Performance and sleepiness as a function of frequency and placement of sleep disruption. Psychophysiology 1986;23:263–271.

27. Bonnet MH, Arand DL: Clinical effects of sleep fragmentation versus sleep deprivation. Sleep Med Rev 2003;7:297–310.

28. Bonnet MH: Acute sleep deprivation. In Kryger MH, Roth T, Dement WC (eds): Principles and Practice of Sleep Medicine, 5th ed. St. Louis: Elsevier, 2011, pp 54–65.

29. Van Dongen HPA, Maislin G, Mullington JM, et al: The cumulative cost of additional wakefulness: dose-response effects of neurobehavioral function and sleep physiology from chronic sleep restriction and total sleep deprivation. Sleep 2003;26: 117–126.

30. Banks S; Dinges DF: Behavioral and physiological consequences of sleep restriction. J Clin Sleep Med 2007;3: 519–528.

31. Donga E, van Dijk M, van Dijk JG, et al: A single night of partial sleep deprivation induces insulin resistance in multiple metabolic pathways in healthy subjects. J Clin Endocrinol Metab 2010;95:2963–2968.

32. Van Cauter E, Spiegel K, Leproult R: Metabolic consequences of sleep and sleep loss. Sleep Med 2008;9(Suppl 1):S23–S28.

33. Spiegel K, Tasali E, Penev P, Van Cauter E: Sleep curtailment in healthy young men is associated with decreased leptin levels, elevated ghrelin levels, and increased hunger and appetite. Ann Intern Med 2004;141:846–850.

34. Spiegel K, Sheridan JF, Van Cauter E: Effect of sleep deprivation on response to immunization. JAMA 2002;288:1471–1472.

Chapter 7

Neurobiology of Sleep

Chapter Points

- Serotonergic neurons in the DRN are active during wake, less active during NREM, and even less active during REM sleep.
- Noradrenergic neurons in the LC are active during wake, less active during NREM sleep, and inactive during REM sleep.
- Histaminergic neurons in the TMN are active during wake and episodes of cataplexy.
- Cholinergic neurons in REM-on areas are active during REM sleep.
- Cholinergic neurons in wake/REM-on areas are active during wake and REM sleep.
- Neurons in the VLPO are active during sleep and inactive during wake. They contain GABA and galanin.
- Hypocretin neurons in the lateral and posterior hypothalamus project to many areas of the brain important for the control of wake and sleep. They stabilize transitions between wake and sleep.
- Hypocretin neurons are absent (or very decreased) in patients with narcolepsy with cataplexy. These patients also have low or undetectable cerebrospinal fluid hypocretin-1.
- The hypotonia of REM sleep is due to a combination of inhibition and dysfacilitation.
- The brainstem regions involved in hypotonia include the subcoeruleus area (sublateral dorsal area), areas of the medulla and interneurons inhibiting the spinal cord motor neurons (glycine and GABA).

In 1930, von Economo published findings of an autopsy study of the brains of patients dying from encephalitis lethargica.[1,2] Von Economo found that patients with damage to the posterior hypothalamus and rostral midbrain often had excessive sleepiness, whereas those with injury to the anterior hypothalamus had unrelenting insomnia. Based on these observations, he hypothesized that the anterior hypothalamus contained neurons that promoted sleep, whereas neurons near the hypothalamus-midbrain junction helped promote wakefulness. Decades later, the importance of those areas of the brain for sleep and wake, respectively, has been increasingly understood. A number of major brain areas involved in control of wake and sleep, their abbreviations,

and major associated neurotransmitters (neuromodulators) are listed in Table 7–1.[3–6]

The term *neurotransmitter* is currently applied to situations in which one presynaptic neuron directly influences another postsynaptic neuron. In **neuromodulation,** a given neurotransmitter regulates the activity of diverse populations of neurons in the central nervous system. Examples of neurotransmitters that are also neuromodulators include acetylcholine (ACh), serotonin (5HT), dopamine (DA), and histamine (HA). Neurons are often characterized with respect to sleep by when they are most active.[3] Some neurons are active during wake, during rapid eye movement (REM) only (REM-on), during REM and wake (wake/REM-on), during non–rapid eye movement (NREM) only (NREM-on), or during NREM and REM sleep (Fig. 7–1). Figure 7–2 shows sections through important brainstem areas involved in the regulation of wake and sleep and identifies important brain regions.

MAJOR BRAIN AREAS IMPORTANT FOR SLEEP AND WAKE

Hypothalamic Areas

Lateral Hypothalamus

Neurons in the lateral and posterior hypothalamus are the sole source of the awake-promoting neuropeptides hypocretin 1 (Hcrt1) and hypocretin 2 (Hcrt2), also known as Orexin A and Orexin B, respectively.[7,8] Hcrt1 can attach to both Hcrt1 and 2 receptors, whereas Hcrt2 attaches only to Hcrt2 receptors. Patients with narcolepsy with cataplexy have loss of 90% or more of Hcrt-producing neurons and have low to undetectable cerebrospinal fluid (CSF) levels of Hcrt1.[9,10] One study of a few patients with narcolepsy without cataplexy found partial loss of Hcrt neurons.[11] Canine narcolepsy is due to a mutation in the gene for the Hcrt2 receptor.

Hcrt neurons send abundant excitatory projections to the dorsal raphe (Hrct1 and Hcrt2 receptors) nucleus, the locus coeruleus (Hcrt1 receptors), and the tuberomammillary nucleus (Hcrt2 receptors) (Fig. 7–3). These areas in turn send inhibitory projections to Hcrt neurons. Hcrt neurons have a strong excitatory effect on the cholinergic neurons of the basal forebrain that contribute to cortical arousal but have no effect on GABAergic sleep-promoting neurons within the ventrolateral preoptic (VLPO) area.

TABLE 7–1		
Brain Areas important for Sleep		
AREA	**ABBREVIATION**	**NEUROTRANSMITTER**
Lateral dorsal tegmentum	LDT	Acetylcholine (ACh)
Pedunculopontine tegmentum	PPT	Acetylcholine (ACh)
Locus coeruleus	LC	Norepinephrine (NE)
Dorsal raphe nucleus	DRN	Serotonin (5HT)
Tuberomammillary nucleus	TMN	Histamine (HA)
Ventrolateral preoptic area	VLPO	Gamma-aminobutyric acid (GABA) Galanin
Lateral posterior hypothalamus	LPH	Hypocretin 1 and 2 (Orexin A, B)

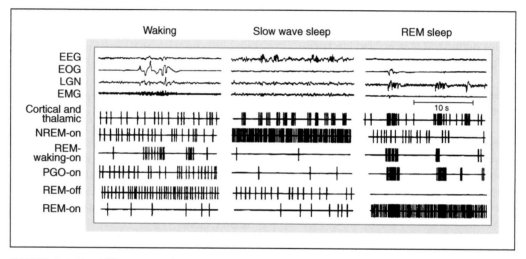

FIGURE 7–1 Activity of different neurons during wake, non–rapid eye movement (NREM), and rapid eye movement (REM) sleep. EEG = electroencephalogram; EMG = electromyogram; EOG = electro-oculogram; LGN = lateral geniculate nucleus; PGO = ponto-geniculo-occipital. *From Rechtschaffen A, Siegel J: Sleep and dreaming. In Kandel E, Schwartz JH, Jessell TM (eds): Principles of Neural Science, 4th ed. New York: McGraw-Hill, 2000, p. 940, Fig. 47–3.*

As is discussed later, Hcrt appears to stabilize transitions between wake and sleep. Hcrt neurons are relatively inactive in quiet waking but are transiently activated during sensory stimulation. Mileykovskiy and coworkers[12] found that Hcrt cells are silent in slow wave sleep and tonic periods of REM sleep, with occasional burst discharge in phasic REM (Fig. 7–4). Hcrt cells discharge in active waking and have moderate and approximately equal levels of activity during grooming and eating and maximal activity during exploratory behavior. The authors of this study concluded that Hcrt cells are activated during emotional and sensorimotor conditions similar to those that trigger cataplexy in narcoleptic animals.

Ventrolateral Preoptic Nucleus

The VLPO is an area in the hypothalamus containing neurons active during sleep. Most sleep-active neurons in the VLPO are believed to be active during both NREM and REM sleep (Fig. 7–5).[13] Many of the VLPO neurons **are activated by** sleep-inducing factors including **adenosine** and **prostaglandin D$_2$.** These neurons are sensitive to warmth, and heating this area of the brain increases their activity and decreases wake. A compact group of VLPO neurons (VLPO cluster) projects to the tuberomammillary nucleus (TMN) and inhibits the neuronal activity of that area. A second group of VLPO neurons is located dorsal and medial to the VLPO cluster neurons and the group is called the *extended VLPO (eVLPO)* by some authors.[14] The eVLPO neurons make up the majority of the projections to the dorsal raphe nucleus (DRN) and locus coeruleus (LC) as well as to the interneurons of the lateral dorsal tegmental/pedunculopontine tegmental (LDT/PPT) region.[14] One study showed a subset of neurons in the eVLPO were more active during REM than NREM.[14] However, most VLPO neurons appear to be active during both NREM and REM. The neurons in the VLPO contain the neurotransmitters/neuromodulators gamma-aminobutyric acid (GABA) and galanin. The VLPO neuronal projections to the DRN, LC, and TMN are inhibitory

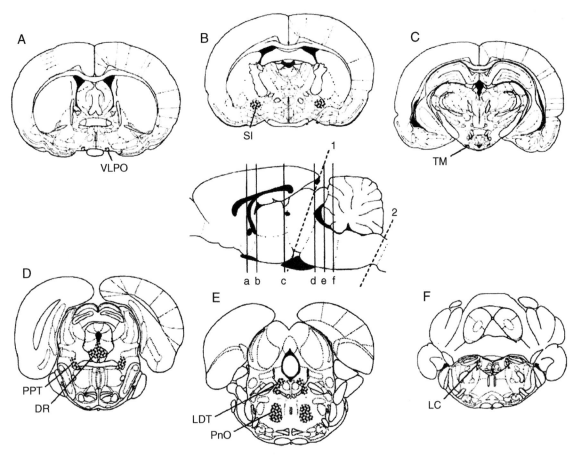

FIGURE 7-2 **A–F,** Major brainstem areas important for sleep in the rat brain at various sections. **Center,** A lateral view of the brain shows locations of the sections depicted (a–f). **A,** Ventrolateral preoptic area (VLPO). **B,** Substantia innominata (SI). **C,** Tuberomammillary nucleus (TM). **D,** Pedunculopontine tegmentum (PPT) and dorsal raphe nucleus (DR). **E,** Lateral dorsal tegmentum (LDT). **F,** Locus coeruleus (LC) and pontine reticular nucleus, oral part (PnO). The PnO in the rat is homologous to the medial pontine reticular formation in the cat. **A–F,** *From Baghdoyan HA, Lydic R: Neurotransmiters and neuromodulators regulating sleep. In Bazi CW, Ballow BA, Sammaritan MR (eds): Sleep and Epilepsy: The Clinical Spectrum. Amsterdam: Elsevier Science, 2002, pp. 17–44.*

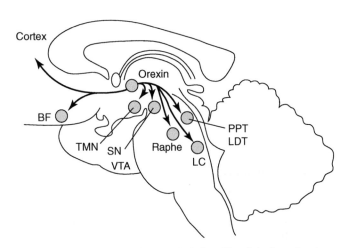

FIGURE 7-3 Orexin (hypocretin) neurons in the lateral hypothalamic area innervate all of the ascending arousal systems, as well as the cerebral cortex. BF = basal forebrain; LC = locus coeruleus; LDT = lateral dorsal tegmental; PPT = pedunculopontine tegmental; SN = substantia nigra; TMN = tuberomammillary nucleus; VTA = ventral tegmental area.

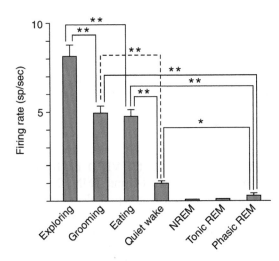

FIGURE 7-4 Orexin (hypocretin) neurons are active during wake and quiet during non–rapid eye movement (NREM) sleep with some activity only during phasic rapid eye movement (REM) sleep. *P < .05, **P < .01 Bonferroni t test. *From Mileykovskiy BY, Kiyashchenko LI, Siegel JM: Behavioral correlates of activity in identified hypocretin/Orexin neurons. Neuron 2005;46:787–798.*

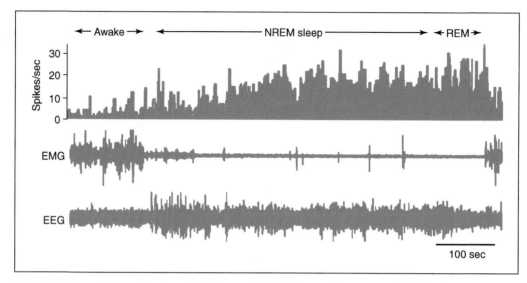

FIGURE 7–5 Neurons of the ventrolateral preoptic (VLPO) are active during both non–rapid eye movement (NREM) and rapid eye movement (REM) sleep. EEG = electroencephalogram; EMG = electromyogram. *From Szymusiak R, Gvilla I, McGinty D: Hypothalamic control of sleep. Sleep Med 2007;8:291–301.*

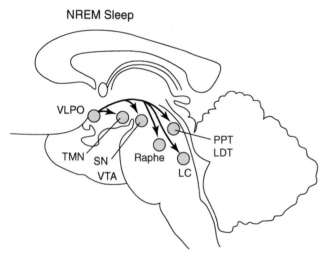

FIGURE 7–6 Inhibitory projections from the ventrolateral preoptic area (VLPO; gamma-aminobutyric acid, galanine) during non–rapid eye movement (NREM) sleep to the tuberomamillary (TMN), the raphe area, locus coeruleus (LC), and pendunculopontine lateral/dorsal tegmentum (PPT/LDT) area, substantia nigra (SN), and ventral tegmental area (VTA). *From Espana RA, Scammell TE: Sleep neurobiology for the clinician. Sleep 2004;27:811–820.*

(Fig. 7–6). The neurons in the VLPO receive inhibitory projections from the DRN, LC and TMN. Destruction of the VLPO impairs sleep. A group of sleep-active neurons in the median preoptic nucleus (MnPO) was described after the identification of the VLPO.[13] Similar to VLPO cells, a subset of MnPO neurons expresses c-Fos and discharges more rapidly during NREM and REM sleep. Interestingly, unlike VLPO neurons, the MnPO cells also fire faster during prolonged wakefulness (which increases sleep pressure). There is no evidence that lesions of the MnPO area impair sleep.

Tuberomammillary Nucleus

Histaminergic neurons are confined to the posterior hypothalamus in the area called the *tuberomammillary nucleus.* TMN neurons project to the cerebral cortex, amygdala, substantia nigra (SN), DRN, LC, and nucleus of the solitary tract. HA acting at H1 receptors is associated with wakefulness, and antihistamines (H1 receptor blockers) cause drowsiness or sleep. Conversely, H3 receptor agonists cause sleepiness possibly by stimulating autoregulatory receptors that decrease HA release. The TMN receives stimulatory input from the lateral hypothalamus (Hcrt). The TMN firing rate is high during wake, lower during NREM, and absent during REM.[3] In contrast to REM sleep, during attacks of cataplexy, TMN neurons have a high firing rate associated with preservation of consciousness.[15] Low CSF HA has been found in patients with narcolepsy with and without low Hcrt.[16,17] The low HA may be a marker rather than a cause of sleepiness because lesions of the TMN have minimal effect on wakefulness. However, this may simply mean that HA is not essential for wakefulness in general. HA may be important at the onset of wakefulness.

Brainstem Regions

Dopamine Regions

Neurons producing dopamine (DA) are abundant in the SN and ventral tegmental area (VTA). Previously, studies **suggested that DA neurons do not change their firing rates substantially across sleep stages.**[3] However, extracellular DA levels are high in several brain regions during wakefulness. Whereas the average rate of firing of the VTA neurons does not change across states, they have burst firing during wake that releases more DA. Recent work has identified DA cells in the ventral periaqueductal gray (vPAG) that are wake active.[18] The vPAG contains DA neurons that are active (express Fos) during wakefulness but not sleep. DA neurons in the vPAG project to and receive input from cholinergic neurons in the LDT area, Orexin neurons, VLPO, and prefrontal cortex. Loss of vPAG DA neurons promotes sleep.

DA agonists acting at D1, D2, and D3 receptors increase waking and decrease NREM and REM sleep. Exactly which DA neurons are important for maintenance of wakefulness is not clear. DA blockers of D1 and D2 receptors can promote sleep. In patients with low DA activity such as in Parkinson's disease, low doses of DA agonists (pramipexole, ropinirole) that bind D2/D3 autoreceptors on DA neurons can actually cause sleepiness by reducing DA signaling. Amphetamines promote wakefulness by increasing DA signaling.

Reticular Formation

The reticular formation is a loose collection of neurons extending from the caudal medulla to the core of the midbrain. Sections above the mid pons produce coma or hypersomnolence. Wakefulness depends on the activity of the ascending reticular activating system (ARAS). This system projects to higher brain centers. One pathway ascends dorsally to the thalamus, and the second ascends ventrally through the lateral hypothalamus and forebrain (Fig. 7–7).

Dorsal RAS

Lateral Dorsal Tegmentum/Pedunculopontine Tegmentum. Neurons in the LDT and PPT areas that are located in the dorsal midbrain and pons make up the majority of the dorsal RAS pathway through the pons and are cholinergic. Some of the neurons are active during wake and REM sleep (wake/REM-on), whereas others are active mainly during REM sleep (REM-on).[3-5] Acetylcholine (ACh) release in the thalamus is high during wake and REM sleep. The cholinergic neurons from the LDT/PPT densely innervate the thalamus (especially the medial and intralaminar thalamic nuclei), lateral hypothalamus, and midbrain. During wake and REM sleep, these cholinergic neurons depolarize thalamic relay neurons, thereby activating thalamocortical signaling and produce fast cortical rhythms. During NREM sleep, these neurons are inactive. REM-on neurons are active during REM sleep but not wake or NREM sleep. Wake/REM-on neurons are active during wake and REM sleep (Table 7–2 and Fig. 7–8).[19] Other cholinergic neurons in the basal forebrain (BF) project to the cortex, hippocampus, and amygdala. The firing rate of these neurons is also high during wake and REM and low during NREM sleep.

TABLE 7–2			
Activity of Brain Areas Important for Wake and Sleep			
	WAKE	**NREM**	**REM**
EEG	Fast, low voltage	Slow, high voltage	Fast, low voltage
LDT/PPT			
Wake-on REM-on	Active	Not active	Active
REM-on	Not active	Not active	Very active
TMN	Active	Reduced	Absent
DRN	Active	Less active	Low activity
LC	Active	Less active	Absent
VLPO*	Not active	Active	Active
Hypocretin	Maximally active	Not active	Not active
Dopaminergic neurons	Activity previously thought not to be sleep state dependent. vlPAG neurons active during wake		

*Some neurons in extended VLPO more active during REM than NREM sleep.
DRN = dorsal raphe nucleus; EEG = electroencephalogram; LC = locus coeruleus; LDT = lateral dorsal tegmentum; NREM = non-rapid eye movement; PPT = pedunculopontine tegmentum; REM = rapid eye movement; TMN = tuberomammilary nucleus; VLPO = ventrolateral preoptic area; vlPAG = ventrolateral periaqueductal gray.
Adapted from Saper CB, Chou TC, Scammell TE: The sleep switch: hypothalamic control of sleep and wakefulness. Trends Neurosci 2001;24:726–731.

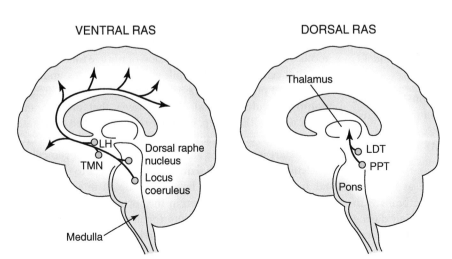

VENTRAL RAS   DORSAL RAS

FIGURE 7–7 Reticular activating system (RAS). The ventral RAS includes neurons from the locus coeruleus, dorsal raphe nuclei, tuberomammillary nucleus (TMN), and lateral hypothalamus (LH). The dorsal RAS includes projections from the lateral dorsal tegmental (LDT) and pedunculopontine tegmental (PPT) areas.

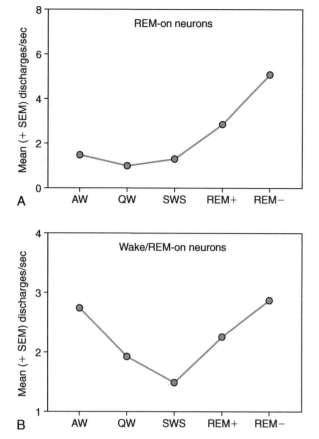

A

B

FIGURE 7–8 Firing rate of rapid eye movement (REM)-on neurons and wake/REM-on neurons in the PPT/LPT area. AW = active wake; QW = quiet wake; REM+ = REM sleep with eye movements; REM− = REM sleep without eye movements; SEM = standard error of the mean; SWS = slow wave sleep. *From Thakkar MM, Strecker RE, McCarley RW: Behavioral state control through differential serotonergic inhibition in the mesopontine cholinergic nuclei: a simultaneous unit recording and microdialysis study. J Neurosci 1998;18:5490–5497.*

Ventral RAS The ventral RAS projects through the lateral hypothalamus terminating on magnocellular neurons in the substantia innominata, medial septum, and diagonal band. These regions contain neurons that project to the cortex. The ascending projections of this branch are joined by input from the TMN and lateral hypothalamus. The ventral RAS is composed of projections from the DRN (5HT) and LC (norepinephrine [NE]).

Dorsal Raphe Nucleus DRN serotonergic neurons are active during wake, less active during NREM, and minimally active during REM sleep.[3] The influences of DRN neurons are mainly stimulatory. They are part of the RAS network (see Table 7–2).

Locus Coeruleus Neurons in the LC utilize NE as the neurotransmitter and innervate wide areas of the brain with chiefly stimulatory effects. LC firing rates are high during wake, lower during NREM, and absent during REM sleep (see Table 7–2).

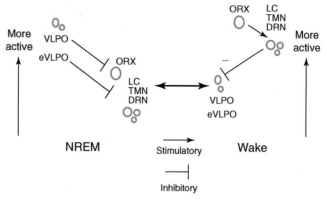

FIGURE 7–9 Non–rapid eye movement (NREM) flip-flop switch. During NREM, the ventrolateral preoptic area (VLPO) inhibits hypocretin neurons as well as the locus coeruleus (LC), tuberomammillary nucleus (TMN), dorsal raphe nucleus (DRN) areas promoting sleep. During wake, the hypocretin neurons stimulate the LC, TMN, and DRN areas, which are active and inhibit the VLPO neurons. eVLPO = extended ventrolateral preoptic area; ORX = Orexin (hypocretin).

Basal Forebrain

Cholinergic neurons in the BF excite cortical pyramidal cells. GABA BF neurons disinhibit cortical neurons. Lesions that destroy BF ACh and GABA neurons increase delta power.

CONTROL OF NREM SLEEP

During NREM sleep, the VLPO neurons are active and inhibit the firing of neurons in the TMN, DRN, and LC (see Table 7–2 and Fig. 7–5). The Orexin neurons do not innervate the VLPO but stimulate the TMN, DRN, or LC more or less depending on the sleep state. Orexin neurons are active during wake. This mutually inhibitory system functions as a flip-flop switch transitioning between the two states (Fig. 7–9; see also Fig. 7–8).[6]

FEATURES OF REM SLEEP

The major tonic and phasic features of REM sleep[3-5] are listed in Box 7–1. The tonic features include electroencephalogram (EEG) desynchronization (reduction in cortical EEG amplitude), theta rhythm generation by the hippocampus (sawtooth wave in the EEG), suppression of muscle tone (atonia), absent thermoregulation, penile erections in males, and constriction of pupils. The phasic features of REM sleep include **ponto-geniculo-occipital (PGO)** waves that precede and occur during REM sleep, irregular respiration and heart rate (sympathetic bursts), and REMs (see Fig. 7–1). The PGO waves start in the pons and transit to the lateral geniculate nucleus (LGN) of the thalamus and from there to the occipital area. PGO waves are believed to be an integral part of REM sleep but are not seen in the cortical EEG. Recording requires electrodes placed into the appropriate brain areas. The density of the PGO waves correlates with the amount of eye movement measured in REM sleep.

BOX 7-1

Characteristics of Rapid Eye Movement Sleep

TONIC FEATURES

1. EEG desynchronization (reduction in cortical EEG amplitude).
2. Theta rhythm generated in hippocampus (saw-tooth waves in EEG).
3. Suppression of muscle tone (atonia).
4. Absent thermoregulation (no shivering).
5. Penile erections in males.
6. Pupils constrict (parasympathetic dominance).

PHASIC FEATURES

1. PGO waves: Precede and occur during REM sleep.
   A. PGO waves arrive in bursts in association with eye movements.
   B. PGO waves originate in pons, travel to LGN of the thalamus and then to the occipital cortex.
2. Contraction of middle ear muscles.
3. Irregular respiration and heart rate.
4. REMs.

EEG = electroencephalogram; LGN = lateral geniculate nucleus; PGO = ponto-geniculo-occipital waves; REM = rapid eye movements.

REM SLEEP

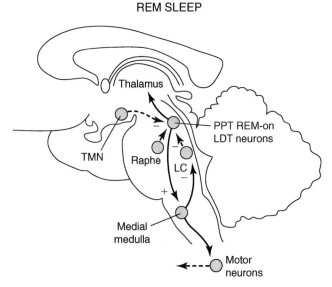

FIGURE 7-10 The rapid eye movement (REM)-on cells of the lateral dorsal tegmentum (LDT) and pedunculopontine tegmentum (PPT) are inhibited during wake and, to a lesser extent, NREM sleep by norepinephrine, serotonin, and histamine from the locus coeruleus (LC), dorsal raphe nucleus (DRN), and tuberomammilary nucleus (TMN), respectively. During REM sleep, these areas (LC, DRN, TMN) are silent, disinhibiting the REM-on neurons. These neurons activate cholinoceptive neurons in the medial medulla that ultimately inhibit the motor neurons (atonia of REM sleep). Note that neurons in the medial medulla feedback and inhibit LC that normally increases motor tone. *From Espana RA, Scammell TE: Sleep neurobiology for the clinician. Sleep 2004;27:811–820.*

Control of REM Sleep

Several models are proposed for the control of REM sleep.[3–6,20–22] In one model, the activity of REM-on neurons in the LDT and PPT nuclei is high whereas that in the mono-aminergic centers is low (TMN, DRN, and LC)[4,5] (Fig. 7–10). Different populations of REM-on cells in the lateral pontine tegmentum (LPT) and PPT stimulate effector cells in the medial pontine reticular formation (mPRF) (or pontine reticular nucleus, oral part [PnO] in the cat). The neurons in the mPRF are cholinoceptive. Infusion of cholinergic ago-nists into this area results in many of the manifestations of REM sleep. Specific areas in the mPRF provide ascending projections resulting in PGO waves and REMs. An area called the *pontine inhibitory area (PIA)* contains nuclei that are responsible for muscle atonia.[4] It is thought that the area below the LC that is called the *subcoeruleus area* (or sublat-eral dorsal [SLD] area by other authors) is the area initiating atonia.

In Figure 7–10, neurons from the LDT/PPT provide an excitatory projection to area in the medial medulla. The neurons in that area project to the motor neurons of the spinal cord. The neurotransmitters GABA and glycine hypo-polarize the motor neurons resulting in the atonia of REM sleep. At the same time, neurons in the medial medulla provide inhibitory projections to the LC. This reduces the normal LC-provided augmentation of muscle activity. Thus, both inhibition and dysfacilitation are important.[3] Other authors hypothesize slightly different atonia mechanisms as discussed later.

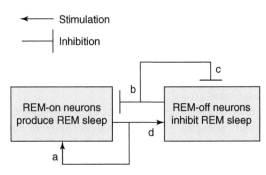

Reciprocal interaction schematic

FIGURE 7-11 Reciprocal interaction model of rapid eye movement (REM) sleep. The REM-on population has positive feedback *(a)*, so that the activity grows. This activity excites the REM-off population *(d)*. The REM-off population then inhibits the REM-on population *(b)*, terminating the REM episodes. The REM-off neurons have negative feedback *(c)*, and as the REM-off activity diminishes, the REM-on population is released from inhibition *(b)* and the activity grows until another REM episode occurs. *From McCarley RW: Neurobiology of REM and NREM sleep. Sleep Med 2007;8:302–330.*

A model (in simplified form) for transitions to and from REM sleep presented by McCarley[5] is illustrated in Figure 7–11. There is reciprocal interaction between REM-off neurons (LC, DRN) and REM-on neurons (LDT, PPT). The REM-on population has positive feedback (see Fig. 7–11, line a) so that the activity increases. This activity excites the REM-off population (see Fig. 7–11, line d). The

REM FLIP FLOP

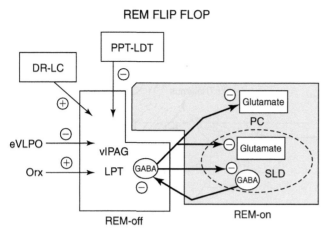

vlPAG ventrolateral   SLD sublateral dorsal   PC precoerulus
       periaqueductal   tegmentum
       gray

FIGURE 7–12 A flip-flop model for rapid eye movement (REM) sleep in which REM-off and REM-on neurons mutually inhibit each other. The gamma-aminobutyric acid (GABA) neurons are inhibitory. DR = dorsal raphe; eVLPO = extended ventrolateral preoptic area; LDT = lateral dorsal tegmentum; LPT = lateral pontine tegmentum; ORX = Orexin (hypocretin); PPT = pedunculopontine tegmentum. *From Fuller PM, Saper CB, Lu J: The pontine REM switch: past and present. J Physiol 2007;584:735–741.*

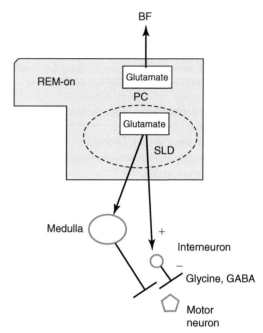

FIGURE 7–13 Postulated mechanisms for rapid eye movement (REM) EEG phenomenon and REM atonia in the flip-flop model of REM sleep. Glutamatergic neurons of the precoerulus (PC) area project to the basal forebrain (BF). Glutamatergic neurons of the sublateral dorsal nucleus (SLD; mesopontine tegmentum) project to the medulla and spinal cord mediating hypotonia. GABA = gamma-aminobutyric acid. *Based on Fuller PM, Saper CB, Lu J: The pontine REM switch: past and present. J Physiol 2007;584:735–741.*

REM-off population then inhibits the REM-on population (see Fig. 7–11, line b), terminating the REM episodes. The REM-off neurons have negative feedback (see Fig. 7–11, line c), and as the REM-off activity diminishes, the REM-on population is released from inhibition and the activity increases until another REM episode occurs. This model provides an explanation for the cycles of NREM and REM sleep that occur during sleep. A more complicated model includes the influence of inhibitory neurons (GABA) in several brain areas.[5]

A different model of control of REM sleep by Lu and Fuller and colleagues[20–22] concentrates on different nuclei as the two parts of reciprocally interacting REM-on and REM-off areas located in the mesopontine tegmentum (Fig. 7–12). GABAergic neurons in the REM-off and REM-on areas mutually inhibit each other. In this REM sleep flip-flop circuit model, the REM-off GABAergic neurons in the ventrolateral periaqueductal gray (vlPAG) and LPT and REM-on GABAergic cells in the SLD tegmental area mutually inhibit each other. The SLD in rats is equivalent to the subcoeruleus area or perilocus coeruleus area in cats. The LDT/PPT and eVLPO provide inhibitory input to the REM-off neurons. Hypocretin (Orexin) neurons provide stimulatory input to the REM-off neurons.

In this model, REM-on glutamatergic neurons in the pre-coeruleus (PC) and medial parabrachial (PB) areas project to the medial septum–BF and activate the hippocampus (theta rhythm of REM sleep) and neocortex (Fig. 7–13). REM-on glutamatergic neurons in the SLD project to glycinergic/GABAergic interneurons in the spinal cord that, in turn, project to anterior horn cell motor neurons inducing muscle atonia. The SLD glutamatergic neurons also project

to a region of the intermediate ventromedial medulla (IVMM) containing neurons that project to the spinal ventral horn. However, it is not known whether this projection is excitatory or inhibitory nor is it known whether these projections are direct (i.e., spinal motor neuron) or indirect (i.e., spinal interneuron). The interneurons hyperpolarize the motorneurons with GABA and glycine. As noted previously, the atonia of skeletal muscles during REM sleep results not only from the inhibition by GABA and glycine at the alpha motor neurons but also from dysfacilitation—loss of 5HT and NE stimulation on motorneurons from monoaminergic nuclei.

In this model, cholinergic and monoaminergic systems may modulate REM sleep by acting on either the REM-off or the REM-on groups or on both simultaneously (not shown). However, the cholinergic and monoaminergic systems are located external to the REM flip-flop switch. Of note, this flip-flop model does not account for the periodicity of alternation between NREM and REM sleep.[5] In addition, neuronal activity in the brainstem on transitions from NREM to REM is a gradual change. The important projections from cholinergic areas to the thalamus by REM-on cells are also not addressed.

Effects of Medications

Given the previous models for NREM and REM sleep, one can see that antihistamines in general cause sleepiness, cholinergic medications tend to increase REM sleep, and serotonergic medications tend to impair sleep.[3,23] However, there are 14 different 5HT receptors and some receptors are autoreceptors. Hence, the effect of serotonergic medications is complex.

As mentioned, while HA in general promotes wake, medications active at H3 autoreceptors may actually augment sleepiness. Thus, actions of medications depend on the specific type of receptor predominantly affected. Some medications work by augmenting the effects of naturally occurring neurotransmitters (neuromodulators). As discussed in Chapter 25, benzodiazepine receptor agonists augment the effect of GABA at GABA-A receptors, thereby promoting sleep.

Adenosine: A Possible Mediator of Sleepiness after Prolonged Wakefulness

The concentration of adenosine in the forebrain increases during prolonged wakefulness and returns to normal after recovery sleep.[4,5,13] It was hypothesized that the accumulation of adenosine might be the mechanism of sleep homeostatic drive build-up. However, adenosine knock-out mice still exhibit the effects of sleep restriction on slow wave sleep (increased activity). Therefore, adenosine is likely not the only substance mediating the build-up of pressure for sleep during prolonged wakefulness. Adenosine receptor antagonists (caffeine) have potent effects on maintaining wakefulness. Caffeine blocks adenosine A1 and A2a receptors.[23] Adenosine binds to A1 receptors on the cholinergic neurons of the BF, decreasing the firing of these neurons. This causes a reduction in cortical arousal. Adenosine also may decrease GABAergic neuronal activity in the same area. These BF GABA neurons may have inhibitory activity with respect to the neurons that promote sleep. The later sleep-promoting neurons are themselves GABAergic and project to areas of the brain associated with wake and inhibit them.

CLINICAL REVIEW QUESTIONS

1. Which of the following brain areas is active during NREM and REM sleep?
   A. TMN.
   B. LC.
   C. DRN.
   D. VLPO.

2. Which of the following brain areas is active during REM sleep?
   A. LDT/PPT.
   B. LC.
   C. DRN.
   D. TMN.

3. Neurons in which of the following areas are active during cataplexy but not REM sleep?

A. LDT/PPT.
B. LC.
C. DRN.
D. TMN.

4. What is the neurotransmitter (neuromodulator) of VLPO neurons?
   A. GABA, galanine.
   B. 5HT.
   C. HA.
   D. NE.

5. Which of the following neurotransmitters/modulators is responsible for the alerting effects of amphetamine?
   A. 5HT.
   B. DA.
   C. NE.
   D. HA.

6. Which of the following is NOT true about hypocretin neurons?
   A. Stabilize wake-sleep transitions.
   B. Active during wake.
   C. Located in the lateral hypothalamus.
   D. Provide inhibitory input to the LC, DRN.

7. What is the major transmitter/neuromodulator of neurons in the DRN?
   A. 5HT.
   B. DA.
   C. NE.
   D. HA.

8. Which of the following brain areas contains neurons active during BOTH wake and REM sleep?
   A. LC.
   B. LDT/PPT.
   C. DRN.
   D. TMN.

9. During REM sleep, neurons in what area are responsible for hypotonia?
   A. Subcoeruleus/sublateral dorsal tegmentum.
   B. LDT/PPT.
   C. LC.
   D. DRN.
   E. TMN.

10. What neurotransmitter(s) is believed to mediate the inhibition of spinal motorneurons (by interneurons)?
    A. GABA/glycine.
    B. Glutamate.
    C. 5HT.
    D. NE.

Answers

1. **D.**

2. **A.**

3. **D.**

4. **A.**

5. **B.**

6. **D.** Stimulatory input to the LC and DRN.

7. **A.**

8. **B.**

9. **A.**

10. **A.**

REFERENCES

1. Von Economo C: Sleep as a problem of localization. J Nerv Ment Dis 1930;71:249–259.
2. Reid A, McCall S, Henry JM, Taubenberger K: Experimenting on the past: the enigma of von Economo's encephalitis lethargica. J Neuropathol Exp Neurol 2001;60:663–670.
3. Espana RA, Scammell TE: Sleep neurobiology for the clinician. Sleep 2004;27:811–820.
4. Siegel JM: The neurobiology of sleep. Semin Neurol 2009;29:277–296.
5. McCarley RW: Neurobiology of REM and NREM sleep. Sleep Med 2007;8:302–330.
6. Saper CB, Chou TC, Scammell TE: The sleep switch: hypothalamic control of sleep and wakefulness. Trends Neurosci 2001;24:726–731.
7. De Lecca L, Kilduff TS, Peyron C, et al: The hypocretins: hypothalamic specific peptides with neuroexcitatory activity. Proc Natl Acad Sci U S A 1998;95:322–327.
8. Sakurai T: Orexins and Orexin receptors: a family of hypothalamic neuropeptides and G protein coupled receptors that regulate feeding behavior. Cell 1998;92:573–585.
9. Nishino S, Ripley B, Overeem S, et al: Hypocretin (Orexin) deficiency in human narcolepsy. Lancet 2003;355:39–40.
10. Thannickal T, Moore RY, Nienhuis R, et al: Reduced number of hypocretin neurons in human narcolepsy. Neuron 2000;27:469–474.
11. Thannickal TC, Nienhuis R, Siegel JM: Localized loss of hypocretin (orexin) cells in narcolepsy without cataplexy. Sleep 2009;32:993–998.
12. Mileykovskiy BY, Kiyashchenko LI, Siegel JM: Behavioral correlates of activity in identified hypocretin/Orexin neurons. Neuron 2005;46:787–798.
13. Szymusiak R, Gvilia I, McGinty D: Hypothalamic control of sleep. Sleep Med 2007;8:291–301.
14. Lu J, Bjorkum AA, Xu M, et al: Selective activation of the extended ventrolateral preoptic nucleus during rapid eye movement sleep. J Neurosci 2002;2:4568–4576.
15. John J, Wu MF, Boehmer LN, Siegel JM: Cataplexy-active neurons in the hypothalamus: implications for the role of histamine in sleep and waking behavior. Neuron 2004;42:619–634.
16. Kanbayhashi T, Kodama T, Kondo H, et al: CSF histamine contents in narcolepsy, idiopathic hypersomnia and obstructive sleep apnea syndrome. Sleep 2009;32:181–187.
17. Nishino S, Sakurai E, Nevisimalov S, et al: Decreased CSF histamines in narcolepsy with and without low CSF hypocretin-1 in comparison to healthy controls. Sleep 2009;32:175–180.
18. Lu J, Jhou TC, Saper CB: Identification of wake-active dopaminergic neurons in the ventral periaqueductal gray matter. J Neurosci 2006;26:193–202.
19. Thakkar MM, Strecker RE, McCarley RW: Behavioral state control through differential serotonergic inhibition in the mesopontine cholinergic nuclei: a simultaneous unit recording and microdialysis study. J Neurosci 1998;18:5490–5497.
20. Lu J, Sherman D, Devor M, Saper CB: A putative flip-flop switch for control of REM sleep. Nature 2006;441:589–594.
21. Fuller PM, Saper CB, Lu J: The pontine REM switch: past and present. J Physiol 2007;584:735–741.
22. Vetrivelan R, Fuller PM, Tong QA, Lu J: Medullary circuitry regulating rapid eye movement sleep and motor atonia. J Neurosci 2009;29:9361–9369.
23. Boutreal B, Koob GF: What keeps us awake. Sleep 2004;27:1181–1194.

Chapter 8

Monitoring Respiration—
Technology and Techniques

Chapter Points

- The recommended sensor to detect apnea is a nasal-oral (oronasal) thermal device.
- The recommended sensor to detect hypopnea is the NP signal (with or without square root linearization).
- The NP signal is proportional to the flow squared. The NP signal tends to underestimate low flow and overestimate high flow. Flattening of the inspiratory portion of the NP tracing is suggestive of airflow limitation and high upper airway resistance.
- Although the most sensitive method to detect respiratory effort is esophageal manometry, RIP is the recommended method used in most clinical studies.
- The RIPsum is an estimate of tidal volume (more accurate when calibrated).
- The relationship between the SpO_2 and the corresponding PaO_2 depends on many factors affecting the position of the oxyhemoglobin saturation curve (including $PaCO_2$, temperature, and abnormal hemoglobin).
- A valid $P_{ET}CO_2$ measurement assumes that the tracing has an alveolar plateau.
- SpO_2 utilizes the absorption of two wavelengths of light while co-oximetry utilizes four wavelengths and can determine the true fraction of oxyhemoglobin when significant amounts of COHb or MetHb are present.

The three major components of respiratory monitoring during sleep include measurement/detection of airflow, measurement/detection of respiratory effort, and measurement of arterial oxygen saturation (SaO_2). Ancillary monitoring may include detection of snoring and recording surrogates of the arterial partial pressure of carbon dioxide ($PaCO_2$) including end-tidal partial pressure of carbon dioxide ($P_{ET}CO_2$) and transcutaneous partial pressure of carbon dioxide ($TcPCO_2$). The techniques employed for respiratory monitoring are discussed in detail in this chapter. The criteria for defining important respiratory events are presented in Chapter 9. The *AASM Manual for the Scoring of Sleep and Associated Events* (hereafter referred to as

the "AASM scoring manual")[1] outlines rules for scoring respiratory events. These are discussed in detail in Chapter 9. The AASM scoring manual[1] recommends specific sensor types and techniques to be used for recording respiration during sleep (Table 8–1). The recommendations are based on consensus and evidence from an accompanying systematic review of the validity and reliability of scoring respiratory events during sleep.[2] This review serves as an update of a previous AASM consensus statement concerning the respiratory definitions and the accuracy of monitoring techniques published in 1999.[3]

TECHNIQUES TO MEASURE AIRFLOW OR TIDAL VOLUME

The techniques used to detect (measure) airflow during sleep studies are listed in Table 8–2. The pneumotachograph (PNT) is the most accurate method to measure airflow during sleep studies (Fig. 8–1).[2,3] This device quantifies airflow by measurement of the pressure drop across a linear (constant) resistance (usually a wire screen)[3]. The relationship between the pressure change, flow rate, and resistance is given by the following equation:

$$\text{Pressure change} = \text{Flow} \times \text{Resistance} \qquad \text{Equation 8–1}$$

The PNT is worn in a mask covering the nose and mouth. Although the PNT is commonly used to measure airflow during sleep research, this device is rarely used during clinical sleep studies.

Thermal devices were the first to be used to monitor airflow during clinical sleep studies.[2,3] These devices actually detect changes in temperature induced by airflow (cooler inspired air, warmer exhaled air). The changes in device temperature result in changes in voltage output (thermocouples) or resistance (thermistors). Thermal sensors are generally adequate to detect an absence of airflow (apnea), but their signal does not vary in proportion to airflow.[4,5] Therefore, thermal sensors are not an ideal means of detecting a reduction in airflow (hypopnea). Figure 8–2 compares thermal sensor estimates of minute ventilation with those using an accurate measurement of tidal volume (the head out of the box plethysmograph).[4] A wide scatter of points illustrates the poor ability of thermal devices to track changes in tidal

TABLE 8–1

American Academy of Sleep Medicine Recommended Sensors

	ADULT	**PEDIATRIC**
Airflow sensor to detect apnea	Recommended: • Nasal-oral thermal (oronasal) sensor Alternative sensor (if recommended sensor signal is unreliable) • Nasal pressure (with or without square root transformation of the signal)	Same as adult except alternative sensors for apnea detection also include the end-tidal PCO_2 signal and summed calibrated respiratory inductance plethysmography signal
Airflow sensor to detect hypopnea	Recommended: • Nasal pressure (with or without square root transformation of the signal) Alternative sensors (if recommended sensor signal is unreliable) • Nasal-oral thermal device • Respiratory inductance plethysmography (calibrated or uncalibrated)	Recommended: same Alternative sensors: Nasal-oral thermal device
Sensor to detect respiratory effort	Recommended: • Esophageal pressure • Respiratory inductance plethysmography (calibrated or uncalibrated) Alternative: • Diaphragmatic or intercostal muscle EMG	Same except muscle EMG not mentioned
Arterial oxygen saturation	Recommended: • Pulse oximetry	Same
Alveolar hypoventilation ($PaCO_2$)	Insufficient evidence to recommend a sensor The following may be used if validated • End-tidal PCO_2 monitoring • Transcutaneous PCO_2 monitoring	Acceptable: End-tidal PCO_2 monitoring Transcutaneous PCO_2 monitoring

EMG = electromyogram; $PaCO_2$ = arterial partial pressure of carbon dioxide; PCO_2 = partial pressure of carbon dioxide.
From Iber C, Ancoli-Israel S, Chesson A, Quan SF for the American Academy of Sleep Medicine: The AASM Manual for the Scoring of Sleep and Associated Events: Rules, Terminology and Technical Specifications, 1st ed. Westchester, IL: American Academy of Sleep Medicine, 2007.

volume (and flow). Figure 8–3 compares thermistor and thermocouple signals in a nose model with a PNT as the gold standard (accurate measure of flow).[5] Note that thermal signals and PNT flow are equal at 1 L/sec (by design). However, as airflow decreases, the thermal signals overestimate flow. This figure illustrates that thermal sensors are not ideal sensors to detect hypopneas (reductions in flow). The same study demonstrated that the thermal sensor signal decreases when the nostrils are large or the thermal sensor is further from the nares. Of note, thermal devices composed of polyvinylidine fluoride (PVDF) film may offer a better estimate of flow[6] (Fig. 8–4). Nasal-oral thermal sensors usually have a portion of the device placed within or just outside the nostrils with another portion over the mouth (detection of oral flow) (Fig. 8–5). A major advantage of thermal sensors is that they can detect both nasal and oral airflow without the need for a cumbersome mask covering the face.

Measurement of nasal pressure (NP) provides an estimate of nasal airflow that is more accurate than one obtained with most thermal sensors.[7–12] NP is measured using a nasal cannula connected to an accurate pressure transducer.

Because the cannula tips are inside the nares and the other side of the pressure transducer is open to the atmosphere, the pressure being measured is actually the pressure drop across the resistance of the nasal inlet associated with nasal airflow. The resistance of the nasal inlet is not a constant (nonlinear). The relationship of NP and flow is given by Equations 8–2 and 8–3.[7,10]

$$NP = K1 \times (Flow)^2 \qquad K1 = constant \qquad \text{Equation 8–2}$$

$$Flow = K2 \times \sqrt{NP}. \qquad K2 = constant \qquad \text{Equation 8–3}$$

Because NP varies with the square of flow, the NP signal tends to underestimate airflow at low flow rates and overestimate flow at high flows (Fig. 8–6). The NP signal is "linearized" by taking the square root (Equation 8–3) and when calibrated, it very closely approximates the flow from a PNT at least over a short period of time (see Fig. 8–6). However, in clinical practice, the NP signal rather than the square root of the signal is most often recorded as an estimate of nasal airflow. Even when linearized, the NP signal may not provide an absolutely accurate estimate of total airflow over the entire night. Changes in cannula position, periods of partial oral

TABLE 8-2
Monitoring Airflow or Tidal Volume

DEVICE	PHYSIOLOGY
PNT	• Pressure drop across PNT = Flow × Resistance • Flow = Pressure difference/Resistance • PNT usually placed in a mask covering the nose and mouth
Nasal-oral thermal device	• Changes in temperature induced by airflow result in changes in resistance (thermistor) or voltage output (thermocouple) • Accurate for the presence or absence of airflow • Can detect nasal and oral airflow • Signal not proportional to flow
NP	• Measures pressure difference across the nares • NP = K1 × (Flow)^2 (K1 and K2 are constants) • Flow = K2 × $\sqrt{NP}$. • Flattening of the inspiratory flow contour detects airflow limitation • Oral breathing not well detected
RIP	• RIPsum is an estimate of tidal volume • Most accurate if calibrated • Time derivative of the RIPsum gives an estimate of flow

NP = nasal pressure; PNT = pneumotachograph; RIP = respiratory inductance plethysmography.

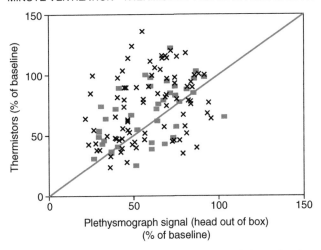

MINUTE VENTILATION - THERMISTOR VS. PLETHYSMOGRAPHY

FIGURE 8-2 Thermistor signals are not a good estimate of changes in minute ventilation (do not accurately track changes in flow or tidal volume). The *dark line* is the line of identity. *Reproduced from Berg S, Haight JSJ, Yap V, et al: Comparison of direct and indirect measurement of respiratory airflow: implications for hypopneas. Sleep 1997;20:60–64.*

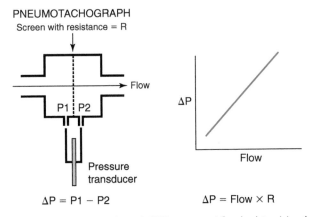

FIGURE 8-1 The pneumotachograph (PNT) measures airflow by determining the pressure drop across a linear (constant) resistance.

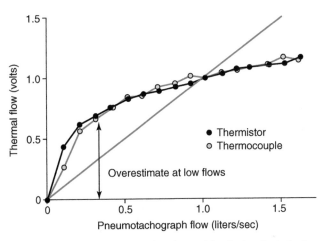

FIGURE 8-3 Thermal devices overestimate the actual flow (underestimate the drop in flow) as flow decreases. The *straight line* is the line of identity. *Reproduced from Farré R, Montserrat JM, Rotger M, et al: Accuracy of thermistors and thermocouples as flow-measuring devices for detecting hypopneas. Eur Respir J 1998;11:179–182.*

flow, and obstruction of the cannula by nasal secretions make the linearized NP signal a less accurate measure of flow over the entire night.[11] Thurnheer and coworkers[11] compared the NP and linearized NP signals ($\sqrt{NP}$.) for detection of respiratory events with the PNT (flowmeter) (Fig. 8–7). The number of apneas and hypopneas per hour of sleep (apnea-hypopnea index [AHI]) was determined using each of the three signals (PNT, NP, and linearized NP). A *hypopnea* was defined as a reduction in signal to 50% or

less of the baseline. The bias (mean difference between AHI values) and limits of agreement (±2 SD [standard deviation] of the differences) were determined by comparing the AHI values detected by the NP versus PNT and the linearized NP versus PNT signals in each patient. The AHI values from both the NP and the linearized NP signals showed excellent agreement with the AHI values determined from the PNT (flowmeter) (Table 8–3; see also Fig. 8–7). The AHI values detected by the NP signal tended to be slightly higher than the linearized NP signal, but the differences were usually small. Of note, when a more stringent criteria was used for NP events (signal reduction to ≤25% of baseline), the NP

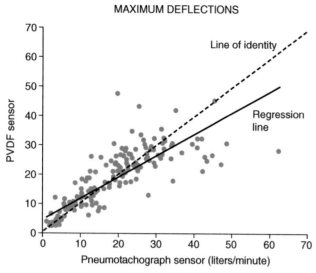

MAXIMUM DEFLECTIONS

FIGURE 8–4 PVDF thermal sensor signals appear to be fairly accurate estimates of airflow. PVDF = polyvinylidene fluoride. *Reproduced from Berry RB, Koch GL, Trautz S, Wagner MH: Comparison of respiratory event detection by a polyvinylidene fluoride film airflow sensor and a pneumotachograph in sleep apnea patients. Chest 2005;128: 1331–1338.*

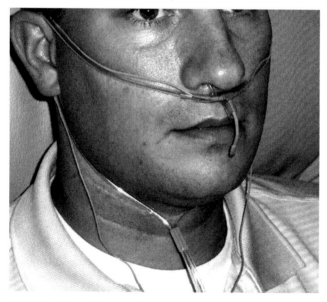

FIGURE 8–5 Use of both nasal pressure and a nasal-oral thermal sensor is recommended to monitor airflow during sleep. Note that the thermal device has an extension over the mouth to detect oral flow.

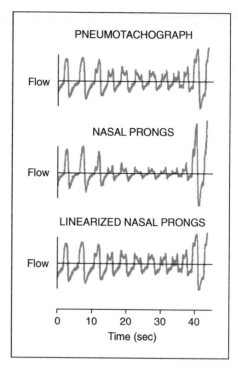

FIGURE 8–6 Simultaneous flow signals during hypopnea from a pneumotachograph, nasal prongs (nasal pressure), and linearized nasal prongs (square root transformation of nasal pressure). The nasal prongs signal decreases more than that of the pneumotachograph during a reduction in airflow. The linearized nasal prongs signal is very similar to that of the pneumotachograph. *Reproduced from Farré R, Rigau J, Montserrat JM, et al: Relevance of linearizing nasal prongs for assessing hypopneas and flow limitation during sleep. Am J Respir Crit Care Med 2001;163:494–497.*

results were essentially identical to the linearized NP results. Recall that NP = K (Flow)^2 and, therefore, if flow drops from 1 to 0.5, the NP signal drops to 0.25 NP. Using an AHI of 5/hr by PNT to diagnose obstructive sleep apnea (OSA), all of the 20 patients in the study would have been correctly classified by the linearized NP signal but there would have been two false positives with the AHI determined by NP (50% drop).

Heitman and colleagues[12] also compared the NP and linearized NP signals with a full-face mask with PTN for

detection of hypopneas during sleep. A hypopnea was defined as either a 50% drop in the device signal or less than a 50% drop in the device signal with an associated arousal or 3% or greater arterial oxygen desaturation. The intermeasurement agreements (kappa) between NP and PNT and linearized NP and PNT signals were both excellent and essentially identical.

In addition to the signal amplitude, the shape (contour) of both the PNT and the NP signals during inspiration provides additional useful information[7,8,13] (Fig. 8–8). During normal unobstructed flow, the inspiratory shape (contour) of the NP signal is round (see Fig. 8–8A), whereas during airflow limitation (a constant or decreased airflow associated with an increasing driving pressure), the shape of the PNT and NP signals is flattened (see Fig. 8–8C). Of note, airflow limitation is characteristically present during obstructive reductions in airflow (hypopnea) or snoring. In contrast, when reductions in airflow are simply due to a fall in inspiratory effort, the NP signal amplitude is reduced but the shape is round. Airflow limitation is usually associated with an increased pressure drop across the upper airway (more negative inspiratory pressure below the site of upper airway narrowing; see Fig. 8–8C).

The most important limitation of the NP technique is that approximately 10% of patients are "mouth breathers" and the NP signal may be misleading. The NP signal may show

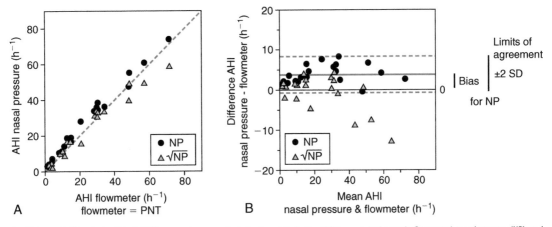

FIGURE 8–7 **A,** The relationship of AHI (apnea + hypopnea index) values detected by PNT (pneumotachograph; flowmeter), nasal pressure (NP), and linearized NP (square root of NP). The linearized NP detects slightly fewer and the NP slightly more events than the PNT. **B,** A Bland-Altman plot shows the differences in the NP AHI and the flowmeter AHI plotted against the mean of the two values for each subject. The mean difference in AHI values (bias) and the spread of the differences (limits of agreement = ± 2 standard deviations [SD]) for the NP AHI values are also shown. A plot of differences in the linearized NP and PNT AHI values is also shown (bias and limits of agreement not shown). **A** and **B,** *Reproduced from Thurnheer R, Xie X, Bloch KE: Accuracy of nasal cannula pressure recordings for assessment of ventilation during sleep. Am J Respir Crit Care Med 2001;146:1914–1919.*

TABLE 8–3

Comparison of Methods for Detection of AHI with the Pneumotachograph (Flowmeter)

DEVICE	BIAS = MEAN DIFFERENCE OF AHI VALUES (AHI DEVICE— AHI PNT) (EVENTS/hr)	LIMITS OF AGREEMENT (± 2 SD OF AHI DIFFERENCES) (EVENTS/hr)
NP (50%)*	3.9	−0.8 to 8.5
NP (25%)†	−0.8	−9 to 9.6
Linearized NP (50%)‡	−0.9	−9.9 to 8.1
RIPsum§	2.6	−3.3 to 8.6
Time derivative RIPsum‖	1.0	−5.6 to 7.6

*NP (50%) hypopnea defined as a drop in NP signal to 50% of baseline with duration ≥ 10 sec.
†NP (25%) hypopnea defined as a drop in NP to 25% of baseline with duration ≥ 10 sec.
‡Linearized NP (50%) hypopnea defined as a drop in square root of NP signal to 50% of baseline with duration ≥ 10 sec.
§RIPsum hypopnea defined by a 50% drop in RIPsum signal with duration ≥ 10 sec.
‖Time derivative of RIPsum hypopnea defined by a 50% drop in signal with duration ≥ 10 sec.
AHI = apnea-hypopnea index; NP = nasal pressure; PNT = pneumotachograph; RIP = respiratory inductance plethysmography; SD = standard deviation.
Adapted from Thurnheer R, Xie X, Bloch KE: Accuracy of nasal cannula pressure recordings for assessment of ventilation during sleep. Am J Respir Crit Care Med 2001;146:1914–1919.

recommends nasal-oral thermal sensors for detection of apnea and NP sensors (with or without square root transformation of the signal) for detection of hypopnea (see Table 8–1).[1] Simultaneous use of both NP and nasal-oral thermal sensors is recommended and has the additional advantage of having a backup sensor if the other airflow detection device fails (see Fig. 8–5).

The AASM scoring manual[1] notes that if the recommended sensor signal is not reliable, the alternative sensor can be used. In adults, the alternative airflow sensor for apnea detection is the NP signal. The alternative sensors for hypopnea detections are oronasal thermal flow and respiratory inductance plethysmography (RIP; discussed later).[14,15] In children, alternative sensors for apnea detection include the exhaled PCO_2 waveform, nasal pressure, and the summed respiratory inductance plethysmography (RIPsum) signal. The alternative sensor for hypopnea detection is the nasal-oral thermal flow sensor.

RIP[13,14] is another method that can be used to detect apnea and hypopnea (Figs. 8–10 and 8–11). The signals from rib cage (RC) and abdominal bands (AB) sensors can be summed in an uncalibrated manner (RIPsum = RC + AB) or as a calibrated signal (RIPsum = a × RC + b × AB) as an estimate of *tidal volume* (not airflow). Here, RC and AB are signals from bands around the rib cage and abdomen and "a" and "b" are calibration factors determined during a calibration procedure. If one takes the time derivative of the RIPsum signal, the result is an estimate of airflow (RIPflow). The RIPsum during apnea has minimal deflections (approximately zero tidal volume) and during hypopnea reduced deflections (reduced tidal volume). In the case of an obstructive apnea (see Fig. 8–10), the RC and AB deflections must nearly exactly cancel each other (paradox). In the case of hypopnea, there is a reduction in the RIPsum signal (low tidal volume) as well as both the RC and the AB signals. In the case of obstructive hypopnea, there may also be paradox

minimal deflections (apparent apnea) while the nasal-oral thermal sensor will continue to show airflow (Fig. 8–9). As a consequence of this phenomenon, events that are actually hypopneas may be misclassified as apnea if the NP signal is used to detect apneas. The AASM scoring manual

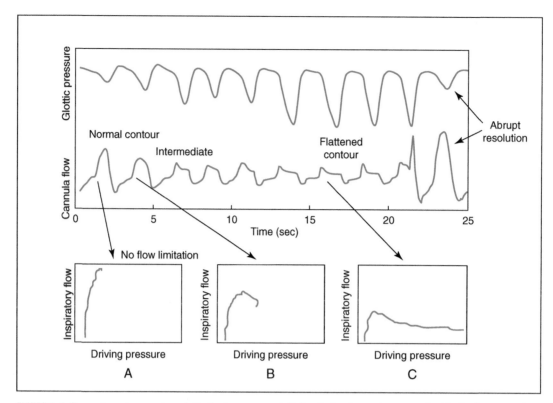

FIGURE 8–8 Changes in nasal pressure (cannula flow) and pressure recorded below the site of upper airway narrowing (glottic refers to supraglottic pressure) during a reduction in airflow. At **A,** the flow is rounded, whereas at **C,** the flattened airflow contour is associated with an increase in pressure drop across the upper airway and airflow limitation. ***A–C,*** *Reproduced from Hosslet J, Normal RG, Ayapa I, Rapoport DM: Detection of flow limitation with a nasal cannula/pressure transducer system. Am J Respir Crit Care Med 1988;157:1481–1467.*

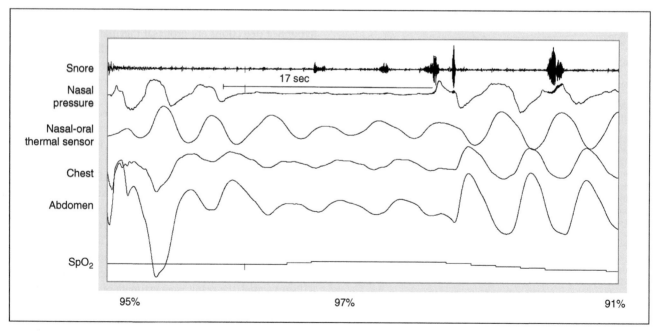

FIGURE 8–9 The nasal pressure signal shows an absence of airflow, whereas the nasal-oral thermal sensor shows continued airflow. This pattern of airflow is due to oral breathing. Nasal-oral thermal sensors are the recommended device for detecting apnea. SpO_2 = pulse oximetry.

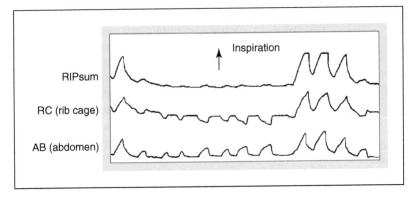

FIGURE 8-10 Obstructive apnea: Respiratory inductance plethysmography signals from the rib cage (RC) and abdominal bands (AB) are summed (RIPsum). The RIPsum is an estimate of tidal volume. Here, tidal volume is essentially zero (apnea) and RC and AB signals show paradox (moving in opposite directions). *Reproduced from Berry RB: Sleep Medicine Pearls, 2nd ed. Philadelphia: Hanley & Belfus, 2003, p. 89.*

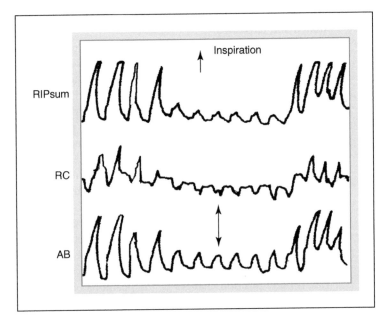

FIGURE 8-11 Obstructive hypopnea: Respiratory inductance plethysmography signals from the rib cage (RC) and abdominal bands (AB) are summed (RIPsum). The RIPsum is an estimate of tidal volume. Here, tidal volume is reduced (hypopnea) and RC and AB signals show paradox (moving in opposite directions). *Reproduced from Berry RB: Sleep Medicine Pearls, 2nd ed. Philadelphia: Hanley & Belfus, 2003, p. 84.*

with chest and abdomen moving in opposite directions (see Fig. 8–11). If a RIPsum signal is not available, one can detect hypopnea by a reduction in the RC and AB RIP signals. RIP is discussed further in the respiratory effort section. In the previously discussed study of Thurnheer and coworkers,[11] detection of apnea-hypopnea by the *calibrated* RIPsum and the time derivative of the RIPsum were compared with the PNT (flowmeter) signal (see Table 8–3). The AHI values obtained from the RIPsum and time derivative of the RIPsum signals showed good agreement with AHI values from the PNT signal.

MEASURING RESPIRATORY EFFORT

Determination of respiratory effort is essential to classify apneas as obstructive (continued respiratory effort), central (absent effort), or mixed (central followed by obstructive portions). The commonly used methods of detecting respiratory effort are listed in Table 8–4. The most sensitive and accurate method of detecting respiratory effort is by measurement of esophageal pressure[1-3,13-15] (Fig. 8–12). Changes

in esophageal pressure are estimates of changes in pleural pressure that occur during respiration (negative intrathoracic pressure during inspiration). Esophageal pressure monitoring can detect rather feeble respiratory efforts even when RC and AB movements are minimal. In addition, the size of the pressure deflections provides an estimate of the magnitude of respiratory effort. As discussed in Chapter 9, detection of respiratory effort–related arousals (RERAs) is most accurately performed with esophageal pressure manometry. Measurement of esophageal pressure can be performed using air-filled balloons, fluid-filled catheters, or catheters with pressure transducers on their tips.[13] The technique does require special equipment and expertise and is routinely performed in only a few sleep centers. In Figure 8–12, note that RC and AB effort belts (here RIP) fail to detect the presence of the progressive increase in inspiratory effort documented by increasing esophageal pressure excursions during an OSA. Some research sleep studies measure supraglottic pressure instead of esophageal pressure using a transducer tip placed just below the tongue base. This allows measurement of the pressure drop across the upper airway.

TABLE 8-4
Measurement of Respiratory Effort

METHOD	SENSORS	COMMENTS
Esophageal pressure deflections	Esophageal balloon Transducer-tipped catheter Fluid-filled catheter	Signal proportional to changes in pleural pressure Sensitive for detection of inspiratory effort Relatively invasive
Intercostal/diaphragm EMG activity	Bipolar recording using surface electrodes	ECG artifact a problem Obtaining a good signal may be difficult in some patients
Chest and abdominal movement	Piezoelectric belts	Relatively inexpensive Signals may not accurately reflect changes in chest and abdominal volume during respiration
Chest and abdominal movement	RIP belts	Inductance varies with cross-sectional area subtended by the belt Can quantify changes in volume when RIP signals are calibrated

ECG = electrocardiogram; EMG = electromyogram; RIP = respiratory impedance plethysmography.

Because this site is below the area of upper airway closure or narrowing in obstructive respiratory events, supraglottic pressure can also be used to detect respiratory effort.

Until recently, the most common method for detecting respiratory effort in clinical sleep studies utilized piezoelectric (PE) sensors connected to bands around the RC and AB. Changes in the tension on the PE transducer as the RC and AB expand and contract produce a voltage that can be measured. The signal from these devices depends on the degree of tension on the transducer. The PE belts are adequate for detection of respiratory effort in most patients but do not really quantify the changes in RC or AB volume. Although relatively inexpensive compared with RIP effort belts, the PE effort belts may provide misleading information (false absence of respiratory effort), especially if not properly positioned and tensioned.

RIP belts provide a more accurate method of detecting changes in RC and AB motion during respiration than PE belts.[3,14,15] The inductance of coils in bands around the RC and AB changes during respiration as the RC and AB expand and contract. The band inductance varies proportionately to the **cross-sectional area** the band encircles. An oscillator is applied to each circuit and changes in inductance are converted into a voltage output. The RIP bands consist of wires attached to a cloth band in a zig-zag pattern. This produces a larger change in inductance for a given change in band circumference.

Recall that if the RIP signals are calibrated, the RIPsum signal = a RC + b AB is an estimate of tidal volume. Here, the constants a and b are determined during a calibration procedure. The accuracy of the RIPsum signal can deteriorate if body position changes or the positions of the bands change during sleep. Stats and associates[15] studied patients

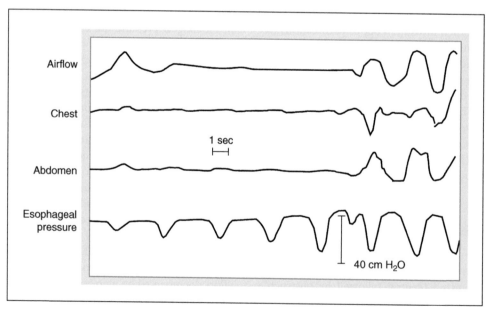

FIGURE 8-12 Esophageal pressure deflections increase during an obstructive apnea that might at first glance appear to be central apnea (absent inspiratory effort). In this patient, the chest and abdomen effort belt signals showed minimal deflections during obstructive apnea. The situation was corrected by increasing the gain of the signals while scoring respiratory events.

with sleep apnea using both **calibrated** RIP belts and esophageal pressure monitoring. In only 9% of patients were obstructive apneas sometimes misclassified as central apneas by the RIP belts. In these instances, esophageal pressure deflections were present when there was no detectable change in the RIP belt signals. Thus, RIP effort belts are not 100% sensitive for detecting respiratory effort. However, if the bands are properly positioned and tensioned (sized), they will detect respiratory effort (if present) in most patients.

The vast majority of sleep centers do not perform RIP belt calibration. It should be noted that the deflections of uncalibrated RIP bands do not always accurately reflect the magnitude of inspiratory effort or always show paradox (see Figs. 8–10 and 8–11) during obstructive apnea and hypopnea. Chest-abdominal paradoxical motion is discussed in detail in Chapter 9.

Respiratory effort can also be measured by recording the respiratory muscle electromyogram (EMG) signal using bipolar surface electrodes.[16-18] The common sites include the intercostal muscles and the diaphragm (Fig. 8–13). Surface diaphragm EMG recording utilizes two electrodes about 2 cm apart horizontally in the seventh and eighth intercostal spaces in the right anterior axillary line. The right side of the body is used to reduce electrocardiogram (ECG) artifact. Intercostal EMG recording often uses the right parasternal area (second and third intercostal spaces in the midaxillary line). Inspiratory EMG activity is noted in the intercostal muscles and the diaphragm during non–rapid eye movement (NREM) sleep. During rapid eye movement (REM) sleep, the intercostal activity is inhibited but diaphragmatic activity persists, although often diminished in amplitude during bursts of eye movements.

The AASM scoring manual[1] recommends use of esophageal manometry or calibrated or uncalibrated RIP belts for detection of respiratory effort during sleep studies in adults and children (see Table 8–1). The measurement of respiratory muscle EMG is listed as an alternative method of detecting respiratory effort in adults.

MEASURING SaO$_2$

Continuous measurement of the arterial partial pressure of oxygen (PaO$_2$) during sleep studies is not feasible. Spot checks of arterial blood gases (ABGs) are only rarely performed during sleep studies and many facilities do not have the capability to process arterial blood samples. Instead of PaO$_2$, SaO$_2$ is estimated during sleep studies by continuous recording of pulse oximetry (SpO$_2$), typically with finger or ear probes. The relationship of SaO$_2$ and the PaO$_2$ is given by the oxyhemoglobin (O$_2$Hb) saturation curve (Fig. 8–14A). The curve is also called the oxyhemoglobin dissociation curve in some texts. The relationship between the SaO$_2$ and the PaO$_2$ is affected by temperature, hydrogen ion concentration, PCO$_2$, and 2,3-diphosphoglycerate (2,3-DPG) concentration. An abnormal hemoglobin[19] (e.g., hemoglobin S in Fig. 8–14B) or changes in acid-base status can influence the relationship of the SaO$_2$ and the PaO$_2$ in the blood. The P$_{50}$ is the PaO$_2$ at which hemoglobin is 50% saturated. Normally, the P$_{50}$ is approximately 26 mm Hg. A higher P$_{50}$ implies a shift to the right, lower oxygen affinity, and a higher PaO$_2$ for a given SaO$_2$.

The total hemoglobin concentration (Hbt) is the sum of concentrations of oxygenated hemoglobin (O$_2$Hb), deoxygenated or reduced hemoglobin (RHB), carboxyhemoglobin

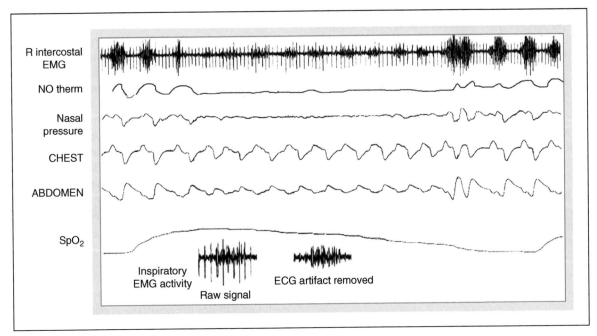

FIGURE 8–13 An obstructive apnea with respiratory effort monitored by both chest and abdominal respiratory inductance plethysmography (RIP) bands and right intercostal electromyogram (EMG). The right intercostal EMG signal shows bursts coincident with inspiratory effort (and movement of chest and abdomen). A blow up of one EMG burst is shown at the bottom of the figure in a raw form and with the electrocardiogram (ECG) artifact minimized. SpO$_2$ = pulse oximetry.

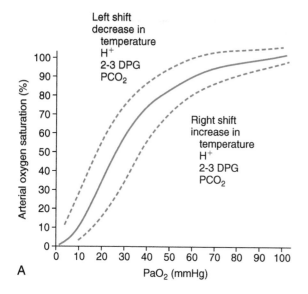

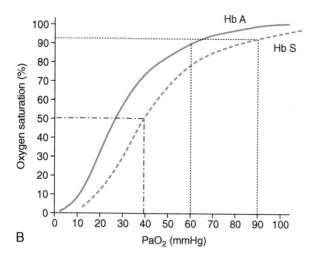

FIGURE 8–14 A, The oxyhemoglobin saturation curve. Changes in body temperature, hydrogen ion concentration, partial pressure of carbon dioxide (PCO_2) and the concentration of 2-3-diphosphoglycerate (2-3 DPG) can shift the curve. **B,** The oxyhemoglobin saturation curve for normal hemoglobin (HbA) and sickle hemoglobin (HbS). PaO_2 = arterial partial pressure of oxygen.

(COHb) and methhemoglobin (metHb) (Equation 8–4). COHb and MetHb do not bind oxygen but shift the oxyhemoglobin saturation curve to the left.[20,21] In addition, they affect the fraction of hemoglobin available for binding to oxygen. The ability of carbon monoxide to bind Hb is about 240 times that of oxygen.

The SaO_2 as defined in Equation 8–5 is often called the *functional saturation*. The arterial oxygen content of the blood (CaO_2) is determined largely by the SaO_2 (Equation 8–6). Here CaO_2 is in mLO_2/mL, Hb is in g/100mL, 1.34 is the mLO_2/g of fully saturated Hb.

$$Hbt = O_2Hb + RHb + COHb + MetHb \qquad \text{Equation 8–4}$$

where O_2Hb = concentration of oxygenated hemoglobin, RHb = concentration of reduced hemoglobin, COHb = concentration of carboxyhemoglobin, MetHb = concentration

of methemoglobin, and Hbt = total hemoglobin concentration.

$$SaO_2 \% = (O_2Hb) \times 100/(O_2Hb + RHb) \qquad \text{Equation 8–5}$$

$$CaO_2 = 1.34\ Hb\ SaO_2 + 0.003\ PaO_2 \qquad \text{Equation 8–6}$$

If COHb or MetHb are present in significant amounts, one can define a fractional saturation based on Equation 8–7. This shows that the fractional hemoglobin oxygen saturation of oxygenated hemoglobin (FO_2Hb) depends on the concentrations of COHb and MetHb as well as RHb. An accurate oxygen-carrying capacity can be computed using Equation 8–5 with SaO_2 replaced by FO_2Hb. FO_2Hb is sometimes referred to as the *fractional saturation*. Using equations similar to Equation 8–7, fractional concentrations can be defined for carboxyhemoglobin (FCOHb), methemoglobin (FMetHb), and reduced hemoglobin (RHb) as the concentration of each entity divided by the total hemoglobin times 100.

$$FO_2Hb(\%) = O_2Hb \times 100/(O_2Hb + RHb + COHb + MetHb)$$

$$= O_2Hb \times 100/Hbt$$

$$\text{Equation 8–7}$$

One should note that the SaO_2 value supplied by some clinical laboratories is determined by a measured PaO_2 and the use of a table or computer program to provide a value for the SaO_2. Accurate measurement of SaO_2 and FO_2Hb depends on the clinical laboratory using a **co-oximeter**. This instrument uses absorption of 4 wavelengths of light to determine the concentrations of oxygenated and deoxygenated hemoglobin as well as COHb and MetHb. Thus, COHb and MetHb can affect the relationship between PaO_2 and SaO_2 (position of the oxyhemoglobin saturation curve) and the relationship between the SaO_2 and the FO_2Hb.

In the sleep center, the major purpose of SpO_2 is not to determine the oxygen-carrying capacity of the blood (depends on FO_2Hb) but to infer changes in PaO_2 due to respiratory events. The oxyhemoglobin saturation curve describes the relationship between O_2Hb and the free hemoglobin ($O_2Hb + RHb$, Hb available for oxygen binding). In this sense, the ability of the SpO_2 to allow correct inference about the PaO_2 depends on the accuracy with which SpO_2 reflects the SaO_2 (rather than the FO_2Hb) and the position of the oxyhemoglobin saturation curve. As discussed later, COHb and MetHb also affect the performance of the 2-wavelength oximeters commonly used in clinical settings.

PULSE OXIMETRY

Pulse oximeters[22] provide an estimate of the SaO_2 by determining the absorption of two wavelengths of light (660 nm [red] and 940 nm [infrared]) by capillary blood. This determines the relative amount of the O_2Hb and RHb. The absorption of radiation at 660 nm is much greater with RHb than with O_2Hb, while O_2Hb absorbs more radiation at 940 nm (Fig. 8–15A). The ability of SpO_2 to determine the SaO_2 is

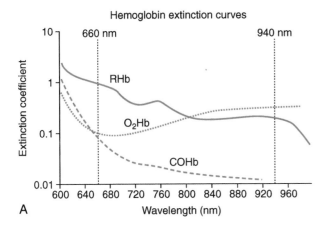

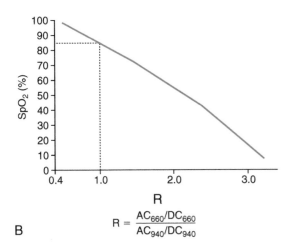

$$R = \frac{AC_{660}/DC_{660}}{AC_{940}/DC_{940}}$$

B

FIGURE 8–15 **A,** Hemoglobin extinction curves for reduced hemoglobin (RHb), oxyhemoglobin (O₂Hb), and carboxyhemoglobin (COHb) at different wavelengths of light. Note that y axis is a log scale. **B,** Empirical curve of the ratio of absorption of radiation at wavelengths of 660 and 940 nm. AC = the pulse added absorption; DC = the steady state or background absorbance. Note at R = 1, the arterial oxygen saturation (SpO₂) is 85%. **A** and **B,** Adapted from Tremper KK, Barker SJ: Pulse oximetry. Anesthesiology 1989;70:108–109.

based on the empirical observation that the ratio (R) of absorbance at the two wavelengths is related to the SaO_2 (see Fig. 8–15B). This relationship (calibration curve) is determined experimentally by determining R at varying SaO_2 for each oximeter. To specifically determine the absorbance of arterial blood, the AC (pulse added absorbance) at each wavelength is divided by the DC (background absorbance) to account for the effect of the absorption of the radiation by venous blood and tissue. SpO_2 is accurate down to about 70%. Whereas values below 70% are often reported, one must keep in mind that they probably do not correspond accurately to the actual SaO_2.

As previously mentioned, the accuracy of SpO_2 can be impaired by the presence of COHb[23] or MetHb,[24] which absorb light at the two wavelengths (660 and 940 nm) used by pulse oximeters. In the case of COHb, the absorption of 660 nm is similar to O_2Hb and causes a falsely elevated SpO_2 estimate of the FO_2Hb. It is estimated that for every 1% of circulating COHb, the pulse oximeter reading is falsely

elevated by about 1% compared with the FO_2Hb. Fortunately, the SpO_2 is closer to the SaO_2 as determined by Equation 8–5 than the FO_2Hb. For example, a typical set of values would be: FO_2Hb = 87%, FRHb = 9%, FCOHb = 4%, SpO_2 = 91%, SaO_2 = 87/(87 + 9) = 90.6%. As noted previously, the oxyhemoglobin saturation curve describes the relationship between the O_2Hb and the "free hemoglobin" (O_2Hb + RHb); hence, the PaO_2 is determined based on the measured SaO_2. As noted previously, COHb can shift the oxygen hemoglobin saturation curve to the left. However, at the levels of COHb typically encountered in the sleep center, this should not significantly affect the PaO_2 that can be inferred from the SpO_2. Conversely, the difference between the SpO_2 and the FO_2Hb is larger and is approximately equal to the concentration of COHb.[20]

MetHb occurs when the normal ferrous state (Fe^{2+}) of the iron moiety in Hb is oxidized to the ferric stage (Fe^{3+}). metHb absorbs nearly equal amounts of red and near-infrared light, giving an R = 1.[24] As the concentration of MetHb increases, the pulse oximeter reads closer and closer to 85%. Therefore, methemoglobinemia may cause the SpO_2 to give a falsely low estimate of the SaO_2 and, hence, the PaO_2. On the other hand methemoglobin shifts the oxyhemoglobin saturation curve to the left and the SaO_2 is less than the FO_2Hb as oxygen does not bind methemoglobin. Methemoglobinemia can occur from medications (e.g., benzocaine, sulfonamides) but is rarely a problem in the sleep center unless a patient has an inherited form of methemoglobinemia (this usually is known before the sleep study).

A number of additional factors can impair the accuracy of SpO_2. These include poor perfusion (patient sleeping on the finger or hand) and nail polish. If the oximetry signal seems to fluctuate widely or inappropriately low or high readings are noted, the probe or probe position should be changed. When in doubt, the technologist can place the probe on her or his own finger as a test of oximeter accuracy.

In summary, multiple factors can affect the value of PaO_2 that can be inferred from a given SpO_2 value measured during a sleep study. If an abnormal relationship between the SpO_2 and the corresponding PaO_2 is suspected based on clinical history (e.g., sickle cell disease or methemoglobinemia) or a surprisingly low SpO_2 is found, one can draw an ABG for measurement of PaO_2 and co-oximetry for measurement of SaO_2, FO_2Hb, metHb, and COHb. This assumes that such a measurement is available and clinically indicated.

SpO₂ AND SLEEP MONITORING

In sleep monitoring, an *arterial oxygen desaturation* is usually defined as a decrease in the SpO_2 of 3% or 4% or more from baseline. Note that the nadir in SaO_2 commonly follows apnea (hypopnea) termination by approximately 6 to 8 seconds (longer in severe desaturations) (Fig. 8–16). This delay is secondary to circulation time and instrumental delay (the oximeter averages over several cycles before producing a reading). Figure 8–16 identifies the apneas and the corresponding nadirs in saturation. Various measures have been

FIGURE 8–16 Apneas are followed by arterial oxygen desaturations. Longer apneas are associated with more severe desaturation. SpO_2 = pulse oximetry.

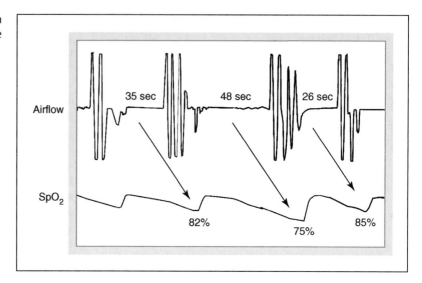

FIGURE 8–17 A long averaging time impairs the ability of oximetry to detect arterial oxygen desaturation. SpO_2 = pulse oximetry. *Reproduced from Jasani R, Sanders MH, Strollo PJ: Diagnostic studies for apnea/hypopnea. In Johnson JT, Gluckman JL, Sanders MH (eds): Management of Obstructive Sleep Apnea. London: Martin Dunitz, 2002, p. 68.*

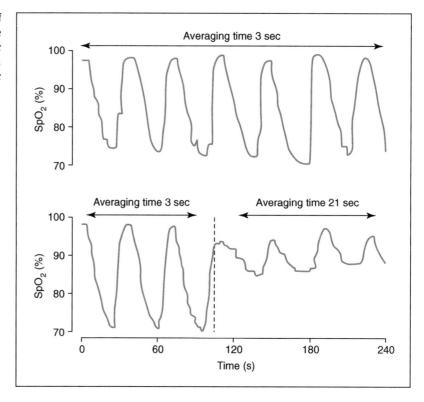

applied to assess the severity of desaturation, including computing the number of desaturations, the average minimum SpO_2 during desaturations, the time below 80%, 85%, 90%, as well as the mean SaO_2 and the minimum saturation during NREM and REM sleep. The time with an $SpO_2 \leq 88\%$ is also commonly determined.

Oximeters may vary considerably in the number of desaturations they detect and their ability to discard movement artifact. As illustrated in Figure 8–17, using long averaging times may dramatically decrease the detection of desaturations.[25,26] Here, the results of identical oximeters monitoring the same patient are shown. The averaging time of one of the oximeters is increased and there are obvious large differences in the results. The ability of oximeters to detect desaturations is especially important in light of the definitions of hypopnea that depend on an associated desaturation.

The AASM scoring manual[1] recommends a maximum averaging time of 3 seconds at a heart rate of 80 bpm. In patients with a slow heart rate, a slightly longer averaging time (at least a 3-beat average) may be needed.

MEASUREMENT OF $PaCO_2$ DURING SLEEP

Documentation of hypoventilation during sleep requires measurement (or estimate) of the $PaCO_2$. The AASM scoring manual[1] defines *sleep-related hypoventilation* in adults as an increase in the $PaCO_2$ during sleep ≥ 10 mm Hg compared with an awake supine value. However, continuous ABG monitoring during polysomnography to determine the $PaCO_2$ is not practical. An ABG sample sometimes is performed at the start or the end of the study. The sample can be used to validate a surrogate measure of $PaCO_2$ such as $P_{ET}CO_2$ or $TcPCO_2$. If an ABG sample is taken just at awakening, it may be used to infer hypoventilation. In children, an arterialized capillary blood gas is often performed rather than an arterial sample. The AASM scoring manual[1] defines *hypoventilation in children* based on a $PaCO_2$ greater than 50 mm Hg for ≥ 25% of total sleep time.

$P_{ET}CO_2$

Capnography[27,28] consists of the continuous measurement of the fraction of CO_2 in exhaled gas. This is usually performed using an infrared sensor and, less commonly, a mass spectrophotometer. The PCO_2 is determined by multiplication of the fraction of CO_2 by (Patm—47 mm Hg). Here, the Patm is the atmospheric pressure (760 mm Hg at sea level) and 47 mm Hg is the partial pressure of H_2O in exhaled gas at body temperature. A schematic tracing of exhaled PCO_2 versus time is shown in Figure 8–18. During initial exhalation, the dead space (PCO_2 = 0) reaches the sensor (phase 1), then a mixture of dead space and alveolar gas (phase 2), and finally, alveolar gas (phase 3). The alveolar plateau occurs because the PCO_2 in the air from the different alveoli differs slightly. The differences are larger (slope of alveolar plateau steeper) in patients with lung disease. The $P_{ET}CO_2$ is an estimate of the mean alveolar PCO_2 (and, therefore, an estimate of the $PaCO_2$). Of note, there is a gradient between the $PaCO_2$ and the $P_{ET}CO_2$ ($PaCO_2$—$P_{ET}CO_2$) with the $PaCO_2$ being typically 2 to 5 mm Hg higher than the $P_{ET}CO_2$ in normal individuals. In lung disease, the gradient can be much larger. In general, the $P_{ET}CO_2$ is a valid estimate of $PaCO_2$ only if an alveolar plateau is present.

The two common methods of capnography are mainstream and side stream. In the mainstream method, the sensor is located directly in the path of exhaled gas. In the side stream method, gas is continually suctioned through a tube to a more remote sensor (in the instrument at bedside). In the side stream approach, nasal cannulas are used to suction exhaled gas from the nares (Fig. 8–19). When no CO_2 is exhaled (during inspiration or apnea), the nasal cannula suctions room air (PCO_2 = 0). In the side stream method, there is a delay in exhaled gas reaching the sensor so the CO_2 tracing is delayed compared with the exhaled airflow (see Fig. 8–19).

The exhaled CO_2 tracing is sometimes used to indicate apnea (absence of exhaled PCO_2). However, this is not recommended for two reasons. First, gas sampled by the nasal cannula may not detect mouth breathing, and second, small expiratory puffs rich in CO_2 may still produce deflections in the exhaled CO_2 trace[29] (Fig. 8–20).

Capnography is used much more frequently during pediatric than in adult sleep studies.[1-3,30] Children may have long periods of obstructive hypoventilation (see Chapter 9) due to high upper airway resistance (airflow limitation without discrete apneas or hypopneas). Other than a mild decrease in the SpO_2, the significance of these events would be underestimated except for the demonstration of an increase in $P_{ET}CO_2$.

TcPCO$_2$ MONITORING

Measurement of $TcPCO_2$[30,31] depends on the fact that heating of capillaries in the skin causes increased capillary blood flow and makes the skin permeable to the diffusion of CO_2. The CO_2 in the capillaries diffuses through the skin and is measured by an electrode at the skin surface. The measured value is corrected for the fact that heat increases the skin CO_2 production as the measured value exceeds the $PaCO_2$ measured at 37°C. Typically, $TcPCO_2$ electrodes are calibrated with a reference gas. A thermostat controls the heating of the membrane-skin interface. It is usually recommended that the probe of most $TcPCO_2$ monitoring devices be moved every 3 to 4 hours to avoid skin irritation/damage.

The response time of newer $TcPCO_2$ units has improved, but in general, the measured PCO_2 may not increase rapidly enough to correlate with short respiratory events. However, $TcPCO_2$ can be a good instrument for documenting trends in the PCO_2 during the night. Figure 8–21 shows trends in the SpO_2 and $TcPCO_2$. Decreases in the SpO_2 occur in association with increases in the $TcPCO_2$ during episodes of REM sleep.

ACCURACY OF $P_{ET}CO_2$ AND TcPCO$_2$

The limitations of both methods for estimating the $PaCO_2$ should be considered by the clinician when interpreting the data. This is especially true if measured values are not consistent with what is occurring clinically with the patient. The measurement of $P_{ET}CO_2$ and $TcPCO_2$ was not found to be accurate for determining changes in $PaCO_2$ during sleep by Sanders and coworkers.[32] $P_{ET}CO_2$ was especially inaccurate

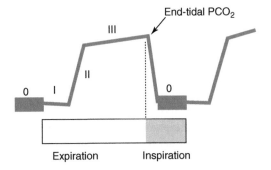

CAPNOGRAPHY - Exhaled CO_2 Versus Time

Phases of exhaled PCO_2

0 Inspiration

I Dead space (no CO_2 exhaled)

II Mixture of dead space and alveolar gas

III Alveolar plateau

FIGURE 8–18 A schematic tracing of exhaled partial pressure of carbon dioxide (PCO_2). The end-tidal PCO_2 is an estimate of the arterial PCO_2.

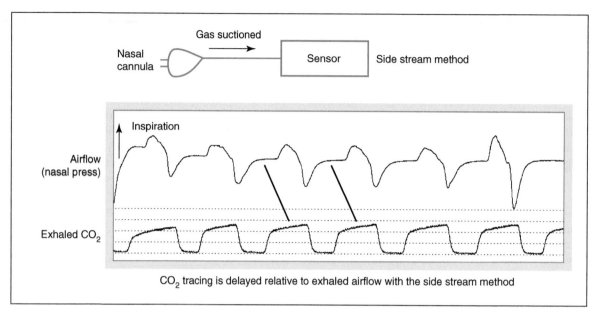

FIGURE 8–19 The CO$_2$ tracing is delayed relative to exhaled airflow in the side stream method.

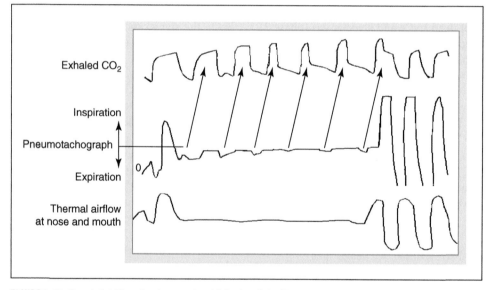

FIGURE 8–20 The exhaled CO$_2$ tracing shows continued deflections during "inspiratory apnea" due to small exhaled puffs of air rich in CO$_2$. *Reproduced from Berry RB: Sleep Medicine Pearls, 2nd ed. Philadelphia: Hanley & Belfus, 2003, p. 90.*

during simultaneous administration of supplemental oxygen or during positive airway pressure treatment. Of note, exhaled gas was sampled from a mask rather than using a nasal cannula. Another investigation found reasonable agreement between the P$_{ET}$CO$_2$ and the TcPCO$_2$ during pediatric polysomnography.[30] Storre and colleagues[31] found reasonable agreement between PaCO$_2$ and TcPCO$_2$ values during noninvasive positive airway pressure titration. The best agreement was between a given PaCO$_2$ value and the corresponding TcPCO$_2$ value about 2 minutes later.

The AASM scoring manual[1] in the respiratory scoring rules for adults states that there was insufficient evidence to recommend a specific method for detecting hypoventilation

during sleep. However, it was stated that P$_{ET}$CO$_2$ or TcPCO$_2$ may be acceptable if validated and calibrated. In the pediatric rules, it states that "acceptable methods for assessing alveolar hypoventilation are either transcutaneous or end-tidal PCO$_2$ monitoring."[1]

Concerning P$_{ET}$CO$_2$ monitoring, the clinician should review the exhaled CO$_2$ tracings to determine whether an alveolar plateau is present. If an alveolar plateau is not present, the P$_{ET}$CO$_2$ value may not be an accurate estimate of PaCO$_2$. Other problems for exhaled PCO$_2$ monitoring include oral breathing and occlusion of the nasal cannula with secretions. If tidal volumes are very small, a true alveolar sample may never reach the sensor. If only a mixture of

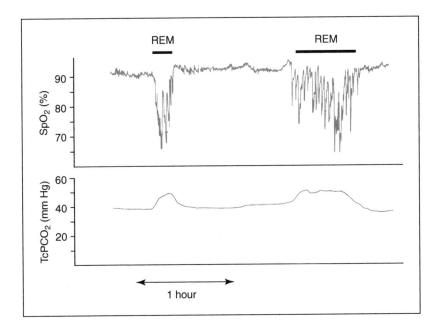

FIGURE 8–21 Trends in the arterial oxygen saturation (SpO$_2$) and transcutaneous partial pressure of carbon dioxide (TcPCO$_2$) during the night. Note the simultaneous increase in transcutaneous PCO$_2$ and the decrease in SpO$_2$ during episodes of rapid eye movement (REM) sleep.

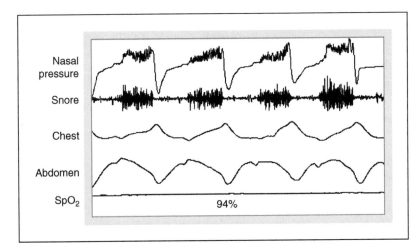

FIGURE 8–22 Snoring noted both in the snore sensor (applied to the neck near the trachea) and as a vibration (oscillation) in the nasal pressure signal. Note that the nasal pressure signal also has a flattened shape. SpO$_2$ = pulse oximetry.

dead space (PCO$_2$ = 0) and alveolar gas is sampled, the P$_{ET}$CO$_2$ value will likely be much lower than the PaCO$_2$.

Concerning TcPCO$_2$ measurement, the actual tracings should also be carefully reviewed. If an abrupt change (offset) in the TcPCO$_2$ tracing is noted, this suggests a measurement artifact is present. Most TcPCO$_2$ devices require calibration at the start of monitoring. Poor application of the sensor or dislodgment of the sensor during sleep can cause a measurement artifact. There is some advantage to the simultaneous use of both P$_{ET}$CO$_2$ and TcPCO$_2$ if tolerated. If the values show reasonable agreement during periods of stable breathing, this increases confidence in their validity. Of course, the goal standard to validate the accuracy of their measurements is a simultaneous ABG measurement.

SNORING SENSORS

Snoring is a sound produced by vibration of upper airway structures. Although snoring sensors are widely used, there is little published evidence to demonstrate the utility of measurement/detection of snoring during sleep. When snoring is present, upper airway narrowing of some degree can be inferred. There is evidence that vibration of different areas of the upper airway causes different sounds. However, the utility of this information remains to be determined. Snore sensors are usually microphones or PE transducers that are usually applied to the neck near the trachea. Microphones can also be attached to the upper chest area or the face. Snoring can also be seen in the NP signal as a rapid oscillation[9,13] in the pressure tracing if an appropriate high-frequency filter setting (100 Hz) is used and the transducer is sufficiently sensitive. Of note, some NP transducers have a choice of output of a filtered or an unfiltered signal. The unfiltered signal must be used to detect snoring. The AASM scoring manual[1] does not provide guidance on use of snoring sensors and the signal is not part of the scoring criteria for respiratory events in adults. Snoring is mentioned in scoring of RERAs in children. Figure 8–22 illustrates an example of snoring. Snoring is visualized in both the snore sensor applied to the neck and the NP signal.

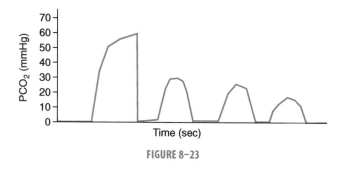

FIGURE 8–23

CLINICAL REVIEW QUESTIONS

1. The sum of the thorax and abdominal band RIP signals (RIPsum) is an estimate of:

   A. Airflow (flow rate).

   B. Tidal volume.

2. Which of the following is NOT true about the nasal pressure signal?

   A. More accurate estimate of flow than most thermal sensors.

   B. Signal is proportional to the flow rate.

   C. Measures the pressure drop across the nasal inlet.

   D. Flattening of the inspiratory flow suggests airflow limitation is present.

   E. NP signal tends to underestimate flow at low flow rates and overestimate flow at high flow rates.

3. Figure 8–23 is a schematic of a tracing of exhaled PCO_2 during a sleep study. The best estimate of the $PaCO_2$ is which of the following?

   A. 60 mm Hg.

   B. Slightly greater than 60 mm Hg.

   C. Slightly lower than 60 mm Hg.

   D. 30 mm Hg.

   E. 25 mm Hg.

4. Which of these can cause a greater than expected PaO_2 for a given SpO_2?

   A. Lower PCO_2.

   B. Lower temperature.

   C. Higher pH (lower hydrogen ion concentration).

   D. Higher PCO_2.

Answers

1. **B.** The deflection in the RIPsum is an estimate of tidal volume. A calibrated RIP signal is a more accurate estimate of tidal volume. The time derivative of the RIPsum signal is an estimate of flow.

2. **B.** The NP signal is proportional to the square of the flow rate. For this reason, a square root transformation of the NP signal is a better estimate of airflow. However, the

clinical importance of using this transformation has not been demonstrated.

3. **B.** The $P_{ET}CO_2$ provides an estimate of the $PaCO_2$ when a plateau is present. There is a gradient between the $P_{ET}CO_2$ and the $PaCO_2$. Usually, the $PaCO_2$ is 2 to 5 mm Hg above the end-tidal value. The exhaled PCO_2 is the mixture of gas from many alveoli. (Rarely, the $P_{ET}CO_2$ is greater than the $PaCO_2$ due to late emptying of alveoli with very high $PaCO_2$ values).

4. **D.** When the oxyhemoglobin saturation curve is shifted to the right, a given SaO_2 is associated with a higher PaO_2. The curve is shifted to the right by an increase in $PaCO_2$ (see Fig. 8–14).

REFERENCES

1. Iber C, Ancoli-Israel S, Chesson A, Quan SF for the American Academy of Sleep Medicine: The AASM Manual for the Scoring of Sleep and Associated Events: Rules, Terminology and Technical Specifications, 1st ed. Westchester, IL: American Academy of Sleep Medicine, 2007.
2. Redline S, Budhiraja R, Kapur V, et al: The scoring of respiratory events in sleep: reliability and validity. J Clin Sleep Med 2007;3:169–200.
3. American Academy of Sleep Medicine Task Force: Sleep-related breathing disorders in adults: recommendation for syndrome definition and measurement techniques in clinical research. Sleep 1999;22:667–689.
4. Berg S, Haight JSJ, Yap V, et al: Comparison of direct and indirect measurement of respiratory airflow: implications for hypopneas. Sleep 1997;20:60–64.
5. Farré R, Montserrat JM, Rotger M, et al: Accuracy of thermistors and thermocouples as flow-measuring devices for detecting hypopneas. Eur Respir J 1998;11:179–182.
6. Berry RB, Koch GL, Trautz S, Wagner MH: Comparison of respiratory event detection by a polyvinylidene fluoride film airflow sensor and a pneumotachograph in sleep apnea patients. Chest 2005;128:1331–1338.
7. Norman RG, Ahmed M, Walsben JA, Rapoport DM: Detection of respiratory events during NPSG: nasal cannula/pressure sensor versus thermistor. Sleep 1997;20:1175–1184.
8. Hosselet J, Normal RG, Ayapa I, Rapoport DM: Detection of flow limitation with a nasal cannula/pressure transducer system. Am J Respir Crit Care Med 1988;157:1461–1467.
9. Hernandez L, Ballester E, Farre R, et al: Performance of nasal prongs in sleep studies. Chest 2001;119:442–450.
10. Farré R, Rigau J, Montserrat JM, et al: Relevance of linearizing nasal prongs for assessing hypopneas and flow limitation during sleep. Am J Respir Crit Care Med 2001;163:494–497.
11. Thurnheer R, Xie X, Bloch KE: Accuracy of nasal cannula pressure recordings for assessment of ventilation during sleep. Am J Respir Crit Care Med 2001;146:1914–1919.
12. Heitman SJ, Atkar RS, Hajduk EA, et al: Validation of nasal pressure for the identification of apneas/hypopneas during sleep. Am J Respir Crit Care Med 2002;166:386–391.
13. Berry RB: Esophageal and nasal pressure monitoring during sleep. In Lee-Chiong TL, Sateia MJ, Caraskadon MA (eds): Sleep Medicine. Philadelphia: Hanley & Belfus, 2002, pp. 661–671.
14. Tobin MJ, Cohen MA, Sackner MA: Breathing abnormalities during sleep. Arch Intern Med 1983;143:1221–1228.
15. Staats BA, Bonekat HW, Harris CD, Offord KP: Chest wall motion in sleep apnea. Am Rev Respir Dis 1984;130:59–63.

16. Bennett JR, Dunroy HMA, Corfield DR, et al: Respiratory muscle activity during REM sleep in patients with diaphragm paralysis. Neurology 2004;61:134–137.

17. White JES, Drinnan MJ, Smithson AJ, et al: Respiratory muscle activity and oxygenation during sleep in patients with muscle weakness. Eur Respir J 1995;8:808–814.

18. Stoohs RA, Blum HC, Knaack L, et al: Comparison of pleural pressure and transcutaneous diaphragmatic electromyogram in obstructive sleep apnea syndrome. Sleep 2005;28:321–329.

19. Wagner MH, Berry RB: A patient with sickle disease and a low baseline sleeping oxygen saturation. J Clin Sleep Med 2007;3:313–315.

20. Toffaletti J, Zijlstra W: Misconceptions in reporting oxygen saturation. Anesth Analg 2007;105:S5–S9.

21. Roughton FJW, Darling RC: The effect of carbon monoxide on the oxyhemoglobin dissociation curve. Am J Physiol 1944;141:17–31.

22. Tremper KK, Barker SJ: Pulse oximetry. Anesthesiology 1989;70:98–108.

23. Barker SJ, Tremper KK: The effects of carbon monoxide inhalation of pulse oximetry and transcutaneous PO_2. Anesthesiology 1987;66:677–679.

24. Barker SJ, Tremper KK, Hyatt J: Effects of methemoglobin on pulse oximetry and mixed venous oximetry. Anesthesiology 1989;7:112–117.

25. Davila DG, Richards KC, Marshall BL, et al: Oximeter performance: the influence of acquisition parameters. Chest 2002;122:1654–1660.

26. Jasani R, Sanders MH, Strollo PJ: Diagnostic studies for apnea/hypopnea. In Johnson JT, Gluckman JL, Sanders MH (eds): Management of Obstructive Sleep Apnea. London: Martin Dunitz, 2002, p. 68.

27. Gravenstein JS, Paulus DA: Clinical perspectives. In Gravenstein JS, Jaffe MB, Paulus DA (eds): Capnography. Cambridge, UK: Cambridge University Press, 2004, pp. 3–12.

28. D'Mello J, Butani M: Capnography. Indian J Anaesthesiol 2002;46:269–278.

29. Berry RB: Sleep Medicine Pearls, 2nd ed. Philadelphia: Hanley & Belfus, 2003, p. 90.

30. Kirk VG, Batuyong ED, Bohn SG: Transcutaneous carbon dioxide monitoring and capnography during pediatric polysomnography. Sleep 2006;29:1601–1608.

31. Storre JH, Steurer B, Kabitz HJ, et al: Transcutaneous PCO_2 monitoring during initiation of noninvasive ventilation. Chest 2007;132:1810–1816.

32. Sanders MH, Kern NB, Costantino JP, et al: Accuracy of end-tidal and transcutaneous PCO_2 monitoring during sleep. Chest 1994;106:472–483.

Chapter 9

Monitoring Respiration—Event Definitions and Examples

- An oronasal thermal sensor is recommended for apnea identification. The nasal pressure signal is recommended for hypopnea identification. An event with absent nasal pressure excursions but persistent oronasal sensor excursions >10% of baseline would not be scored as an apnea.
- In adults, an event may be an RERA or a hypopnea based on which hypopnea definition is being used.
- Hypoventilation in adults is defined as an increase in the $PaCO_2$ of 10 mm Hg or greater from an awake supine value.
- Hypoventilation in children is defined as a PCO_2 greater than 50 mm Hg for 25% or more of the total sleep time by either $P_{ET}CO_2$ monitoring or $TcPCO_2$ monitoring.
- Obstructive apneas and hypopnea in children are defined based on two missed breaths rather than an absolute time duration.
- Respiratory rules for children are used for patients younger than 18 years. Adult respiratory scoring rules may be used for children aged 13 years or older.
- In children, central apneas have absent inspiratory effort throughout the **entire duration** of the event and one of the following is met:
  1. The event lasts 20 seconds or longer.
  2. The event lasts 2 breaths (or the duration of 2 breaths as determined by the baseline breathing pattern) AND is associated with an arousal, an awakening, or a 3% or greater desaturation.

RESPIRATORY EVENTS IN ADULTS

History of Respiratory Event Definitions

To understand the origins of the current respiratory event definitions, a historical perspective is helpful. The apnea-hypopnea index (AHI) is the number of apneas and hypopneas per hour of sleep. This metric is often used to make the diagnosis of sleep apnea and to grade the severity. Definitions of apnea have been relatively standard (typically absent or nearly absent airflow for ≥10 sec), but varying definitions

of hypopnea (reductions in airflow) have resulted in a "floating metric."[1] Early studies of patients with obstructive sleep apnea (OSA) focused on obstructive apnea,[2] hence, the name of the syndrome. However, it soon became obvious that reductions in airflow (hypopnea) also had clinical significance. The importance of *hypopnea,* defined as a reduction in airflow associated with a 4% or greater desaturation, was emphasized by Block and coworkers.[3] Gould and colleagues[4] noted that some patients fit the clinical picture of OSA but the majority of their respiratory events were hypopneas rather than apneas. They defined hypopnea as a 50% reduction in respiratory inductance plethysmography (RIP) belt deflections lasting greater than 10 seconds and proposed the term the "sleep hypopnea syndrome." Others have used the term the "obstructive sleep apnea hypopnea syndrome." A landmark paper on the incidence of obstructive sleep apnea (Wisconsin cohort study) defined hypopnea as a discernible reduction in the amplitude of calibrated RIP plus an arterial oxygen desaturation of 4% or more.[5] The Sleep Heart Health Study,[6] a large multicenter population-based investigation, defined hypopneas as a decrease in airflow or thoracoabdominal excursion of at least 30% of baseline for 10 seconds or more accompanied by a 4% or more decrease in oxygen saturation.[5] Airflow was monitored with an oronasal thermal sensor and respiratory effort with RIP belts. Using this definition of hypopnea, the study found associations between an increase in the AHI and cardiovascular morbidity.

The widespread use of nasal pressure (NP) monitoring allowed recognition of more subtle and more frequent changes in airflow during sleep than was possible with thermal devices.[7] It was also recognized that reductions in airflow from obstructive events not associated with desaturations could be associated with consequences such as arousal from sleep and sleep fragmentation (upper airway resistance syndrome).[8] Therefore, definitions of hypopnea based on flow and arousal were proposed. In order to standardize definitions of respiratory events, a consensus statement was published in 1992 ("Chicago criteria").[9] Criteria for an obstructive apnea/hypopnea event (OAHE) was presented with no differentiation between obstructive apnea and hypopnea because "both events have similar pathophysiology." An OAHE was defined as a 50% or greater reduction in airflow from baseline lasting 10 seconds or longer using a valid measure of breathing OR any discernible reduction in airflow using a valid measure of breathing during sleep when associated with either an arousal or a 3% or greater arterial oxygen desaturation. Valid measures of breathing included a pneumotachograph, NP, RIPsum (or simultaneous reduction in both chest and abdominal RIP band signals). A 3% rather than a 4% desaturation was recommended based on reanalysis of Wisconsin cohort data showing similar associations with important outcomes using either 3% or 4% desaturations. A *respiratory effort–related arousal (RERA)* was defined as an event lasting 10 seconds or longer with a pattern of progressively more negative esophageal pressure terminated by a sudden change in pressure to a less negative pressure and arousal.

The choice of the definition of apnea and hypopnea can make a significant difference in the AHI and, therefore, a significant difference in the incidence of OSA.[10-12] Ideal definitions of AHI would identify a population with symptoms and with an increased risk of adverse outcomes (if untreated). As previously noted, AHI values based on hypopnea definitions requiring an associated desaturation in large population studies have shown that increases in AHI are associated with cardiovascular morbidity. Another consideration in choosing a definition of hypopnea is the desire to have a high interscorer reliability. Whitney and associates[10] reviewed the results when three experienced scorers analyzed the sleep studies of 20 randomly selected patients using different definitions of hypopnea. The sleep studies had been performed using a thermal sensor for airflow. Hypopnea was defined as a reduction in the nasal-oral thermal flow signal or the chest and abdominal RIP excursions to 70% of baseline or lower for a duration of 10 seconds or longer. There was a very large range of resulting AHIs (Table 9–1). Using a definition of hypopnea based entirely on a reduction in flow magnitude, there was a reasonably high interscorer reliability (see Table 9–1). However, inclusion of a desaturation criteria in the hypopnea definition did significantly improve the interscorer reliability for identifying these events. One rationale for not including arousal in hypopnea definitions is that scoring of arousals has relatively low interscorer reliability (see Table 9–1). However, the reliability of scoring hypopneas with a definition using a combination of flow and either arousal or desaturation resulted in only slightly lower interscorer reliability than flow plus desaturation alone. Of note, the method used to define a reduction in flow (nasal-oral thermal sensor versus RIP or NP) and the patient population studied may affect the changes in the AHI produced by varying definitions of hypopnea. Tsai and coworkers[12] defined *AHI-A* as a discernible reduction in thoracoabdominal deflection (RIP) of 10 seconds or longer associated with a 4% or greater arterial oxygen desaturation and *AHI-B* as a discernible reduction in thoracoabdominal deflection longer than 10 seconds plus either a 4% or greater desaturation OR an arousal. They found AHI-B was, on average, only about 2 events/hr greater than AHI-A. However, depending on the AHI cutoff criteria, AHI-B did diagnose more patients as having OSA.

TABLE 9–1

Effects of Varying Hypopnea Definitions on Interscorer Reliability and Apnea-Hypopnea Index (Events by Three Scorers)*

	MEAN EVENTS/HR			ICC
AHI #1 Hypopnea = 30% reduction in airflow	25.9	32.9	27.4	0.74
AHI #2 Hypopnea = 30% reduction in airflow + 3% desaturation	11.35	9.97	10.8	0.97
AHI #3 Hypopnea = 30% reduction in airflow + 4% desaturation	6.08	5.38	5.75	0.99
AHI #4 Hypopnea = 30% reduction in airflow + 3% desaturation OR arousal	14.11	14.58	14.06	0.95
AHI #5 Hypopnea = 30% reduction in airflow + 4% desaturation OR arousal	9.75	10.78	10.05	0.94
Arousal index	13.5	20.63	17.31	0.54

*Hypopnea is defined as a reduction in nasal-oral thermal flow or chest and abdominal RIP excursions to 70% of baseline for 10 seconds or longer.
AHI = apnea-hypopnea index; ICC = intraclass correlation, a measure of interscorer reliability; RIP = respiratory inductance plethysmography.
Adapted from Whitney CW. Gottleib DJ, Redline S, et al: Reliability of scoring respiratory disturbance indices and sleep staging. Sleep 1998;21:749–757.

A clinical practice parameter published by the American Academy of Sleep Medicine (AASM) recommended a definition of hypopnea similar to the one used in the population-based studies (30% reduction in flow + ≥4% desaturation).[13] The rationale for the choice was that large population-based studies had shown an increased risk of cardiovascular consequences associated with an increased AHI based on this hypopnea definition. The Centers for Medicaid and Medicare Services (CMS) subsequently adopted this practice parameter definition of hypopnea for establishing criteria for continuous positive airway pressure (CPAP) reimbursement (http://www.cmshhs.gov/mcd/viewdecisionmemoasp?id= 204 2008).

The recently published AASM scoring manual[14] provides definitions of apnea, hypopnea, and RERAs. There are different respiratory scoring rules for adults and children. An accompanying review[15] discussed the evidence for the new respiratory rules. In the following sections, the AASM scoring manual definitions for apnea, hypopnea, and RERA events are presented (Table 9–2). Although the new criteria are expected to standardize terminology, the hypopnea controversy will likely continue. A recent study by Ruehland and colleagues[16] found that compared with a diagnosis of OSA based on Chicago criteria, using the AASM recommended definition of hypopnea would result in 40% of patients being classified as not having OSA. If the AASM alternative hypopnea definition was used, 25% of the patients diagnosed with OSA by the Chicago criteria would be classified as negative for OSA.

TABLE 9–2

Adult Respiratory Event Rules

Apnea	Score apnea when **all** of the following are met:
	• Oronasal thermal sensor (or alternative) drops by ≥90% of baseline.
	• Duration ≥ 10 sec.
	• At least 90% of events duration must meet apnea amplitude reduction criteria.
	Classification
	  1. Obstructive: continued or increased inspiratory effort for duration of apnea.
	  2. Mixed
	    • Initially absent inspiratory effort in the first portion of the event.
	    • Resumption of inspiratory effort during second portion of event.
	  3. Central: Absent inspiratory effort for duration of apnea.
	(Desaturation NOT needed to score an apnea.)

Hypopnea recommended	All criteria must be met: • NP excursions (or alternative sensor) drop by ≥30% of baseline amplitude. • Duration ≥ 10 sec. • At least 90% of duration must meet hypopnea amplitude criteria. • ≥4% arterial oxygen desaturation from pre-event baseline.
Hypopnea alternative	All criteria must be met: • NP excursions (or alternative sensor) drop by ≥50% of baseline amplitude. • Duration ≥ 10 sec. • At least 90% of duration must meet hypopnea amplitude criteria. • ≥3% arterial oxygen desaturation from pre-event baseline **OR** arousal.
RERA	• A sequence of breaths lasting at least 10 sec. • Increasing respiratory effort or flattening of the NP waveform. • Followed by an arousal from sleep. • Does not meet criteria for an apnea or hypopnea.
Hypoventilation*	• Increase in $PaCO_2$ or validated surrogate ≥10 mm Hg above a supine awake value.

*For adults, hypoventilation is based on the $PaCO_2$. No other sensor was recommended for documentation of hypoventilation. It was stated that $P_{ET}CO_2$ or $TcPCO_2$ may be used as surrogate measures of $PaCO_2$ if there is demonstration of reliability and validity.
NP = nasal pressure; $PaCO_2$ = arterial partial pressure of carbon dioxide; $P_{ET}CO_2$ = end-tidal carbon dioxide pressure; RERA = respiratory effort–related arousal; $TcPCO_2$ = transcutaneous carbon dioxide pressure.
From Iber C, Ancoli-Israel S, Chesson A, Quan SF for the American Academy of Sleep Medicine: The AASM Manual for the Scoring of Sleep and Associated Events: Rules, Terminology and Technical Specifications, 1st ed. Westchester, IL: American Academy of Sleep Medicine, 2007.

The term *respiratory disturbance index*[17] (RDI) is used by some sleep centers and publications. In many sleep centers, the terms RDI and AHI mean the same thing. However, the 2005 AASM practice parameters for indications for polysomnography (PSG) defined the RDI as equal to the AHI + RERA index. Here, the RERA index is the number of RERAs/hr of sleep. The 1992 Consensus statement of the AASM recommended making a diagnosis of OSA based on the number of apneas/hypopneas obstructive events + RERAs/hr of sleep and also presented severity criteria based on this metric.[9] However, the term RDI was not specifically used. Of note, the term RDI was not defined in the AASM scoring manual. It is important to note the definition of RDI when reading sleep study reports or publications concerning sleep apnea.

Recommended Respiratory Sensors in Adults[14]

The sensors and methods for respiratory monitoring are discussed in detail in Chapter 8. The recommended sensor for apnea detection is a thermal flow sensor at the nose and mouth (oronasal thermal sensor). If the thermal signal is inadequate, the NP signal may be used. The recommended sensor for hypopnea detection is NP with or without a square root transformation. If the NP signal is inadequate, either the oronasal thermal signal or the RIP signal (calibrated or uncalibrated) may be used. Whether the RIP sum signal or both chest and abdomen RIP signals are to be used was not specified. The sensors recommended for detecting respiratory effort include esophageal manometry or RIP (calibrated or uncalibrated). An alternative sensor for detection of respiratory effort is diaphragmatic/intercostals EMG. The sensor for detection of arterial oxygen desaturation is pulse oximetry. It is recommended that oximeters use a maximal averaging time of 3 seconds at a heart rate of 80 bpm or greater. At lower heart rates, most oximeters choose the averaging time based on heart rate and average at least 3 pulses. The recommended sensor for detection of an RERA (see later) is esophageal manometry. Flattening in the NP signal or RIP are alternative sensors that may be used.

Definition of Apnea (AASM Scoring Manual)[14]

Sensor: The recommended sensor for apnea detection is a thermal flow sensor at the nose and mouth.

Apnea Scoring Rules in Adults (AASM Scoring Manual)[14]

Apnea Rule: Score an apnea when all of the following criteria are met:

1. There is a **drop** in the peak thermal sensor excursion by ≥90% of baseline.
2. The duration of the event lasts at least 10 seconds.
3. At least 90% of the event's duration meets the amplitude reduction criteria for apnea.

Apnea Types
1. Score a respiratory event as an OBSTRUCTIVE apnea if it meets apnea criteria and is associated with **continued or increased inspiratory effort** throughout the entire period of absent airflow.
2. Score a respiratory event as a CENTRAL apnea if it meets apnea criteria and is associated with **absent inspiratory effort** throughout the entire period of absent airflow.
3. Score a respiratory event as a MIXED apnea if it meets apnea criteria and is associated with **absent inspiratory effort** in the **initial part** of the event, followed by **resumption of inspiratory effort** in the **second part** of the event.

Figure 9–1 presents examples of obstructive, central, and mixed apneas using esophageal pressure to detect respiratory effort. Figure 9–2 presents examples of the corresponding events using chest and abdominal RIP belts.

The nasal-oral thermal sensor and not the NP signal is used to score apnea. Absent NP signal excursions do not meet criteria for scoring apnea if nasal-oral thermal sensor excursions are still present and do not meet criteria for scoring an apnea. In the event shown in Figure 9–3, NP excursions are absent for greater than 10 seconds. However, the event is not scored as an apnea because the thermal signal is not decreased by 90% of baseline. The combination of absent NP excursions and persistent nasal-oral thermal sensor excursion is likely due to oral breathing. Also note that the apnea criteria do NOT depend on the presence of either arterial oxygen saturation (SaO_2) or arousal. The AASM scoring manual states that if the oronasal thermal signal is not functioning, one then uses the NP signal to score apnea. Although not specifically recommended by the AASM scoring manual, one could also use the RIPsum signal.

Hypopnea Scoring Rules in Adults[14]

In the AASM scoring manual, two hypopnea definitions are presented (a recommended hypopnea definition and an alternate hypopnea definition).

Hypopnea (Recommended)
Score a hypopnea if all of the following criteria are met:

1. The NP signal excursions (or those of the alternative hypopnea sensor) **drop by ≥30% of baseline.**

2. The duration of this drop occurs for a period of at least 10 seconds.
3. There is a **4% or greater desaturation from the pre-event baseline.**
4. At least **90% of the event's duration** must meet the amplitude reduction of criteria.

This recommended hypopnea definition is essentially the definition recommended by the 2001 AASM Clinical Practice Parameter[13] and later accepted by CMS. As discussed previously, evidence for the use of this definition includes the fact that a similar definition was used in the Wisconsin Cohort Study and the Sleep Heart Health Study and that an increased AHI based on this hypopnea definition was associated with an increased risk of cardiovascular morbidity in those studies. In addition, as previously mentioned, definitions of hypopnea using changes in SaO_2 tend to have high interscorer reliability. The respiratory event illustrated in Figure 9–4 meets the *recommended* criteria for a hypopnea because the NP signal excursions are essentially zero for over 10 seconds and the event is associated with an SaO_2 of 4% or greater.

Hypopnea (Alternative)
Score a hypopnea if all of the following criteria are met:

1. The NP signal excursions (or those of the alternative hypopnea sensor) **drop by ≥50% of baseline.**
2. The duration of this drop occurs for a period of at least 10 seconds.
3. There is a **≥3% desaturation** from the pre-event baseline *or the event is associated with an arousal.*
4. At least 90% of the event's duration must meet the amplitude reduction of criteria for hypopnea.

The alternative definition of hypopnea is similar to the 1999 AASM Task Force Consensus definition of an obstructive apnea/hypopnea event. The use of 3% rather than 4% is based on the fact that reanalysis of some of the large studies using a 3% desaturation–based instead of a 4% desaturation-based hypopnea definition found similar results.[9] The definition recognizes that some reduction in airflow events are not associated with a drop in the SaO_2 of 4% or greater but are associated with arousal. Frequent respiratory arousals in the absence of significant desaturation can result in fragmented sleep and daytime sleepiness. However, interscorer reliability of scoring hypopneas with a definition based on either desaturation or arousals is slightly lower than with the scoring of events associated only with desaturations (see Table 9–1).

Event Duration Rules[14]

A. Event duration (apnea or hypopnea) is measured from the **nadir preceding** the first breath that is clearly reduced to the **beginning of the first breath** that approximates the baseline breathing amplitude (Fig. 9–5).
B. When the baseline amplitude cannot be easily determined (underlying breathing variability is large), events

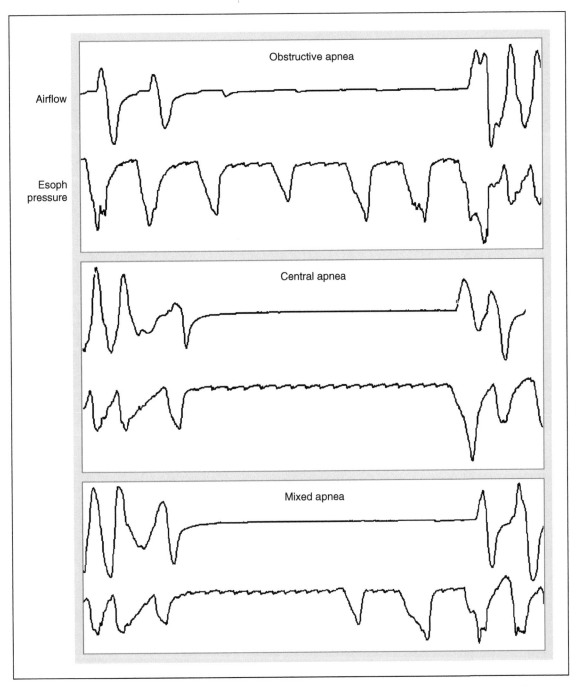

FIGURE 9–1 Examples of obstructive, central, and mixed apnea. Airflow was recorded using a pneumotachograph in a mask over the nose and mouth and respiratory effort by esophageal pressure monitoring. The frequent small deflections in the esophageal pressure are cardiac artifact.

can also be terminated when either there is a **sustained increase in breathing amplitude** or, in the case in which a desaturation has occurred, there is **event-associated resaturation of at least 2%.**

Clarification of Event Duration Criteria for Apneas and Hypopneas

The AASM scoring manual steering committee publishes responses to questions about the scoring rules and clarifications as frequently asked questions (FAQs) (http://www. aasmnet.org/Resources/PDF/FAQsScoringManual.pdf). In response to a question concerning event duration, the FAQ R11 stated that the amplitude criteria to define events need last for only 9 contiguous seconds. For example, if 9 contiguous seconds of an event has a 90% or greater drop in nasal-oral thermal sensor excursions, the event is scored as an apnea even if, based on the event duration rules, the event lasts for longer than 10 seconds. Of note, an apnea or a hypopnea is NOT scored unless the event duration is 10 seconds or longer.

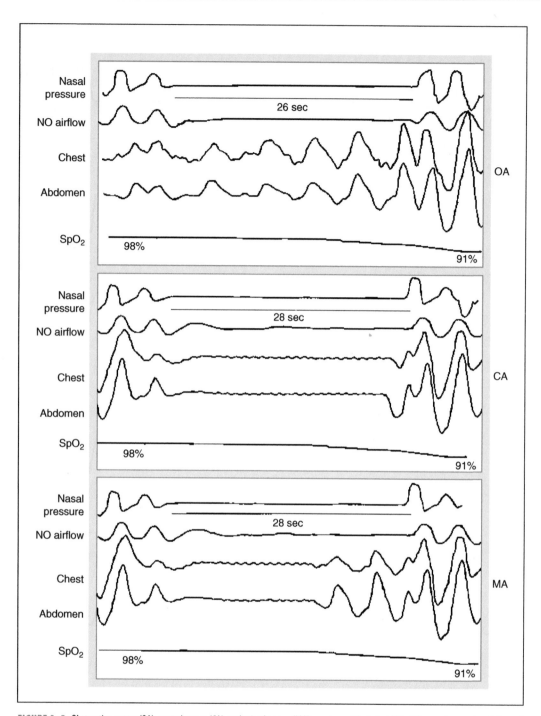

FIGURE 9–2 Obstructive apnea (OA), central apnea (CA), and mixed apnea (MA) events are illustrated. NO airflow = the nasal-oral thermal airflow sensor signal; chest and abdomen = RIP belt signals; SpO₂ = pulse oximetry.

RERA Rule in Adults (AASM Scoring Manual)[14]

Score an RERA, if there is a sequence of breaths lasting at least 10 seconds characterized by increasing respiratory effort or flattening of the NP waveform leading to an arousal from sleep when the sequence of breaths does not meet criteria for an apnea or a hypopnea (Fig. 9–6).

RERA Detection

As noted previously, the preferred sensor for the detection of RERAs is esophageal manometry, although NP and RIP

can be used.[14] As discussed in Chapter 8, flattening of the NP signal is associated with airflow limitation and usually increasingly negative esophageal pressure (or supraglottic pressure). Arousal often follows a crescendo increase in esophageal pressure deflections (at least during non–rapid eye movement [NREM] sleep) as seen in Figure 9–7. However, respiratory arousal can also occur after a long period of airflow limitation and relatively constant but increased esophageal pressure deflections. Whereas both hypoxia and hypercapnia may drive inspiratory effort during

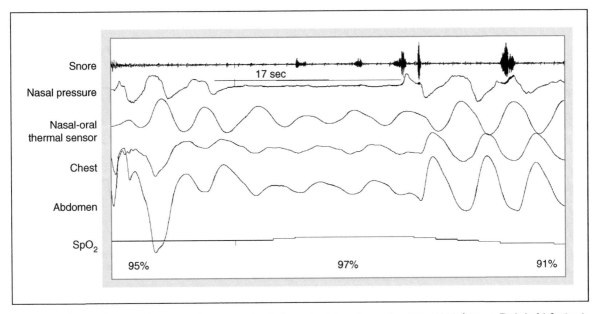

FIGURE 9–3 This event is not scored as an apnea because excursions in the nasal-oral thermal sensor do not meet criteria for apnea. The lack of deflections in the nasal pressure signal is likely due to oral breathing during the event. The event would meet criteria for hypopnea using either the recommended or the alternate American Academy of Sleep Medicine (AASM) criteria. SpO_2 = pulse oximetry.

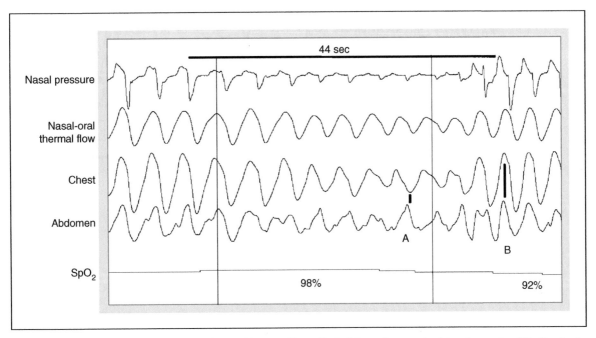

FIGURE 9–4 An event meeting the recommended definition of hypopnea. The amplitude of the nasal pressure signal drops by more than 30% of baseline for well over 9 contiguous seconds and the event duration is longer than 10 seconds. In addition, the event is associated with a greater than 4% desaturation. Note the paradox in the chest and abdomen tracings at *A* during the event but not at *B* after the event. SpO_2 = pulse oximetry. The *vertical lines* are 30 seconds apart.

obstructive respiratory events, it is the magnitude of the inspiratory effort (magnitude of esophageal pressure excursion) and the threshold for arousal that determine whether arousal occurs.[18] During experimental mask occlusion in normal subjects, arousal usually occurs when esophageal pressure deflections (negative pressure) reaches 20 to 30 cm H_2O. However, snorers and patients with OSA may not arouse until esophageal pressures reach 40 to 80 cm H_2O.

This implies a decrease in arousability (high arousal threshold) in these groups.

Because esophageal pressure monitoring is infrequently used, RERA detection is usually based on flattening of the NP signal (flow limitation arousal).[14,19] After arousal, there is usually a sudden change in the NP contour from flat to round (see Fig. 9–7). Ayappa and colleagues[19] compared arousal associated with flow limitation (FLA) and arousal

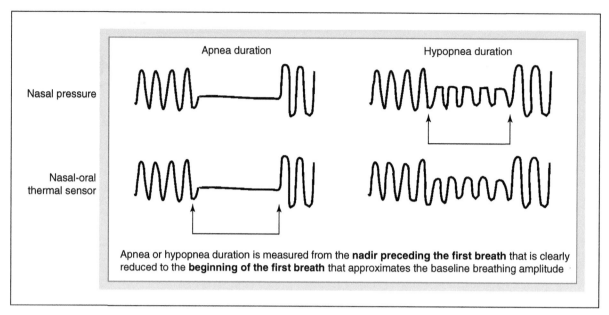

FIGURE 9–5 Event duration rules. Note that the oronasal thermal sensor is used to define the apnea duration and the nasal pressure signal the hypopnea duration.

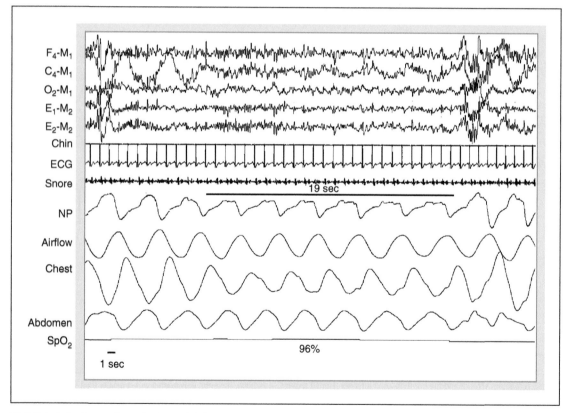

FIGURE 9–6 Respiratory effort–related arousal (RERA). Flattening of nasal pressure for more than 10 seconds followed by an arousal. There is no desaturation so it would not qualify as a hypopnea (by the recommended definition). The drop in flow is not 50% of baseline so the event would not qualify as a hypopnea (alternative definition). ECG = electrocardiogram; NP = nasal pressure; SpO$_2$ = pulse oximetry.

associated with increased respiratory effort by esophageal manometry (RERAs). The FLA index and RERA index were highly correlated (Fig. 9–8). However, a few FLA events were noted with flow limitation but without an increase in respiratory effort. Some RERAs (esophageal pressure manometry) were noted without flow limitation. Thus, although flow limitation (NP flattening) and high respiratory effort most often occur together, this is not invariably true. Fortunately, the majority of RERAs will be detected with NP monitoring.

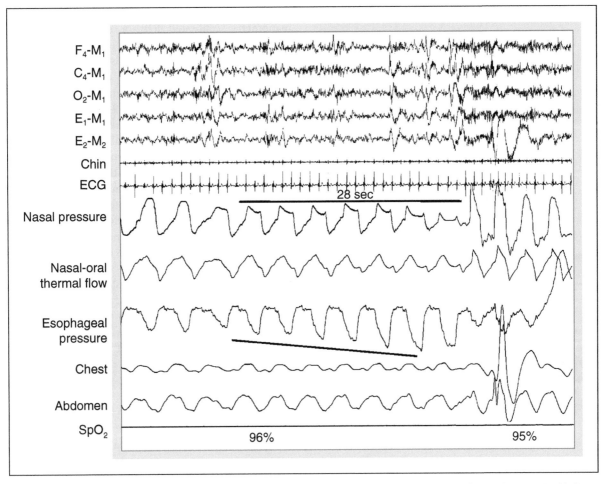

FIGURE 9–7 RERA. The event demonstrates increasing respiratory effort by esophageal pressure *(slanted line)* and flattening of the nasal pressure signal for longer than 10 seconds followed by an arousal. After the event termination, there is a decrease in esophageal pressure excursions and the nasal pressure contour becomes round. The event is not associated with a desaturation and is not a hypopnea by the recommended hypopnea scoring rule. The event also is not associated with a 50% drop in the nasal pressure excursions. Therefore, the event is not a hypopnea using the alternative hypopnea scoring rule. ECG = electrocardiogram; SpO₂ = pulse oximetry.

Hypopnea or RERA?

Of note, if the *recommended* definition of hypopnea is used, some obstructive events that would otherwise meet criteria for the alternate definition of hypopnea would be scored as RERAs. Such an event would be associated with an arousal but not 4% or greater desaturation and have NP flattening for 10 seconds or longer with drop in the excursions of the NP signal by 50% or more from baseline (Fig. 9–9). Note that part of the RERA definition is that the event **does not meet criteria for a hypopnea.**

Relationship of Arousal and Respiratory Event

The AASM scoring manual did not specify a maximum time interval from respiratory event termination until arousal initiation for the arousal to be considered respiratory. FAQ R19 states "The scoring manual does not specify the time requirement linking arousals and respiratory event. When arousals do occur with respiratory events, they usually occur within 5 seconds of airway opening." Arousals associated with respi-

ratory event termination can occur slightly before, concurrent with, or after event termination.[20]

Scoring Apneas and Hypopneas during Wake

In some cases, apneas and hypopneas may begin during an epoch scored as sleep but end in an epoch scored as wake (or vice versa). Scoring manual FAQ R10 states "**If any portion of either the apnea or hypopnea occurs during an epoch that is scored as sleep, then the corresponding respiratory event can be scored and included in the computation of the AHI.** However, if the apnea or hypopnea occurs entirely during an epoch scored as wake, it should not be scored or counted toward the apnea-hypopnea index because of the difficulty of defining a denominator in that situation."

Classification of Hypopneas

The AASM scoring manual recommends that hypopneas not be classified (obstructive, central, or mixed) without a

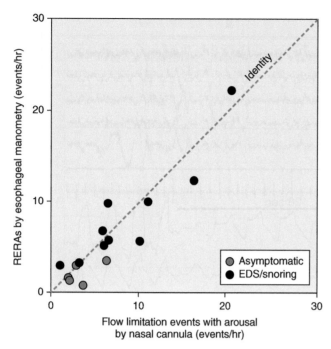

FIGURE 9–8 Flow limitation arousals and respiratory effort–related arousals (RERAs) by esophageal monitoring (events/hour) were highly correlated, although not identical. *Reproduced from Ayappa I, Norman RG, Krieger AC, et al: Non-invasive detection of respiratory effort–related arousals (RERAs) by a nasal cannula/pressure transducer system. Sleep 2000;23:763–771.*

quantitative assessment of ventilatory effort (esophageal manometry, calibrated RIP, or diaphragmatic/intercostal electromyography [EMG]). Of course, an accurate measure of airflow (PNT or NP) would also be needed. The AASM scoring manual did not provide definitions for hypopnea types. However, a possible scheme for defining types of hypopneas is presented in Table 9–3 and Figure 9–10. One can define an *obstructive hypopnea* as one due to an increase in upper airway resistance (usually with increased respiratory effort). A *central hypopnea* would be due to a reduction in respiratory effort with a proportionate decrease in airflow. A *mixed hypopnea* would be characterized by both increased upper airway resistance (NP flattening and airflow limitation) and decreased respiratory effort (decreased esophageal pressure excursions). In the absence of esophageal pressure monitoring, the shape of the NP tracing (or PNT) can provide some clues (see Table 9–3). The presence of a flattened NP tracing, snoring, or chest-abdominal paradox suggests airflow limitation (increased upper airway resistance), whereas a rounded shape without snoring is consistent with a lack of airflow limitation. Even with sophisticated monitoring equipment, it may be difficult to precisely classify some hypopneas.

Chest-Abdominal Paradox

During normal inspiration, the rib cage expands and the diaphragm contracts, moving the abdominal contents

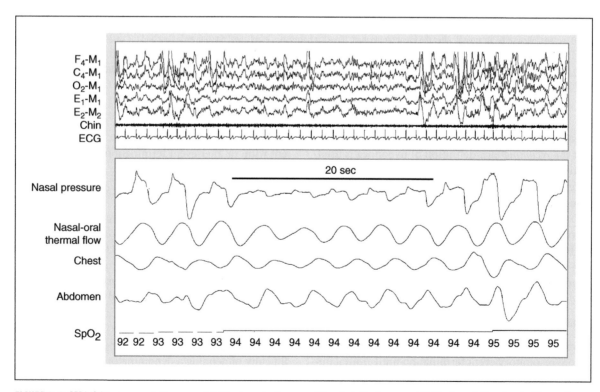

FIGURE 9–9 RERA if the recommended hypopnea definition is used or hypopnea if the alternative hypopnea definition is used. Note that the 20 second arrow is the duration of the 50% drop in NP excursions. However, the event duration as defined by the event duration rules would be longer (nadir preceding first breath that is clearly reduced to the beginning of the first breath that approximates baseline breathing). The event duration would begin one breath earlier and end one breath later than the 20 second line. ECG = electrocardiogram; SpO_2 = pulse oximetry.

TABLE 9–3

Idealized Findings in Hypopnea

TYPE	PNT/NP AMPLITUDE/SHAPE	CHEST/ABDOMEN DEFLECTIONS	ESOPHAGEAL PRESSURE DEFLECTIONS	UPPER AIRWAY RESISTANCE	SNORE
Central	Decreased amplitude Round shape	Decreased No paradox	Decreased	Normal	None
Obstructive	Decreased amplitude Flattened shape	Variable Paradox common	Increased	Increased Airflow limitation	Present
"Mixed"	Decreased amplitude Flattened shape	Decreased Paradox common	Decreased	Increased Airflow limitation	May be present

NP = nasal pressure; PNT = pneumotachogram.

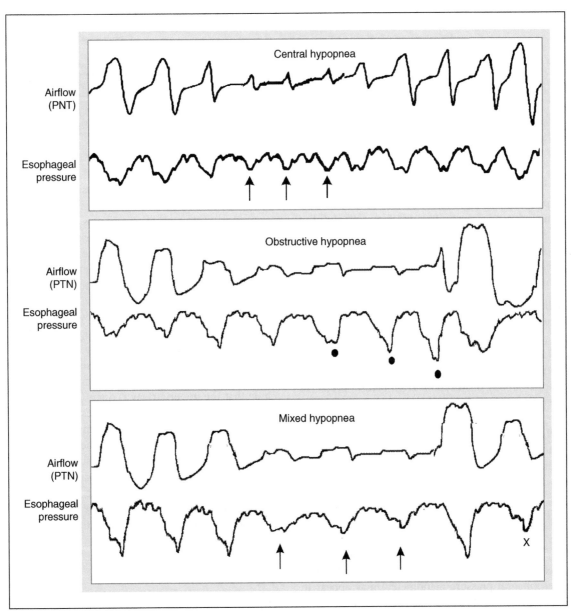

FIGURE 9–10 Examples of central, obstructive, and mixed hypopneas with an accurate measure of airflow (pneumotachograph [PNT]) and esophageal pressure monitoring. In central and mixed hypopnea, the esophageal excursions decrease *(up arrows)*. In mixed hypopnea, airflow limitation is present (flattened airflow), and in central hypopnea, the airflow contour is round. In obstructive hypopnea, the esophageal pressure excursions are increased *(black circles)* for at least part of the event.

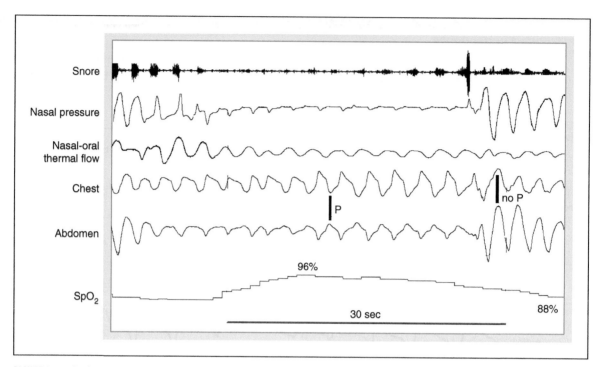

FIGURE 9-11   An obstructive hypopnea with paradox (P) in chest and abdominal movement during the respiratory event but not during less obstructed breathing (no P). SpO$_2$ = pulse oximetry.

downward; the abdomen also moves outward. During chest-abdomen paradox, the chest moves outward and the abdomen inward or vice versa. Paradox is most helpful at identifying high upper airway resistance when it is present during the obstructive event and NOT present during unobstructed breathing (Fig. 9–11; see also Fig. 9–4).

Conditions in which paradox may occur[21]:

1. Loss of diaphragm tone/weakness: The abdomen is sucked inward as the rib cage expands during inspiration.
2. Loss of accessory muscle tone: Destabilizes the rib cage so it may be sucked inward when the diaphragm contracts (abdomen expands).
3. Partial upper airway obstruction: High pleural pressures can overcome mechanisms maintaining rigidity of thorax—parts are sucked inward. This is common in children with more pliable chest walls.
4. Complete upper airway obstruction: The total volume of respiratory system does not change—when the abdomen expands (diaphragm contracts) the chest volume must decrease.

False Classification of Apneas as Central

As discussed in Chapter 8, even with RIP, an obstructive apnea (by esophageal pressure manometry) may appear to be a central apnea.[22,23] In Figure 9–12, the RIP rib cage and abdominal band tracings are nearly flat but persistent respiratory effort is definitely noted in the esophageal pressure tracing. Although misclassification of a few events is unlikely to have major clinical consequences, proper adjustment

of chest and abdominal bands (position and tightness) is crucial to avoid significant errors in event classification. Computer software often adjusts sensitivity with an "autogain" to avoid large breaths being off-scale. However, this may decrease the gain so that small efforts are not recognized. In Figure 9–13, with an increase in the gain (size) of chest and abdominal tracings, the event is clearly not a central apnea.

Regarding central apneas, it is worth noting that the upper airway can actually close during a central apnea.[24] This should not be surprising, considering the obstructive portion of mixed apneas. Some have proposed that the observation of cardiac oscillations in airflow tracings allows one to conclude that the upper airway is open (Fig. 9–14).[25] However, a study by Morrell and associates[26] found that during ventilator-induced central apneas in dogs, cardiac oscillations could be present in the flow tracings even if the airway was noted to be closed by direct visualization. The appearance of cardiac oscillations in the airflow tracings is rarely noted in obstructive apnea. Therefore, the presence of cardiac oscillations in the flow may be a clue that a central apnea is present but one may not be able to infer that the upper airway is indeed open.

Hypoventilation in Adults[14]

Hypoventilation during wakefulness is usually defined as an arterial partial pressure of carbon dioxide (PaCO$_2$) equal to or greater than 45 mm Hg. During sleep, there may be periods of time in which the SpO$_2$ is reduced without associated events that meet criteria for apnea or hypopnea. Such

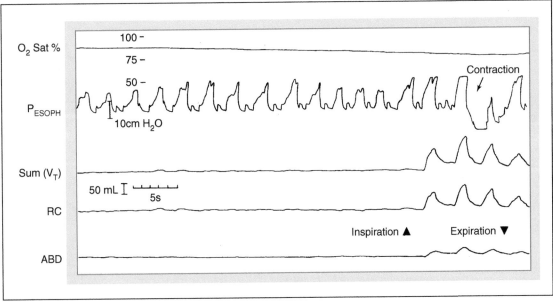

FIGURE 9–12   An obstructive apnea appears to be a central apnea based on the rib cage (RC) and abdominal (ABD) respiratory inductance plethysmography (RIP) tracings. The true nature of the event is shown by the persistent esophageal pressure (P_{ESOPH}) deflections. *Data from Tobin MJ, Cohen MA, Sackner MA: Breathing abnormalities during sleep. Arch Intern Med 1983;143:1221–1228.*

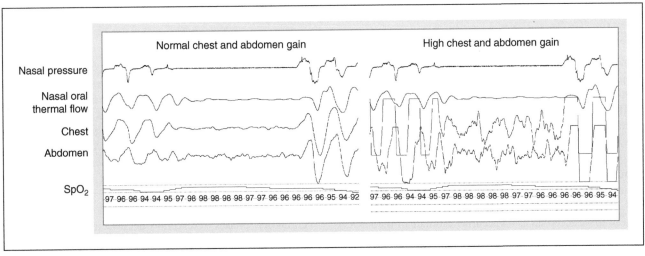

FIGURE 9–13   Left, The event may at first appear to be a central apnea. However, with an increase in gain in the chest and abdomen tracings, the obstructive nature of the event is apparent. **Right,** The many small fluctuations in the chest and abdomen tracings are due to cardiac oscillations that are readily apparent only at the high gain. SpO_2 = pulse oximetry.

periods of arterial oxygen desaturation are sometimes termed "hypoventilation." However, this is presumptive without direct measurement of $PaCO_2$ or a surrogate. The AASM scoring manual provides criteria for hypoventilation during sleep and discourages use of the term "hypoventilation" without documentation of an elevated $PaCO_2$.

Hypoventilation Rule (AASM Scoring Manual[14])
Score hypoventilation during sleep if there is a ≥10 mm Hg increase in $PaCO_2$ during sleep in comparison with an **awake supine value.**

The AASM scoring manual also notes that persistent oxygen desaturation in the absence of apnea or hypopnea is

not sufficient to document hypoventilation. It is observed that finding an increase in the $PaCO_2$ obtained immediately upon awakening is suggestive of sleep hypoventilation. The manual concluded that sufficient evidence was not available to recommend a sensor to document hypoventilation. The manual also states that both end-tidal carbon dioxide pressure ($P_{ET}CO_2$) and transcutaneous carbon dioxide pressure ($TcPCO_2$) may be used as surrogate measures of $PaCO_2$ if demonstrated to be reliable and valid.

Continuous arterial blood gas monitoring during PSG is not practical (or well tolerated) and arterial blood gas testing is most often performed at the start (to validate a surrogate measure of PCO_2) or on awakening often at study

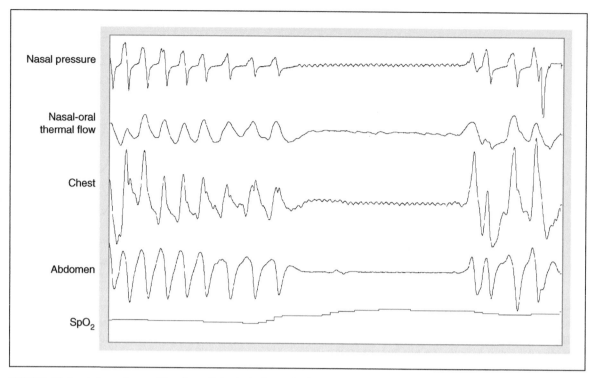

FIGURE 9–14 A central apnea is seen with cardiac oscillations in the chest and airflow channels. The oscillations are also seen in the nasal pressure signal. There is controversy about whether this means that the upper airway is open or closed. As discussed previously, the upper airway can close during central apnea. SpO_2 = pulse oximetry.

termination (to provide evidence for hypoventilation during sleep). In children, an arterialized capillary blood gas rather than an arterial sample is often performed.

The most common approaches to documenting hypoventilation during sleep monitoring include measurement of $P_{ET}CO_2$ or $TcPCO_2$. These methods are discussed in Chapter 8. Figure 9–15 presents a tracing from a patient with a neuromuscular disorder. The awake $P_{ET}CO_2$ was 43 mm Hg, but during sleep, the $P_{ET}CO_2$ reached the mid 70s. As discussed in Chapter 8, a $P_{ET}CO_2$ tracing should show an alveolar plateau to be accepted as an accurate estimate of the $PaCO_2$. In Figure 9–15, many of the breaths are not associated with a good alveolar plateau. The last 2 breaths illustrate a desired alveolar plateau. It should also be noted that the $PaCO_2$ typically exceeds the $P_{ET}CO_2$ by 4 to 6 mm Hg in normal individuals. The difference can be increased in patients with lung disease.

Cheyne-Stokes Breathing Rule[14]

Score Cheyne-Stokes breathing (CSB) if there are at least three consecutive cycles of cyclic crescendo and decrescendo change in breathing amplitude and **at least one** of the following:

1. Five or more central apneas or hypopneas per hour of sleep.
2. The cyclic crescendo and decrescendo change in breathing amplitude has a duration of at least 10 consecutive minutes.

CSB is characterized by central apnea or hypopnea at the nadir of respiratory effort (Fig. 9–16) as well as an intervening pattern of crescendo-decrescendo ventilation (flow or tidal volume) between apneas/hypopneas. CSB is most commonly noted in patients with systolic congestive heart failure (CHF) but can occur after stroke or with diastolic heart failure. When CSB is associated with systolic CHF, a few other characteristic PSG findings are of interest. First, the cycle time (time from the onset of one apnea to the next apnea) is usually approximately 50 to 60 seconds with long ventilatory phases (crescendo-decrescendo) between the central apneas.[27] If associated arousals are present, they are often at the zenith of respiratory effort. In addition, due to low cardiac output, there is a long circulation time and the nadir in desaturation is delayed relative to the event termination. Figure 9–17 presents a schematic showing the differences between central apnea in primary (idiopathic) central apnea and CSB.

Respiratory Parameters Reported in PSG (Adults)[14,17]

The following is a list of respiratory parameters that are recommended for presentation in a PSG report. Of note, the RDI was not defined in the AASM scoring manual but is added for completeness. Not all sleep centers report an RDI. Two definitions of the RDI in common use are presented here. The sleep study report should specify the RDI definition (if reported) and the definition of hypopnea (recommended or alternative) that was used for scoring the sleep study.

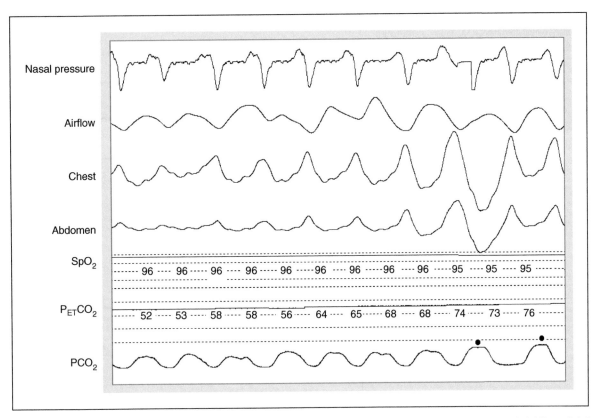

FIGURE 9–15 Documentation of an increased partial pressure of carbon dioxide (PCO_2) during sleep. Note the alveolar plateaus *(black circles)*. PCO_2 = exhaled PCO_2 waveform tracing; $P_{ET}CO_2$ = most recent end-tidal reading; SpO_2 = pulse oximetry.

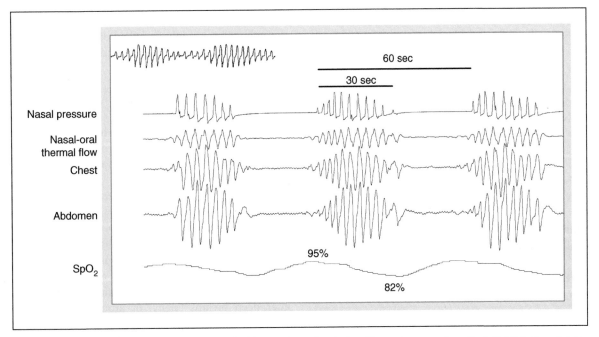

FIGURE 9–16 Cheyne-Stokes respiration with a crescendo-decrescendo pattern of respiration with central apneas at the nadir of effort. Note the nadir in the pulse oximetry (SpO_2) is very delayed following the end of the apneas. **Top left corner,** A tracing of Cheyne-Stokes breathing with a hypopnea at the nadir.

FIGURE 9–17 Differences between Cheynes-Stokes breathing and idiopathic (primary) central sleep apnea (CSA). SaO_2 = arterial oxygen saturation; SpO_2 = pulse oximetry.

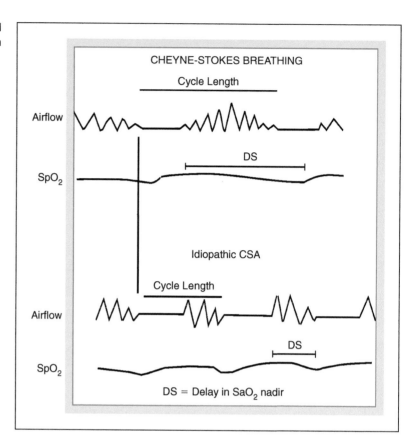

1. AH = number of apneas + number of hypopneas.
2. Number of obstructive, central, and mixed apneas.
3. Number of hypopneas.
4. AHI = number of apneas and hypopneas per hour of sleep

$$60 \times AH / TST \text{ (total sleep time [min])}$$

5. AHI during supine and nonsupine sleep.
6. AHI NREM and AHI rapid eye movement (REM).
7. OD = number of arterial oxygen desaturations.
8. Oxygen desaturation index (ODI) = (OD × 60)/TST (min).
9. Number of RERAs.
10. RERA index = (number of RERAs) × 60/TST (min)
11. RDI
    Definition #1 RDI = AHI
    Definition #2 RDI = AHI + RERA index

RESPIRATORY EVENT SCORING RULES IN CHILDREN

The AASM scoring manual provides separate rules for the scoring of respiratory events in children. The rules are based on a systematic review of the literature in children. Although many of the rules are similar to those in adults, there are differences. In children 13 years or older, the sleep specialist has the option to use adult rules. The sensors for monitoring respiration in children are very similar to those for monitoring adults (Table 9–4). In children, it is very common for some respiratory sensors to fail during monitoring. For example, sensors might be pulled off by the child or the NP cannula may be dislodged or occluded with secretions.

Ages for Which Pediatric Scoring Rules Should Be Used

Criteria for respiratory events during sleep for infants and children can be used for children younger than 18 years. An individual sleep specialist may choose to score children ≥13 **years of age** using adult criteria.

In adult patients, a 10-second breathing pause (minimum apnea duration) is approximately 2 missed breaths (at a respiratory rate of 12 breaths/min). In children, the respiratory rates are much faster and obstructive apneas shorter than 10 seconds can have physiologic significance. Therefore, the 2 missed breath rule is used for apneas in children. Short central apneas are common in children and are often seen after deep breaths (sighs) or arousals. Therefore, central apneas must be longer (≥20 sec) or associated with physiologic significance to be scored. If a central apnea is greater in duration than 2 missed breaths but less than 20 seconds, it must be associated with arousal, desaturation, or awakening to be scored. The respiratory scoring rules for children are listed in Table 9–4.

TABLE 9-4

Pediatric Respiratory Rules

Obstructive apnea	• Duration at least 2 missed breaths or equivalent duration. • >90% fall in signal for ≥90% of event duration. • Continued or increased inspiratory effort. • Event duration is from the end of last normal breath to the beginning of first breath achieving baseline amplitude.
Mixed apnea	• Duration at least 2 breaths or equivalent duration. • >90% fall in signal for ≥90% of event duration. • Absent inspiratory effort in the initial portion of the event, followed by resumption of inspiratory effort before the end of the event.
Central apnea	• Absent inspiratory effort. • Duration ≥ 20 sec. OR duration at least 2 missed breaths **AND** associated with arousal, awakening, or ≥3% desaturation.
Hypopnea	• NP signal falls by ≥50% from baseline. • Duration at least 2 missed breaths (or equivalent duration). • Fall lasts ≥90% of the event duration. • Arousal, awakening, or ≥3% desaturation occurs.

RERA	• All of the following in NP:
	  a. Discernible but <50% fall in signal.
	  b. Flattening of NP.
	  c. The event accompanied by snoring, noisy breathing, elevation in the end-tidal PCO_2 or transcutaneous PCO_2, or increased WOB.
	  d. Duration at least 2 breath cycles.
	• All of the following when using esophageal pressure:
	  a. Progressive increase in respiratory effort.
	  b. Snoring, noisy breathing, increased end-tidal or transcutaneous PCO_2, increased WOB.
	  c. Duration at least 2 breath cycles.

Hypoventilation	≥25% of the total sleep time with a PCO_2 > 50 mm Hg. ($P_{ET}CO_2$ or $TcPCO_2$ are acceptable.)
Periodic breathing	There are >3 episodes of central apnea lasting >3 sec separated by no more than 20 sec of normal breathing.

NP = nasal pressure; PCO_2 = partial pressure of carbon dioxide; $P_{ET}CO_2$ = end-tidal carbon dioxide pressure; RERA = respiratory effort–related arousal; $TcPCO_2$ = transcutaneous carbon dioxide pressure; WOB = work of breathing.
From Iber C, Ancoli-Israel S, Chesson A, Quan SF for the American Academy of Sleep Medicine: The AASM Manual for the Scoring of Sleep and Associated Events: Rules, Terminology and Technical Specifications, 1st ed. Westchester, IL: American Academy of Sleep Medicine, 2007.

Recommended Sensors in Children by AASM Scoring Manual[14]

As in adults, the recommended sensor to score an apnea is an oronasal thermal sensor. The alternative apnea sensors differ somewhat from those in adults and include NP, exhaled CO_2, or the summed signal of calibrated RIP. The recommended sensor for hypopnea is NP. The alternative sensor for hypopnea is a oronasal thermal sensor. Although not recommended, one could use the RIPsum as well. For detection of respiratory effort, recommended methods include esophageal manometry and RIP (calibrated or uncalibrated). For alveolar hypoventilation, acceptable signals are $P_{ET}CO_2$ and $TcPCO_2$.

Apnea Rules for Children[14]

Obstructive Apnea

Score an event as an OBSTRUCTIVE apnea if it meets all of the following criteria:

1. *Event lasts at least 2 breaths* (or the duration of 2 breaths as determined by baseline breathing pattern).
2. The event is associated with a >90% fall in the signal amplitude for ≥90% of the entire respiratory event compared with pre-event baseline amplitude.
3. The event is associated with continued or increased respiratory effort throughout the entire period of decreased airflow.
4. The **duration of the apnea** is measured from the end of the last normal breath to the beginning of the first breath that achieved the pre-event baseline inspiratory excursions.

Mixed Apnea

Score a respiratory event as a MIXED apnea if it meets both criteria 1 and 2 for obstructive apnea, and it is associated with absent inspiratory effort in the initial portion of the

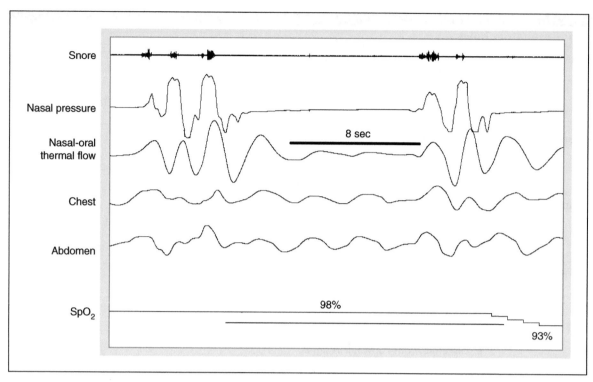

FIGURE 9–18 A short obstructive apnea in a 7-year-old child. There is a fall in the nasal-oral thermal flow of greater than 90% and continued inspiratory efforts are noted. Even though the event duration is short, it was followed by an arterial oxygen desaturation. Of note, a desaturation is NOT necessary to score an obstructive apnea. SpO$_2$ = pulse oximetry.

event followed by resumption of inspiratory effort before the end of the event.

Central Apnea

Score a respiratory event as a CENTRAL apnea if it is associated with absent inspiratory effort throughout the **entire duration** of the event and one of the following is met:

1. The event lasts 20 seconds or longer.
2. The event lasts 2 breaths (or the duration of 2 breaths as determined by the baseline breathing pattern) AND is associated with an arousal, an awakening, or a 3% or greater desaturation.

An example of a short obstructive apnea (only 2 breaths in duration based on thermal sensor) is shown in Figure 9–18. Examples of two possible central events are shown in Figure 9–19. In the top event, there is an absence of airflow with absent inspiratory effort. However, the duration is only 11 seconds and because it was not associated with an arousal (following the event) or an arterial oxygen desaturation, it would NOT be scored as a central apnea. The lower central event meets criteria for scoring a central apnea.

The AASM scoring manual presents only a single hypopnea definition for children (versus the recommended and alternative definitions in adults). The hypopnea definition for children is similar to the alternative adult definition except that the duration must be at least the equivalent of 2 missed breaths.

Hypopnea Rule (Children)[14]

Score a hypopnea if **all** the following criteria are met:

1. The event is associated with a ≥50% **fall in the amplitude** of the **NP** or alternative signal compared with the pre-event baseline excursion.
2. The event lasts at least 2 missed breaths (or the duration of 2 missed breaths as determined by baseline breathing pattern) from the end of the last normal breathing amplitude.
3. The fall in NP signal amplitude must last for ≥90% of the entire respiratory event compared with the signal amplitude preceding the event.
4. The event is associated with an arousal, awakening, or 3% or greater desaturation.

The AASM scoring manual stated that if the NP signal is not functioning, the oronasal thermal signal can be used to score hypopnea.

RERA Rules for Children[14]

Score an RERA if the conditions in either 1 or 2 are met (+ an arousal occurs):

1. Using a NP sensor, ALL must be met:
   a. Discernible fall in amplitude of signal but it is less than 50% in comparison with baseline.
   b. Flattening of NP waveform.

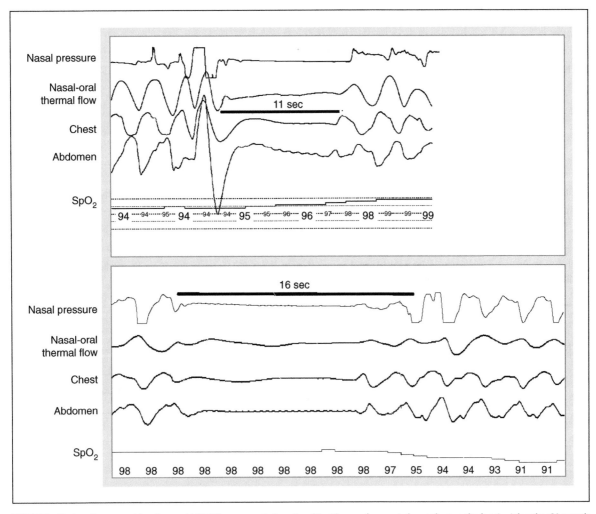

FIGURE 9–19 A respiratory event in a 6-year-old child. The *upper central event* would not be scored as a central apnea because the duration is less than 20 seconds and there is no associated arousal or desaturation. The *bottom central event* would be scored as a central apnea because it is longer than 2 missed breath cycles and is associated with an arterial oxygen desaturation. SpO$_2$ = pulse oximetry.

c. The event is accompanied by snoring, noisy breathing, elevation in P$_{ET}$CO$_2$ or TcPCO$_2$, or visual evidence of increased work of breathing.

d. The duration of the event is at least 2 breath cycles (or duration of 2 breath cycles as determined by baseline breathing pattern).

2. Using an esophageal pressure sensor. ALL must be met:

a. Progressive increase in inspiratory effort during the event.

b. The event is accompanied by snoring, noisy breathing, elevation in P$_{ET}$CO$_2$ or TcPCO$_2$, or visual evidence of increased work of breathing.

c. The duration of the event is at least 2 breath cycles (or duration of 2 breath cycles as determined by baseline breathing pattern).

The AASM scoring manual stated that an RERA cannot be scored without an adequate NP or esophageal manometry signal.

Hypoventilation Rule for Children[14]

Score the presence of **sleep-related hypoventilation when >25% of the total sleep time** as measured by the TcPCO$_2$ and/or the P$_{ET}$CO$_2$ is spent with a PaCO$_2$ >50 mm Hg.

The AASM scoring manual noted that the P$_{ET}$CO$_2$ signal often malfunctions (dislodged or occluded with nasal secretions) during pediatric PSG or provides falsely low values in patients who have marked nasal obstruction, are obligate mouth breathers, or are receiving either supplemental oxygen or CPAP during the PSG. As previously noted, it is essential to obtain an **alveolar plateau** in the PCO$_2$ signal for the P$_{ET}$CO$_2$ value to be considered valid. As discussed earlier, the TcPCO$_2$ value is good for illustrated trends in PaCO$_2$ but a time lag in change in the TcPCO$_2$ values is noted after acute changes in respirations (slow response time).

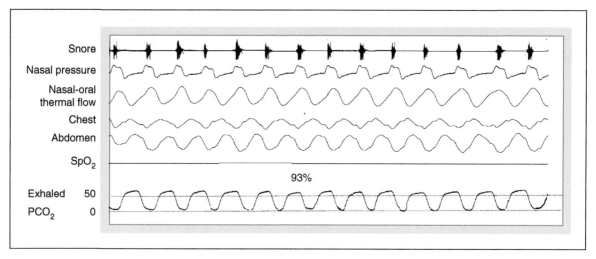

FIGURE 9–20 Obstructive hypoventilation. The end-tidal partial pressure of carbon dioxide (PCO_2) is greater than 50 mm Hg and there is evidence of snoring and flattening of the nasal pressure. A very mild drop in the pulse oximetry (SpO_2) is noted.

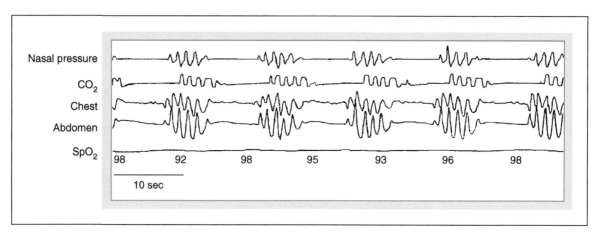

FIGURE 9–21 Periodic breathing in a newborn infant (43 wk conceptual age). Note the lag in the end-tidal PCO_2 tracing (CO_2) compared with the nasal pressure tracing. SpO_2 = pulse oximetry.

Obstructive Hypoventilation

Obstructive hypoventilation[29,30] is a term used to describe the periods during which there is evidence of hypoventilation (increased $P_{ET}CO_2$) without discrete events but associated with evidence of upper airway narrowing (snoring, NP flattening, chest-abdominal paradox). Figure 9–20 presents an example of obstructive hypoventilation in a 6-year-old child. Although this term is not specifically defined in the AASM scoring manual, it is widely used.

Periodic Breathing Rule for Children[14]

Score periodic breathing if there are more than three episodes of central apnea that last longer than 3 seconds separated by no more than 20 seconds of normal breathing.

Figure 9–21 presents a 60-second tracing from a newborn term infant. The central apneas are longer than 3 seconds, there are more than three central apneas, and the breathing between the central apneas is less than 20 seconds. This meets criteria for periodic breathing. This is a normal breathing pattern in preterm and term infants.

Respiratory Parameters Reported in PSG (Children)

Many sleep centers report respiratory events in children somewhat differently than those in adults. The differences include reporting the central AHI and obstructive AHI separately and reporting data concerning the $P_{ET}CO_2$ and/or $TcPCO_2$. Specifically, the maximum $P_{ET}CO_2$ and time spent greater than 50 mm Hg (absolute time or as % TST) are typically reported. Not all sleep centers report an RDI. The RDI should be defined if included in the report.

1. A + H = number (#) of apneas + number of hypopneas.
2. Number of obstructive apneas, central apneas, mixed apneas, and hypopneas.
3. AHI = number of apneas and hypopneas/hr of sleep

$$60 \times AH / TST \text{ (min)}$$

4. Obstructive AHI = (# obstructive apneas + # mixed apneas + # hypopneas) × 60/TST (min).
5. Central AHI = number of central apneas × 60/TST (min).

6. AHI during supine and nonsupine sleep.
7. AHI NREM and AHI REM.
8. OD = number of arterial oxygen desaturations.
9. ODI = (OD × 60)/TST (min).
10. # RERA = number of RERAs.
11. RERA index = number of RERAs × 60/TST (min).
12. RDI
    Definition #1 RDI = AHI
    Definition #2 RDI = AHI + RERA index
13. Time with $P_{ET}CO_2$ or $TcPCO_2$ greater than 50 mm Hg (as total minutes or as % TST).

CLINICAL REVIEW QUESTIONS

1. Hypoventilation during wakefulness for adults is defined as a $PaCO_2 \geq 45$ mm Hg. Hypoventilation during sleep is defined as:

   A. $PaCO_2 \geq 5$ mm Hg above an awake supine value.

   B. $PaCO_2 \geq 10$ mm Hg above an awake supine value.

   C. $P_{ET}CO_2 \geq 5$ mm Hg above the wake value.

   D. $P_{ET}CO_2 \geq 10$ mm Hg above the wake value.

2. In the table, which group (A, B, C, or D) is correct for recommended and alternate definitions of hypopnea in adults and hypopnea in children? NP = nasal pressure excursions.

	CHANGE IN NP FROM BASELINE	DESATURATION
A. Adult hypopnea (recommended)	Drop of ≥30%	≥4%
Adult hypopnea (alternate)	Drop of ≥30%	≥4% (or arousal)
Child hypopnea	Drop of ≥50%	≥3% (or arousal)
B. Adult hypopnea (recommended)	Drop of ≥30%	≥4%
Adult hypopnea (alternate)	Drop of ≥50%	≥3% (or arousal)
Child hypopnea	Drop of ≥30%	≥3% (or arousal)
C. Adult hypopnea (recommended)	Drop of ≥30%	≥4%
Adult hypopnea (alternate)	Drop of ≥50%	≥ 3% (or arousal)
Child hypopnea	Drop of ≥30%	≥3% (or arousal)
D. Adult hypopnea (recommended)	Drop of ≥30%	≥4%
Adult hypopnea (alternate)	Drop of ≥50%	≥3% (or arousal)
Child hypopnea	Drop of ≥50%	≥3% (or arousal)

3. In children, hypoventilation is defined by which of the following?

   A. $PaCO_2 \geq 50$ mm Hg for ≥10% of total sleep time.

   B. $PaCO_2 > 50$ mm Hg for ≥25% of total sleep time.

   C. $PaCO_2 \geq 50$ mm Hg for ≥25% of total sleep time.

   D. $PaCO_2 < 55$ mm Hg for ≥25% of total sleep time.

4. At what **age and above** can adult scoring rules be used at the discretion of the clinician?

   A. 12 years.

   B. 13 years.

   C. 14 years.

   D. 16 years.

5. According to the AASM scoring manual, score periodic breathing in children if:

   A. >3 episodes, central apnea lasting >3 seconds, separated by no more than 20 seconds.

   B. >3 episodes, central apnea lasting >3 seconds, separated by no more than 10 seconds.

   C. >3 episodes, central apnea lasting >2 seconds, separated by no more than 20 seconds.

   D. >3 episodes, central apnea lasting >5 seconds, separate by no more than 20 seconds.

Answers

1. **B.** The AASM scoring manual defines hypoventilation based on the arterial $PaCO_2$ of ≥10 mm Hg above the waking value. The $P_{ET}CO_2$ or $TcPCO_2$ can be used to define hypoventilation only when it has been validated as an estimate of the patient's ventilation.

2. **D**

3. **B**

4. **B**

5. **A**

REFERENCES

1. Redline S, Sander M: Hypopnea, a floating metric: implications for prevalence, morbidity estimates, and case finding. Sleep 1997;20:1209–1217.
2. Guilleminault C: State of the art: sleep and control of breathing. Chest 1978;73:293–299.
3. Block AJ, Boysen PG, Wynne JW, et al: Sleep apnea, hypopnea, and oxygen desaturation in normal subjects: a strong male predominance. N Engl J Med 1979;330:513–517.
4. Gould GA, Whyte KF, Rhind GB, et al: The sleep hypopnea syndrome. Am Rev Respir Dis 1988;137:895–898.
5. Young T, Palta M, Dempsey J, et al: The occurrence of sleep-disorders breathing among middle-aged adults. N Engl J Med 1993;28:1230–1235.
6. Neito FJ, Young TB, Lind BK, et al: Association of sleep disorders breathing, sleep apnea, and hypertension in a large community based study. JAMA 2000;283:1829–1836.
7. Norman RG, Ahmed M, Walsben JA, Rapoport DM: Detection of respiratory events during NPSG: nasal cannula/pressure sensor versus thermistor. Sleep 1997;20:1175–1184.

8. Guilleminault C, Stoohs R, Clerk A, et al: A cause of excessive daytime sleepiness: the upper airway resistance syndrome. Chest 1993;104:781–787.

9. American Academy of Sleep Medicine Task Force: Sleep-related breathing disorders in adults: recommendation for syndrome definition and measurement techniques in clinical research. Sleep 1999;22:667–689.

10. Whitney CW, Gottlieb DJ, Redline S, et al: Reliability of scoring respiratory disturbance indices and sleep staging. Sleep 1998;21:749–757.

11. Redline S, Kapur VK, Sanders MH, et al: Effects of varying approaches for identifying respiratory disturbances on sleep apnea assessment. Am J Respir Crit Care Med 2000;161: 369–374.

12. Tsai WH, Flemons WW, Whitelaw WA, Remmers JE: A comparison of apnea-hypopnea indices derived from different definitions of hypopnea. Am J Respir Crit Care Med 1999; 159:43–48.

13. Meoli AL, Casey KR, Clark RW: Clinical practice review committee-AASM. Hypopnea in sleep disordered breathing in adults. Sleep 2001;24:469–470.

14. Iber C, Ancoli-Israel S, Chesson A, Quan SF for the American Academy of Sleep Medicine: The AASM Manual for the Scoring of Sleep and Associated Events: Rules, Terminology and Technical Specifications, 1st ed. Westchester, IL: American Academy of Sleep Medicine, 2007.

15. Redline S, Budhiraja R, Kapur V, et al: The scoring of respiratory events in sleep: reliability and validity. J Clin Sleep Med 2007;3:169–200.

16. Ruehland WR, Rochford PO, O'Donoghue FJ, et al: The new AASM criteria for scoring hypopneas: impact on the apnea hypopnea index. Sleep 2009;32:150–157.

17. Kushida CA, Littner MR, Morgenthaler T, et al: Practice parameters for the indications for polysomnography and related procedures: an update for 2005. Sleep 2005;28:499–521.

18. Berry RB, Gleeson K: Respiratory arousal from sleep: mechanisms and significance. Sleep 1997;20:654–675.

19. Ayappa I, Norman RG, Krieger AC, et al: Non-invasive detection of respiratory effort–related arousals (RERAs) by a nasal cannula/pressure transducer system. Sleep 2000;23: 763–771.

20. Younes M: Role of arousals in the pathogenesis of obstructive sleep apnea. Am J Respir Crit Care Med 2004;169:623–633.

21. Hirshkowitz M, Kryger M: Respiratory monitoring during sleep. In Principles and Practice of Sleep Medicine, 3rd ed. Philadelphia: Elsevier, 2005, pp. 1378–1393.

22. Staats BA, Bonekat HW, Harris CD, Offord KP: Chest wall motion in sleep apnea. Am Rev Respir Dis 1984;130:59–63.

23. Tobin MJ, Cohen MA, Sackner MA: Breathing abnormalities during sleep. Arch Intern Med 1983;143:1221–1228.

24. Badr SM, Toiber F, Skatrud JB, Dempsey J: Pharyngeal narrowing/occlusion during central apnea. J Appl Physiol 1995;78:1806–1815.

25. Ayappa I, Norman RG, Rapoport DM: Cardiogenic oscillations on the airflow signal during continuous positive airway pressure as a marker of central apnea. Chest 1999;116:660–666.

26. Morrell MJ, Badr MS, Harms CA, Dempsey JA: The assessment of upper airway patency during apnea using cardiac oscillation in the airflow signal. Sleep 1995;18:651–668.

27. Hall MJ, Xie A, Rutherford R, et al: Cycle length of periodic breathing in patients with and without heart failure. Am J Respir Crit Care Med 1996;154:376–381.

28. Grigg-Damberger M, Gozal D, Marcus CL, et al: The visual scoring of sleep and arousal in infants and children: development of polygraphic features, reliability, validity, and alternative methods. J Clin Sleep Med 2007;3:201-240.

29. Rosen C, D'Andrea L, Haddad G: Adult criteria for obstructive sleep apnea do not identify children with severe obstruction. Am Rev Respir Dis 1992;146:1231–1234.

30. Sheldon SH, Glaze DG: Sleep in neurologic disorders. In Sheldon SH, Ferber R, Kryger M (eds): Principles and Practice of Pediatric Sleep Medicine. Philadelphia: Elsevier, 2005, pp. 279–280.

Chapter 10

Sleep and Respiratory Physiology

Chapter Points

- Mechanisms of hypoxemia include high altitude, hypoventilation, $\dot{V}/\dot{Q}$ mismatch, and shunt.
- If hypoxemia is due to hypoventilation alone, the A-a gradient [alveolar PO_2 (PAO_2) – arterial PO_2 (PaO_2)] is normal.
- Alveolar hypoventilation with a normal A-a gradient suggests that a disorder of ventilatory control or respiratory muscle strength is present.
- Patients with alveolar hypoventilation due to parenchymal lung disease have an increased A-a gradient (usually >25).
- The $PaCO_2$ = constant × [CO_2 production/alveolar ventilation]. If everything else remains the same, a 50% decrease in alveolar ventilation causes a doubling of the $PaCO_2$.
- For a given minute ventilation (tidal volume × respiratory rate), the alveolar ventilation is lower with a pattern of higher respiratory rate and smaller tidal volume.
- Increases in the dead space–to–tidal volume ratio (V_D/V_T) from a high V_D and/or a low V_T reduce the alveolar ventilation for a given minute ventilation.
- OVD is characterized by a reduced FEV_1/FVC and normal or increased lung volumes (TLC, FRC, RV). If the VC is reduced, this is secondary to a high RV.
- RVD is characterized by a normal FEV_1/FVC ratio and a reduced VC and TLC.
- The most common pulmonary function test abnormality in patients with simple obesity is a reduced ERV (low FRC relative to the RV).
- Muscle weakness can cause RVD but must be fairly severe (MIP < 60 cm H_2O).
- An increased serum HCO_3 is a clue that chronic hypoventilation may be present (especially if >27 mEq/L).
- The hydrogen ion concentration (pH) is determined by the ratio $PaCO_2/HCO_3$. Compensatory mechanisms attempt to normalize the ratio.

The goal of this chapter is to present a brief overview of aspects of respiratory physiology useful for the sleep physician. Most patients who have arterial oxygen desaturation in the sleep center do so from apnea or hypopnea. However, patients with respiratory disorders may have sleep-related arterial oxygen desaturation and/or hypoventilation without a significant number of discrete apnea or hypopnea events. These abnormalities in gas exchange can occur because the normal effects of sleep on ventilation and oxygenation are magnified by abnormal function of the lung, chest wall, respiratory muscles, or ventilatory control centers. The effects of lung disease on breathing during sleep are discussed in more detail in Chapters 21 and 22.

ARTERIAL BLOOD GASES

Alveolar hypoventilation during wakefulness is defined as an arterial partial pressure of carbon dioxide ($PaCO_2$) of 45 mm Hg or higher. If the sleeping $PaCO_2$ is ≥10 mm Hg above the awake value, *nocturnal hypoventilation* is said to be present. *Hypoxemia* is defined as a low arterial partial pressure of oxygen (PaO_2) relative to predicted values. A PaO_2 less than 55 mm Hg while breathing room air is considered severe and an indication for chronic 24-hour supplemental oxygen therapy. Milder degree of hypoxemia can be identified by comparing a PaO_2 with a predicted value for age. A simple estimate of a normal predicted PaO_2 is 105 – ½ age (yr).

The alveolar gas equation[1] (Equation 10–1) allows one to compute the alveolar (ideal) partial pressure of oxygen (PAO_2) from the fractional concentration of oxygen in inspired gas (FIO_2), which is 0.21 when breathing room air, and the $PaCO_2$. The respiratory exchange ratio (R) is the CO_2 elimination divided by the O_2 uptake. At steady state, R is equal to the respiratory quotient (RQ), which equals the CO_2 production/O_2 consumption ($\dot{V}CO_2/\dot{V}O_2$). R is usually assumed to be 0.8.[1] In Equation 10–1, FIO_2 = 0.21 (breathing room air), P_B is the barometric pressure (760 mm Hg at sea level), and PH_2O is the partial pressure of water vapor (47 mm Hg at 37°C).

Computation of the PAO_2 and the A-a gradient

$$PAO_2 = FIO_2(P_B - PH_2O) - PaCO_2/R$$

$$R = \dot{V}CO_2/\dot{V}O_2 \text{ (assumed to be 0.8)}$$

$$\dot{V}CO_2 = CO_2 \text{ elimination} \quad \dot{V}O_2 = O_2 \text{ uptake}$$

Equation 10–1

Breathing room air, Equation 10–1 becomes Equation 10–2. The A-a gradient (Equation 10–3) is the difference between the ideal PAO_2 and the actual (measured) PaO_2. Equation 10–4 gives the predicted A-a gradient (usually <25 mm Hg).

$$\text{(room air)} \quad PAO_2 = 0.21(760 - 47) - PaCO_2/0.8$$
$$= 150 - PaCO_2/0.8$$

Equation 10–2

$$\text{A-a gradient} = PAO_2 - PaO_2$$

Equation 10–3

Predicted estimate of normal A-a gradient = $4 + age\ (yr)/4$

For example, for a 48-year-old, A-a gradient = 16

Equation 10–4

The major causes of hypoxemia are listed in Table 10–1. Causes of hypoxemia include a low FIO_2, a low P_B (high altitude), hypoventilation (increased $PaCO_2$), and incomplete oxygenation of the blood by the lung (ventilation-perfusion [$\dot{V}/\dot{Q}$] mismatch or shunt). In $\dot{V}/\dot{Q}$ mismatch, some alveoli are underventilated for their blood flow (low $\dot{V}/\dot{Q}$) and blood is incompletely oxygenated. This can be overcome by increasing the FIO_2, thereby increasing the effective oxygen flow to underventilated alveoli. If shunt is causing hypoxemia, blood completely bypasses the alveoli. The deoxygenated blood mixes with oxygenated blood to give a lower than ideal PaO_2. Raising the FIO_2 has no effect on shunted blood. Most patients with lung disease also have defects in CO_2 excretion. This may not result in alveolar hypoventilation because the patient may compensate by increasing the minute ventilation (discussed later).

Hypoxemia can occur simply as a consequence of hypoventilation. For example, a patient with normal lungs may have an increased $PaCO_2$ due to muscle weakness or abnormal ventilatory control. In this case, the PaO_2 is fairly close to the ideal (PAO_2) computed from the alveolar gas equation (Equation 10–1) using the known $PaCO_2$. The A-a gradient (Equation 10–3) in such patients is normal. Lung disease severe enough to cause an increased $PaCO_2$ is always associated with an increased A-a gradient.

Box 10–1 presents examples of use of the alveolar gas equation (Equation 10–1). In a patient with amyotrophic lateral sclerosis (ALS; Example 1), an arterial blood gas reveals a PaO_2 of 60 and $PaCO_2$ of 65 mm Hg. The computed A-a gradient is 8.7 mm Hg (normal). Hypoxemia is due to hypoventilation. In Example 2, a patient with chronic obstructive pulmonary disease has evidence of both hypoxemia and hypercapnia and the A-a gradient is increased. The hypoxemia is due to both $\dot{V}/\dot{Q}$ mismatch and hypoventilation. In patients with hypoventilation of unclear etiology, calculating an A-a gradient can provide an important clue as to whether the hypoventilation is due to lung disease or due totally to hypoventilation. A normal A-a gradient in a patient with hypoventilation would suggest a disorder of ventilatory control or muscle weakness.

OXYGEN TRANSPORT AND SATURATION

The majority of the oxygen-carrying capacity of the blood is due to oxygen bound to hemoglobin (Hb) with a small fraction of dissolved oxygen (Equation 10–5).[1] When fully saturated, a gram of Hb carries about 1.34 mL/dL of oxygen (1 dL = 100 mL).

Oxygen content of arterial blood (CaO_2 [mL O_2/100 mL])

$$CaO_2 = 1.34\ mL/g \times Hb\ (g/100\ mL) \times SaO_2 + 0.003\ PaO_2$$

Equation 10–5

TABLE 10–1

Major Causes of Hypoxemia

	A-a GRADIENT	RESPONDS TO SUPPLEMENTAL OXYGEN
Low FIO_2, low P_B	Normal	Yes
Hypoventilation	Normal	Yes
$\dot{V}/\dot{Q}$ mismatch	Increased	Yes
Shunt	Increased	No

A-a = alveolar-arterial; FIO_2 = fractional concentration of oxygen in inspired gas; P_B = barometric pressure; $\dot{V}/\dot{Q}$ = ventilation-perfusion (ratio).

BOX 10–1

Examples of Computation of the Alveolar Partial Pressure of Oxygen and the A-a Gradient

EXAMPLE 1: HYPOVENTILATION DUE TO AMYOTROPHIC LATERAL SCLEROSIS (NORMAL A-a GRADIENT)

Laboratory: PaO_2 = 60 mm Hg and $PaCO_2$ = 65 mm Hg (breathing room air)

$PAO_2 = 150 - 65/0.8 = 68.7$

A-a gradient = $PAO_2 - PaO_2 = 68.7 - 60 = 8.7$ (normal)

EXAMPLE 2: HYPOVENTILATION DUE TO CHRONIC OBSTRUCTIVE PULMONARY DISEASE (INCREASED A-a GRADIENT)

Laboratory: PaO_2 = 50 mm Hg and $PaCO_2$ = 55 mm Hg

$PAO_2 = 150 - 55/0.8 = 81$

A-a gradient = $PAO_2 - PaO_2 = 81 - 50 = 31$ (increased)

A-a = alveolar-arterial; $PaCO_2$ = arterial partial pressure of carbon dioxide; PAO_2 = alveolar partial pressure of oxygen; PaO_2 = arterial partial pressure of oxygen.

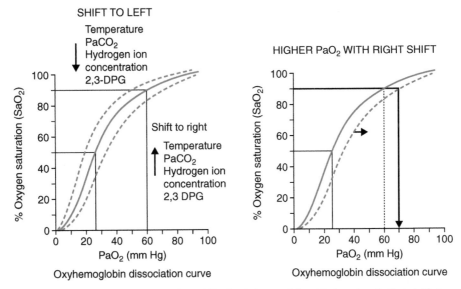

FIGURE 10–1 **Left,** The shift in the oxygen hemoglobin dissociation curve left or right depends on the illustrated factors. **Right,** A shift to the right increases the arterial partial pressure of oxygen (PaO₂) for a given arterial oxygen saturation (SaO₂). 2,3-DPG = 2,3-diphosphoglycerate; PaCO₂ = arterial partial pressure of carbon dioxide.

$$SaO_2 = 100 \times O_2Hb/(O_2Hb + RHb) \qquad \text{Equation 10–6}$$

The arterial oxygen saturation (SaO₂) is usually expressed as the ratio of oxygenated hemoglobin (O₂Hb) to the total amount of Hb that can bind oxygen (Equation 10–6). The amount of hemoglobin that can bind oxygen is the sum of O₂Hb and deoxygenated (reduced) hemoglobin (RHb). The SaO₂ value for a given PaO₂ depends on the position of the oxygen-hemoglobin saturation curve (also called the oxygen-hemoglobin dissociation curve)[1] (Fig. 10–1). At the usual body temperature and pH, a PaO₂ of 60 mm Hg corresponds to approximately an SaO₂ of 90%. A left shift results in a lower PaO₂ being associated with a given SaO₂ and vice versa. A shift to the left can occur with decreasing temperature, hydrogen ion concentration [H⁺], PaCO₂, or level of 2,3-diphosphoglycerate (2,3-DPG). Abnormal Hbs can also result in a different relationship between the SaO₂ and the PaO₂. For example, in patients with sickle cell disease (SCD), the PaO₂ for a given SaO₂ is higher due to the rightward shift of the O₂Hb saturation curve for hemoglobin S (HbS) compared with hemoglobin A (HbA).[2] The position of the O₂Hb dissociation curve is often defined by the P₅₀, which is the PaO₂ corresponding to an SaO₂ of 50%. For HbA, the P₅₀ is 26 mm Hg but is 42 to 56 mm Hg in SCD patients.[2] The net effect is a rightward shift in the O₂Hb dissociation curve for HbS. This means that for a given SaO₂, the PaO₂ is higher in SCD patients than would be expected based on the normal O₂Hb dissociation curve. The amount of right shift varies considerably between SCD patients and can be influenced by transfusion with blood (HbA) (Fig. 10–2).

Table 10–2 presents some useful PaO₂ and associated saturations. For PaO₂ values of 30, 40, and 60 mm Hg, the corresponding SaO₂ is 60%, 75%, and 90% values, respectively. The SaO₂ is measured noninvasively during sleep

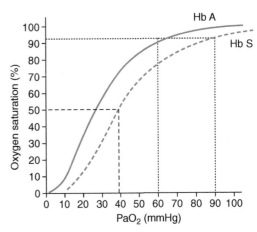

FIGURE 10–2 A patient with sickle hemoglobin (Hb S) will have a higher arterial partial pressure of oxygen (PaO₂) associated with a given SaO₂. Hb A = hemoglobin A.

TABLE 10–2

Typical SaO₂ Values for Given PaO₂ (Assumes Normal pH)

PaO₂ (MM HG)	SaO₂ (%)
30	60
40	75
60	90

PaO₂ = arterial partial pressure of oxygen; SaO₂ = arterial oxygen saturation.

studies by pulse oximetry[3] (SpO₂) to detect arterial oxygen desaturation and hypoxemia.

At normal PaO₂ levels, only a small amount of oxygen is dissolved in the blood and most of the oxygen-carrying capacity depends on the amount of Hb bound to oxygen.

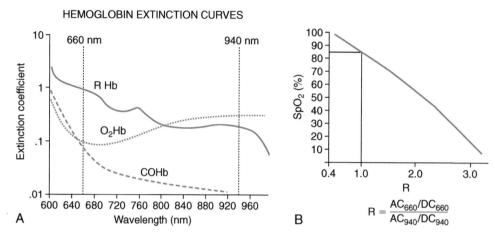

FIGURE 10–3 **A,** Hemoglobin extinction curves for reduced hemoglobin (R Hb), oxyhemoglobin (O₂Hb), and carboxyhemoglobin (COHb) at different wavelengths of light. Note that the y axis is a log scale. **B,** Empirical curve of the ratio of absorption of radiation (R) at wavelengths of 660 and 940 nm. AC = pulse added absorption; DC = steady state or background absorbance; SpO₂ = pulse oximetry. **A and B,** *Adapted from Temper KK, Barker SJ: Pulse oximetry. Anesthesiology 1989;70:98–108.*

However, determining the oxygen-carrying capacity of Hb is complicated by the fact that both carboxyhemoglobin (COHb) and methemoglobin (MetHb) are forms of circulating Hb that do not bind oxygen. Carboxyhemoglobin occurs when carbon monoxide (CO) binds to Hb. Smokers have increased carboxyhemoglobin. MetHb occurs when the normal ferrous state (Fe^{2+}) of the iron moiety in Hb is oxidized to the ferric stage (Fe^{3+}). Significant methemoglobinemia can occur after exposure to certain medications but is uncommon in the sleep center. The sum of the fractional concentrations of O_2Hb, RHb, COHb, and MetHb equal 100% (Equation 10–7). The true fraction of hemoglobin bound to oxygen (FO_2Hb) is given by Equation 10–8 and depends on the fraction (%) of carboxyhemoglobin (FCOHb) and methemoglobin (FMetHb) as well as the fraction of reduced hemoglobin (FRHb).[4–6]

$$FO_2Hb + FRHb + FCOHb + FMetHb = 100\%$$

Equation 10–7

or

$$FO_2Hb = O_2Hb \times 100/(O_2Hb + RHb + COHb + MetHb)$$

$$FO_2Hb = O_2Hb \times 100/Hb_t$$

Equation 10–8

where O_2Hb, RHb, COHb, and MetHb are the concentrations of the types of Hb and equal the total Hb concentration (Hb_t). For example, if the $FO_2Hb = 85\%$, $FCOHb = 8\%$, $FMetHb = 1\%$, then the FRHb is 6%. Using these numbers and Equation 10–6, the SaO_2 equals $85 \times 100/(85 + 6)$ or 93%, which is considerably higher than FO_2Hb of 85%. The FO_2Hb and the amount of Hb are the main determinants of the blood's oxygen-carrying capacity. When significant COHb or MetHb is present, Equation 10–5 should have SaO_2 replaced by FO_2Hb. The difference between the SaO_2 and the FO_2Hb (in %) at normal PO_2 values is approximately equal to the sum of FCOHb and FMetHb.[4] The FO_2Hb is sometimes called the fractional saturation and the SaO_2 the functional or effective saturation. Of note, the PaO_2 depends on

the SaO_2, not the FO_2Hb. That is, the oxyhemoglobin saturation curve expresses the ratio of oxygenated Hb to the total Hb available for oxygen binding. Neither COHb nor MetHb binds oxygen. However, the position of the oxyhemoglobin saturation curve is shifted to the left by the presence of COHb or MetHb.[4,7]

The previous four fractions of Hb can be accurately measured by co-oximeters that measure the absorption of 4 or more wavelengths of electromagnetic radiation by blood.[1,5] This is possible because the four forms of Hb differ in their absorption for the different wavelengths of radiation. In contrast, pulse oximetry[3] uses only two wavelengths: 660 nm (red) and 940 nm (infrared) to measure the O_2Hb and RHb. The absorption of radiation at 660 nm is much greater with RHb than O_2Hb, whereas O_2Hb absorbs more radiation at 940 nm (Fig. 10–3A). SpO_2 is based on the empirical observation that the ratio (R) of absorbance at the 2 wavelengths is related to the oxygen saturation (see Fig. 10–3B). This relationship (calibration curve) is calculated experimentally by determining R at varying oxygen saturations. To specifically determine the absorbance of arterial blood, the AC (pulse added absorbance) at each wavelength is divided by the DC (background absorbance) to account for the effect of the absorption of the radiation by venous blood and tissue. COHb has about the same absorbance at 660 as O_2Hb and, if present, increases the measured SpO_2 value. In normal individuals, FCOHb is 2% or less but can be 8% or more in cigarette smokers. Patients with SCD often have FCOHb values of 4% or more due to production of CO from chronic hemolysis. Based on a canine experiment,[3] it has been estimated that a pulse oximeter sees COHb as 90% O_2Hb and 10% RHb. For example, from the values $FO_2Hb = 85\%$, $COHb = 4\%$, $MetHb = 0\%$, $RHb = 11\%$, one can estimate the SpO_2 as 88.6% ($85 + 0.9 \times 4$). This is essentially the same as the SaO_2 computed from Equation 10–6 for these values. Thus, the SpO_2 is a much better estimate of the SaO_2 than the FO_2Hb is. In patients who are heavy smokers, it is important to remember that the SpO_2 may overestimate the FO_2Hb.

TABLE 10–3
Different Patterns of Breathing with Changing Dead Space and Tidal Volume

		V_D/V_T	V_D (ML)	V_T (ML)	RR (BPM)	MV (L/MIN)	ALVEOLAR VENTILATION (L/MIN)	$PaCO_2$ (MM HG)
A	Normal	0.3	200	600	10	6.0	4.0	40
B	Low V_T, same MV	0.5	200	400	15	6.0	3.0	53
C	High V_D	0.42	300	700	10	7.8	4.0	40
D	High V_D, low V_T	0.75	300	500	20	10.0	4.0	40

Notes:
B. Low V_T; even with higher RR and similar MV, the alveolar ventilation is decreased.
C. High V_D is compensated by an increase in V_T; with a higher MV, a normal alveolar ventilation is obtained.
D. High V_D, low V_T results require much higher MV to achieve a normal alveolar ventilation.
$PaCO_2 = K\ VCO_2/(RR \times V_T)(1 - V_D/V_T)$
Assume $K \times \dot{V}CO_2 = 160$
K = constant = 0.863; MV = minute ventilation; $PaCO_2$ = arterial partial pressure of carbon dioxide; RR = respiratory rate; $\dot{V}CO_2$ = carbon dioxide production;
V_D = dead space; V_T = tidal volume.

If a patient has a lower than expected SpO_2 while awake in the sleep center, a number of possibilities should be considered including a faulty oximetry probe, poor signal quality due to poor perfusion, a shift in the O_2Hb saturation curve due to the factors illustrated in Figure 10–1 or an abnormal Hb. If oximetry issues are ruled out, an arterial blood gas is needed to determine whether hypoxemia is really present. In this situation, co-oximetry analysis could also determine whether significant COHb or MetHb is present and determine a true SaO_2 and the fraction of Hb that is oxygenated. Sometimes, the SaO_2 reported with an arterial blood gas is simply determined from the measured PaO_2 and a nomogram. If clinically indicated, analysis with a co-oximeter will provide more accurate information.

DETERMINANTS OF $PaCO_2$

The $PaCO_2$ is related to the $\dot{V}CO_2$ and the alveolar ventilation ($\dot{V}_A$) (Equation 10–9). For a given $\dot{V}CO_2$, if the $\dot{V}_A$ doubles, the $PaCO_2$ decreases by half. The $PaCO_2$ will increase if the $\dot{V}_A$ decreases or the $\dot{V}CO_2$ increases (Equation 10–9). The $\dot{V}_A$ equals the minute ventilation ($\dot{V}_E$) minus the dead space ventilation ($\dot{V}_D$). The $\dot{V}_D$ is "wasted ventilation". The $\dot{V}_E$ = the respiratory rate (RR) × tidal volume (V_T) (Equation 10–10). The $\dot{V}_D$ can be written as the product of the RR and the dead space (V_D). The dead space includes the anatomic dead space (no alveoli) and overventilated areas of the lung (high $\dot{V}/\dot{Q}$ units). The equation for $PaCO_2$ can be written so that $PaCO_2$ depends on the minute ventilation ($V_T \times RR$) and the V_D/V_T ratio (Equation 10–11).

$$PaCO_2 = K\ \frac{\dot{V}CO_2}{\dot{V}_A} \qquad \text{Equation 10–9}$$

K = constant

$$\dot{V}_A = \dot{V}_E - \dot{V}_D \qquad \text{Equation 10–10}$$

$$= RR \times V_T - RR \times V_D$$

$$K\ \frac{\dot{V}CO_2}{RR \times V_T\left(1 - V_D/V_T\right)} \qquad \text{Equation 10–11}$$

K = constant

For the same minute ventilation, breathing with a low V_T and high RR increases the V_D/V_T ratio, decreases the $\dot{V}_A$, and increases the $PaCO_2$ (Table 10–3). The normal V_D/V_T ratio in % is 24.6 + 0.17 × age (yr). For example, a 40-year-old individual would have a V_D/V_T of about 31% or a ratio of 0.31. The anatomic V_D is approximately equal to a person's weight in pounds. The physiologic V_D equals the anatomic V_D + the effect of high $\dot{V}/\dot{Q}$ lung units. In lung disease, the physiologic V_D is increased and higher than normal minute ventilation is needed to produce the same alveolar ventilation (and $PaCO_2$). Patients who have a rapid shallow breathing pattern are predisposed to hypoventilation because this is an inefficient method of breathing. However, patients with muscle weakness or a stiff chest wall (high work of breathing) may utilize a pattern of ventilation with a small V_T and high RR to avoid respiratory muscle fatigue.

NORMAL CHANGES IN VENTILATION DURING SLEEP

The changes in arterial blood gases during normal sleep are summarized in Figure 10–4. During sleep, the metabolic rate falls (hence, decreased CO_2 production), but this is offset by a proportionately greater fall in minute ventilation with the result that the $PaCO_2$ increases slightly. The fall in ventilation is due to increased upper airway resistance and decreased chemosensitivity as well as the loss of the wakefulness stimulus to breathe.[8-11] The result is that the $PaCO_2$ rises and the PaO_2 falls slightly.

Because of the normal position on the flat portion of the O_2Hb dissociation curve, there is little change in the SaO_2 as a result of the fall in PO_2 associated with sleep (Fig. 10–5). If the baseline awake PaO_2 is lower, the fall in SaO_2 will be

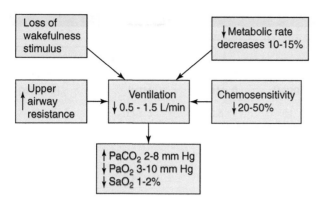

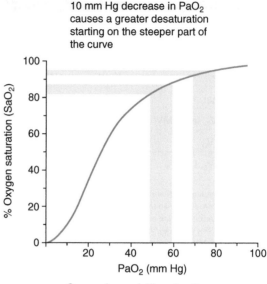

FIGURE 10–4 Changes in ventilation and gas exchange with normal sleep. The loss of wakefulness stimuli and reduced ventilatory drive + increased upper airway resistance result in a reduction in minute ventilation. Although the metabolic rate and CO_2 excretion are lower, the net effect is a mild increase in the arterial partial pressure of carbon dioxide ($PaCO_2$) and decrease in the arterial pressure of oxygen (PaO_2). SaO_2 = arterial oxygen saturation. *From Mohsenin V: Sleep in chronic obstructive pulmonary disease: sleep and respiration. Semin Respir Crit Care Med 2005;26:109–115.*

FIGURE 10–5 The same drop in arterial partial pressure of oxygen (PaO_2) causes a greater drop in the arterial oxygen saturation (SaO_2) if the starting point is on the steeper slope of the oxygen-hemoglobin saturation curve.

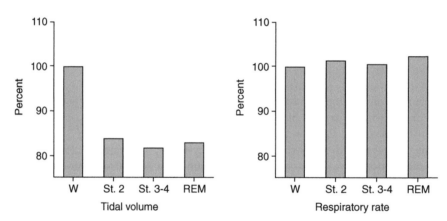

FIGURE 10–6 The fall in minute ventilation with sleep is due to a fall in tidal volume (V_T) with no significant change in respiratory rate (RR). REM = rapid eye movement; St. 2 = stage N2; St. 3-4 = stage 3-4 (stage N3); W = wake. *From Krieger J: Respiratory physiology: breathing in normal subjects. In Kryger MH, Roth T, Dements WC (eds): Principles and Practice of Sleep Medicine. Philadelphia: Elsevier, 2005, pp. 232–255.*

greater for the same drop in PaO_2. In patients with lung disease and a lower awake PO_2, even a normal sleep-related drop in PO_2 will be associated with a larger decrease in the SaO_2.

The change in ventilation with sleep is due to a fall in V_T with minimal change in the RR[9] (Fig. 10-6). During the transition from wake to stage N1 and early stage N2, the ventilation can be slightly irregular. However, in stable stage N2 and stage N3, the V_T and RR are nearly constant. During rapid eye movement (REM) sleep, ventilation is irregular with periods of decreased V_T associated with bursts of eye movements.[12] The FRC decreases from wake to sleep.[13] In some individuals, there may be a further decrease from non–rapid eye movement (NREM) to REM sleep.[14]

TESTS OF VENTILATORY CONTROL

The major chemoreceptors are the carotid body (responding to PaO_2 and $PaCO_2$) and the medullary chemoreceptors (responding to changes in the $[H^+]$ that occurs with changes in $PaCO_2$).[15–17] Hypercapnic hypoxemia creates the greatest stimulus.[15–17]

The sensitivity of the chemoreceptors and ventilatory control centers to changes in arterial blood gases can be determined by measuring the ventilatory responses to rises in $PaCO_2$ (hypercapnic ventilatory response [HCVR]) and falls in PaO_2 (hypoxic ventilatory response [HOVR]).[9,10] These are measured by rebreathing methods. The end-tidal partial pressure of carbon dioxide ($P_{ET}CO_2$) and end-tidal partial pressure of oxygen ($P_{ET}O_2$) are determined on a breath-by-breath basis (assumed to be alveolar values) and plotted against the ventilation at that time on a breath-by-breath basis. A line is then drawn to fit the points. The HCVR is measured under hyperoxic conditions (minimizing the effect of peripheral chemoreceptors) and the HOVR is measured under eucapnic conditions ($PaCO_2$ kept constant by removal of some of the CO_2 from the system).[16,17] The slope of the HCVR is a measure of sensitivity to hypercapnia (Fig. 10–7A). However, the position of the curve—that is, set point or base point—is also important. The slope of the HOVR (see Fig. 10–7B) is not constant and analysis is more complex. However, if expressed as ventilation versus the SaO_2 (SpO_2 is measured), the slope is linear (see Fig. 10–7C).

If a person has a normal ventilatory control center but abnormal lungs, high airway resistance, or abnormal thoracic cage, the slope of the ventilatory response to CO_2 will be lower (see Fig. 10–7A). Thus, measuring ventilation in a patient with a high airway resistance or low respiratory system compliance is not an ideal method to test the neural drive to breathe. The mouth occlusion pressure (P0.1)—the mouth pressure measured 0.1 second after the start of inspiration (unexpected airway occlusion)—can be used instead of ventilation as a better index of drive. Pressures at 0.1 second are before voluntary changes in pressure can occur. Because there is no flow during occlusion, the P0.1 is not affected by airway resistance. However, maintaining adequate ventilation with a high airway resistance may require a compensatory increase in ventilatory drive (increased P0.1). The P0.1 response to hypercapnia or hypoxemia is determined during rebreathing with intermittent airway occlusion (measurement of P0.1). The P0.1 values are plotted versus PCO_2, PO_2, or SaO_2 depending on the test.

During sleep, the HCVR and HOVR are reduced during NREM compared with wake and decreased in REM sleep compared with NREM sleep (Fig. 10–8).[10,11] Figure 10–9 shows the breath-by-breath values of the ventilatory response to $PaCO_2$ in an obstructive sleep apnea (OSA) patient before

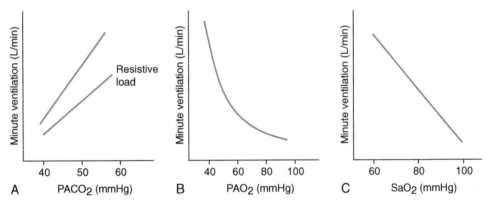

FIGURE 10–7 Schematic representation of the hypercapnic ventilatory response **(A)** and the hypoxic ventilatory response **(B** and **C)**. If the hypercapnic response is performed with a resistive load, the slope is lower. This illustrates that this testing depends not simply on the ventilatory control centers but also on the resistance and compliance of the respiratory system. $PACO_2$ = alveolar partial pressure of carbon dioxide (estimated from end-tidal values during the rebreathing test); PAO_2 = alveolar partial pressure of oxygen (estimated from end-tidal values during the rebreathing test); SAO_2 = arterial oxygen saturation (actually SpO_2 from oximetry).

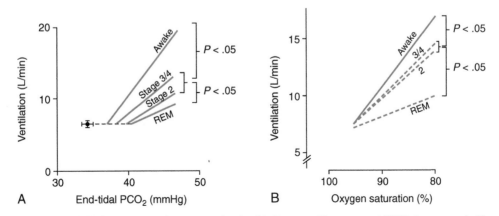

FIGURE 10–8 A, The hypercapnic ventilatory response is reduced during non–rapid eye movement (NREM) sleep compared with wake and decreased in rapid eye movement (REM) sleep compared with NREM sleep. PCO_2 = partial pressure of carbon dioxide. **B,** The hypoxic ventilatory response is also decreased during NREM compared with wake and REM compared with NREM. **A** and **B,** *From Douglas NJ, White DP, Weil JV, et al: Hypercapnic ventilatory response in sleeping adults. Am Rev Respir Dis 1982;126:286–289.*

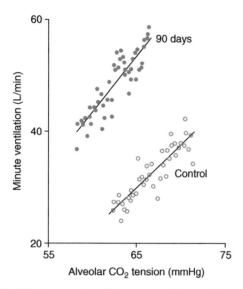

FIGURE 10–9 The hypercapnic ventilatory response before and after continuous positive airway pressure (CPAP) treatment. The slope did not change but the curve shifted to the left. Alveolar CO_2 = estimated $PACO_2$ from end-tidal sample of exhaled gas during rebreathing test. *From Berthon-Jones M, Sullivan CE: Time course of change in ventilatory response to CO_2 with long-term CPAP therapy for obstructive sleep apnea. Am Rev Respir Dis 1987;135:144–147.*

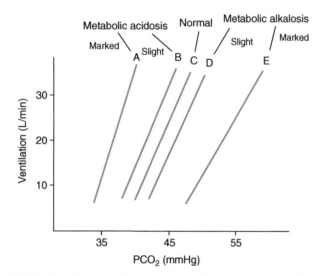

FIGURE 10–10 Changes in the hypercapnic ventilatory response with metabolic acidosis and alkalosis. The slope did not change but the position of the curve shifted left or right. PCO_2 = partial pressure of carbon dioxide. *From Oren A, Whipp BJ, Wasserman K: Effects of chronic acid-base changes on the rebreathing hypercapnic ventilatory response in man. Respiration 1991;58:181–185.*

(control) and after continuous positive airway pressure (CPAP) treatment.[18] The slope did not change but the set point (baseline $PaCO_2$) decreased and the position of the curve shifted to the left. At any given $PaCO_2$, the ventilation is higher. A shift in curve position without a change in slope can be seen with changes in HCO_3 due to chronic metabolic acidosis or alkalosis[19,20] (Fig. 10–10). One explanation for the parallel shift in the hypercapnic ventilatory response curve

after CPAP treatment is that the patients on CPAP no longer developed an elevated nocturnal $PaCO_2$ and, therefore, no longer accumulated HCO_3 at night to compensate (see next section). A fall in the serum HCO_3 would be associated with a leftward shift in the ventilatory response (see Fig. 10–10).

ACID-BASE PHYSIOLOGY

Some basic information regarding acid-base physiology can be useful in evaluating patients with sleep-related breathing disorders. The relationship of the pH ($-\log [H^+]$) to the serum HCO_3 and $PaCO_2$ is given by the logarithmic version of the Henderson-Hasselbalch equation (Equation 10–12). A nonlogarithmic form of the Henderson-Hasselbalch equation relates the $[H^+]$ to the ratio of the $PaCO_2$ and HCO_3 (Equation 10–13).[21]

$$pH = 6.10 + \log(HCO_3/0.03 \times PaCO_2) \quad pH = -\log[H^+]$$

Equation 10–12

$$[H^+] = 24 \frac{PaCO_2}{[HCO_3]} \quad \begin{array}{l} [H^+] \text{ in nanomoles/L} = 10^{-9} \text{ moles/L} \\ HCO_3 \text{ in mEq/L} \end{array}$$

Equation 10–13

If a change in $PaCO_2$ occurs, the body attempts to compensate by changing the HCO_3 in the same direction, thereby minimizing the change in the $PaCO_2$–to–HCO_3 ratio (Fig. 10–11). However, compensation is never complete (pH remains below or above 7.4). Of note, at a pH of 7.40, the $[H^+]$ is 40 nanomoles/L. In order to use the nonlogarithmic form of the Henderson-Hasselbalch equation (Equation 10–13), one can use the fact that around a pH of 7.40, when the pH increases (decreases) by 0.01 unit above or below 7.4, the $[H^+]$ decreases (increases) by approximately 1 nanomol/L below or above 40 (Box 10–2). It is worth remembering that a lower pH is associated with a higher $[H^+]$. For example, a pH of 7.35 corresponds to an $[H^+]$ of 45 and a pH of 7.45 corresponds to an $[H^+]$ of 35 nanomol/L. Box 10–2 presents examples of acute and chronic respiratory acidosis.

In evaluating the acid-base status of an arterial blood gas, a few simple rules are helpful. More comprehensive rules exist but a useful rule is that for every 10 mm Hg the $PaCO_2$ increases or decreases, the HCO_3 increases or decreases about 1 mEq/L acutely and 3 to 4 mEq/L chronically. If a patient's $PaCO_2$ increased from 40 to 60 mm Hg after chronic renal compensation, the HCO_3 would be expected to increase by 6 to 8 mEq/L. Similarly, the pH would be expected to decrease by approximately 0.03 (Fig. 10–11). Assuming a baseline HCO_3 of 24 mEq/L, this would result in a HCO_3 around 30 mEq/L. Noting electrolyte results can be helpful when evaluating obese patients with severe sleep apnea. If such a patient has chronic respiratory acidosis (high $PaCO_2$), he or she will usually have a high HCO_3 (or serum CO_2). An elevated HCO_3 in the absence of a reason to have a metabolic alkalosis (e.g., diuretic) is a clue that respiratory acidosis could be present. The utility of an elevated HCO_3 for identifying patients with the obesity hypoventilation syndrome is discussed in Chapter 15.

ACID BASE CHANGES

Goal keep the PCO_2/HCO_3 ratio unchanged

	Primary	Compensation
Respiratory acidosis	Increased PCO_2	Increased HCO_3
Respiratory alkalosis	Decreased PCO_2	Decreased HCO_3
Metabolic acidosis	Decreased HCO_3	Decreased PCO_2
Metabolic alkalosis	Increased HCO_3	Increased PCO_2

General rule: for every 10 mmHg change in PCO_2 the HCO_3 changes by 3-4 chronically and 1 meq/L acutely

Or pH changes by .08 acutely or .03 chronically

FIGURE 10–11 The major acid-base changes. For primary respiratory changes, there is renal compensation, and for metabolic changes, there is respiratory compensation. PCO_2 = partial pressure of carbon dioxide.

BOX 10–2

Using the Henderson-Hasselbalch Equation (Approximate [H⁺] values corresponding to different pH values near 7.40)

[H⁺] (NANOMOLES/L)	PH
30	7.50
35	7.45
40	7.40
45	7.35
50	7.30

Sample calculations: $[H^+] = 24\, PaCO_2/HCO_3$

Normal $\quad 40 = \dfrac{24\,(40)}{24} \quad pH = 7.40\,Normal$

Acute hypoventilation $\quad 48 = \dfrac{24\,(50)}{25} \rightarrow 7.32$

Chronic hypoventilation $\quad 44 = \dfrac{25\,(50)}{27} \rightarrow 7.36$

$PaCO_2$ = arterial partial pressure of carbon dioxide.

PULMONARY FUNCTION TESTING

Pulmonary function testing is often needed to evaluate patients with a low awake PaO_2 (or SaO_2) or to determine the etiology of unexpected daytime hypoventilation or dyspnea on exertion. Sometimes pulmonary function testing is ordered after a sleep study reveals an unexplained low sleeping baseline SaO_2 without discrete apneas or hypopneas. Therefore, some knowledge of pulmonary function testing can be very useful for the sleep clinician.

The patterns of impairment in lung disease include obstructive ventilatory dysfunction (OVD) and restrictive ventilatory dysfunction (RVD).[22-25] Disorders with an OVD pattern of impairment include asthma, chronic bronchitis, and emphysema. The term *chronic obstructive pulmonary disease (COPD)* is used because patients typically have a mixture of chronic bronchitis and emphysema in variable proportions. Patients with asthma usually have a significant component of reversible airflow obstruction. Patients with COPD have a mixture of chronic bronchitis and emphysema and may also have some improvement after inhaled bronchodilator. *Chronic bronchitis* is a clinical diagnosis based on a history of sputum production, but the term is often used for COPD patients with OVD who do not have a significant component of emphysema. The RVD disorders are divided into extrinsic RVD (involvement of the chest wall, pleura, or muscle weakness) and intrinsic RVD (lung parenchymal disorders such as interstitial lung disease) (Box 10–3).

Spirometry, lung volume determination, and measurement of the diffusing capacity for carbon monoxide (D_LCO) are an essential part of the evaluation of all patients with lung disease or hypoventilation. Nomenclature of the lung volumes is illustrated in Figure 10–12. The total lung capacity (TLC) is the lung volume at maximal inspiration, residual volume (RV) is the lung volume at maximal expiration, and the functional residual capacity (FRC) is the end-expiratory lung volume. The RV is about 25% of TLC and FRC is approximately 40% to 45% of TLC. The expiratory reserve volume (ERV) and inspiratory capacity compose about one third and two thirds of the vital capacity (VC). Recognition of either OVD or RVD can help guide further evaluation. In addition, if lung function abnormalities are documented, the severity as well as response to treatment can also be assessed.

Spirometry is a measurement of exhaled volume versus time (Fig. 10–13). Spirometry cannot measure absolute lung volumes (TLC, FRC, RV), but it is widely available. Spirometry is also a convenient method to follow the course of lung disease. The most important parameters include the forced expiratory volume in 1 second (FEV_1), the forced vital

BOX 10–3

Patterns of Pulmonary Function Abnormality

OVD

A reduction in flow rates often with an increase in absolute lung volumes (increase RV > TLC)
1. Asthma
2. Chronic bronchitis
3. Emphysema

RVD

A reduction in the total lung capacity with or without a reduction in other lung volumes
1. Intrinsic RVD—due to parenchymal lung disease (e.g., interstitial lung disease)
2. Extrinsic RVD—due to chest wall, pleural disease, or muscle weakness

OVD = obstructive ventilatory dysfunction; RVD = restrictive ventilatory dysfunction.

capacity (FVC), and the FEV_1/FVC ratio. OVD is associated with a reduced FEV_1/FVC ratio, whereas the ratio is normal or increased in RVD (see Table 10–5). OVD processes are associated with reductions in airflow, hence, a reduced FEV_1. In very mild disease, the FEV_1 may be normal but the FEV_1/FVC reduced. The RVD pattern of spirometry is characterized by a normal FEV_1/FVC ratio and a reduced FVC.

Bronchodilator testing is performed by administering inhaled bronchodilator to a patient who has not used a bronchodilator before the study. American Thoracic Society criteria[21] for a significant bronchodilator response include an increase in the FEV_1 or FVC by 12% AND an absolute increase of at least 200 mL. A large improvement of 15% to 40% is suggestive of asthma. However, asthmatics may not have an acute bronchodilator response but may improve with chronic bronchodilator therapy. Patients with COPD typically have no response (predominant emphysema) or a modest response of 10% to 15% (predominant chronic bronchitis).

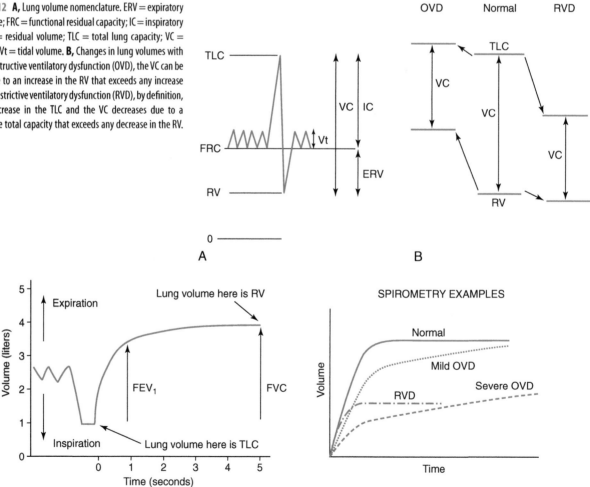

FIGURE 10–12 **A,** Lung volume nomenclature. ERV = expiratory reserve volume; FRC = functional residual capacity; IC = inspiratory capacity; RV = residual volume; TLC = total lung capacity; VC = vital capacity; Vt = tidal volume. **B,** Changes in lung volumes with disease. In obstructive ventilatory dysfunction (OVD), the VC can be decreased due to an increase in the RV that exceeds any increase in the TLC. In restrictive ventilatory dysfunction (RVD), by definition, there is a decrease in the TLC and the VC decreases due to a decrease in the total capacity that exceeds any decrease in the RV.

FIGURE 10–13 **Left,** Spirometry records exhaled volume versus time. **Right,** Typical patterns of obstructive ventilatory dysfunction (OVD) and restrictive ventilatory dysfunction (RVD) are noted. OVD is characterized by a reduced forced expiratory volume in 1 second–to–forced vital capacity (FEV_1/FVC) ratio. Either OVD or RVD can result in a reduced vital capacity—but with different alternations in the total lung capacity (TLC) and residual volume (RV) (see Fig. 10–12).

Lung volume testing by helium dilution or body plethysmography is used to determine the FRC. The patient then performs a slow VC maneuver and the inspiratory capacity (IC) and ERV are determined (see Fig. 10–12A). Then the TLC and RV are computed (TLC = FRC + IC and RV = FRC – ERV). Note that the VC equals the difference between the TLC and the RV. Changes in either the TLC, the RV, or both can decrease the VC.

By definition, RVD is associated with a reduced TLC. Ideally, a spirometric diagnosis of RVD should always be confirmed by documenting a reduced TLC. In OVD, the TLC is normal or increased. The RV in OVD is usually increased (airtrapping) more than the TLC, and this can result in a decrease in the VC. In RVD, the TLC is decreased more than the RV, and this results in a decrease in the VC (see Fig. 10–12B).

The FRC is the resting end-expiratory volume and is the volume at which the outward recoil of the chest wall is balanced by the inward lung elastic recoil. The inspiratory activity (diaphragm, intercostals, sternocleidomastoid) is required to reach TLC and expiratory muscle activity is required (abdominal muscles) to reach RV. In OVD, the RV is the first lung volume to be significantly affected (due to airtrapping). In advanced OVD, the RV is increased much more than the FRC and TLC. In severe OVD, the FRC and TLC can also be increased.

The DLCO is a noninvasive method to assess the ability of the lung to transfer gas (Table 10–4). As might be expected, obstructive diseases that affect the alveoli (emphysema) are associated with a reduced DLCO. OVD due to asthma or chronic bronchitis is usually associated with a relatively normal DLCO. Disorders causing RVD that affect the lung parenchyma (alveolar filling or interstitial lung disease) are associated with a reduced DLCO. Of note, early in these disorders, the DLCO may be reduced even though the FVC and TLC are still in the normal range. In extrinsic RVD (respiratory muscle weakness or chest wall/pleural disorders), the DLCO is relatively normal because the alveoli are not directly affected by the disorder. The diffusing capacity depends on the effective surface area for gas transfer, the pulmonary blood volume, and the Hb. CO diffuses across the alveoli and binds to Hb. The diffusing capacity must be corrected for anemia if this is present. Destruction of the effective surface area for diffusion occurs with emphysema or parenchymal lung disorders causing RVD. Pulmonary vascular diseases that reduce the pulmonary blood volume can reduce the diffusing capacity. Table 10–5 presents a summary of pulmonary function findings and normal ranges. Of note, the pattern of near normal spirometry and a decreased diffusing capacity can occur with emphysema, interstitial lung disease, pulmonary vascular disease, or anemia. Some patients with emphysema have minimal abnormalities in airflow but a reduced diffusing capacity. Some patients with early manifestations of disorders of the lung causing RVD can have a reduction in the diffusing capacity while the FVC and TLC are still normal.[22] The situation is especially common in lung disease due to medications (e.g., amiodarone, chemotherapy agents). In pulmonary

TABLE 10–4

Clinical Use of the Diffusing Capacity

	DIFFUSING CAPACITY NORMAL	DIFFUSING CAPACITY REDUCED
OVD	Asthma Chronic bronchitis COPD—predominant chronic bronchitis	Emphysema COPD with emphysema
RVD	Extrinsic RVD	Intrinsic RVD
Normal or near-normal spirometry		Anemia Emphysema Interstitial lung disease Pulmonary vascular disease

COPD = chronic obstructive pulmonary disease; OVD = obstructive ventilatory dysfunction; RVD = respiratory ventilatory dysfunction.

TABLE 10–5

Patterns of Pulmonary Function

	NORMAL	OVD	INTRINSIC RVD	EXTRINSIC RVD
FEV_1	80–120% of predicted	Decreased	Decreased	Decreased
FVC	80–120% of predicted	Normal to decreased	Decreased	Decreased
FEV_1/FVC	>0.70	**Decreased**	**Normal**	**Normal**
TLC	80–120% of predicted	Normal to increased	**Decreased**	**Decreased**
DLCO	≥75–80% of predicted (corrected for hemoglobin)	Normal—asthma, bronchitis Reduced—significant emphysema	Decreased	Normal to mildly decreased

Note: Mixed OVD + RVD = decreased FEV_1/FVC ratio and reduced TLC.
DLCO = diffusing capacity for carbon monoxide; FEV_1 = forced expiratory volume in 1 second; FVC = forced vital capacity; OVD = obstructive ventilatory dysfunction; RVD = restrictive ventilatory dysfunction; TLC = total lung capacity.

vascular disease (e.g., scleroderma), reduction in the diffusing capacity can occur in association with minimal changes in spirometry. A mixed pattern of OVD and RVD can occur and is characterized by a reduced FEV_1/FVC ratio in combination with a reduced TLC (normal or increased in OVD). Severity criteria for OVD and RVD are somewhat arbitrary,[22-26] but some commonly used criteria are listed in Appendix 10–1.

OBESITY

Because a significant percentage of patients with OSA have obesity, it is useful to understand the typical pulmonary function findings in this condition (Fig. 10–14). In obesity, the FRC is either reduced or reduced in relation to the RV. Therefore, in simple obesity, the most common pulmonary function finding is a reduced ERV. Usually, the TLC and RV are normal, as is the VC. In contrast, the obesity hypoventilation syndrome may be associated with reductions in the TLC and VC (see Fig. 10–14). The finding of a reduced TLC in a patient with severe obesity and OSA could be a clue that the obesity hypoventilation syndrome might be present.

MUSCLE STRENGTH

Muscle Forces

The muscle forces needed to reach different lung volumes are illustrated in Figure 10–15. The lung recoil is inward at all lung volumes. The resting point of the chest wall is approximately 65% to 70% of TLC (Fig. 10–16). At lung volumes above FRC but below the resting point of the chest wall, chest wall recoil is outward (thereby assisting tidal breathing). At TLC, the chest wall recoils inward and at RV outward. Inspiratory muscle weakness causes a low TLC. Expiratory muscle weakness causes an increased RV.

Typically, muscle weakness affects both the inspiratory muscles (diaphragm and intercostal muscles) and the expiratory muscles (abdominal muscles) at the same time. This results in a pattern of low TLC, high RV, and low VC. Note that at FRC, no muscle force is needed. One might predict that patients with muscle weakness would have a normal FRC. However, owing to chronic changes in the chest wall and lungs in patients with chronic neuromuscular disorders, the FRC is usually decreased. Most individuals with a normal chest wall and lungs can reach TLC with pleural pressures of –20 to –30 cm H_2O. If the chest wall and lungs are normal, significant muscle weakness must occur before the lung volumes and the VC change.

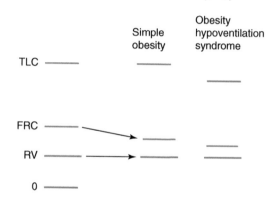

CHANGES WITH SIMPLE OBESITY AND THE OBESITY HYPOVENTILATION SYNDROME (OHS)

FIGURE 10–14 Typical lung volume changes in simple obesity and in patients with the obesity hypoventilation syndrome. In simple obesity, the most common finding is a reduced expiratory reserve volume (ERV = FRC – RV) due to a low-normal or low functional residual capacity (FRC). In the obesity hypoventilation syndrome, the total lung capacity (TLC) and vital capacity (VC) are decreased (VC = TLC – RV). RV = residual volume.

FIGURE 10–15 Summary of the muscle forces needed at the different lung volumes. At total lung capacity (TLC), inspiratory muscles are needed to overcome inward lung elastic recoil and inward recoil of the chest wall (CW). At residual volume (RV), expiratory muscles (along with lung recoil) are needed to balance the outward recoil of the chest wall. At functional residual capacity (FRC), no muscle forces are needed.

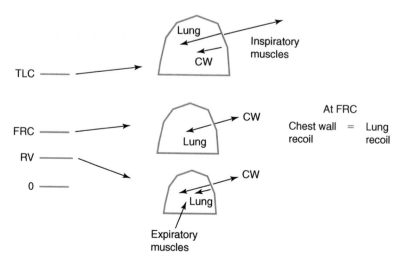

RESPIRATORY SYSTEM STATIC FORCES

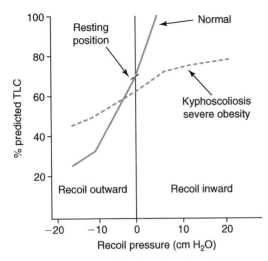

FIGURE 10–16 The neutral point of the chest wall (resting position) is approximately 65% to 70% of total lung capacity (TLC). At higher volumes, the chest wall recoils inward, and at lower volumes, outward. Note that in kyphoscoliosis or moderate to severe obesity, the resting point is shifted to lower lung volumes and the slope (compliance = Δ volume/Δ pressure) is decreased.

Maximum Inspiratory Pressure and Maximum Expiratory Pressure

Although the maximum inspiratory pressure (MIP) and maximum expiratory pressure (MEP) are often said to be the most sensitive tests of respiratory muscle strength, measurement of these parameters requires patient cooperation and special expertise.[27] The apparatus to measure the MIP and MEP consists of a mouthpiece with a small orifice (typically 1 mm × 15 mm) to provide a leak and an accurate pressure transducer. The leak is required to prevent the patient from using cheek muscles to perform the maneuvers. The MIP is usually performed at RV, and the MEP is performed at TLC. Unfortunately, the published normal ranges are wide and vary considerably between studies. In general, the pressures decrease with age, they are higher in men than in women, and the MEP exceeds the MIP in normal individuals. For clinically significant changes in the FVC to begin to occur, the MIP is usually less than 60 cm H_2O. An MEP less than 60 cm H_2O is associated with a reduced ability to cough and clear secretions. An American College of Chest Physicians (ACCP) Consensus group recommended noninvasive positive-pressure ventilation (NPPV) for progressive neuromuscular disorders when the MIP was less than 60 cm H_2O (or FVC < 50% of predicted).[28] One can be more confident of the finding of a reduced MIP when it is associated with a reduction in the VC. Studies of VC and MIP in patients with neuromuscular disorders have found that reduction in VC exceeds that predicted by loss of muscle strength.[29] This is thought to be due to alterations in the mechanical properties of the chest wall or lung. Thus, the VC is usually reduced when clinically significant muscle weakness is present. Of special interest is the fact that performance of FVC testing in the supine position was also found to be a very sensitive

test of diaphragmatic weakness.[30] In this posture, the chest wall muscles are less effective and any weakness in the diaphragm is more evident.

CLINICAL REVIEW QUESTIONS

1. What is the most commonly reduced lung volume in obesity?
   A. ERV.
   B. FRC.
   C. TLC.
   D. RV.

2. Which of the following changes occur from wake to sleep?
   A. Reduced V_T, unchanged RR.
   B. Unchanged V_T, increased RR.
   C. Unchanged minute ventilation, increased RR.
   D. Reduced V_T, increased RR.

3. Which of the following is associated with an increase in $PaCO_2$?
   A. Decreased alveolar ventilation.
   B. Decreased V_D/V_T ratio.
   C. Decreased dead space.
   D. Decreased CO_2 production.

4. Which of the following would be most consistent with a stable patient with muscle weakness and hypoventilation?
   A. $PaCO_2 = 60$, $PaO_2 = 55$ mm Hg.
   B. $PaCO_2 = 60$, $PaO_2 = 70$ mm Hg.
   C. $PaCO_2 = 50$, $PaO_2 = 50$ mm Hg.
   D. $PaCO_2 = 50$, $PaO_2 = 60$ mm Hg.

5. A patient has weak expiratory muscle weakness but fairly normal inspiratory muscle weakness. Which lung volume would be affected the most?
   A. TLC.
   B. FRC.
   C. RV.

6. A patient has stable hypoventilation with a $PaCO_2$ of 70 mm Hg. What would the expected serum HCO_3 be, assuming a normal HCO_3 value is 24 mEq/L?
   A. 34.
   B. 28.
   C. 26.
   D. 40.

7. The relative hypercapnic ventilatory response is:
   A. Wake > NREM > REM.
   B. Wake > REM > NREM.
   C. Wake > NREM = REM.

8. Chronic metabolic alkalosis is associated with which of the following phenomenon?

   A. Increased $PaCO_2$, shift in hypercapnic ventilatory response line to the right.

   B. Decreased $PaCO_2$, shift in hypercapnic ventilatory response curve to the left.

   C. Increased $PaCO_2$, shift in hypercapnic ventilatory response line to the left.

   D. Decreased $PaCO_2$, shift in hypercapnic ventilatory response line to the right.

9. What column (A, B, or C) lists the correct expected PO_2 values for the SaO_2 values?

		A	B	C
$SaO_2 = 60\%$	PO_2	40	30	30
$SaO_2 = 75\%$	PO_2	60	40	40
$SaO_2 = 90\%$	PO_2	75	60	80

10. The following pulmonary function test results are most consistent with:

    A. RVD intrinsic.

    B. RVD extrinsic.

    C. OVD-predominant asthmatic bronchitis.

    D. OVD-predominant emphysema.

	PREBRONCHODILATOR	% PREDICTED	POSTBRONCHODILATOR	% CHANGE
FEV_1 (L)	1.61	48	1.86	18
FVC (L)	3.32	75	3.93	18
FEV_1/FVC	0.48			
TLC	7.13	111		
FRC	4.71	132		
RV	3.72	188		
D_LCO	21.85	78		

(For normal ranges, see Table 10–5.)

Answers

1. **A.** FRC is reduced, but can be low normal in some patients while the ERV is reduced.

2. **A.**

3. **A.**

4. **B.** (normal A-a gradient).

5. **C.**

6. **A.** The $PaCO_2$ is increased by 30 mm Hg so the additional HCO_3 would be 3 × (3 to 4) or a 9 to 12 mEq/L increase. The expected HCO_3 would be around 33–36 mEq/L.

7. **A.**

8. **A.** (see Fig. 10–10).

9. **B.**

10. **C.** OVD, predominant asthmatic bronchitis. The FEV_1/FVC is decreased, there is a response to bronchodilator, and the D_LCO is at the lower limits of normal.

REFERENCES

1. West JB, Wagner P: Ventilation, blood flow, and gas exchange. In Murray JF, Nadel JA (eds): Textbook of Respiratory Medicine, 3rd ed. Philadelphia: WB Saunders, 2000, pp. 55–89.

2. Seakins M, Gibbs WN, Milner PF, et al: Erythrocyte Hb-S concentration—an important factor in low oxygen affinity of blood in sickle cell anemia. J Clin Invest 1973;52: 422–432.

3. Temper KK, Barker SJ: Pulse oximetry. Anesthesiology 1989; 70:98–108.

4. Toffaletti J, Zijlstra W: Misconceptions in reporting oxygen saturation. Anesth Analg 2007;105:S5–S9.

5. Barker SJ, Temper KK: The effects of carbon monoxide inhalation of pulse oximetry and transcutaneous PO_2. Anesthesiology 1987;66:677–679.

6. Barker SJ, Tremper KK, Hyatt J: Effects of methemoglobin on pulse oximetry and mixed venous oximetry. Anesthesiology 1989;7:112–117.

7. Roughton FJW, Darling RC: The effect of carbon monoxide on the oxyhemoglobin dissociation curve. Am J Physiol 1944;141: 17–31.

8. Mohsenin V: Sleep in chronic obstructive pulmonary disease. sleep and respiration. Semin Respir Crit Care Med 2005;26: 109–115.

9. Krieger J: Respiratory physiology: breathing in normal subjects. In Kryger MH, Roth T, Dements WC (eds): Principles and Practice of Sleep Medicine. Philadelphia: Elsevier, 2005, pp. 232–255.

10. Douglas NJ, White DP, Weil JV, et al: Hypercapnic ventilatory response in sleeping adults. Am Rev Respir Dis 1982;126: 758–762.

11. Douglas NJ, White DP, Weil JV, et al: Hypoxic ventilatory response decreases during sleep in normal men. Am Rev Respir Dis 1982;125:286–289.

12. Gould GA, Gugger M, Molloy J, et al: Breathing pattern and eye movement density during REM sleep in humans. Am Rev Respir Dis 1988;138:874–877.

13. Hudgel DW, Devadda P: Decrease in functional residual capacity during sleep in normal humans. J Appl Physiol 1984;57; 1319–1322.

14. Muller NLP, Francis W, Gurwitz D, et al: Mechanism of hemoglobin desaturation during rapid eye movement sleep in normal subjects and in patients with cystic fibrosis. Am Rev Respir Dis 1980;121:463–469.

15. Caruana-Montaldo B, Gleeson K, Zwillich CW: The control of breathing in clinical practice. Chest 2000;117:205–225.

16. Rebuck A, Slutsky AS: Measurement of ventilatory responses to hypercapnia and hypoxia. In Hornbein TF (ed): Regulation of Breathing. New York: Marcel Dekker, 1981, pp. 745–772.

17. Berger JA: Control of breathing. In Murray JF, Nadel JA (eds): Textbook of Respiratory Medicine, 3rd ed. Philadelphia: WB Saunders, 2000, pp. 179–196.

18. Berthon-Jones M, Sullivan CE: Time course of change in ventilatory response to CO_2 with long-term CPAP therapy for obstructive sleep apnea. Am Rev Respir Dis 1987;135: 144–147.

19. Oren A, Whipp BJ, Wasserman K: Effects of chronic acid-base changes on the rebreathing hypercapnic ventilatory response in man. Respiration 1991;58:181–185.

20. Javaheri S, Shore NS, Burton R, et al: Compensatory hypoventilation in metabolic alkalosis. Chest 1982;81:296–301.

21. Effros R, Widell JL: Acid-base balance. In Murray JF, Nadel JA (eds): Textbook of Respiratory Medicine, 3rd ed. Philadelphia: WB Saunders, 2000, pp. 155–178.

22. American Thoracic Society: Lung function testing: selection of reference values and interpretative strategies. Am Rev Respir Dis 1991;144:1202–1218.

23. Miller WF, Scacci R, Gast LR (eds): Laboratory Evaluation of Pulmonary Function. Philadelphia: JB Lippincott, 1987, pp. 106–109.

24. Crapo RO: Pulmonary function testing. N Engl J Med 1994; 331:25.

25. Pellegrino R, Viegi G, Brusasco V, et al: Interpretative strategies for lung function tests. Eur Respir J 2005:26:948–968.

26. Rabe KF, Hurd S, Anzueto A, et al: Global Initiative for Chronic Obstructive Lung Disease. Global strategy for the diagnosis, management, and prevention of chronic obstructive pulmonary disease: GOLD executive summary. Am J Respir Crit Care Med 2007;176:532–555.

27. ATS/ERS statement of respiratory muscle testing. Am J Respir Crit Care Med 2002;166:518–624.

28. American College of Chest Physicians: Clinical indications for noninvasive positive pressure ventilation in chronic respiratory failure due to restrictive lung disease, COPD, and nocturnal hypoventilation. Chest 1999;116:521–534.

29. De Troyer A, Borenstein S, Cordier R: Analysis of lung volume restriction in patients with respiratory muscle weakness. Thorax 1980;35:867–873.

30. Lechtzin N, Wiener CM, Shade DM, et al: Spirometry in the supine position improves the detection of diaphragmatic weakness in patients with amyotrophic lateral sclerosis. Chest 2001;121:436–442.

Severity Criteria for Pulmonary Function Testing

OVD

FEV_1 >60 to <80% predicted	Mild
FEV_1 40–60% of predicted	Moderate
FEV_1 < 40% of predicted	Severe

RVD

TLC or VC > 70% to <80% predicted	Mild
TLC or VC 60–70% predicted	Moderate
TLC or VC < 50% predicted	Severe

DLCO

DLCO 60–80% predicted	Mild
DLCO 40% to <60% predicted	Moderate
DLCO < 40% predicted	Severe

Notes:

1. Severity criteria are arbitrary, the above are fairly simple to use.
2. Most severity scales for OVD use postbronchodilator FEV_1.
3. The global initiative for lung disease (GOLD) criteria for COPD severity differ: < 0.70; mild, FEV_1 > 80% of predicted; moderate, FEV_1 50–80% of predicted; severe, FEV_1 30–50% of predicted; very severe, FEV_1 < 30% of predicted or FEV_1 < 50% of predicted and severe symptoms.
4. RVD severity criteria for intrinsic RVD usually are commonly based on the worst classification for the TLC and DLCO. A TLC moderate but DLCO severe would be considered severe or FEV_1 < 50% of predicted and severe symptoms.

COPD = chronic obstructive pulmonary disease; DLCO = diffusing capacity for carbon monoxide; FEV_1 = forced expiratory volume in 1 second; OVD = obstructive ventilatory dysfunction; RVD = restrictive ventilatory dysfunction; TLC = total lung capacity; VC = vital capacity.

Severity Criteria for Pulmonary Function Testing

Chapter 11

Cardiac Monitoring during Polysomnography

Chapter Points

- Score sinus tachycardia during sleep for a sustained heart rate > 90 bpm for adults.
- Score sinus bradycardia during sleep for a sustained heart rate < 40/min for ages 6 through adult.
- Score asystole for cardiac pauses > 3 seconds for ages 6 through adult.
- Score WCT for a rhythm lasting a minimum of 3 consecutive beats at a rate > 100/min with a QRS duration ≥ 120 msec (0.12 sec).
- Score NCT for a rhythm lasting a minimum of 3 consecutive beats at a rate > 100/min with a QRS duration < 120 msec (0.12 sec).
- Score Afib if there is an irregularly irregular ventricular rhythm associated with replacement of consistent P waves by rapid oscillations that vary in size, shape, and timing.
- When the heart rate is ~ 150, consider aflutter with 2/1 block.
- Change to 10-second window to better visualize ECG.
- Sustained WCT (>30 sec) should be treated as an emergency and it is likely ventricular tachycardia (especially in patients with known coronary artery disease). Emergency procedures in the sleep center should be activated.
- In lead II, the P wave should be upright.
- It is essential that the technologist or ordering physician document the presence of a pacemaker. It is also helpful to know whether the patient has known Afib.
- A sudden run of wider complex beats < 100 bpm (e.g., 60–70 bpm) is not WCT (by definition > 100 bpm). Among other considerations, determine whether the patient has a pacemaker. Pacemaker spikes may be better visualized with a high filter of 100 Hz with the 60-Hz notch filter off.

The purpose of this chapter is to discuss the aspects of electrocardiographic (ECG) monitoring relevant to polysomnography. For a detailed discussion of the ECG and related disorders, the reader is referred to reference 1. The normal ECG recording is composed of several different waveforms.

Each waveform represents a different electrical event during the contraction of the heart. The waveforms include the P wave, QRS complex, and T wave (Fig. 11–1). The *P wave* represents atrial depolarization (right atrium followed by left). The *QRS complex* represents ventricular depolarization. By convention, if the first deflection is negative, the deflection is called a *Q wave*. The first positive deflection is called the *R wave*. The negative deflection following the R wave is called the *S wave*. If a single negative deflection occurs, it is termed the *QS wave*. The second positive deflection following an S wave is called the *R′ wave* (Fig. 11–2). The entire QRS duration should be less than 0.12 second. The *T wave* represents ventricular repolarization. The *U wave* is a small wave that follows the T wave. It may be absent or very small and is usually in the same direction as the T wave but approximately 10% of its amplitude.

The *PR interval* is the time from the **start** of the P wave to the first part of the QRS complex (see Fig. 11–1). The PR interval varies with heart rate (shorter with faster heart rate) but is normally 0.12 to 0.2 second in duration. The time from the start of the QRS until the end of the T wave is the *QT interval*. The QT shortens with increases in heart rate. The *RR interval* is the time between successive QRS complexes. The heart rate in beats per minute (bpm) is 60/RR interval (sec). The corrected *QT duration (QTc)* is based on heart rate and is given by the formula

$$QTc = (QT\ interval)/\sqrt{RR}\ interval\ (sec)$$

Normal QTc < 0.44 sec

A prolonged QT (Fig. 11–3) can occur with congenital long QT syndromes, medications including antibiotics (erythromycin, clarithromycin, levofloxacin), antipsychotics (haloperidol, risperidone), tricyclic antidepressants, antiarrhythmic medications (amiodarone, sotalol), and electrolyte abnormalities (hypokalemia, hypomagnesemia). A life-threatening complication of a long QT is the development of polymorphic ventricular tachycardia (torsades de pointes).

The *ST interval* is the time interval from the end of the QRS complex (J point) to the start of the T wave. The ST is usually isoelectric (zero potential as identified by the T-P segment) but can be slightly up-sloping. The ST segment can be changed by ischemia (ST depression), acute myocardial infarction (ST elevation), or pericarditis (ST elevation).

The standard ECG uses 12 leads. In standard ECG recording, electrodes are placed on the right and left arms (RA, LA) and left leg (LL). A ground is placed on the right leg (RL). Leads I, II, and III are then recorded as (I LA+/RA–, II LL+/RA–, III LL+/LA–) (Fig. 11–4). These leads plus an additional three frontal plane leads (aVF, aVR, aVL) are depicted in Figure 11–5. In the standard ECG, transverse plane electrodes are also recorded (precordial leads). The precordial

leads V_1 (fourth intercostal space to the right of the sternum), V_2 (fourth intercostal space to the left of the sternum), V_4 (fifth intercostal space on the midclavicular line), V_3 (midpoint on a straight line between V_2 and V_4), V_5 (lateral to V_4 and on the anterior axillary line), and V_6 (lateral to V_5 on the midaxillary line) are depicted in Figure 11–6. Each precordial lead is recorded against linked left arm, left leg, and right arm electrodes, with the right leg as ground.

ECG RECORDING DURING POLYSOMNOGRAPHY

In most sleep centers, a single ECG lead is recorded during sleep monitoring. Monitoring of a single ECG lead is most useful for determining the cardiac rhythm and the heart rate. Determination of the QRS axis requires multiple frontal plane electrodes. In addition, accurate determination of ST changes requires both frontal and precordial electrodes. The QRS duration in a single lead may not reflect the widest value if part of the QRS is isoelectric in that particular lead. Multiple precordial leads are also needed for differentiation of

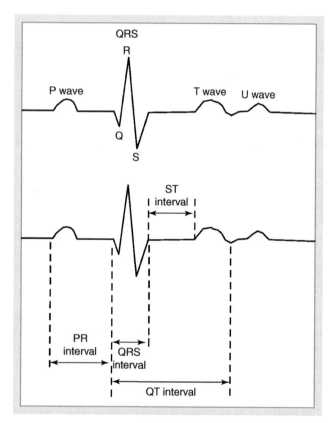

FIGURE 11–1 Nomenclature of ECG waves and intervals. *From Wagner GS (ed): Marriott's Practical Electrocardiography, 9th ed. Philadelphia: Williams & Wilkins, 1994, pp. 11–13.*

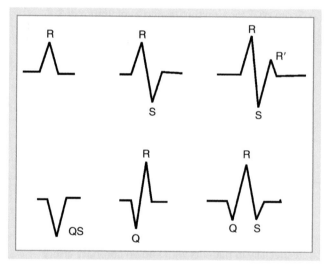

FIGURE 11–2 Nomenclature of the QRS complex. *Adapted from Wagner GS (ed): Marriott's Practical Electrocardiography, 9th ed. Philadelphia: Williams & Wilkins, 1994, pp. 11–13.*

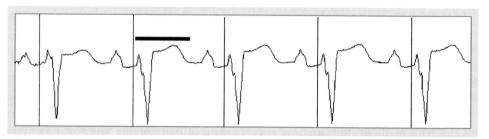

FIGURE 11–3 Long QT. The *vertical gray lines* are 1-second apart and the *black bar* marks the QT interval which is 0.55 second. The RR interval is approximately 1 second, so that the QTc = 0.55 (prolonged). The patient was taking risperidone, which can prolong the QT interval. The patient also appears to have ST elevation and a wide QRS. A 12 lead ECG is needed to assess the significance of these findings. The patient was asymptomatic.

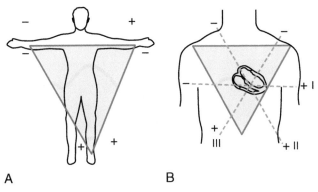

FIGURE 11–4 A, The three leads I, II, and III. **B,** The three leads are moved so that they intersect at the heart. Lead II is in a heart base–to–apex direction.

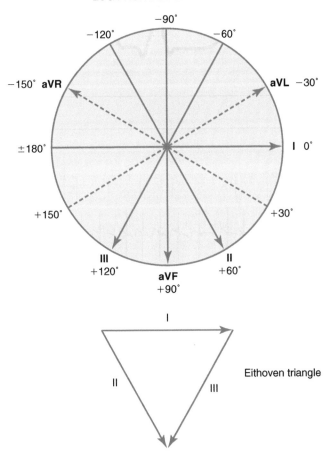

ECG FRONTAL PLANE LEADS

Eithoven triangle

FIGURE 11–5 Electrocardiogram (ECG) frontal plane leads.

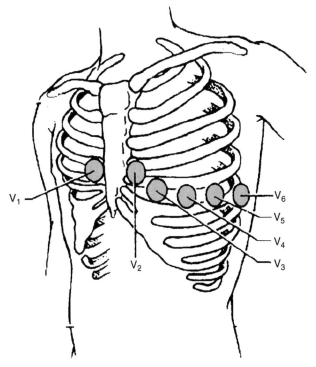

FIGURE 11–6 Placement of the precordial leads V_1 to V_6. *Adapted from Drew BJ, Califf RM Funk M, et al: Practice standards for electrocardiographic monitoring in hospital settings. Circulation 2004;110:2721–2746.*

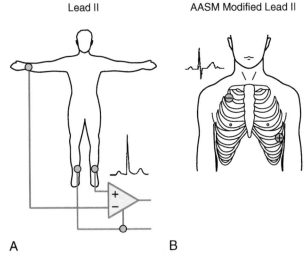

FIGURE 11–7 A, Standard ECG lead II. **B,** Modified lead II recommended for sleep recording by the American Academy of Sleep Medicine (AASM) scoring manual. *From Iber C, Ancoli-Isreal S, Chesson A, Quan SF for the American Academy of Sleep Medicine: The AASM Manual for the Scoring of Sleep and Associated Events: Rules, Terminology and Technical Specifications, 1st ed. Westchester, IL: American Academy of Sleep Medicine, 2007, p. 39.*

the causes of wide-complex tachycardia (WCT). Some sleep centers record three or more cardiac electrodes. The American Academy of Sleep Medicine (AASM) scoring manual[2,3] recommends use of a modified lead II with the negative torso electrode placed parallel with the right leg and below the right shoulder and the positive electrode parallel to the left leg (hip) on the lower left chest rib cage around the sixth to seventh intercostal spaces (Fig. 11–7). The exact intercostal level was not specified in the AASM scoring manual. Because

the main purpose is detecting the cardiac rhythm, a precise location is not essential.

In the standard and modified lead II, the P wave, R wave, and T wave are upright (Fig. 11–8). Examples of abnormal P wave, ST elevation, and a peaked T wave are also shown in this figure. A digital polysomnography (PSG) recording

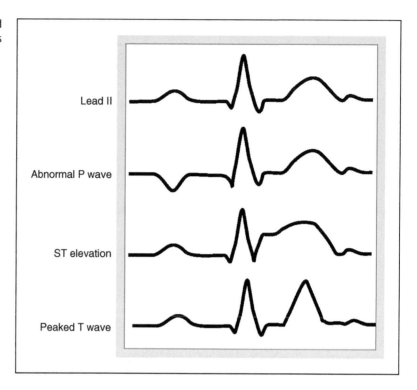

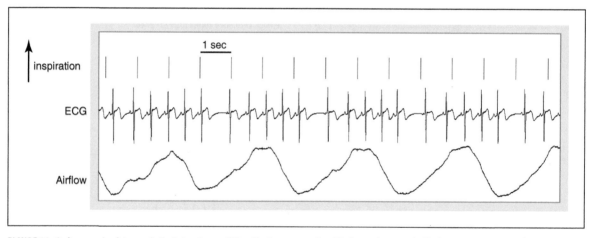

FIGURE 11–9 An example of sinus arrhythmia in a 5-year-old boy. The heart rate varies with the respiratory cycle. The heart rate increases with inspiration and decreases with expiration. The average heart rate is approximately 100 bpm. The electrocardiogram (ECG) was recording during a period of low arterial oxygen saturation.

viewed in a 10-second window corresponds to a traditional ink pen recording at a paper speed of 30 mm/sec. The traditional ECG paper speed used for recording was 25 mm/sec. Therefore, a 10-second PSG window provides a view similar to a standard ECG and is useful to observe the details of the ECG tracing. Most PSG software also has tools allowing measurement of durations and intervals of interest. The AASM scoring manual recommends that the ECG signal be acquired with a sampling rate of 500/sec (a sampling rate of 200/sec is acceptable). The recommended low- and high-frequency filter settings for display of the signal are 0.3 and 70 Hz, respectively.

A simple way to estimate heart rate is to count the number of QRS complexes in 10 seconds and then multiply by 6 for beats per minute. If the rhythm is irregular, a longer interval of 20 to 30 seconds should be used for a more accurate estimate of the average heart rate.

SINUS RHYTHM AND NORMATIVE DATA FOR HEART RATE

Normal sinus rhythm is associated with an upright P wave, R wave, and T wave in lead II. Each P wave is followed by a QRS complex with a relatively constant PR interval. If there is significant variability in heart rate with respiration, this is often called a *sinus arrhythmia* (Fig. 11–9). In a sinus arrhythmia, the heart rate increases with inspiration and decreases during expiration. Traditionally, *sinus bradycardia* is defined as a heart rate less than 60 bpm and *tachycardia* greater than 100 bpm. However, the heart rate normally decreases during sleep. The lowest heart rate in normal adults is usually during non–rapid eye movement (NREM) sleep when there is an increase in parasympathetic tone and a decrease in sympathetic tone. A review of the evidence that formed the basis for the AASM cardiac scoring rules by Caples and coworkers[2] reports unpublished data from the Sleep Heart Health Study cohort of 2067 adult individuals. The individuals in the analysis had an apnea-hypopnea index (AHI) lower than 5/hr and were not taking cardiac or antihypertensive medications. The 95% confidence interval based on mean ± 2 standard deviations (SD) for heart rate during sleep found a minimum normative value of 43 bpm in men and 47.5 bpm in women. The maximum normative values for heart rate were 80.8 bpm for men and 84.7 bpm for women. Based on this information, the new AASM cardiac scoring rules define **sinus bradycardia during sleep as a sustained heart rate less than 40 bpm for adults and children 6 years and older** (Table 11–1). Here, "sustained" means longer than 30 seconds in duration.[4] It should be noted that normal individuals, especially endurance-conditioned athletes, often exhibit heart rates less than 40 bpm during sleep. The AASM cardiac scoring rules also define **sinus tachycardia during sleep in adults as a sustained heart rate greater than 90 bpm** (see Table 11–1).

Defining normal heart rate limits is more complex in children in whom the heart rate is faster than in adults. The heart rate in normal children during wakefulness undergoes a large decrease with age[5-7] (Table 11–2). Scant information

---

TABLE 11–1

Cardiac Scoring Rules (AASM)

- Score *sinus tachycardia during sleep* for a sustained heart rate > 90 bpm for adults.

- Score *sinus bradycardia during sleep* for a sustained heart rate < 40/min for ages 6 through adult.

- Score *asystole* for cardiac pauses *greater* than 3 seconds for ages 6 years through adult.

- Score *wide-complex tachycardia* for a rhythm lasting a minimum of 3 consecutive beats at a rate > 100/min with a QRS duration ≥ 120 msec (0.12 sec).

- Score *narrow-complex tachycardia* for a rhythm lasting a minimum of 3 consecutive beats at a rate > 100/min with a QRS duration < 120 msec (0.12 sec).

- Score *atrial fibrillation* if there is an irregularly irregular ventricular rhythm associated with replacement of consistent P waves by rapid oscillations that vary in size, shape, and timing.

Note: The term *sustained* was defined in an FAQ from the AASM Scoring Manual committee to be > 30 sec. Sustained wide-complex tachycardia and sustained narrow-complex tachycardia are present for > 30 sec.
AASM = American Academy of Sleep Medicine; FAQ = frequently asked question.
Adapted from Anonymous: Scoring Manual FAQs. Available at http://www.aasmnet.org/Resources/PDF/FAQScoringManual.pdf
From Iber C, Chesson A, Ancoli-Israel S, et al: The Scoring of Sleep and Associated Events: Rules, Terminology and Technical Specifications, 1st ed. Westchester, IL: American Academy of Sleep Medicine, 2007.

TABLE 11–2

Normal Heart Rate during Wakefulness in Children

AGE	MINIMUM	MAXIMUM	MEAN	2ND–98TH PERCENTILE	NO. OF SUBJECTS
<1 day	88	168	123	93–154	189
1–2 days	57	170	123	91–159	179
3–6 days	87	166	129	91–166	181
1–3 wk	96	188	148	107–182	119
1–2 mo	114	204	149	121–179	112
3–5 mo	101	188	141	106–186	109
6–11 mo	100	176	134	109–169	138
1–2 yr	68	165	119	89–151	191
3–4 yr	68	145	108	73–137	210
5–7 yr	60	139	100	65–133	226
8–11 yr	51	145	91	62–130	233
12–15 yr	51	133	85	60–119	247

Adapted from Davignon A, Rautaharju P, Boiselle E, et al: Normal ECG standards for infants and children. Pediatr Cardiol 1979;1:133–152.

is available for normative heart rates in children during sleep. As in adults, one would expect a lower heart rate in sleep than during wakefulness. The Cleveland Children's Sleep and Health Study[6] (CCHS) in a group of children aged 8 to 11 years (AHI < 5/hr) reported the mean ± 2 SD heart rate during sleep was 73 ± 10 bpm overall, 70 ± 9 bpm in boys, and 75 ± 9 bpm in girls. These values represented a 20% reduction from waking values. A 95% lower confidence limit of 51 bpm in boys and 57 bpm in girls was found. The corresponding upper limits for boys and girls were 89 bpm and 94 bpm, respectively. A recent study analyzed data from the CCHS study and the Tucson Children's Assessment of Sleep Apnea (TUCASA) study.[7] The study concluded that sleeping heart rates in children are lower than wake and decrease significantly with age. African American ethnicity, female sex, and obesity were associated with faster heart rates. The AASM scoring manual did not provide rules for scoring the heart rate in children because of the age dependence and scant data.

CONDUCTION SYSTEM

A brief review of the cardiac conduction system (Fig. 11–10) is useful for understanding the terminology of premature beats and block. The electrical impulse during normal sinus rhythm starts with an impulse from the sinoatrial (SA) node located high in the right atrium near the entry of the superior vena cava. The SA node is the major cardiac pacemaker because the cells there have the highest intrinsic rate. The impulse is conducted through atrial muscle without special fibers until it reaches the atrioventricular (AV) node located at the bottom of the right atrium near the interatrial septum. The next part of the specialized conducting system is the bundle of His (common bundle). The bundle splits into a right bundle and a left bundle. The left bundle then splits into

left anterior and right posterior fascicles. The Purkinje fibers then transmit the signal to myocardial cells. Purkinje cells have both pacemaking capability and the ability to rapidly conduct electrical impulses. Impulses conducted via the normal pathway produce a narrow QRS complex and coordinated right and left ventricular contraction. Impulses originating in the AV node or His bundle (together termed the *AV junction*) usually have a rate of 40 bpm and result in a normal QRS duration. Impulses beginning below the separation of the common bundle result in wide QRS complexes. Of note, if an impulse reaches the normal AV junction during a relatively refractory period, it may be conducted with a wide QRS (aberrant conduction). If an impulse arrives at the AV junction very early during a refractory period, it may not be conducted at all. This phenomenon does not represent heart block but is simply a reflection that the AV node does have a refractory period that depends on a number of factors including the heart rate.

In summary, normally electrical impulses begin in the SA node, traverse the AV node, and are transmitted out to the ventricles by the Purkinje system via the left and right bundles. When the P wave is not present or is not conducted, slower pacemakers in the heart may function to continue regular ventricular rhythm. Rhythms from pacemakers in junctional areas (AV node and His bundle) usually have a narrow QRS complex with a rate approximately 40 to 60 bpm (junctional or nodal rhythm). If the rhythm originates from a pacemaker in the ventricles, the QRS is wide and the rate is slow (idioventricular rhythm). If the sinus node activity slows sufficiently, one of the other pacemakers may cause ventricular capture (so-called escape rhythms). The junctional and idioventricular rates can increase above the typical values in some circumstances. The terms *accelerated junctional rhythm* and *accelerated idioventricular rhythm (AVIR)* are used to describe these rhythms.

Bundle branch block (BBB) is due to dysfunction of either the right or the left bundles (RBBB or LBBB) and results in a wide QRS. The type of BBB is best identified using a 12-lead ECG. RBBB and LBBB produce characteristic patterns in leads I, V_1, and V_6. The pattern in lead II is variable. The other cause of a widened QRS commonly encountered in sleep centers is a ventricular pacemaker with the lead in the right ventricle. This gives a pattern of an LBBB because the right ventricle depolarized slightly before the left.

BRADYCARDIA AND AV BLOCK DURING SLEEP

The common causes of a slow heart rate during sleep are listed in Table 11–3. A slow heart rate during sleep (sustained heart rate < 40 bpm) can be a normal variant, associated with the effects of medications, high parasympathetic tone, or associated with disease of the conduction system (SA node, AV node). Cyclic increases and decreases in heart rate are commonly associated with untreated obstructive sleep apnea (OSA). This phenomenon is often called *tachycardia-bradycardia cycles*. However, in many patients, the lower heart rate is typically greater than 40 bpm and the high heart

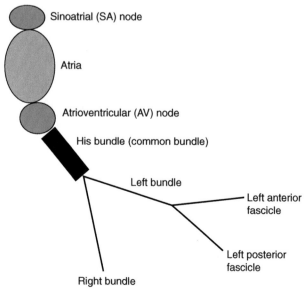

FIGURE 11–10 The normal cardiac conduction system.

<table>
</table>

TABLE 11-3

Causes of a Slow Heart Rate

- Sinus bradycardia
- Sinus pauses (>3 sec)
- Sinus node disorder (sick sinus syndrome)
- AV block
- Medications
- Increased parasympathetic (vagal) tone

AV = atrioventricular.

rate may not exceed 90 bpm. The heart rate typically accelerates at apnea termination owing to withdrawal of vagal tone and an increase in sympathetic activity. The slowing of the heart rate at event onset is thought to be due to vagal tone. Typically, the heart rate slows, then speeds up toward the end of the obstructive events with a sudden increase in heart rate at apnea termination. Some PSG computer programs provide a moving time average heart rate based on the ECG. Others simply record a heart rate output of the oximeter, which is a moving time average (Fig. 11-11).

Sinus Pause/Asystole

The AASM scoring manual recommends **scoring asystole if a sinus pause is greater than 3 seconds in duration for ages 6 years through adult**[4] (Fig. 11-12; see also Table 11-1). The

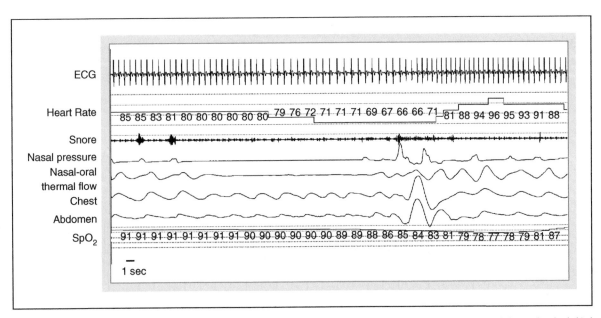

FIGURE 11-11 The heart rate during an obstructive apnea. The heart rate signal is the output of the oximeter (a moving time average) that tends to lag behind the actual change in heart rate. Changes in the heart rate can be noted by changes in the RR interval, which widen at apnea onset then narrow at apnea termination. ECG = electrocardiogram; SpO$_2$ = pulse oximetry.

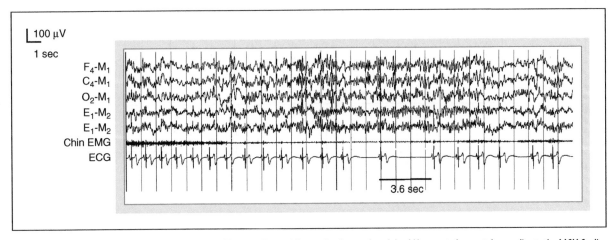

FIGURE 11-12 Three sinus pauses in a 30-second tracing. The second pause is longer than 3 seconds and should be reported as asystole according to the AASM Cardiac Scoring Rules. ECG = electrocardiogram; EMG = electromyogram.

review paper providing evidence for scoring rules quotes normative data in young healthy subjects[2] that found sinus pauses to be longer in males (range 1.20–2.06 sec) than in females (1.08–1.92 sec). In trained athletes, up to 37% had sinus pauses between 2 and 3 seconds. A study of a cohort of 40- to 79-year-old individuals found the longest pause during sleep to be 2 seconds.[8] For this reason, sinus pauses of 3 seconds or longer are scored as asystole.

Of note, a common cause of apparent sinus pause is a nonconducted premature atrial impulse. This is discussed in the section on "Premature Beats" (PBs).

AV Block

AV block is classified into three types[1] based on ECG characteristics that correlate with the location of the abnormality in the conducting system or the influences of changes in autonomic tone.

1. **First-degree AV block** is defined as a prolongation of PR interval longer than 0.20 second (Fig. 11–13). The normal PR interval is usually 0.12 to 0.20 second. A prolonged PR interval was found in between 0.5% and 2% of healthy middle-aged males.

2. **Second-degree AV block** is defined when one or more (but not all) of atrial impulses fail to reach the ventricle because of abnormal conduction.

   a. Mobitz type I (Wenckebach): A pattern of AV block in which there are varying PR intervals. Usually, there is progressive prolongation of the PR interval until a P wave is not conducted (Fig. 11–14). This is typical of a block in the AV node, which is capable of variations in conduction time. This type of second-degree AV block is generally thought to be benign.

   b. Mobitz type II: A pattern of AV block in which the PR intervals are nearly constant (Fig. 11–15). It is often seen in the setting of BBB.

3. **Third-degree AV block (complete AV block):** None of the atrial impulses are conducted to the ventricles (Fig. 11–16). One can often see both P waves and QRS complexes, but they have no fixed relationship (AV dissociation).

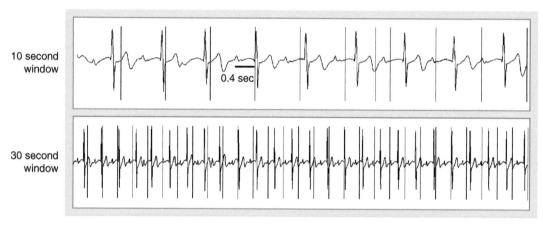

FIGURE 11–13 First-degree atrioventricular (AV) block. **Top,** A 10-second window shows a prolonged PR interval. **Bottom,** A 30-second window. One can see the difficulty in noting the abnormality unless viewed in a 10-second window.

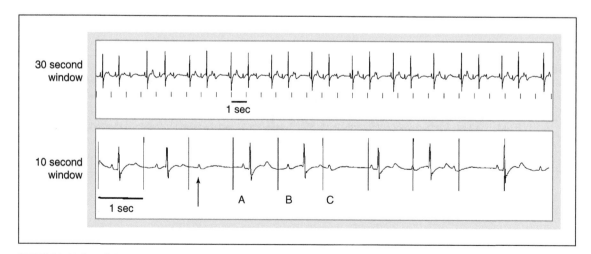

FIGURE 11–14 Second-degree AV block type I (Wenckebach) viewed in 30-second and 10-second windows. Arrow shows nonconducted P wave. *A,* Note that the PR interval at *B* is longer than at *A.* At *C,* P wave without a QRS.

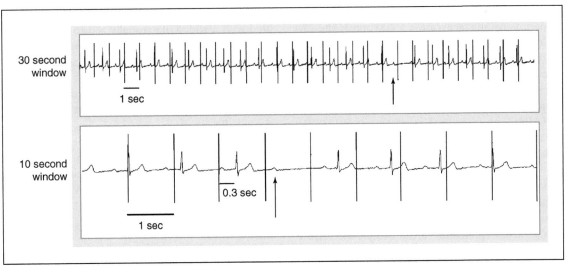

FIGURE 11–15 Second-degree AV block, Mobitz II. The PR interval is constant but some P waves *(up arrows)* are not conducted (no associated QRS).

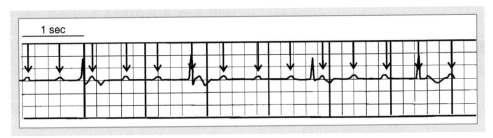

FIGURE 11–16 Third-degree AV block. The *down arrows* show P waves with a PP interval that is fairly constant. The P waves have no fixed relationship to the QRS (AV dissociation). Because the QRS is narrow, this means the pacemaker is in the AV junction—so-called junctional rhythm. Here, the junction rate is slow at approximately 33 bpm.

The term *AV dissociation* means that the atrial and ventricular rhythms have no relationship. This can occur with third-degree block. However, other causes include an intrinsic ventricular rhythm that is faster than the sinus rhythm (RR interval is shorter than PP interval).

Aberrant Conduction

When cardiac tissue responds to a stimulus, the reaction is followed by a refractory period (dormant interval) during which it cannot respond to a similar stimulus. The refractory period of cardiac conducting paths is proportional to the length of the preceding cycle (RR interval). Thus, a long preceding cycle in combination with a short immediate cycle predisposes to the cardiac conduction system being in a refractory state. A wide QRS can occur even if the beat originates in a supraventricular location (SA node or AV junction). This occurs for three reasons[1]: (1) a refractory right or left bundle fascicle, (2) anomalous supraventricular activation, or (3) a paradoxical critical rate.[1] In the first case, the impulse transverses the bundle of His but finds either the right or the left bundle refractory. In the second case, the impulse bypasses the AV node, arises in the AV node in an eccentric location, or is abnormally conducted due to diseased junctional fibers such that the impulse does not

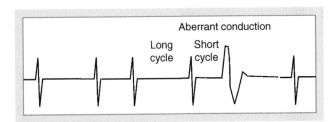

FIGURE 11–17 A schematic example of atrial fibrillation with irregular RR intervals and normal QRS duration. The fifth beat has a wide QRS duration due to aberrant conduction. The immediate cycle is short and the preceding cycle is long. These factors predispose to aberrant conduction.

reach the left and right fascicles at the same time. In the third case, a critical rate occurs above which part of the ventricular conducting system is refractory. A preceding long RR interval and a short current RR interval increases the chance of aberrant conduction. Figure 11–17 shows an example of a beat with aberrant conduction when the preceding cycle is long and the current cycle is short.

Premature Beats

PBs are QRS complexes not originating in the SA node that occur earlier than the next expected sinus beat. These can occur as a single PB, a pair of PBs (couplet of PBs), three PBs (by convention, nonsinus tachycardia > 100 bpm). The PBs can also follow every normal beat (bigeminy), every second sinus beat (trigeminy), or every third sinus beat (quadrigeminy) (Table 11–4).

The characteristics of PBs are listed in Table 11–5. Supraventricular premature beats (SVPBs) are either atrial premature beats (APBs), or junctional premature beats (JPBs). Although exceptions occur, SVPBs usually have a narrow QRS complex and the QRS morphology resembles that of the normal sinus beats. In the case of APBs, there is usually a visible abnormal P wave (sometimes called *P'*) (Fig. 11–18). The abnormal P wave may be negative in lead II or have a different morphology than the sinus P waves. The APBs are also known as PACs (premature atrial complexes). The P wave can be hidden in the preceding T wave. SVPBs usually reset the SA node and the next sinus beat occurs less than two PP intervals after the last normal P wave (Fig. 11–19). If the SVPB is aberrantly conducted, the QRS can be wide.

Ventricular premature beats (VPBs) invariably are associated with a wide QRS (usually > 0.16 sec) and are not preceded by an abnormal P wave. There is usually a compensatory pause following the VPB with the next P wave occurring about two PP intervals after the last normal P wave (Fig. 11–20). VPBs originate in a ventricular focus and can be conducted retrograde via the AV node to the atria. The retrograde P wave can be seen deforming the VPBs or following the beat. When all VPBs have the same morphology, they are said to be unifocal (unimorphic or monomorphic). If VPBs originate from multiple ventricular areas, they are usually of different morphology (polymorphic VPBs).

TACHYCARDIAS DURING SLEEP

The scoring criteria for narrow-complex tachycardia (NCT) and WCT are listed in Table 11–1. In both cases, there must be **3 or more beats with rate greater than 100 bpm.** Note that this differs **from sinus tachycardia during sleep, which must have a sustained (>30 sec) rate of greater than 90 bpm.** The common causes of tachycardias seen during sleep studies are shown in Table 11–6. Tachycardias are divided into NCT and WCT. With a single ECG lead, it is not possible to determine whether a WCT originates from a ventricular focus rather than a supraventricular focus with aberrant conduction. Therefore, the AASM scoring manual recommends scoring a WCT rather than a ventricular tachycardia (VT). However, most WCTs are VT.

Narrow-Complex Tachycardia

NCT is characterized by a QRS duration shorter than 0.12 second, with 3 or more beats and a heart rate greater than 100 bpm (Fig. 11–21). The major types of narrow complex tachycardias are listed in Table 11–6. The term *paroxysmal supraventricular tachycardia (PSVT)* is used to describe a diverse group of rhythms characterized by regular rhythm and narrow QRS, when the morphology does not otherwise allow identification of atrial fibrillation (Afib) or atrial flutter.

TABLE 11–4	
Premature Beat Terminology	
1 beat	A PB
2 beats	A pair or couplet
3 beats	Nonsustained rhythm (nonsustained tachycardia if rate > 100 bpm)
>30 sec	Sustained rhythm
PB follows every normal sinus beat	Bigeminy
PB follows every second normal beat	Trigeminy
PB follows every third normal beat	Quadrigeminy
PB = premature beat.	

TABLE 11–5		
Characteristics of Premature Beats		
	SVPBS	**VPBS ALSO KNOWN AS PVCS**
QRS complex	Normal duration (usually), resembles sinus beats Wide QRS can occur (aberrant conduction)	Wide QRS
Source of rhythm	Atria: APB Junctional (AV node + His)	Ventricles
Compensatory pause	No (usually): SA node discharged (reset)	Compensatory pause: sinus node not reset
P wave	Atrial: P wave premature and abnormal Junctional: none	Usually none Retrograde P wave can occur
Exceptions	APB: P wave can be obscured in preceding T wave	May appear < 0.12 sec in a given lead if part of wave is isoelectric in that lead
APB = atrial premature beat; AV = atrioventricular; PVCs = premature ventricular complexes; SA = sinoatrial; SVPB = supraventricular premature beat; VPBs = ventricular premature beats.		

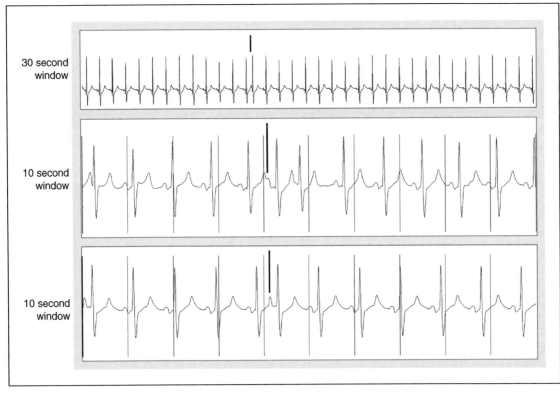

FIGURE 11–18 Atrial premature beats (APBs) are shown with *dark lines* that are over the abnormal P wave. Note that the QRS intervals are normal in duration and have the same morphology as the QRS in the sinus beats.

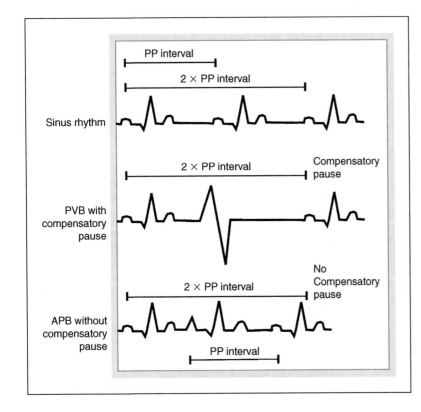

FIGURE 11–19 Schematic representation of a premature ventricular beat (PVB) with compensatory pause and an atrial premature beat (APB) without pause.

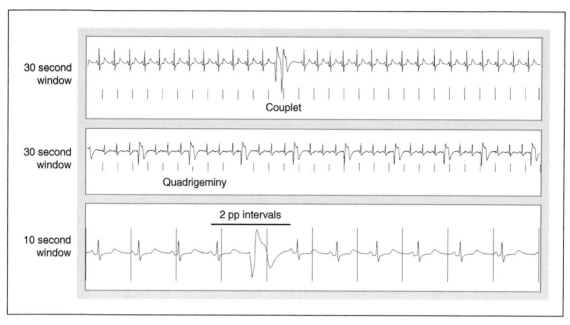

FIGURE 11–20 Tracings of PVBs illustrate a couplet, quadrigeminy, and the compensatory pause.

TABLE 11–6
Common Tachycardias during Sleep
SINUS TACHYCARDIA DURING SLEEP
Rate > 90 sec for ≥ 30 sec.
NARROW-COMPLEX TACHYCARDIA
≥3 consecutive beats, rate > 100 bpm, QRS duration < 0.12 sec

• PSVT: usually regular, rate 120–240 bpm
  • Ectopic atrial tachycardia
  • Ectopic nodal tachycardia
  • AV nodal re-entrant tachycardia, AV re-entrant tachycardia

• Afib: irregular atrial activity, ventricular activity irregular, rate variable
• Aflutter: flutter waves 280–300 bpm, ventricular response is variable (2/1 block ventricular rate ~ 150, 4/1 block ventricular rate ~ 70)
• MAT: irregular RR intervals, with three or more P wave morphologies (atrial rate 100–250 bpm)
WIDE-COMPLEX TACHYCARDIA
≥3 beats, rate > 100 bpm, QRS duration > 0.12 sec
• Ventricular tachycardia: usually regular
• PSVT usually regular
• SVT with aberrant conduction: usually regular
• Afib with aberrant conduction: regular, irregular
• Aflutter with aberrant conduction: often irregular
Afib = atrial fibrillation; Aflutter = atrial flutter; AV = atrioventricular; MAT = multifocal atrial tachycardia; PSVT = paroxysmal supraventricular tachycardia.

The etiology of PSVT could be a rapidly firing ectopic focus in the atria or nodal area or via re-entrant mechanisms in the AV nodal areas. AV re-entrant tachycardia is due to an accessory path outside the AV node (Wolff-Parkinson-White), and AV nodal re-entrant tachycardia is due to a conduction loop through the nodal area. The reader is referred to reference 1 for further reading on this topic. PSVT has regular RR intervals, and Afib has irregular RR intervals. Atrial flutter can have regular or irregular RR intervals. Both Afib and atrial flutter, which are discussed later, can result in a ventricular rate greater than 100 bpm and narrow QRS complexes. When a burst of NCT is short, it is often not possible to differentiate between PSVT and Afib.

Afib and Atrial Flutter

Afib and atrial flutter can present as either NCT or WCT in the sleep center. However, patients may also exhibit a ventricular rate less than 100 bpm due to the effects of medications on the AV node or intrinsic AV node disease. In the case of Afib with an average ventricular response less than 100 bpm, the rhythm is called *Afib with a controlled ventricular rate*. If the average heart rate exceeds 100 bpm, the rhythm is termed *Afib with a rapid ventricular response (Afib with RVR)*. The hallmark of Afib is that it is an irregular rhythm (Fig. 11–22). This occurs due to irregular conduction via the AV node. In atrial flutter, the saw-tooth–shaped flutter waves (called *F waves*) usually have a frequency of 250 to 300 bpm and are often discernible (Fig. 11–23). The ventricular rate can be regular (fixed AV block) or irregular (variable AV conduction). **An NCT of 150 bpm should**

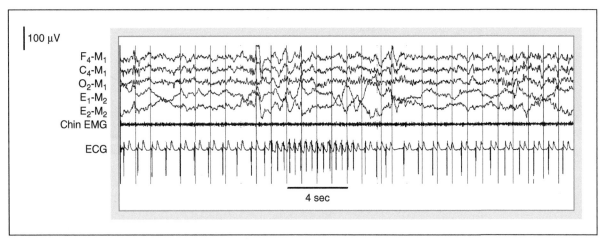

FIGURE 11–21 Narrow-complex tachycardia in a 30-second window. ECG = electrocardiogram; EMG = electromyogram.

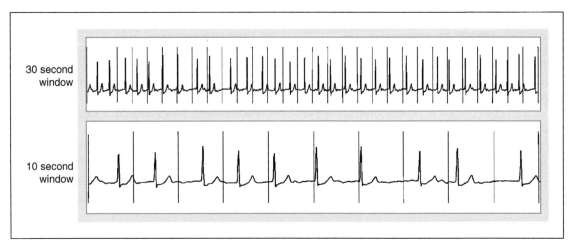

FIGURE 11–22 Atrial fibrillation. Absence of P waves and irregularly irregular RR intervals. The average rate is approximately 64 bpm. This is an example of atrial fibrillation with a controlled ventricular response. Therefore, although abnormal, this would not qualify for narrow-complex tachycardia.

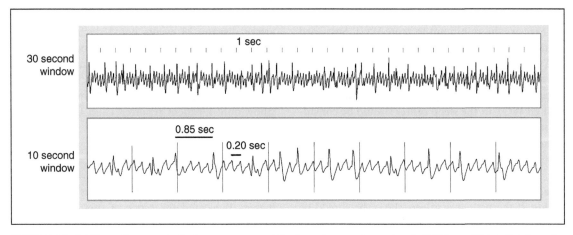

FIGURE 11–23 Atrial flutter. The saw-tooth–like flutter waves are noted. They have a frequency of approximately 60/0.20 sec = 300/min. Note that owing to variable block, the ventricular response is variable. For the RR interval of 0.85 sec, the rate is 70 bpm (4/1 block).

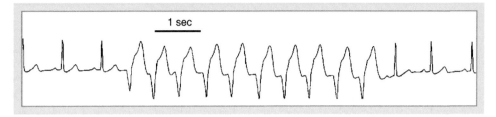

FIGURE 11–24 Nonsustained wide-complex tachycardia (WCT). The WCT is most likely ventricular tachycardia based on probability. From a single ECG lead, differentiating supraventricular tachycardia with aberrant conduction (SVTAC) from ventricular tachycardia (VT) is not possible.

always trigger the suspicion of atrial flutter with 2/1 block. In this circumstance, the flutter waves may be hidden by the preceding T wave. A sinus tachycardia with a heart rate of 150 bpm in the absence of an extreme situation such as hypotension or exercise is unlikely. The ventricular response to atrial flutter may also be approximately 70 bpm (4/1 block). Sometimes, the AV block can be variable resulting in an atrial flutter with irregular RR intervals (see Fig. 11–23). Multifocal atrial tachycardia (MAT), also known as multifocal atrial rhythm if the rate is less than 100 bpm, is characterized by at least three different P wave morphologies and has an irregular PP and RR interval. MAT is often seen in association with an exacerbation of chronic obstructive pulmonary disease (therefore, it is uncommon in the sleep center). Atrial fibrillation and MAT are the two rhythms characteristically associated with irregular RR intervals.

Wide-Complex Tachycardia

WCT is characterized by a QRS of 0.12 sec or greater (Fig. 11–24; see also Table 11–6). The two causes are VT (or Vtach) originating in the ventricles or supraventricular tachycardia with aberrant conduction (SVTAC) originating from the atria or junctional areas. Even with multiple ECG leads, differentiating VT from SVTAC is difficult. The lead V_1 has been used in emergency settings and intensive care units to help distinguish VT from SVTAC. However, this is beyond the scope of the sleep disorders center. At least three wide complexes are the minimum to score WCT. Sustained WCT is usually defined as longer than 30 seconds and nonsustained WCT as less than 30 seconds. VT accounts for up to 80% of cases of WCT in unselected populations. It accounts for 95% of cases in patients with previous myocardial infarction. **Sustained WCT in the sleep center should be considered VT until proved otherwise.**

If sustained WCT occurs in the sleep center in an out-of-hospital setting, the emergency medical services (EMS) should be called (911) and emergency equipment including an automated external defibrillator (AED) should be brought to the bedside. If the patient is asleep, she or he should be gently awakened and assessed for chest pain or shortness of breath. If the sleep center is within the hospital, an emergency code is usually called for rapid response.

For nonsustained ventricular tachycardia (NSVT), the clinical setting and condition of the patient dictate the actions. A symptomatic patient would require EMS activation (outpatient setting) or transfer to the emergency department or evaluation of the patient by an in-house on-call physician. An asymptomatic patient would usually require notification of the primary physician or physician on call for the sleep center. In order to be accredited by the AASM, a sleep center must have clearly specified written procedures for handling cardiac emergencies. In some sleep centers, it is a policy to wake the patient up if recurrent NSVT is noted to check for symptoms.[9]

Patients with NSVT require a cardiac evaluation if this has not been recently performed. NSVT in patients with structural heart disease has a poor prognosis without intervention. A typical evaluation includes echocardiography (evaluation for cardiomyopathy and valvular heart disease), Holter monitoring, and stress testing to rule out coronary artery disease.[9]

ADVERSE EVENTS DURING PSG

An investigation by Mehra and Strohl[10] collected information from 16,084 sleep studies and found that the incidence of serious adverse events during nocturnal PSG was very low at 0.35% and the incidence of death within 2 weeks of an adverse event was 0.006%. A total of 56 events were noted. These included 1 death due to VT in a patient with coronary artery disease, 28 events noted during the study (due to arrhythmias), and another 28 events noted after the study by the scoring technologist (complex ventricular arrhythmias). In the latter cases, the referring physician was notified of the problem. Of the 28 nonfatal events noted during the sleep study, only 1 patient reported chest pain and shortness of breath.

PACEMAKERS AND WIDE-COMPLEX QRS

A detailed discussion of ECG patterns from BBBs and pacemakers is beyond the scope of this chapter. However, an example is presented here to emphasize a few points. The sudden appearance of wide complexes on the ECG can cause panic in the sleep center. Sometimes, the fact that the rate is

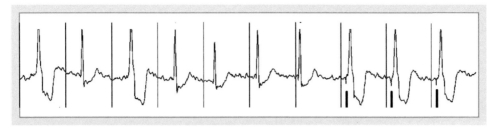

FIGURE 11-25 Atrial fibrillation with ventricular pacer activity. A 10-second window is shown. Although only the pacer spikes of the last 3 wide beats are visualized, all the wide beats have the same morphology and are all paced beats. Note that the 3-beat run of paced beats follows a long pause in ventricular activity (pacemaker activated when rate dipped below a cutoff). The *dark upright bars* mark the pacer spikes. These were not well visualized until the 60-Hz filter was turned off and 100 Hz was used for the high filter.

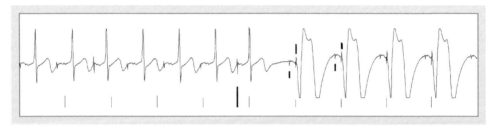

FIGURE 11-26 A dual-chamber pacemaker. On the *left,* the atrial pacer spikes are noted with a narrow QRS showing normal conduction of the atrial impulse to the ventricles. The *longer vertical black line* marks an atrial pacer spike. On the *right,* both atrial and ventricular pacer spikes are noted and the QRS is wide. The atrial impulse is not conducted normally and the ventricular pacer is activated, leading to a wide QRS. The *small vertical black lines* mark pacer spikes.

less than 100 (often 60 or 70) is missed in the excitement. However, in the prestudy evaluation, it is always helpful if the sleep technologist asks the patient whether he or she has a pacemaker. As mentioned previously, a ventricular pacemaker with the pacing lead in the right ventricle will produce wide-paced beats with an LBBB morphology. Pacer spikes are often difficult to see. Using a high-frequency filter of 100 Hz rather than the AASM-recommended high-frequency filter setting of 70 Hz AND turning off the 60-Hz filter may help in visualizing pacer spikes.

Figure 11-25 shows a single-chamber ventricular pacemaker in a patient in Afib with AV nodal dysfunction. When the ventricular rate falls below a cutoff value, the ventricular pacer fires producing a wide-complex QRS. Figure 11-26 shows a tracing with a patient with a dual-chamber pacer (one atrial and one ventricular lead). On the left portion of the tracing, only the atrial pacer lead is activated. On the right, both atrial and ventricular leads are pacing. This produces a wide QRS.

If all beats have a wide QRS and the patient does not have a pacemaker, the patient likely has a BBB. From lead II alone, one cannot accurately tell whether an LBBB or an RBBB is present. In precordial lead V_1 (see Fig. 11-6), an RBBB usually is manifested by a QRS with an "M or rSR" pattern (small initial upward deflection, downward deflection, larger upward deflection). LBBB in V_1 is usually manifested by a "QS or rS" pattern. The "QS" pattern is a single wide downward deflection (see Fig. 11-2). The "rS" pattern has a small initial upward deflection followed by a wider downward deflection. However, accurate diagnosis of a BBB requires a 12-lead ECG. One can simply comment in the sleep study report that a wide QRS appeared to be present.

REFERENCES

1. Wagner GS (ed): Marriott's Practical Electrocardiography, 9th ed. Philadelphia: Williams & Wilkins, 1994.
2. Caples SM, Rosen CLK, Shen WK, et al: The scoring of cardiac events during sleep. J Clin Sleep Med 2007;3:147–154.
3. Iber C, Ancoli-Isreal S, Chesson A, Quan SF for the American Academy of Sleep Medicine: The AASM Manual for the Scoring of Sleep and Associated Events: Rules, Terminology and Technical Specification, 1st ed. Westchester, IL: American Academy of Sleep Medicine, 2007.
4. Anonymous: Scoring Manual FAQs. Available at http://www.aasmnet.org/Resources/PDF/FAQScoringManual.pdf
5. Davignon A, Rautaharju P, Boiselle E, et al: Normal ECG standards for infants and children. Pediatr Cardiol 1979;1: 133–152.
6. Rosen CL, Quan SF, Xue W, et al: Pediatric heart rate data during sleep from ethnically diverse cohorts. Sleep 2006;29:88–89.
7. Archbold KH, Johnson NL, Goodwin JL, et al: Normative heart rate parameters during sleep for children aged 6 to 11 years. J Clin Sleep Med 2010;6:47–50.
8. Bjerregaard P: Mean 24 hour heart rate and pauses in healthy subjects 40–79 years of age. Eur Heart J 1983;4:44–51.
9. Gamaldo C, Sala RE, Collop NA: Complex arrhythmia during a sleep study—what to do? J Clin Sleep Med 2009;5:171–173.
10. Mehra R, Strohl KP: Incidence of serious adverse events during nocturnal polysomnography. Sleep 2004;27:1379–1383.

Monitoring of Limb Movements and Other Movements during Sleep

Chapter Points

- A significant LM has a duration from 0.5 to 10 seconds and a minimum amplitude 8 μV above the baseline resting EMG.
- The minimum number of LMs to define a PLM series (and, hence, LMs are PLMs) is four. The period length between LMs in a PLM series is 5 to 90 seconds (onset to onset).
- If the onset of two LMs is separated by < 5 seconds, they are counted as 1 LM.
- LMs are not considered part of a PLM series if they occur from 0.5 second before the start of a respiratory event to 0.5 second after the respiratory event. That is, LMs associated with respiratory events are not counted.
- PLMD is diagnosed when PLMS is present, RLS is not present, and there is a clinical sleep disturbance or complaint of daytime fatigue, and PLMS and the sleep complaint are not better explained by another disorder. PLMS is common and usually asymptomatic. PLMD is uncommon.
- ALMA and HFT occur at a faster rate than PLMs and often occur at sleep-wake transitions. They are felt to have no clinical significance.
- The EMG changes associated with the RBD (REM sleep without atonia) can occur in the chin EMG, chin EMG and limb EMG, or limb EMG alone. The changes include a sustained elevation of the chin EMG activity and TMA in either the chin EMG, the limb EMG, or both.
- The diagnosis of RBD requires BOTH finding REM without atonia AND either PSG documentation OR a history of dream-enacting behavior. In addition, absence of REM-related epileptiform activity (rare) is required to diagnose the RBD.
- Bruxism can occur in any stage of sleep and wake and a rhythmic pattern may be seen in the EEG or chin EMG derivations. The diagnosis of bruxism requires at least two episodes of audible sound of teeth grinding—diagnosis not based on EEG/EMG findings alone. If no sounds are audible, one might simply comment that a pattern typical of bruxism was observed.
- The frequency of rhythmic movement disorder movements is 0.5 to 2 Hz. The amplitude of movements must be at least twice the background. Video PSG is extremely helpful in making the diagnosis and documenting the type (e.g., head banging, body rocking).

A number of movement disorders are classified in the International Classification of Sleep Disorders, 2nd edition (ICSD-2), as *sleep-related movement disorders*[1] (Table 12–1). The restless legs syndrome (RLS) and periodic limb movement disorder (PLMD) are discussed in detail in Chapter 23. This chapter discusses monitoring of limb movements (LMs) and also the scoring rules for periodic limb movements in sleep (PLMS), bruxism, the rhythmic movement disorder (RMD), and the rapid eye movement (REM) sleep behavior disorder (RBD). The chapter also covers three LM patterns considered to be benign conditions: alternating leg movement activity (ALMA), hypnagogic foot tremor (HFT), and excessive fragmentary myoclonus (EFM). These three LM patterns are listed in the ICSD-2 under "Isolated Symptoms and Apparently Normal Variants."

LIMB MONITORING TECHNIQUES

Recording of limb muscle electromyogram (EMG) activity in polysomnography (PSG) is used to document the presence and frequency of LMs.[2,3] The EMG activities of the right anterior tibialis (RAT) and left anterior tibialis (LAT) muscles are routinely monitored. However, in patients with suspected RBD, arm muscle EMG activity is also recorded because this disorder is associated with abnormal EMG activity during REM sleep in the arms and legs as well as the chin derivations. The classic periodic leg movement (PLM) consists of

TABLE 12-1

Sleep-Related Movement Disorders (ICSD-2)

- Restless legs syndrome
- Periodic limb movement disorder
- Sleep-related leg cramps
- Sleep-related bruxism
- Sleep-related rhythmic movement disorder
- Sleep-related movement disorder, unspecified
- Sleep-related movement disorder due to drug or substance
- Sleep-related movement disorder due to medical condition

ICSD-2 = International Classification of Sleep Disorders, 2nd ed.
Data from American Academy of Sleep Medicine: ICSD-2 International Classification of Sleep Disorders, 2nd ed. Diagnostic and Coding Manual. Westchester, IL: American Academy of Sleep Medicine, 2005.

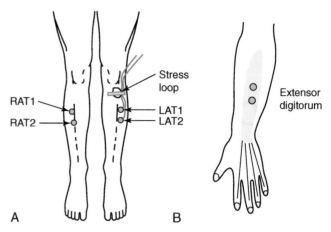

FIGURE 12-1 A, Placement of electrodes for monitoring right (RAT) and left anterior tibialis (LAT) electromyogram (EMG) activity (RAT, LAT). **B,** Placement of electrodes for monitoring the activity of forearm muscles (extensor digitorum).

extension of the big toe, dorsiflexion at the ankle, and sometimes flexion at the knee and hip—similar to the movement associated with the Babinski reflex. The PSG finding of PLMs is a very common finding and usually not associated with symptoms. However, PLMs can result in sleep disturbance of the patient or bed partner.

Leg EMG is recorded using bipolar AC amplifiers with surface electrodes using methods similar to those used to record chin EMG activity. The electrodes should have an impedance less than 10 KΩ (<5 KΩ is preferred). The recommended low- and high-frequency filter display settings are 10 Hz and 100 Hz, respectively. Use of a 60-Hz notch filter is discouraged. Having the patient move the left and right legs (wiggle toes) is part of the biocalibration series. In electroencephalogram (EEG) derivations that use a 35-Hz high-frequency filter, turning off the 60-Hz filter has relatively little effect. However, given the 100-Hz high-frequency filter setting used for leg EMG recording, turning off the 60-Hz filter will significantly increase signal amplitude if 60-Hz contamination is present. This can be minimized by low electrode impedance.[2,3]

Separate EMG electrodes are placed along the long axis of the belly of the anterior tibialis muscle around the middle of the muscle (Fig. 12-1). The American Academy of Sleep Medicine (AASM) scoring manual[3] recommends that the electrodes be placed either 2 to 3 cm apart or one third the length of the anterior tibialis muscle, whichever is shorter. As discussed later, because voltage amplitude criteria are used to identify significant LMs, the relaxed leg EMG activity should be less than ± 5 µV. Both legs should be monitored for the presence of LMs. Using a separate channel (tracing) for each leg is strongly preferred. Combining electrodes from the two legs to give a single recorded channel may suffice for some clinical settings, though it should be recognized that this strategy may reduce the number of detected LMs. Movements of the upper limbs may be sampled if clinically

indicated. The extensor digitorum is commonly monitored. The muscle is on the lateral/dorsal aspect of the forearm and is an extensor of the digits (see Fig. 12-1). Placement of the electrodes to monitor the extensor digitorum is along the long axis of the belly of the muscle separated by a few centimeters. The location of the muscle can be determined by having the patient extend the arm with the palm down and then make a fist (opening and closing the hand). During biocalibration, the patient is asked to extend the digits to check for signal adequacy.

CRITERIA FOR LMS AND PLMS

In the following discussion, **individual leg (limb) movements are denoted by LM, individual periodic leg movements as PLMs,** and the PSG finding of periodic limb movements in sleep by **PLMS.** Although leg movements (RAT, LAT EMG) are typically monitored, the term *periodic limb movements* is used to be more inclusive. Scoring criteria for PLMs proposed by Coleman[2] were widely used and included in the International Classification of Sleep Disorders, 1st edition[4] (ICSD-1). Subsequently, a task force of the American Sleep Disorders Association published recommendations for recording and scoring LMs[5] using similar scoring criteria and providing many illustrative tracings of LMs. The ICSD-2 used these criteria for defining PLMs.[4] Significant LMs were 0.5 to 5 seconds in duration with an amplitude at least one quarter of the LM amplitude during biocalibration.[1] Subsequently, the scoring criteria were revised by the World Association of Sleep Medicine (WASM) in collaboration with the International Restless Legs Syndrome Study Group (IRLSSG).[6] The major change was extending the maximum duration of LMs to 10 seconds and using voltage amplitude criteria. These criteria for scoring LMs and PLMs are identical with the recommendations of the recently published AASM scoring manual.[3,7] Of note, the resting anterior tibialis EMG activity should be less than ± 5 µV.

The current criteria for determining a significant LM event are listed in Table 12–2. In the new criteria, a significant LM has a duration from 0.5 to 10 seconds with a **minimum amplitude 8 µV above the resting leg EMG.** The *time of onset* is the time at which the amplitude increased to 8 µV above baseline resting activity, and the *end of the LM (offset)* is defined as the START of a period lasting at least 0.5 second during which the EMG does not exceed 2 µV above resting EMG (Fig. 12–2). Use of voltage criteria based on an absolute increase in microvolts above the resting baseline requires a stable resting EMG for the relaxed anterior tibialis muscle. The absolute signal should be no greater than 10 µV between negative and positive deflections (±5 µV).

The AASM scoring manual also provides rules for defining a PLM series (Table 12–3), that is, criteria for identifying a LM as a PLM. The minimum number of consecutive LMs

to define a PLM series is 4 consecutive LMs. The time from onset of one LM to the onset of the next LM is 5 to 90 seconds. LMs on different legs separated by less than 5 seconds between LM onsets are counted as a single LM. Figure 12–3 presents a 90-second segment of left and right anterior tibial EMG tracings.

LMs ASSOCIATED WITH RESPIRATORY EVENTS ARE NOT SCORED

An LM should **not** be scored if it occurs during a **period from 0.5 second before an apnea or hypopnea to 0.5 second after an apnea or hypopnea** (LMs associated with respiratory events are not scored).[3] The scoring rules did not provide information about scoring LMs associated with respiratory

---

TABLE 12–2

Rules Defining a Significant Leg Movement Event

1. **Minimum** duration of an LM event is 0.5 sec.

2. **Maximum** duration of an LM event is 10 sec.

3. The minimum amplitude of an LM event is an 8-µV increase in EMG voltage above resting EMG.

4. The timing of the onset of an LM event is defined as the point at which there is an 8-µV increase in EMG above resting EMG.

5. The timing of the **ending of an LM event** is defined as the **START** of a period lasting at least 0.5 sec during which the EMG does not exceed 2 µV above resting EMG.

EMG = electromyogram; LM = leg movement.
From Iber C, Ancoli-Israel S, Chesson A, Quan SF for the American Academy of Sleep Medicine: The AASM Manual for the Scoring of Sleep and Associated Events: Rules, Terminology and Technical Specification, 1st ed. Westchester, IL: American Academy of Sleep Medicine, 2007, pp. 41–42.

TABLE 12–3

Rules Defining a Periodic Leg Movement Series*

1. The minimum number of consecutive LM events to define a PLM series is **4 LMs.**

2. The minimum period length between LMs (defined as the time between onsets of consecutive LMs) to include them as part of a PLM series is **5 sec.**

3. The maximum period length between LMs (defined as the time between onsets of consecutive LMs) to include them as part of a PLM series is **90 sec.**

4. LMs on two different legs separated **by < 5 sec between movement onsets** are counted as a **single** LM.

*Criteria for LMs to be considered PLMs.
Note: It is understood that PLMS means that the LMs occur during sleep.
LM = leg movement; PLM = periodic leg movement.
From Iber C, Ancoli-Israel S, Chesson A, Quan SF for the American Academy of Sleep Medicine: The AASM Manual for the Scoring of Sleep and Associated Events: Rules, Terminology and Technical Specification, 1st ed. Westchester, IL: American Academy of Sleep Medicine, 2007, pp. 41–42.

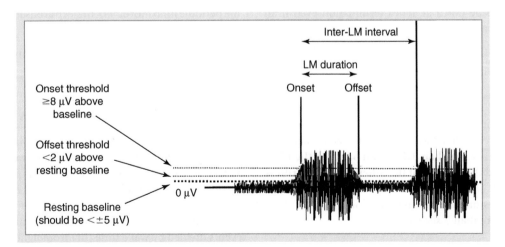

FIGURE 12–2 Criteria for onset and offset of leg movements (LMs). The time of onset is the time at which the amplitude increased to 8 µV above the baseline resting activity. The end of the LM (offset) is defined as the START of a period lasting at least 0.5 second during which the EMG does not exceed 2 µV above the resting EMG. *Adapted from Zucconi M, Ferri R, Allen R, et al: The official World Association of Sleep Medicine (WASM) Standards for Recording and Scoring Periodic Leg Movements in Sleep (PLMS) and Wakefulness (PLMW) developed in collaboration with a task force from the International Restless Legs Syndrome Study Group (IRLSSG). Sleep Med 2006;7:175–183.*

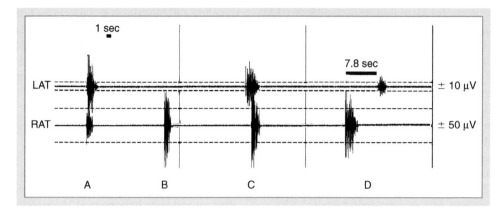

FIGURE 12–3 A 90-second tracing of the left anterior tibilais (LAT) and right anterior tibialis (RAT) EMGs. The *broken lines* in the LAT tracing are +10 μV amplitude lines. The *dark bars* are durations in seconds. According to the scoring rules, a total of 5 periodic limb movements (PLMs) are shown. In group *A,* there is 1 PLM. In group *B,* there is 1 PLM. In group *C,* there is 1 PLM because limb movements (LMs) whose onset is separated by less than 5 seconds are considered as 1 LM. In group *D,* there are 2 PLMs.

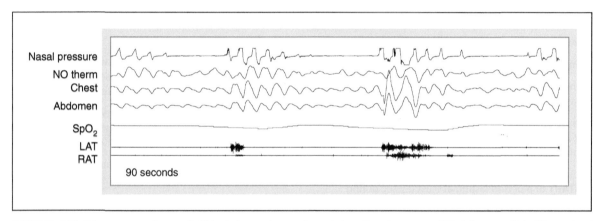

FIGURE 12–4 The LMs are not counted as part of a PLM series because they occur in association with respiratory events. LAT = left anterior tibialis; NO = nasal-oral thermal flow; RAT = right anterior tibialis; SpO₂ = pulse oximetry.

effort–related arousals (RERAs). However, some clinicians would extend the previous rule to RERAs. It is not uncommon for LMs to be noted at apnea termination even if an associated cortical arousal is not present. In Figure 12–4, the leg EMG bursts associated with respiratory events are not scored as LMs or PLMs.

ASSOCIATION OF AROUSALS WITH PLM

According to the AASM scoring manual, an arousal and PLM should be considered associated with each other (Fig. 12–5) when there is **less than 0.5 second between the END of one event and the ONSET of the other event, regardless of which is first.** This recommendation differs from previous criteria, which required the arousal to follow the onset of the PLM by not more than 3 seconds.

PERIODIC LIMB MOVEMENTS IN SLEEP

Of note, the term PLMS implies that PLMs occur during sleep. The AASM scoring manual[3] recommends reporting the number of PLMS and the periodic limb movement in

sleep index (PLMSI), which is the number of PLMs per hour of sleep. The number of PLMs associated with arousal and the periodic limb movement in sleep arousal index (PLMSAI) should also be reported.

PLMSI = 60 × number of PLMs/TST (min)

PLMSAI = 60 × number of PLMs with arousal/TST (min)

PERIODIC LIMB MOVEMENTS IN WAKE

The AASM scoring manual did not recommend criteria for scoring periodic limb movements during wake (PLMW). The WASM in collaboration with the IRLSSG[6] published recommendations for PLMW. The criteria for PLMW events is the same as for PLMS events except that the patient is awake (Fig. 12–6). The *PLMW index* is defined as the number of PLMW events divided by wake time (hr) from lights out to lights on while the patient is in bed. That is, time when the patient is out of bed or sitting on the side of the bed is not included. Of note, frequent PLMW events are highly suggestive of the RLS. If PLMW events are noted, the patient history should be reviewed to determine if RLS symptoms are reported.

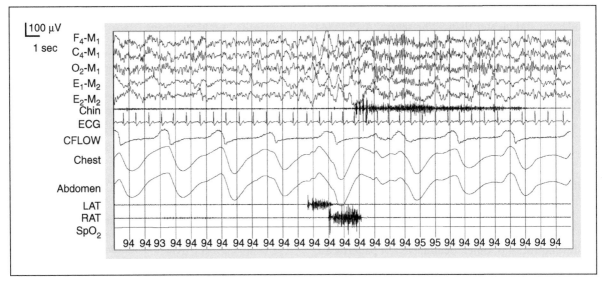

FIGURE 12–5 A LM (part of a PLM series) is associated with an arousal. Note that the LM on the LAT tracing and the LM on the RAT tracing are counted as a single LM. CFLOW = positive airway pressure device flow signal; ECG = electrocardiogram; LAT = left anterior tibialis; RAT = right anterior tibialis; SpO$_2$ = pulse oximetry.

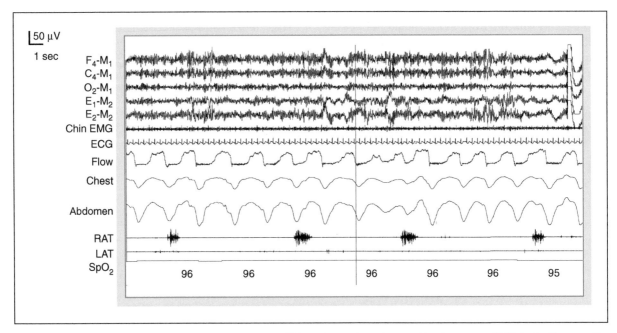

FIGURE 12–6 PLMs in wake. A 60-second tracing with the patient in stage W during the start of a continuous positive airway pressure (CPAP) titration. Flow = machine flow (CFLOW). PLMs in wake are noted. The patient reported severe symptoms of the restless legs syndrome. ECG = electrocardiogram; EMG = electromyogram; LAT = left anterior tibialis; RAT = right anterior tibialis; SpO$_2$ = pulse oximetry.

SUGGESTED IMMOBILIZATION TEST

The Suggested Immobilization Test (SIT) was developed to help make the diagnosis of the RLS.[8] The test detects and counts PLMW. The patient sits with the legs outstretched and attempts to keep the legs still for 30 minutes to an hour. EMG recording of the left and right anterior tibialis muscles is performed. The test is often administered in the evening. The combination of rest and monitoring in the evening worsens RLS. In one study of the SIT, patients with RLS had significantly more PLMW than controls (76.1/hr vs. 26.9/hr). In

this study, using a PLMW index of 40/hr to diagnose RLS, the sensitivity and specificity were 81% and 81%, respectively (compared with RLS clinical criteria based on history).

CLINICAL SIGNIFICANCE OF PLMS

PLMS is discussed in more detail in Chapter 23. There are no widely accepted criteria for what constitutes a normal, mildly, moderately, or severely increased PLMSI. In the ICSD-1,[4] the following severity scheme was recommended:

PLMSI less than 5/hr normal, 5 to 25 mild, 25 to less than 50/hr moderate, and greater than 50/hr severe. A PLMSAI greater than 25/hr was identified as severe. It has been recognized that most patients with PLMS in the absence of the RLS are usually asymptomatic. Approximately 80% to 90% of patients with RLS will have PLMs on a given sleep study.[9] The PLMD (clinical sleep disturbance or daytime fatigue due to PLMS without RLS) is thought to be rare. The new AASM scoring manual does not provide a scheme for grading severity of the PLM index. The ICSD-2 requires a PLM index of 15/hr in adults and 5/hr in children as criteria for the diagnosis of the PLMD (Table 12–4).[1]

OTHER LMS DURING SLEEP

In the following sections, other identifiable LM patterns are discussed, including ALMA, HFT, and EFM. To date, the presence of these patterns does not appear to be associated with clinically significant disorder. However, ALMA and HFT are fairly common and are sometimes confused with PLMs.

Of note, PLMS during REM sleep (stage R) is uncommon except in patients with the RBD. PLMs should not be confused with transient muscle activity in the leg EMG that can occur during stage R. Transient muscle activity is discussed in a later section.

ALTERNATING LEG MUSCLE ACTIVATION

ALMA[7,10–12] is characterized by EMG bursts that alternate between the legs (Fig. 12–7). Because there have been no reported clinical consequences of this pattern, it is believed

TABLE 12–4
Periodic Leg Movement Disorder Diagnostic Criteria (ICSD-2)*
A. PLMs present—LMs meet criteria to be PLMs i. 0.5–10 sec in duration. ii. Amplitude > 8 µV above baseline. iii. In a sequence of four or more movements. iv. Onsets of consecutive LMs ≥ 5 and ≤ 90 sec.
B. PLM index > 15/hr adults and > 5/hr in children ("in most cases").
C. There is a clinical sleep disturbance or complaint of daytime fatigue.
D. The PLMs and clinical sleep disturbance are not better explained by another current sleep disorder or medical, neurologic, or psychiatric disorder.

Notes:
1. A diagnosis of RLS excludes PLMD.
2. If PLMs are present **without** a sleep complaint, they can simply be noted as a PSG finding.
3. If only the bed partners' sleep is disturbed, this is not sufficient to make a diagnosis of PLMD.
*Updated according to the AASM scoring manual.
AASM = American Academy of Sleep Medicine; LMs = leg movements; PLMD = periodic leg movement disorder; PLMs = periodic leg movements; PSG = polysomnography; RLS = restless leg syndrome.
Data from American Academy of Sleep Medicine: ICSD-2 International Classification of Sleep Disorders, 2nd ed. Diagnostic and Coding Manual. Westchester, IL: American Academy of Sleep Medicine, 2005; and Iber C, Ancoli-Israel S, Chesson A, Quan SF for the American Academy of Sleep Medicine: The AASM Manual for the Scoring of Sleep and Associated Events: Rules, Terminology and Technical Specification, 1st ed. Westchester, IL: American Academy of Sleep Medicine, 2007, pp. 41–42.

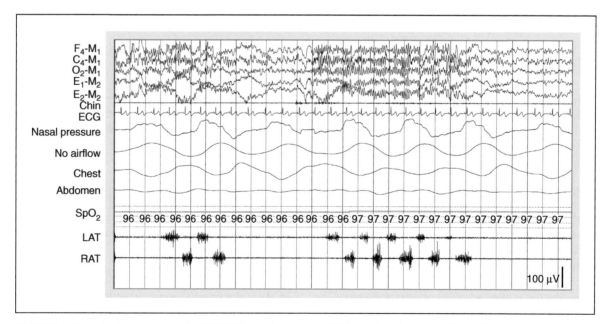

FIGURE 12–7 Alternating leg movement activity (ALMA). A 30-second tracing shows EMG bursts alternating between the legs. ECG = electrocardiogram; LAT = left anterior tibialis; RAT = right anterior tibialis; SpO₂ = pulse oximetry.

to be a benign finding. ALMA can often occur in association with arousals or at sleep-wake transitions.

The usual range of duration of ALMA EMG bursts is 100 to 500 msec (see Fig. 12–7). The AASM scoring manual criteria for ALMA are listed in Table 12–5. ALMA consists of short EMG bursts that alternate between the legs and are higher in frequency than PLMs. The minimum frequency of ALMAs is 0.5 Hz, meaning that the onsets can be separated by no more than 2 seconds (in contrast, individual PLMs are separated by a **minimum** of 5 sec).

HYPNAGOGIC FOOT TREMOR

HFT[7,11,13] is a phenomenon characterized by a pattern of leg EMG bursts that is more rapid than those seen with PLMs. The usual range for the duration of HFT bursts is 250 to 1000 msec. The pattern may be seen during wakefulness or associated with arousal from sleep (Fig. 12–8). Unlike ALMA, the EMG bursts of HFT do not alternate between the legs. The maximum time period between onset of HFT EMG bursts is 3.3 seconds. The AASM scoring manual criteria for HFT are listed in Table 12–6.

A summary of criteria for scoring PLMs, ALMAs, and HFTs is shown in Table 12–7 for comparison.

EXCESSIVE FRAGMENTARY MYOCLONUS

EFM[7,11,13,14] (Fig. 12–9) is defined by a characteristic EMG pattern in the leg tracings consisting of very brief EMG bursts (<150 msec). It is thought to be a benign phenomenon. It most cases, no movements are visible, or if present, they are much like the small twitchlike movements of the

---

TABLE 12–5

Scoring Criteria for Alternating Leg Movement Activity

These rules define ALMA:

1. **Four ALMAs** is the minimum number of **discrete and alternating** bursts of leg muscle activity needed to score an ALMA series.

2. The **minimum frequency** of alternating EMG bursts in ALMA is **0.5 Hz** (≤2 sec duration between bursts).

3. The **maximum frequency** of alternating EMG bursts in ALMA is **3.0 Hz** (≥0.33 sec duration between bursts).

ALMA = alternating leg movement activity; EMG = electromyogram.
From Iber C, Ancoli-Israel S, Chesson A, Quan SF for the American Academy of Sleep Medicine: The AASM Manual for the Scoring of Sleep and Associated Events: Rules, Terminology and Technical Specification, 1st ed. Westchester, IL: American Academy of Sleep Medicine, 2007, pp. 41–42.

TABLE 12–6

Scoring Criteria for Hypnagogic Foot Tremor

These rules define HFT:

1. The **minimum** number of bursts needed to mask a train of bursts in HFT is **4**.

2. The **minimum frequency** of the EMG bursts of HFT is **0.3 Hz** (≤3.3 sec between onset of bursts).

3. The **maximum frequency** of the EMG bursts of HFT is **4 Hz** (≥0.25 sec between onset of bursts).

EMG = electromyogram; HFT = hypnagogic foot tremor.
From Iber C, Ancoli-Israel S, Chesson A, Quan SF for the American Academy of Sleep Medicine: The AASM Manual for the Scoring of Sleep and Associated Events: Rules, Terminology and Technical Specification, 1st ed. Westchester, IL: American Academy of Sleep Medicine, 2007, pp. 41–42.

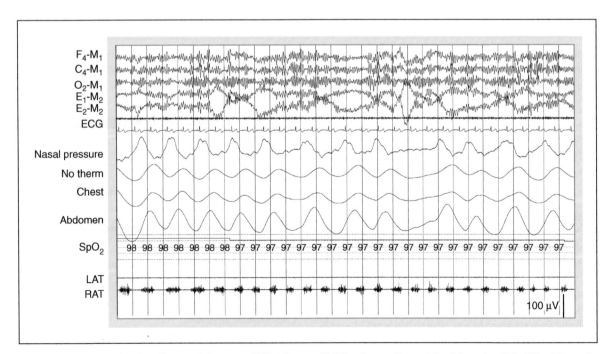

FIGURE 12–8 A 30-second tracing of hypnagogic foot tremor (HFT) during stage W. ECG = electrocardiogram; LAT = left anterior tibialis; RAT = right anterior tibialis; SpO₂ = pulse oximetry.

TABLE 12-7

Comparison of Periodic Leg Movements, Alternate Leg Movement Activity, and Hypnagogic Foot Tremor Events

	LMS, PLMS	ALMA	HFT
EMG burst duration	0.5–10 sec	100–500 msec	250–1000 msec
Number of bursts in a series	4	4	4
Minimum frequency (1/sec)	0.01	0.5	0.3
Maximum frequency (1/sec)	0.2	3	4
Minimum time between onsets (sec)	5	0.33	0.25
Maximum time between onsets (sec)	90	2.0	3.3
Sleep present	Yes	Not required	Not required

ALMA = alternating leg movement activity; EMG = electromyogram; HFT = hypnagogic foot tremor; LMs = leg movements; PLMs = periodic leg movements.

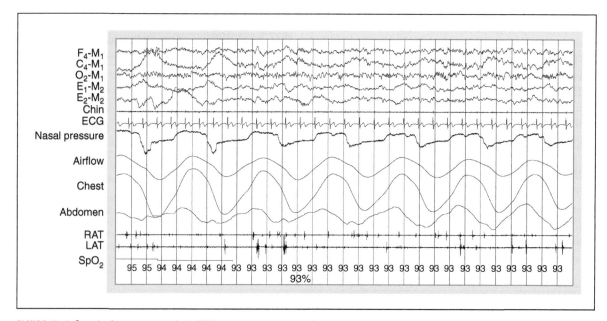

FIGURE 12-9 Excessive fragmentary myoclonus (EFM). A 30-second epoch with fragmentary myoclonus during non–rapid eye movement (NREM) sleep. In this patient, 30 minutes of similar activity were noted meeting criteria for EFM. ECG = electrocardiogram; LAT = left anterior tibialis; RAT = right anterior tibialis; SpO₂ = pulse oximetry.

fingers and toes seen intermittently during REM sleep in normal individuals. To qualify for EFM, the EMG pattern often seen during REM sleep must also be seen during non–rapid eye movement (NREM) sleep (Table 12–8).

BRUXISM

Bruxism is a grinding or clinching of the teeth[1,3,7] (Fig. 12–10). It is associated with characteristic rhythmic muscle artifact in the EEG (rhythmic EMG activity of the scalp muscle underlying the EEG electrodes) and chin EMG activity. During sleep, jaw contractions are either tonic (jaw clinching) or phasic (intermittent bursts of activity) termed *rhythmic masticatory muscle activity (RMMA)*. Of note, a diagnosis of bruxism consists of more than detection of RMMA—there must be audible tooth grinding (Table 12–9).

TABLE 12-8

Scoring Criteria for Excessive Fragmentary Myoclonus

These rules define EFM:
1. The usual maximum EMG burst duration seen in EFM events is **150 msec.**

2. At least **20 minutes of NREM sleep with EFM** must be recorded.

3. At least **5 EMG potentials/min** must be recorded.

Note: Twitchlike movements in fingers, toes, and corner of mouth may be seen but no gross movements.
EFM = excessive fragmentary myoclonus; EMG = electromyogram; NREM = non–rapid eye movement.
From Iber C, Ancoli-Israel S, Chesson A, Quan SF for the American Academy of Sleep Medicine: The AASM Manual for the Scoring of Sleep and Associated Events: Rules, Terminology and Technical Specification, 1st ed. Westchester, IL: American Academy of Sleep Medicine, 2007, pp. 41–42.

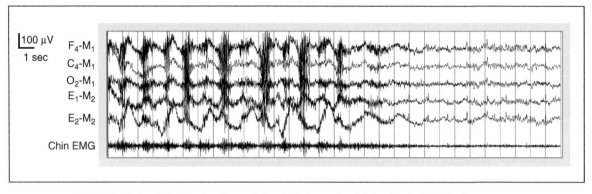

FIGURE 12–10 An episode of bruxism. The sound of tooth grinding was heard during the episode. EMG = electromyogram.

TABLE 12–9
Sleep-Related Bruxism (ICSD-2)
A. The patient reports or is aware of tooth grinding sounds or tooth clenching during sleep.

B. One of more of the following is present:
  i. Abnormal wear of teeth.
  ii. Jaw muscle discomfort, fatigue, or pain and jaw lock upon awakening.
  iii. Masseter muscle hypertrophy upon voluntary forceful clenching.

C. The jaw muscle activity is not better explained by another current sleep disorder, medical or neurologic disorder, medication use, or substance use disorder.
PSG Criteria (not listed as essential ICSD-2 criteria but outlined in explanatory text in the ICSD-2 manual): • At least 25 individual bursts/hr of sleep or • Four bruxism episodes/hr of sleep. • There should also be at least two audible tooth grinding episodes per sleep recording session in the absence of abnormal EEG (epilepsy).

EEG = electroencephalogram; ICSD-2 = International Classification of Sleep Disorders, 2nd ed; PSG = polysomnography.
Adapted from American Academy of Sleep Medicine: ICSD-2 International Classification of Sleep Disorders, 2nd ed. Diagnostic and Coding Manual. Westchester, IL: American Academy of Sleep Medicine, 2005.

TABLE 12–10
Scoring Manual Rules for Bruxism
1. Bruxism may consist of brief (phasic) or sustained (tonic) elevations of chin EMG activity that are at least **twice the amplitude of the background EMG.**
2. Brief elevations of chin EMG activity are scored as bruxism if they are **0.25–2 sec in duration** and if **at least three such elevations occur in a regular sequence.**
3. Sustained elevations of chin EMG activity are scored as bruxism if the **duration > 2 sec.**
4. A period of at least 3 sec of stable background chin EMG must occur before a new episode of bruxism can be scored.
5. Bruxism can be scored reliably by audio in combination with PSG by a **minimum of two audible tooth grinding episodes/night of PSG in the absence of epilepsy.**

EMG = electromyogram; PSG = polysomnography.
From Iber C, Ancoli-Israel S, Chesson A, Quan SF for the American Academy of Sleep Medicine: The AASM Manual for the Scoring of Sleep and Associated Events: Rules, Terminology and Technical Specification, 1st ed. Westchester, IL: American Academy of Sleep Medicine, 2007, pp. 41–42.

Bruxism is common in childhood (14–17%) and less prevalent in teenagers (12%), middle-aged adults (8%), and older adults (3%). Bruxism tends to occur in families. Approximately 20% to 50% of patients have at least one family member with a history of bruxism.

PSG Characteristics of Bruxism

Bruxism can occur in any stage of sleep or at arousal from sleep. It is most common in stage N1 and N2 and least common during REM sleep. The ICSD-2 recommends audio monitoring and monitoring of at least one masseter muscle for the diagnosis of bruxism. PSG criteria were not listed as essential diagnostic criteria for bruxism in the ICSD-2.

However, in the explanatory text, PSG criteria included at least 25 individual bursts/hr of sleep or 4 bruxism episodes/hr of sleep. It was also stated that there should also be at least two episodes in which tooth grinding is heard on audio monitoring in the absence of epilepsy. The AASM scoring manual provides updated scoring criteria for bruxism (Table 12–10). The scoring rules indicate that the chin EMG activity must be at least twice the amplitude of the background EMG. At least three elevations of EMG activity that are 0.25 to 2 seconds in duration should be present. For **sustained EMG** elevations to be scored as bruxism, the duration must be **more than 2 seconds**.

Whereas rhythmic EMG activity in the chin electrodes can often be noted during bruxism episodes, such activity is often more prominent if EMG recording over the masseter muscles is performed. In some patients, bruxism may actually be more apparent from muscle artifact in the EEG and electro-oculogram (EOG) derivations than in the chin EMG.

TABLE 12–11
Prevalence of Rhythmic Movements

AGE	FREQUENCY OF RMs
9 mo	59% of infants reported to have some type of RM • Body rocking (43%) • Head banging (22%) • Head rolling (24%)
18 mo	33% have some type of RM
5 yr	5% still have some type of RM

RMs = rhythmic movements.
From American Academy of Sleep Medicine: ICSD-2 International Classification of Sleep Disorders, 2nd ed. Diagnostic and Coding Manual. Westchester, IL: American Academy of Sleep Medicine, 2005.

TABLE 12–12
Sleep-Related Rhythmic Movement Disorder (ICSD-2)

A. The patient exhibits repetitive, stereotyped, and rhythmic movement behaviors.
B. The movements involve large muscle groups.
C. The movements are predominantly sleep related, occurring near nap or bedtime, or when the individual appears drowsy or sleepy.
D. The behaviors result in a significant complaint manifested by at least one of the following: i. Interference with normal sleep. ii. Significant impairment of daytime function. iii. Self-inflicted bodily injury that requires medical treatment (or would result in injury if preventable measures were not used).
E. The rhythmic movements are not better explained by another current sleep disorder, medical or neurologic disorder, mental disorder, medication use, or substance use disorder.

CLINICAL SUBTYPES OF RMD

• Body rocking type
• Head banging type
• Head rolling type
• Other type: body rolling, leg rolling, leg banging
• Combined type: involves one or more subtypes.

ICSD = International Classification of Sleep Disorders, 2nd ed; RMD = rhythmic movement disorder.
Adapted from American Academy of Sleep Medicine: ICSD-2 International Classification of Sleep Disorders, 2nd ed. Diagnostic and Coding Manual. Westchester, IL: American Academy of Sleep Medicine, 2005.

In Figure 12–10, one can see rhythmic contractions of the chin EMG and also muscle artifact in the EEG and EOG derivations. During this episode, loud tooth grinding was heard.

RHYTHMIC MOVEMENTS AND THE SLEEP-RELATED RHYTHMIC MOVEMENT DISORDER

Rhythmic movements (RMs) are common in normal infants and children[15–17] (Table 12–11). Without significant evidence of consequences, the movements alone would not be considered a disorder. The term *rhythmic movement disorder (RMD)* implies consequences are present. The ICSD-2 terminology is *sleep-related rhythmic movement disorder (SRRMD)*.[1] The ICSD-2 diagnostic criteria for the SRRMD are listed in Table 12–12. Adverse consequences in making the diagnosis of SRRMD include interference with normal sleep, daytime sleepiness or sleep disturbance, and bodily injury to the patient (or potential bodily injury if preventive measures were not taken).

Several clinical subtypes of RMD are noted including body rocking type, head banging type, head rolling type, and combined type.

PSG Findings in RM

The literature concerning RM varies[1,15–17] with some references stating that RMs occur at sleep-wake transitions,[16] whereas others state that RMs are more common in stage N2.[1] The ICSD-2 manual[1] states that RM usually occurs during stage N2, can occur during N3, or occurs only in stage R. In some patients, RMs occur primarily during sleep-wake transitions. In most patients, the EEG shows normal activity between episodes of rhythmic behavior (although often obscured by movement artifact).

The AASM scoring manual[3] provides criteria for scoring RMs (Table 12–13). The frequency of movements is between 0.5 and 2.0 Hz. **At least four movements must be present** to define a cluster of RMs. The minimum amplitude of individual bursts is twice the background EMG activity

TABLE 12–13
Scoring Rules for the Polysomnography Features* of the Rhythmic Movement Disorder

These rules defines the PSG characteristics of RMD 1. The minimum frequency for scoring RMD is 0.5 Hz.
2. The maximum frequency for scoring RMD is 2.0 Hz.
3. The minimum number of individual movements required to make a cluster of rhythmic movements is **four.**
4. The minimum amplitude of an individual rhythmic burst is twice the background EMG activity.

**Note:* To be considered a DISORDER, a related complaint in addition to the body movements must be present.
EMG = electromyogram; RMD = rhythmic movement disorder.
From Iber C, Ancoli-Israel S, Chesson A, Quan SF for the American Academy of Sleep Medicine: The AASM Manual for the Scoring of Sleep and Associated Events: Rules, Terminology and Technical Specification, 1st ed. Westchester, IL: American Academy of Sleep Medicine, 2007, pp. 41–42.

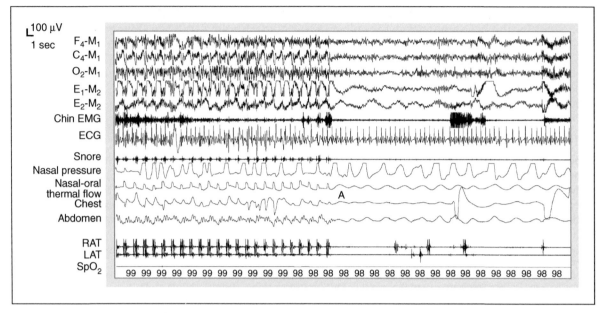

FIGURE 12–11 Head banging, a form of rhythmic movement (RM) disorder. A 60-second tracing of a 5-year-old child. The RMs are seen as rhythmic activity in multiple tracings—especially prominent here in the leg tracings and E_1-M_2. This is stage W with RM stopping at point *A*. ECG = electrocardiogram; EMG = electromyogram; LAT = left anterior tibialis; RAT = right anterior tibialis; SpO_2 = pulse oximetry.

(Fig. 12–11). The scoring manual recommends that bipolar surface electrodes be placed to record large muscle group involvement. However, time-synchronized video PSG is necessary to make the diagnosis of RMD. For most patients, no treatment for SRRMD is needed. In others with violent movements, bed padding may be necessary. The disorder can persist into childhood and adulthood. In some studies, an association between RMD and attention deficit hyperactivity disorder has been found in school-age children.[16]

RBD: SCORING PSG FEATURES

The RBD requires PSG evidence of REM sleep without atonia and either video PSG showing dream-enacting behavior or a compatible clinical history of episodes of dream-enacting behavior (Table 12–14).[1,3,7,18] The sustained muscle activity of the chin EMG or transient muscle activity of the chin or leg EMG is interrupted by episodes of dream-enacting behavior. The AASM scoring manual presents a system for defining excessive sustained chin EMG activity or excessive transient muscle activity in the chin or leg EMG derivations[1,18–21] (Table 12–15). Figure 12–12 is a 30-second tracing with periods of sustained chin EMG activity as well as excessive transient muscle activity in the leg EMG. *Sustained chin EMG activity* is defined as an epoch of REM sleep with at least 50% of the epoch having a chin amplitude greater than the minimum amplitude in NREM sleep. *Excessive transient muscle activity in the leg EMG* is defined as an epoch having at least 5 of the 10 sequential 3-second miniepochs containing bursts of transient muscle activity. Excessive transient muscle activity bursts are 0.1 to 5.0 seconds in duration and at least four times as high in amplitude as the background EMG activity. Figure 12–13 presents a 30-second

TABLE 12–14

Rapid Eye Movement Sleep Behavior Disorder (ICSD-2)

A. Presence of REM sleep without atonia: the EMG finding of excessive amounts of sustained or intermittent elevation of submental EMG tone or excessive phasic submental or (upper or lower) limb EMG twitching.

B. At least one of the following is present:
   i. Sleep-related injurious, potentially injurious, or disruptive behavior by history.
   ii. Abnormal REM sleep behavior documented during PSG monitoring.

C. Absence of EEG epileptiform activity during REM sleep unless RBD can be clearly distinguished from any concurrent REM sleep-related seizure disorder.

D. The sleep disturbance is not better explained by another sleep disorder, medical or neurologic disorder, mental disorder, or substance use disorder.

EMG = electromyogram; ICSD = International Classification of Sleep Disorders, 2nd ed; PSG = polysomnography; RBD = rapid eye movement sleep behavior disorder; REM = rapid eye movement.
From American Academy of Sleep Medicine: ICSD-2 International Classification of Sleep Disorders, 2nd ed. Diagnostic and Coding Manual. Westchester, IL: American Academy of Sleep Medicine, 2005.

epoch of stage R (REM) with typical low-amplitude chin EMG activity but excessive transient muscle activity in the leg EMG derivations.

In frequently asked questions (FAQ) M1 (http://www.aasmnet.org/Resources/PDF/FAQsScoringManual.pdf), the following question was asked: "In scoring the PSG features of RBD, how many epochs of REM sleep must show

TABLE 12–15

Scoring Rules for the Polysomnography Features* Associated with the Rapid Eye Movement Sleep Behavior Disorder

RULES

1. The PSG characteristics of RBD are characterized **by either or both** of the following features:
   a. Sustained muscle activity in REM sleep in the **chin EMG.**
   b. Excessive transient muscle activity during REM in **the chin or limb EMG.**

DEFINITIONS

Sustained muscle activity in REM sleep is defined as an epoch of REM sleep with at least 50% of the duration of the epoch having a chin EMG amplitude greater than the minimum amplitude in NREM.

Excessive transient muscle activity in REM sleep: In a 30-second epoch of REM sleep divided into 10 sequential 3-sec miniepochs, at least five (50%) of the miniepochs contain bursts of transient muscle activity. In RBD, excessive transient muscle activity bursts are 0.1–5.0 sec in duration and at least four times as high in amplitude as the background EMG activity.

Note: PSG features ALONE are not sufficient to diagnose RBD.

EMG = electromyogram; NREM = non–rapid eye movement; PSG = polysomnography; RBD = rapid eye movement sleep behavior disorder; REM = rapid eye movement.

From Iber C, Ancoli-Israel S, Chesson A, Quan SF for the American Academy of Sleep Medicine: The AASM Manual for the Scoring of Sleep and Associated Events: Rules, Terminology and Technical Specification, 1st ed. Westchester, IL: American Academy of Sleep Medicine, 2007, pp. 41–42.

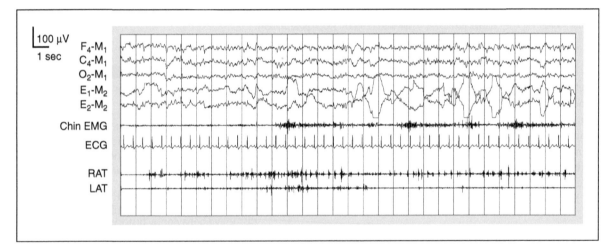

FIGURE 12–12 A 30-second tracing of stage R with transient muscle activity seen in the right anterior tibialis (RAT) and left anterior tibialis (LAT). Sustained muscle activity in the chin electromyogram (EMG) is noted in the last two thirds of the epoch. The RAT and LAT activity also meets criteria for excessive transient muscle activity. ECG = electrocardiogram.

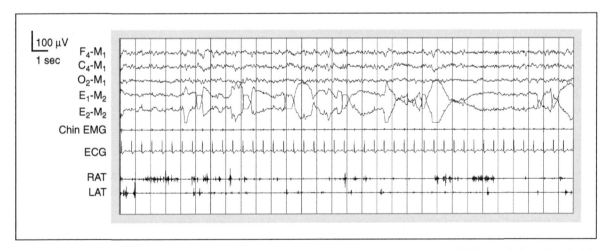

FIGURE 12–13 Another 30-second epoch in the same patient presented in Figure 12–12. Here, the chin electromyogram (EMG) is typical of stage R but the right anterior tibialis (RAT) and left anterior tibialis (LAT) show excessive transient muscle activity. ECG = electrocardiogram.

either sustained or excessive transient muscle activity for REM sleep as a whole to be considered compatible with RBD? The answer was "the manual has deliberately not specified this as there are little normative data. Clinicians are encouraged to read the relevant section of the supporting paper[7] to help them decide how to address this issue in their own laboratories." Certainly, a relatively large number of epochs with sustained or excessive transient EMG activity would be suggestive of RBD. Conversely, fewer epochs with intense EMG activity associated with characteristic body movements would also be suggestive of a diagnosis of RBD. In summary, patients with RBD can have characteristic findings in the chin EMG, limb EMGs (e.g., RAT and LAT), or both. Clinical correlation is needed. The RBD is discussed in more detail in Chapter 28.

CLINICAL REVIEW QUESTIONS

1. Frequent LMs during wake as documented by the anterior tibial derivations is most suggestive of:
   A. PLMD.
   B. PLMS.
   C. RLS.

2. A diagnosis of PLMD requires:
   A. Adult PLMSI > 5/hr, pediatric PLMSI > 5/hr.
   B. Adult PLMSI > 15/hr, pediatric PLMSI > 15/hr.
   C. Adult PLMSI > 10/hr, pediatric PLMSI > 5/hr.
   D. Adult PLMSI > 15/hr, pediatric PLMSI > 5/hr.

3. The duration of a significant LM is:
   A. 0.5–5 sec.
   B. 0.5–10 sec.
   C. 1–10 sec.
   D. 0.5–15 sec.

4. According to the AASM scoring manual, the minimum amplitude of a significant LM is:
   A. 25% of the baseline leg EMG.
   B. 50% of the baseline leg EMG.
   C. >8 µV above baseline limb EMG activity.
   D. >10 µV above baseline limb EMG activity.

5. A diagnosis of EFM requires that fragmentary myoclonus be present for at least:
   A. 20 min of REM sleep.
   B. 10 min of NREM sleep.
   C. 20 min of NREM sleep.
   D. 10 min of REM sleep.

6. A diagnosis of SRRMD requires:
   A. Movements must occur during sleep.
   B. Behaviors result in a significant complaint (impaired daytime function, bodily injury, interference with normal sleep).
   C. The minimum and maximum frequency of movements must be 1–3 Hz.

Answers

1. **C.** The diagnosis of RLS is based on clinical history but frequent LMs during wake (as during a prolonged sleep latency) are suggestive of the diagnosis.

2. **D.**

3. **B.**

4. **C.**

5. **C.**

6. **B.** To be diagnosed as a "disorder," complaints must be present. Frequency of movements is 0.5–2 Hz. Movements can occur during sleep-wake transitions.

REFERENCES

1. American Academy of Sleep Medicine: ICSD-2 International Classification of Sleep Disorders, 2nd ed. Diagnostic and Coding Manual. Westchester, IL: American Academy of Sleep Medicine, 2005.
2. Coleman RM: Periodic movements in sleep (nocturnal myoclonus) and restless legs syndrome. In Guilleminault C (ed): Sleeping and Waking Disorders: Indications and Techniques. Boston: Butterworths, 1982, pp. 265–295.
3. Iber C, Ancoli-Israel S, Chesson A, Quan SF for the American Academy of Sleep Medicine: The AASM Manual for the Scoring of Sleep and Associated Events: Rules, Terminology and Technical Specification, 1st ed. Westchester, IL: American Academy of Sleep Medicine, 2007, pp. 41–42.
4. American Sleep Disorders Association: International Classification of Sleep Disorders, 1st ed. Rochester, MN: American Sleep Disorders Association, 1990, pp. 65–68.
5. American Sleep Disorders Association: Recording and scoring leg movements. The Atlas Task Force. Sleep 1993;16:748–759.
6. Zucconi M, Ferri R, Allen R, et al: The official World Association of Sleep Medicine (WASM) Standards for Recording and Scoring Periodic Leg Movements in Sleep (PLMS) and Wakefulness (PLMW) developed in collaboration with a task force from the International Restless Legs Syndrome Study Group (IRLSSG). Sleep Med 2006;7:175–183.
7. Walters AS, Lavigne G, Hening W, et al: The scoring of movements in sleep. J Clin Sleep Med 2007;3:155–167.
8. Montplaisir J, Boucher S, Nicholas A, et al: Immobilization tests and periodic leg movements in sleep for the diagnosis of restless legs syndrome. Mov Disord 1998;13:324–329.
9. Montplaisir J, Boucher S, Poirer G, et al: Clinical, polysomnographic, and genetic characteristics of restless legs syndrome: a study of 133 patients diagnosed with the new standard criteria. Mov Disord 1997;12:61–65.
10. Chervin RD, Consens FB, Kutluay E: Alternating leg muscle activation during sleep and arousals: a new sleep-related motor phenomenon? Mov Disord 2003;18:551–559.
11. Berry RB: A woman with rhythmic foot movements. J Clin Sleep Med 2007;3:749–751.
12. Constantino FI, Iero I, Lanuzza B, et al: The neurophysiology of the alternating leg muscle activation (ALMA) during study of one patient before and after treatment with pramipexole. Sleep Med 2006;7:63–71.

13. Broughton R, Tolentino MA, Krelina M: Excessive fragmentary myoclonus in NREM sleep: a report of 38 cases. Electroencephalogr Clin Neurophysiol 1985;6:123–133.

14. Vetrugno R, Piazzi G, Provini F, et al: Excessive fragmentary hypnic myoclonus: clinical and neurophysiological findings. Sleep Med 2001;3:73–76.

15. Hoban TF: Rhythmic movement disorder in children. CNS Spectr 2003;8:135–138.

16. Stepanova I, Nevsimalova S, Hanusova J: Rhythmic movement disorder in sleep persisting into childhood and adulthood. Sleep 2005;28:851–857.

17. Kohyama J, Matsukura F, Kimura K, Tachibana N: Rhythmic movement disorder: polysomnographic study and summary of reported cases. Brain Dev 2002;24:33–38.

18. Lapierre O, Montplaisir J: Polysomnographic features of REM sleep behavior disorder: development of a scoring method. Neurology 1992;43:1371–1374.

19. Consens F, Chervin RD, Koeppe RA, et al: Validation of polysomnographic score for REM sleep behavior disorder. Sleep 2005;28:993–997.

20. Sforza E, Krieger J, Petiau C: REM sleep behavior: clinical and physiopathological findings. Sleep Med Rev 1997;1:57–69.

21. Eisensehr I, Lindeiner H, Jager M, Noachtar S: REM sleep behavior disorder in sleep-disordered patients with versus without Parkinson's disease: is there a need for polysomnography? J Neurol Sci 2001;186:7–11.

Chapter 13

Polysomnography, Portable Monitoring, and Actigraphy

Chapter Points

- PSG is indicated for evaluation of suspected OSA and for PAP titration. PSG is indicated for preoperative evaluation for planned surgery (to treat OSA or snoring), and postoperatively to document surgical effectiveness.
- PSG is indicated to document effectiveness of oral appliance treatment of OSA. The practice parameters for oral appliance therapy state that a diagnostic study should be performed if an oral appliance is planned for snoring or suspected OSA.
- PSG is indicated for evaluation of OSA patients being treated with CPAP or an oral appliance in whom symptoms have returned (PSG using CPAP or OA).
- PSG is indicated **if there is a clinical suspicion of OSA** in patients with heart failure, coronary artery disease, recent or past stroke or transient ischemic attack, and neuromuscular disorders.
- A repeat PSG is indicated if an initial study is negative but there is a high index of suspicion for OSA.
- A PSG is indicated if there is weight loss (>10%) of an OSA patient on CPAP to determine whether CPAP is still indicated.
- A PSG is indicated in a patient using CPAP after weight gain (>10%) to determine whether higher pressure is needed.
- A PSG is **NOT** indicated for evaluation of the restless legs syndrome, insomnia, uncomplicated parasomnias, COPD, or a patient doing well on CPAP treatment.
- Attended PM can be used as an alternative to PSG to diagnose OSA when there is a high pretest probability and to determine the effectiveness of therapy. Attended PM (type 3) is indicated if treatment is urgent and PSG is delayed or the patient cannot have a PSG in the sleep center owing to immobility or safety issues.

- An unattended PM (type 3) is indicated to diagnose OSA in patients with a high probability of having moderate to severe OSA—IF combined with a comprehensive sleep evaluation and significant co-morbid medical disorders or sleep disorders that would benefit from PSG are excluded. A negative PM study should be followed by a PSG in most cases (to be studied by PM, there must be a high probability of having moderate to severe OSA).
- Review of the raw PM data is essential to verify adequate technical quality of a study and to determine whether the respiratory events were properly scored.
- The AASM PMGs recommended at a minimum airflow, respiratory effort, and oxygen saturation should be monitored.
- Qualified providers should either place the PM sensors or instruct the patients to avoid a high proportion of technically inadequate studies.
- Selection of the PM device should take into account the setting in which it will be used and whether the patient will place the sensors without assistance at home.

POLYSOMNOGRAPHY

The American Academy of Sleep Medicine (AASM) practice parameters[1-6] outline the indications for polysomnography (PSG) (Tables 13–1 to 13–4 and Appendix 13–1). PSG is the standard test for diagnosis of suspected sleep-related breathing disorders (SRBDs), narcolepsy (when combined with a multiple sleep latency test [MSLT]), positive airway pressure (PAP) titration, and evaluation of parasomnias (under certain conditions).[2,6] PSG is also indicated to document the efficacy of prior surgical treatment and determine the efficacy of oral appliance (OA) treatment (PSG while wearing the OA).[2,6] The 2005 practice parameters for

TABLE 13-1
Indications for Polysomnography (Sleep-Related Breathing Disorders)
DIAGNOSTIC PSG
• Diagnosis of suspected sleep-related breathing disorders (OSA, central sleep apnea).
• Preoperative PSG before planned surgery for **snoring or OSA** (**attended** cardiorespiratory [type 3 PM] study is also acceptable).
REPEAT PSG
• Repeat PSG is indicated if the initial PSG was negative + there is a high clinical suspicion for OSA.
• After ≥ 10% **weight loss** in a patient on CPAP to see whether CPAP is still needed (if clinically indicated).
FOLLOW-UP PSG (NON-PAP TREATMENT)
• After surgery for moderate to severe OSA—usually 3–6 mo after surgery (most would also study patients with mild OSA).
• After previous surgery for OSA if symptoms return.
• After adequate adjustment of oral appliance for OSA (all severities*) (PSG using OA).
*Amended by practice parameters for oral appliance treatment to include all severities of OSA.[6] Cardiorespiratory study = four channels, airflow, effort (or two effort channels), oxygen saturation, and ECG or heart rate. ECG = electrocardiogram; OSA = obstructive sleep apnea; PAP = positive airway pressure; PM = portable monitoring; PSG = polysomnography.

TABLE 13-2
Indications for Polysomnography (Positive Airway Pressure Titration and Treatment)
PAP TITRATION
• Patients: AHI ≥ 15/hr with or without symptoms, AHI ≥ 5/hr with symptoms.
• Full night of PSG titration.
• Split study—if at least 3 hr remain for titration • AHI > 40 during 2 hr of monitoring in the initial diagnostic portion. • AHI 20–40 special clinical circumstances (long apnea/severe desaturation). • 3 hr remain for PAP titration. • Repeat PSG for PAP titration if inadequate PAP titration portion of study
REPEAT PSG ON CPAP
• After ≥ 10% weight gain to determine whether CPAP is adequate (if clinically indicated).
• Clinical symptoms return in patient on CPAP (consider PSG + MSLT if narcolepsy is suspected).
REPEAT PSG ON CPAP NOT INDICATED
• Routine follow-up of a patient doing well on PAP treatment.
Type 3 (cardiorespiratory study) = four channels, airflow, effort (or two effort channels), oxygen saturation, and ECG or heart rate. AHI = number of apneas + hypopneas/hr of sleep. AHI = apnea-hypopnea index; CPAP = continuous positive airway pressure; ECG = electrocardiogram; MSLT = multiple sleep latency test; OSA = obstructive sleep apnea; PAP = positive airway pressure; PSG = polysomnography. From Kushida CA, Morgenthaler T, Littner MR, et al: Practice parameters for the treatment of snoring and obstructive sleep apnea with oral appliances: an update for 2005. Sleep 2006;29:240–243.

PSG stated that **attended** cardiorespiratory pulmonary studies (airflow + effort or two effort channels, oximetry, and electrocardiogram [ECG] or heart rate) are an acceptable alternative to PSG for diagnosis of obstructive sleep apnea (OSA) in patients with high pretest probability of OSA[2,7] or for determining the adequacy of prior surgery for OSA or effectiveness of current OA treatment.[2,6,7] In 2007, the AASM published *Clinical Guidelines for the Use of Portable Monitoring in Evaluation of Adult Patients with OSA*[8] (hereafter referred to as PMGs). The PMGs state that **unattended** portable monitoring (PM) "may be" acceptable to monitor patients with a high probability of having moderate to severe OSA, **if monitoring is performed according to the guidelines**. Unattended PM monitoring is also acceptable for assessing the efficacy of non-PAP treatment of OSA. The Centers for Medicare and Medicaid Services (CMS) now recognize a diagnosis of OSA by unattended PM as acceptable for reimbursement of continuous positive airway pressure (CPAP) treatment[9] and considers unattended PM studies reimbursable provided certain conditions are met.[10]

PSG for Patients with SRBDs (see Table 13-1)

PSG is the standard diagnostic study for evaluation of a suspected SRBD. A diagnostic study may be repeated if the initial study was negative for sleep apnea and there is a high clinical index of suspicion for this disorder. PSG should be performed **preoperatively** for planned surgery to treat **snoring or suspected OSA**.[1,2] PSG is indicated for snoring because an appreciable number of patients will also have OSA. A PSG is indicated after surgery for OSA (after surgical healing) to document effectiveness. The practice parameters specify "in moderate to severe OSA," although most clinicians would perform a PSG after surgery for mild OSA as well.

Determination of the presence of OSA is indicated for planned OA treatment of snoring or suspected OSA.[6] The type of diagnostic procedure was not specified in the practice parameters for OAs. However, PSG is always indicated to diagnose OSA. PSG is indicated after adjustment of an OA for OSA (not for primary snoring) to document efficacy. The 2007 practice parameters for PSG recommended a sleep study with the patient using an OA for treatment of moderate to severe OSA to document efficacy.[2] In a subsequent practice parameter on OA treatment of OSA, a PSG to document efficacy was recommended for **OSA of all severities.**[6]

TABLE 13–3

Indications for Polysomnography in Nonrespiratory Sleep Disorders

NARCOLEPSY

PSG INDICATED

• Before MSLT for diagnosis of suspected narcolepsy.

PARASOMNIAS OR SEIZURE DISORDER

PSG INDICATED

• Nocturnal seizure is suspected (undiagnosed).

• Presumed parasomnia/nocturnal seizure disorder does not respond to conventional treatment.

• Presumed parasomnia is injurious to the patient or others (or is potentially injurious) or follows trauma or with forensic (legal) implications.

• Presumed parasomnia has atypical features (stereotypic behavior, frequent events per night, atypical age of onset).

PSG NOT INDICATED

• Typical, noninjurious behavior for which clinical evaluation is sufficient.

• Known seizure disorder patient without nocturnal complaints.

SLEEP-RELATED MOVEMENT DISORDER

PSG INDICATED

• For suspected periodic limb movement disorder.

PSG NOT INDICATED

• Evaluation and treatment of RLS.

INSOMNIA

PSG NOT INDICATED (Patients Complaining of Insomnia)

• Routine evaluation of transient insomnia, chronic insomnia, or insomnia associated with psychiatric disorders.

PSG INDICATED (Patients Complaining of Insomnia)

• Sleep-related breathing disorder is suspected.

• Periodic limb movement disorder is suspected.

• Initial diagnosis is uncertain.

• Treatment of insomnia fails (behavioral or pharmacologic).

• Precipitous arousals occur with violent or dangerous behavior.

MSLT = multiple sleep latency test; PSG = polysomnography; RLS = restless legs syndrome.

TABLE 13–4

Summary of Circumstances in Which Polysomnography Is NOT Indicated

• Routine evaluation of a patient doing well on CPAP treatment.

• Evaluation of asthma or chronic lung disease (unless OSA is suspected).

• Routine evaluation of insomnia.

• Evaluation and treatment of RLS (unless the periodic limb movement disorder is suspected).

• Evaluation of uncomplicated parasomnias for which a clinical diagnosis is sufficient.

• Evaluation of a circadian rhythm sleep disorder.

CPAP = continuous positive airway pressure; OSA = obstructive sleep apnea; RLS = restless legs syndrome.

diagnostic PSG is indicated to determine whether CPAP is still needed. This assumes the test is clinically indicated based on evaluation of the patient's overall clinical status and the likelihood of weight loss maintenance.

The 2005 practice parameters for PSG also mentioned a number of circumstances in which SRBDs are very common.[2] However, PSG is NOT routinely indicated in those circumstances **unless a clinical evaluation** reveals a reasonable suspicion for SRBD. The disorders discussed included patients with **systolic or diastolic heart failure**, **recent or past stroke or transient ischemic attack (TIA)**, **coronary artery disease**, and **tachyarrhythmias or bradyarrhythmias**. Most clinicians would also place resistant hypertension or pulmonary hypertension of unknown etiology in this category as well. The clinician should recognize that many patients with significant OSA do not complain of daytime sleepiness. A history of snoring and gasping would suggest a PSG is indicated. It should also be noted that some patients with OSA complain of insomnia. The practice parameters do list **neuromuscular diseases** as a group of disorders in which PSG is indicated for evaluation of sleep-related symptoms. Routine evaluation of **chronic lung disease** is not an indication for PSG unless coexistent OSA is suspected. Nocturnal oximetry is a useful tool for determining whether nocturnal oxygen desaturation is occurring in a patient with chronic obstructive pulmonary disease (COPD). A saw-tooth pattern is suggestive of sleep apnea.

PSG Titration and PSG on CPAP (see Table 13–2)

A PSG for PAP titration is the standard procedure to select a level of pressure for treatment.[1,2,11] The titration can be performed on a separate night after a diagnostic PSG or during the second part of the night during a split (partial-night) study. A split sleep study is recommended when (1) the diagnostic portion shows an apnea-hypopnea index (AHI) greater than 40/hr with at least 2 hours of monitoring, (2) there is an AHI of 20 to 40 with special clinical

For patients with prior effective surgical treatment (documented by PSG), the PSG may be repeated at a later time if symptoms of sleep apnea return. For a patient using an OA as treatment for OSA, the PSG may also be repeated while the patient wears the OA if the patient's symptoms return. If a patient on CPAP **loses more than 10% of body weight**, a

circumstances such as severe desaturation or arrhythmia thought due to OSA, and (3) at least 3 hours remain for the PSG titration.[1,2,11,12] If the PSG titration does not last at least 3 hours or is not adequate, a repeat PSG titration is indicated. PSG PAP titration techniques and PAP treatment are discussed in Chapter 19. Of note, financial constraints may require use of less stringent split study criteria.

PSG is **NOT** recommended in patients on CPAP treatment who are doing well. If the patient is being treated on CPAP and is NOT doing well, a repeat PSG study on CPAP is indicated.[2] However, before this expensive procedure, it is essential to document adequate objective adherence and to optimize treatment and the mask interface. PSG is also indicated if a patient on CPAP **gains more than 10% of body weight** to determine whether the pressure is adequate. However, a repeat PSG titration may not be clinically indicated.

PSG Indications: Nonrespiratory Disorders

PSG Indicated (see Tables 13–3 and 13–4)
A PSG preceding an MSLT is indicated for evaluation of suspected **narcolepsy** or to help differentiate narcolepsy from **idiopathic hypersomnia**.[1–3] PSG is indicated for evaluation of suspected periodic limb movement disorder but NOT the restless legs syndrome (RLS; a clinical diagnosis). A PSG with extended (and bilateral) electroencephalogram (EEG) derivations and video monitoring is indicated to evaluate (1) nocturnal behavior possibly due to seizures, (2) atypical parasomnia behavior (frequent episodes each night, stereotypic behavior, or behavior unusual for age), (3) nocturnal behavior/parasomnia that has resulted in injury to the patient or others (or has the potential to do so), (4) presumed parasomnia or nocturnal seizure disorder that does not respond to conventional treatment, or (5) if there are legal/forensic implications of nocturnal behavior.[2] The practice parameters recommend looking at events in a 10-second window to observe for seizure activity and consultation with a physician with expertise in reading clinical EEGs if necessary.

PSG NOT Indicated (see Tables 13–3 and 13–4)
PSG is not indicated for evaluation of insomnia (unless OSA is suspected) or unless insomnia does not respond to usual treatment. PSG is not indicated for diagnosis of depression or insomnia with depression.[2,4] The practice parameters for use of PSG[4] in evaluation of insomnia state "PSG is indicated when initial diagnosis is uncertain, treatment fails (behavioral or pharmacologic), or precipitous arousals occur with violent or injurious behavior (Guideline)."

Although the PSG finding of a short rapid eye movement (REM) latency is common in depression, this finding is not sufficiently sensitive or specific to warrant a PSG in evaluating patients with suspected depression. A PSG is NOT indicated for (1) typical uncomplicated and noninjurious parasomnias when the diagnosis is clearly delineated or (2) patients with known seizure disorders who have no

nocturnal complaints. Table 13–4 is a summary of the circumstances in which PSG is not indicated.

Approach to the Sleepy Patient on PAP Treatment

If a patient with OSA continues to have daytime sleepiness on adequate PAP treatment (documented adequate adherence and adequate control of respiratory events), there are two options. As discussed in Chapter 18 on medical treatment of OSA, an alerting agent such as modafinil may be added.[13] If there is a suspicion of narcolepsy in addition to OSA, a nocturnal PSG on PAP treatment (documenting adequate treatment) followed by an MSLT on PAP can be performed (see Chapters 14 and 24). If unambiguous cataplexy is present, the patient likely has narcolepsy and the MSLT is simply confirmatory. It is essential that adequate PAP treatment for OSA be confirmed before expensive testing. This includes documentation of adequate objective adherence. Many PAP devices also have the ability to record residual AHI. A high residual AHI would be an indication for an adjustment in pressure (empirical increase) or a PSG PAP titration.[1,2] The PAP device estimate of residual AHI is not always accurate, but a high value has a reasonable positive predictive value that the residual AHI is indeed elevated.[14] A surprising number of patients (up to 15%) on chronic PAP treatment are not adequately treated (AHI > 10/hr).[15,16]

Approach to Reading the PSG
Before the PSG is read, a review of the clinical history with special attention to symptoms of sleep apnea, narcolepsy, RLS, and medications is very useful. The amount of chronic alcohol intake and the medications actually taken before the sleep study should be noted. The presence of underlying lung disease may help explain a low awake arterial oxygen saturation (SaO_2) or low baseline sleeping SaO_2. A clinical history of pacemaker insertion or known atrial fibrillation is also very helpful in providing a useful interpretation of ECG findings. If a PAP titration is planned for a patient currently using CPAP, the current treatment pressure level should be noted. During the reading of the PSG, a return to the clinical history may be helpful (Table 13–5).

All digital PSG systems have a view that shows graphical summary information of the entire night (Fig. 13–1 and Table 13–6). It is often useful to look at the big picture before going through the data in smaller time windows. The biocalibrations are often helpful in noting the appearance of eyes-open wake in a given patient and whether the patient produces an alpha rhythm with eye closure (see Chapters 3 and 4).

PORTABLE MONITORING (HOME SLEEP TESTING, OUT OF CENTER SLEEP TESTING)

PM, also called home sleep testing (HST) or out of center sleep testing (OCST), has been the subject of intense interest

TABLE 13-5		
Historical Elements to Review Based on Polysomnography Findings		
EEG/EOG/EMG		
• Long sleep latency—?history of insomnia		
• Short REM latency—?history of symptoms of narcolepsy, cataplexy, or depression		
• Alpha sleep—?chronic pain syndrome or psychiatric disorders		
• Persistent eye movements during stage N2—?SSRI medication		
• Increased spindle activity—?benzodiazepines (regular medication or special medication before sleep study)		
• Transient muscle activity (chin EMG) activity during stage R—?SSRI treatment, history of dream enactment		
• Arousals from stage N3 with body movement—?history of NREM parasomnia		
• Body movement and speech during REM sleep—?history suggestive of RBD		
RESPIRATION		
• Low awake SaO$_2$—?presence of lung disease		
• Low sleeping baseline SaO$_2$—?presence of lung disease		
• Cheyne-Stokes breathing—?history of congestive heart failure		
• Ataxic breathing, low respiratory rate—?history of potent opiates		
• Delay in SaO$_2$ nadir after respiratory events—?decreased cardiac output		
LEG MONITORING		
• Frequent LMs during wake—?symptoms of RLS		
• High PLM index—can be seen associated with OSA, PAP titration, RLS		
• Increased transient muscle activity during REM sleep—?SSRI medications, history of dream enactment		
ECG		
• Tachycardia in sleep (>90 bpm)—?anxiety, stimulants		
• Bradycardia in sleep (<40 bpm)—?beta blocker, ?known cardiac disorder		
• Atrial fibrillation—?previously documented		
• Pacemaker—?if wide complex QRS with normal rate (e.g., 60–80)		
? = consult history for relevant items. ECG = electrocardiogram; EEG = electroencephalogram; EMG = electromyogram; EOG = electro-oculogram; LMs = limb movements; NREM = non–rapid eye movement; PAP = positive airway pressure; PLM = periodic limb movement; RBD = rapid eye movement sleep behavior disorder; REM = rapid eye movement; RLS = restless legs syndrome; SaO$_2$ = arterial oxygen saturation; SSRI = selective serotonin reuptake inhibitor.		

recently.[17,18] The tests are not always performed in the home; hence, the terms HST or PM are not ideal but are used in much of the literature on this subject. The term PM is used in this chapter. In the past, PM has been used to diagnose OSA in settings in which access to PSG is limited or delayed.

The traditional classification of monitoring devices for the diagnosis of sleep apnea was originated by Ferber and colleagues (Table 13–7).[19-21] This classification was used for the Tri-Society PM evidence review,[22] executive summary,[23] and practice parameters for the PM.[7] The original classification used "level I, II, III, and IV" to refer to different classes of monitoring but currently the terminology is "type 1, 2, 3, and 4." The Centers for Medicare and Medicaid Services (CMS) has a different classification for monitoring (Table 13–8).[9] The CMS terminology defines the respiratory disturbance index (RDI) as the total number of apneas and hypopneas per hour of **monitoring time.** Therefore, the index determined by PM (no EEG) would be an RDI using the CMS definition. CMS also refers to PM as HST.

Developments in the Use of PM

Important developments in the history of PM are listed in Table 13–9. AASM practice parameters in 1994,[20] 1997,[1] and 2005[2] specified a limited role for **attended** PM. However, unattended PM was widely used in locales in which access to PSG was very limited. On the basis of a Tri-Society evidence review for the use of PM,[22] practice parameters published in 2003[7] stated that certain type 3 PM devices used in the **attended** setting could be used to rule in or rule out OSA.[7] Before 2008, the National Carrier Determination (NCD) 240.4 on CPAP treatment specified a diagnosis of

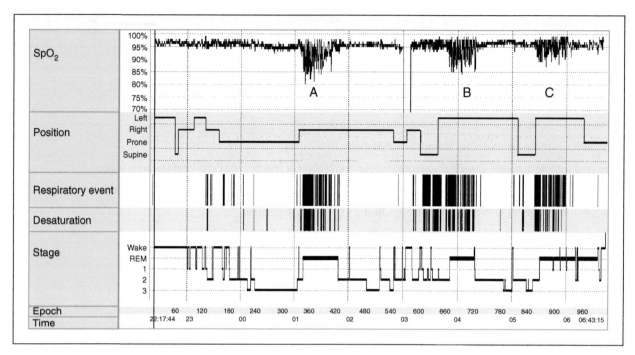

FIGURE 13–1 Summary view shows three periods of significant arterial oxygen desaturations (A, B, and C) during rapid eye movement (REM) sleep. In addition, the summary view shows that no supine REM sleep was recorded. SpO$_2$ = pulse oximetry.

TABLE 13–6

Special Elements of Polysomnography to Note during Interpretation

Technologist comments—especially for epochs of abnormal EEG or ECG or notable body movements.

Biocalibrations—observe adequacy of tracings, sensor function, production of alpha with eye closure, nature of eyes-open wakefulness, correct polarity of nasal pressure and chest and abdominal belts.

Overnight summary view—the big picture of SaO$_2$ and hypnograms
• REM-associated OSA.
• Postural OSA.

Alternate between 30- and 90-second windows to observe sleep and respirations.

10-second window for suspicious or abnormal EEG or ECG activity.

ECG = electrocardiogram; EEG = electroencephalogram; OSA = obstructive sleep apnea; REM = rapid eye movement; SaO$_2$ = arterial oxygen saturation.

OSA must be made by attended PSG for subsequent CPAP treatment to be reimbursed. There were several requests for CMS to revise the policy to include PM (HST) devices. The evaluation of PM changed from an analysis of accuracy of PM compared with PSG to an analysis of PM's ability to identify OSA patients who would benefit from treatment. In 2007, the AASM published clinical guidelines for the use of unattended PM[8] (PMGs) (Appendix 13–2). In a 2008 ruling, CMS issued a decision allowing patients to qualify for CPAP treatment on the basis of a diagnosis by HST provided certain guidelines are followed.[9] The specific rules vary according to local carrier determinations (LCDs; see

Appendix 13–3, for example). In general, a physician Board-certified or Board-eligible (BC/BE) in sleep medicine or associated with a sleep center accredited by the AASM or the Joint Commission is allowed to interpret the HSTs. The durable medical equipment (DME) providers are not allowed to perform HST on patients that they will provide with PAP equipment. In 2009, CMS published a decision stating that PM testing itself would be reimbursable.[10] The reimbursement fees vary between locales but are very modest. The AASM now offers accreditation for OCST.

Accuracy of PMs

The analysis of agreement between measurements from different devices is complex.[22,24] A systematic review of agreement between PSG and ambulatory sleep studies was published in 2003.[22] At that time, the best evidence for agreement between PM and PSG was for type 3 PM studies in the attended setting. The analysis focused on comparison of AHI values. However, the major issue is ability of the PM-derived AHI to correctly classify patients as having OSA and identifying those patients who would benefit from treatment. For example, AHI results of 30/hr versus 60/hr would both be consistent with severe sleep apnea even though the AHI values were quite different. Conversely, AHI results of 3 versus 13 would classify the patient as either being normal or having mild OSA. Numerous studies have compared the AHIs derived from PSG and PM devices. There are a number of reasons why the AHIs from PSG and PM might differ (Table 13–10). In general, studies comparing PSG and PM have either used simultaneous monitoring with PSG and PM in the sleep center or compared PSG in the sleep center with unattended PM on a different night at home. Both approaches

TABLE 13–7

Classification of Portable Monitoring*

	TYPE 1: ATTENDED PSG	TYPE 2: UNATTENDED PSG	TYPE 3: MODIFIED PORTABLE SLEEP APNEA TESTING	TYPE 4: CONTINUOUS SINGLE OR DUAL BIOPARAMETER RECORDING
Measures (channels)	Minimum of seven channels including ECG, EEG, EOG, chin EMG, airflow, respiratory effort, oxygen saturation	Minimum of seven channels including EEG, EOG, chin EMG, heart rate or ECG, airflow, respiratory effort, oxygen saturation	Minimum of four, including ventilation (at least two channels of respiratory movement or respiratory movement and airflow), heart rate or ECG, and oxygen saturation	Minimum of one oxygen saturation, flow, or chest movement
Body position	Documented or objectively measured	Possible	Possible	No
Leg movement	EMG or motion sensor desirable but optional	Optional	Optional	No
Personnel interventions	Possible	No	No	No

*Levels I, II, III, and IV monitoring are now termed types 1, 2, 3, and 4.
ECG = electrocardiogram; EEG = electroencephalogram; EMG = electromyogram; EOG = electro-oculogram; PSG = polysomnography.
From Ferber R, Millman R, Coppola M, et al: ASDA standards of practice: portable recording in the assessment of obstructive sleep apnea. Sleep 1994;17:378–392.

TABLE 13–8

Centers for Medicare and Medicaid Services Classification of Portable Monitoring

HCPCS CODE	TYPE	SETTING	MONITORING
G0398	2	Unattended	Minimum of seven channels including EEG, EOG, EMG, ECG/heart rate, oxygen saturation, anterior tibial EMG
G0399	3	Unattended	Minimum of four channels and must record ventilation, oximetry, and ECG or heart rate
G0400	4	Unattended	Minimum of three channels, and one must be airflow
	—	Unattended	Minimum of three channels including peripheral arterial tonometry, actigraphy, and oximetry

2011 Codes for PM Studies
95800 Sleep study, unattended, simultaneous recording; heart rate, oxygen saturation, respiratory analysis (e.g., by airflow or peripheral arterial tone), and **sleep time**;
95801 Sleep study, unattended, simultaneous recording; minimum of heart rate, oxygen saturation, and respiratory analysis (e.g., by airflow or peripheral arterial tone);
95806 Sleep study, simultaneous recording of ventilation, respiratory effort, ECG or heart rate, and oxygen saturation, unattended by a technologist.
Note: Some durable medical equipment (DMAC) providers still use G codes. The entire area is in flux. The reader should consult the CMS website or their local DMAC provider for the latest information.
ECG = electrocardiogram; EEG = electroencephalogram; EMG = electromyogram; EOG = electro-oculogram; HCPCS = Healthcare Common Procedure Coding System.

are problematic. In either case, even if the same type of sensors are used and the same number of events are identified, the two devices would still give different AHI values as monitoring time (PM) would exceed total sleep time (PSG). For example, if both methods detect 70 apneas and hypopneas, dividing by 5 hours of total sleep time (TST; AHI = 14/hr) will give a higher index than dividing by 7 hours of monitoring time (AHI = 10/hr). It is also possible that the oximeters used in different systems could differ in their ability to detect desaturations. Comparing PM and PSG AHI values during simultaneous recording reduces the effects of night-to-night variability. However, this does not mimic how

the devices are actually used. The different nights–different locations approach mimics real world conditions. However, if the different nights approach is used to compare PSG and PM, the AHI values could differ simply due to night-to-night variability in the AHI.

In general for milder OSA, the amounts of REM and supine sleep are the major determinants of the AHI. These patients have elevated AHI mainly in the supine position or during REM sleep. Table 13–11 presents the effect of different proportions of REM and supine sleep on the overall AHI (assuming certain AHI values in different conditions). In milder OSA patients, night-to-night differences in the

TABLE 13–9

History of Recent Developments in Portable Monitoring (Home Sleep Testing)

1994 Practice Parameter for Portable Monitoring[20]	Type 2 or type 3 PM is an acceptable alternative to PSG in the following circumstances: 1. Patients with severe clinical symptoms of OSA and when initiation of treatment is urgent and PSG is not readily available. 2. Patient unable to be studied in sleep laboratory. 3. Diagnosis already established by PSG and treatment initiated and the purpose is to evaluate response to treatment.
Tri-Society (ACCP, ATS, AASM) 2003 Evidence Review (Chest)[22] Executive Summary[23] (Am J Respir Crit Care Med) PM Practice Parameters (Sleep)[24]	**Attended** type 3 studies may be used to rule in or rule out OSA provided certain limitations are met. These include manually scoring the records, using the device in patients without significant co-morbid conditions, not using type 3 devices for PAP titrations or split-night studies, and symptomatic patients who have a negative type 3 study should have a PSG. Type 2, type 4 studies not recommended.
2004 CMS Decision	Insufficient evidence to recommend unattended type 2, 3, 4 PM.
2005 AASM Practice Parameters for PSG and Related Procedures[2]	**Attended** cardiorespiratory study (type 3) is an acceptable alternative to PSG if: • High pretest probability of OSA. • A negative type 3 study with patients with high pretest probability of OSA is followed by a PSG. Here, type 3 is defined as airflow, effort, oximetry, and ECG or heart rate. **Attended** cardiopulmonary study acceptable: • Preoperative for planned surgery for snoring or OSA. • After surgery for OSA—moderate to severe. • To document effectiveness of an OA. • After surgical or dental treatment of OSA and symptoms return. Attended cardiorespiratory study NOT recommended for PAP titration.
AASM Portable Monitoring Task Force 2006–2007	Clinical Guidelines for Unattended Monitoring 2007[6]
CMS 240.4 Final decision 2008–2009[9,10]	Unattended HST permitted • Type 3 (four channels with ventilation, oximetry, ECG or heart rate). • Type 4 (three channels, one airflow) • PAT type: three channels including PAT, actigraphy, SpO_2.
Local Carrier Determinations	• Restrictions on who can perform and interpret HST. • May require monitoring of airflow. • Set Fee schedule. • Most have followed AASM Clinical Guidelines for unattended monitoring.

AASM = American Academy of Sleep Medicine; ACCP = American College of Chest Physicians; ATS = American Thoracic Society; CMS = Centers for Medicare Services; ECG = electrocardiogram; HST = home sleep testing; OA = oral appliance; OSA = obstructive sleep apnea; PAP = positive airway pressure; PAT = peripheral arterial tonometry; PM = portable monitoring; PSG = polysomnography; SpO_2 = pulse oximetry.

TABLE 13–10

Reasons for Difference in Apnea-Hypopnea Index by Polysomnography versus Portable Monitoring

PM AHI > PSG AHI	PSG AHI > PM AHI
• Respiratory events scored when patient actually awake. • Ethanol intake? • More sleep/more REM sleep at home. • Night-to-night variability. • Variability in human scoring.	• Monitoring time > TST (i.e., 10/5 < 10/2). • Less supine time at home. • PM sensors dislodged during the night. • Different sensors. • Different scoring (hypopnea with arousals only with PSG). • Night-to-night variability. • Variability in human scoring.

AHI = apnea-hypopnea index; PM = portable monitoring; PSG = polysomnography; REM = rapid eye movement; TST = total sleep time.

proportions of REM and supine sleep are a significant source of night-to-night variability. A study by Smith and associates[25] found that patients tend to sleep more in the supine position in the sleep center. During this study, PSG and PM were simultaneously recorded in the sleep center and PM was also performed on a separate night at home (Table 13–12). Differences in the AHI during simultaneous monitoring were likely due to the effect of using monitoring time versus TST to compute the AHI. During PM monitoring at home, less supine sleep also contributed to differences in the AHI. To compensate for night-to-night variability, many PM devices now have the ability to monitor multiple nights. One study suggested that night-to-night variability in the home might be less than in the sleep center (Fig. 13–2).[26]

A Bland-Altman plot[27] is a commonly used method to display agreement between two measuring devices. The

TABLE 13–11

Effects of Different Proportions of Supine and Rapid Eye Movement Sleep on the Total Apnea-Hypopnea Index

		SUPINE NREM	NONSUPINE NREM	SUPINE REM	NONSUPINE REM
Assumed AHI (#/hr) in different conditions		5	2	30	10
PROPORTIONS OF DIFFERENT CONDITIONS OF FOUR NIGHTS AND THE RESULTING AHI	**OVERALL AHI**	**SUPINE NREM (%TST)**	**NONSUPINE NREM (%TST)**	**SUPINE REM (%TST)**	**NONSUPINE REM (%TST)**
Night 1	6.8	40	40	10	10
Night 2	4.2	20	60	0	20
Night 3	3.3	30	65	0	5
Night 4	9.7	70	10	20	0

Note: The AHI was highest on night 4 because the amount of supine REM sleep (as %TST) was the highest on that night.
AHI = apnea-hypopnea index; NREM = non–rapid eye movement; REM = rapid eye movement; TST = total sleep time.

TABLE 13–12

Illustration of the Importance of Less Supine Sleep at Home

	PSG	PM IN LABORATORY DURING PSG	UNATTENDED PM AT HOME
AHI (#/hr)	25.7 ± 12.2	19.5 ± 16	13.7 ± 13
	Based on TST 4.0 ± 1.6 hr	Based on monitoring time 7.3 ± 0.8 hr	Based on monitoring time 8.2 ± 0.8 hr
% supine time median		**49**	**26**
AHI supine		22 ± 19	24 ± 21

PSG by Embla, PM = Embletta (nasal pressure, chest and abdominal belts, SpO$_2$, actigraph).
Values shown as mean ± SD.
Note: Computation of AHI based on a mean of 4 hours with PSG and 7.3 hours with PM in the sleep laboratory.
Note: At home, much less supine time was recorded.
AHI = apnea-hypopnea index; PM = portable monitoring;
PSG = polysomnography; SpO$_2$ = pulse oximetry; TST = total sleep time.
From Smith LA, Chong DW, Vennelle M, et al: Diagnosis of sleep-disordered breathing in patients with chronic heart failure: evaluation of a portable limited sleep study system. J Sleep Res 2007;16:428–435.

difference in paired values (measurement device 1 – measurement device 2) is plotted on the y axis and the average of the pair of values (device 1, device 2) is plotted on the x axis. Santos-Silva and coworkers[28] compared AHI values determined by a type 3 device (Stardust by Philips-Respironics) at home with those determined by PSG. A Bland-Altman plot of the data is illustrated in Figure 13–3. In this study, diagnostic agreement between AHI values was 83% (defined as either both AHI values > 30/hr or AHI values differing by < 10/hr).

Clinical Use of PM

Indications for Attended PM

PM is rarely used in the attended setting. The indications for PM as stated in various practice parameters is shown in Table 13–9. In 1994 and 1997 practice parameters,[2,20] **attended** type 2 or 3 PMs were stated to be acceptable alternatives when treatment of OSA is urgent and PSG is delayed, the patient is unable to be studied in the sleep center (safety or immobility), or the diagnosis of OSA is already established and the purpose is to evaluate the response to treatment.[1] The 2003 practice parameters for the use of portable monitoring added that certain PMs may be used in the **attended** setting to rule in or to rule out OSA.[7] The 2005 practice parameters for PSG stated that attended cardiorespiratory studies (type 3 PM) are an acceptable alternative to PSG for diagnosis of OSA in patients with a high probability of OSA as long as a negative PM study was followed by PSG. Attended cardiorespiratory studies were also said to be acceptable for preoperative evaluation for planned surgery for snoring or OSA. After surgery, attended cardiorespiratory studies were acceptable to document surgical effectiveness in patients with moderate to severe OSA. A specific statement concerning the use of attended cardiorespiratory studies in patients being considered for an OA treatment of snoring or suspected sleep apnea was not made in any of the practice parameters. The practice parameters for OAs did state that "the presence or absence of OSA must be determined before initiating treatment with oral appliances to identify those patients at risk due to complications of sleep apnea and to provide a baseline to establish the effectiveness of subsequent treatment."[6]

If a high probability of OSA is present, an attended cardiorespiratory study would be acceptable based on the 2005 practice parameters.[2] In the attended setting, cardiorespiratory studies are acceptable to document the effectiveness of an OA (after adequate adjustment) or in OSA patients treated with surgery or an OA when symptoms return.

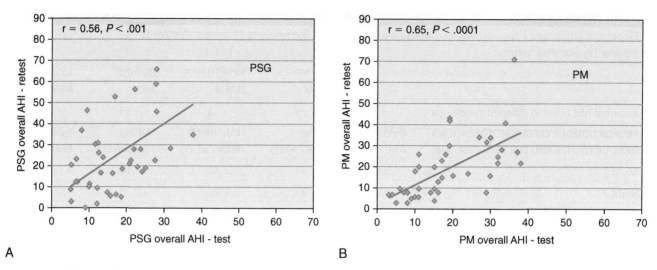

FIGURE 13-2 **A,** The apnea-hypopnea index (AHI) on nights 1 and 2 (test vs. retest) in the sleep center with polysomnography (PSG). **B,** The AHI on nights 1 and 2 (test vs. retest) at home with portable monitoring (PM). There was less difference between the two nights with PM compared with PSG. Note the considerable night-to-night variability using both PSG and PM. *From Levendowski D, Steward D, Woodson BT, et al: The impact of obstructive sleep apnea variability measured in-lab versus in-home on sample size calculations. Int Arch Med 2009;2:1–8.*

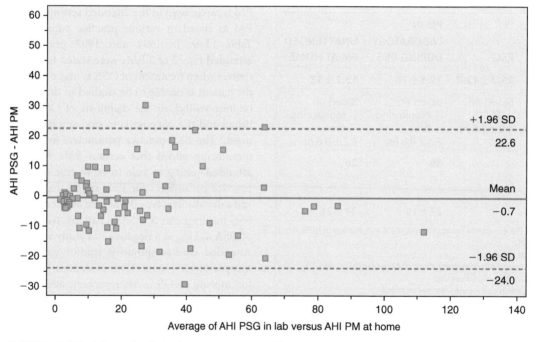

FIGURE 13-3 A Bland-Altman plot of pairs of apnea-hypopnea index (AHI) values (device 1, device 2). The difference (AHI PSG − AHI PM) is plotted on the y axis against the average on the x axis [(device 1 + device 2)/2]. The confidence limits are + 1.96 standard deviations (SDs). The mean difference (bias) is near zero. There tended to be more scatter at the higher AHI values. PM = portable monitoring; PSG = polysomnography. *From Santos-Silva R, Truksians V, Truksina E, et al: Validation of a portable monitoring system for the diagnosis of obstructive sleep apnea syndrome. Sleep 2009;32;629–636.*

Indications for Unattended PM

PM is most often used in the unattended setting. The recent AASM PMGs[8] (see Appendix 13–2) state that **unattended PM "may"** be indicated for diagnosis of OSA in patients with a high pretest probability or for documenting the efficacy of non-PAP treatments for OSA—**IF** guidelines for patient selection and procedures for PM performance and

interpretation are followed[8] (Table 13–13). In brief, PM must be combined with a comprehensive sleep evaluation by a qualified physician, patients must have a high probability of **moderate to severe OSA**, there must be an absence of medical co-morbid conditions that degrade the accuracy of PM (severe lung disease, neuromuscular disease, and congestive heart failure). Patients with co-morbid sleep

TABLE 13-13

Indications for Use of Unattended Portable Monitoring

- PM must be combined with a **comprehensive sleep evaluation.**

- Patient has a high pretest probability of moderate to severe OSA.

- No co-morbid medical conditions that may degrade PM accuracy
  - Severe pulmonary disease.
  - Neuromuscular disease.
  - Congestive heart failure.

- No clinical suspicion of other sleep disorders
  - CSA.
  - Narcolepsy.
  - PLMD.
  - Parasomnias.
  - Circadian rhythm sleep disorders.

- Not for screening asymptomatic populations.

- Patients who cannot have PSG due to immobility, safety, or critical illness.

- Unattended PM may be used to monitor response to non-PAP treatments for sleep apnea (oral appliances, surgery, weight loss).

- Unattended PM in patient's home is permitted when all guidelines are followed.

CSA = central sleep apnea; OSA = obstructive sleep apnea; PAP = positive airway pressure; PLMD = periodic limb movement disorder; PM = portable monitoring; PSG = polysomnography.

disorders (e.g., narcolepsy) requiring PSG should also be excluded. A minimum of airflow, respiratory effort, and oxygen saturation must be measured (type 3 PM). The same sensors and respiratory definitions recommended for PSG in the AASM scoring manual should be used if possible. The raw data must be reviewed and the PSG interpreted by a qualified sleep physician. A follow-up visit with the patient to discuss results is indicated. If a PM study is negative or technically inadequate, a PSG should be ordered to avoid a false-negative PM result. The following sections discuss recommended patient selection and methodology for PM.

Patient Selection for PM

Ideally, each patient should be seen by a BC/BE sleep physician before PM testing. If this is not possible, an evaluation can be performed with questionnaires before or at the time of testing. Review of the medical record to exclude patients with co-morbidities that degrade PM accuracy is also important. In the PMGs, these include patients with severe pulmonary disease, neuromuscular disease, or congestive heart failure (CHF). The rationale is that such patients may exhibit hypoventilation without discrete respiratory events or Cheyne-Stokes breathing (common in severe systolic CHF). However, one can argue that if PM devices use the same

sensors that are used for PSG (the recommendation), then PM and PSG should have similar ability to detect central apnea, Cheyne-Stokes breathing, or hypoventilation (manifested by a low SaO_2 without discrete events).[29] The counterargument is that such patients will likely need a PSG PAP titration. In this case, a split-sleep study may be more cost effective than PM followed by a PSG titration. PM also would miss arrhythmias because pulse rate obtained from the oximeter rather than an ECG tracing is usually recorded. The AASM PMGs state that PM "may" be used in the unattended setting and can be used to document the effectiveness of non-PAP treatment IF PM guidelines are followed. Examples would include a study with the patient wearing an OA (after suitable adjustment) or after previous upper airway surgery.

Recommended PM Methodology

The PMGs[8] recommend monitoring at a minimum airflow, respiratory effort, and SaO_2 (Table 13-14). The recommended sensors for PM are the same as those recommended for PSG in the AASM scoring manual.[29] Note that CMS uses the metric RDI rather than AHI for PM [(apneas + hypopneas)/monitoring time]. RDI usually means AHI + RERA index. Adequately trained personnel should either place the monitoring equipment on the patient or train them on the application of the sensors. This is essential to avoid a high percentage of technically inadequate studies. The PM data must be viewed in the raw form, and if automated scoring is used, it must be edited for accuracy. A physician must look at the raw data as well as the data summary before making an interpretation. It was recommended that PSG be interpreted by a BC/BE sleep physician or a physician associated with an accredited sleep center.

For quality assurance, standard operating procedures for the PM process must exist. To verify adequate scoring, interrater reliability on scoring of PM studies should be performed on a routine basis and documented. If PM is inadequate technically or if the study results are negative in a patient with a high pretest probability of having OSA, an attended PSG should be performed. The reader may wish to review the AASM accreditation standards for OOC sleep testing on the website (www.aasmnet.org).

Types of PM Devices

Numerous devices are available for PM (Fig. 13-4). Devices having more sensors provide more information but are more difficult for patients to place. It is always a trade off between information and complexity of sensor application. Tracings from a typical PM device (type 3) are shown in Figures 13-5 and 13-6. Figure 13-5 shows a tracing from a device that monitors airflow using both an oronasal thermal device and nasal pressure. Respiratory effort is monitored by chest and abdominal respiratory inductance plethysmography (RIP) bands. An oximetry channel and derived heart rate are also recorded as well as body position. Figure 13-6 shows a tracing from a different PM device that monitors airflow by nasal pressure (with or without oronasal thermistor) and

TABLE 13–14

Recommended Portable Monitoring Methodology

Parameters to be monitored	• Monitor at least three parameters: airflow, effort, and oximetry.

Sensors	• Same sensors as for PSG
	  • Airflow (ideally two sensors)
	    • Apnea—oronasal thermal device.
	    • Hypopnea—nasal pressure.
	  • Respiratory effort—RIP
	  • Pulse oximetry with adequate averaging time and motion artifact rejection.

Personnel and setting	• PM should be performed by AASM accredited sleep center
	  • Policy and procedures.
	  • Quality assurance program.
	  • Interscorer reliability program.
	• Experienced sleep technician/technologist either places sensor or directly educates the patient on sensor application.

Device	• Display of raw data is available for manual scoring and editing. • Scoring criteria according to AASM scoring manual. • PSG should be performed when PM is technically inadequate or fails to establish diagnosis of OSA in patients with high pretest probability.
BC/BE SP or physician on staff of AASM accredited sleep center	• Review of raw data by BC/BE SP and interpretation.
Follow-up	• If PM study is technically inadequate or fails to establish a diagnosis of OSA in a patient with a high pretest probability, a diagnostic PSG should be performed. • Follow-up visit with MD or trained health care provider after PM testing to discuss results of test with the patient and plan treatment.

AASM = American Academy of Sleep Medicine; BC/BE SP = Board-certified/Board-eligible sleep physician; OSA = obstructive sleep apnea; PM = portable monitoring; PSG = polysomnography; RIP = respiratory inductance plethysmography.

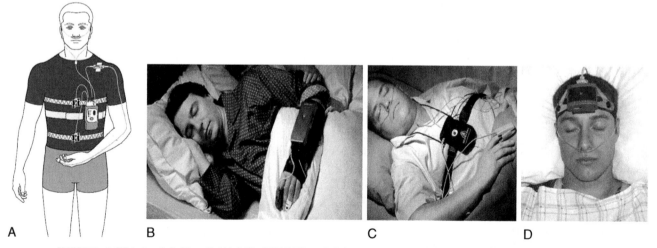

FIGURE 13–4 PM devices. **A,** Embletta (Embla). **B,** WatchPAT 100 (Itamar). **C,** Stardust II (Philips-Respironics). **D,** ARES (Advanced Brain Monitoring).

effort by two RIP belts. The device also records SaO$_2$, body position by a position sensor in the device, and actigraphy to enable elimination of periods of wake/artifact from the final index time (the monitoring time used for AHI calculation). One useful feature is that the device provides XFlow, which is an estimate of total flow derived by differentiating the sum of the chest and abdominal RIP bands. If the airflow sensors fail (become dislodged), the XFlow signal provides

a backup (Fig. 13–7). The downside is that the two RIP bands are more difficult to place than a single effort band. Disposable band material is available for the RIP bands.

Peripheral Arterial Tonometry

Unique PM devices that detect respiratory events by recording changes in sympathetic tone (rather than airflow) using peripheral arterial tonometry (PAT) are also available.[30,31]

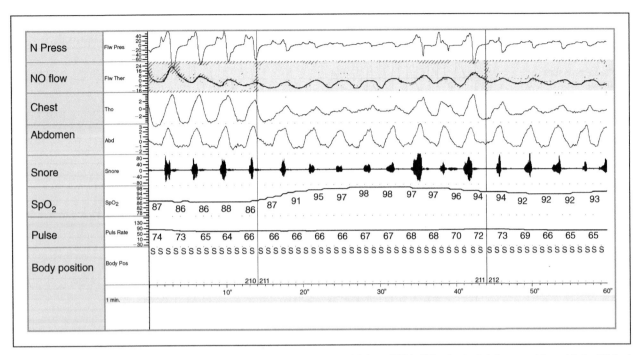

FIGURE 13–5 A 60-second tracing shows an obstructive hypopnea recorded with a type 3 PM device (PDX by Philips-Respironics). An oronasal thermal device (NO flow) and nasal pressure (N Press), chest and abdominal respiratory inductance plethysmography (RIP) bands, snoring, oximetry, pulse rate (from the oximeter), and body position (S = supine) are recorded. SpO$_2$ = pulse oximetry.

Devices using this technology (WatchPAT 100, 200, Itamar Medical) are worn on the wrist. The devices have two probes—a PAT probe and an oximetry probe—worn on separate digits. The PAT signal is a measure of the blood volume in the digit. Increases in sympathetic tone stimulate alpha receptors on the digital blood vessels, causing constriction. A reduction in blood flow to the digits decreases the finger tip volume and the PAT signal. Because surges in sympathetic tone follow respiratory event termination, the combination of a decrease in PAT signal, a fall in pulse oximetry (SpO$_2$) followed by an increase, and an increase in heart rate allows determination of respiratory events (Fig. 13–8). Nonrespiratory arousals would not reduce the SpO$_2$. The device has a built-in actigraphy to help with estimation of an appropriate index time (used to compute an event index). Recently, the combination of actigraphy and the PAT signal has been used to determine estimates of wake, non–rapid eye movement (NREM) sleep, and REM sleep because the sympathetic tone characteristics of these sleep stages differ. Newer models also have a body position sensor and a snore sensor. The device has been validated with several studies. The device cannot be used in patients on alpha blockers (e.g., terazosin) and with patients in atrial fibrillation. Another downside is that the PAT probes are relatively expensive. The national carrier determination for HST recognizes "3 channels of monitoring including PAT, oximetry, and actigraphy" as a valid PM method. However, not all LCDs will allow reimbursement for PAT studies. The device does not fall within recommended PMGs. Recently, the ability to edit events in the program analyzing the information has been improved. New 2011 procedure codes for PM devices now include PAT devices (see Table 13–8).

Practical Considerations in PM

A systematic approach is indicated to avoid a high percentage of technically inadequate PM studies. The choice of the device (Table 13–15) and method of device application (Table 13–16) are major considerations. Devices with more sensors provide more information but are more difficult to apply. The software should provide accurate autoscoring to minimize the amount of event editing required. If the software is similar to that used for PSG, this may be an advantage to reduce training costs. The durability of the device and cost of expendables (e.g., nasal cannula) should be considered.

PM devices can be placed in the sleep center or in the home by a technologist (see Table 13–16). Alternatively, the patient can be trained on the device and apply the device himself or herself at home. PM devices are typically either returned to the sleep center the following day or mailed if patients live a distance from the center. Device loss can be a major expense. The application of the PM device by a technologist in private homes is expensive and has safety issues. Therefore, having patients come to the sleep center is recommended if possible. The more complex the PM device, the less likely patients can apply it themselves. Adequate training is essential. One option is to have patients practice in the sleep center, and if they are unable to successfully attach the device, they can simply wear the device home. It is also possible to give patients the option of wearing the device home or applying it themselves. In a study by Golpe and colleagues,[32] setup of PM device in the patient's home resulted in 7% of inadequate studies whereas having the patients

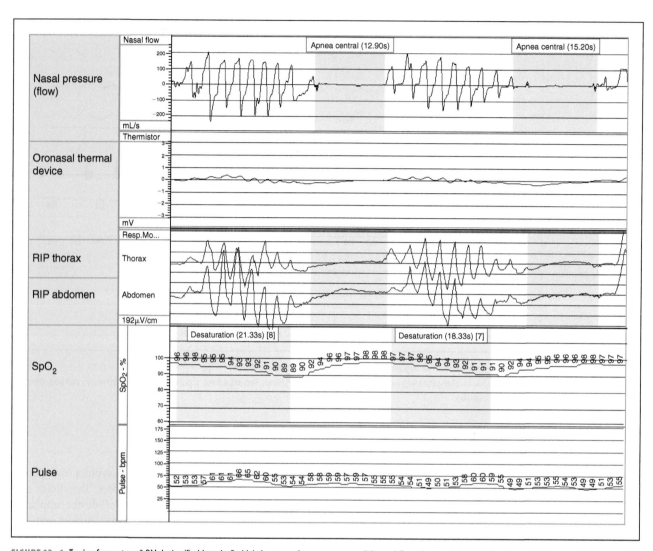

FIGURE 13–6 Tracing from a type 3 PM device (Embletta by Embla) shows nasal pressure, oronasal thermal flow, chest and abdominal respiratory inductance plethysmography (RIP) channels, oximetry (SpO₂), and pulse. Body position and actigraphy were also recorded but are not shown. The illustrated event is a central apnea of the Cheyne-Stokes type. This was an unexpected finding. The patient had no history of known congestive heart failure but did report nocturnal dyspnea.

apply the devices themselves had 33% inadequate studies. This study used a five-channel device recording oronasal airflow, wrist actigraphy, body position, and SaO₂. In our experience, patients have difficulty applying some types of oximeter probes as well as chest and abdominal belts. Other common problems include dislodgment of either the nasal cannula or the oximeter probe as well as pulling leads out of the PM device during body movement. Patients can be trained to apply tape at strategic points to reduce these events. The selection of the device to be used must take into account how the setup will be delivered.

It is also useful to have patients complete a brief sleep diary to record their estimate of how long they slept and if the night of sleep was fairly typical. An occasional patient will sleep very poorly with the device attached. **If minimal sleep is recorded, a false-negative study is likely.** Devices that can record more than one night provide another monitoring night opportunity and may also reduce the influence of night-to-night variability.

Integration of PM into the Overall Patient Care Algorithm

Diagnosis of OSA using PM is only the first part of the process if the study is positive. It is expected that in populations with a high probability of OSA, a high percentage of PM tests will be positive. If PAP is chosen for treatment, there are several alternative pathways to proceed (Table 13–17).[33–35] The standard approach would be to perform a PSG PAP titration and subsequent PAP treatment. Patients could also use an auto-PAP (autotitrating, autoadjusting, positive airway pressure [APAP]) device at home for 3 days or more and information obtained could be used to select a pressure for chronic CPAP treatment.[33,35] APAP devices automatically provide the lowest effective pressure during the night. Commonly, the 90th or 95th percentile pressure is chosen for treatment with a fixed pressure (CPAP). The use of APAP devices is discussed in Chapter 19. A third possible approach is starting CPAP at a pressure derived using prediction equations with subsequent

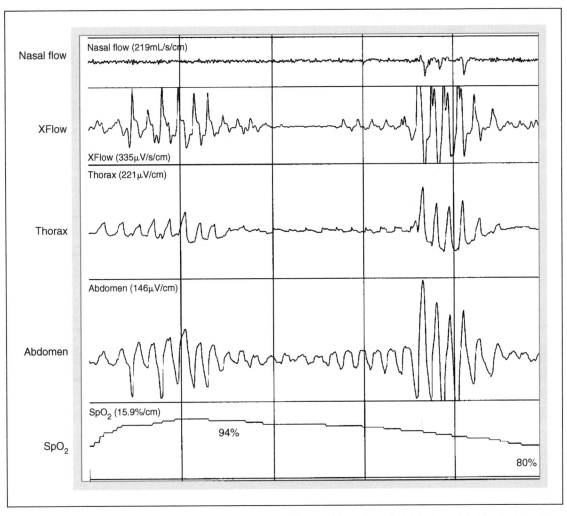

FIGURE 13–7 In this tracing from an Embletta, the nasal flow channel is inadequate (likely nasal cannula dislodged or occluded) but the derived XFlow (derivative of thorax and abdomen RIP bands) provides a reasonable estimate of flow. SpO_2 = pulse oximetry.

adjustment based on oximetry, symptoms, or machine estimates of residual AHI.[13,33-35] Finally, **simply treating the patient with an auto-PAP** (autoadjusting) eliminates the need for titration. These approaches are discussed in Chapter 19 (PAP treatment). If a high percentage of PM studies are positive, a reasonable question to consider is the relative cost-benefit of algorithms using PM for diagnosis compared with one using split PSG. Issues of cost and reimbursement will vary between settings (VA Health Care System vs. private sector). If a large number of PM studies need to be repeated or validated by a PSG to eliminate false negatives, any cost savings from using PM will be reduced. Currently, in the United States, unattended autotitration is not reimbursed. In addition, whereas APAP devices cost DME companies more, insurance carriers reimburse them at the CPAP level. These conditions limit the application of alternative diagnostic treatment pathways to special settings such as the VA Health Care System. The very modest reimbursement for PM studies also discourages routine use of these studies.

Overall Approach to Using PSG and PM

An overall approach to using a combination of PSG and PM is presented in Figure 13–9.

Economic factors at present limit this approach but wider use may be practical in the future. A clinical evaluation determines whether there is a high probability of OSA, if other sleep disorders are present, or whether complicating issues are present that will likely require a PSG titration. Patients with a high probability of OSA undergo PM, and if OSA is diagnosed, they can have APAP treatment or APAP titration followed by CPAP treatment. If the PM is negative, a PSG can be performed. If other sleep disorders are suspected or there are complicating factors such as CHF (Cheyne-Stokes possible), narcotics, obesity hypoventilation possible (supplemental oxygen or massive obesity), a PSG with split study if indicated is performed. Although PM can often diagnose Cheyne-Stokes breathing, a PSG titration will likely be needed.

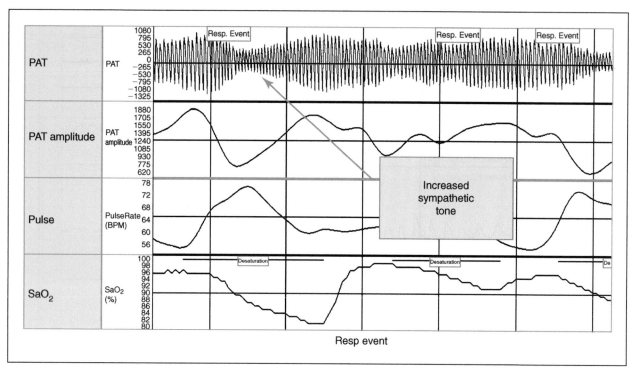

FIGURE 13–8 Peripheral arterial tonometry (PAT) detection of a respiratory event. The PAT signal falls (increased sympathetic tone) associated with an increase then a decrease in pulse and an arterial oxygen desaturation. SaO_2 = arterial oxygen saturation.

TABLE 13–15

Practical Considerations in Portable Monitoring—Choice of Device

- More complex PM devices provide backup sensors and more information—but are more difficult to place.

- Multiple-night recording ability may reduce night-to-night variability effects.

- An automatic scoring program that is accurate and easily editable is essential given low reimbursement for technical component.

- Ease of device setup is essential—if patient is to self-apply device.

- Efficient device use requires ability to
  - Clean device and reprogram easily.
  - "Rapid device turnaround" requires a systematic approach.

- Methods of dealing with device damage or loss
  - Patient signing responsibility contract.
  - Warranty options.

PM = portable monitoring.

TABLE 13–16

Method of Device Setup and Return

SLEEP CENTER SETUP

- Advantages
  - Controlled environment
  - Technologist can place device

- Disadvantages
  - Travel cost for patients (two round trips unless device mailed back)

IN-HOME SETUP

Technologist Travels to Home

- Advantages
  - Lower % technically inadequate studies (compared with patient sensors at home)

- Disadvantages
  - Travel costs
  - Technologist safety issues

Mail Device to Patient

- Requires simple device

- Higher percentage of failed studies

TABLE 13-17

Positive Airway Pressure Treatment after Portable Monitoring Diagnosis of Obstructive Sleep Apnea

- PSG PAP titration followed by CPAP treatment

- Autotitration followed by CPAP treatment

- CPAP on empirically determined pressure
  - Adjustment on basis of residual snoring/apnea
  - Adjustment on basis of bed partner observations
  - Adjustment based on pulse oximetry
  - Adjustment based on device estimate of residual AHI

- Treatment with APAP device

APAP = autotitrating, autoadjusting positive airway pressure;
AHI = apnea-hypopnea index; CPAP = continuous positive airway pressure;
PAP = positive airway pressure; PSG = polysomnography (see Chapter 19).

ACTIGRAPHY

Actigraphy utilizes a portable device (the actigraph) usually worn on the wrist that records movement over an extended period of time (Fig. 13–10). Sleep-wake patterns are estimated from the pattern of movement. Software is available to estimate TST and wake time from the data. The estimates of TST and wake time are more accurate in normal individuals than in patients with sleep disorders. However, the sleep-wake pattern of actigraph data is extremely valuable in documenting patterns of sleep and wake. AASM practice parameters have been published in 2005 and most recently in 2007.[36,37] The temporary Healthcare Common Procedure Coding System (HCPCS) code for actigraphy was 0089T. In 2009, actigraphy received a current procedural terminology (CPT) code. The new code is 95803—actigraphy testing, recording, analysis, interpretation, and report (minimum of 72 hr–14 consecutive days of recording). Medical practices often set fees for actigraphy in the $250 to $300 range.

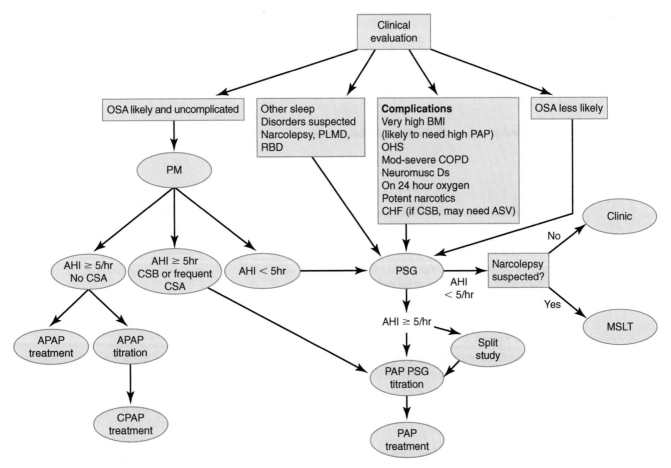

FIGURE 13–9 Systematic approach to using combination of polysomnography (PSG) and portable monitoring (PM) to evaluate patients. AHI = apnea-hypopnea index; APAP = autoadjusting, autotitrating positive airway pressure; ASV = adaptive servo-ventilation, a treatment for CSA or CSB; BMI = body mass index; CHF = congestive heart failure; COPD = chronic obstructive pulmonary disease; CPAP = continuous positive airway pressure; CSA = central sleep apnea; CSB = Cheyne-Stokes breathing; MSLT = multiple sleep latency test; OSA = obstructive sleep apnea; PAP = positive airway pressure; PLMD = periodic limb movement disorder; RBD = rapid eye movement sleep behavior disorder.

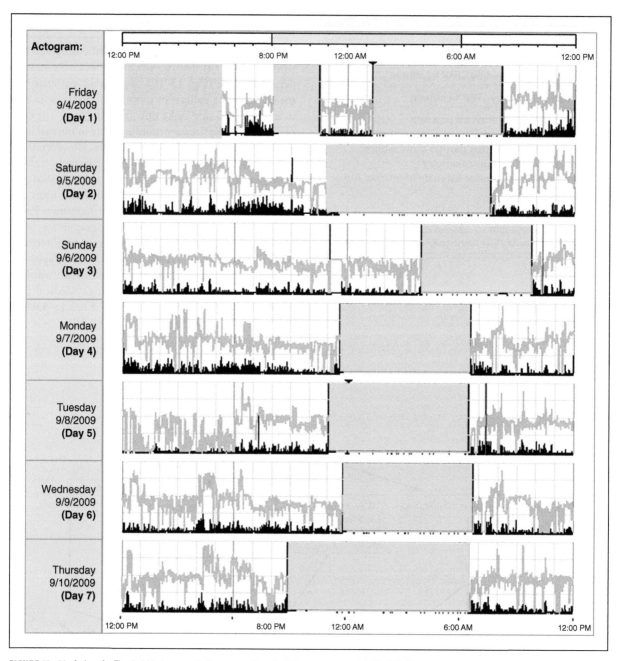

FIGURE 13–10 Actigraphy. The *dark black* represents the amount of activity (when present = wake). The *light blue* represents periods of low activity identified as sleep. The *light gray* represents ambient light detection. This patient had irregular bedtimes.

However, at this writing, actigraphy is still not reimbursed by most insurance plans or Medicare. Studies of actigraphy have usually compared the results with that of PSG or sleep logs. However, actigraphy does not measure sleep (EEG) or the subjective experience of sleep (sleep logs).

Indications

The indications for actigraphy are listed in Table 13–18. Actigraphy provides a fairly accurate estimate of sleep patterns in normal, healthy adult populations and in patients suspected of certain sleep disorders. Actigraphy is indicated to assist in the evaluation of patients with advanced sleep

phase syndrome (ASPS), delayed sleep phase syndrome (DSPS), and shift work disorder. In addition, there is some evidence to support the use of actigraphy in the evaluation of patients suspected of jet lag disorder and non–24-hour sleep-wake syndrome (including that associated with blindness). Actigraphy is also useful for documenting the response to treatment in circadian disorders.

When PSG is not available, actigraphy is indicated to estimate TST in patients with OSA.[37] In patients with insomnia and hypersomnia, there is evidence to support the use of actigraphy in the characterization of circadian rhythms and sleep patterns/disturbances. In assessing response to therapy, actigraphy has proved useful as an outcome measure

TABLE 13-18

Indications for Actigraphy

1. Assess the sleep-wake patterns of normal individuals. (Standard)

2. To assist in evaluation of suspected circadian rhythm sleep disorders.
   - Advanced sleep phase—Indicated. (Guideline)
   - Delayed sleep phase—Indicated. (Guideline)
   - Shift work disorder—Indicated. (Option)
   - Free-running circadian rhythm sleep disorder (non-24 hr)—Indicated. (Option)
   - ISWR—Indicated. (Option)
   - Jet lag disorder—Not indicated for diagnosis. (Guideline)

3. When PSG is not available, actigraphy provides an estimate of total sleep time in OSA. When used with respiratory monitoring, actigraphy may improve the accuracy in assessing severity (AHI). (Standard)

4. Actigraphy is indicated to characterize **circadian rhythm patterns or sleep disturbance** in individuals with **insomnia**, including insomnia with depression. (Option)

5. Actigraphy is indicated to determine circadian pattern and estimate average daily sleep time in individuals complaining of hypersomnia. (Option)

6. Actigraphy is useful in assessing **response to therapy** in
   - Circadian rhythm sleep disorders.
   - Insomnia.

7. Actigraphy is useful
   A. Characterizing sleep and circadian rhythm patterns as well as treatment outcomes among **older individuals living in the community**, especially if used in conjunction with other measures such as sleep diaries/caregiver observations.
   B. Characterizing sleep and circadian rhythm patterns and documenting treatment outcome in **older nursing home residents.**
   C. Delineating sleep patterns and documenting treatment responses in **normal infants and children and in special pediatric populations** (PSG difficult and difficult to interpret).

AHI = apnea-hypopnea index; ISWR = irregular sleep wake rhythm; OSA = obstructive sleep apnea; PSG = polysomnography.

in patients with circadian rhythm disorders and insomnia. In older adults (community dwelling and nursing home residents), sleep monitoring can be difficult. Actigraphy is indicated for characterizing sleep and circadian patterns and to document treatment responses. Similarly, in normal infants and children, as well as special pediatric populations, actigraphy has proved useful for delineating sleep patterns and documenting treatment responses.

Actigraphy in OSA

If the number of events detected by PM was divided by a better estimate of TST than the monitoring time, this might improve the estimate of the AHI. However, patients with OSA by the very nature of the disorder have periodic movements at the end of respiratory events. Hedner and associates[38] validated a special actigraphic system optimized for use in OSA patients. The device was compared with PSG on an epoch-by-epoch basis. The overall sensitivity and specificity to identify sleep were 89% and 69%, respectively. The agreement ranged from 86% in the normal subjects to 86%, 84%, and 80% in the patients with mild, moderate, and severe OSA, respectively. There was a tight agreement between the mean values of actigraphy and PSG in determining mean sleep efficiency, TST, and sleep latency. Whereas for most individuals, the difference between the PSG and the actigraphy was relatively small, for some, there was a substantial disagreement. Another study did not find good agreement between actigraphic and PSG estimates of TST.[39] Elbaz and coworkers[40] used actigraphy combined with respiratory monitoring and found a better estimate of the AHI than use of time in bed. The utility of actigraphy with PM remains to be determined. However, it certainly allows elimination of large portions of the night in which wake is obvious.

Patients with Hypersomnia

Practice parameters on use of PSG/MSLT to diagnose narcolepsy stated that sleep logs may be obtained for 1 week before to assess sleep-wake schedules. Not all patients can keep accurate sleep logs. Therefore, actigraphy could be potentially useful to document sleep patterns before MSLT. However, current practice parameters for actigraphy[37] do not list evaluation of sleep before MSLT as an indication.

Actigraphy in Insomnia

The practice parameters for actigraphy did not recommend testing as a routine evaluation of patients with insomnia. However, actigraphy was said to be "useful" in documenting sleep-wake patterns.[37] Therefore, documenting sleep patterns rather than the absolute amount of sleep and wake is likely the best use of the actigraph. In insomnia patients, periods of low activity in which patients lay quietly in bed but are awake may be scored as sleep by actigraphy software. When performing actigraphy, it is essential to require patients to complete a sleep log (lights off, lights on, out of bed, actigraph off for shower, and so on, estimated TST; and sleep latency). This information enables a correct interpretation of actigraphic tracings. For example, total absence of movement usually indicates that the actigraph has been removed (shower, swimming), but here patient logs are essential to verify device removal. Many modern wrist actigraph devices also provide the capability of recording the amount of ambient light. This is useful in patients with circadian rhythm sleep disorders in whom light exposure may either exacerbate or improve the underlying disorder. Some actigraphy devices also have event markers that the patient can press when getting in bed, trying to sleep, or after awakening in the morning.

Sleep logs and actigraphy provides complementary information. In a study of patients with insomnia undergoing treatment, Vallières and Morin[41] compared findings from

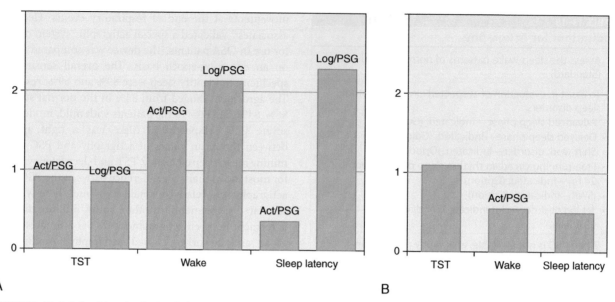

FIGURE 13–11 A, A plot of the ratios of actigraphic/polysomnography (Act/PSG) and sleep log/PSG estimates of total sleep time (TST), wake, and sleep latency from the data of a study by Vallières and Morin in patients with insomnia. Both Act and sleep logs slightly underestimated the TST but overestimated wake time. Sleep logs overestimated sleep latency and Act underestimated sleep latency (laying in bed still but awake). **B,** A plot of Act/PSG ratios (all three bars) for TST, wake, and sleep latency from a study of older insomniacs by Sivertsen and coworkers. Act slightly overestimated TST but underestimated wake and sleep latency. **A,** Data from Vallières A, Morin CM: Actigraphy in assessment of insomnia. Sleep 2003;26:902–906; **B,** data from Sivertsen B, Omvki S, Havik OE, et al: A comparison of actigraphy and polysomnography in older adults: treatment of chronic primary insomnia. Sleep 2006;29:1353–1358.

actigraphy and sleep logs with PSG (Fig. 13–11A). Both actigraphy and sleep logs underestimated TST and overestimated wake time. Actigraphy underestimated the sleep latency whereas sleep logs overestimated the sleep latency. They found actigraphy to be more sensitive at detecting treatment effects than sleep logs. In contrast, Sivertsen and coworkers[42] found different results in a group of older adults treated for primary insomnia (expected to have more wake time). Actigraphy slightly overestimated TST and underestimated wake (see Fig. 13–11B). In this study, actigraphy provided a better estimate of TST than of wake time.

CLINICAL REVIEW QUESTIONS

1. A 45-year-old man referred to the sleep laboratory with a long history of snoring, witnessed apnea, and daytime sleepiness. The physical examination shows a body mass index (BMI) of 31 kg/m², very crowded upper airway, and neck circumference of 17 inches. An unattended PM (type 3) sleep study found an AHI of 3.5 events/hr with the lowest SaO_2 being 89%. The patient reports he did not sleep that well (worried about pulling out wires from PM device). Which of the following would you do next?

   A. Repeat PM (type 3).
   B. Attended PSG.
   C. Tell the patient that he doesn't have OSA.
   D. Refer him for an OA or upper airway surgery to treat primary snoring.

2. A 40-year-old man was referred to the sleep center with a long history of loud snoring, witnessed apnea, and daytime sleepiness. The physical examination shows a BMI of 31 kg/m², and a very long, swollen uvula. His neck is 18 inches in circumference. The patient is otherwise healthy. Which of the following would you do next?

   A. PM (type 3 airflow, effort, SaO_2, heart rate).
   B. Attended PSG.
   C. Nocturnal oximetry.
   D. Treatment with APAP.
   E. Refer him for an OA or surgery to treat primary snoring.

3. A 40-year-old man was referred to the sleep center with a history of loud snoring that bothers his wife. The patient denies daytime sleepiness. His wife has never noted breathing pauses. The patient has been evaluated by an ear-nose-throat (ENT) physician who recommends upper airway surgery for snoring. On examination, he has a long uvula but a minimally crowded upper airway. His neck circumference is 15 inches and his BMI is 22 kg/m². Which of the following do you recommend?

   A. Proceed to have the upper airway surgery.
   B. Schedule for a PSG.
   C. Schedule for oximetry (type 4 PM).
   D. Schedule an unattended type 3 PM study.

4. You are asked to follow a 50-year-old woman who was diagnosed with OSA about 2 years ago at another sleep

center. She was placed on CPAP at 8 H$_2$O. Her initial symptoms of snoring and daytime sleepiness have resolved, and she reports using her CPAP nightly. She is otherwise healthy. There has been no change in her weight (BMI = 31 kg/m^2), her menopause status (post-menopausal), or medications (for hypertension). Which of the following do you recommend?

A. Clinical follow-up in 1 year or sooner if symptoms recur.

B. Verify CPAP compliance objectively from machine information.

C. Order a PSG on CPAP.

D. Order a diagnostic PSG to see if CPAP is still needed.

5. A 35-year-old man with OSA had palatal surgery performed 3 months ago for OSA (preoperative AHI was 25/hr). He reports that his snoring is much improved and that his daytime sleepiness is better as well. Physical examination shows a well-healed palatal scar. Which of the following do you recommend?

A. PSG.

B. Nocturnal oximetry.

C. Clinical follow-up only.

D. PSG if symptoms return.

6. A 55-year-old man was recently diagnosed with CHF. He has been treated with a beta blocker, angiotensin-converting enzyme inhibitor, and diuretic, but continues to have nocturnal dyspnea and frequent awakenings. He reports only mild snoring that is unchanged. On physical examination, he has minimal upper airway crowding but has basilar crackles and 1+ pedal edema. Which of the following do you recommend?

A. Increased diuretic dose.

B. PSG.

C. Trial of a hypnotic to consolidate sleep.

D. Unattended type 3 PM.

7. A 75-year-old man recently had a left-sided cerebrovascular accident and now has mild right hemiparesis. Per spouse, there is no snoring or witnessed apnea. He complains of insomnia and frequent nocturnal arousals. Physical examination is notable for the hemiparesis and moderate obesity. Which of the following do you recommend?

A. SpO$_2$.

B. PSG.

C. Unattended cardiorespiratory sleep study (level 3).

D. Cognitive behavior therapy for insomnia.

E. Empirical trial of a hypnotic.

8. A 16-year-old boy with Duchenne's muscular dystrophy complains of frequent episodes of nocturnal dyspnea and frequent awakenings. He is wheelchair-bound and

has extreme muscle weakness. Physical examination shows diffuse muscle atrophy and weakness, obesity. Arterial blood gases on room air show arterial partial pressure of oxygen (PaO$_2$) = 65 mm Hg, SaO$_2$ = 92%, arterial partial pressure of carbon dioxide (PaCO$_2$) = 46 mm Hg. Which of the following do you recommend?

A. Empirical nocturnal low-flow O$_2$.

B. Nocturnal SpO$_2$ arterial oxygen saturation monitoring.

C. PSG.

D. Hypnotic.

9. A 45-year-old woman has complaints of poor sleep with frequent nocturnal arousals. Her husband says that she kicks her legs at night. Only mild snoring and no witnessed apneas are reported. The patient DENIES symptoms of the RLS. Which of the following is recommended?

A. PSG.

B. Unattended type 3 PM study.

C. Sleep diary for 2 weeks.

D. Empirical treatment with a hypnotic.

E. Actigraphy

10. A 60-year-old woman is complaining of severe difficulty initiating and maintaining sleep. This has not improved with several hypnotics and cognitive behavioral therapy for insomnia. Her husband reports mild snoring and no breathing pauses. She has coronary artery disease and has recently undergone an angioplasty with two stents. The patient also has a long history of hypertension and diabetes mellitus. Her medications include clopidogrel and aspirin. Physical examination shows moderate obesity and a slightly crowded oropharynx. Which of the following do you recommend?

A. Ask the patient whether she snores and/or has daytime sleepiness.

B. PSG.

C. SpO$_2$.

D. Actigraphy.

E. Cognitive behavioral therapy.

11. A PM test is performed for insomnia and the results are listed here. The patient reports loud snoring but no daytime sleepiness. What do you recommend?

Monitoring time: 7 hr.

AHI (based on monitoring time) = 3/hr.

Events: 13 obstructive apneas, 8 hypopneas.

Desaturations: 70, with oxygen desaturation index (ODI) of 10/hr, lowest SpO$_2$ = 83%.

A. PSG.

B. Evaluate raw tracings.

C. Treatment for snoring.

D. Inform the patient that OSA is not present.

Answers

1. **B.** PM can give false-negative results, especially if the patient sleeps very poorly. Because there is a high index of suspicion, a PSG should be ordered. Patients with a high pretest probability for OSA but a negative PM study should have a full night PSG.

2. **A or B.** This patient has a high pretest probability of having OSA. A PM study is indicated in combination with a comprehensive sleep evaluation if PM is performed according to AASM PMGs. Of course, ordering a PSG is also indicated and is the gold standard. Treatment of snoring by either surgery or an OA should not be undertaken if OSA is ruled out. Unlike snoring, a posttreatment PSG or PM is indicated if OSA is present.

3. **B.** A PSG (or **attended** type 3 PM) should be performed before upper airway surgery for snoring or OSA. If significant OSA is present, other treatments might be considered. The study will also document as baseline (for comparison with postoperative PSG). Note that the practice parameter for PSG 2005 does specify that either a PSG or an attended type 3 (cardiorespiratory) study be performed. Note that an **unattended** type 3 study can be used for non-PAP treatment follow-up. It should be used as a diagnostic study only if there is a high probability of OSA. In this case, the patient is not high probability (no witnessed apnea, no increased neck circumference).

4. **B.** Follow-up PSG or an **attended** cardiorespiratory (type 3) sleep study is NOT routinely indicated in patients treated with CPAP whose symptoms continue to be resolved with CPAP treatment. It is good clinical practice to objectively document CPAP adherence (patients often overestimate their use). In the absence of significant weight loss, there is no reason to believe that CPAP is no longer needed.

5. **A.** After upper airway surgery for OSA, a PSG or **attended** level 3 study is indicated routinely to assess treatment results (after surgical healing). AASM PMGs state that an **unattended** type 3 PM "may" be indicated if performed following AASM guidelines. Improvement in symptoms is unreliable as is SpO$_2$ monitoring for the diagnosis of OSA in this setting.

6. **B.** A large percentage of patients with systolic or diastolic heart failure have some form of SRBD. A PSG is indicated if they have nocturnal symptoms suggestive of SRBDs (disturbed sleep, nocturnal dyspnea, snoring) or if they remain symptomatic despite optimal medical management of CHF. The current patient reported frequent awakenings and nocturnal dyspnea on treatment. Of note, many patients **with CHF and OSA or CSA do NOT report daytime sleepiness.**

7. **B.** Patients with history of stroke or TIAs should be evaluated for symptoms and signs of sleep apnea. If there is **suspicion of sleep apnea,** the patients should undergo a PSG. There is a high incidence of CSA or OSA after CVA. Given that the symptoms are suspicious (frequent nocturnal arousals) but do not fall into the "high probability of moderate to severe OSA" category, an unattended PM type 3 is not indicated. SpO$_2$ is not sensitive enough in this situation. Before treating insomnia, OSA should be ruled out with a PSG.

8. **C.** According to the AASM practice parameters, for patients with neuromuscular disorders and sleep-related symptoms, PSG is routinely indicated to evaluate symptoms of sleep disorders that are not adequately diagnosed by obtaining a sleep history, assessing sleep hygiene, and reviewing sleep diaries. The main concern here is nocturnal hypoventilation. Noninvasive PAP ventilation (not supplemental oxygen) is indicated for nocturnal hypoventilation. In this setting, SpO$_2$ can be useful and some would argue that this is also a correct answer. However, PSG can determine whether OSA, nocturnal hypoventilation, or a combination is present.

9. **A.** PSG is indicated when a diagnosis of PLMD is considered because of complaints by the patient or an observer of repetitive limb movements during sleep and frequent awakenings, fragmented sleep, difficulty maintaining sleep, or EDS. A PSG is NOT indicated for diagnosis of RLS. Of note, some patients with OSA also have leg kicks at night. A PM study would not be indicated because it does not address the leg movements. PLMD is thought to be uncommon. In this setting, actigraphy might be useful if the OSA and PLMD are ruled out. Empirical treatment with hypnotics is not recommended until the nature of the disturbance is identified.

10. **B.** Patients with coronary artery disease should be evaluated for symptoms and signs of sleep apnea. If there is suspicion of sleep apnea, the patients should undergo a sleep study. Answer A could also be considered as being correct. However, whereas snoring and EDS are cardinal symptoms of OSA, some patients complain of insomnia. PSG is not routinely indicated for insomnia. **However, in cases that do not respond to treatment, especially in high-risk settings, a PSG is probably the safest course.** Note that the practice parameters do NOT say that an unattended type 3 PM study is indicated in this situation. If the TST is much less than the monitoring time, PM may also underestimate the AHI. The practice parameters for using PSG to evaluate insomnia[4] state "Polysomnography is indicated when initial diagnosis is uncertain, treatment fails (behavioral or pharmacologic), or precipitous arousals occur with violent or injurious behavior. (Guideline)"

11. B. There is an inconsistency between the ODI of 10/hr and the AHI of 3/hr. The technical adequacy of the oximetry and flow tracings should be determined. In many cases, the ODI is more accurate than the AHI. The other explanation for the above findings is that the automated scoring did not pick up respiratory events where a desaturation is present. Scoring may need to be manually edited. Whereas a PSG could be indicated, the first issue is to determine whether the PM study already performed can provide an accurate estimate of breathing abnormalities.

REFERENCES

1. Standards of Practice Committee Task Force: Practice parameters for the indications of polysomnography and related procedures. Sleep 1997;20:406–422.
2. Kushida CA, Littner MR, Morgenthaler T, Alessi CA: Practice parameters for the indications for polysomnography and related procedures: an update for 2005. Sleep 2005;28:499–521.
3. Littner MR, Kushida C, Wise M, et al: Practice parameters for clinical use of the multiple sleep latency test and the maintenance of wakefulness test. Sleep 2005;28:113–121.
4. Littner M, Kramer M, Kapen S, et al: Practice parameters for using polysomnography to evaluate insomnia: an update. Sleep 2003;26:754–760.
5. Morgenthaler TI, Lee-Chiong T, Alessi C, et al: Practice parameters for the clinical evaluation and treatment of circadian rhythm sleep disorders. Sleep 2007;30:1445–1459.
6. Kushida CA, Morgenthaler T, Littner MR, et al: Practice parameters for the treatment of snoring and obstructive sleep apnea with oral appliances: an update for 2005. Sleep 2006;29:240–243.
7. Chesson A, Berry RB, Pack A: Practice parameters for the use of portable monitoring devices in the investigation of suspected sleep apnea in adults. Sleep 2003;26:907–913.
8. Collop NA, Anderson WM, Boehlecke B, et al: Clinical guidelines for the use of unattended portable monitors in the diagnosis of obstructive sleep apnea in adult patients. Portable Monitoring Task Force of the American Academy of Sleep Medicine. J Clin Sleep Med 2007;3:737–747.
9. Department of Health and Human Services Centers for Medicare and Medicaid Services: Decision Memo for Continuous Positive Airway Pressure (CPAP) Therapy for Obstructive Sleep Apnea (OSA). CAG#0093R. March 2008. Available at http://www.cmshhs.gov/mcd/viewdecisionmemo.asp?id=204 2008
10. Centers for Medicare and Medicaid Services, 2009: Decision memo for sleep testing for obstructive sleep apnea (CAG-00405N). Available at http://www.cmshhs.gov/mcd/viewdecisionmemo.asp?id_227 2009
11. Gay P, Weaver T, Loube D, et al: Evaluation of positive airway pressure treatment for sleep related breathing disorders in adults. Sleep 2006;29:381–401.
12. Kushida CA, Littner MR, Hirshkowitz M, et al: Practice parameters for the use of continuous and bilevel positive airway pressure devices to treat adult patients with sleep-related breathing disorders. Sleep 2006;29:375–380.
13. Morgenthaler TI, Kapen S, Lee-Chiong T, et al: Practice parameters for the medical therapy of obstructive sleep apnea. Sleep 2006;29:1031–1035.
14. Desai H, Patel A, Patel P, et al: Accuracy of auto-titrating CPAP to estimate the residual apnea-hypopnea index in patients with obstructive sleep apnea on treatment with auto-titrating CPAP. Sleep Breath 2009;13:383–390.
15. Baltzan MA, Kassissia I, Elkholi O, et al: Prevalence of persistent sleep apnea in patients treated with continuous positive airway pressure. Sleep 2006;29:557–563.
16. Pittman SD, Pillar G, Berry RB, et al: Follow-up assessment of CPAP efficacy in patients with obstructive sleep apnea using an ambulatory device based on peripheral arterial tonometry. Sleep Breath 2006;10:123–131.
17. Chediak AD: Why CMS approved home sleep testing for CPAP coverage. J Clin Sleep Med 2008;4:16–18.
18. Collop NA: Portable monitoring for the diagnosis of obstructive sleep apnea. Curr Opin Pulm Med 2008;14:525–529.
19. Ferber R, Millman R, Coppola M, et al: ASDA standards of practice: portable recording in the assessment of obstructive sleep apnea. Sleep 1994;17:378–392.
20. American Sleep Disorders Association: ASDA Standards of Practice. Practice parameters for the use of portable recording in the assessment of obstructive sleep apnea. Sleep 1994;17:372–377.
21. Littner MR: Portable monitoring in the diagnosis of the obstructive sleep apnea syndrome. Semin Respir Crit Care Med 2005;26:56–67.
22. Flemons WW, Littner MR, Rowley JA, et al: Home diagnosis of sleep apnea: a systematic review of the literature: an evidence review cosponsored by the American Academy of Sleep Medicine, the American College of Chest Physicians, and the American Thoracic Society. Chest 2003;124:1543–1579.
23. Executive summary on the systematic review and practice parameters for portable monitoring in the investigation of suspected sleep apnea in adults. Am J Respir Crit Care Med 2004;169:1160–1163.
24. Flemons W, Littner M: Measuring agreement between diagnostic devices. Chest 2003;124:1535–1542.
25. Smith LA, Chong DW, Vennelle M, et al: Diagnosis of sleep-disordered breathing in patients with chronic heart failure: evaluation of a portable limited sleep study system. J Sleep Res 2007;16:428–435.
26. Levendowski D, Steward D, Woodson BT, et al: The impact of obstructive sleep apnea variability measured in-lab versus in-home on sample size calculations. Int Arch Med 2009;2:1–8.
27. Bland JM, Altman DG: Measuring agreement in method comparison studies. Stat Methods Med Res 1999;8:135–160.
28. Santos-Silva R, Truksians V, Truksina E, et al: Validation of a portable monitoring system for the diagnosis of obstructive sleep apnea syndrome. Sleep 2009;32:629–636.
29. Iber C, Ancoli-Israel S, Chesson AJ, Quan S for the American Academy of Sleep Medicine: The AASM Manual for the Scoring of Sleep and Associated Events: Rules, Terminology and Technical Specification, 1st ed. Westchester, IL: American Academy of Sleep Medicine, 2007.
30. Bar A, Pillar G, Dvir I, et al: Evaluation of a portable device based on peripheral arterial tone for unattended home sleep studies. Chest 2003;123:695–703.
31. Ayas NT, Pittman S, MacDonald M, White DP: Assessment of a wrist-worn device in the detection of obstructive sleep apnea. Sleep Med 2003;4:435–442.
32. Golp R, Jimenex A, Carpizo R: Home sleep studies in the assessment of sleep apnea/hypopnea syndrome. Chest 2002;122:1156–1161.
33. Masa JF, Jimenez A, Duran J, et al: Alternative methods of titrating continuous positive airway pressure. Am J Respir Crit Care Med 2004;170:1218–1224.
34. Fitzpatrick MF, Alloway CED, Wakeford TM, et al: Can patients with obstructive sleep apnea titrate their own continuous positive airway pressure? Am J Respir Crit Care Med 2003;167:716–722.
35. Berry RB, Hill G, Thompson L, Mclarin V: Portable monitoring and autotitraton versus polysomnography for the diagnosis and treatment of sleep apnea. Sleep 2008;31:1423–1431.

36. Littner MR, Kushida DA, Anderson WM, et al: Standards of Practice Committee of the American Academy of Sleep Medicine: practice parameters for the role of actigraphy in the study of sleep and circadian rhythms: an update for 2002. Sleep 2003;26:337–341.

37. Morgenthaler T, Alessi C, Friedman L, et al: Practice parameters for the use of actigraphy in the assessment of sleep and sleep disorders: an update for 2007. Sleep 2007;30:519–529.

38. Hedner J, Pillar G, Pittman SD, et al: A novel adaptive wrist actigraphy algorithm for sleep-wake assessment in sleep apnea patients. Sleep 2004;27:1560–1566.

39. Penzel T, Kesper K, Pinnow I, et al: Peripheral arterial tonometry, oximetry and actigraphy for ambulatory recording of sleep apnea. Physiol Meas 2004;25:1025–1036.

40. Elbaz M, Roue GM, Lofaso F, Quera Salva MA: Utility of actigraphy in the diagnosis of obstructive sleep apnea. Sleep 2002;25:527–531.

41. Vallières A, Morin CM: Actigraphy in assessment of insomnia. Sleep 2003;26:902–906.

42. Sivertsen B, Omvki S, Havik OE, et al: A comparison of actigraphy and polysomnography in older adults: treatment of chronic primary insomnia. Sleep 2006;29:1353–1358.

AASM Practice Parameters for Polysomnography (Selected Statements)

4.1.3.1 Polysomnography is routinely indicated for the diagnosis of sleep-related breathing disorders (SRBDs). (Standard)

4.1.3.2 Polysomnography is indicated for positive airway pressure (PAP) titration in patients with SRBDs. (Standard)

4.1.3.3 A preoperative clinical evaluation that includes polysomnography or an attended cardiorespiratory (type 3) sleep study is routinely indicated to evaluate for the presence of obstructive sleep apnea (OSA) in patients before they undergo upper airway surgery **for snoring or OSA.** (Standard)

4.1.3.4 Follow-up polysomnography or an attended cardiorespiratory (type 3) sleep study is routinely indicated for the assessment of treatment results in the following circumstances: (Standard)

1. After good clinical response to oral appliance treatment in patients with moderate to severe OSA.*
2. After upper airway surgery in patients with moderate to severe OSA, to ensure therapeutic benefit.
3. After surgical or dental treatment of patients with SRBDs whose symptoms return despite a good initial response to treatment.

4.1.3.5 Follow-up polysomnography is routinely indicated for the assessment of treatment results in the following circumstances: (Standard)

1. After substantial weight loss (e.g., 10% of body weight) has occurred in patients on continuous positive airway pressure (CPAP) for treatment of SRBDs to ascertain whether CPAP is still needed at the previously titrated pressure.
2. After substantial weight gain (e.g., 10% of body weight) has occurred in patients previously treated with CPAP successfully, who are again symptomatic despite the continued use of CPAP, to ascertain whether pressure adjustments are needed.

3. When clinical response is insufficient or when symptoms return despite a good initial response to treatment with CPAP. In these circumstances, testing should be devised with consideration that a concurrent sleep disorder may be present (e.g., OSA and narcolepsy).

4.1.3.6 Follow-up polysomnography or a cardiorespiratory (type 3) sleep study is NOT routinely indicated in patients treated with CPAP whose symptoms continue to be resolved with CPAP treatment. (Option)

4.1.3.7 A multiple sleep latency test is not routinely indicated for most patients with SRBDs. A subjective assessment of excessive daytime sleepiness should be obtained routinely. When an objective measure of daytime sleepiness is also required, previously published practice parameters should be consulted. (Standard)

4.1.3.8 Patients with systolic or diastolic heart failure should undergo polysomnography if **they have nocturnal symptoms suggestive of SRBDs** (disturbed sleep, nocturnal dyspnea, snoring) or if they remain symptomatic despite optimal medical management of congestive heart failure (CHF). (Standard)

4.1.3.9 Patients with coronary artery disease should be evaluated for symptoms and signs of sleep apnea. **If there is suspicion of sleep apnea,** the patients should undergo a sleep study. (Guideline)

4.1.3.10 Patients with history of stroke or transient ischemic attacks should be evaluated for symptoms and signs of sleep apnea. If there is suspicion of sleep apnea, the patients should undergo a sleep study. (Option)

4.1.3.11 Patients referred for evaluation of significant tachyarrhythmias or bradyarrhythmias should be questioned about symptoms of sleep apnea. A sleep study is indicated if questioning results in a **reasonable suspicion that OSA or central sleep apnea (CSA)** is present. (Guideline)

Polysomnography in Other Medical Disorders

4.2.3.1 For patients with **neuromuscular disorders and sleep-related symptoms,** polysomnography is routinely indicated to evaluate symptoms of sleep disorders that are

---

*Amended in Practice Parameters for Oral Appliance treatment[6] to include mild, moderate, and severe OSA.

not adequately diagnosed by obtaining a sleep history, assessing sleep hygiene, and reviewing sleep diaries. (Standard)

4.2.3.2 Polysomnography is not indicated to diagnose **chronic lung disease.** (Standard)

Alternate Tools

4.2.5.1 Nocturnal oximetry may be helpful or sufficient in assessing a disorder in which the only or principal clinical issue is the level of hypoxemia and when determining sleep stages or assessing sleep apnea is not necessary. (Standard)

4.3 Narcolepsy

4.3.3.1 Polysomnography and a multiple sleep latency test performed on the day after the polysomnographic evaluation are routinely indicated in the evaluation of suspected narcolepsy. (Standard)

4.4 Parasomnias and Seizure Disorders

4.4.1.1 A clinical history of any parasomnia must describe and characterize the behaviors in detail with special emphasis on age of onset, time of night, frequency, regularity, and duration of episodes. (Standard)

4.4.1.2 Common, uncomplicated, noninjurious parasomnias, such as typical disorders of arousal, nightmares, enuresis, sleeptalking, and bruxism, can usually be diagnosed by clinical evaluation alone. (Standard)

4.4.1.3 A clinical history, neurologic examination, and a routine electroencephalogram (EEG) obtained while the patient is awake and asleep are often sufficient to establish the diagnosis and permit the appropriate treatment of a sleep-related seizure disorder. The need for a routine EEG should be based on clinical judgment and the likelihood that the patient has a sleep-related seizure disorder. (Option)

4.4.3.5 Polysomnography may be indicated when the presumed parasomnia or sleep-related seizure disorder does not respond to conventional therapy. (Option)

4.4.3.6 Polysomnography is not routinely indicated in cases of typical, uncomplicated, and noninjurious parasomnias when the diagnosis is clearly delineated. (Option)

4.4.3.7 Polysomnography is not routinely indicated for patients with a seizure disorder who have no specific complaints consistent with a sleep disorder. (Option)

4.4.4.1 The minimum channels required for the diagnosis of parasomnia or sleep-related seizure disorder include sleep-scoring channels (EEG, electro-oculogram [EOG], chin electromyogram [EMG]); EEG using an expanded bilateral montage; and EMG for body movements (anterior tibialis or extensor digitorum). Audiovisual recording and documented technologist observations during the period of study are also essential. (Option)

4.4.4.2 Interpretation of polysomnography with video and extended EEG montage requires skills in both sleep medicine and seizure recognition. Polysomnographers and electroencephalographers who are not experienced or trained in recognizing and interpreting both polysomnographic and EEG abnormalities should seek appropriate consultation or should refer patients to a center where this expertise is available. (Option)

4.4.4.3 A paper speed of at least 15 mm/sec and preferably 30 mm/sec is recommended to enhance the recognition of seizure activity. In digital EEG recordings, the sampling rate must be adequate to identify brief paroxysmal discharges. (Option)

4.5 Restless Legs Syndrome and Periodic Limb Movement Disorder

4.5.3.1 Polysomnography is indicated when a diagnosis of periodic limb movement disorder is considered because of complaints by the patient or an observer of repetitive limb movements during sleep and frequent awakenings, fragmented sleep, difficulty maintaining sleep, or excessive daytime sleepiness. (Standard)

4.5.3.2 Polysomnography is not routinely indicated to diagnose or treat restless legs syndrome, except where uncertainty exists in the diagnosis. (Standard)

4.5.4.1 The minimum channels required for the evaluation of periodic limb movements and related arousals include EEG, EOG, chin EMG, and left and right anterior tibialis surface EMG. Respiratory effort, airflow, and oximetry should be used simultaneously if sleep apnea or upper-airway resistance syndrome is suspected to allow a distinction to be made between inherent periodic limb movements and those limb movements associated with respiratory events. (Standard)

4.5.4.2 Intraindividual night-to-night variability exists in patients with periodic limb movement sleep disorder, and a single study might not be adequate to establish this diagnosis. (Option)

4.6 Depression with Insomnia

4.6.3.1 Neither a polysomnogram nor a multiple sleep latency test is routinely indicated in establishing the diagnosis of depression. (Standard)

4.7 Circadian Rhythm Sleep Disorders

4.7.3.1 Polysomnography is not routinely indicated for the diagnosis of circadian rhythm sleep disorders. (Standard)

From Kushida CA, Littner MR, Morgenthaler T, Alessi CA: Practice parameters for the indications for polysomnography and related procedures: an update for 2005. Sleep 2005;28:499–521.

Clinical Guidelines for the Use of Unattended Portable Monitors in the Diagnosis of Obstructive Sleep Apnea in Adult Patients

1.1 Portable monitoring (PM) for the diagnosis of obstructive sleep apnea (OSA) should be performed only in conjunction with a *comprehensive sleep evaluation.* Clinical sleep evaluations using PM must be supervised by a practitioner with Board certification in Sleep Medicine or an individual who fulfills the eligibility criteria for the Sleep Medicine Certification Examination. In the absence of a comprehensive sleep evaluation, there is no indication for the use of PM.

1.2 Provided that the recommendations of 1.1 have been satisfied, PM **may be** used as an alternative to polysomnography (PSG) for the diagnosis of OSA in patients with a high pretest probability of moderate to severe OSA. PM should NOT be used in patient groups described in 1.2.1, 1.2.2, and 1.2.3 (those with co-morbidities, other sleep disorders, or for screening).

1.2.1 PM is not appropriate for the diagnosis of OSA in patients with significant co-morbid medical conditions that may degrade the accuracy of PM, including, but not limited to, moderate to severe pulmonary disease, neuromuscular disease, or congestive heart failure (CHF).

1.2.2 PM is not appropriate for the diagnostic evaluation of OSA in patients suspected of having other sleep disorders, including central sleep apnea, periodic limb movement disorder (PLMD), insomnia, parasomnias, circadian rhythm disorders, or narcolepsy.

1.2.3 PM is not appropriate for general screening of asymptomatic populations.

1.3 PM **may be indicated** for the diagnosis of OSA in patients for whom in-laboratory PSG is not possible by virtue of immobility, safety, or critical illness.

1.4 PM **may be indicated** to monitor the response to non–continuous positive airway pressure (CPAP) treatments for OSA, including oral appliances, upper airway surgery, and weight loss.

2.1 At a minimum, the PMs must record airflow, respiratory effort, and blood oxygenation. The type of biosensors used to monitor these parameters for in-laboratory PSG are recommended for use in PMs.

2.2 The sensor to detect apnea is an oronasal thermal sensor and to detect hypopnea is a nasal pressure transducer. Ideally, PMs should use both sensor types.

2.3 Ideally, the sensor for identification of respiratory effort is either calibrated or uncalibrated inductance plethysmography.

2.4 The sensor for the detection of blood oxygen is pulse oximeter with appropriate signal averaging time and accommodation for motion artifact.

3. Methodology for Portable Monitoring

3.1 PM testing should be performed under the auspices of an American Academy of Sleep Medicine (AASM)–accredited comprehensive Sleep Medicine Program with policies and procedures for sensor application, scoring, and interpretation of PM. A quality/performance improvement program for PM including interscorer reliability must be in place to ensure accuracy and reliability.

3.2 An experienced sleep technician, sleep technologist, or appropriately trained health care practitioner must perform the application of PM sensors or directly educate the patient in correct application of sensors.

3.3 PM devices must allow for the display of raw data for manual scoring or editing of automated scoring by a trained and qualified sleep technician/technologist. Evaluation of PM data must include review of the raw data by a Board-certified sleep specialist or an individual who fulfils the eligibility criteria for sleep medicine certification.

3.4 Scoring criteria should be consistent with current published AASM standards for scoring apneas and hypopneas.

3.5 Due to the known rate of false-negative PM tests, in-laboratory polysomnography (PSG) should be performed in cases where PM is technically inadequate or fails to establish the diagnosis of OSA in patients with a high pretest probability.

3.6 A follow-up visit with a physician or other appropriately trained and supervised health care provider should be performed on all patients undergoing PM to discuss the results of the test.

3.7 Unattended PM can be used with the parameters above in the patient's home.

From Collop NA, Anderson WM, Boehlecke B, et al: Clinical guidelines for the use of unattended portable monitors in the diagnosis of obstructive sleep apnea in adult patients. Portable Monitoring Task Force of the American Academy of Sleep Medicine. J Clin Sleep Med 2007;3:737–747.

First Coast Services Durable Medical Area Contractor (DMAC Region I)

Local Carrier Determinations for Polysomnography and Sleep Testing (L29949)—Excerpts

Prior to ordering the tests, the patient must have a face-to-face clinical evaluation by a physician. The evaluation must include:

1. A sleep history and physical examination including, but not limited to, snoring, daytime sleepiness, observed apneas, choking or gasping during sleep, morning headaches; and
2. Epworth sleepiness scale; and
3. Physical examination that documents body mass index, neck circumference, and a focused cardiopulmonary and upper airway evaluation.

Accreditation

All centers billing sleep studies must maintain proper certification/accreditation documentation on file that indicates it is accredited by the American Academy of Sleep Medicine (AASM) or that it is accredited as a sleep laboratory by the Joint Commission.

Physician Training/Certification

All sleep tests must be reviewed and the tests must be interpreted by either:

1. A Diplomate of the American Board of Sleep Medicine (ABSM) OR
2. A Diplomate in Sleep Medicine by a member board of the American Board of Medical Specialties (ABMS) OR
3. An active physician staff member of an AASM-accredited sleep center or sleep laboratory OR
4. An active physician staff member of a Joint Commission–accredited sleep laboratory.

Home Sleep Testing

Type 1 PSG is covered when used to aid the diagnosis of OSA in beneficiaries who have clinical signs and symptoms indicative of OSA if performed attended in a sleep laboratory facility. Type 1 devices are capable of recordings of all of the physiologic parameters and signals defined for PSG. The recording is furnished in a sleep laboratory facility in which a technologist is physically present to supervise the recording during sleep time and has the ability to intervene if needed. Minimal requirements include recording of electro-encephalogram (EEG), electro-oculogram (EOG), chin electromyogram (EMG), anterior tibialis EMG, electrocardiogram (ECG), airflow, respiratory effort, and oxygen saturation. Body position must be documented or objectively measured. Trained personnel must be in constant attendance and able to intervene.

A type 2 sleep testing device is covered when used to aid the diagnosis of OSA in beneficiaries who have clinical signs and symptoms indicative of OSA if performed unattended in or out of a sleep laboratory facility or attended in a sleep laboratory facility. Type 2 devices are portable devices that may measure the same channels as type 1 testing, except that a heart-rate monitor can replace the ECG. This device has a minimum of seven channels (e.g., EEG, EOG, EMG, ECG-heart rate, airflow, respiratory effort, and oxygen saturation—this type of device monitors sleep staging). A sleep technician is not necessarily in constant attendance in type 2 studies but is needed for preparation.

A type 3 sleep testing device is covered when used to aid the diagnosis of OSA in beneficiaries who have clinical signs and symptoms indicative of OSA if performed unattended in or out of a sleep laboratory facility or attended in a sleep laboratory facility. Type 3 devices monitor and record a minimum of four channels and must record ventilation or airflow, heart rate or ECG, and oxygen saturation. A sleep technician is not necessarily in constant attendance in type 3 studies but is needed for preparation.

A type 4 sleep testing device measuring three or more channels, one of which is airflow, is covered when used to aid the diagnosis of OSA in beneficiaries who have signs and symptoms indicative of OSA if performed unattended in or out of a sleep laboratory facility or attended in a sleep laboratory facility. Type 4 devices must include airflow as one of the required three channels. Other measurements may include oximetry and heart rate. A sleep technician is not necessarily in constant attendance in type 4 studies but is needed for preparation.

PAT. A sleep testing device measuring three or more channels that include actigraphy, oximetry, and peripheral arterial tone is covered when used to aid the diagnosis of OSA in beneficiaries who have signs and symptoms indicative of OSA if performed unattended in or out of a sleep laboratory facility or attended in a sleep laboratory facility. A sleep technician is not necessarily in constant attendance in such studies but is needed in preparation.

Chapter 14

Subjective and Objective Measures of Daytime Sleepiness

- The ESS measures self-rated average sleep propensity (chance of dozing) over eight common situations. The scale ranges from 0 to 24 with 10 or less being considered normal.
- The MSLT objectively measures the tendency to fall asleep (MSL) and the propensity to have SOREMPs.
- The MSLT consists of five naps spaced every 2 hours beginning about 1.5 to 3 hours after the wake-up time.
- The MSLT should be preceded by a PSG to detect causes of sleepiness such as sleep apnea and to verify adequate sleep before the MSLT. MSLT findings are not considered reliable if less than 360 minutes of sleep is recorded.
- The MSLT diagnostic criteria for narcolepsy include an MSL of 8 minutes or less and 2 or more SOREMPs. However, a negative MSLT does NOT rule out narcolepsy because the sensitivity of the MSLT for diagnosing narcolepsy is only approximately 70% to 80%.
- The MSLT diagnostic criteria for idiopathic hypersomnia include an MSL of less than 8 minutes and 0 to 1 SOREMPs in five naps.
- Up to 6% of untreated patients with OSA will have an MSLT meeting criteria for narcolepsy.
- If narcolepsy in addition to OSA is suspected, patients should have a PSG on CPAP to document good treatment and adequate sleep and a subsequent MSLT on CPAP. This assumes that OSA has been well treated with CPAP for a period of time (e.g., documented CPAP adherence).
- Medications that may affect MSLT sleep latency (stimulants, sedatives) or the number of SOREMPs (REM-suppressant medications) should be withdrawn for 10 days to 2 weeks preceding testing if possible.
- The MWT objectively quantifies a patient's ability to remain awake in a situation predisposing to sleep (dimly lighted room, sitting on a bed). The 40 minute MWT is recommended. Each MWT nap is terminated after 40 minutes if no sleep has been recorded; after

3 consecutive epochs of stage N1, or after a single epoch of any other sleep stage (N2, N3, or R). The sleep latency is defined as the time from lights out until the **first epoch of any stage of sleep.**

Excessive daytime sleepiness (EDS) is defined as sleepiness that occurs in a situation when an individual would usually be expected to be awake and alert. EDS is said to affect at least 5% of the general population. Causes of EDS include sleep deprivation/inadequate sleep, a number of sleep disorders (obstructive sleep apnea [OSA], narcolepsy, and idiopathic hypersomnia), sleep disturbance from medical conditions, and medication side effects. The periodic limb movement disorder can be associated with EDS but is a fairly uncommon disorder. Depression and mood disorders are common but are more likely to be associated with insomnia complaints than with EDS. However, up to 15% of depressed patients may complain of daytime sleepiness. The degree of sleepiness can be assessed by **subjective** and **objective** measures of sleepiness.

SUBJECTIVE MEASURES

Questionnaires such as the Stanford Sleepiness Scale or the Epworth Sleepiness Scale (ESS)[1,2] are measures of self-rated symptoms of sleepiness. The Stanford Sleepiness Scale (Table 14–1) measures subjective feelings of sleepiness ("fogginess, beginning to lose interest in staying awake"). A score above 3 is considered sleepy. In contrast, the ESS measures self-rated average sleep propensity (chance of dozing) over eight common situations that almost everyone encounters. The propensity to fall asleep is rated as 0, 1, 2, or 3 where 0 corresponds to never and 3 to a high chance of dozing (Table 14–2). The maximum score is 24 and normal is assumed to be 10 or less. ESS scores of 16 or greater are associated with severe sleepiness.

The ESS correlates roughly with the severity of OSA (apnea-hypopnea index [AHI]) (Table 14–3)[2,3] and improves (lower score) after continuous positive airway pressure

TABLE 14-1

Stanford Sleepiness Scale

DEGREE OF SLEEPINESS	SCALE RATING
Feeling active, vital, alert, or wide awake	1
Functioning at high levels, but not at peak; able to concentrate	2
Awake, but relaxed; responsive but not fully alert	3
Somewhat foggy, let down	4
Foggy; losing interest in remaining awake; slowed down	5
Sleepy, woozy, fighting sleep; prefer to lie down	6
No longer fighting sleep, sleep onset soon; having dreamlike thoughts	7
Asleep	X

TABLE 14-2

Epworth Sleepiness Scale

SITUATION: "USUAL WAY OF LIFE IN RECENT TIMES"	CHANCE OF DOZING SCORE 0, 1, 2, 3*
Sitting and reading	0–3
Watching TV	0–3
Sitting, inactive in a public place (e.g., a theater or a meeting)	0–3
As a passenger in a car for an hour without a break	0–3
Lying down to rest in the afternoon when circumstances permit	0–3
Sitting talking to someone	0–3
Sitting quietly after a lunch without alcohol	0–3
In a car, while stopped for a few minutes in traffic	0–3
Total	0–24
*0 = would NEVER doze	0–10 normal
1 = SLIGHT chance of dozing	
2 = MODERATE chance of dozing	
3 = HIGH chance of dozing	

TABLE 14-3

Epworth Sleepiness Scale Scores in Mild, Moderate, and Severe Obstructive Sleep Apnea

SEVERITY OF OSA (AHI)	MEAN AHI (MEAN ± SD)	TOTAL NUMBER OF SUBJECTS	ESS (MEAN ± SD)	RANGE OF ESS
Mild OSA (AHI ≥ 5–15)	8.8 ± 2.3	22	9.5 ± 3.3	4–16
Moderate OSA (AHI > 15–30)	21.1 ± 4.0	20	11.5 ± 4.2	5–20
Severe OSA (AHI > 30)	49.5 ± 9.6	13	16.0 ± 4.4	8–23

AHI = apnea-hypopnea index; ESS = Epworth Sleepiness Scale; OSA = obstructive sleep apnea; SD = standard deviation.
Adapted from Johns MW: A new method for measuring daytime sleepiness: The Epworth Sleepiness Scale. Sleep 1991;14:540–545.

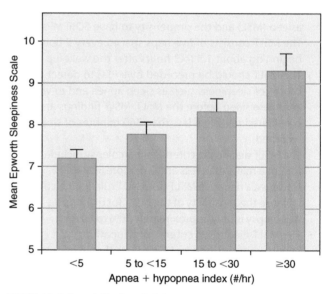

FIGURE 14-1 Epworth Sleepiness Scale increases with worsening obstructive sleep apnea (OSA) severity as measured by the apnea-hypopnea index (events/hr). *From Gottlieb DJ, Whitney CW, Bonekat WH, et al: Relation of sleepiness to respiratory disturbance index. Am J Respir Crit Care Med 1999;159:502–507.*

(CPAP) treatment.[4] However, as noted in Table 14–3, there is a wide range of ESS scores at any level of OSA severity. A large study by Gottlieb and coworkers[3] found a modest correlation between the ESS and OSA severity in a large population-based study of 1824 subjects. The degree of daytime sleepiness in the population was relatively mild (Fig. 14–1). Johns[2] reported a significant negative correlation between the ESS and the **mean sleep latency (MSL)** on the multiple sleep latency test (MSLT; an objective measure of sleepiness discussed in the next section) in a group of sleepy patients. However, Benbadis and colleagues[5] found no correlation between the MSLT findings and the ESS. Sangal and associates[6] found a statistically significant but low negative correlation between the ESS and the sleep latency (higher ESS associated with lower sleep latency) on the maintenance of wakefulness test (MWT) and MSLT in a large group of narcolepsy patients. A scatter plot of ESS versus sleep latency on the MSLT is shown in Figure 14–2. There was also a

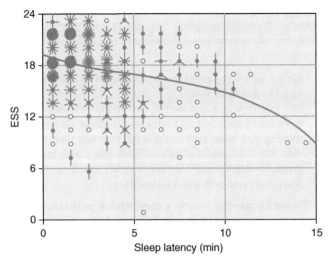

FIGURE 14–2 Scatter plot of Epworth Sleepiness Scale (ESS) score versus mean sleep latency on the multiple sleep latency test (MSLT) in 522 drug-free patients with narcolepsy. The *line* represents a quadratic fit. *From Sangal RB, Mitler MM, Sangal JM: Subjective sleepiness ratings (Epworth Sleepiness Scale) do not reflect the same parameter of sleepiness as objective sleepiness (maintenance of wakefulness test) in patients with narcolepsy. Clin Neurophysiol 1999;110:2131–2135.*

BOX 14–1

Indications for Use of the Multiple Sleep Latency Test

MSLT INDICATED

- Confirmation of suspected narcolepsy (Standard).
- Suspected idiopathic hypersomnia (Option)—to help differentiate idiopathic hypersomnia from narcolepsy.

MSLT NOT INDICATED (STANDARD)

- Routine evaluation of patients with OSA.
- Change in sleepiness in OSA after CPAP treatment.
- Evaluation of sleepiness in medical or neurologic conditions (other than narcolepsy).
- Evaluation of sleepiness in insomnia.

REPEAT MSLT INDICATED (STANDARD)

- Initial MSLT affected by extraneous/unusual conditions.
- Appropriate study conditions not present during initial testing.
- Ambiguous or uninterpretable findings.
- Clinical suspicion of narcolepsy not confirmed by an earlier MSLT.

AASM Levels of recommendation: Standard > Guideline > Option.
AASM = American Academy of Sleep Medicine; CPAP = continuous positive airway pressure; MSLT = multiple sleep latency test; OSA = obstructive sleep apnea.
From Littner MR, Kushida C, Wise M, et al: Practice parameters for clinical use of the multiple sleep latency test and the maintenance of wakefulness test. Sleep 2005;28:113–121.

modest correlation between the sleep latencies as determined by the MSLT and MWT. Of interest, the correlation between the MSLT and the MWT latencies (r = 0.52, $P <$ .001) was stronger than correlations between the ESS and the MWT or the MSLT latencies (r = –0.29, P < .001 and r = –0.27, P < .001, respectively).[6]

OBJECTIVE MEASURES

Multiple Sleep Latency Test

The MSLT[7–12] is used to support a diagnosis of narcolepsy and/or quantify the degree of daytime sleepiness. The MSL (lights out to sleep onset) is a measure of the degree of daytime sleepiness. **The sleep latency is the time from lights out to the beginning of the first epoch of any stage of sleep.** The test is terminated if no sleep occurs within 20 minutes of lights out (maximum sleep latency is 20 min). After sleep onset, the MSLT continues for **15 minutes of clock time.** If rapid eye movement (REM) sleep occurs within this time period, a sleep-onset rapid eye movement period (SOREMP) is said to have occurred. The MSLT criteria used to support a diagnosis of narcolepsy are an MSL of 8 minutes or less and 2 or more SOREMPs.[13] Many factors can alter the findings of the MSLT and considerable clinical judgment is needed to avoid an error in interpretation. The MSLT may be used in the **research** setting as an objective measure of daytime sleepiness of a given population of interest or to assess a response to treatment. The **clinical** indications for the use of the MSLT (Box 14–1) are outlined by the current American Academy of Sleep Medicine (AASM) practice

parameters concerning the use of the MSLT[10] and prior guidelines published by this organization.[8,9]

A standard-level recommendation states "the MSLT is a validated objective measure of the ability or tendency to fall asleep." As mentioned previously, the sleep latency is the parameter that reflects the degree of daytime sleepiness. The MSLT is indicated for evaluation of patients with suspected narcolepsy or idiopathic hypersomnia, but NOT for evaluation of OSA patients before or after treatment, or to quantify sleepiness in patients with insomnia, medical, or neurologic disorders (other than narcolepsy). The practice parameters also outlined conditions under which a repeat MSLT is indicated. These include a prior MSLT with unusual conditions or if the initial MSLT was negative in a patient with a strong clinical suspicion of narcolepsy (see Box 14–1).

MSLT Protocol

A standardized MSLT protocol performed by an experienced sleep technologist (Boxes 14–2 and 14–3) is required to obtain accurate testing results. A four-nap MSLT is not reliable for the diagnosis of narcolepsy unless 2 SOREMPs have occurred after four naps. Even then, a five-nap MSLT is suggested because the physician reading the study may disagree with the technologist's assessment of SOREMPs. A technologist experienced in performing the MSLT is essential.[8–11] The

BOX 14–2

Multiple Sleep Latency Test Protocol—Part 1

- A PSG during the patient's normal major sleep period MUST precede the MSLT.
- A minimum of 360 min of sleep during the PSG is required for a valid MSLT.
- Five nap opportunities at 2-hr intervals.
- Initial nap 1.5–3 hr after termination of nocturnal PSG.
- MSLT should NOT follow a split-sleep study.
- Sleep log may be obtained for 1 wk before the MSLT to assess sleep-wake schedule.

IMPORTANT CONSIDERATIONS

- Stimulants, stimulant-like medications, and REM-suppressing medications should be stopped 2 wk before the MSLT (or at least a time period > five times the medication half-life).
- Other medications should be adjusted as needed to minimize sedating or stimulating properties.
- Room temperature should be adjusted for patient comfort.
- Study room should be dark and quiet during testing.
- Drug screening is usually performed on the morning of the MSLT (or after if clinically indicated).
- Smoking should be stopped at least **30 min** before each nap.
- Patient must **abstain from caffeinated beverages** and **avoid unusual exposure to bright light.**
- Avoid vigorous physical activity. Stimulating activity should cease at least **15 min** before naps.
- Recommended montage: frontal, central, and occipital EEG derivations, left and right EOG, mental/submental EMG, and ECG.

ECG = electrocardiogram; EEG = electroencephalogram; EMG = electromyogram; EOG = electro-oculogram; MSLT = multiple sleep latency test; PSG = polysomnography; REM = rapid eye movement.
From Littner MR, Kushida C, Wise M, et al: Practice parameters for clinical use of the multiple sleep latency test and the maintenance of wakefulness test. Sleep 2005;28:113–121.

BOX 14–3

Multiple Sleep Latency Test Protocol—Part 2

NAP PROTOCOL

- Before each nap, patient should be asked if he or she needs to go to the bathroom.
- Biocalibration instructions*: (1) Lie quietly with your eyes open for 30 sec, (2) close both eyes for 30 sec, (3) without moving your head, look to the right, then left, then right, then left, right, and then left, (4) blink eyes slowly for five times, (5) clinch or grit your teeth tightly together.
- Start every nap with these instructions:

"Please lie quietly, assume a comfortable position, keep your eyes closed and try to fall asleep."
After these instructions, bedroom lights are turned off.

- A nap is terminated after 20 min if sleep does not occur.
- MSLT continues for **15 min of clock time** after sleep onset (to detect SOREMP).
- Between naps, the patient is **out of bed and prevented from sleeping** (observation by staff).
- A light breakfast is recommended at least 1 hr before the first trial. A light lunch is recommended immediately after the second nap. (**Meals before nap 1 and after nap 2.**)

MSLT DEFINITIONS AND REPORT

DEFINITIONS

- **Sleep latency**—time from lights off to the start of the first epoch of any stage of sleep (including stage N1). If no sleep is noted, the sleep latency is recorded as 20 min.
- **REM latency**—time from the beginning of the first epoch of sleep to the beginning of the first epoch of REM sleep.

MSLT REPORT

- Start and stop times of each nap.
- Sleep latency of each nap and MSL for the MSLT.
- Number of SOREMPs (>15 sec of REM sleep in any 30-sec epoch).
- Events that represent a deviation from the standard MSLT protocol.

*The standard in most sleep centers is to ask for the patient to look up and down as well as right and left.
MSL = mean sleep latency; MSLT = multiple sleep latency test; REM = rapid eye movement; SOREMPs = sleep-onset rapid eye movement periods.
From Littner MR, Kushida C, Wise M, et al: Practice parameters for clinical use of the multiple sleep latency test and the maintenance of wakefulness test. Sleep 2005;28:113–121.

technologist is required to accurately score sleep in real time. Of note, **polysomnography (PSG) must precede the MSLT.** This is required to rule out causes of sleepiness such as sleep apnea and to document an adequate amount of sleep preceding the MSLT. An adequate total sleep time during the PSG is needed for valid MSLT results. **At least 360 minutes of sleep must be recorded for the MSLT findings to be reliable.** A very high percentage of REM sleep (% of total sleep time) on the PSG should alert the physician to the possibility of REM rebound. This might be a clue to the recent withdrawal of a REM-suppressing medication or prior sleep deprivation. A sleep diary for 1 to 2 weeks before the MSLT may be helpful in documenting the adequacy of preceding sleep. Preceding sleep deprivation can result in shortened sleep latency.[11,12] Some patients may need a total sleep time longer than 360 minutes during the PSG and during the weeks before the MSLT to normalize the MSL.[12,14] A urine drug screen may help identify surreptitious medication use that can affect the MSLT results. Cigarette smoking should stop at least 30 minutes before each nap (Table 14–4). Vigorous physical activity should be avoided and any stimulating activity stopped at least 15 minutes before each nap. The patient should be asked whether she or he needs to use the bathroom before the nap is scheduled to begin. Between

TABLE 14–4

Multiple Sleep Latency Test Timetable: Before Testing

–2 weeks	Stop REM suppressing medications, stimulants, and stimulant-like medications.
–(1–2 wk)	Keep sleep diary and obtain adequate sleep and regular routine.
–1 day	PSG during regular sleep period precedes MSLT.
–30 min	Stop tobacco smoking.
–15 min	Stop stimulating activity.
–10 min	Comfortable clothing, visit restroom if needed.
–5 min	Calibration series.
–30 sec	Assume comfortable position for sleep.
–5 sec	**"Please lie quietly, assume a comfortable position, keep your eyes closed and try to fall asleep."**
0 sec	Lights out

MSLT = multiple sleep latency test; PSG = polysomnography; REM = rapid eye movement.

TABLE 14–5

Multiple Sleep Latency Facts*

MSL (MIN)	(MEAN ± SD)
Normal	10.4 ± 4.3 (four naps)
	11.6 ± 5.2 (five naps)
Narcolepsy	3.1 ± 2.9
Idiopathic hypersomnia	6.2 ± 3.0
Sleep apnea	7.2 ± 6.0
PROPORTION OF POPULATIONS WITH SHORT MSLS	

- 30% of normal individuals have an MSL < 8 min.
- 16% of normal individuals have an MSL < 5 min.
- 16% of patients with narcolepsy have an MSL > 5 min.

*MSLT MSL in normal and patient groups.
MSL = mean sleep latency; MSLT = multiple sleep latency test; SD = standard deviation.
Data from Littner MR, Kushida C, Wise M, et al: Practice parameters for clinical use of the multiple sleep latency test and the maintenance of wakefulness test. Sleep 2005;28:113–121; Arand D, Bonnet M, Hurwitz T, et al: A review by the MSLT and MWT Task Force of the Standards of Practice Committee of the AASM. The clinical use of the MSLT and MWT. Sleep 2005;28:123–144; and Aldrich MS, Chervin RD, Malow BA: Value of the multiple sleep latency test (MSLT) for the diagnosis of narcolepsy. Sleep 1997;20:620–629.

naps, the subject should be out of bed and observed in order to prevent sleep between the naps. A light breakfast was recommended at least one hour before the first nap and a light lunch immediately after the second nap. A typical MSLT schedule might include wake-up 6:00–7:00 AM, breakfast, nap 1 at 9:00 AM, nap 2 at 11:00 AM, light lunch, nap 3 at 1:00 PM, nap 4 at 3:00 PM, nap 5 at 5:00 PM.

Other MSLT Considerations

Although not specifically addressed in the recent AASM practice parameters, it is usual practice to have patients change out of night clothes before nap testing begins. This was the recommendation in earlier published guidelines for the MSLT.[8,9] As untreated OSA can be associated with MSLT findings consistent with narcolepsy,[15] adequate treatment of sleep apnea (for a sufficient time period to allow for symptom improvement) should precede MSLT evaluation for narcolepsy. If narcolepsy is suspected in a patient being treated for sleep apnea (e.g., with CPAP or an oral appliance), PSG is usually performed on CPAP/oral appliance treatment. The PSG documents adequate treatment of sleep apnea and at least one night of adequate sleep before the MSLT. Although not addressed in the recent MSLT practice parameters, the 1992 AASM MSLT guidelines stated "To determine the concurrent presence of narcolepsy after treatment of the obstructive sleep apnea syndrome by CPAP, the MSLT should be performed with the patient using the CPAP device." In this case, recording of machine flow is often performed in addition to electroencephalogram (EEG), electro-oculogram (EOG), chin electromyogram (EMG), and electrocardiogram (ECG). It is also worth mentioning that if unequivocal

cataplexy is present in a patient with OSA, a diagnosis of concurrent narcolepsy can be made in the absence of confirmatory MSLT findings (see Chapter 24).

MSL Values in Normal Populations and Patients

Traditional gradations of the MSL considered a value less than 5 minutes to denote severe sleepiness and a value less than 10 minutes to denote pathologic sleepiness.[8,9] A normal MSL was often stated to be greater than 15 minutes (10–15 was termed a *gray zone*). However, a recent large systematic review and meta-analysis of MSLT studies found the average MSL in normal individuals to be just above 10 minutes[11] (Table 14–5), with many normal individuals having an MSL less than 10 minutes.

The MSL values for studies of groups of patients with the major sleep disorders associated with daytime sleepiness published from a large analysis[11] are listed in Table 14–5. Patients with narcolepsy had the shortest MSL. The sleep latency of patients with idiopathic hypersomnia and OSA is usually between 5 and 10 minutes. Of interest, up to 30% of normal populations have an MSL of 8 minutes or less. An MSL value of 8 minutes or less is part of the International Classification of Sleep Disorders, 2nd edition (ICSD-2) criteria for diagnosis of narcolepsy and **less than 8 minutes** for the diagnosis of idiopathic hypersomnia.[13] Previously, a sleep latency of less than 5 minutes was the criterion.[8,9,12] The ICSD-2[13] chose an MSL of 8 minutes rather than 5 minutes as a diagnostic criteria to improve the sensitivity of the MSLT for the diagnosis of narcolepsy.[12] About 16% of narcoleptics have an MSL greater than 5 minutes and 16% of normal controls have an MSL below 5 minutes.[11,13]

Factors Affecting the MSLT MSL

A number of factors can affect the sleep latency during the MSLT (Box 14–4). The time of day of the nap affects the sleep latency. Of note, the shortest sleep latency tends to be in the third or fourth nap (early afternoon)[7] (Fig. 14–3). The MSL for a five-nap MSLT is slightly higher than that for a four-nap MSLT. The sleep latency on the last nap is often the highest and may reflect anticipation of the end of the test ("anticipation of leaving the sleep center"). Interpretation of the MSLT can be problematic in shift workers or late sleepers. The MSL increases with increasing age (Fig. 14–4). The normative MSLT results for children are discussed in a later section. Medications (stimulants or sedatives) that could affect the MSL should be withdrawn 2 weeks before the MSLT if this is medically practical. Abrupt withdrawal before the study should also be avoided.

Number of SOREMPs

The occurrence of REM sleep within 15 minutes of sleep onset (SOREMP) is more specific for the diagnosis of narcolepsy than an MSL of 8 minutes or less. Studies of normal populations have found 0 to 1 SOREMPs in five naps.[7,11] However, SOREMPs can occur in normal individuals with prior sleep or REM sleep deprivation, in untreated OSA, and when there is a circadian phase delay (Box 14–5). Patients with depression or other psychiatric disorders can also have a short REM latency. In general, **the number of MSLT SOREMPs increases as the sleep latency decreases.**[11] Those disorders associated with SOREMPs during the MSLT may also be associated with a short **nocturnal** REM latency.[12]

BOX 14–4

Factors Known to Affect the MSL

- Age.
- MSL on five-nap MSLT > four-nap MSLT.
- Shift work, delayed sleep phase (circadian factors).
- Medications affecting MSL (stimulants or sedating medications).
- Prior sleep deprivation or fragmentation.

MSL = mean sleep latency; MSLT = multiple sleep latency test.

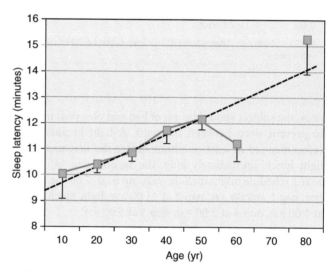

FIGURE 14–4 Effects of age on the mean sleep latency (MSL) during the MSLT in normal individuals. The MSL increases with age. A linear regression is shown. *From Arand D, Bonnet M, Hurwitz T, et al: A review by the MSLT and MWT Task Force of the Standards of Practice Committee of the AASM. The clinical use of the MSLT and MWT. Sleep 2005;28:123–144.*

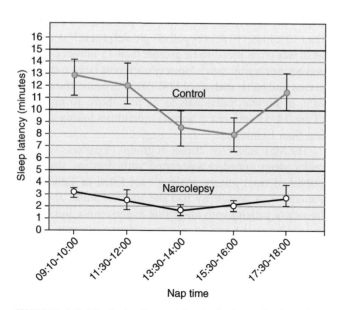

FIGURE 14–3 Variation in sleep latency during the day in control and narcolepsy patients. Note the naps in the afternoon have the shortest sleep latency. *From Richardson GS, Carskadon MA, Flagg W: Excessive daytime sleepiness in man: multiple sleep latency measurements in narcoleptic and control subjects. Electroencephalogr Clin Neurophysiol 1978;45:621–627.*

BOX 14–5

Causes of Sleep-Onset Rapid Eye Movement Periods

Narcolepsy
Untreated OSA
Prior sleep and REM sleep deprivation/fragmentation
Depression
Acute withdrawal of REM-suppressing medications (tricyclic antidepressants, serotonin reuptake inhibitors, lithium)
Delayed circadian phase

OSA = obstructive sleep apnea; REM = rapid eye movement.

TABLE 14-6

Multiple Sleep Latency Test Findings in Patients Evaluated for Daytime Sleepiness

	NARCOLEPSY WITH CATAPLEXY	NARCOLEPSY WITHOUT CATAPLEXY*	SLEEP-RELATED BREATHING DISORDER
N	106	64	1251
MSL < 5 min	87%	81%	39%
MSL < 8 min	93%	97%	63%
≥2 SOREMPs	74%	91%	7%
≥2 SOREMPs + MSL < 5 min	67%	75%	4%
≥ 2 SOREMPs + MSL < 8 min	71%	91%	6%
SOREMP on PSG	33%	24%	1%

*Diagnosis made in patients with narcolepsy without cataplexy by repeat MSLT (if necessary).
MSL = mean sleep latency; MSLT = multiple sleep latency test; PSG = nocturnal polysomnography; SOREMPs = sleep-onset rapid eye movement periods.
From Aldrich MS, Chervin RD, Malow BA: Value of the multiple sleep latency test (MSLT) for the diagnosis of narcolepsy. Sleep 1997;20:620–629.

Utility of the MSLT for Diagnosis of Narcolepsy

A recent review of the MSLT[11] that analyzed available study data found that 2 or more SOREMPs were associated with a **sensitivity of 0.78 and specificity of 0.93** for the diagnosis of narcolepsy. Aldrich and coworkers[12] published their MSLT findings on a large number of patients with suspected narcolepsy (Table 14–6). If an initial MSLT was not diagnostic but narcolepsy was suspected clinically, repeat MSLT testing was performed. The study showed that patients with OSA can have a very short sleep latency and 2 or more SOREMPs (although the proportion of OSA patients is much lower compared with narcolepsy).[12] In this study, about 63% of patients with sleep-related breathing disorders have an MSL less than 8 minutes whereas only 7% had 2 or more SOREMPs. The study also showed that a significant proportion of patients with a narcolepsy + cataplexy can have a negative MSLT.

Normative MSLT Findings in Children and Adolescents

Limited normative MSLT information for children and adolescents exists. The majority of what is known on this topic comes from the work of Carskadon and colleagues.[16,17] Table 14–7 presents sleep latency data from children and preadolescents (Tanner stages I–V) as well as older adolescents.[16] Of note, the older adolescents in this study had a sleep period of 10:00 PM to 8:00 AM. The sleep latency of children and preadolescents was significantly longer than that of adolescents. Of note, many children who no longer take daily naps **may not sleep at all during any MSLT nap.** Therefore, the adult criteria of an MSL of 8 minutes or less for a diagnosis of narcolepsy in adults may not identify children with narcolepsy. For example, a 10-year-old child with an MSL of 12 minutes or less is considered to have evidence of daytime sleepiness. Many adolescents go to bed later (and wake up earlier on school days) so the data listed in Table 14–7 may

TABLE 14-7

Multiple Sleep Latency Test Findings in Children and Adolescents

STAGE OF DEVELOPMENT	MEAN SLEEP LATENCY (MIN)	STANDARD DEVIATION
Tanner stage 1	19.0	1.8
Tanner stage 2	18.5	2.1
Tanner stage 3	16.5	2.8
Tanner stage 4	15.5	3.3
Tanner stage 5	16.1	1.5
Older adolescents	15.7	3.5

From Carskadon M: The second decade. In Gulleminault C (ed): Sleeping and Waking Disorders—Indications and Techniques. Boston: Butterworths, 1982, pp. 99–125.

not apply to them. With such a compressed weekday sleep period, they would be expected to have a shorter sleep latency than is shown in Table 14–7.

In addition to having a shorter sleep latency, adolescents frequently have a delayed circadian phase, with most teenagers having bedtimes between 10:30 to 11:00 PM or later. In one study of the MSLT in 10th graders (26 subjects), 2 SOREMPs was seen in 16% of the participants and one REM episode was noted in 48%.[17] The majority of the SOREMPs were in the morning naps. Therefore, one must be cautious in making the diagnosis of narcolepsy in adolescents based on **SOREMPs that occur only in the first two naps.**

Clinical Examples of MSLTs

Clinical Example #1 The results of a typical five-nap MSLT are presented in tabular form to illustrate specific points (see

TABLE 14-8

Nap 1

Epoch	30	31	32	33	34	35	36	37	38	39
Stage	LO	W	W	W	1	2	2	2	3	3
Epoch	40	41	42	43	44	45	46	47	48	49
Stage	W	1	2	3	R	R	W	1	2	2
Epoch	50	51	52	53	54	55	56	57	58	59
Stage	R	R	1	1	2	2	2	3	3	3
Epoch	60	61	62	63	64	65	66	67	68	69
Stage	3	3	3	3						

LO = lights out; R = rapid eye movement; W = wake.

TABLE 14-10

Nap 3

Epoch	30	31	32	33	34	35	36	37	38	39
Stage	LO	W	W	1	1	2	2	2	3	3
Epoch	40	41	42	43	44	45	46	47	48	49
Stage	W	1	2	3	W	1	W	1	2	2
Epoch	50	51	52	53	54	55	56	57	58	59
Stage	2	2	3	3	3	3	3	W	1	1
Epoch	60	61	62	63	64	65	66	67	68	
Stage	1	W	W							

LO = lights out; W = wake.

TABLE 14-9

Nap 2

Epoch	30	31	32	33	34	35	36	37	38	39
Stage	LO	W	W	W	W	W	W	W	W	W
Epoch	40	41	42	43	44	45	46	47	48	49
Stage	W	W	W	W	W	W	W	W	W	W
Epoch	50	51	52	53	54	55	56	57	58	59
Stage	W	W	W	W	W	W	W	W	W	W
Epoch	60	61	62	63	64	65	66	67	68	69
Stage	W	W	W	W	W	W	W	W	W	W
Epoch	70	71								
Stage	W									

LO = lights out; W = wake.

TABLE 14-11

Nap 4

Epoch	30	31	32	33	34	35	36	37	38	39
Stage	LO	W	W	W	1	2	2	W	W	W
Epoch	40	41	42	43	44	45	46	47	48	49
Stage	R	R	W	3	W	1	W	1	2	2
Epoch	50	51	52	53	54	55	56	57	58	59
Stage	2	2	3	3	3	3	3	W	1	1
Epoch	60	61	62	63	64	65	66	67	68	
Stage	1	W	W	W						

LO = lights out; R = rapid eye movement; W = wake.

TABLE 14-12

Nap 5

Epoch	30	31	32	33	34	35	36	37	38	39
Stage	LO	W	W	W	W	2	W	1	2	3
Epoch	40	41	42	43	44	45	46	47	48	49
Stage	W	1	2	3	R	R	W	1	2	2
Epoch	50	51	52	53	54	55	56	57	58	59
Stage	2	R	R	R	1	2	3	W	1	1
Epoch	60	61	62	63	64	65	66	67	68	
Stage	1	W	W	W	W					

LO = lights out; R = rapid eye movement; W = wake.

Tables 14-8 to 14-12). In the tables, the lights out time (LO) is assumed to be **at the end of the epoch listed.** The epochs are 30 seconds in duration. The light gray shading marks the sleep latency, and the dark gray the REM latency.

Nap 1 In nap 1, the sleep latency is 1.5 minutes (start of epoch 34-start of epoch 31) and the REM latency is 10 epochs or 5 minutes (start of epoch 44-start of epoch 34). The MSLT continues for 15 minutes of clock time after sleep onset to start of epoch 64 (start of epoch 34 + 30 epochs = to start of epoch 64) (Table 14-8).

Nap 2 In nap 2, no sleep occurs for 20 minutes after LO. The nap is terminated and the sleep latency is 20 minutes (start of epoch 31 + 40 epochs = start of epoch 71) (Table 14-9).

Nap 3 In nap 3, the sleep latency is 1 minute (start of epoch 33-start of epoch 31). Even if there is intervening wake, the test continues for 15 minutes of clock time (30 epochs) after the start of sleep (start of 33 + 30 = start of epoch 63). In this nap, no stage R (REM sleep) was noted (Table 14-10).

Nap 4 In nap 4, the sleep latency is 1.5 minutes. Although stage W occurs after sleep onset, the REM latency is still the time from the start of sleep until the start of stage R [(epoch 40-epoch 34) = 6 epochs or 3.0 min]. The MSLT continues for 30 epochs after the start of sleep (start of epoch 34 + 30 = start of epoch 64) (Table 14-11).

Nap 5 In nap 5, the first epoch of sleep is epoch 35. The sleep latency is 4 epochs or 2 minutes (start of epoch 35-start of

TABLE 14-13

Example of a Multiple Sleep Latency Test Report

NAPS	LIGHTS OUT	LIGHTS ON	SLEEP LATENCY (MIN)	REM (YES OR NO)	REM LATENCY (MIN)
1	8:10 am	8:24:30 am	1.5	1	5.0
2	10:05 am	10:25 am	20.0	0	N/A
3	12:05 pm	12:21 pm	1.0	0	N/A
4	2:06 pm	2:22:30 pm	1.5	1	3.0
5	4:08 pm	4:15 pm	2.0	1	4.5
			Mean: 5.2	SOREMPs: 3	

N/A = not applicable; REM = rapid eye movement; SOREMP = sleep-onset rapid eye movement period.

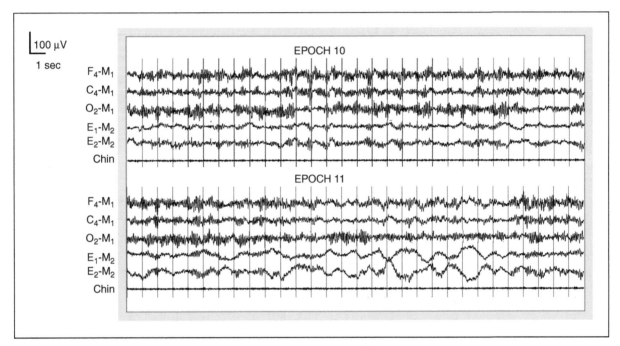

FIGURE 14-5   Two 30-second epochs of sleep during an MSLT. Lights out was at the end of epoch 9. Epochs 10 and 11 are stage W.

epoch 31 = 4 epochs). The first epoch of stage R is epoch 44. Therefore, the REM latency is 9 epochs or 4.5 minutes. The MSLT continues for 30 epochs after sleep onset until the start of epoch 65 (start of epoch 35 + 30 = start of epoch 65) (Table 14–12).

A summary of the data from these naps appears in Table 14–13.

The typical MSLT report summarizes the reason for performing the test, pertinent findings on the preceding PSG, associated findings from the sleep diary and urine drug screen, and a interpretation of the MSLT findings. The time of the start of each nap should also be specified along with any unusual circumstances or deviations from the standard protocol.

Clinical Example #2 Thirty-second epochs during an MSLT (epoch numbers 10–15) are shown in Figures 14–5 to 14–7.

LO is assumed to have occurred at the end of epoch 9. Because epoch 12 is the first epoch of sleep (stage N1), the sleep latency is 1 minute. The REM latency is determined by the time from the start of epoch 12 to the start of REM sleep. The first epoch of REM sleep is epoch 15. Therefore, the REM latency is 3 epochs or 1.5 minutes.

Maintenance of Wakefulness Test

The MWT was designed to test the patient's ability to stay awake.[10,11,18] The recent AASM practice parameters[10] regarding the MWT state:

1. The MWT is a validated objective measure of the ability to stay awake for a defined time. (Standard)
2. The MWT is used in association with clinical history to assess the ability to maintain wakefulness. (Standard)

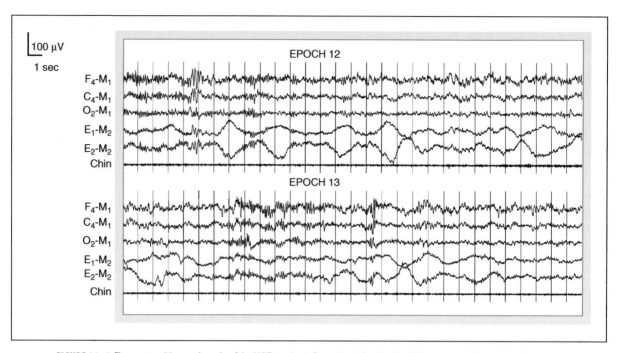

FIGURE 14–6   The next two 30-second epochs of the MSLT starting in Figure 14–5. Epochs 12 and 13 are stage N1. Epoch 12 is sleep onset.

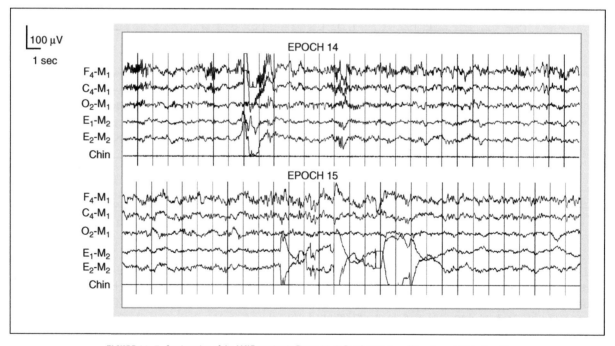

FIGURE 14–7   Continuation of the MSLT starting in Figure 14–5. Epoch 14 is stage N2 and epoch 15 is stage R.

3. The MWT 40-minute protocol is recommended when the sleep clinician requires objective data to assess an individual's ability to remain awake. (Option)

Although the MWT has been used in both the 20-minute and the 40-minute versions,[18–20] the longer test was recommended by the AASM practice parameters. The MWT has been used to assess the effects of sleep disturbance and treatment on the ability of patients to stay awake as reflected by the MSL.[11,18–20] The study is believed to assess different information than can be attained with the MSLT.[21] For example, some patients with a short MSLT sleep latency may have a normal MWT sleep latency. In research, the MWT is often used to document the effects of treatment from alerting agents.[22] The AASM practice parameters for the use of the MWT list specific indications as summarized in the following paragraph.[10]

Specific Indications for the Use of the MWT

The AASM practice parameters for the use of the MWT list specific indications[10]:

1. The MWT 40-minute protocol may be used to assess an individual's ability to remain awake when his or her ability to remain awake constitutes a public or personal safety issue. (Option)
2. The MWT may be indicated in patients with excessive sleepiness to assess response to treatment. (Guideline)

MWT Protocol

The MWT protocol recommended by the AASM practice parameters[10] is outlined in Table 14–14. The 40-minute nap protocol is recommended. A **four-nap protocol** is standard. Note that the **sleep latency is defined as the time from LO to the start of any epoch of sleep.** The requirement of a preceding PSG is left up to the clinician. In contrast to the MSLT, during the MWT, the patient sits upright in bed (head and shoulders comfortably supported) and the instruction before LO is "Please sit still and remain awake for as long as possible. Look directly ahead of you, and do not look directly at the light." Of note, it is essential that the testing individual be observed and not allowed to use extreme measures (hitting, moving in bed) to maintain alertness.

Each MWT nap lasts a maximum of 40 minutes after LO. **The nap is terminated if no sleep has occurred in 40 minutes or if three consecutive epochs of stage N1 are noted or any single epoch of other stages of sleep.** A low-intensity light is present behind the patient's head just out of the visual field (usually a nightlight). The MWT definitions and recommended information to be included in the MWT report are listed in Table 14–15.

MWT Normative Data

Normative data for the MWT from a systematic review of MWT studies are displayed in Table 14–16. Using the 40-minute MWT, 59% of patients were able to stay awake for 40 minutes on each nap. The 95% lower confidence limit was 8 minutes (97.5% had MSL > 8 min). Conversely, these data do little to set a standard for individuals in whom alertness is essential for personal and public safety. Certainly, staying awake for all trials is an appropriate expectation for individuals requiring the highest level of safety. Therefore, whereas a MSL less than 8 minutes is abnormal, an MSL of 8 to 40 minutes is of uncertain significance. A "normal" MWT finding is no guarantee of what will happen in the work environment. The ability to maintain alertness (different than the ability to maintain wakefulness) may depend on adherence to treatment, prior total sleep time, medication side effects, and circadian factors. Of note, **the sleep latency on the MWT increases with age similar to the sleep latency on the MSLT.**[11]

Relationship between the MSLT and the MWT

Some of the differences in MSLT and MWT protocols are outlined in Table 14–17. When Sangal and associates[21]

TABLE 14–14

Maintenance of Wakefulness Test Protocol

- Four trials of MWT 40-min protocol are recommended.
- Four trials at 2-hr intervals.
- MWT begins 1.5–3 hr after the patient's usual wakeup time (0900 or 1000 hr).
- Performance of a PSG is not required—need decided by clinician based on clinical circumstances.
- Sleep log not required—need decided by clinician based on clinical circumstances.

ROOM CONDITIONS

- Light source positioned behind the subject's head such that it is just out of his or her field of vision and should deliver an illuminance of 0.10–0.13 lux at the corneal level (a 7.5-W night light can be used, placed 1 ft off the floor and 3 ft laterally removed from the subject's head).
- Room temperature for patient comfort.
- Subject seated in bed, the back and head supported by a bedrest (bolster pillow) such that the neck is not uncomfortably flexed or extended.

OTHER CONSIDERATIONS

- Drug screening **may be indicated.** If ordered, it is usually performed on the morning of MWT (timing can be changed by clinician).
- Conventional recording montage for MWT includes frontal, central, occipital EEG as well as right and left EOGs, chin EMG, ECG.

MWT NAP PROTOCOL

- The patient should be asked if she or he needs to go to the bathroom.
- Biocalibration instructions: (1) Lie quietly with your eyes open for 30 sec, (2) close both eyes for 30 sec, (3) without moving your head, look to the right, then left, then right, then left, right, and then left, (4) blink eyes slowly for five times, (5) clinch or grit your teeth tightly together.
- Light breakfast is recommended at least 1 hr before the first trial.
- A light lunch is recommended immediately after termination of the second/noon trial.
- **Instructions: "Please sit still and remain awake for as long as possible. Look directly ahead of you, and do not look directly at the light."**
- Trials are ended after 40 min if no sleep occurs, or after unequivocal sleep, defined as three consecutive epochs of stage 1 sleep or one epoch of any other sleep stage.
- Patients are not allowed to use extraordinary measures to stay awake such as singing or slapping the face.

ECG = electrocardiogram; EEG = electroencephalogram; EMG = electromyogram; EOG = electro-oculogram; MWT = maintenance of wakefulness test; PSG = polysomnography.
From Littner MR, Kushida C, Wise M, et al: Practice parameters for clinical use of the multiple sleep latency test and the maintenance of wakefulness test. Sleep 2005;28:113–121.

TABLE 14-15

Maintenance of Wakefulness Test Definitions and Maintenance of Wakefulness Test Report

DEFINITIONS

- Sleep onset defined as the time from lights out to the first epoch of > 15 sec of cumulative sleep in a 30-sec epoch.
- If no sleep, MSL reported at 40 min.

MWT REPORT

- Start and stop times for each trial.
- Sleep latency.
- Total sleep time.
- Stages of sleep achieved for each trial.
- MSL—arithmetic mean of the four trials.

MSL = mean sleep latency; MWT = maintenance of wakefulness test.

TABLE 14-16

Normative Data for Maintenance of Wakefulness Test (40-min Naps)

MSL (mean ± SD)	30.4 ± 11.2 min (mean ± SD)
MSL upper limit 95% confidence limits	40 min
MSL lower limit 95% confidence limits	8 min
MSL > 8 min	97.5% of normal individuals
MSL = 40 min (able to stay awake during all naps)	59% of normal individuals

MSL = mean sleep latency; SD = standard deviation.
From Arand D, Bonnet M, Hurwitz T, et al: A review by the MSLT and MWT Task Force of the Standards of Practice Committee of the AASM. The clinical use of the MSLT and MWT. Sleep 2005;28:123–144.

TABLE 14-17

Comparisons of Multiple Sleep Latency Test and Maintenance of Wakefulness Test

	MSLT	MWT
Naps/trials	5	4
Nap/trial times	2-hr intervals starting 1.5–3 hr after PSG ends.	2-hr intervals starting 1.5–3 hr after wakeup time.
Preceding PSG	Required.	If clinically indicated.
Sleeping posture	Ad lib, supine, lateral.	Sitting up in bed with head supported.
End test	• No sleep for 20 min after start of study. • After 15 min from onset of first stage of sleep ("clock time").	• No sleep for 40 min after start of study. • After first epoch of unequivocal sleep (three consecutive epochs of stage N1 or a single epoch of any other stage of sleep).
Sleep latency	First epoch of sleep.	First epoch of sleep (15 consecutive sec in a 30-sec epoch).
REM periods	Monitoring for 15 min of clock time after sleep onset to detect SOREMPs.	N/A Amount of all stages of sleep specified in report.
Additional considerations	Sleep logs "may be obtained" for 1 wk before MSLT. Stop cigarette smoking at least 30 min before nap. Abstain from caffeine day of study. Stop stimulating activities including vigorous activity for at least 15 min before nap	No guidance. No guidance. No guidance. No guidance.

MSLT = multiple sleep latency test; MWT = maintenance of wakefulness test; N/A = not applicable; PSG = polysomnography; REM = rapid eye movement; SOREMPs = sleep-onset rapid eye movement periods.

---

administered both the MSLT and the MWT to a group of patients with EDS, the correlation between the MSL on the two tests was significant but low ($r = 0.41$, $P < .001$). Several individuals did not fall asleep during the MWT but had some degree of daytime sleepiness as assessed by the MSLT. Table 14–18 illustrates classifications of a group of OSA patients by MSL (low or high) on a four-nap MSLT and MWT. The study found that 15% of the patients were sleepy (MSLT MSL low) but able to stay awake (MWT MSL high) (Fig. 14–8 and Table 14–8).

MSLT and MWT Changes with Treatment Both the MSLT and the MWT have been used to assess the efficacy of treatment in patients with disorders of daytime sleepiness such as OSA and narcolepsy.[19-23] In one study by Poceta and coworkers,[19] the MWT sleep latency increased from 18 to 31 minutes in a group of patients with OSA after adequate CPAP treatment.

TABLE 14–18

Comparison of Multiple Sleep Latency Test and Maintenance of Wakefulness Test in Sleep Apnea Patients (N = 170)*

Sleep apnea	MWT MSL low	MWT MSL high
MSLT MSL high	15%	34%
MSLT MSL low	36%	**15%**

Note: 15% of patients were in the sleepiest group by MSLT, but by MWT were in the group better at maintaining wake.
*Cutoff low and high MSLT and MWT based on median values for the studies (7.5-min MSL on the MSLT and 30-min MSL on the MWT).
MSL = mean sleep latency; MSLT = multiple sleep latency test; MWT = maintenance of wakefulness test.
From Sangal RB, Thomas L, Mitler MM: Maintenance of wakefulness test and multiple sleep latency test: measurements of different abilities in patients with sleep disorders. Chest 1992;101:898–902.

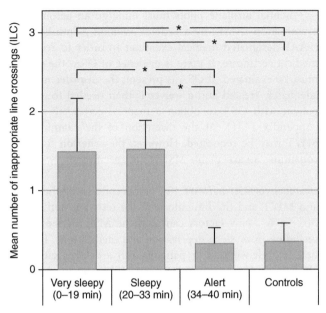

FIGURE 14–9 The mean number of inappropriate line crossings (ILCs) in four groups of patients divided by the MWT sleep latency. The very sleepy and sleepy groups had significantly more ILCs than the alert and control groups (*$P < .05$). *From Philip P, Sagaspe P, Taillard J, et al. Maintenance of wakefulness test, obstructive sleep apnea syndrome and driving risk. Ann Neurol 2008;64:410–416.*

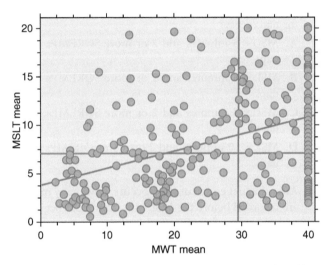

FIGURE 14–8 MSL (min) on the MSLT versus MSL on the maintenance of wakefulness test (MWT). The *vertical* and *horizontal lines* divide MSLT and MWT into low and high quadrants. The *horizontal line* is the median sleep latency of the MSLT (7.5 min). The *vertical line* is the median sleep latency on the MWT (30 min). *From Sangal RB, Thomas L, Mitler MM: Maintenance of wakefulness test and multiple sleep latency test: measurements of different abilities in patients with sleep disorders. Chest 1992;101: 898–902.*

A recent meta-analysis of patients with mild to moderate OSA undergoing CPAP treatment found an improvement in the ESS (subjective sleepiness) by 1.2 points and an improvement in the sleep latency on the MWT (2.1 min). A significant change in the sleep latency by the MSLT was not detected.[20] Another meta-analysis that included patients with severe OSA found an improvement in the ESS of 2.94 points more than placebo for the entire group.[4] For patients with AHI greater than 30 or ESS greater than 11, the ESS improved by 4.75 points. The MWT and MSLT data were pooled and the MSL improved by 0.93 minutes with CPAP.

Sangal and associates[21] found an improvement in objective daytime sleepiness with the MWT but not the MSLT in a group of sleepy patients undergoing treatment. Thus, a few studies have suggested that the MWT might be more robust than the MSLT in documenting an improvement in sleepiness after treatment. However, in a large study of the effect of modafinil on daytime sleepiness in patients with narcolepsy, the sleep latency on both the MWT and the MSLT significantly improved compared with placebo at a dose of 400 mg daily.[23] The increases in MSL were around 2 minutes using both tests. However, of interest, the improvement at a modafinil dose of 200 mg was significant only for the MWT.

The MSLT and MWT Assessment of Safety or "Fit for Duty" The MSL on an MSLT or MWT required for a person to safely pursue an occupation critically dependent on alertness has not been standardized. Furthermore, the ability to stay awake is not the same as maintaining alertness. Studies using driving simulators have attempted to provide a performance-based test of alertness.[24,25] Test results showed decreased alertness in patients with OSA and in patients with narcolepsy, as compared with a control group. However, the simulator results did not correlate with MSLT results, and in one study half of each group performed as well as controls.[24] A study of untreated OSA patients found an MWT MSL less than 19 minutes was associated with impairment on a driving simulator.[25] The same group extended this work by testing patients with OSA during actual 90-minute driving sessions on the road with a driving instructor intervening if necessary (the test car had two steering wheels).[26] Inappropriate line crossing was determined by video recording. Two groups "very sleepy" with an MWT MSL less than 19 minutes and "sleepy" with a MSL of 20 to 33 minutes had significantly higher line crossings than controls and patients with mild sleepiness (MWT MSL 34–40 min) (Fig. 14–9).

Potential airplane pilots must undergo an aeromedical examination (AME) by a Federal Aviation Administration (FAA)–designated medical examiner in order to receive a medical certificate. If there is evidence of OSA, the patient must be evaluated. If OSA is present, the disorder must be adequately treated and a waiver is then needed to allow a patient with OSA to obtain a medical certificate and fly (Appendix 14–1). At the discretion of the examiner, an MWT may be requested. However, the criterion for what constitutes an acceptable MSL is not specified.

Limitations of MSLT and MWT Key points concerning the MSLT and MWT and the limitations of the tests are outlined in Box 14–6. Many factors can alter the MSL on the MSLT including prior sleep deprivation and medications. Evaluation of shift workers or patients with a delayed circadian phase is problematic. The MSL by MSLT and the MSL by MWT do not separate groups of normal individuals from groups with sleep disorders causing EDS. Considerable overlap in the MSL values occurs. If a patient is taking an antidepressant that is known to suppress REM sleep, this makes the MSLT interpretation problematic if fewer than 2 SOREMPs are noted. Conversely, discontinuation of antidepressant medication must be done cautiously. Weaning the antidepressant is recommended rather than abrupt discontinuation. Close patient follow-up and coordination of care with the physician who prescribed the medication. In some patients with severe depression, the risks may outweigh the potential benefits. If patients have significant OSA, this disorder must be effectively treated (objective CPAP adherence documented) before a MSLT evaluation to diagnose narcolepsy. Finally, a negative MSLT result does not rule out narcolepsy and a significant proportion of patients with narcolepsy and cataplexy may have a negative study on any given day.[12]

CLINICAL REVIEW QUESTIONS

1. Which of the following are the MSLT diagnostic criteria for narcolepsy?
   A. MSL < 5 minutes and 2 or more SOREMPs in five naps.
   B. MSL < 8 minutes and 2 or more SOREMPs in five naps.
   C. MSL ≤ 8 minutes and 2 or more SOREMPs in five naps.
   D. MSL < 10 minutes and 2 or more SOREMPs in five naps.

2. After the first epoch of sleep occurs, how many minutes are recorded before the MSLT is terminated (beginning with the start of the first epoch of sleep)?
   A. 15 minutes of clock time.
   B. 15 minutes of sleep.
   C. Until the first epoch of unequivocal REM sleep.
   D. 20 minutes of clock time.

3. After lights out, how many minutes of continuous wake are allowed before an MSLT nap is terminated (maximum sleep latency)?
   A. 15 minutes.
   B. 20 minutes.
   C. 10 minutes.
   D. 40 minutes.

4. Which of the following is true concerning the MWT?
   A. A 20-minute test is recommended.
   B. A PSG must precede testing.
   C. A 40-minute test is recommended.
   D. The patient is supine during testing.

5. Which of the following are true about the recommended MSLT protocol?
   A. PSG (required), patient out of bed between naps and observed to prevent sleep (required).
   B. Sleep diary for 1 to 2 weeks before MSLT (required).

BOX 14–6

Key Points and Limitations of Multiple Sleep Latency Test and Maintenance of Wakefulness Test

1. Proper interpretation of an MSLT requires analysis of the preceding nocturnal sleep study, a careful medication history, and knowledge of the sleep habits (diary) for at least 1 wk preceding the MSLT.
2. Previous sleep deprivation (sleep restriction) can affect the MSL.
3. No validated normal MSLT findings exist outside of the usual testing hours of 0800 to 1800. Therefore, evaluation of shift workers or patients with a delayed circadian phase is problematic.
4. Due to large standard deviations, MSLs determined by the MSLT and MWT do not separate normal populations from those with sleep disorders such as narcolepsy.
5. MSLT diagnostic criteria are not validated for patients younger than 8 years of age.
6. Antidepressants are widely used but are highly problematic for MSLT.
7. As a diagnostic test for narcolepsy, the MSLT is specific if OSA and other causes of SOREMPs are ruled out. However, a significant percentage of false-negative MSLTs can occur (sensitivity ~70%).
8. A small but clinically significant proportion of untreated OSA patients can have 2 or more SOREMPs on the MSLT. Therefore, if OSA is present, this should be adequately treated before the MSLT can be used to support a diagnosis of narcolepsy.
9. MWT results cannot be assumed to necessarily reflect a patient's ability to maintain alertness during real-life conditions.

MSL = mean sleep latency; MSLT = multiple sleep latency test; MWT = maintenance of wakefulness test; OSA = obstructive sleep apnea; SOREMPs = sleep-onset rapid eye movement periods.

C. Urine drug screen (required).

D. Stop cigarette smoking 30 minutes before a nap (optional).

6. About what percentage of normal individuals will have an MSL ≤ 8 minutes?

   A. 10%.

   B. 20%.

   C. 30%.

   D. 40%.

7. An 18-year-old male is evaluated for daytime sleepiness. He falls asleep in morning classes routinely but denies cataplexy (emotionally induced muscle weakness). The patient's normal sleep period is from midnight (or later on weekends) until approximately 6 am (weekdays) and 10 to 11 am on weekends. An MSLT is performed with naps at 8 am, 10 am, 12 noon, 2 pm, and 4 pm. The results include an MSL of 8 minutes and 2 SOREMPs (8 am and 10 am naps). The patient was off from school for 1 week before the sleep study. What is the most likely diagnosis?

   A. Narcolepsy without cataplexy.

   B. Idiopathic hypersomnia.

   C. Insufficient sleep syndrome.

   D. Insufficient sleep syndrome and delayed sleep phase.

8. A 20-year-old female pharmacy student is evaluated for falling asleep in class. She also reports that when she hears a very funny joke that her mouth drops open and she has difficulty keeping her head upright. The patient sleeps about 7.0 hours/night. The MSLT was preceded by an unremarkable PSG. MSLT results include an MSL of 5 minutes and 1 SOREMP in five naps. A urine drug screen was declined. What is the most likely diagnosis?

   A. Idiopathic hypersomnia.

   B. Narcolepsy with cataplexy.

   C. Insufficient sleep syndrome.

   D. Occult drug abuse.

9. A 40-year-old policeman is evaluated for falling asleep on the job. He denies cataplexy (emotionally induced weakness). A PSG finds an AHI of 25/hr with many obstructive apneas. An MSLT is performed and shows an MSL of 4 minutes and 2 SOREMPs. What is the most likely diagnosis?

   A. Narcolepsy without cataplexy.

   B. OSA.

   C. OSA and narcolepsy.

   D. Insufficient sleep syndrome.

10. A lawyer regularly flies an airplane for recreation on the weekends. During an FAA medical evaluation, a history of snoring was noted. Subsequently, a PSG showed moderate to severe OSA. After treatment with CPAP, the patient remained somewhat sleepy and began taking modafinil (alerting agent). To receive medical clearance for a pilot's license, a PSG (to document adequate CPAP) with a subsequent MWT was ordered. The PSG found an AHI of 3/hr on CPAP treatment. The patient took his usual modafinil before the MWT and the MSL on four naps was 40 minutes. What do you recommend?

    A. Medical clearance (assuming continued treatment adherence).

    B. Denial of medical clearance.

    C. Increase modafinil dose and repeat MWT.

    D. Objective download of CPAP use.

11. All of the following concerning the MWT protocol are true EXCEPT:

    A. The patient is seated upright in bed.

    B. A preceding PSG is not required.

    C. The MWT is stopped after 3 consecutive epochs of stage N1 or any single epoch of any other stage of sleep (N2, N3, R).

    D. Four naps lasting up to 40 minutes is recommended (40-min protocol).

    E. The study is stopped after the first epoch of any stage of sleep.

Answers

1. **C.**

2. **A.**

3. **B.**

4. **C.**

5. **A.** A urine drug screen and sleep diary for 1 to 2 weeks preceding the MSLT are optional. The practice parameters stated that they "may" be helpful. However, most sleep centers include a drug screen and sleep diary as part of their MSLT protocol. Cigarette smoking should stop 30 minutes before a nap (required, not optional). The patients should be out of bed between naps.

6. **C.** 30%.

7. **D.** The fact that only the morning naps show SOREMPs and the history of a delayed sleep phase suggest that the SOREMPs are due to a circadian phase delay. The patient likely was sleeping for 6 hours or less on week nights. The MSL of 8 minutes likely was longer than expected as the patient likely obtained more sleep when not waking up early to attend school.

8. **B.** The MSLT had only 1 SOREMP. However, the MSLT is only about 70% to 80% sensitive. The patient gives a

history consistent with cataplexy and, therefore, likely has narcolepsy with cataplexy. If cataplexy is present in a patient with a normal neurologic examination, the MSLT is considered confirmatory (see Chapter 24). Drug abuse is an important consideration. On questioning, the patient admitted to exposure to "second-hand marijuana smoke" from her boyfriend. For this reason, she declined a urine drug screen. The patient did have mildly insufficient sleep, but this is not uncommon in students.

9. **B.** About 6% of patients with untreated OSA will have an MSLT meeting criteria for narcolepsy. Sleep apnea should be treated before an MSLT is performed. If daytime sleepiness persists on adequate treatment and narcolepsy is suspected, a PSG on treatment (or after surgical treatment) followed by an MSLT can be used to support a diagnosis of narcolepsy (the patient has both OSA and narcolepsy). Note that if the patient had unequivocal cataplexy, then the correct answer is C (both OSA and narcolepsy are present).

10. **A and D?** The use of an MWT to clear a patient for duty where alertness is essential is an area of controversy. A normal MWT does not ensure the patient will perform safely (i.e., adhere to treatment and obtain adequate sleep). The required sleep latency cutoff is poorly defined. The use of a patient's usual stimulant medication before the MWT seems reasonable but is not included in the MWT practice parameters. In this case, the patient maintained wakefulness during the entire test. A CPAP download showed excellent adherence. A recommendation for medical clearance was reported with the stipulation that the patient demonstrate continued adherence to treatment.

11. **E.** Although the sleep latency is defined as the time from lights out to the first epoch of any stage of sleep, the study is terminated after 3 consecutive epochs of stage N1 or a single epoch of any other stage of sleep (N2, N3, R).

REFERENCES

1. Johns MW: A new method for measuring daytime sleepiness: The Epworth Sleepiness Scale. Sleep 1991;14:540–545.
2. Johns MW: Sleepiness in different situations measured by the Epworth Sleepiness Scale. Sleep 1994;17:703–710.
3. Gottlieb DJ, Whitney CW, Bonekat WH, et al: Relation of sleepiness to respiratory disturbance index. Am J Respir Crit Care Med 1999;159:502–507.
4. Patel SR, White DP, Malhotra A, et al: Continuous positive airway pressure therapy in a diverse population with obstructive sleep apnea. Arch Intern Med 2003;163:565–571.
5. Benbadis SR, Mascha E, Perry MC, et al: Association between the Epworth Sleepiness Scale and the multiple sleep latency test in a clinical population. Ann Intern Med 1999;130:289–292.
6. Sangal RB, Mitler MM, Sangal JM: Subjective sleepiness ratings (Epworth Sleepiness Scale) do not reflect the same parameter of sleepiness as objective sleepiness (maintenance

of wakefulness test) in patients with narcolepsy. Clin Neurophysiol 1999;110:2131–2135.
7. Richardson GS, Carskadon MA, Flagg W: Excessive daytime sleepiness in man: multiple sleep latency measurements in narcoleptic and control subjects. Electroencephalogr Clin Neurophysiol 1978;45:621–627.
8. Carskadon MA: Guidelines for the multiple sleep latency test. Sleep 1986;9:519–524.
9. Standards of Practice Committee, American Sleep Disorders Association: The clinical use of the multiple sleep latency test. Sleep 1992;15:268–276.
10. Littner MR, Kushida C, Wise M, et al: Practice parameters for clinical use of the multiple sleep latency test and the maintenance of wakefulness test. Sleep 2005;28:113–121.
11. Arand D, Bonnet M, Hurwitz T, et al: A review by the MSLT and MWT Task Force of the Standards of Practice Committee of the AASM. The clinical use of the MSLT and MWT. Sleep 2005;28:123–144.
12. Aldrich MS, Chervin RD, Malow BA: Value of the multiple sleep latency test (MSLT) for the diagnosis of narcolepsy. Sleep 1997;20:620–629.
13. American Academy of Sleep Medicine: International Classification of Sleep Disorders, 2nd ed. Diagnostic and Coding Manual. Westchester, IL: American Academy of Sleep Medicine, 2005, pp. 81–90.
14. Janjua T, Samp T, Cramer-Bornemann MC, et al: Clinical caveat: prior sleep deprivation can affect the MSLT for days. Sleep Med 2003;4:69–72.
15. Chervin RD, Aldrich MS: Sleep onset REM periods during multiple sleep latency tests in patients evaluated for sleep apnea. Am J Respir Crit Care Med 2000;161:426–431.
16. Carskadon M: The second decade. In Gulleminault C (ed): Sleeping and Waking Disorders—Indications and Techniques. Boston: Butterworths, 1982, pp. 99–125.
17. Carskadon MA, Wolfson AR, Acebo C, et al: Adolescent sleep patterns, circadian timing, and sleepiness at a transition to early school days. Sleep 1998;21:871–881.
18. Doghramji K, Mitler MM, Sangal RB, et al: A normative study of the maintenance of wakefulness test (MWT). Electroencephalogr Clin Neurophysiol 1997;103:554–562.
19. Poceta JS, Timms RM, Jeong D, et al: Maintenance of wakefulness test in obstructive sleep apnea syndrome. Chest 1992;101:893–902.
20. Marshall NS, Barnes M, Travier N, et al: Continuous positive airway pressure reduced daytime sleepiness in mild to moderate obstructive sleep apnea: a meta-analysis. Thorax 2006;61: 430–434.
21. Sangal RB, Thomas L, Mitler MM: Maintenance of wakefulness test and multiple sleep latency test: measurements of different abilities in patients with sleep disorders. Chest 1992;101: 898–902.
22. Sangal RB, Thomas L, Mitler M: Disorders of excessive sleepiness: treatment improves the ability to stay awake but does not reduce sleepiness. Chest 1992;102:699–703.
23. Randomized Trial of modafinil as a treatment for the excessive daytime somnolence of narcolepsy: US Modafinil in Narcolepsy Multicenter Study Group. Neurology 2000;54:1166–1175.
24. George CFP, Boudreau AC, Smiley A: Comparison of simulated driving performance in narcolepsy and sleep apnea patients. Sleep 1996;19:711–717.
25. Sagaspe P, Taillard J, Chaumet G, et al: Maintenance of wakefulness test as a predictor of driving performance in patients with untreated obstructive sleep apnea. Sleep 2007;30:327–330.
26. Philip P, Sagaspe P, Taillard J, et al: Maintenance of wakefulness test, obstructive sleep apnea syndrome and driving risk. Ann Neurol 2008;64:410–416.

Federal Aviation Administration Policy Concerning Fitness to Fly in Sleep Apnea Patients

Examiners may re-issue an airman medical certificate under the provisions of an Authorization, if the applicant provides the following:

- An Authorization granted by the FAA; and
- A current report (performed within last 90 days) from the treating physician that references the present treatment, whether this has eliminated any symptoms, and with specific comments regarding daytime sleepiness.
- If there is any question about response to or compliance with treatment, then a Maintenance of Wakefulness Test (MWT) will be required.

The Aeromedical Examiner must defer to the Aerospace Medical Certification Division (AMCD) or Region if:

- There is any question concerning the adequacy of therapy;
- The applicant appears to be non-compliant with therapy;
- The MWT demonstrates sleep deficiency; or
- The applicant has developed some associated illness, such as right-sided heart failure.

Authorization for Special Issuance of a Medical Certificate (Authorization), valid for a specified period, may be granted to a person who does not meet the established medical standards if the person shows to the satisfaction of the Federal Air Surgeon that the duties authorized by the class of medical certificate applied for can be performed without endangering public safety during the period in which the Authorization would be in force.

Available at http://flightphysical.com/AASI/AASI-Sleep-Apnea.htm

Obstructive Sleep Apnea Syndromes: Definitions, Epidemiology, Diagnosis, and Variants

Chapter Points

- Risk factors for the presence of OSA include obesity, male gender, older age, and postmenopausal status (not on HRT). Hypothyroidism, acromegaly, cigarette smoking, and chronic alcohol use are also considered risk factors but the evidence is less compelling.
- A significant proportion of patients diagnosed with OSA based on an increased AHI do not complain of daytime sleepiness.
- A high Mallampati (or modified Mallampati) score for the upper airway is a predictor of the presence of OSA.
- Patients with habitual snoring, witnessed apnea or gasping, hypertension, and a large neck circumference are at increased risk for having OSA.
- Questionnaires are not sufficiently sensitive or specific to obviate the need for objective testing to determine the presence or absence of OSA.
- In patients with milder OSA, the amount of supine and REM sleep may have a large impact on the overall AHI.
- The two groups of patients with OSA who have daytime hypercapnia are those with the OHS and the combination of obstructive airways disease (COPD) and OSA.
- Approximately 80% of patients with the OHS have OSA. The other 20% have sleep-related worsening of daytime hypercapnia and hypoxemia with relatively few discrete apneas or hypopneas.
- Patients with OSA and obstructive airway disease (COPD) may have severe arterial oxygen desaturation during sleep and daytime hypercapnia.
- Pediatric patients with OSA often present with a different symptom complex than that of adults. Common manifestations include daytime hyperactivity, labored breathing during sleep, diaphoresis, and paradoxical chest movement. Enuresis can also be a manifestation of pediatric OSA.
- The age range of highest prevalence of pediatric OSA patients is typically from 2 to 8 years when hypertrophy of the adenoids and tonsils occurs.
- The values of respiratory indices considered to be diagnostic of pediatric OSA vary but are typically an obstructive AI > 1/hr or obstructive AHI > 1–2/hr. The decision to treat is based on symptoms as well as PSG findings.

HISTORY AND DEFINITIONS

The obstructive sleep apnea (OSA) syndrome was first recognized as a significant health problem only over the last half of the 20th century. In 1956, Burwell and coworkers[1] used the term *pickwickian syndrome* to describe individuals with obesity, hypersomnolence, hypercapnia, cor pulmonale, and erythrocytosis. The term *pickwickian* was based on the character Fat Boy Joe from Charles Dickens' *The Posthumous Papers of the Pickwick Club* (1837), who was markedly obese and tended to fall asleep uncontrollably during the day. The current terminology describing such individuals is the *obesity hypoventilation syndrome (OHS)*. We now know that such patients represent only 10% to 15% of the total number of patients with OSA. Guilleminault and colleagues[2] described the OSA syndrome in patients with daytime sleepiness and obstructive apneas on polysomnography (PSG). An apnea index of 5/hr or greater was considered abnormal.[3] An *apnea* was defined as absent airflow at the nose and mouth for 10 seconds or more. Obstructive apneas are secondary to airway closure at a supraglottic location that reverses at apnea termination often associated with a brief awakening (arousal).[4] Obstructive apneas are followed by a fall in arterial oxygen saturation (SaO_2) of varying severity. It was soon realized the episodes of reduced airflow and tidal volume (hypopneas) that are the result of upper airway narrowing are also clinically significant.[5,6] Patients with primarily hypopneas had the same symptoms, arousals, and arterial oxygen desaturation as patients with obstructive apneas. The term *obstructive sleep apnea hypopnea syndrome (OSAHS)* has been used to be more inclusive. However, many clinicians still use the term *obstructive sleep apnea (OSA)* to refer to the syndrome and the term *OSA* is used in this chapter with the understanding that patients may have variable amount of apneas and hypopneas. As discussed in Chapter 8, the definition of hypopnea has varied considerably.[7,8] The American Academy of Sleep Medicine (AASM) scoring manual[9] recommends scoring apnea on the basis of an oronasal thermal sensor and hypopnea on the basis of nasal pressure monitoring. The recommended hypopnea definition requires a 30% reduction in nasal pressure signal for 10 seconds or longer in association with a 4% or greater arterial oxygen desaturation. The alternative definition of hypopnea requires a 50% or greater reduction in the nasal pressure signal associated with **either an arousal or a 3% or greater arterial oxygen desaturation.** Patients with OSA have **variable proportions of obstructive, mixed, and central apneas** as well as hypopneas.

Diagnostic Criteria

As discussed in Chapter 8, the *apnea-hypopnea index (AHI)* is defined as the number of apneas and hypopneas per hour of sleep. The respiratory disturbance index (RDI) is the number of apneas, hypopneas, and respiratory effort–related arousals (RERAs) per hour of sleep (RDI = AHI + RERA index). RERAs are events associated with increased respiratory effort (as evidenced by esophageal pressure manometry or flattening of the nasal pressure signal) for 10 seconds or longer that are associated with arousal but do not meet criteria for hypopnea[9] (see Chapter 8). Whereas the recent AASM scoring manual defines RERAs, the manual does not define the term *RDI*. The Centers for Medicare and Medicaid Services (CMS) guidelines[10] regarding reimbursement criteria for continuous positive airway pressure (CPAP) define the RDI as the number of respiratory events per hour of monitoring time. This definition refers to the respiratory event index obtained from portable monitoring (PM) devices that do not record sleep. To add to the confusion, some publications and sleep centers use the term *RDI* as the number of apneas and hypopneas per hour of sleep. Therefore, careful attention to the respiratory event definition is required when reading the literature or a sleep study interpretation.

A commonly used diagnostic criteria for OSA syndrome has been an AHI ≥ 5/hr **associated with symptoms** or an AHI ≥ 15/hr with or without associated symptoms.[11,12] Some

---

BOX 15–1

International Classification of Sleep Disorders, 2nd Edition, Criteria for Obstructive Sleep Apnea

Diagnosis = A + B + D or C + D

A. At least one of the following applies:
  i. Complaints of unintentional sleep episodes during wakefulness, daytime sleepiness, unrefreshing sleep, fatigue, or insomnia.
  ii. Awakenings with breath-holding, gasping, or choking.
  iii. Bed partner reports loud snoring and/or breathing interruptions during the patient's sleep.
B. Polysomnography shows the following:
  i. Scoreable respiratory events (apneas + hypopneas + RERAs)/hr of sleep ≥ 5/hr.
  ii. Evidence of respiratory effort during all or a portion of each respiratory event (in the case of RERAs, respiratory effort is best detected by esophageal manometry).

OR

C. Polysomnography shows the following:
  i. Scoreable respiratory events (apneas + hypopneas + RERAs)/hr of sleep ≥ 15/hr.
  ii. Evidence of respiratory effort during all or a portion of each respiratory event.
D. The disorder is not better explained by another current sleep disorder, medical or neurologic disorder, medication use, or substance use disorder.

RERAs = respiratory effort–related arousal.
From American Academy of Sleep Medicine: ICSD-2 International Classification of Sleep Disorders, 2nd ed. Diagnostic and Coding Manual. Westchester, IL: American Academy of Sleep Medicine, 2005.

---

diagnostic criteria have used the RDI ([apneas + hypopneas + RERAs]/hour of sleep) instead of the AHI. The International Classification of Sleep Disorders, 2nd edition (ICSD-2), criteria for a diagnosis of the OSA syndrome in adults[13] (Box 15–1) requires either scoreable respiratory events (apneas, hypopneas, or RERAs) of 5/hr or greater with associated symptoms or scoreable respiratory events of 15/hr or greater with or without symptoms. Of note, the ICSD-2 criteria mentions only scoreable respiratory events (apneas, hypopneas, RERAs) per hour of sleep and does not define the parameter "RDI."

EPIDEMIOLOGY OF OSA

Prevalence and Progression

Prevalence is defined as the proportion of a population with a condition. The prevalence of OSA depends on the defining RDI or AHI criteria, the definition of hypopnea, the method used to detect airflow, and presence or absence of a requirement that symptoms be present. The Wisconsin-based cohort study of state employees younger than 65 years of age found a prevalence of sleep-disordered breathing (SDB) defined as an AHI of 5/hr or greater (with hypopneas based on a definition of discernible change in airflow and ≥ 4% desaturation) to be 9% in women and 24% in men.[14] The *sleep apnea syndrome*, defined as the presence of both SDB and self-reported sleepiness, was present in 2% of women and 4% of men. Bixler and associates[15] found a 17% and 7% prevalence of an AHI greater than 5/hr in and 15/hr in men, respectively. Higher prevalence rates may be present in referral or clinical populations. It is estimated that in Western countries, up to 5% of the population have an undiagnosed OSA syndrome (elevated AHI and symptoms).[16] Another publication in 1997 presented data that 93% of women and 82% of men with moderate to severe OSA were undiagnosed.[17] There is also evidence that OSA severity can progress with time. Analysis of 8-year follow-up of 282 participants of the Wisconsin cohort study showed a mean increase in the AHI from 2.6 events/hr to 5.1.[16] In obese individuals with a body mass index (BMI) over 30, the mean AHI increased from 4.8/hr to 10.1/hr. However, not all studies of untreated patients with OSA have also shown progression in AHI severity.

Risk Factors

A number of population-based studies have documented several risk factors for the presence of OSA (Table 15–1).[16] Of these, the most consistent findings have been the presence of obesity and male gender.[16,18]

Obesity

An association between AHI and obesity has been documented in many studies.[16–21] Peppard and coworkers[19] followed the effects of weight change on AHI. A 10% weight gain predicted an approximate 32% increase in the AHI. A 10% weight loss predicted a 26% reduction in the AHI. A 10% increase in weight was associated with a sixfold increase

TABLE 15–1

Risk Factors for Obstructive Sleep Apnea

RISK FACTOR	EVIDENCE
Obesity—present in roughly 70% of OSA	+++
Male sex	+++
Aging	++
Postmenopausal state	++
Black race	+ (some studies)
Alcohol	++
Smoking	+

OSA = obstructive sleep apnea.
Adapted from Malhotra A, White DP: Obstructive sleep apnea. Lancet 2002;360:237–245.

in the risk of developing moderate to severe OSA. Other studies have documented a decrease in the AHI with weight loss.[22,23] Whether the type of obesity or areas of excess fat (neck vs. abdomen) are important is currently under investigation. Davies and colleagues[21] found that neck circumference correlated with AHI better than general obesity. Prediction models for OSA have used neck circumference as a predictor.[24] However, a recent study found neck circumference to correlate best with AHI in women whereas abdominal girth correlated better in men.[25]

Male Sex

In the Wisconsin cohort study by Young and associates,[14,16] men had about twice the incidence of the OSA **syndrome** compared with women (4% vs. 2%) (AHI ≥ 5/hr + symptoms). Bixler and coworkers[26] found the prevalence of OSA defined as an AHI greater than 10/hr + symptoms to be 3.9% in men and 1.2% in women ($P = .0006$). Analysis of the Sleep Heart Health data also showed the risk of OSA in men was greater (odds ratio 1.5).[27] Further discussion of the effect of gender on the pathophysiology of OSA is contained in Chapter 16.

Age

The prevalence of OSA appears to be higher in the elderly than in middle-aged populations. The prevalence of a chronic nonfatal disease would increase as cases accumulate even if the incidence (new cases/yr) was constant or declining. Ancoli-Israel and colleagues[28] studied 427 community-dwelling elderly age 65 years or older using limited channel ambulatory monitoring. A prevalence of OSA, defined as an AHI greater than 10/hr, was found to be 62%. Here, hypopneas were based on changes in flow (based on two channels of respiratory inductance plethysmography) independent of changes in the SaO_2 (no oximetry). This is a prevalence of about three times that in middle-aged populations. There is evidence from the Sleep Heart Health Study that the SDB prevalence increases from age 40 to around 60.[27] After that, the prevalence appears to plateau (Fig. 15–1). In older adults, the AHI may be less correlated with excessive sleepiness and increased cardiovascular risk. Enright and coworkers[29] studied a large group of subjects over age 65 with questionnaires and echocardiography, ultrasound of the carotids, and an electrocardiogram. Snoring was very common but, interestingly, reported snoring seemed to decrease after age 75. Loud snoring, observed apneas, and daytime sleepiness were not associated with hypertension or the prevalence of cardiovascular disease. Conversely, decreased snoring reports could be secondary to a lower frequency of having a bed partner or hearing deficits in the elderly. It is possible that the presence of OSA in the elderly population has different implications.[30]

Postmenopausal Status

Conventional wisdom is that postmenopausal women have a greater incidence of OSA than premenopausal women. However, the confounders of increased age and often

FIGURE 15-1 The prevalence of obstructive sleep apnea (OSA) tends to increase with age but levels off after age 65 years. AHI = apnea-hypopnea index. *From Young T, Shahar E, Nieto FJ, et al: Predictors of sleep disordered breathing in community dwelling adults: the Sleep Heart Health Study. Arch Intern Med 2002;162:895.*

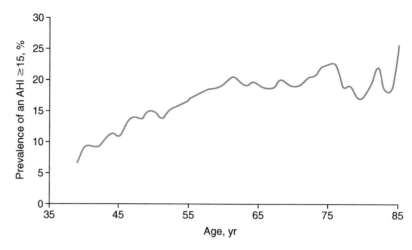

increased BMI in the postmenopausal group complicate the analysis. An analysis of the Wisconsin cohort study of the risk of having an AHI greater than 15 (adjusted for age and body habitus) found an odds ratio of 3.5 for greater risk in postmenopausal compared with premenopausal women.[31] Another frequently quoted study found a greater risk but included men in the control group.[26] The Sleep Heart Health Study analysis of women older than 50 years found that the prevalence of an AHI greater than 15/hr in women on hormone replacement therapy (HRT) was approximately half that of the nonusers.[32] There was a higher prevalence of SDB in non-HRT users even when other factors such as age and BMI were considered. The risk was especially high in the 50- to 59-year-old group. Thus, it appears that postmenopausal women are at increased risk of developing OSA if they are not on HRT treatment.

Ethnicity

One study found that OSA is more common in African American than in white populations.[33] However, this finding was not present in another study that controlled for differences in age and BMI.[27] An investigation by Redline and associates[34] found an increase in the risk of having OSA greater in African Americans than in whites only for those younger than age 25 years. Ip and coworkers[35] found a similar prevalence of OSA in a Chinese population as in whites. The fact that OSA is common in Asian areas where obesity is much less common has led to the hypothesis that craniofacial characteristics of the Asian population might predispose to OSA.[36] Whereas increasing BMI was still associated with an increased prevalence of OSA in the study of Chinese patients, the association was not as strong as that typically seen in white populations. The lack of obesity in Asian patients should certainly not discourage evaluation for possible sleep apnea.

Smoking

Analysis of data for the Wisconsin sleep cohort data by Wetter and colleagues[37] found that current cigarette smokers are at a greater risk for sleep apnea than never smokers.

Heavy smokers were at the greatest risk. Of interest, former smokers did not have an increased risk. Therefore, smoking cessation should be considered in all patients with OSA.

Alcohol Intake

Most studies of acute ingestion of alcohol in patients with snoring or OSA have found an increase in the AHI.[38,39] Alcohol does suppress REM sleep and, in this sense, could reduce the longer events associated with REM sleep during the early part of the night. However, more severe desaturations and presumably longer events do occur in some patients in the early portion of the night if bedtime alcohol is consumed.[38] Block and associates[40] found effects of alcohol on breathing in normal men but not women. Stradling and coworkers[20] found alcohol consumption to be associated with the presence of OSA in a group of middle-aged men. However, definite epidemiologic evidence for a worsening of OSA with chronic alcohol consumptions is lacking. It seems likely that consumption of alcohol (or abstinence from alcohol) could significantly change the AHI in individual patients. Alcohol could also prolong respiratory events. In a study of the effect of alcohol on the arousal response to mask occlusion in normal subjects, ethanol ingestion delayed the time to arousal during non–rapid eye movement (NREM) sleep.[41] Most occlusions were preformed in the early part of the night when the alcohol level would have been higher. Considering the very common use of alcohol, relatively little is known about its effects on breathing during sleep.

Hypothyroidism

Hypothyroidism has been thought to be associated with sleep apnea.[42-44] However, there are no large cohort studies evaluating the prevalence of sleep apnea in hypothyroid subjects versus euthyroid patients. Pelttari and coworkers[43] examined 26 patients with hypothyroidism and 188 euthyroid control subjects, finding that 50% of hypothyroid patients and 29% of control subjects had significant respiratory events. If hypothyroidism is found in a patient with OSA, continued effective treatment is indicated until restoration of the euthyroid condition.[44] Even then, one would need a sleep study to demonstrate that treatment of OSA was not needed. Whereas some physicians order thyroid function tests on all OSA patients, this is not cost effective. Winkelman and colleagues[45] reviewed the results of 255 consecutive patients suspected of having OSA in whom thyroid function studies were ordered. Hypothyroidism was present in only 1.6% of patients and the frequency did not differ between those documented to have OSA and those who did not. Thyroid testing is recommended only for high-risk groups (women > 60 yr) and if there are clinical signs or symptoms suggesting possible hypothyroidism.[46] Postmenopausal women with OSA or OSA patients without predisposing OSA risk factors might warrant thyroid studies. The reason hypothyroidism exacerbates OSA is unclear and possibly multifactorial. Upper airway muscle myopathy, narrowing of the upper airway by mucoprotein deposition in the tongue (macroglossia), and abnormalities in ventilatory control are possible mechanisms.

Acromegaly

Growth hormone excess resulting in acromegaly is also associated with sleep apnea. Grunstein and associates[46] noted that 60% of unselected patients with acromegaly had sleep apnea. Weiss and coworkers[47] found that 75% of a group with acromegaly had OSA. Independent predictors of OSA included increased activity of acromegaly (higher growth hormone), older age, and an increased neck circumference. Potential pathophysiologic mechanisms of the association between acromegaly and OSA include macroglossia and increased muscle mass of the upper airway. Patients with acromegaly may have central as well as obstructive apnea.[46] Therefore, alterations in ventilatory control may also play a role. Patients with acromegaly **without** sleep apnea may also have daytime sleepiness as a direct manifestation of growth hormone excess. The daytime sleepiness may improve after effective treatment of the acromegaly.[48]

DIAGNOSIS OF OSA

Recent clinical guidelines for the evaluation, management, and long-term care of OSA in adults recommended that high-risk populations for OSA be questioned in detail concerning symptoms of OSA.[49] However, certain basic sleep questions were recommended for all patients as part of a general history and physical examination (Table 15–2). The comprehensive sleep examination questions the patient concerning the typical manifestations of OSA. A number of populations with a high prevalence of OSA have been identified including patients with refractory hypertension, congestive heart failure, and recent or past cerebrovascular accident or transient ischemic attack (see Table 15–2).

OSA Symptoms and Key Historical Points

The patient or bed partner frequently reports excessive daytime sleepiness, loud habitual snoring, gasping/choking or witnessed apnea, personality change, morning headache,

---

TABLE 15–2

Recommendations for Evaluation of General Medical Patients and Populations at High Risk for Obstructive Sleep Apnea

HIGH-RISK PATIENTS FOR OSA	ROUTINE QUESTIONS AND OBSERVATIONS	COMPREHENSIVE SLEEP EXAMINATION QUESTIONS
Obesity (BMI > 30)	Obesity?	Witnessed apneas?
Congestive heart failure	Retrognathia?	Snoring?
Atrial fibrillation	Daytime sleepiness?	Gasping/choking at night?
Refractory hypertension	Snoring?	Nonrefreshing sleep?
Type 2 diabetes	Breathing pauses?	Total sleep amount?
Nocturnal arrhythmias	Hypertension?	Sleep fragmentation?
CVA		Nocturia?
Pulmonary hypertension		Morning headaches?
High-risk driving populations		Decreased concentration?
Preoperative for bariatric surgery		Memory loss?
		Decreased libido?
		Irritability?

BMI = body mass index; CVA = cerebrovascular accident; OSA = obstructive sleep apnea.
From Epstein LJ, Kristo D, Strollo PJ, et al: Clinical guideline for the evaluation, management and long-term care of obstructive sleep apnea in adults. J Clin Sleep Med 2009;5:263–276.

BOX 15–2

Common Symptoms and Manifestations of Obstructive Sleep Apnea

Symptoms	Nocturnal Behavior
Excessive daytime sleepiness	Loud habitual snoring
Nonrestorative sleep	Choking, gasping during sleep
Frequent awakenings	Breathing pauses/witnessed apnea
Morning headaches	Body movements, restlessness in bed
Dry mouth in the morning	
Personality change	
Intellectual changes	
Erectile dysfunction	
Nocturia	

---

or nonrestorative sleep (Box 15–2). Patients may also report a progression of symptoms with recent weight gain or nasal congestion. The Epworth Sleepiness Scale (ESS), a subjective estimate of the propensity to doze off in eight situations, is often (but not invariably) increased (see Chapter 14). The range of the scale is 0 to 24 with greater than 10 indicating excessive daytime sleepiness.[50] Data in Table 15–3 taken from one of the first descriptions of the ESS show that the

TABLE 15-3				
Epworth Sleepiness Scale Scores in Mild, Moderate, and Severe Obstructive Sleep Apnea				
	MEAN AHI (MEAN ± SD)	**TOTAL NUMBER OF SUBJECTS**	**ESS (MEAN ± SD)**	**RANGE OF ESS**
Mild OSA (AHI > 5–15)	8.8 ± 2.3	22	9.5 ± 3.3	4–16
Moderate OSA (AHI > 15–30)	21.1 ± 4.0	20	11.5 ± 4.2	5–20
Severe OSA (AHI > 30)	49.5 ± 9.6	13	16.0 ± 4.4	8–23

AHI = apnea-hypopnea index; ESS = Epworth Sleepiness Scale; OSA = obstructive sleep apnea; SD = standard deviation.
From Johns MW: Daytime sleepiness, snoring, and obstructive sleep apnea. The Epworth Sleepiness Scale. Chest 1993;103:30–36.

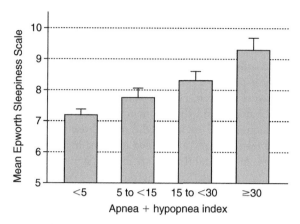

FIGURE 15-2 Epworth Sleepiness Scale increases with worsening OSA severity as measured by the apnea-hypopnea index. However, note that the mean value is lower than expected given the severity of OSA. Note the relative mild daytime sleepiness even with severe OSA. These results are from a population-based study. Sleep clinic populations may manifest greater sleepiness. *From Gottlieb DJ, Whitney CW, Bonekat WH, et al: Relation of sleepiness to respiratory disturbance index. Am J Respir Crit Care Med 1999;159:502–507.*

score increases with severity of OSA (the AHI), but there was a wide range of scores at any AHI range.[50] Other studies have confirmed that the correlation between the AHI and subjective or objective sleepiness, although statistically significant, is low (correlation coefficient in the range of 0.4–0.5).[51,52] The wide variability in symptoms is likely due in part to different individual susceptibility to sleep fragmentation or other factors contributing to symptoms of daytime sleepiness such as medications or reduced sleep time. A number of population-based studies have found that a substantial percentage of patients with OSA do not report daytime sleepiness, and the absence of sleepiness should not discourage a further evaluation. However, patients with more severe OSA do have, on average, greater daytime sleepiness (Fig. 15–2). It is important to remember that two patients with the same AHI can have vastly different degrees of daytime sleepiness or arterial oxygen desaturation. Severe desaturation, even in the absence of daytime sleepiness, could put the patient at risk for a number of adverse cardiovascular consequences of sleep apnea.

A number of investigations have studied the effect of gender on presenting symptoms of OSA.[53–55] In general, men and women report many of the same symptoms. However, women may report more insomnia and less witnessed apnea. Women with OSA are also more likely to complain of depression, morning headache, awakenings, and fatigue.[55] It is important to remember that patients with central sleep apnea may present with many of the same symptoms as OSA. Historical elements that may alert the clinician to possible central apnea include congestive heart failure or the use of potent narcotics. Patients with congestive heart failure can have either OSA, Cheyne-Stokes breathing, or a combination of OSA and central sleep apnea. Patients with narcotics often have central apneas at baseline or when

BOX 15-3

Obstructive Sleep Apnea Physical Examination—Key Elements in Patients Suspected of Having Obstructive Sleep Apnea

Increased BMI*
Presence of nasal obstruction
Increased Mallampati or modified Mallampati score*
High-arched palate (narrow airway)
Retrognathia
Increased neck circumference (>17 inches in men, >16 inches in women)
Evidence of right heart failure (JVD, pedal edema)

*Independent predictor of the presence of OSA.
BMI = body mass index; JVD = jugular venous distention; OSA = obstructive sleep apnea.
From Nuckton TJ, Glidden DV, Brownder WS, Claman DM: Physical examination: Mallampati score as an independent predictor of obstructive sleep apnea. Sleep 2006;29:903–908.

undergoing a positive airway pressure (PAP) titration (see Chapter 21).

Physical Examination

The physical examination of patients with suspected OSA should target abnormalities known to be associated with the syndrome (Box 15–3). These include measurement of BMI and systemic blood pressure as well as careful examination of the nose, ears, and oropharynx.[56–58] Observation of the oropharynx usually reveals a crowded upper airway and examination of the patient's face in profile may reveal retrognathia (Figs. 15–3 and 15–4). Measurement of neck circumference and observation of signs of right heart failure may also be

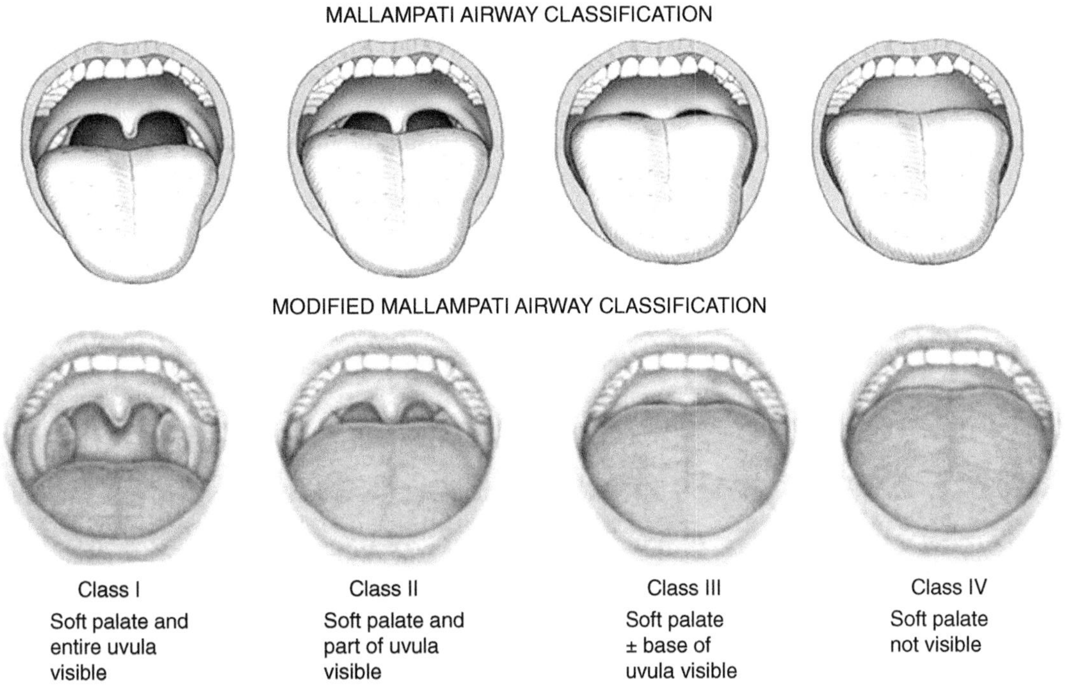

MALLAMPATI AIRWAY CLASSIFICATION

MODIFIED MALLAMPATI AIRWAY CLASSIFICATION

| Class I | Class II | Class III | Class IV |
| Soft palate and entire uvula visible | Soft palate and part of uvula visible | Soft palate ± base of uvula visible | Soft palate not visible |

FIGURE 15–3 Mallampati and modified Mallampati airway classification. In the Mallampati maneuver, patients are instructed not to emit sounds but to open the mouth as wide as possible and protrude the tongue as far as possible. In the modified Mallampati, the patient is instructed to open the mouth as wide as possible without emitting sounds. *Mallampati reproduced from Friedman M, Tanyeri H, La Rosa M, et al: Clinical predictors of obstructive sleep apnea. Laryngoscope 1999;109:1901–1907; and modified Mallampati reproduced with permission from Nuckton TJ, Glidden DV, Brownder WS, Claman DM: Physical examination: Mallampati score as an independent predictor of obstructive sleep apnea. Sleep 2006;29:903–908.*

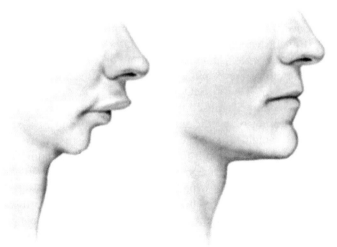

FIGURE 15–4 A patient with severe retrognathia on the **left** and orthognathia (normal) on the **right.** *From Friedman M, Tanyeri H, La Rosa M, et al: Clinical predictors of obstructive sleep apnea. Laryngoscope 1999;109:1901–1907.*

revealing. A neck size greater than 17 inches in men and 16 inches in women suggests the possibility of OSA. However, a smaller neck circumference does not rule out OSA.

The Mallampati (MP) score of the upper airway was developed to predict the risk of difficult endotracheal intubation (see Fig. 15–3). The patient's oropharynx is examined with tongue protruded. The modified Mallampati score (MMP), also called the Friedman score,[56] is similar but the patient simply opens the mouth *without* saying "ah" or tongue protrusion. Friedman and coworkers[56] found that the

MMP, tonsil size, and BMI were reliable predictors of OSA. Zonato and colleagues[57] found a significant correlation between the AHI and the MMP and BMI. Although retrognathia (see Fig. 15–4) was not correlated with AHI, this abnormality was more frequent in patients with severe OSA as compared with snorers. Nuckton and associates[58] analyzed over 30 variables reflecting airway anatomy, body habitus, symptoms, and medical history and found the MMP and MP to be independent predictors of the presence and severity of OSA. The variables associated with an increased risk of OSA in their study included increased neck circumference, witnessed apnea, and hypertension.

Laboratory Testing in OSA

Laboratory testing in patients with OSA is usually not indicated apart from routine health maintenance unless a particular problem such as hypothyroidism is suspected. In patients with severe nocturnal hypoxemia, polycythemia (increased hematocrit) may be present. An unexplained elevation in the serum CO_2 (composed primarily of HCO_3) on electrolyte testing is suggestive of chronic compensation for hypercapnia (in the absence of evidence of causes of metabolic alkalosis).[59,60] Pulmonary function testing, chest radiography, and arterial blood gas testing are indicated in patients with a low awake SaO_2 or suspected hypoventilation to eliminate pulmonary causes of impaired gas exchange.[60]

Prediction of the Presence of OSA

A number of clinical indices and questionnaires have been developed to predict the presence of OSA based on symptoms, signs, and measurements. Although they have some success, they are neither satisfactorily sensitive nor specific enough to be a substitute for objective documentation of the presence of OSA by a sleep study. An adaptation of a prediction rule developed by Flemons and coworkers[24,61] used an adjusted neck circumference (Table 15–4) to classify patients as low, moderate, or high probability. The population in which the prediction value was developed was predominantly male, hypopneas were defined as a reduction in airflow associated with a 3% or greater desaturation, and the presence of OSA was defined by an AHI greater than 10/hr. Netzer and colleagues[62] studied the utility of the Berlin Questionnaire (Appendix 15–1) to predict whether patients were high or low risk for having OSA. The questionnaire consists of three categories: category 1 concerns snoring and witnessed apnea, category 2 concerns being sleepy/tired/fatigued more than three or four times a week or nodding

off while driving a vehicle, and category 3 concerns the presence of hypertension. After questionnaire completion, patients were studied by PM. The Berlin Questionnaire identified patients with an AHI ≥ 5/hr (based on assignment to the high-risk group) with a sensitivity of 0.86 and a specificity of 0.77. The STOP-BANG (snoring, tired, observed apnea, [blood] pressure, body mass index, age, neck circumference, gender) Questionnaire is a screening tool (Appendix 15–2) that has been used for preoperative evaluation to detect sleep apnea. A study of 2467 patients found sensitivities of 84%, 92%, and 100% for AHI cutoffs of greater than 5/hr, greater than 15/hr, and greater than 30/hr.[63,64]

Diagnostic Testing for Suspected Sleep Apnea

Attended PSG is the gold standard to determine whether OSA is present and to classify the severity.[65] Figure 15–5 presents an obstructive apnea during REM sleep. Box 15–4 lists the classic PSG findings in patients with OSA. The abnormality in the sleep architecture varies with severity. Patients with severe OSA usually have a high arousal index, increased wake after sleep onset (WASO) and stage N1 sleep, and decreases in stage N3 or stage R sleep. A typical classification of OSA severity based on the AHI (or RDI in some sleep centers) is 5 to fewer than 15/hr mild, 15 to 30 moderate, and greater than 30/hr severe OSA. Whereas the AHI (RDI) is the most widely used index for classification of severity, it is also important to characterize the severity of arterial oxygen desaturation. A widely accepted standard for the characterization of the severity of desaturation does not exist. It is common to present the number of desaturations (usually defined as a drop in the $SaO_2 > 4\%$), the lowest SaO_2, the average SaO_2 at desaturation, and the time below various saturations. For example, a commonly used metric is the time at or below an SaO_2 of 88%.

PSG can diagnose OSA either with an entire night of monitoring or by the initial diagnostic portion of a split (partial-night) study. The second part of the study is used as a PAP titration. CMS formerly required a minimum of 2 hours of sleep (not monitoring) during the diagnostic portion to qualify a patient for reimbursement of CPAP treatment. Currently, if less than 2 hours of monitoring is performed, the number of events to qualify the patient should be the same as if 2 hours of sleep had been recorded. For example, if an AHI of 15/hr qualifies a patient for CPAP (symptoms not required) a total number of apneas and hypopneas must equal 30 or more[10] (Box 15–5).

Because the AHI is often higher in the supine position[66,67] and during REM sleep,[68–70] presentation of the AHI for those conditions in the sleep study report may be useful. The diagnosis of postural OSA is usually made when the AHI-supine is greater than twice the AHI-nonsupine.

Some clinicians define REM-associated OSA as a normal AHI during NREM sleep associated with an elevated AHI during REM sleep. Other clinicians use the term to denote patients with an AHI-REM/AHI-NREM greater than 2. There is also an interaction between body position and sleep

TABLE 15–4
Prediction of Obstructive Sleep Apnea
NC = measure neck circumference (cm)
A. If hypertension present, +4
B. If habitual snoring present, +3
C. If gasping or choking present, +3
Adjusted neck circumference = NC + A + B + C
<43 cm (17 inches) low probability 43–48 cm (17–19 inches) moderate probability >48 cm (19 inches) high probability
From Flemons WW: Obstructive sleep apnea. N Engl J Med 2002;347:498–504.

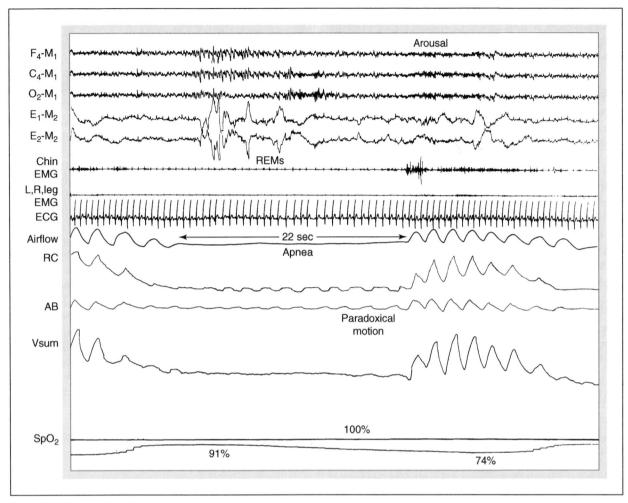

FIGURE 15–5 An obstructive apnea during rapid eye movement (REM) sleep. The longest respiratory event duration and most severe arterial oxygen desaturation are usually during REM sleep (especially supine REM sleep). Note the slowing of the heart rate at the start of the apnea and speeding at apnea termination. Here Vsum is the sum of rib cage (RC) and abdominal (AB) respiratory inductance plethysmograph bands. ECG = electrocardiogram; EMG = electromyogram; SpO_2 = pulse oximetry.

stage. The AHI tends to be higher during supine than during nonsupine REM sleep.[69] Patients with a mild to moderate overall AHI are more likely to have REM-related OSA. An occasional patient with REM-related OSA may exhibit very severe arterial oxygen desaturation and long apneas during REM sleep but a relatively normal AHI-NREM. A study by Kass and coworkers[70] identified a group of patients with overall AHI less than 10/hr but AHI-REM greater than 15/hr who had objective evidence of daytime sleepiness. Other studies have not demonstrated a relationship between the AHI-REM and sleepiness.[71,72] A recent large population-based analysis of the Sleep Heart Health Study cohort found a relationship between the AHI-NREM but not the AHI-REM and daytime sleepiness.[73] However, treatment decisions in an individual patient with REM-related OSA should be individualized. In patients with milder OSA, there can be considerable night-to-night variability in the AHI. The best advice is to **"treat the patient not the AHI."** If a patient with REM-related OSA is symptomatic and the overall AHI is 5/hr or greater, it is reasonable to offer treatment. However,

one should carefully consider other causes of daytime sleepiness (narcolepsy, insufficient sleep). Conversely, if a patient is completely asymptomatic with an overall AHI of 15/hr or less, conservative therapy may suffice.

Cyclic variation in heart rate is typically noted during the repeated episodes of obstructive events.[74,75] The heart rate slows at the start of the events and increases at event termination (Fig. 15–6). Often, the heart rate remains between 60 and 100 bpm. A standard part of most PSG reports is to present the maximum and minimum heart rate along with notations of abnormalities (premature ventricular contractions, atrial fibrillation, sinus pauses).

There are many formats for summarizing respiratory event results of PSG in OSA patients. However, given the importance of REM sleep and supine sleep, the AHI is often presented for those situations (Table 15–5). Note that the patient in Table 15–5 has a much higher AHI during supine and REM sleep. It is also important to present the amount of supine sleep (% of total sleep time supine) during the recording period. The longest respiratory events and most severe

BOX 15–4

Polysomnographic Findings in Obstructive Sleep Apnea

EEG FINDINGS

Increased WASO and stage N1
Reduced stage N3
Reduced stage R (REM sleep)
Increased respiratory arousals

RESPIRATORY FINDINGS

Snoring
Obstructive, mixed apneas, and central apneas
Obstructive hypopneas
AHI: mild 5 to <15/hr, moderate 15–30/hr, severe > 30/hr
AHI supine > 2 × AHI nonsupine – postural OSA
AHI REM > AHI NREM common
Apnea duration REM > NREM

ARTERIAL OXYGEN DESATURATION

Lowest SaO$_2$ during REM sleep
Longest REM periods in the early morning hours typically have the worst desaturation

CYCLIC VARIATION IN HEART RATE

Slowing of heart rate at apnea onset and speeding at event termination

AHI = apnea-hypopnea index; EEG = electroencephalogram; NREM = non–rapid eye movement; OSA = obstructive sleep apnea; REM = rapid eye movement; SaO$_2$ = arterial oxygen saturation; WASO = wake after sleep onset.

BOX 15–5

Excerpt from CMS Transmittal 96RNCD: A Clarification of Apnea-Hypopnea Index and Respiratory Disturbance Index for NCD 240.4 (CPAP)

- A positive test for obstructive sleep apnea (OSA) is established if either of the following criteria using the apnea-hypopnea index (AHI) or respiratory disturbance index (RDI) are met:
  - AHI or RDI greater than or equal to 15 events per hour of sleep or continuous monitoring, respectively, or
  - AHI or RDI greater than or equal to 5 and less than or equal to 14 events per hour of sleep or continuous monitoring, respectively, with documented symptoms of excessive daytime sleepiness, impaired cognition, mood disorders or insomnia, or documented hypertension, ischemic heart disease, or history of stroke.
- The AHI is equal to the average number of episodes of apnea and hypopnea per hour of sleep.
- The RDI is equal to the average number of respiratory disturbances per hour of continuous monitoring.
- If the AHI or RDI is calculated based on less than 2 hours of continuous recorded sleep, the total number of recorded events to calculate the AHI or RDI during sleep testing is at least the number of events that would have been required in a 2-hour period.

RDI refers to home sleep testing.
Available at https://www.cms.gov/transmittals/downloads/R96NCD.pdf

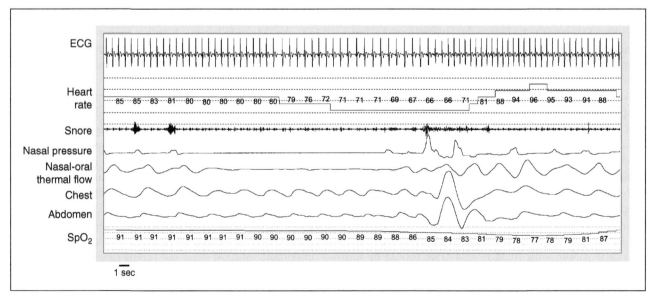

FIGURE 15–6 The heart rate during an obstructive apnea. The heart rate signal is the output of the oximeter (a moving time average) that tends to lag behind the actual change in heart rate. Changes in the heart rate can be noted by changes in the RR interval, which widens at apnea onset then narrows at apnea termination. ECG = electrocardiogram; SpO$_2$ = pulse oximetry.

TABLE 15-5

Typical Presentation of Respiratory Events

	TOTAL				
TST (min)	360				
NREM (min)	290				
REM sleep (min)	70				
% supine	16				
	TOTAL	SUPINE	NONSUPINE	NREM	REM
TST in condition	360	60	300	290	70
OA (#)	24	14	10	4	20
MA (#)	5	5	0	0	5
CA (#)	2	1	1	1	1
Hypopnea (#)	24	19	5	20	4
Total (#)	55	39	16	25	30
AHI (#/hr)	9.2	39.0	3.2	5.2	25.7

AHI = apnea-hypopnea index; CA = central apnea; MA = mixed apnea; NREM = non–rapid eye movement; OA = obstructive apnea; REM = rapid eye movement; TST = total sleep time.

arterial oxygen desaturation typically occur during REM sleep in the second part of the night. Split- or partial-night sleep studies (initial part diagnostic, second part PAP titration) are frequently used in severe patients (by AHI). However, because there is often minimal REM sleep during the diagnostic portion, the severity of arterial oxygen desaturation based on a split study may be dramatically underestimated. A full night of diagnostic monitoring provides the best estimate of the typical severity of arterial oxygen desaturation. Chapter 16 discusses the pathophysiology of OSA and the determinants of severity of desaturation. But briefly, a low baseline awake SaO_2, long apnea time (long apnea duration with short intra-apnea ventilation), and a low expiratory reserve volume (ERV) are associated with more severe arterial oxygen desaturation (Box 15–6).[76] A recent large study of the Wisconsin cohort found that a higher BMI was associated with more severe arterial oxygen desaturation independent of age, gender, sleeping position, baseline SaO_2, and event duration.[77] A higher BMI had a greater effect on desaturation during REM than during NREM sleep. In addition, a fall in tidal volume had a greater effect on arterial oxygen desaturation when the BMI was higher. The predicted change in the SaO_2 was also higher in the supine position than in the lateral position, in men than in women, and in smokers than in nonsmokers. Another study found that obstructive events in the supine position tended to be longer, were associated with more severe desaturation, and were more likely to be associated with an arousal at event termination.[66] Respiratory events during REM sleep tend to be of longer duration and associated with more significant arterial oxygen desaturation during REM sleep.[68] Apnea duration during REM sleep does

BOX 15-6

Severity of Associated Arterial Oxygen Desaturation

FACTORS ASSOCIATED WITH SEVERE DESATURATION

Low awake SaO_2
Long apnea time (long apnea duration, short ventilatory period between apneas)
Low ERV (FRC – RV)
  Low FRC—obesity
  High RV—obstructive lung disease

GROUPS WITH SEVERE DESATURATION

Severe obesity
Obesity-hypoventilation syndrome
OSA + COPD (overlap syndrome)

COPD = chronic obstructive pulmonary disease; ERV = expiratory reserve volume; FRC = functional residual capacity; OSA = obstructive sleep apnea; RV = residual volume; SaO_2 = arterial oxygen saturation.

not appear different between supine and nonsupine REM sleep, although supine REM sleep is associated with the worse desaturation. Figure 15–7 illustrates the effects of various apnea durations on desaturation.

Portable Monitoring

The use of PM, also known as home sleep testing (HST) or out of center sleep testing (OCST), is discussed in detail in Chapter 13. PM is most appropriate when PSG is difficult

FIGURE 15-7 Variable arterial oxygen desaturation in a patient with severe OSA. Note as expected longer apnea resulted in more severe arterial oxygen desaturation. SpO$_2$ = pulse oximetry. *From Berry RB: Sleep Medicine Pearls, 2nd ed. Philadelphia: Hanley & Belfus, 2003, p. 86.*

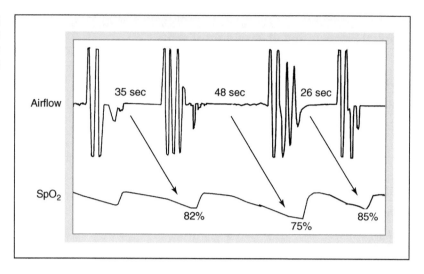

due to immobility or safety issues, when there is a delay in obtaining a PSG due to access or availability and the clinical situation is urgent, when there is a high probability of OSA, when complicated co-morbidities are not present, and when coexisting sleep disorders that may benefit from PSG are not present.[78] It should be remembered that the AHI derived from testing without electroencephalogram (EEG) provides a number of events per hour of monitoring time, not total sleep time. For example, if PSG and PM both identify 100 events, the total sleep time is 6 hours, and the monitoring time is 7 hours, then the AHI PSG = 100/6 and the AHI PM = 100/7. Therefore, the AHI by PM will likely be less than by PSG, even if similar numbers of respiratory events are detected. There is also the concern for a false-negative PM study. This phenomenon is more likely if the patient does not sleep well during PM with the result that monitoring time greatly exceeds total sleep time. If there is a high index of suspicion for OSA but the PM is negative for OSA, a PSG should be performed.[78]

VARIANTS OF SNORING AND OSA

Primary (Simple) Snoring

Whereas snoring is a cardinal symptom of OSA, not all snorers have OSA. *Simple or primary snoring* is defined as the presence of snoring without associated symptoms of insomnia, daytime sleepiness, or sleep disruption (Box 15-7). Although a PSG is not necessary unless OSA is suspected, the PSG characteristics of simple snoring would include evidence of snoring on the PSG as detected by audio recording, snore sensor, or vibration in the nasal pressure signal (or technologist report of snoring) AND the **absence** of a significant number of apneas, hypopneas, or RERAs. Sleep architecture is usually normal.

Snoring may be defined as a vibratory, sonorous noise made during inspiration and, less commonly, expiration.[79] It is associated with a vibration (fluttering) of the soft palate and other pharyngeal structures. Snoring is difficult to

BOX 15-7

Snoring (Simple or Primary Snoring) (ICSD-2)

1. Audible snoring noises are reported by an observer.
2. The patient has no complaints of insomnia, excessive daytime sleepiness, or sleep disruption that are attributable to snoring.

From American Academy of Sleep Medicine: ICSD-2 International Classification of Sleep Disorders, 2nd ed. Diagnostic and Coding Manual. Westchester, IL: American Academy of Sleep Medicine, 2005.

quantify but may be described on the basis of intensity or vibratory qualities. It is associated with a narrowing of the upper airway and evidence of airflow limitation. Any process that narrows the upper airway, increases nasal resistance, or decreases upper airway muscle tone typically worsens snoring. Thus, nasal congestion, the supine posture, and ethanol or hypnotics may have this effect. There is a definite male predominance, although a considerable number of women also snore. Simple snoring is common and tends to increase with age. Some studies have suggested that up to 60% of men and 40% of women older than age 40 are habitual snorers. Snoring can be detected with snore microphones and high-frequency oscillations can sometimes be seen in the nasal pressure signal if appropriate high-filter settings are used (e.g., 100 Hz). Chapter 8 discusses methods to detect snoring. Snoring may be associated with paradoxical breathing and high esophageal pressure deflections. Snoring intensity is loudest in slow wave sleep and softest in REM sleep. A possible association between primary (simple) snoring and cardiovascular disease is still debated. One problem with many population studies that addressed this topic is that PSG was not performed to rule out sleep apnea. A recent study by Lee and associates[80] found that heavy snoring (defined as the presence of snoring for > 50% of the night) was associated with increased carotid atherosclerosis independent of other risk factors such as nocturnal hypoxemia and OSA severity. In addition, patients with heavy snoring are at risk for developing OSA as they age or if significant weight gain occurs.

Although not every snorer needs a sleep study, evaluation is recommended if the patient has a moderate to high likelihood of having OSA, is symptomatic, or if a surgical intervention is being considered. A PSG is also needed before an oral appliance is made for snoring to rule out significant OSA.[65] **If significant sleep apnea is present, this may change the treatment approach.** If upper airway surgery or an oral appliance is used for treatment, a sleep study postoperatively or with the oral appliance in place is needed to document treatment efficacy. Some surgical interventions such as laser-assisted uvuloplasty (LAUP) are indicated for treatment of snoring but not OSA.[81] Surgical treatments for snoring and OSA are discussed in detail in Chapter 18. Of note, if the patient has unsuspected moderate to severe OSA, then PAP is the treatment of choice.[12,49]

The treatment options for simple snoring are similar to those for mild OSA. These include weight loss, the side sleep position, treatment of nasal congestion, upper airway surgery, an oral appliance, and avoidance of alcohol. Although nasal CPAP is effective for snoring, this treatment is usually reserved for patients with OSA.[82] Chapter 20 provides an overview of treatments for snoring and OSA.

Upper Airway Resistance Syndrome

Guilleminault and coworkers[83] identified a group of patients who exhibited subjective and objective (multiple sleep latency test [MSLT]) daytime sleepiness but did not have an AHI of 5/hr or greater (thermal devices measured airflow). The group was defined by having a respiratory arousal index greater than 10/hr using esophageal pressure monitoring. The respiratory arousal events were not associated with desaturation or a change in thermal device–detected airflow. The symptom of sleepiness responded to CPAP treatment. The mean arousal index of the group was 33/hr (range 16–52) and the mean maximally negative esophageal pressure nadir was –37 cm H_2O. There has been controversy as to whether the upper airway resistance syndrome (UARS) is a distinct entity or simply a milder form of OSA.[84,85] The ICSD-2 does not contain a separate diagnostic category for UARS.

As discussed in Chapter 8, esophageal manometry and nasal pressure monitoring each identify many (but not all) of the same events. However, it is possible that use of esophageal pressure monitoring would identify a few patients missed by nasal pressure monitoring. For example, a patient arousing easily might develop relatively high inspiratory effort (esophageal pressure excursions) before airflow changed significantly. If PSG is performed using nasal pressure and if an RDI of 5/hr or greater (RDI = apneas + hypopneas + RERAs/hr of sleep) is used to define OSA, then most patients who would meet criteria for UARS as defined previously would also be diagnosed as having OSA. Furthermore, if the alternative definition of hypopnea is used (considers

arousals as well as desaturation), most RERAs will be classified as hypopneas.[86,87]

Obesity Hypoventilation Syndrome

Most patients with the OSA do not have daytime hypoventilation. Two groups of OSA patients who do present with hypoventilation include those with OHS and the overlap syndrome (a combination of chronic obstructive pulmonary disease [COPD] and OSA). Those obese patients (BMI > 30 kg/m²) with daytime hypoventilation (partial pressure of carbon dioxide [PCO_2] ≥ 45 mm Hg) that is not secondary to lung disease or muscle weakness are said to have OHS (Box 15–8).[88-92] These patients were previously referred to as "pickwickian." It is important to recognize whether a patient has OHS as well as OSA because this group has a high incidence of complications if not properly treated. Nowbar and colleagues[90] studied the outcomes of obese patients admitted to a medical service. Of those who had hypoventilation, the 18-month mortality was 23% compared with 9% in the group with equivalent obesity but no hypoventilation. Of interest, only 6% of the hypoventilation group received treatment for the hypoventilation!

Diagnosis of OHS

The definitive diagnosis of hypoventilation requires an arterial blood gas while awake with a PCO_2 of 45 mm Hg or greater. However, an arterial blood gas is rarely performed on a morbidly obese patient with severe OSA unless they have daytime hypoxemia or present with respiratory failure. Fortunately, an elevated serum HCO_3 (primarily HCO_3) is a very useful clue that a patient with OSA should be tested for

---

BOX 15–8

Obesity Hyperventilation Syndrome

- Daytime PCO_2 > 45 + BMI > 30 kg/m² + no lung disease
- Suspect OHS if HCO_3 > 27 mEq/L (especially without reason for metabolic alkalosis)
- High mortality if untreated
- 80–90% of OHS patients have OSA
- Severe nocturnal desaturation
- 100% sleep-related hypoventilation (worsening of daytime hypercapnia)
- Cor pulmonale—common
- Treatment
  - CPAP—daytime PCO_2 may improve, the addition of oxygen may be needed
  - BPAP—recommended for moderate to severe hypercapnia or persistent low SaO_2 on CPAP
  - BPAP + oxygen
  - Tracheostomy + oxygen—repeated respiratory failure and nonadherence to PAP

BMI = body mass index; BPAP = bilevel positive airway pressure; CPAP = continuous positive airway pressure; OHS = obesity hyperventilation syndrome; OSA = obstructive sleep apnea; PAP = positive airway pressure; PCO_2 = partial pressure of carbon dioxide.

hypoventilation. The serum CO_2 is included on routine metabolic or electrolyte laboratory panels. The elevated HCO_3 in OHS patients represents renal compensation for chronic respiratory acidosis (elevated arterial partial pressure of carbon dioxide [$PaCO_2$]). However, an elevated HCO_3 could also be due to metabolic alkalosis. Mokhlesi and associates[59] found that 20% of 410 patients referred to a sleep center to rule out OSA had OHS. In this study, only 3% of OHS patients had an HCO_3 less than 27 mEq/L but 50% of patients with an HCO_3 of 27 or greater had OHS. The authors concluded that patients with both OSA and an HCO_3 greater than 27 mEq/L should undergo arterial blood gas testing. Other clues that OHS may be present include a borderline awake SaO_2 (90–92%) or evidence of significant cor pulmonale.

Patients with the OHS are a heterogeneous group.[89] The causes of hypoventilation include nocturnal upper airway obstruction (OSA), decreased respiratory system compliance from obesity, and intrinsic or acquired abnormalities in ventilatory drive.[91] Patients with OHS have very increased levels of leptin. This is a protein produced mainly by adipose tissue that is a ventilatory stimulant and interacts with the hypothalamus to inhibit eating. OHS patients are believed to have "leptin resistance" or perhaps "central leptin deficiency".[92] Most OHS patients will have OSA (80–90%) and severe arterial oxygen desaturation.[88,92] However, up to 20% of OHS patients have an AHI of 5/hr or less but exhibit both daytime hypercapnia and severe sleep-related hypoventilation and arterial oxygen desaturation. One study characterized the patients on the basis of their response to PAP treatment.[89] Some OHS patients could be adequately treated with CPAP alone. Opening the upper airway with CPAP during sleep restored adequate oxygenation. Others still had hypoventilation despite the absence of apnea or hypopnea. Some with persistent airflow limitation responded to higher levels of CPAP (decreasing the upper airway resistance). Presumably, they could not compensate for a high upper airway resistance even if apnea and hypopnea were not present. Some patients required the addition of supplemental oxygen along with CPAP.[92,93] Another group of patients required either nasal bilevel positive airway pressure (BPAP) or mechanical ventilation with or without oxygen. The group of OHS patients who manifest hypoventilation without significant OSA are likely to have abnormal ventilatory control or very decreased respiratory system compliance due to massive obesity. The relative importance of OSA, abnormal ventilatory control, and decreased respiratory system compliance varies between individuals with OHS. Of note, patients with severe OHS who are not treated or do not comply with treatment have a high mortality.[90,94]

Treatment of OHS

Piper and coworkers[95] performed a randomized trial that compared CPAP and BPAP for treatment of patients with OHS. Patients with significant residual desaturation ($SaO_2 <$ 80% for > 10 min) on a level of CPAP that eliminated obstructive events, an acute rise in PCO_2 greater than 10 mm Hg during REM sleep, or an increase in PCO_2 greater than 10 mm Hg in the morning compared with the afternoon were excluded. An equivalent reduction in daytime PCO_2 was noted at 3 months in patients randomized to CPAP or BPAP. Adherence to the treatment modalities was also not significantly different. In the BPAP group, the mean inspiratory positive airway pressure (IPAP) and expiratory positive airway pressure (EPAP) levels used were 16 and 10 cm H_2O, respectively, and the spontaneous mode of BPAP was employed. A few patients in both groups required supplemental oxygen in addition to PAP. As noted, the most severe OHS patients were excluded from this study and were treated with noninvasive positive-pressure ventilation (NPPV; BPAP) outside of the study protocol.

OHS patients may require high levels of EPAP to prevent obstructive apnea and this tends to limit the available range of pressure support unless very high IPAP levels are used. In a study of the effect of NPPV in OHS patients by Berger and colleagues,[89] EPAP values up to 14 cm H_2O and IPAP values up to 25 cm H_2O were needed. The mean IPAP and EPAP values were 18 and 8 cm H_2O, respectively. OHS patients may present with acute respiratory failure.[96,97] The treatment of choice is PAP (usually BPAP and oxygen). Very severe patients may require temporary endotracheal intubation and mechanical ventilation. Tracheostomy can be life-saving in patients noncompliant with PAP treatment who have repeated bouts of hypercapnic respiratory failure.

For stable chronic OHS patients, treatment with PAP may reduce the daytime PCO_2 as well as reduce apnea and hypopnea and nocturnal desaturation. Berthon-Jones and Sullivan[98] showed chronic CPAP treatment of OSA patients with daytime hypoventilation resulted in a leftward shift in the ventilatory response to carbon dioxide (ventilation plotted vs. PCO_2) during the day without a change in slope (Fig. 15–8). The PCO_2 set point is lowered and there is higher ventilation at any given PCO_2. A study by Mokhlesi and associates[99] found that **the amount of improvement in the daytime PCO_2 is critically dependent on adherence**. There was considerable variability but the PCO_2 dropped by about 3 mm Hg for every hour of nightly adherence and reached a plateau with longer than 4.5 hours of use.

In summary, the treatment of OHS patients may require CPAP or BPAP with or without the need for supplemental oxygen. Although CPAP is often sufficient for some patients, most clinicians would use BPAP if the hypoventilation is moderate to severe. Adequate treatment can improve daytime as well as nocturnal gas exchange and prevent apneas and hypopneas. It is of interest that a fair number of OHS patients do not complain of significant daytime sleepiness. OHS patients may present with acute on chronic respiratory failure. Moderate to severe OHS patients have a poor prognosis if they do not receive appropriate treatment or are not adherent to treatment.

Overlap Syndrome

Patients with the OSA and COPD may have daytime hypoventilation and severe nocturnal oxygen desaturation.

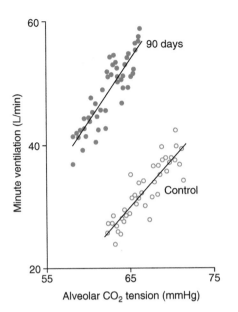

FIGURE 15–8 The ventilatory response to hypercapnia at baseline and after 90 days of continuous positive airway pressure (CPAP) treatment in OSA patients with daytime hypercapnia. The slope did not change but the curves shifted to lower alveolar partial pressure of carbon dioxide ($PACO_2$) and the set point (baseline $PACO_2$) decreased. *From Berthon-Jones M, Sullivan CE: Time course of change in ventilatory response to CO_2 with long-term CPAP therapy for obstructive sleep apnea. Am Rev Respir Dis 1987;135: 144–147.*

An epidemiologic study found that patients with mild COPD have no higher incidence of OSA than the general population.[100] However, because both COPD and OSA are common, the combination is common even if by chance. Of interest, those patients with both airway obstruction and sleep apnea in this study had worsened arterial oxygen desaturation. An early study of a group of patients with OSA and hypoventilation found that the presence of COPD was associated with hypoventilation.[101] Of note, patients with COPD alone rarely retain CO_2 until the forced expiratory volume in 1 second (FEV_1) is below 1.0 L or 40% of predicted. However, patients with OSA and mild to moderate COPD may retain CO_2.[101,102] Patients with the overlap syndrome tend to have particularly severe arterial oxygen desaturation at night. They are often assumed to simply have COPD and are treated with nocturnal oxygen alone. This may incompletely reverse the nocturnal hypoxemia and worsen the CO_2 retention during sleep.[103] The long-term outcome of patients with the overlap syndrome may worsen if upper airway obstruction is not addressed.[104] Proper treatment usually requires CPAP or BPAP and supplemental oxygen if needed.[104,105] The daytime PCO_2 may improve in some patients with adequate treatment of upper airway obstruction during sleep. Aggressive treatment of the underlying COPD with smoking cessation and bronchodilators may also be helpful in improving gas exchange both during the day and at night. More information about the overlap syndrome is contained in Chapter 22.

TABLE 15–6		
Differences Between Children and Adults with Obstructive Sleep Apnea		
	CHILDREN	**ADULTS**
CLINICAL FINDINGS		
Peak age	Preschool (4–6 yr)	60–70
Sex ratio	M = F age < 13 yr M > F if older children included	M > F
Etiology	Adenotonsillar hypertrophy	Obesity/upper airway structural shape
Weight	Variable: failure to thrive to obese	Obese
Excessive daytime sleepiness	Less common	Common
Neurobehavioral	Hyperactivity, developmental delay	Impaired vigilance
POLYSOMNOGRAPHY		
Definition of abnormal	Any obstructive apnea OAHI > 1.0–1.4	AHI ≥ 5/hr
Obstruction pattern	Obstructive hypoventilation Apnea during REM sleep	Obstructive apnea/ hypopnea Higher AHI in REM sleep
Sleep architecture	Normal	Reduced stages N3 and R
Sleep stage with OSA	REM	REM > NREM
Cortical arousal	Low rates < 50% of apneas	High rates 60–80% of apnea/ hypopnea

AHI = apnea-hypopnea index; NREM = non–rapid eye movement; OAHI = obstructive apnea-hypopnea index; OSA = obstructive sleep apnea; REM = rapid eye movement.

PEDIATRIC OSA

The major differences in the presentation and characteristics of OSA between children and adults are listed in Table 15–6.[106–110] Although very obese children or those with structural upper airway abnormalities can present with symptoms similar to those of adults, the typical history in childhood OSA is one of hyperactivity or developmental delay[111] combined with abnormal sleep behaviors observed by the parents. These nocturnal behaviors include snoring, labored breathing, diaphoresis, paradoxical chest movement, or frequent movements during sleep. Pediatric patients may also have enuresis as a manifestation of OSA. Barone and associates,[112] using a case-controlled study, found obesity and enuresis to be associated with sleep apnea but not with each other.

Epidemiology of Pediatric OSA

A 2008 review concluded that the prevalence of "always" snoring in children ranged from 1.5% to 6%.[108] Reports of "habitual snoring" ranged from 5% to 12%. The prevalence of parent-reported apneic events ranged from 0.2% to 4%. Using questionnaires filled out by parents, the prevalence of OSA has been estimated to be 4% to 11%. The prevalence by diagnostic studies has been estimated to be 1% to 4% (reported range 0.1–13%). Evidence suggests that pediatric OSA is more common among children who are heavier. Studies considering younger children (<13 yr) have generally found an equal prevalence of OSA in boys and girls. In a majority of studies including older children, a male predominance was found.[108] There may be a higher prevalence among African Americans compared with whites. The age range in which pediatric OSA is most common is said to be from 4 to 6 years (or 2 to 8 according to some authors).[106,108] This is the time that hypertrophy of the tonsils occurs.

Although pediatric patients with OSA typically present with complaints of hyperactivity and behavioral problems rather than daytime sleepiness, the presence of daytime sleepiness may be greater than previously appreciated.[113,114] First, pediatric patients in the age range for adenotonsillar hypertrophy rarely self-report sleepiness. Questionnaires have been developed to assess parental report of their children's sleepiness. However, parental report likely underestimates objective daytime sleepiness. Obesity also appears to affect the likelihood of pediatric OSA being associated with objective sleepiness. Gozal and Kheirandish-Gozal[114] found that obese children tended to be more sleepy (based on a MSLT mean sleep latency [MSL] ≤ 12 min) at **any given level of OSA**. Of interest, in over 50% of cases with documented objective sleepiness, the parents did not report excessive daytime sleepiness.

Diagnosis

The ICSD-2 criteria[13] for the diagnosis of pediatric OSA are listed in Box 15–9. The criteria emphasize parental observations as well as PSG findings. In pediatric sleep monitoring, any scoreable obstructive apnea of a duration equal to two respiratory cycles is considered abnormal. Many pediatric sleep reports separate the central from obstructive apnea-hypopnea index (OAHI). The values of the obstructive apnea index (OAI; obstructive apneas/hr of sleep) or OAHI needed to diagnose pediatric OSA remains somewhat controversial. Table 15–7 presents normative values from two publications. Most clinicians make the diagnosis of pediatric OSA based on an **obstructive** apnea index (OAI) greater than 1/hr or an OAHI greater than 1 to 2/hr. However, the decision to treat a given patient depends on symptoms. No widely accepted severity ranges are available, but many centers treat patients

BOX 15–9

Diagnostic Criteria for the Pediatric Obstructive Sleep Apnea Syndrome (ICSD-2)

A. The caregiver reports snoring, labored/obstructed breathing, or both during the child's sleep

B. The caregiver of the child reports observing at least one of the following:
   i. Paradoxical inward rib cage motion during inspiration
   ii. Movement arousals
   iii. Diaphoresis
   iv. Neck hyperextension during sleep
   v. Excessive daytime sleepiness, hyperactivity, or aggressive behavior
   vi. Slow rate of growth
   vii. Morning headaches
   viii. Secondary enuresis

C. Polysomnography recording demonstrates one or more scoreable respiratory events per hour (i.e., apnea or hypopnea of at least two respiratory cycles in duration)

D. Polysomnography recording demonstrates either i or ii
   i. At least one of the following is observed:
      a. Frequent arousals from sleep associated with increased respiratory effort
      b. Arterial oxygen desaturation in association with the apneic episodes
      c. Hypercapnia during sleep
      d. Markedly negative esophageal pressure swings
   ii. Periods of hypercapnia, desaturation, or hypercapnia with desaturation during sleep associated with snoring, paradoxical inward rib cage motion during inspiration, and at least one of the following:
      a. Frequent arousals from sleep
      b. Markedly negative esophageal pressure swings

E. The disorder is not better explained by another current sleep disorder, medical or neurologic disorder, mediation use, or substance use disorder

From American Academy of Sleep Medicine: ICSD-2 International Classification of Sleep Disorders, 2nd ed. Diagnostic and Coding Manual. Westchester, IL: American Academy of Sleep Medicine, 2005.

with an OAHI of 2 to 5/hr. An AHI of 10/hr is considered moderate to severe in children. Most apnea in pediatric patients occurs during REM sleep. However, the most common pattern in pediatric sleep monitoring is "obstructive hypoventilation" (Fig. 15–9). This pattern consists of long periods of airflow limitation, increased inspiratory effort, increased end-tidal partial pressure of carbon dioxide ($P_{ET}CO_2$), and variable amounts of arterial oxygen desaturation. Traditional monitoring (thermistor flow) often demonstrates few changes except for an elevation in $P_{ET}CO_2$ and perhaps no or mild drops in the SaO_2. Paradoxical motion of the chest and abdomen may be noted (chest moving inward during inspiration). Nasal pressure monitoring shows

TABLE 15-7

Normative Respiratory Values for Children Ages 1 to 18

VALUE	BECK AND MARCUS*	ULIEL ET AL†
Obstructive AHI (#/hr)	≤1.4	
Obstructive AI (#/hr)	0 (any obstructive apnea is considered abnormal)	1
Central apnea index (#/hr)	≤0.4	0.9
Time with SaO_2 < 89 or 90% (%TST)	0% TST < SaO_2 of 90%	0% TST < SaO_2 of 89%
SaO_2 nadir	≥91%	≥89 Baseline sleeping SaO_2 > 92%
Time $P_{ET}CO_2$ ≥ 50 mm Hg	<25%	
Time $P_{ET}CO_2$ > 45 mm Hg		<10%
Periodic limb movement index (#/hr)	≤4.3	

AHI = apnea-hypopnea index; AI = apnea index; $P_{ET}CO_2$ = end-tidal carbon dioxide pressure; SaO_2 = arterial oxygen saturation; TST = total sleep time.
*Beck SE, Marcus SL: Pediatric polysomnography. Sleep Med Clin 2009;4:393–406.
†Uliel S, Tauman R, Greenfield M, et al: Normal polysomnography respiratory values in children and adolescents. Chest 2004;125:872–878.

airflow limitation (flattening) and reduced but stable flow. This common pattern is the reason that $P_{ET}CO_2$ is an integral part of most pediatric sleep studies. The AASM scoring manual states that sleep-related hypoventilation in children should be scored when the PCO_2 > 50 mm Hg for ≥25% of the total sleep time using transcutaneous or end-tidal measurement of the PCO_2.[9] However, a PSG study of normal children by Uliel and coworkers[115] recommended that $P_{ET}CO_2$ greater than 45 mm Hg for longer than 10% of total sleep time be considered abnormal.

Although the major cause of OSA in children is adenotonsillar hypertrophy, tonsil size does not correlate with findings on sleep studies. One child with large tonsils may be without symptoms while another with modest tonsil enlargement may have significant symptoms. Other upper airway characteristics are likely responsible. With the obesity epidemic in children, obesity is becoming a major risk factor for OSA in children. Indeed, very obese children may present with symptoms similar to those of adults (daytime sleepiness).

Tonsillectomy and adenoidectomy (TNA) is considered the treatment of choice in patients with pediatric sleep apnea (even if obese). A PSG is recommended before TNA to avoid unnecessary surgery and to triage patients to appropriate postsurgical care. Patients with a high AHI, extremes of body weight, severe oxygen desaturation, cor pulmonale, daytime hypoventilation, young age, and congenital craniofacial abnormalities are at an increased risk for postoperative complications. In high-risk patients, TNA should be performed in the hospital with appropriate postoperative monitoring.[105,116] The efficacy of TNA is much lower than expected and a postoperative PSG is recommended.[117,118] Even if TNA is initially successful, symptoms of OSA can recur in later life. The surgical treatment of OSA in pediatric patients is

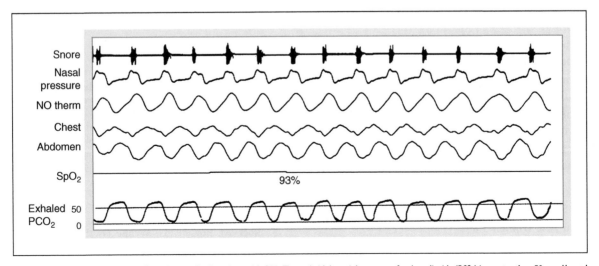

FIGURE 15-9 Obstructive hypoventilation in a pediatric patient with OSA. The end-tidal partial pressure of carbon dioxide (PCO_2) is greater than 50 mm Hg and there is evidence of flattening of the nasal pressure (airflow limitation). A very mild drop in the pulse oximetry (SpO_2) is noted.

discussed in more detail in Chapter 20. Patients with significant residual OSA following TNA can be treated with weight loss, CPAP, or other surgical procedures.

CLINICAL REVIEW QUESTIONS

1. Of the following, what is the best documented risk factor for OSA?
   A. Cigarette smoking.
   B. Alcohol consumption.
   C. Postmenopausal status.
   D. Obesity.

2. Which of the following is NOT **always** true about patients with the OHS?
   A. Daytime $PCO_2 \geq 45$ mm Hg.
   B. BMI > 30 kg/m^2.
   C. Worsening PCO_2 and PO_2 with sleep.
   D. AHI ≥ 5/hr.

3. Which of the following symptoms is less typical of pediatric patients with OSA?
   A. Diaphoresis and labored breathing during sleep.
   B. Hyperactivity or behavioral problems.
   C. Adenotonsillar hypertrophy of variable severity.
   D. Daytime sleepiness.

4. Which of the following is the ICSD-2 criterion for diagnosis of OSA in adults?
   A. (Apneas + hypopneas + RERAs)/hr = 5/hr.
   B. (Apneas + hypopneas + RERAs)/hr = 15/hr.
   C. (Apneas + hypopneas + RERAs)/hr = 5/hr + symptoms
   D. (Apneas + hypopneas + RERAs)/hr = 5/hr + symptoms OR (Apneas + hypopneas + RERAs)/hr ≥ 15/hr.

5. Which of the following group of symptoms in a patient would indicate a good candidate for portable monitoring?
   A. Snoring, witnessed apnea, daytime sleepiness, hypertension.
   B. Snoring, witnessed apnea, congestive heart failure, daytime sleepiness.
   C. Snoring, no witnessed apnea, nonrestorative sleep, no daytime sleepiness.
   D. Snoring, daytime sleepiness, neuromuscular disorder.

6. What is the approximate prevalence of OSA defined as an AHI ≥ 5/hr associated with symptoms?
   A. Men 10% Women 5%
   B. Men 4% Women 2%
   C. Men 2% Women 1%
   D. Men 4% Women 4%

7. Which of the following combinations has the highest probability of having OSA?
   A. Snoring, no witnessed apnea, hypertension.
   B. Snoring, daytime sleepiness, no witnessed apnea.
   C. Snoring, witnessed apnea, hypertension.
   D. No snoring, no witnessed apnea, daytime sleepiness.

Answers

1. **D.** Obesity is the best documented risk factor of those listed.

2. **D.** Approximately 20% of OHS patients do not have OSA but simply have daytime hypoventilation that worsens during sleep.

3. **D.** Daytime sleepiness is not a major complaint of pediatric OSA patients. However, sleepiness may not be recognized. Obese pediatric OSA patients are more likely to report sleepiness.

4. **D.** This option most completely describes the criteria for adult OSA.

5. **A.** This describes a patient with a high probability of moderate to severe OSA who does not have co-morbid medical disorder such as congestive heart failure or a neuromuscular disorder. Patient C may well have sleep apnea but is not considered to have a high probability of having OSA based on lack of witnessed apnea.

6. **B.** This answer describes the findings of the Wisconsin study by Young and associates. The prevalence likely varies with the population being studied and the prevalence may well be increasing owing to the obesity epidemic.

7. **C.** Snoring, witnessed apnea, and hypertension were found to be major risk factors for the presence of OSA. Although daytime sleepiness is a cardinal symptom of OSA, many OSA patients do not report sleepiness.

REFERENCES

1. Burwell C, Robin E, Whaley R, Bickelman A: Extreme obesity associated with alveolar hypoventilation—a pickwickian syndrome. Am J Med 1956;21:811–818.
2. Guilleminault C, Tilikan A, Dement WC: The sleep apnea syndromes. Annu Rev Med 1976;27:465–484.
3. Gulleminault C: Obstructive sleep apnea: the clinical syndrome and historical perspective. Med Clin North Am 1985;69:1187–1203.
4. Remmers JE, Degroot WJ, Sauerland EK, et al: Pathogenesis of upper airway occlusion during sleep. J Appl Physiol 1978;44:931–938.
5. Block AJ, Boysen PG, Wynne JW, Hunt LA: Sleep apnea, hypopnea, and oxygen desaturation in normal subjects. N Engl J Med 1979;300:513–517.
6. Gould GA, Whyte KF, Rhind GB, et al: The sleep hypopnea syndrome. Am Rev Respir Dis 1988;137:895–898.

7. Redline S, Sander M: Hypopnea, a floating metric: implications for prevalence, morbidity estimates, and case finding. Sleep 1997;20:1209–1217.
8. Redline S, Kapur VK, Sanders MH, et al: Effects of varying approaches for identifying respiratory disturbances on sleep apnea assessment. Am J Respir Crit Care Med 2000;161:369–374.
9. Iber C, Ancoli-Israel S, Chesson A, Quan SF, for the American Academy of Sleep Medicine: The AASM Manual for Scoring of Sleep and Associated Events: Rules, Terminology and Technical Specifications, 1st ed. Westchester, IL: American Academy of Sleep Medicine, 2007.
10. Revision of NCD240.4 CPAP Therapy for OSA. Transmittal R96 (recent revision). Available at https://www.cms.gov/transmittals/downloads/R96NCD.pdf
11. American Academy of Sleep Medicine Task Force: Sleep-related breathing disorders in adults: recommendation for syndrome definition and measurement techniques in clinical research. Sleep 1999;22:667–689.
12. Loube DI, Gay PC, Strohl KP, et al: Indications for positive airway pressure treatment of adult obstructive sleep apnea patients. A consensus statement. Chest 1999;115:863–866.
13. American Academy of Sleep Medicine: ICSD-2 International Classification of Sleep Disorders, 2nd ed. Diagnostic and Coding Manual. Westchester, IL: American Academy of Sleep Medicine, 2005.
14. Young T, Palta M, Leder R, et al: The occurrence of sleep-disordered breathing among middle-aged adults. N Engl J Med 1993;328:1230–1235.
15. Bixler E, Vgontzas A, Ten Have T, et al: Effects of age on sleep apnea in men. Am J Respir Crit Care Med 1998;157:144–148.
16. Young T, Peppard PE, Gottlieb DJ: Epidemiology of obstructive sleep apnea. Am J Respir Crit Care Med 2002;165:1217–1239.
17. Young T, Evans L, Finn L, Palta M: Estimation of the clinically diagnosed proportion of sleep apnea syndrome in middle aged men and women. Sleep 1997;20:705–709.
18. Malhotra A, White DP: Obstructive sleep apnea. Lancet 2002;360:237–245.
19. Peppard PE, Young T, Palta M, et al: Longitudinal study of moderate weight change and sleep-disordered breathing. JAMA 2000;284:3015–3021.
20. Stradling JR, Crosby JH: Predictors and prevalence of obstructive sleep apnea and snoring in 1001 middle aged men. Thorax 1991;46:85–90.
21. Davies RJ, Ali NJ, Stradling JR: Neck circumference and other clinical features in the diagnosis of the obstructive sleep apnoea syndrome. Thorax 1992;47:101–105.
22. Smith PL, Gold AR, Meyers DA, et al: Weight loss in mildly to moderately obese patients with obstructive sleep apnea. Ann Intern Med 1985;103:850–855.
23. Schwartz AR, Gold AR, Schubert N, et al: Effect of weight loss on upper airway collapsibility in obstructive sleep apnea. Am Rev Respir Dis 1991;144:494–498.
24. Flemons WW: Obstructive sleep apnea. N Engl J Med 2002;347:498–504.
25. Simpson L, Mukherjee S, Cooper MN, et al: Sex differences in the association of regional fat distribution with the severity of obstructive sleep apnea. Sleep 2010;33:467–474.
26. Bixler E, Vgontzas A, Ten Have T, et al: Prevalence of sleep disordered breathing in women. Am J Respir Crit Care Med 2001;163:608–613.
27. Young T, Shahar E, Nieto FJ, et al: Predictors of sleep disordered breathing in community dwelling adults: the Sleep Heart Health Study. Arch Intern Med 2002;162:893–900.
28. Ancoli-Israel S, Klauber MR, Kripke DF: Sleep disordered breathing in a community dwelling elderly. Sleep 1991;14:486–495.
29. Enright PL, Newman AB, Wahl PW, et al: Prevalence and correlates of snoring and observed apneas in 5,201 older adults. Sleep 1996;19:531–538.
30. Young T: Sleep-disordered breathing in older adults. Is it a condition distinct from that in middle-aged adults? Sleep 1996;19:529–530.
31. Young T, Finn L, Austin D, Peterson A: Menopausal status and sleep disordered breathing in the Wisconsin Sleep Cohort Study. Am J Respir Crit Care Med 2003;167:1181–1185.
32. Shahar E, Redline S, Young T, et al for the Sleep Heart Health Study Research Group: Hormone replacement therapy and sleep disordered breathing. Am J Respir Crit Care Med 2003;167;1186–1192.
33. Ancoli-Israel S, Klauber M, Stepnowksy C, et al: Sleep-disordered breathing in African-American elderly. Am J Respir Crit Care Med 1995;152:1946–1949.
34. Redline S, Tishler PV, Hans MG, et al: Racial differences in sleep-disordered breathing in African-Americans and Caucasians. Am J Respir Crit Care Med 1997;153:186–192.
35. Ip M, Lam B, Lauder I, et al: A community study of sleep disordered breathing in middle-aged Chinese men in Hong Kong. Chest 2001;119:62–69.
36. Li KK, Kushida C, Powell NB, et al: Obstructive sleep apnea syndrome: a comparison between Far-East Asian and white men. Laryngoscope 2000;110:1689–1693.
37. Wetter DW, Young TB, Bidwell TR, et al: Smoking as a risk factor for sleep-disordered breathing. Arch Intern Med 1994;154:2219–2224.
38. Issa FG, Sullivan CE: Alcohol, snoring, and sleep apnea. J Neurol Neurosurg 1982;45:353–359.
39. Scanlan MF, Roebuck T, Little PJ, et al: Effect of moderate alcohol upon obstructive sleep apnea. Eur Respir J 2000;16:909–913.
40. Block AJ, Hellard DW, Slayton PC: Effect of alcohol ingestion on breathing and oxygenation during sleep. Analysis of the influence of age and sex. Am J Med 1986;80:595–600.
41. Berry RB, Bonnet MH, Light RW: Effect of ethanol on the arousal response to airway occlusion during sleep in normal subjects. Am Rev Respir Dis 1982;145:445–452.
42. Grunstein RR, Sullivan CE: Sleep apnea and hypothyroidism: mechanisms and management. Am J Med 1988;85:775–779.
43. Pelttari L, Rauhala E, Polo O, et al: Upper airway obstruction in hypothyroidism. J Intern Med 1994;236:177–181.
44. Lin CC, Tsan KW, Chen PJ: The relationship between sleep apnea syndrome and hypothyroidism. Chest 1992;102:1663–1667.
45. Winkelman JW, Goldman H, Piscatelli N, et al: Are thyroid function tests necessary in patients with suspected sleep apnea? Sleep 1996;19:790–793.
46. Grunstein RR, Ho KY, Sullivan CE: Sleep apnea in acromegaly. Ann Intern Med 1991;115:527–532.
47. Weiss V, Sonka K, Pretl M, et al: Prevalence of the sleep apnea syndrome in acromegaly population. J Endocrinol Invest 2000;23:515–519.
48. Astrom C, Christensen L, Gjerris F, et al: Sleep in acromegaly before and after treatment with adenomectomy. Neuroendocrinology 1991;53:328–331.
49. Epstein LJ, Kristo D, Strollo PJ, et al: Clinical guideline for the evaluation, management and long-term care of obstructive sleep apnea in adults. J Clin Sleep Med 2009;5:263–276.
50. Johns MW: Daytime sleepiness, snoring, and obstructive sleep apnea. The Epworth Sleepiness Scale. Chest 1993;103:30–36.
51. Bennett LS, Langford BA, Stradling JR: Sleep fragmentation indices as predictors of daytime sleepiness and nCPAP response in obstructive sleep apnea. Am J Respir Crit Care Med 1998;158:778–786.

52. Gottlieb DJ, Whitney CW, Bonekat WH, et al: Relation of sleepiness to respiratory disturbance index. Am J Respir Crit Care Med 1999;159:502–507.

53. Walker RP, Durazo Arvizu R, Wachter B, Gopalsami C: Preoperative differences between male and female patients with sleep apnea. Laryngoscope 2001;111:1501–1505.

54. Shepertycky MR, Bano K, Kryger MH: Differences between men and women in the clinical presentation of patients diagnosed with obstructive sleep apnea syndrome. Sleep 2005;28:309–314.

55. Quintana-Gallego E, Carmona-Bernal C, Capote F, et al: Gender differences in obstructive sleep apnea syndrome: a clinical study of 1166 patients. Respir Med 2004;98: 984–989.

56. Friedman M, Tanyeri H, La Rosa M, et al: Clinical predictors of obstructive sleep apnea. Laryngoscope 1999;109:1901–1907.

57. Zonato A, Bittencour LR, Martiho FL, et al: Association of systematic head and neck physical examination with the severity of obstructive apnea-hypopnea syndrome. Laryngoscope 2003;113:973–980.

58. Nuckton TJ, Glidden DV, Brownder WS, Claman DM: Physical examination: Mallampati score as an independent predictor of obstructive sleep apnea. Sleep 2006;29:903–908.

59. Mokhlesi B, Taulaimat A, Baibussowitsch I, et al: Obesity hypoventilation syndrome: prevalence and predictors in patients with obstructive sleep apnea. Sleep Breath 2007; 11:117–124.

60. Berry RB, Sriram P: Evaluation of hypoventilation. Semin Respir Crit Care Med 2009;30:303–314.

61. Flemons W, Whitelaw WA, Bryant R, Remmers JE: Likelihood ratios for a sleep apnea clinical prediction rule. Am J Respir Care Med 1994;150:1279–1285.

62. Netzer NC, Stoohs RA, Netzer CM, et al: Using the Berlin questionnaire to identify patients at risk for the sleep apnea syndrome. Ann Intern Med 1999;131:485–491.

63. Ong TH, Raudha S, Fook-Chong S, et al: Simplifying STOP-BANG: use of a simple questionnaire to screen for OSA in an Asian population. Sleep Breath 2010;14:371–376; Epub 2010;April 26.

64. Chung F, Yegneswaran B, Liao P, et al: STOP questionnaire: a tool to screen patients for obstructive sleep apnea. Anesthesiology 2008;108:812–821.

65. Kushida CA, Littner MR, Morgenthaler T, et al: Practice parameters for the indications for polysomnography and related procedures. An update for 2005. Sleep 2005;28: 499–521.

66. Oksenberg A, Khamaysi I, Silverberg DS, Tarasiuk A: Association of body position with severity of apneic events in patients with severe nonpositional obstructive sleep apnea. Chest 2000;118:1018–1024.

67. Oksenberg A, Silverberg DS, Arons E, Radwan H: Positional vs nonpositional obstructive sleep apnea patients: anthropomorphic, nocturnal polysomnographic, and multiple sleep latency test data. Chest 1997;112:629–639.

68. Findley LJ, Wihoit SC, Surrat PM: Apnea duration and hypoxemia during REM sleep in patients with obstructive sleep apnea. Chest 1985;87:432–436.

69. Oksenberg A, Arons E, Nasser K, et al: REM-related obstructive sleep apnea: the effect of body position. J Clin Sleep Med 2010;6:343–348.

70. Kass JE, Akers SM, Bartter TC, et al: Rapid-eye-movement–specific sleep-disordered breathing: a possible cause of daytime sleepiness. Am J Respir Crit Care Med 1996;154: 167–169.

71. Haba-Rubio J, Janssens JP, Rochat T, et al. Rapid eye movement related disordered breathing: clinical and polysomnographic features. Chest 2005;128:3350–3357.

72. Punjabi NM, Bandeen-Roche K, Marx JJ, et al: The association between daytime sleepiness and sleep-disordered breathing in NREM and REM sleep. Sleep 2002;25:307–314

73. Chami HA, Baldwin CM, Silverman A, et al: Sleepiness, quality of life, and sleep maintenance in REM versus non-REM sleep-disordered breathing. Am J Respir Crit Care Med 2010;181:997–1002.

74. Zwillich C, Devlin T, White D, et al: Bradycardia during sleep apnea. Characteristics and mechanisms. J Clin Invest 1982;69:1286–1292.

75. Bonsignore MR, Romano S, Marrone O, et al: Different heart rate patterns in obstructive sleep apnea during NREM sleep. Sleep 1997;20:1167–1174.

76. Bradley TD, Martinez D, Rutherford R, et al: Physiological determinants of nocturnal arterial oxygenation in patients with obstructive sleep apnea. J Appl Physiol 1985;59: 1364–1368.

77. Peppard PE, Ward NR, Morrell MJ: The impact of obesity on oxygen desaturation during sleep disordered breathing. Am J Respir Crit Care Med 2009;180:788–793.

78. Collop NA, Anderson WM, Boehlecke B, et al: Clinical guidelines for the use of unattended portable monitors in the diagnosis of obstructive sleep apnea in adult patients. Portable Monitoring Task Force of the American Academy of Sleep Medicine. J Clin Sleep Med 2007;3:737–747.

79. Hoffstein V: Snoring. Chest 1996;109:201–222.

80. Lee SA, Amis TC, Byth K, et al: Heavy snoring as a cause of carotid atherosclerosis. Sleep 2008;31:1207–1213.

81. Littner M, Kushida CA, Hartse SE, et al: Practice parameters for the use of laser-assisted uvulopalatoplasty: an update 2000. Sleep 2001;24:603–619.

82. Berry RB, Block AJ: Positive nasal airway pressure eliminates snoring as well as obstructive sleep apnea. Chest 1984;85: 15–20.

83. Guilleminault C, Stoohs R, Clerk A, et al: A cause of excessive daytime sleepiness: the upper airway resistance syndrome. Chest 1993;104:781–787.

84. Douglas NJ: Upper airway resistance syndrome is not a distinct syndrome. Am J Respir Crit Care Med 2000;161: 1413–1416.

85. Guilleminault C, Chowdhuri S: Upper airway resistance syndrome is a distinct syndrome. Am J Respir Crit Care Med 2001;161:1412–1413.

86. Masa JF, Corral J, Teran J, et al: Apnoeic and obstructive nonapnoeic sleep respiratory events. Eur Respir J 2009;34: 156–161.

87. Cracowski C, Pépin JL, Wuyam B, Lévy P: Characterization of obstructive nonapneic respiratory events in moderate sleep apnea syndrome. Am J Respir Crit Care Med 2001;164: 944–948.

88. Rapoport DM, Sorkin B, Garay SM, Goldring RM: Reversal of the "Pickwickian syndrome" by long-term use of nocturnal nasal-airway pressure. N Engl J Med 1982;307:931–933.

89. Berger KI, Ayappa I, Chatr-Amontri B, et al: Obesity hypoventilation syndrome as a spectrum of respiratory disturbances during sleep. Chest 2001;120:1231–1238.

90. Nowbar S, Burkart KM, Gonzales R, et al: Obesity-hypoventilation in hospitalized patients: prevalence, effects, and outcome. Am J Med 2004;116:1–7.

91. Pérez de Llano LA, Golpe R, Piquer MO, et al: Clinical heterogeneity among patients with obesity hypoventilation syndrome: therapeutic implications. Respiration 2008;75:34–39.

92. Piper AJ, Grunstein RR: Obesity hypoventilation syndrome: mechanisms and management. Am J Respir Crit Care Med 2011;183:292–298.

93. Banerjee D, Yee BJ, Piper AJ, et al: Obesity hypoventilation syndrome: hypoxemia during continuous positive airway pressure. Chest 2007;131:1678–1684.

94. Budweiser S, Riedl SG, Jörres RA, et al: Mortality and prognostic factors in patients with obesity-hypoventilation syndrome undergoing noninvasive ventilation. J Intern Med 2007;261:375–383.

95. Piper AJ, Wang D, Yee BJ, et al: Randomized trial of CPAP vs bilevel support in the treatment of obesity hypoventilation syndrome without severe nocturnal desaturation. Thorax 2008;63:395–401.

96. Shivaram U, Cash ME, Beal A: Nasal continuous positive airway pressure in decompensated hypercapnic respiratory failure as a complication of sleep apnea. Chest 1993;104:770–774.

97. Piper AJ, Sullivan CE: Effects of short-term NIPPV in the treatment of patients with severe obstructive sleep apnea and hypercapnia. Chest 1994;105:434–440.

98. Berthon-Jones M, Sullivan CE: Time course of change in ventilatory response to CO_2 with long-term CPAP therapy for obstructive sleep apnea. Am Rev Respir Dis 1987;135:144–147.

99. Mokhlesi B, Tulaimat A, Evans AT, et al: Impact of adherence with positive airway pressure therapy on hypercapnia in obstructive sleep apnea. J Clin Sleep Med 2006;2:57–62.

100. Sander MH, Newman AB, Haggerty CL, et al: Sleep and sleep disordered breathing in adults with predominantly mild obstructive airway disease. Am J Respir Crit Care Med 2003;167:7–14.

101. Bradley TD, Rutherford R, Lue F, et al: Role of diffuse airway obstruction in the hypercapnia of obstructive sleep apnea. Am Rev Respir Dis 1986;134:920–924.

102. Chan CS, Grunstein RR, Bye PTP, et al: Obstructive sleep apnea with chronic airflow limitation: comparison of hypercapnic and eucapnic patients. Am Rev Respir Dis 1989;140:1274–1278.

103. Goldstein RS, Ramcharan V, Bowes G, et al: Effect of supplemental nocturnal oxygen on gas exchange in patients with severe obstructive lung disease. N Engl J Med 1984;310:425–429.

104. Fletcher EC, Schaaf JW, Miller J, Fletcher JG: Long-term cardiopulmonary sequelae in patients with sleep apnea and chronic lung disease. Am Rev Respir Dis 1987;135:525–533.

105. Sampol G, Sagalés MT, Roca A, et al: Nasal continuous positive airway pressure with supplemental oxygen in coexistent sleep apnea-hypopnea syndrome and severe chronic obstructive pulmonary disease. Eur Respir J 1996;9:111–116.

106. Marcus CL. Sleep-disordered breathing in children. Am J Respir Crit Care Med 2001;164:16–30.

107. American Academy of Pediatrics: Clinical practice guideline: diagnosis and management of childhood obstructive sleep apnea syndrome. Pediatrics 2002;109:704–712.

108. Lumeng JC, Chervin RD: Epidemiology of pediatric OSA. Proc Am Thorac Soc 2008;5:242–252.

109. Katz ES, D'Ambrosio CM: Pediatric obstructive sleep apnea syndrome. Clin Chest Med 2010;31:221–234.

110. Carroll JL, Loughlin GM: Obstructive sleep apnea in infants and children: diagnosis and management. In Ferber R, Kryger M (eds): Principles and Practice of Sleep Medicine in the Child. Philadelphia: WB Saunders, 1995, pp. 193–230.

111. Chervin RD, Archbold KH, Dillon JE, et al: Inattention, hyperactivity, and symptoms of sleep-disordered breathing. Pediatrics 2002;109:449–456.

112. Barone JG, Hanson C, DaJusta DG, et al: Nocturnal enuresis and overweight are associated with obstructive sleep apnea. Pediatrics 2009;124:e53–e59.

113. Chervin RD, Weatherly RA, Ruzicka DL, et al: Subjective sleepiness and polysomnographic correlates in children scheduled for adenotonsillectomy vs other surgical care. Sleep 2006;29:495–503.

114. Gozal D, Kheirandish-Gozal L: Obesity and excessive daytime sleepiness in prepubertal children with obstructive sleep apnea. Pediatrics 2009;123:13–18.

115. Uliel S, Tauman R, Greenfield M, et al: Normal polysomnography respiratory values in children and adolescents. Chest 2004;125:872–878.

116. Rosen GM, Muckle RP, Mahowald MW, et al: Postoperative respiratory compromise in children with obstructive sleep apnea syndrome: can it be anticipated? Pediatrics 1994;93:784–788.

117. Brietzke SE, Gallagher D: The effectiveness of tonsillectomy and adenoidectomy in the treatment of pediatric obstructive sleep apnea/hypopnea syndrome: a meta-analysis. Otolaryngol Head Neck Surg 2006;134:979–984.

118. Friedman M, Wilson M, Chang HW: Updated systematic review of tonsillectomy and adenoidectomy for treatment of pediatric obstructive sleep apnea/hypopnea syndrome. Otolaryngol Head Neck Surg 2009;140:800–808.

Berlin Questionnaire

Please choose the correct response to each question.

Category 1

1. Do you snore?
   a. Yes*
   b. No
   c. Don't know

If you snore:

2. Your snoring is:
   a. Slightly louder than breathing
   b. As loud as talking
   c. Louder than talking*
   d. Very loud—can be heard in adjacent rooms*

3. How often do you snore?
   a. Nearly every day*
   b. 3–4 times/wk*
   c. 1–2 times/wk
   d. 1–2 times/mo
   e. Never or nearly never

4. Has your snoring ever bothered other people?
   a. Yes*
   b. No
   c. Don't know

5. Has anyone noticed that you quit breathing during your sleep?
   a. Nearly every day*
   b. 3–4 times/wk*
   c. 1–2 times/wk
   d. 1–2 times/mo
   e. Never or nearly never

Category 2

6. How often do you feel tired or fatigued after your sleep?
   a. Nearly every day*
   b. 3–4 times/wk*
   c. 1–2 times/wk
   d. 1–2 times/mo
   e. Never or nearly never

7. During your waking time, do you feel tired, fatigued, or not up to par?
   a. Nearly every day*
   b. 3–4 times/wk*
   c. 1–2 times/wk
   d. 1–2 times/mo
   e. Never or nearly never

8. Have you ever nodded off or fallen asleep while driving a vehicle?
   a. Yes*
   b. No

If yes:

9. How often does this occur?
   a. Nearly every day
   b. 3–4 times/wk
   c. 1–2 times/wk
   d. 1–2 times/mo

Category 3: Somnolence

One or more of the following are present:
   a. Frequent somnolence or fatigue despite adequate "sleep"
   b. Falls asleep easily in a nonstimulating environment (e.g., watching TV, reading, riding in or driving a car) despite adequate "sleep"
   c. [Parent or teacher comments that child appears sleepy during the day, is easily distracted, is overly aggressive, or has difficulty concentrating][†]
   d. [Child often difficult to arouse at usual awakening time][†]

Scoring:

If two or more items in category 1 are positive, category 1 is positive.
If two or more items in category 2 are positive, category 2 is positive.
If one or more items in category 3 are positive, category 3 is positive.
High risk of OSA: Two or more categories scored as positive.
Low risk of OSA: Only one or no category positive.

---

*Items are considered positive.
†Pediatric questions.
OSA = obstructive sleep apnea.

STOP-BANG Scoring Model

1. **S**noring
Do you snore loudly (louder than talking or loud enough to be heard through closed doors)? Yes No

2. **T**ired
Do you often feel *t*ired, fatigued, or sleepy during daytime? Yes No

3. **O**bserved
Has anyone *o*bserved you stop breathing during your sleep? Yes No

4. Blood **p**ressure
Do you have or are you being treated for high blood *p*ressure? Yes No

5. **B**MI
*B*MI > 35 kg/m² ? Yes No

6. **A**ge
*A*ge older than 50 yr old? Yes No

7. **N**eck circumference
*N*eck circumference > 40 cm? Yes No

8. **G**ender
*G*ender male? Yes No

High risk of OSA: Answering yes to three or more items.
Low risk of OSA: Answering yes to less than three items.

BMI = body mass index; OSA = obstructive sleep apnea.

Chapter 16

Pathophysiology of Obstructive Sleep Apnea

Chapter Points

- Patients with OSA have a positive critical pressure during sleep. A positive intraluminal pressure is needed to keep the airway patent.
- Patients with OSA have airway occlusion or severe narrowing during sleep because of a variable combination of factors including unfavorable upper airway anatomy, inadequate upper airway muscle compensation, and instability in ventilatory control. Whereas a high arousal threshold may prolong respiratory events, a low arousal threshold may predispose to instability in ventilatory control.

Traits Contributing to Obstructive Sleep Apnea

ANATOMIC/ PHYSIOLOGIC TRAIT	APNEA PREDISPOSITION
Upper airway anatomy	Small pharyngeal airway
Upper airway motor control	Poor muscle response during sleep
Ventilatory control stability	High loop gain
Arousal threshold	Low arousal threshold

From White DP: The pathogenesis of obstructive sleep apnea. Am J Respir Cell Mol Biol 2006;34:1–6.

- The reasons for the greater prevalence of OSA in men than in women are incompletely understood. Men have longer upper airways and this may predispose to upper airway collapse.
- The activity of phasic upper airway muscles (e.g., genioglossus—tongue protruder) increases with each inspiration. The activity of tonic upper airway muscles is constant (does not vary with respiration). However, the activity level of tonic muscles can vary with sleep state (wake > NREM > REM). The activity of phasic upper airway muscles is controlled by central pattern generators, sleep state (wakefulness stimuli, NREM, REM), and negative-pressure stimulation of upper airway mechanoreceptors. More negative upper airway

pressure is associated with increased upper airway inspiratory activity in the genioglossus.
- Upper airway muscle activity falls with sleep onset and the decrease is greater in patients with OSA than in normal individuals. During wake, increased upper airway muscle activity in patients with OSA may compensate for unfavorable anatomy.
- The arousal stimulus during obstructive apnea and hypopnea appears to be proportional to the magnitude of inspiratory effort (esophageal pressure excursions). Hypercapnia and hypoxemia may cause increasing respiratory effort, but arousal occurs when the level of effort reaches an arousal threshold.
- The arousal threshold to respiratory stimuli during NREM sleep is increased in patients with OSA compared with normal individuals (higher inspiratory effort is needed to trigger arousal).
- Factors associated with more severe arterial oxygen desaturation include a higher BMI, low awake SaO_2 or PaO_2, longer respiratory events/shorter period of ventilation between events, and a smaller ERV.

PATHOGENESIS OF UPPER AIRWAY OBSTRUCTION

Multiple factors determine upper airway patency during sleep (Table 16–1).[1-9] Different factors may be more or less important in a given individual. Patients with obstructive sleep apnea (OSA) tend to have small upper airways either secondary to a small bony enclosure or due to increased soft tissue surrounding the airway.[10,11] In general, a short and posteriorly placed mandible, a long dependent palate, a large tongue, nasal obstruction, and thick lateral pharyngeal walls, and/or pharyngeal fat all predispose to upper airway collapse during sleep. Most studies have suggested that the shape of the upper airways of OSA patients differs from that of normal individuals and is narrower in the lateral dimension.[10-12] A study comparing the passive properties of the upper airway during general anesthesia in normal individuals with those of OSA patients found that the upper airways of OSA patients are narrower and more collapsible.[13]

Airflow through the pharynx shows various degrees of airflow limitation during sleep. Inspiratory flow limitation is defined by an increase in the pressure drop across the upper airway (more negative supraglottic and intrathoracic pressure) without a corresponding increase in flow rate (Fig. 16–1). This alinearity in the pressure-flow relationship

TABLE 16–1	
Factors Determining Upper Airway Patency	
OPEN UPPER AIRWAY	**CLOSED UPPER AIRWAY**
PASSIVE FACTORS	
• Larger, stiffer upper airway (P_{CRIT} 0 or negative) • Large bony enclosure • Less soft tissue (thinner lateral pharyngeal walls) • Higher lung volume • Lateral decubitus posture	• Smaller, more compliant upper airway (positive P_{CRIT}) • Small bony enclosure • More soft tissue • Lower lung volume • Supine posture
UPPER AIRWAY MUSCLE FACTORS	
• High upper airway muscle activity • Large upper airway muscle response to negative pressure	• Low upper airway muscle activity • Low upper airway muscle response to negative upper airway pressure
VENTILATORY CONTROL STABILITY	
STABLE VENTILATORY DRIVE	FLUCTUATING VENTILATORY DRIVE

• Low loop gain
  • Low controller gain
  • Low plant gain
• High arousal threshold
	• High loop gain
	  • High controller gain
	  • High plant gain
	• Low arousal threshold

P_{CRIT} = passive closing pressure of the upper airway.	

during inspiration is commonly caused by narrowing of a hypotonic upper airway in response to the increasingly negative intraluminal pressure developed during inspiration.[14,15] In Figure 16–2, the first three breaths do not show airflow limitation and airflow has a round shape. The fourth breath, which occurs after sleep onset, demonstrates airflow limitation with a constant flow during the time when the inspiratory pressure (supraglottic pressure) as reflected by esophageal pressure is becoming more negative (increased pressure difference across the upper airway).

The pharynx is not rigid and pharyngeal resistance is not constant. The nonrigid portions of the pharynx tend to become increasingly narrow with more negative inspiratory pressure. The collapsibility of the upper airway and tendency for closure can be defined by the pharyngeal passive closing pressure (P_{CRIT}).[16,17] The P_{CRIT} values for normal people, snorers, patients with obstructive hypopneas, and patients with obstructive apnea are plotted in Figure 16–3.[14] As upper airway dysfunction increases (normal → snorers → apnea), the P_{CRIT} is progressively more positive. During sleep, a positive pressure is needed to keep the airway open ($P_{CRIT} > 0$) in patients with sleep apnea. In normal patients, the airway does not collapse unless a negative mask pressure is applied.

The P_{CRIT} is determined by applying various positive or negative mask pressures (Pmask) and determining the inspiratory flow rate. In patients with OSA, flow decreases as mask pressure decreases from a more positive pressure (Fig. 16–4). The mask pressure at which flow is zero is P_{CRIT}. The inverse of the slope is the effective resistance (Δ pressure/Δ flow) and is called the *upstream resistance (Rus)*. The equation relating flow ($\dot{V}$max), mask pressure, and P_{CRIT}

$$\dot{V}max = (Pmask - P_{CRIT})/R_{us}$$

Pus = Pmask in Starling resistor model

Equation 16–1

The relationship between flow and mask pressure can be modeled using a Starling resistor (Fig. 16–5) using Pus

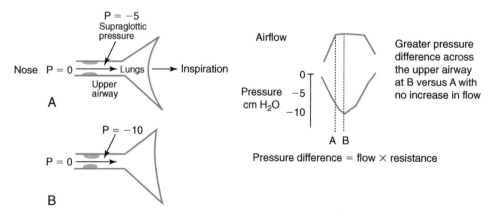

FIGURE 16–1 A higher pressure (P) difference across the upper airway (more negative supraglottic pressure) at B compared with A does not increase airflow. This is an example of airflow limitation. The effective resistance has increased with more negative supraglottic pressure.

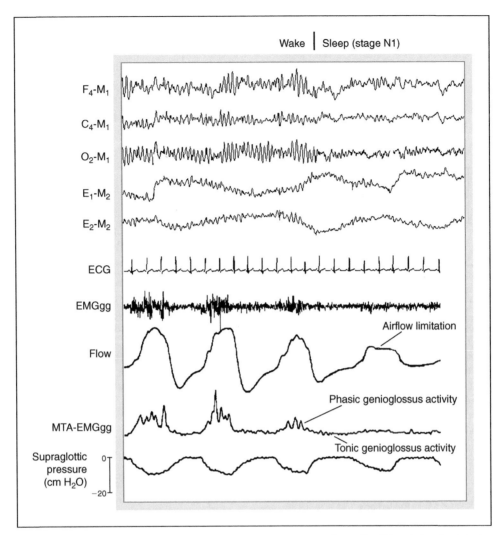

FIGURE 16–2 With sleep onset, there is a fall in genioglossus activity and inspiratory effort and flow. This results in airflow limitation (flat flow). Note the phasic (inspiratory) increase in genioglossus activity during stable breathing preceding sleep. ECG = electrocardiogram; EMGgg = genioglossus electromyogram; MTA-EMGgg = rectified moving time average of EMGgg. *Adapted from Berry RB: OSAHS definitions, epidemiology, and consequences. In Carney P, Berry RB, Geyer JD (eds): Clinical Sleep Disorders, 1st ed. Philadelphia: Lippincott Williams & Wilkins, p. 261.*

(upstream pressure) = Pmask. This consists of a collapsible segment between rigid tubes.[16] As long as the intraluminal pressure within any point of the collapsible segment is less than P_{CRIT}, the relationship in Figure 16–4 will hold. Creating more negative pressure downstream from the collapsible segment will not increase flow. When the intraluminal pressure along the entire collapsible segment is less than the P_{CRIT}, no flow occurs.

During wakefulness, upper airway muscle activity maintains an open upper airway even if the airway is anatomically narrow. Some upper airway muscles such as the genioglossus (GG; tongue protruder) and palatoglossus show increased activity with inspiration (phasic activity) (see Fig. 16–2), whereas others such as the tensor veli palatini (a muscle of the palate) show tonic (constant) activity.[18-20] Activation of phasic upper airway muscles is triggered slightly before the

muscles of the respiratory pump. This allows for a stable upper airway during inspiratory flow. The inspiratory activity of the GG muscle is affected by (1) negative intraluminal pressure via effects on upper airway mechanoreceptors in the laryngeal area, (2) central pattern generators in the brainstem, and (3) influences of sleep state (wakefulness stimulus).[1-6] The activity of the phasic upper airway muscles (GG) but not the tonic palatal muscles relates closely to pharyngeal pressure. The activity of tonic upper airway muscles appears to be more sleep state–dependent (wake > non–rapid eye movement [NREM] > rapid eye movement [REM]).[18,20]

The effects of negative upper airway pressure on the GG are mediated through a reflex neural pathway. The pathway starts with upper airway mechanoreceptors and travels through the superior laryngeal nerve to sensory brainstem

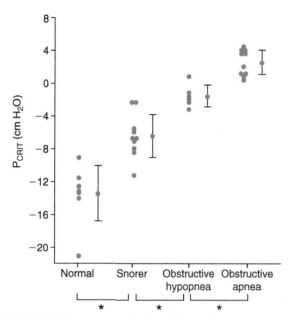

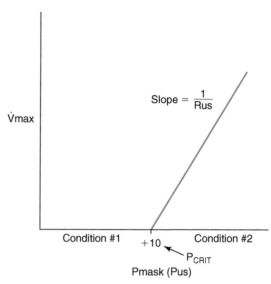

FIGURE 16-3 This figure compares the values of pharyngeal passive closing pressure of the upper airway (P_{CRIT}) for normal subjects, snorers, and patients with obstructive hypopnea and obstructive apnea. The data are presented as both individual values and means ± standard deviation (SD) for the four groups. Note the progressive increase in the mean pharyngeal P_{CRIT} with increasing levels of pharyngeal collapsibility and airway obstruction ($P < .01$). *From Gleadhill IC, Schwartz AR, Schubert N, et al: Upper airway collapsibility in snorers and in patients with obstructive hypopnea and apnea. Am Rev Respir Dis 1991;143:1300–1303.*

FIGURE 16-4 The relationship between the flow rate ($\dot{V}max$) and various mask pressures (Pmask) in a sleeping patient. When Pmask falls below P_{CRIT}, no flow is noted (Condition #1). When Pmask exceeds P_{CRIT} (Condition #2), the flow depends on the pressure difference (Pmask – P_{CRIT}) and the slope of the line is the inverse of the upstream resistance (Rus). In the Starling model, the Pmask is considered the upstream pressure (Pus)—see Figure 16–5. *From Gold AR, Schwartz AR: The pharyngeal critical pressure. Chest 1996;100:1077–1088.*

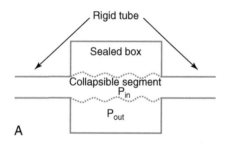

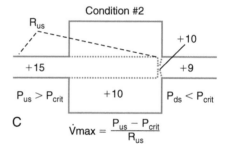

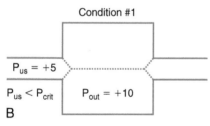

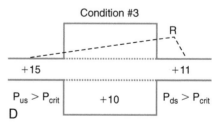

FIGURE 16-5 **A,** Starling resistor model with pharynx assumed to be a collapsible segment with rigid tubes on the upstream and downstream sides. The intraluminal pressure (P_{in}) and extraluminal pressure (P_{out}) are shown. **B,** The upstream pressure (P_{us}) is less than critical closing pressure (P_{crit}). No airflow occurs. P_{out} is the pressure surrounding the collapsible segment of the upper airway. **C** and **D** represent the addition of +15 cm H_2O pressure to the upstream side of the collapsible segment (P_{us}). **C,** The P_{us} is greater than the P_{crit} and airflow depends on the resistance of the upstream resistance (R_{us}). The collapsible segment collapses or flutters to maintain the intraluminal pressure at its downstream end at +10 cm H_2O. If flow stops, the pressure along the entire collapsible segment suddenly becomes +15 cm H_2O and flow temporarily resumes until pressure reaches +10 cm H_2O and the process repeats. The pressure downstream (P_{ds}) from the collapsible segment is less than P_{crit}. **D,** The R_{us} is lower, such that the pressure drop across the collapsible segment is less than P_{crit} ($P_{ds} > P_{crit}$) and flow is not limited by the collapsible segment but depends on the resistance of the entire tube. $\dot{V}max$ = flow rate. *Adapted from Gold AR, Schwartz AR: The pharyngeal critical pressure. Chest 1996;100:1077–1088.*

nuclei (nucleus of the solitary tract [NTS]). Neurons in the NTS then stimulate hypoglossal motoneurons in the brainstem that innervate the GG via the hypoglossal nerve.

Greater upper airway inspiratory muscle activity occurs with more negative upper airway pressure. Hypoxia and hypercapnia could potentially modulate (increase) upper airway muscle activity via effects on the central pattern generators or indirectly by augmenting ventilatory drive/inspiratory effort, generating more negative upper airway pressure (higher suction pressure). Pillar and coworkers[21] administered exogeneous CO_2 to normal individuals during NREM sleep and found no significant augmentation of GG activity. The epiglottic negative pressure was not significantly different between baseline and CO_2 inhalation. Thus, hypercapnia was not associated with more negative upper airway pressure or an increase in GG activity. This study was performed with subjects in the lateral sleep position. In contrast, during monitoring in the supine position, Lo and colleagues[8] did find that exogenous CO_2 administration augmented GG activity. The administration of continuous positive airway pressure (CPAP) did not change the slope of the GG response to hypercapnia. However, upper airway pressure was not measured. The etiology of the effect of posture is not clear. With sleep onset, the loss of the wakefulness stimulus on upper airway muscles causes a decrement in their activity. This may be mediated in part by a loss of serotonergic or noradrenergic excitatory modulation of upper airway motor neuron activity.[5]

At the onset of NREM sleep, the activity of both phasic and tonic upper airway muscles decreases[18,19,22,23] and upper airway resistance increases[24] (see Fig. 16–2). With stable sleep, the activity of the GG may actually return to waking or higher than wakefulness levels as upper airway pressure becomes increasingly negative[25] (Fig. 16–6). If upper airway activity is favorable or upper airway muscle activity has "compensatory effectiveness," stable ventilation will be maintained. Compensatory effectiveness requires a sufficient increase in upper airway muscle activity (stimulated by hypercapnia and negative upper airway pressure) and that the increase in muscle activity is effective in maintaining upper airway patency.[26]

Patients with OSA tend to have higher than normal awake basal GG activity.[27–29] The higher activity is believed to be compensation for an intrinsically narrow or more collapsible

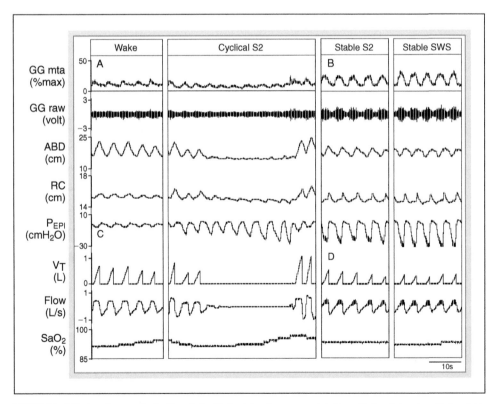

FIGURE 16–6 Tracings from a patient with periods of both obstructive apnea and stable ventilation during sleep. During stable stage N2 sleep without apneas (Stable S2), high genioglossus activity (B) is noted associated with more negative epiglottic pressure (P_{EPI}) (D). Note that the genioglossus activity is higher than during wakefulness. During slow wave sleep (SWS; stage N3), the genioglossus activity is higher than stage N2 and P_{EPI} is more negative. The inspiratory activity of the moving time average of the genioglossus (GG mta) is higher at B than at A because epiglottic pressure (P_{EPI}) is more negative at D than at C. ABD = abdominal band; Cyclical S2 = stage N2 with repeated obstructive apneas; RC = chest band; SaO_2 = arterial oxygen saturation; V_T = tidal volume. *From Jordan AS, White DP, Lo YL, et al: Airway dilator muscle activity and lung volume during stable breathing in obstructive sleep apnea. Sleep 2009;32:361–368.*

upper airway. Most patients with OSA also have a greater than normal fall in GG activity with sleep onset.[29] A reflex activation of the GG muscle to a sudden brief pulse of negative pressure can be demonstrated.[30] The response of the GG and palatal muscles to negative pressure is reduced during sleep.[30-32] During wake, patients with OSA have a greater response in GG activity to a sudden negative pressure pulse than normal subjects.[33] The greater response to negative pressure and higher basal GG activity allow the upper airway to remain open during wakefulness. In contrast, the response of the palatal muscles to negative pressure may be impaired in OSA patients.[34] Despite evidence for higher basal upper airway muscle activity during wakefulness, the upper airways of OSA patients are still more collapsible than those of normal persons.[35] With sleep onset, the wakeful stimulus to GG activity is no longer present and upper airway muscle activity falls in normal individuals and patients with OSA. However, as noted previously, OSA patients have a greater than normal fall in upper airway muscle activity.[29] Owing to unfavorable anatomy, the residual upper airway activity is not sufficient to maintain an open upper airway. In Figures 16–6 and 16–7, a fall in GG activity as the patient returns to sleep is associated with an obstructive apnea. Posture also has important effects on airway patency,[36] and some patients with OSA have apnea or hypopnea only in the supine position.

During upper airway obstruction, phasic GG activity increases proportionately to esophageal pressure deflections (reflecting increased respiratory drive) (see Figs. 16–6 and 16–7).[9,37,38] Stimulation of chemoreceptors by hypoxia and hypercapnia increase inspiratory drive and esophageal pressure deflections increase. At apnea termination, both GG and palatal muscles are preferentially augmented and the upper airway opens.[9,37,38] Although it was once assumed that increasing GG activity during obstructive apnea or hypopnea was driven entirely by hypoxia and hypercapnia, a study of the effect of upper airway local anesthesia suggests that mechanoreceptor stimulation (from increasingly negative pressure below the site of obstruction) plays an important role in the augmentation of GG activity.[37] In Figure 16–8, the top panels (Pre-lidocaine) show a progressive increase in GG activity during apnea. After topical lidocaine anesthesia of the upper airway, the GG activity is markedly diminished. This implies that mechanoreceptor stimulation from increasingly negative pressure below the site of obstruction results in augmentation of GG activity.

Traditionally, a concept of a balance between negative inspiratory pressure tending to collapse the airway and upper airway muscle dilating forces was assumed to determine the state of the airway. However, more recently, the concept of passive collapse at sleep onset (including return to sleep after termination of respiratory events) has gained

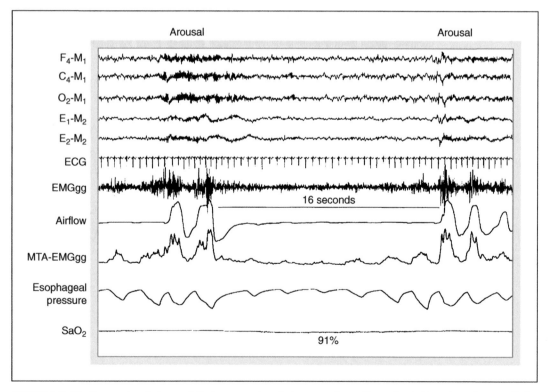

FIGURE 16–7 After the arousal, genioglossus activity decreases as the patient returns to sleep and is associated with an obstructive apnea. During the obstructive apnea, the moving time average of the genioglossus muscle (MTA-EMGgg) progressively increases and esophageal pressure swings also progressively increase. However, the airway does not open until there is a large increase in genioglossus activity associated with an arousal. ECG = electrocardiogram; EMGgg = electromyogram of the genioglossus muscle; SaO$_2$ = arterial oxygen saturation.

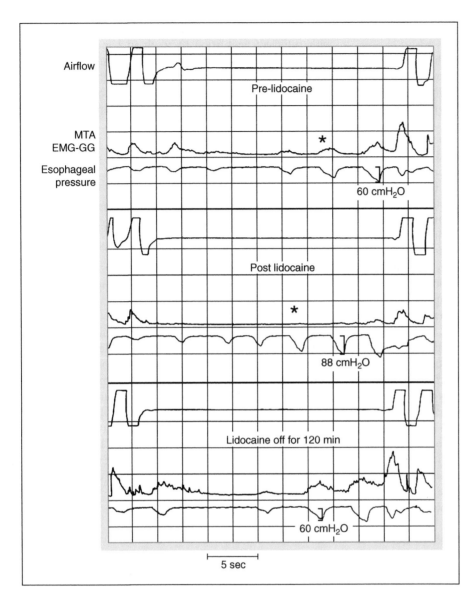

FIGURE 16–8 Genioglossus activity increases with increasing inspiratory effort during an obstructive apnea (*). Topical lidocaine to the upper airway greatly reduces the increase in genioglossus activity (*). After anesthesia has worn off, genioglossus activity returns to baseline. EMG-GG = electromyogram of the genioglossus muscle; MTA = moving time average. *From Berry RB, McNellis M, Kouchi K, Light RW: Upper airway anesthesia reduces genioglossus activity during sleep apnea. Am J Respir Crit Care Med 1997;156: 127–132.*

favor. In fact, at sleep onset, the ventilatory drive decreases and supraglottic pressure may initially decrease (less negative) in some patients (although resistance increases). Upper airway closure has also been documented during central apnea in which there is no inspiration or negative collapsing forces.[39] Therefore, suction pressure during obstruction may help keep the airway closed but is not necessary for the onset of airway occlusion. Cyclic variations in ventilatory drive can induce obstructive or central apneas at the nadir in drive.[40] Thus, even if ventilatory drive to the respiratory pump muscles decreases, the simultaneous reduction of neural drive to the upper airway muscles can result in airway narrowing or collapse.

LUNG VOLUME EFFECTS

Upper airway size also has a dependence on lung volume with decreasing airway size as lung volume decreases.[41,42]

The upper airways of patients with OSA have greater lung volume dependence than normal individuals.[41] The lung volume dependence of the upper airway may be mediated via passive distending forces due to a downward tension on upper airway structures during inspiration ("tracheal tug").[43] Another way of thinking of the tracheal tug is a decrease in extramural pressure surrounding the airway. Any fall in end-expiratory volume (functional residual capacity [FRC]) would then reduce upper airway size. FRC is known to decrease during sleep,[44] and this would tend to predispose to airway closure. Morrell and coworkers[45] demonstrated a progressive fall in end-expiratory retropalatal cross-sectional area as well as end-expiratory lung volume in the breaths leading up to obstructive apnea. Heinzer and colleagues[46] found that an increase in lung volume (induced by extrathoracic pressure) resulted in a lower level of CPAP required to prevent airflow limitation.

VENTILATORY CONTROL AND OSA

Ventilatory instability tends to occur when there is high ventilatory drive. Hypoxia and hypercapnia from apnea coupled with arousal at apnea termination results in a large increase in ventilation. The increased ventilation postapnea may reduce the arterial partial pressure of carbon dioxide ($PaCO_2$), and this coupled with a return to sleep reduces ventilatory drive. The cycles of increased and decreased ventilatory drive predispose to subsequent upper airway closure and help perpetuate repetitive cycles of respiration and apnea.[2,40] As ventilatory drive fluctuates, both upper airway muscle and diaphragmatic activity may fluctuate with apnea or hypopnea tending to occur at the nadir of ventilatory drive. If the patient falls asleep rapidly after arousal, the $PaCO_2$ may be near or below the apneic threshold, the level of $PaCO_2$ below which ventilation is no longer triggered during sleep.[47] If the $PaCO_2$ falls below the apneic threshold, a central apnea will occur. If the upper airway is closed at the time of resumption of inspiratory effort, an obstructive apnea will occur. This is the etiology of mixed apnea (initial central portion, terminal obstructive portion).[48] Alternatively, an obstructive hypopnea or obstructive apnea may occur as ventilatory drive and upper airway muscle activity fall but the $PaCO_2$ remains above the apneic threshold.[49]

Patients with a small difference between the sleeping $PaCO_2$ and the apneic threshold would be more likely to have a central apnea on return to sleep.[47,50] Of note, obstructive apnea may occur before the nadir if inspiratory effort is reached. If one monitors esophageal pressure in patients with OSA, the nadir in deflections in some patients can occur two or three breaths into the apnea (Fig. 16–9).

Recently, the concept of loop gain has been applied to explain ventilatory instability. Loop gain characterizes the response to a perturbation. For example, a patient with a high loop gain may respond to a mild elevation in $PaCO_2$ with sufficient ventilation to result in hypocapnia ("overshoot") rather than simply bringing the system back to the original state (eucapnia). Patients with high loop gain are predisposed to ventilatory instability. High loop gain may be due to high controller gain (high hypercapnic ventilatory response) or high plant gain (large decrease in $PaCO_2$ for a given increase in ventilation). Plant gain is increased when there is hypercapnia, a low dead space, and a low FRC.[1,2]

$$\text{Loop gain} = \text{response to disturbance} / \text{the disturbance}$$
$$\text{Loop gain} = \text{controller gain (chemosensitivity)} \times \text{plant gain}$$
$$\text{Controller gain} = \text{change in ventilation per change in } PaCO_2 \text{ (reaching chemoreceptors)}$$
$$\text{Plant gain} = \text{change in } PaCO_2 \text{ per change in ventilation}$$

Equation 16–2

Younes and associates[51] found that chemical control is more unstable in severe compared with milder OSA patients. Wellman and colleagues[52] subsequently reported that loop gain measured during NREM sleep was an important predictor of apnea severity (respiratory disturbance index), but only in patients with intermediate collapsibility of the pharyngeal airway. Individuals with extreme airway collapsibility will have obstructive events regardless of loop gain. Thus, it would appear that ventilatory control instability may play an important role in the pathophysiology of airway obstruction in some patients with OSA.

STAGE R EFFECTS

The obstructive events are longest and arterial oxygen desaturation the most severe during REM sleep. Many patients

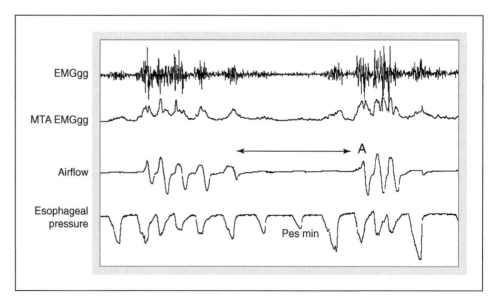

FIGURE 16–9 An obstructive apnea *(double-ended arrow)* associated with a fall in genioglossus activity. Note that the minimum effort does not occur until the second obstructed effort. A = timing of arousal; EMGgg = electromyogram of the genioglossus muscle; MTA = moving time average; (Pes) min = minimum esophageal pressure deflection during apnea.

have obstructive events only during REM sleep or the apnea-hypopnea index (AHI) is much higher during REM sleep. However, the reason for the susceptibility for apnea during REM sleep remains unclear. During REM sleep, ventilation is irregular even in normal persons. REM sleep without phasic eye movements is called "tonic REM" and with eye movements "phasic REM." There tends to be more respiratory irregularity during periods of bursts of eye movements (phasic REM)[53,54] (Fig. 16–10). During phasic REM, there are often periods of reduced airflow, tidal volume (V_T), and respiratory effort. The eye movement bursts are markers of brainstem phasic REM activity that affects respiration. Because periods of REM sleep are longest and the REM density (number of eye movements per time) highest during the early morning hours, it is not surprising that this is the time of the greatest changes in ventilation during sleep in patients with lung disease and OSA.[53,55] One study in normal individuals did not find a significant change in ventilation between early and late REM sleep periods because an increase in respiratory rate compensated for fall in V_T.[54] However, patients with OSA or lung disease are more susceptible to the phasic changes of REM sleep and V_T falls with either no change in respiratory rate or a change insufficient to maintain ventilation.[55] During REM sleep, there is generalized muscle hypotonia and the muscles of respiration other than the diaphragm are less active.[55] Although the diaphragm is not affected by the generalized tonic muscle hypotonia of REM sleep, periodic decrements in diaphragmatic activity (inspiratory effort) do occur and are often associated with bursts of eye movements (Fig. 16–11).[55] The decrements in diaphragmatic activity are associated with reduced V_T. Upper airway muscles are also affected during REM sleep. In normal persons during REM sleep, GG tonic activity is reduced but phasic activity can still be detected if intramuscular

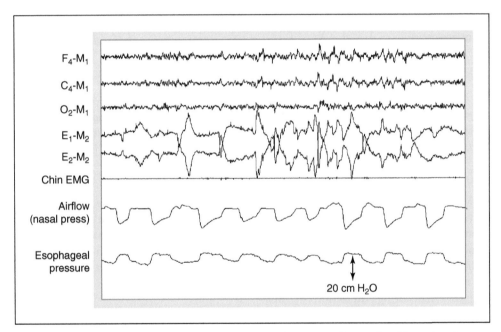

FIGURE 16–10 A period of reduced airflow associated with decreased inspiratory effort as reflected by esophageal pressure deflections during REM sleep (stage R). The reduced airflow occurs during a prolonged burst of eye movements. Note that the airflow profile is flat during inspiration, suggesting the presence of airflow limitation. EMG = electromyogram.

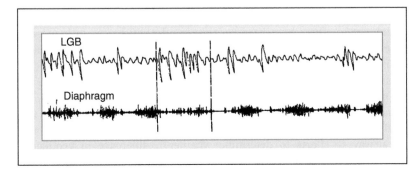

FIGURE 16–11 Recording from the lateral geniculate body (LGB) and diaphragm of a cat during rapid eye movement (REM) sleep. The deflections in the LGB tracing are pontogeniculo-occipital (PGO) waves that occur during bursts of eye movements. These phasic REM changes can be associated with fractionation or decrement in the diaphragmatic electromyogram (EMG) noted *between the dashed lines*. *From Orem J: Neuronal mechanisms of respiration in REM sleep. Sleep 1980;3:251–267.*

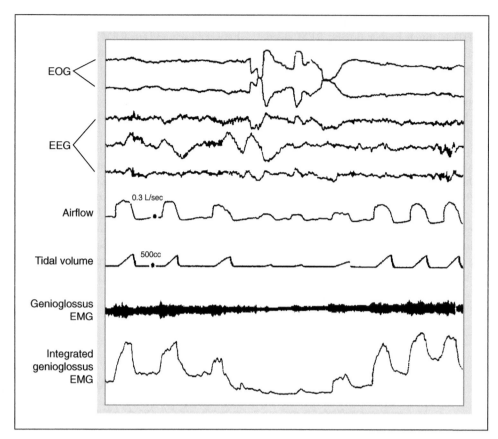

FIGURE 16–12 Reduction in genioglossus activity during bursts of eye movements in REM sleep (stage R). EEG = electro-encephalogram; EMG = electromyogram; EOG = electro-oculogram. *From Wiegand L, Zwillich CW, Wiegand D, White DP: Changes in upper airway muscle activation and ventilation during phasic REM sleep in normal men. J Appl Physiol 1991;71:488–497.*

electromyogram (EMG) electrodes are used (Fig. 16–12). During bursts of eye movements, diaphragmatic and GG phasic activity are often decreased.[56]

As noted previously, many patients have obstructive apnea only during REM sleep (REM-related OSA). However, two studies found no greater collapsibility (P_{CRIT}) of the upper airway during REM than during NREM sleep.[36,57] This variance with clinical experience could be due to REM-associated manifestations that do not affect the P_{CRIT} measurement. These might include changes in lung volume during prolonged reductions in ventilation or impairment of the ability of the airway to compensate for increasing resistance. Jordan and coworkers[58] studied OSA patients who could maintain upper airway patency during some periods of NREM sleep. Stable breathing during stage N2 was compared with cyclic REM sleep (with apneas). The end-expiratory lung volume and peak GG EMG did not differ. During REM sleep, the relationship between the negative epiglottic pressure (P_{EPI}) and the phasic GG activity also did not differ from stage N2 sleep. However, P_{EPI} was much less negative and the tonic GG activity was lower during REM sleep (Fig. 16–13). Perhaps lower GG tonic activity during REM sleep makes the upper airway susceptible to closure especially at end-exhalation when the upper airway size is the smallest. Eckert and associates[59] did not find that

patients with OSA had more REM-induced changes in upper airway muscle activity than normal subjects. Therefore, the normal REM-associated changes in respiratory physiology may have greater impact on patients with susceptible upper airway anatomy. More investigations in this area of inquiry are needed.

GENDER AND OSA

A number of investigations have sought to determine the pathophysiology of the higher incidence of OSA in men than in women. Men have longer upper airways and this is believed to predispose them to pharyngeal collapse.[60] Of note, postmenopausal women have longer upper airways than premenopausal women.[61] One study found that men also have more fat around their upper airway than women.[62] There have been no clear gender differences in loop gain, upper airway collapsibility (P_{CRIT}), or pharyngeal muscle activation.[63–65] Pillar and associates[65] found that men developed more hypopnea due to resistive loading. Because no difference in upper airway muscle activation was noted, the increased tendency for male upper airway narrowing was believed to be due to **anatomic factors**. There have been efforts to determine whether a difference in ventilatory control between men and women could explain the higher

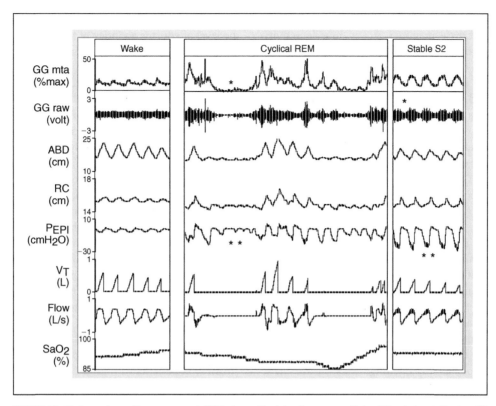

FIGURE 16–13 Comparing rapid eye movement (REM) sleep with obstructive apneas with breathing during stable stage N2 sleep (S2). The tonic (expiratory) genioglossus (GG) EMG is much lower (*) and the epiglottic pressure (P_{EPI}) is much less negative (**). ABD = abdominal band; mta = moving time average; RC = chest band; SaO_2 = arterial oxygen saturation; V_T = tidal volume. *From Jordan AS, White DP, Lo YL, et al: Airway dilator muscle activity and lung volume during stable breathing in obstructive sleep apnea. Sleep 2009;32:361–368.*

prevalence of OSA in men. Loop gain is not different between men and women.[63] As previously noted, the apneic threshold is the sleeping $PaCO_2$ at which ventilation is no longer triggered (see Chapter 21). Men have a **smaller difference between their sleeping $PaCO_2$ and their apneic threshold**, predisposing them to central apnea or hyponea after periods of hyperventilation.[66,67] In summary, no clear explanation for the gender difference in the prevalence of OSA has been found. Anatomic differences (longer upper airway length) or increased upper airway susceptibility to resistive loading or falling ventilatory drive in men may be possible explanations.

MECHANISMS OF APNEA TERMINATION AND AROUSAL

Obstructive apnea or hypopnea termination is often associated with cortical arousals. The relationship between these two phenomena is still the subject of investigation (Box 16–1). During obstructive apnea or hypopnea during NREM sleep, upper airway muscle activity increases proportional to inspiratory effort. Studies by Reemers and coworkers[9] suggested that airway opening does not occur until there is a preferential increase in upper airway muscle activity

BOX 16–1

Respiratory Arousal Mechanisms

- The arousal stimulus during obstructive apnea and hypopnea appears to be proportional to the magnitude of inspiratory effort (esophageal pressure excursions).
- Hypercapnia, hypoxemia, and negative pressure stimuli during obstructive respiratory events result in increasing respiratory effort. However, arousal occurs when the level of effort reaches an arousal threshold.
- The arousal threshold to respiratory stimuli during NREM sleep is increased in patients with OSA compared with normal individuals (higher inspiratory effort is needed to trigger arousal).
- A higher arousal threshold may predispose to longer respiratory events, but a low arousal threshold may contribute to ventilatory instability.
- Obstructive apneas and hypopneas are longer during REM than during NREM sleep. In contrast, normal individuals arouse from experimental mask occlusion more rapidly in REM than in NREM sleep.
- The mechanisms responsible for obstructive event termination and respiratory arousal have similar time courses but may be independent parallel processes. In some studies, 20–40% of obstructive event terminations are not associated with cortical arousal.

(compared with the diaphragm) (see Figs. 16–6 and 16–7). The preferential increase in upper airway muscle activity was believed to be due to associated arousal. One problem with this concept is that not all event terminations are associated with cortical arousal (e.g., 60–80% of event terminations are associated with arousal). Sometimes, obstructive event termination is associated with signs of cortical activation, although the electroencephalogram (EEG) changes may not always meet American Academy of Sleep Medicine (AASM) criteria.[68] For example, a delta burst may be seen at apnea termination. O'Malley and coworkers[69] suggested that by using frontal electrodes, one could detect arousal in the majority of events. Even when cortical arousal cannot be detected, some have hypothesized a state change at the level of the brainstem.[70] These are sometimes referred to as *subcortical or autonomic arousals* because changes in sympathetic tone, heart rate, or blood pressure can occasionally be detected in the absence of cortical changes meeting criteria for arousal.

Younes[71] has challenged the concept that arousal is an essential component of upper airway opening. His work found that arousal may precede, coincide with, follow, or not occur with upper airway opening. Thus, in this view, arousal may be associated with event termination, but what opens the airway is a sufficient augmentation of upper airway muscle activity by chemical and mechanical stimuli. Thus, Younes hypothesizes that airway opening and arousal are two separate independent phenomena that occur in parallel with similar time courses during obstructive respiratory events. Upper airway muscle activity is progressively augmented until an upper airway opening threshold is reached and the airway opens. Likewise, during obstructive events, the arousal stimulus (proportional to the level of inspiratory effort[70,72,73]) increases until the arousal threshold is reached and arousal occurs. If augmentation of upper airway muscle activity is brisk, the required degree of muscle augmentation is not excessive, and the arousal threshold is high, the airway could reopen without arousal (the patient remains asleep). Evidence for this concept is that most patients with OSA have some periods of the night without events and, thus, are able to maintain upper airway patency without arousal. However, this concept does not explain event termination during REM sleep when upper airway muscles do not necessarily augment during the event (see Fig. 16–13). In addition, whereas phasic upper airway muscles augment with increasing inspiratory drive (and more negative upper airway pressure), tonic upper airway muscles do not. Tonic muscles increase their activity with a state change (arousal). Thus, arousal may play a role in termination of some obstructive events. Even if arousal is not essential to upper airway opening, repeated arousals are thought to contribute to daytime sleepiness (along with the associated hypoxemia).[74,75]

The mechanisms that contribute to respiratory arousal are also of interest and still incompletely understood. Whereas hypercapnia and hypoxia drive the increase in respiratory effort, the level of effort rather than individual values of hypoxia or hypercapnia seems to trigger arousal.[70,72,73] Thus, the level of effort is an index of the combined arousal stimulus. Studies have suggested that information from upper airway mechanoreceptors may contribute to the arousal stimulus.[76,77] In NREM sleep, arousal appears to occur when inspiratory effort reaches an "arousal threshold." Normal subjects tend to arouse during mask occlusion when suction pressure reaches –20 to –40 cm H_2O. In contrast, many patients with OSA arouse only after esophageal pressure reaches –60 to –80 cm H_2O.[70,73,78] The increased arousal threshold in OSA patients is probably due in part to chronic sleep deprivation or hypoxemia. Withdrawal of CPAP for even three nights has been shown to increase the arousal threshold in OSA.[78] However, chronic CPAP treatment does not restore the arousal threshold to normal. Patients with OSA could have an intrinsically increased respiratory arousal threshold. Another possible explanation for an elevated arousal threshold is damage to mechanoreceptors from years of snoring or to chemoreceptors from repetitive nightly stimulation. Support for this idea comes from studies showing that upper airway sensation is impaired in patients with OSA.[79] A study of respiratory-related evoked potentials (RREPs) in patients with mild OSA suggested that there is a sleep-specific blunted cortical response to inspiratory occlusion.[80] At least in these milder patients, there was no evidence of impaired mechanoreceptor function because the RREP was normal during wakefulness. One study found that the prolongation in event duration that occurs overnight in patients with OSA is secondary to a blunting of the cortical response as the level of inspiratory effort at apnea termination increased during the night.[81] Another study found that the within-night variation in the arousal threshold followed the cycles of NREM sleep[82] with a higher arousal threshold associated with higher EEG delta power (deeper sleep). Sforza and colleagues[83] studied the within-night changes in the arousal threshold associated with respiratory events and found that the arousal threshold tended to peak during the first 3 hours of sleep, plateau, and then decrease slightly in the last hour of sleep. They did find a mild increase in apnea duration over the night. The authors concluded that their findings showed the arousal threshold was not dependent on sleep fragmentation (which should have continued to worsen during the entire night) and might reflect circadian or homeostatic rhythms. Another explanation is that greater delta power (sleep depth) occurs in the early part of the night[82] and greater sleep depth delayed arousal.

It is worth noting that the apnea duration (time to arousal) depends on both the arousal threshold and the rate of increase in inspiratory effort (respiratory response to arousal).[70] For example, the addition of supplemental oxygen results in longer apneas (reduction in rate of augmentation in inspiratory effort) but event termination occurs at similar levels of esophageal pressure (similar arousal threshold).[70] If one believes that airway opening is independent of arousal, a similar scheme can still be invoked with the determinants of event duration being the rate of upper airway muscle augmentation and the airway opening threshold.

In REM sleep, the arousal mechanisms are less well understood. Esophageal pressure deflections do not show a steady increase (see Fig. 16–13). However, normal subjects arouse more quickly from mask occlusion during REM sleep than during NREM sleep.[70,84] In contrast, patients with OSA have the longest apneas and most severe desaturation during REM sleep.[85]

The reasons for the delayed arousal (longer event duration) during REM sleep in OSA patients are not known. The slower and erratic augmentation of respiratory drive that occurs during REM sleep could delay arousal and event termination even if the arousal threshold is similar to that of NREM sleep.[86] Conversely, there could be an increase in the arousal threshold during REM compared with NREM sleep in some OSA patients with chronic REM sleep fragmentation. Certainly, some OSA patients exhibit a tremendous increase in eye movements during REM sleep on the first night on CPAP. This may be evidence of prior REM sleep fragmentation or deprivation. Prior sleep disturbance could increase the arousal threshold. Zavodny and coworkers[87] found evidence that sleep fragmentation from acoustic stimuli impaired the arousability to resistive loading in stage N2 sleep but not in REM sleep. An effect of sleep fragmentation was seen during early REM sleep. However, because most REM sleep occurred in the second part of the night, sleep fragmentation did not impair arousal when REM sleep for the entire night was analyzed. Thus, to date, there is no compelling evidence that sleep fragmentation increases either respiratory event duration or the respiratory arousal threshold during REM sleep.

UPPER AIRWAY SENSATION

There is evidence that upper airway sensation is impaired in patients with OSA.[79] This could be due to years of trauma from snoring. It is unclear whether damage to upper airway mechanoreceptors could be playing a role in the pathogenesis of OSA in some patients.

ARTERIAL OXYGEN DESATURATION

Patients with a similar AHI may have vastly different degrees of arterial oxygen desaturation. Box 16–2 lists factors determining the severity of arterial oxygen desaturation. Studies of breath-holding in normal subjects suggest that the rate of fall in the SaO_2 is inversely proportional to the baseline SaO_2 and to the lung volume (oxygen stores) at the start of breath-hold.[88] The rate of fall is disproportionately higher at low lung volumes secondary to increases in ventilation-perfusion mismatch. A study of OSA patients by Bradley and associates[89] found that the severity of nocturnal arterial oxygen desaturation was related to several factors, including the awake supine arterial partial pressure of oxygen (PaO_2), the percentage of sleep time spent in apnea, and the expiratory reserve volume (ERV). Patients with a baseline PaO_2 of 55 to 60 mm Hg are on the steep part of the oxyhemoglobin saturation curve (Fig. 16–14). A small fall in PaO_2 results

BOX 16–2

Factors Associated with More Severe Arterial Oxygen Desaturation

- Higher BMI
  - More effect during REM than NREM sleep.
  - More effect supine > lateral sleep.
  - More effect men > women.
- Lower baseline awake supine PaO_2 or SaO_2
- Lower ERV (FRC – RV).
  - Low FRC—obesity.
  - High RV—obstructive airways disease (COPD).
- Longer event duration.
- Greater change in V_T (hypopnea).
- Short ventilatory period between apnea.
- REM sleep versus NREM sleep (REM events are also longer).
- Supine versus lateral position.

BMI = body mass index; COPD = chronic obstructive pulmonary disease; ERV = expiratory reserve volume; FRC = functional residual capacity; NREM = non–rapid eye movement; PaO_2 = arterial partial pressure of oxygen; REM = rapid eye movement; RV = residual volume; SaO_2 = arterial oxygen saturation; V_T = tidal volume.

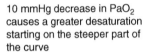

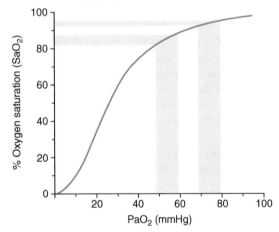

Oxygen-hemoglobin Saturation Curve

FIGURE 16–14 The same drop in the arterial partial pressure of oxygen (PaO_2) causes a bigger drop in the SaO_2 on the steeper part of the oxygen-hemoglobin saturation curve.

in significant desaturation. Whereas apnea duration is an obvious factor in the severity of desaturation, the length of the ventilatory period between events is also important. Some patients do not completely resaturate between events because they quickly return to sleep and the airway closes again. Long event duration and short periods between apneas mean the percentage of total sleep time spent in apnea is high. A small ERV is associated more with severe arterial

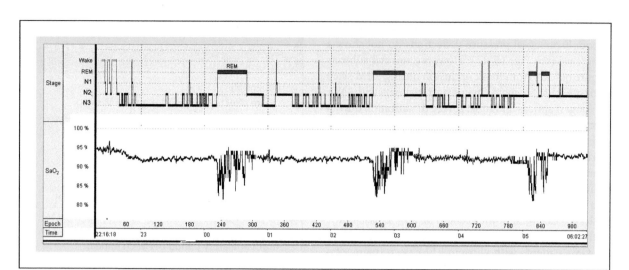

FIGURE 16–15 A total night view shows the hypnogram with rapid eye movement (REM) sleep shown by *horizontal bars*. The patient had almost no events except during REM sleep, but during REM sleep, the desaturation was significant. SaO_2 = arterial oxygen saturation.

oxygen desaturation during respiratory events. The ERV is the difference between the functional residual capacity (FRC; end-expiratory volume) and the residual volume (RV). A small ERV is usually due to a low FRC, a high RV, or both. In obesity, the FRC is reduced. A lower FRC is associated with lower oxygen stores before a respiratory event. Tidal breathing at low lung volumes results in substantial small airway closure (below the closing volume). This increases the amount of ventilation-perfusion mismatch (no ventilation reaches some alveoli). A high RV is usually due to airtrapping associated with obstructive airways disease. The presence of obstructive airway disease also causes more ventilation-perfusion mismatch (see Chapter 10). Low oxygen stores at the start of apnea and ventilation-perfusion mismatch both contribute to a more rapid and more severe drop in the SaO_2 during apnea or reduced ventilation (hypopnea).

Clinically, the groups of OSA patients with severe desaturation include patients with a low PaO_2 for any reason (severe obesity, daytime hypoventilation, and chronic obstructive pulmonary disease [COPD]). In fact, some patients can have significant desaturation after events as short as 10 to 15 seconds. The severity of desaturation also depends on sleep stage. As noted previously, in most OSA patients, the longest apneas and most severe desaturations occur in REM sleep (Fig. 16–15).[85] Some studies also have suggested that at equivalent apnea length, the severity of desaturation is worsened in obstructive compared with central apnea.[90] A recent large study of the Wisconsin cohort found that a higher BMI was associated with oxygen desaturation severity independent of age, gender, sleeping position, baseline SaO_2, and event duration.[91] A higher body mass index (BMI) had a greater effect on desaturation in REM than in NREM sleep. In addition, a fall in V_T had a greater effect on arterial oxygen desaturation when the BMI was higher. The predicted change in the SaO_2 was also higher in the supine position than in the lateral position, in men than in women, and in smokers

than in nonsmokers. Another study found that obstructive events in the supine position tended to be longer, were associated with more severe desaturation, and were more likely to be associated with an arousal at event termination.[92]

As previously mentioned, REM sleep is associated with more severe desaturation than NREM sleep.[85,93] Oksenberg and coworkers also found that supine REM sleep is associated with more severe arterial oxygen desaturation than nonsupine REM sleep. This was not due to longer event duration.[93] Thus, one would expect the most severe arterial oxygen desaturation to usually occur during supine REM sleep.

CLINICAL REVIEW QUESTIONS

1. Which of the following factors may help explain the greater prevalence of OSA in men than in women?

    A. Longer upper airway length in men.

    B. Higher P_{CRIT} (more positive) in men.

    C. Less pharyngeal muscle activation.

    D. Higher loop gain in men than in women.

2. Breathing through the nose rather than the mouth causes more negative supraglottic airway pressure during inspiration (e.g., –6 cm H_2O with nasal breathing, –2 cm H_2O with oral breathing). Which route of breathing is associated with greater phasic activity of the GG muscle?

    A. Oral breathing route.

    B. Nasal breathing route.

3. Which of the following would NOT predispose to upper airway narrowing or closure?

    A. Falling ventilatory drive.

    B. Higher FRC.

    C. Less negative upper airway pressure.

    D. Higher P_{CRIT}.

4. Higher BMI is associated with worse arterial oxygen desaturation in OSA patients.

   Which of the following is true about the effect of BMI on desaturation?
   A. REM > NREM.
   B. Lateral position > supine.
   C. Women > men.

5. Which of the following is NOT true about REM compared with NREM sleep?
   A. Higher P_{CRIT}.
   B. Longer apneas.
   C. Lower tonic upper airway muscle activity.
   D. More severe arterial oxygen desaturation.

6. The arousal stimulus (and arousal threshold) is best related to which of the following?
   A. Hypoxemia.
   B. Hypercapnic.
   C. Hypoxia and hypercapnia.
   D. Level of inspiratory effort.

Answers

1. **A.** Longer upper airway length in men. No clear difference in the P_{CRIT}, upper airway muscle activation, or loop gain have been demonstrated in men compared with women.

2. **B.** Negative upper airway pressure augments phasic upper airway muscle activity.

3. **B.** Upper airway size decreases with falling lung volume. A higher FRC would not predispose to airway closure or narrowing.

4. **A.** BMI has more effect on desaturation in men compared with women and supine compared with lateral sleep.

5. **A.** Studies have not found a higher P_{CRIT} during REM sleep.

6. **D.**

REFERENCES

1. Eckert DJ, Malhotra A: Pathophysiology of adult obstructive sleep apnea. Proc Am Thorac Soc 2008;5:144–153.
2. White DP: Pathogenesis of obstructive and central sleep apnea. Am J Respir Crit Med 2005;172:1363–1370.
3. White DP: Sleep apnea. Proc Am Thorac Soc 2006;3:124–128.
4. White DP: The pathogenesis of obstructive sleep apnea. Am J Respir Cell Mol Biol 2006;34:1–6.
5. Jordan AS, White DP: Pharyngeal motor control and pathogenesis of obstructive sleep apnea. Respir Physiol Neurobiol 2008;160:1–7.
6. Horner RL: Motor control of pharyngeal musculature and implications for the pathogenesis of obstructive sleep apnea. Sleep 1996;19:827–853.
7. Badr MS: Pathophysiology of upper airway obstruction during sleep. Clin Chest Med 1998;19:21–32.
8. Lo Y, Jordan AS, Malhotra A, et al: Genioglossal muscle response to CO_2 stimulation during NREM sleep. Sleep 2006;29:470–477.
9. Remmers JE, Degroot WJ, Sauerland EK, et al: Pathogenesis of upper airway occlusion during sleep. J Appl Physiol 1978;44:931–938.
10. Schwab RJ, Gefter WB, Hoffman EA, et al: Dynamic upper airway imaging during wake respiration in normal subjects and patients with sleep disordered breathing. Am Rev Respir Dis 1993;148:1385–1400.
11. Schwab RJ, Pasirstein M, Pierson R, et al: Identification of upper airway anatomic risk factors for obstructive sleep apnea with volumetric magnetic resonance imaging. Am J Respir Crit Care Med 2003;168:522–530.
12. Leiter JC: Upper airway shape: is it important in the pathogenesis of obstructive sleep apnea? Am J Respir Crit Care Med 1996;153:894–898.
13. Isono S, Remmers JE, Tanakka A, et al: Anatomy of pharynx in patients with obstructive sleep apnea and normal subjects. J Appl Physiol 1997;82:1319–1326.
14. Clark SA, Wilson CR, Satoh M, et al: Assessment of inspiratory flow limitation invasively and noninvasively during sleep. Am Respir Crit Care Med 1998;158:713–722.
15. Berry RB: Nasal and esophageal pressure monitoring. In Lee-Chiong TL, Sateia MJ, Caraskadon MA (eds): Sleep Medicine. Philadelphia: Hanley & Belfus, 2002, pp. 661–671.
16. Gold AR, Schwartz AR: The pharyngeal critical pressure. Chest 1996;100:1077–1088.
17. Gleadhill IC, Schwartz AR, Schubert N, et al: Upper airway collapsibility in snorers and in patients with obstructive hypopnea and apnea. Am Rev Respir Dis 1991;143:1300–1303.
18. Tangel DJ, Messanotte WS, Sandberg EJ, White DP: Influences of NREM sleep on activity of tonic vs. inspiratory phasic muscles in normal men. J Appl Physiol 1992;73:1058–1066.
19. Tangel DJ, Mezzanotte WS, White DP: Influences of NREM sleep on activity of palatoglossus and levator palatini muscles in normal men. J Appl Physiol 1995;78:689–695.
20. Malhotra A, Pillar G, Fogel RB, et al: Genioglossal but not palatal muscle activity relates closely to pharyngeal pressure. Am J Respir Crit Care Med 2000;162:1058–1062.
21. Pillar G, Malhotra A, Fogel RB, et al: Upper airway muscle responsiveness to rising PCO_2 during NREM sleep. J Appl Physiol 2000;89:1275–1282.
22. Worsnop C, Kay C, Pierce R, et al: Activity of respiratory pump and upper airway muscles during sleep onset. J Appl Physiol 1998;85:908–920.
23. Tangel DJ, Messanotte WS, White DP: Influence of sleep on tensor palatini EMG and upper airway resistance in normal men. J Appl Physiol 1991;70;2574–2581.
24. Hudgel DW, Martin RJ, Johnson B, Hill P: Mechanics of the respiratory system and breathing pattern during sleep in normal humans. J Appl Physiol 1984:56:133–137.
25. Basner RC, Ringler J, Schwartzstein RM, et al: Phasic electromyographic activity of the genioglossus increases in normals during slow-wave sleep. Respir Physiol 1991;83:189–200.
26. Younes M: Contributions of upper airway mechanics and control mechanisms to severity of OSA: Am J Respir Crit Med 2003;163:645–658.
27. Mezzanotte WS, Tangel DJ, White DP: Waking genioglossal electromyogram in sleep apnea patient versus normal controls (a neuromuscular compensatory mechanism). J Clin Invest 1992;89:1571–1579.

28. Fogel RB, Malhotra A, Pillar G, et al: Genioglossal activation in patients with obstructive sleep apnea versus controls subjects. Am J Respir Crit Care Med 2001;164:2025–2030.
29. Mezzanotte WS, Tangel DJ, White DP: Influence of sleep onset on upper-airway muscle activity in apnea patients versus normal controls. Am J Respir Crit Care Med 1996;153:1880–1887.
30. Horner RL, Innes JA, Morrell MJ, et al: The effect of sleep on reflex genioglossus muscle activation by stimuli of negative airway pressure in humans. J Physiol (Lond) 1994;476:141–151.
31. Wheatley JR, Tangel DJ, Mezzanotte WS, White DP: Influence of sleep on response to negative airway pressure of tensor palatini muscle and retropalatal airway. J Appl Physiol 1993;75:2117–2124.
32. Wheatley JR, Mezzanotte WS, Tangel DJ, White DP: The influence of sleep on genioglossal muscle activation by negative pressure in normal men. Am Rev Respir Dis 1993;148:597–605.
33. Berry RB, White DP, Roper J, et al: Awake negative pressure reflex response of the genioglossus in OSA patients and normal subjects. J Appl Physiol 2003;94:1875–1882.
34. Mortimore IL, Douglas NJ: Palatal muscle EMG response to negative pressure in awake sleep apneic and control subjects. Am J Respir Crit Care Med 1997;156:867–873.
35. Malhotra A, Pillar G, Edwards J, et al: Upper airway collapsibility: measurement and sleep effects. Chest 2001;120:156–161.
36. Penzel T, Moller M, Becker HF, et al: Effect of sleep position and sleep stage on the collapsibility of the upper airways in patients with sleep apnea. Sleep 2001;24:90–95.
37. Berry RB, McNellis M, Kouchi K, Light RW: Upper airway anesthesia reduces genioglossus activity during sleep apnea. Am J Respir Crit Care Med 1997;156:127–132.
38. Carlson DM, Onal E, Carley DW, et al: Palatal muscle electromyogram activity in obstructive sleep apnea. Am J Respir Crit Care Med 1995;152:1319–1322.
39. Badr MS, Toiber F, Skatrud JB, et al: Pharyngeal narrowing/occlusion during central apnea. J Appl Physiol 1995;78:1806–1815.
40. Onal E, Burrows DL, Hart RH, Lopata M: Induction of periodic breathing during sleep causes upper airway obstruction in humans. J Appl Physiol 1986;61:1438–1443.
41. Hoffstein V, Zamel N, Phillipson EA: Lung volume dependence of cross-sectional area in patients with obstructive sleep apnea. Am Rev Respir Dis 1984;130:175–178.
42. Stanchina ML, Malhotra A, Fogel RB, et al: The influence of lung volume on pharyngeal mechanics, collapsibility, and genioglossus muscle activation during sleep. Sleep 2003;26:851–856.
43. Van de Graaff WB: Thoracic influences on upper airway patency. J Appl Physiol 1988;65:2124–2131.
44. Hudgel DW, Devadda P: Decrease in functional residual capacity during sleep in normal humans. J Appl Physiol 1984;57:1319–1322.
45. Morrell MJ, Arabi Y, Zahn B, Badr MS: Progressive retropalatal narrowing preceding obstructive apnea. Am J Respir Crit Care Med 1998;158:1974–1981.
46. Heinzer RC, Stanchina ML, Malhotra A, et al: Lung volume and continuous positive airway pressure requirement in obstructive sleep apnea. Am J Respir Crit Care Med 2005;172:114–117.
47. Dempsey JA, Skatrud JB: A sleep-induced apneic threshold and its consequences. Am Rev Respir Dis 1986;133:1163–1170.
48. Iber C, Davies SF, Chapman RC, Mahowald MM: A possible mechanism for mixed apnea in obstructive sleep apnea. Chest 1986;89:800–805.
49. Badr MS, Kawak A: Post-hyperventilation hypopnea in humans during NREM sleep. Respir Physiol 1996;103:137–145.
50. Dempsey J: Crossing the apneic threshold. Causes and consequences. Exp Physiol 2004;90:13–24.
51. Younes M, Ostrowski M, Thompson W, et al: Chemical control stability in patients with obstructive sleep apnea. Am J Respir Crit Care Med 2001;163:1181–1190.
52. Wellman A, Jordan AS, Malhotra A, et al: Ventilatory control and airway anatomy in obstructive sleep apnea. Am J Respir Crit Care Med 2004;170:1225–1232.
53. Gould GA, Gugger M, Molloy J, et al: Breathing pattern and eye movement density during REM sleep in humans. Am Rev Respir Dis 1988;138:874–877.
54. Neilly JB, Gaipa EA, Maislin G, Pack A: Ventilation during early and later rapid-eye-movement sleep. J Appl Physiol 1991;71:1201–1215.
55. Becker HF, Piper AJ, Flynn WE, et al: Breathing during sleep in patients with nocturnal desaturation. Am J Respir Crit Care Med 1999;159:112–118.
56. Wiegand L, Zwillich CW, Wiegand D, White DP: Changes in upper airway muscle activation and ventilation during phasic REM sleep in normal men. J Appl Physiol 1991;71:488–497.
57. Boudewyns A, Punjabi N, Van de Heyning PH, et al: Abbreviated method for assessing upper airway function in obstructive sleep apnea. Chest 2000;118:1031–1041.
58. Jordan AS, White DP, Lo YL, et al: Airway dilator muscle activity and lung volume during stable breathing in obstructive sleep apnea. Sleep 2009;32:361–368.
59. Eckert DJ, Malhotra A, Lo YL, et al: The influence of obstructive sleep apnea and gender on genioglossus activity during rapid eye movement sleep. Chest 2009;135:957–964.
60. Malhotra A, Huang Y, Fogel RB, et al: The male predisposition to pharyngeal collapse: importance of airway length. Am J Respir Crit Care Med 2002;166:1388–1395.
61. Malhotra A, Huang Y, Fogel R, et al: Aging influences on pharyngeal anatomy and physiology: the predisposition to pharyngeal collapse. Am J Med 2006;119:72.e9–72.e14.
62. Whittle AT, Marshall I, Mortimore IL, et al: Neck soft tissue and fat distribution: comparison between normal men and women by magnetic resonance imaging. Thorax 1999;54:323–328.
63. Jordan AS, Wellman A, Edwards JK, et al: Respiratory control stability and upper airway collapsibility in men and women with obstructive sleep apnea. J Appl Physiol 2005;99:2020–2027.
64. Rowley JA, Zhou X, Vergine I, et al: Influence of gender on upper airway mechanics: upper airway resistance and Pcrit. J Appl Physiol 2001;91:2248–2254.
65. Pillar G, Malhotra A, Fogel R, et al: Airway mechanics and ventilation in response to resistive loading during sleep: influence of gender. Am J Respir Crit Care Med 2000;162:1627–1632.
66. Rowley JA, Zhou XS, Diamond MP, Badr MS: The determinants of the apnea threshold during NREM sleep in normal subjects. Sleep 2006;29:95–103.
67. Zhou XS, Shahabuddin S, Zahn BR, et al: Effect of gender on the development of hypocapnic apnea/hypopnea during NREM sleep. J Appl Physiol 2000;89:192–199.
68. Iber C, Ancoli-Israel S, Chesson A, Quan SF for the American Academy of Sleep Medicine: The AASM Manual for Scoring of Sleep and Associated Events: Rules, Terminology and Technical Specifications, 1st ed. Westchester, IL: American Academy of Sleep Medicine, 2007.
69. O'Malley EB, Norman RG, Farkas DF, et al: The addition of frontal EEG leads improves detection of cortical arousal following obstructive respiratory events. Sleep 2003;26:435–439.
70. Berry RB, Gleeson K: Respiratory arousal from sleep. Mechanisms and significance. Sleep 1997;20:654–675.
71. Younes M: Role of arousal in the pathogenesis of obstructive sleep apnea. Am J Respir Crit Care Med 2004;169:623–633.

72. Gleeson K, Zwillich CW, White DP: The influence of increasing ventilatory effort on arousal from sleep. Am Rev Respir Dis 1990;142:295–300.
73. Kimoff RJ, Cheong TH, Olha AE, et al: Mechanisms of apnea termination in obstructive sleep apnea. Role of chemoreceptor and mechanoreceptor stimuli. Am J Respir Crit Care Med 1994;149:707–714.
74. Bennett LS, Langford BA, Stradling JR, Davies RJ: Sleep fragmentation indices as predictors of daytime sleepiness and nCPAP response in obstructive sleep apnea. Am J Respir Crit Care Med 1998;158:778–786.
75. Roehrs T, Zorick F, Wittig R, et al: Predictors of objective level of daytime sleepiness in patients with sleep-related breathing disorders. Chest 1989;95:1202–1206.
76. Berry RB, Kouchi KG, Bower JL, Light RW: Effect of upper airway anesthesia on obstructive sleep apnea. Am J Respir Crit Care Med 1995;151:1857–1861.
77. Cala SJ, Sliwinski P, Cosio MG, Kimoff RJ: Effect of topical upper airway anesthesia on apnea duration through the night in obstructive sleep apnea. Appl Physiol 1996;81:2618–2626.
78. Berry RB, Kouchi KG, Der DE, et al: Sleep apnea impairs the arousal response to airway occlusion. Chest 1996;109:1490–1496.
79. Kimoff RJ, Sforza E, Champagne V, et al: Upper airway sensation in snoring and obstructive sleep apnea. Am J Respir Crit Care Med 2001;164:250–255.
80. Gora J, Trinder J, Pierce R, Colrain IM: Evidence of a sleep-specific blunted cortical response to inspiratory occlusions in mild obstructive sleep apnea syndrome. Am J Respir Crit Care Med 2002;166:1225–1234.
81. Montserrat JM, Kosmas EN, Cosio MG, Kimoff RJ: Mechanism of apnea lengthening across the night in obstructive sleep apnea. Am J Respir Crit Care Med 1996;154:988–993.
82. Berry RB, Asyali MA, McNellis MI, Khoo MC: Within-night variation in respiratory effort preceding apnea termination and EEG delta power in sleep apnea. J Appl Physiol 1998;85:1434–1441.
83. Sforza E, Krieger AJ, Petiau C: Arousal threshold to respiratory stimuli in OSA patients: evidence of a sleep dependent temporal rhythm. Sleep 1999;22:69–75.
84. Issa FG, Sullivan CE: Arousal and breathing responses to airway occlusion in healthy sleeping adults. J Appl Physiol 1983;55:1113–1119.
85. Findley LJ, Wihoit SC, Surrat PM: Apnea duration and hypoxemia during REM sleep in patients with obstructive sleep apnea. Chest 1985;87:432–436.
86. Berry RB: Dreaming about an open upper airway. Sleep 2006;29:429–430.
87. Zavodny J, Roth C, Bassetti CL, et al: Effects of sleep fragmentation on the arousability to resistive loading in NREM and REM sleep in normal men. Sleep 2006;29:525–532.
88. Findley LJ, Ries AL, Tisi GM, Wagner PD: Hypoxemia during apnea in normal subjects: mechanisms and impact of lung volume. J Appl Physiol 1983;55:1777–1783.
89. Bradley TD, Martinez D, Rutherford R, et al: Physiological determinants of nocturnal arterial oxygenation in patients with obstructive sleep apnea. J Appl Physiol 1985;59:1364–1368.
90. Series F, Cormier Y, La Forge J: Influence of apnea type and sleep stage on nocturnal postapneic desaturation. Am Rev Respir Dis 1990;141:1522–1526.
91. Peppard PE, Ward NR, Morrell MJ: The impact of obesity on oxygen desaturation during sleep disordered breathing. Am J Respir Crit Care Med 2009;180:788–793.
92. Oksenberg A, Khamaysi I, Silverberg DS, Tarasiuk A: Association of body position with severity of apneic events in patients with severe nonpositional obstructive sleep apnea. Chest 2000;118:1018–1024.
93. Oksenberg A, Arons E, Nasser K, et al: REM-related obstructive sleep apnea: the effect of body position. J Clin Sleep Med 2010;6:343–348.

Chapter 17

Consequences of Obstructive Sleep Apnea and the Benefits of Treatment

Chapter Points

- The nocturnal consequences of OSA vary with severity. Possible changes include episodic hypercapnia, hypoxia, negative intrathoracic pressure, increases in pulmonary and systemic pressure, cyclic slowing then speeding of heart rate, and surges of sympathetic tone at event termination. Most studies show that the cardiovascular consequences are most closely related to the severity of hypoxemia.
- Patients with untreated OSA often have elevated post-awakening AM blood pressure, high daytime sympathetic tone, and decreased heart rate variability.
- The best evidence of increased mortality in untreated OSA is for men, with moderate to severe OSA, with an approximate age range of 60 years (40–70 in other studies).
- Observational studies suggest that OSA patients effectively treated with CPAP have normal survival, all other factors being equal.
- The severity of daytime sleepiness increases with higher AHI but there is substantial variability. Other PSG indices such as the arousal index do not have significantly higher correlations with subjective or objective sleepiness than the AHI.
- OSA patients are at increased risk for motor vehicle accidents (especially if there is a history of sleepiness at the wheel). Effective CPAP treatment can reduce the risk of motor vehicle accidents.
- Patients with OSA may fail to have a fall in blood pressure with sleep (nondippers). Clinical cohorts with hypertension or resistant hypertension have a high prevalence of OSA. Although investigations differ, effective CPAP treatment likely is associated with a small decrease in 24-hour blood pressure.
- OSA in the absence of lung disease or diastolic dysfunction is associated with **daytime** pulmonary hypertension in 20% to 40% of patients. The

pulmonary hypertension is usually of a mild nature (unless other factors are present).
- Untreated OSA is associated with nocturnal arrhythmia, although the incidence is low. In some cases, effective treatment will improve arrhythmias.
- Untreated OSA is associated with an increased incidence of recurrence of Afib after cardioversion.
- Observational studies suggest that untreated OSA is associated with a higher risk of adverse outcomes in patients with CAD.
- Untreated OSA is associated with a higher incidence of stroke. In stroke patients, CPAP treatment of OSA can reduce mortality.
- Untreated OSA can worsen nocturia and CPAP treatment can improve this manifestation.
- Pediatric OSA has significant neurobehavioral consequences that can be improved with treatment.

This chapter reviews the consequences of untreated obstructive sleep apnea (OSA) and the benefits of treatment. Many of the studies discussed are cross-sectional population-based investigations looking for associations between the *prevalence* of a cardiovascular consequence (e.g., hypertension) at a given time with the severity/presence of OSA (various levels of apnea-hypopnea index [AHI]). Prevalence is the amount of disease in a given population. Others follow a population over a period of time and determine the amount of new cases (*incidence* of a given disease). These studies determine the risk of developing consequences at various levels of AHI. The results of population-based studies may also vary depending on the group to be evaluated. It is always worth noting that investigations of clinic-based versus asymptomatic individuals randomly selected may well be different.

Considering the effects of continuous positive airway pressure (CPAP) treatment on consequences of untreated

OSA, it is important to understand that observational studies are less convincing than randomized controlled trials. There is always the concern that patients who adhered to CPAP treatment are somehow more compliant with other medical therapy as well and, therefore, more likely to have better outcomes. A study by Platt and colleagues[1] found CPAP users were more adherent in taking lipid-lowering medications. However, another study by Villar and coworkers[2] found that patients adherent or nonadherent to CPAP did not differ in their adherence to medication. Both of these studies relied on prescriptions filled or patient report, so actual medication use could differ. There are a number of ethical and experimental considerations to designing a study to prove a benefit of CPAP treatment on cardiovascular outcomes. With the widespread knowledge of CPAP, it is difficult to design a study with effective blinding and a satisfactory control treatment (e.g., subtherapeutic CPAP).[3]

PATHOPHYSIOLOGY

During normal non–rapid eye movement (NREM) sleep, there is a decrease in metabolic rate, sympathetic nerve activity, blood pressure, and heart rate, whereas vagal tone increases compared with wakefulness.[4,5] OSA changes this normal pattern considerably[4-6] (Fig. 17–1). Cycles of hypoxia and CO_2 retention elicit changes in sympathetic and parasympathetic activity. Hypoxia and hypercapnia increase ventilatory drive and obstructed inspiratory efforts create negative intrathoracic pressure (sometimes reaching –80 cm H_2O). The negative pressure increases venous return to the right side of the heart (increased right ventricular [RV] preload) and the hypoxia causes pulmonary vasoconstriction (increased RV afterload). The right ventricle may dilate and the septum bulge into the left ventricle, impairing left ventricular (LV) filling and decreasing stroke volume. Negative intrathoracic pressure increases the transmural pressure

across the left ventricle walls and increases the effective afterload. The cycles of increased sympathetic tone[6] (Fig. 17–2) increase systemic vascular resistance. Arousal at apnea termination is associated with a large increase in sympathetic tone and decreased vagal tone with the result that blood pressure and heart rate increase. High sympathetic tone is still present during wakefulness (see Fig. 17–2) and associated with impaired vagally mediated heart rate variability. Intermittent hypoxia causes oxygen free radical production and activates inflammatory pathways that can predispose to atherosclerosis and thrombosis.

MORTALITY

In patients with OSA, frequent coexisting conditions such as hypertension and obesity make analysis of the impact of OSA on survival difficult. It is unlikely that a randomized long-term trial of treatment of OSA versus observation is now possible for ethical reasons. Most of the information we have about mortality and OSA is from retrospective studies or prospective observational studies. Some of the studies are from **clinical cohorts** that would be expected to have a higher prevalence of disease, but such studies are subject to referral bias. Other studies are from large population-based cohorts that are free of referral bias but have a relatively low number of patients with severe OSA. Some studies have analyzed all-cause mortality and others looked at cardiovascular mortality.

An early retrospective study by He and associates[7] showed a decreased survival in untreated patients with an apnea index (AI) greater than 20/hr. Patients with an AI greater than 20/hr who were treated with tracheostomy or CPAP did not have a decreased survival. The causes of death in the patients were not documented. Lavie and coworkers[8] reviewed the results on 1620 patients diagnosed with OSA between 1976 and 1988. Fifty-seven patients had died by

FIGURE 17–1 Pathophysiology of the effects of obstructive sleep apnea (OSA) on the cardiovascular system. BP = blood pressure; HR = heart rate; LV = left ventricular; PCO_2 = arterial partial pressure of carbon dioxide; PNA = parasympathetic nervous system; PO_2 = arterial partial pressure of oxygen; SNA = sympathetic nervous activity. *From Bradley TD, Floras JS: Obstructive sleep apnea and its cardiovascular consequences. Lancet 2009;373:82–93.*

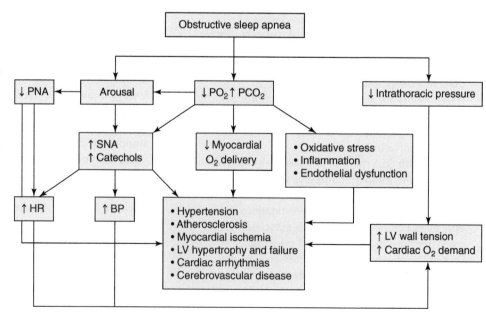

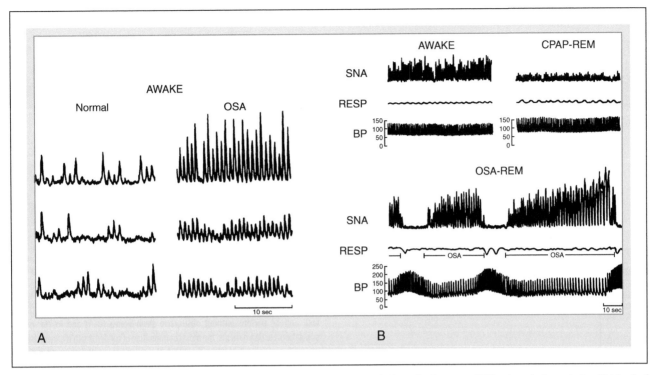

FIGURE 17-2 **A,** Recordings of sympathetic nerve activity (SNA) during wakefulness in patients with obstructive sleep apnea (OSA) and matched controls show high levels of SNA in awake patients with sleep apnea. **B,** Recording of arterial blood pressure (BP) and SNA in the same subject awake, during rapid eye movement (REM) sleep with obstructive apnea (OSA-REM), and during REM sleep on continuous positive airway pressure (CPAP-REM). *A and B, From Somers VK, Dyken ME, Clary MP, Abboud FM: Sympathetic neural mechanisms in obstructive sleep apnea. J Clin Invest 1995;96:1897–1904.*

1990 with 53% of the deaths due to respiratory and cardiovascular causes. Excess mortality was noted in men of 30 to 50 years of age with OSA but not in patients older than 70 years of age. Lavie and colleagues[9] later published results of a sleep clinic cohort (1991–2000) consisting of 14,589 patients and found that the hazard of mortality was higher in male patients with moderate and severe OSA compared with the general population. The results were significant for patients younger than 50 years of age. Another analysis of a similar cohort sought to determine the factors associated with mortality in OSA patients.[10] The study found that the risk of mortality in patients with OSA was increased by the presence of co-morbidities. For patients younger than 62 years, increased mortality was associated with the presence of heart failure or diabetes mellitus. For OSA patients older than 62 years, predicators of increased mortality included chronic obstructive pulmonary disease, congestive heart failure, and diabetes mellitus.[10] Older patients (age > 65 years) with mild to moderate OSA appear to be resistant to the adverse effects of OSA on mortality.[11]

Marshall and associates[12] found an increase in all-cause mortality associated with moderate to severe OSA in a population-based study. Marin and coworkers[13] studied a **clinic population of men** and found an increase of fatal and nonfatal cardiovascular events for severe OSA compared with normal individuals, snorers, patients with mild OSA, and patients with OSA on CPAP treatment (Fig. 17–3). Yaggi and colleagues[14] published data on another cohort referred to a sleep clinic and found an increased mortality in severe

OSA patients. Young and associates[15] published results from the Wisconsin Sleep Cohort and found that severe OSA patients had an increased risk of all-cause mortality. The results of this study were adjusted for gender. Punjabi and coworkers[16] published results on a large population cohort from the Sleep Heart Health Study. There was an increase in mortality for the severe OSA patients who were male and aged 40 to 70 years. In this study, statistical corrections for the effects of age, BMI, and gender (when appropriate) were performed.

Summarizing the results, there is strong evidence for an increased mortality in untreated middle-aged **male patients** with severe OSA (Table 17–1). Indeed, two clinic-based population studies included only or predominantly men. Conversely, the Wisconsin Cohort data did not show a sex difference in the increased mortality associated with severe OSA. However, relatively few patients had severe OSA in this study. It seems likely that women with untreated severe OSA also have increased mortality, but the evidence for this increased mortality is not as strong as that for men. There is also the controversy about whether patients who are not sleepy have an increased risk of cardiovascular morbidity. Evidence from the Sleep Heart Health Study[16] found that adverse outcomes correlated more with measures of oxygenation than with sleepiness (or impaired sleep), suggesting that intermittent hypoxemia rather than indices of sleep fragmentation is associated with increased mortality. Conversely, the Wisconsin-based cohort[15] found an increase in cardiovascular mortality with severe OSA that was present

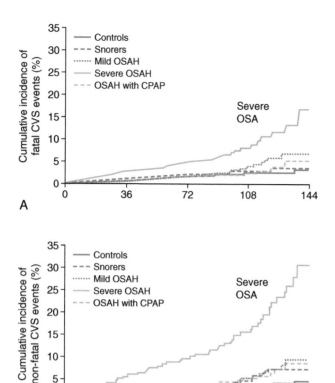

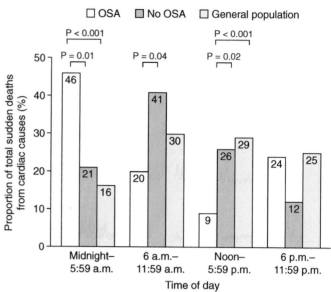

FIGURE 17–4 Day-night pattern of sudden death from cardiac causes in 78 persons with and 34 persons without obstructive sleep apnea (OSA) and in the general population. For OSA patients, the most common time of sudden death is during the sleep period. In normal individuals without OSA, the most common time of sudden death is in the morning. *From Gami AS, Howard DE, Olson EJ, Somers VK: Day-night pattern of sudden death in obstructive sleep apnea. N Engl J Med 2005;352:1206–1214.*

FIGURE 17–3 Cumulative incidence of fatal **(A)** and nonfatal **(B)** cardiovascular events (CVS) in controls, snorers, and patients with mild or severe obstructive sleep apnea (OSA). The patients with OSA treatment with continuous positive airway pressure (CPAP) are also shown. Patients with severe OSA had increased cumulative adverse events. OSAH = obstructive sleep apnea-hypopnea. **A** *and* **B,** *From Marin JM, Carrizo S, Vicente E, Agusti AGN: Long term cardiovascular outcomes in men with obstructive sleep apnea-hypopnea with or without treatment with continuous positive airway pressure: an observational study. Lancet 2005;365:1046–1053.*

irrespective of symptoms of sleepiness. The controversy continues, but it seems likely that the severity of oxygen desaturation due to OSA is the major factor associated with increased cardiovascular morbidity.

The time of sudden death appears to be different for patients with OSA. Gami and colleagues[17] found that for patients with OSA, the relative risk of sudden death from cardiac causes from midnight to 6 AM was 2.57 (95% confidence interval 1.87–3.52) compared with other times during the day. People with OSA have a peak in sudden death from cardiac causes during the sleeping hours, which contrasts strikingly with the nadir of sudden death from cardiac causes during this period in people without OSA and in the general population. In patients without sleep apnea, the risk of sudden death was greatest in the morning hours **after awakening** (Fig. 17–4).[17]

EXCESSIVE DAYTIME SLEEPINESS AND NEUROCOGNITIVE DYSFUNCTION

Excessive daytime sleepiness is a cardinal manifestation of OSA. However, the severity of this symptom is extremely

variable. Chronic sleep deprivation and/or fragmentation from respiratory events is believed to be the major cause of sleepiness, although hypoxemia may also play a role. Normal individuals subjected to experimental sleep fragmentation without hypoxemia develop subjective and objective daytime sleepiness.[18,19] Attempts at finding abnormalities demonstrated on polysomnography that correlate highly with subjective or objective sleepiness have not been very successful. Johns[20] found the Epworth Sleepiness Scale (subjective sleepiness) to correlate with the respiratory distress index (RDI) in a group of 165 patients with OSA (r = 0.439) and slightly less with the minimum arterial oxygen saturation (SaO_2; r = –0.404). Guilleminault and associates[21] found no polysomnographic variable to be significantly correlated with sleepiness as assessed by the multiple sleep latency test (MSLT). Roehrs and coworkers[19] analyzed data from 466 patients using multiple regression analysis and found daytime sleepiness as assessed by the MSLT had a slightly higher correlation with the respiratory arousal index (r = –0.36) than indices of hypoxemia (r = –0.34). Cheshire and colleagues found the arousal index to correlate with impaired cognitive function testing but not objective daytime sleepiness.[22] Bennett and associates[23] found that the AHI, cortical arousal index (central and frontal electroencephalogram [EEG]), sleep disturbance based on a neural network model, and a body movement index correlated with objective daytime sleepiness. The correlation between excessive sleepiness and the indices of sleep disturbance was only slightly higher than the correlation between sleepiness and the AHI. The body movement index (based on video recording rather than EEG) and the neural network had the highest correlation coefficients.

TABLE 17–1

Increased Mortality and Obstructive Sleep Apnea

AUTHOR	SELECTION	PARTICIPANTS	FINDINGS
Punjabi, 2009[16] Population-based	Sleep Heart Health Cohort	6441 patients Average f/u 8.2 yr Severe OSA N = 341	Severe OSA AHI > 30/hr associated with increased mortality only in men 40–70 yr old. Measures of sleep-related hypoxemia but not sleep fragmentation were associated with increased mortality.
Marin, 2005[13] Clinical cohort—sleep clinic recruited	Snorers, OSA, and matched control population	MEN ONLY 264 healthy men 337 simple snorers 403 untreated mild to moderate OSA 235 severe OSA untreated 372 OSA treated with CPAP	Men with severe OSA AHI > 30/hr had increased incidence of fatal (MI, CVA) and nonfatal adverse cardiovascular events (MI, CVA, CABPG, coronary angiography) compared with control group, mild OSA group, and CPAP group. Odds ratio fatal CVE 2.87 Odds ratio nonfatal CVE 3.17 Severe group treated with CPAP did not have increased risk compared with normal men.
Yaggi, 2005[14] Clinical cohort	Patients referred to sleep clinic PSG for diagnosis Adjustments for age, sex, race, smoking status, BMI, DM, Afib, HTN	1022 patients (77% male) 697 had OSA	OSA (AHI > 5/hr) was associated with increased risk of death from any cause.
Lavie, 2005[9] Clinical cohort	Patients referred to sleep clinic	N = 14,589 372 deaths after median f/u of 4.6 yr	RDI > 30/hr males had higher mortality but only in males aged < 50 yr.
Young, 2008[15] Population-based	18-yr mortality f/u PSG at baseline Adjustments for age, gender, BMI, DM, cholesterol, mean BP	N = 1522 Severe OSA N = 63	All-cause mortality higher in severe OSA (AHI > 30/hr) vs. no OSA even when CPAP-treated patients eliminated. The results were not changed based on the presence or absence of sleepiness.
Marshall, 2008[12] (Busselton Health Study) Population-based	Prospective observational Home sleep testing 14-yr f/u Adjustments for age, gender, BMI, DM, cholesterol, mean BP	397 participants moderate to severe OSA N = 18 380 free from MI and CVA at baseline 18 AHI > 15/hr 77 AHI 5 to <15/hr 285 no OSA	Moderate to severe OSA (AHI > 15/hr) had greater risk of all-cause mortality compared with no OSA. Mild OSA had no increased risk.

Afib = atrial fibrillation; AHI = apnea-hypopnea index; BMI = body mass index; BP = blood pressure; CABPG = coronary artery bypass grafting; CPAP = continuous positive airway pressure; CVA = cerebrovascular accident; CVE = complex ventricular event; DM = diabetes mellitus; f/u = follow-up; HTN = hypertension; OSA = obstructive sleep apnea; PSG = polysomnography; RDI = respiratory distress index.

Routine EEG analysis based on sleep staging or EEG arousals may not be sensitive enough to detect all the adverse effects of respiratory disturbance. For example, noncortical arousals from respiratory events or other causes may result in daytime sleepiness.[24] It may also be possible that long periods of airflow limitation with high respiratory effort without discrete arousal could be associated with symptoms. This pattern commonly occurs in children with OSA who develop behavioral changes and impaired school performance without frequent discrete arousals.[25,26] Findings from

the Sleep Heart Health Study show an increase in sleepiness with higher AHI, but the relationship is weak.[27] There is also evidence from several studies that hypoxemia may be a factor associated with impaired cognition in patients with OSA.[28] For many patients, a number of factors other than OSA contribute to daytime sleepiness including insufficient sleep and medication side effects. There is also considerable individual variability in the ability to tolerate sleep fragmentation. Therefore, it should not be surprising that there is only a modest correlation between the AHI and subjective or objective measures. Of note, studies of heart failure patients with OSA often show a large proportion do not complain of daytime sleepiness.[29] It should also be noted that effective treatment of sleepy OSA patients (e.g., CPAP) does not always abolish daytime sleepiness.

AUTOMOBILE ACCIDENTS AND SLEEP APNEA

The true increase in risk of patients with OSA having an automobile accident is difficult to determine. However, published studies have found a two to three times greater risk in untreated patients with OSA.[30-32] Clearly, not all patients with sleep apnea are at high risk of having an auto accident. It appears that the presence of sleep apnea plus a history of a previous accident (or frequent falling asleep at the wheel) identifies a group of patients with especially high risk. The decision of whether to report a patient with OSA to a motor vehicle licensing agency is a difficult one. A balance between patient confidentiality and protection of the public is required. A committee of the American Thoracic Society has issued the following recommendations[33]: "In those jurisdictions in which conditions such as excessive daytime sleepiness caused by sleep apnea may be construed as reportable events, we recommend reporting to licensing bureaus if: (a) the patient has excessive daytime sleepiness, sleep apnea, and a history of a motor vehicle accident or equivalent level of clinical concern; and (b) one of the following circumstances exists: (i) the patient's condition is untreatable or is not amenable to expeditious treatment (within 2 months of diagnosis) or (ii) the patient is not willing to accept treatment or is unwilling to restrict driving until effective treatment has been instituted." The committee also noted that it is the physician's responsibility to notify every patient with sleep apnea that driving when sleepy is unsafe. Some form of written documentation that the patient understands this warning is prudent. A statement concerning sleep apnea and commercial motor vehicle operators by a joint task force of the American College of Chest Physicians, the American College of Occupational and Environmental Medicine, and the National Sleep Foundation[34] provides guidance concerning the evaluation, treatment, and return to work of drivers with suspected or known OSA.

It is concerning that large financial tort settlements have been brought successfully against some physicians for failure to report a person with a medical condition who was subsequently involved in a serious traffic accident. Each state has its own laws, and local medical societies have guidelines. However, in the end, the decision rests with the judgment of the treating physician. In some states, reporting is done to a health agency rather than directly to the motor vehicle licensing agency. Note that reporting does not always result in the loss of the patient's license.

To date, there is no objective test that can quantify a patient's degree of driving impairment. The use of the maintenance of wakefulness test (MWT) and MSLT were discussed in Chapter 14. The MWT is the appropriate test to assess the ability to stay awake. However, MWT results may not generalize to the real world in which sleep deprivation and other factors are operative. There have been promising attempts at developing protocols using driving simulators,[35,36] but results in a simulator may not correlate with driving performance. A study of untreated OSA patients[36] found an MWT mean sleep latency (MSL) less than 19 minutes was associated with impairment on a driving simulator. The same group extended this work by testing patients with OSA during actual 90-minute driving sessions on the road with a driving instructor intervening if necessary (the test car had two steering wheels).[37] Inappropriate line crossing was determined by video recording. Two groups "very sleepy" with a MWT MSL less than 19 minutes and "sleepy" with a MSL 20 to 33 minutes had significantly more line crossings than controls and patients with mild sleepiness (MWT MSL 34–40 min).

Studies have shown improved performance on driver simulators after CPAP treatment of OSA.[38] In addition, studies have also shown that the risk of traffic accidents does appear to be reduced with nasal CPAP therapy (if patients are compliant).[39,40] The evidence for a reduction in motor vehicle accidents with effective OSA treatment was recently summarized by Tregear and coworkers[40] in a systematic review with meta-analysis.

ARTERIAL HYPERTENSION

Normal persons and many patients with hypertension but without sleep apnea have a nocturnal fall in blood pressure. However, 20% to 40% of patients with OSA fail to have the normal nocturnal fall in systemic blood pressure ("nondippers").[41] During obstructive apnea, blood pressure tends to rise slightly and then to rise abruptly at apnea termination (Fig. 17–5) secondary to arousal from sleep and restoration of breathing associated with sympathetic activation and parasympathetic withdrawal.

There is continued controversy about whether OSA can cause daytime (diurnal) as well as nocturnal hypertension. Animal models of simulated OSA suggest that it can.[42] Several studies have found that OSA is very common in adult populations with hypertension (>30%).[43] This association does not prove causality because patients with hypertension and OSA share common, potentially causative, factors such as obesity. Carlson and coworkers[44] found that age, obesity, and sleep apnea were independent and additive risk factors for the presence of hypertension. The Sleep Heart Health Study, a large population-based investigation, found an increased risk of having self-reported hypertension when OSA was present (Table 17–2).[45]

A prospective study of the Wisconsin cohort found an increase in AHI predicted the development of hypertension in the following 4 years (**increased incidence**) after adjusting for confounding factors such as obesity, age, and smoking (Table 17–3).[46] In contrast to these findings, a recent analysis of the Sleep Heart Health data found that there was no relationship between the AHI and the risk of incident hypertension (risk of developing hypertension in the next 5 yr) when

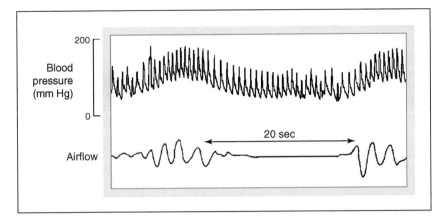

FIGURE 17–5 This tracing shows the swings in arterial blood pressure associated with obstructive sleep apnea (respiratory effort tracing not shown). At apnea termination, there is a steep increase in blood pressure that coincides with increased sympathetic activity. *From Berry RB: Sleep Medicine Pearls, 2nd ed. Philadelphia: Hanley & Belfus, 2003, p. 191. Reproduced with permission.*

TABLE 17–2

Cardiovascular Disease and Obstructive Sleep Apnea Sleep Heart Health Study—Risk of Self Reported Cardiovascular Disease (Prevalence)

	QUARTILE				P
	I	II	III	IV	
AHI (#/hr)	0–1.3	1.4–4.4	4.5–11.0	>11.0	
CAD*	1.0	0.92 (0.71–1.20)	1.20 (0.93–1.54)	1.27 (0.99–1.62)	.004
CHF*	1.0	1.13 (0.54–2.39)	1.95 (0.99–3.83)	2.38 (1.22–4.62)	.002
Stroke*	1.0	1.15 (0.72–1.83)	1.42 (0.91–2.21)	1.58 (1.02–2.46)	.03
APNEA-HYPOPNEA INDEX CATEGORY					
AHI (#/hr)	<1.5	1.5–4.9	5–14.9	15–29.9	≥30	
HTN†	1.0	1.07 (0.91–1.26)	1.20 (1.01–1.42)	1.25 (1.0–1.56)	1.37 (1.03–1.83)	.005

CAD = coronary artery disease; CHF = congestive heart failure; HTN = hypertension.
Values are risk (95% confidence interval).
*Data from Shahar E, Whitney CW, Redline S, et al: Sleep-disordered breathing and cardiovascular disease. Am J Respir Crit Care Med 2001;163:19–25.
†Data from Nieto FJ, Young TB, Lind BK, et al: Association of sleep disordered breathing, sleep apnea, and hypertension in a large community-based study. JAMA 2000;283:1829–1836.

TABLE 17–3

Risk of Incident Hypertension in Obstructive Sleep Apnea (Wisconsin Cohort—Population-Based)*

	QUARTILE				P
	I	II	III	IV	
AHI (#/hr)	0	0.1–4.9	5.0–14.9	>15	
Relative risk (CI)	1.0	1.42 1.13–1.78	2.03 1.29–3.17	2.89 1.46–5.64	.002

*Based on laboratory measure of blood pressure at baseline versus follow-up in 4 years (incident HTN).
CI = confidence interval; HTN = hypertension.
From Peppard PE, Young T, Palta M, Skatrud J: Prospective study of the association between sleep-disordered breathing and hypertension. N Engl J Med 2000;342:1378–1384.

the risk was adjusted for obesity.[47] There was a trend for a relationship when the AHI was greater than 30/hr. One problem with the Sleep Heart Health Study is that the population contained relatively few patients with severe OSA. In summary, patients with OSA are likely at risk of developing hypertension. The risk is most significant with severe OSA and is confounded by the presence of obesity.

Even if sleep apnea does not cause daytime hypertension, it may well worsen the physiologic impact of the disorder or impair treatment efficacy. For example, Verdeechia and coworkers[48] found that hypertensive patients who failed to have a 10% nocturnal fall in blood pressure had greater LV hypertrophy. Studies have also documented an increase in mortality among nondippers.[49] Studies of populations with resistant hypertension have found a high prevalence of OSA.[50] Therefore, the possibility of the presence of OSA should be considered in all patients with resistant hypertension. One study found that CPAP treatment was helpful in patients with resistant hypertension who had OSA.[51]

If sleep apnea is effectively treated, does hypertension improve? This question has been approached by a number of studies that have determined the effect of nasal CPAP on nocturnal and daytime blood pressure in patients with OSA. Becker and colleagues[52] found that effective treatment of sleep apnea with nasal CPAP for 9 weeks or more lowered both nocturnal and daytime blood pressure by approximately 10 mm Hg using a placebo-controlled (sham CPAP)

FIGURE 17–6 A, Time course of mean arterial blood pressure (MAP) before *(dark black circles)* and on treatment *(gray circles)* with therapeutic nasal continuous positive airway pressure (nCPAP). On average, 7.2 hours were recorded during the night. **B,** Time course of MAP before *(closed circles)* and on treatment *(open circles)* with subtherapeutic nCPAP. Note the decreased blood pressure on CPAP but not subtherapeutic CPAP. *From Becker HF, Jerrentrup A, Ploch T, et al: Effect of nasal continuous positive airway pressure treatment on blood pressure in patients with obstructive sleep apnea. Circulation 2003;107:68–73.*

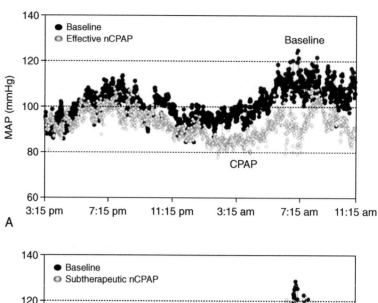

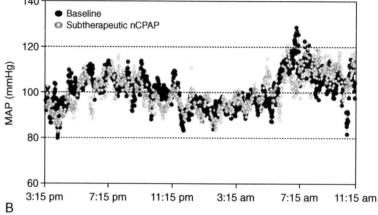

study design (Fig. 17–6). Other investigations have shown smaller[53,54] or no effects on daytime blood pressure.[55,56] These conflicting results may reflect inadequate CPAP treatment (poor adherence), too short a treatment interval, or less severe sleep apnea populations.

A meta-analysis of 12 randomized trials of the effect of CPAP on blood pressure found that CPAP did significantly reduce 24-hour blood pressure by about 2 mm Hg. Results were greatest in patients with more severe OSA and better use of CPAP.[57] Of note, ambulatory blood pressure monitoring can cause awakenings and change what it is trying to measure.[58] The study of Becker and colleagues[52] used beat-to-beat blood pressure with a finger probe rather than a periodically inflating cuff. In general, most hypertensive patients with sleep apnea will still continue to require antihypertensive medications when treated with CPAP. However, 24-hour control of blood pressure may improve on CPAP treatment.

PULMONARY HYPERTENSION

Both hypoxemia and acidosis cause constriction of the pulmonary arteries. Hence, it is not surprising that episodes of pulmonary hypertension occur during obstructive apnea in patients with OSA (Fig. 17–7).[59,60] For patients with normal daytime arterial partial pressure of oxygen (PaO_2), the

pulmonary pressures usually return to normal. Pulmonary hypertension is often defined as a mean pulmonary artery pressure greater than 25 mm Hg. The term pulmonary **arterial** hypertension is reserved for disorders of the pulmonary arteries that result in pulmonary hypertension. Of note, diastolic dysfunction (high pulmonary venous pressures and LV end-diastolic pressure) also results in increased pulmonary arterial pressure. It has been said that OSA patients with normal daytime blood gases usually have normal or only mildly increased daytime pulmonary pressures.[60,61] The presence of coexistent chronic obstructive pulmonary disease (COPD) or LV diastolic dysfunction does appear to increase the prevalence and severity of daytime pulmonary hypertension. However, the presence of COPD is not obligatory.[61,62] Some OSA patients may have an increased vascular response to nocturnal episode acidosis and hypoxemia. In the absence of lung disease or elevated LV end-diastolic pressure, the incidence of pulmonary hypertension in OSA patients has been estimated to be 20% to 40%.[60] Sajkov and associates[62] described a group of patients with OSA with mean pulmonary pressures up to 26 mm Hg (their normal <20 mm Hg) and pulmonary systolic pressures up to 40 mm Hg. The affected group seemed to have a greater increase in pulmonary pressures in response to an increase in cardiac output or hypoxemia. The authors hypothesized that remodeling of the pulmonary vascular bed (possibly due to OSA) was

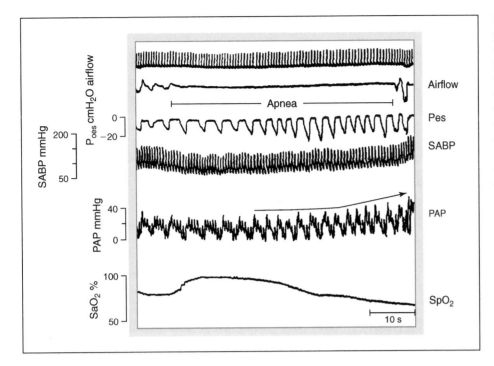

FIGURE 17–7 Increase in systolic blood pressure (SABP) and pulmonary pressure (PAP) during obstructive apnea. Note the progressively negative esophageal pressure (P$_{oes}$). There is cyclic variation in the PAP due to cycles of negative pressure in the chest, **but the overall trend is upward (arrow).** Hypoxemia and acidosis (hypercapnia) cause pulmonary arterial vasoconstriction. SaO$_2$ = arterial oxygen saturation; SpO$_2$ = pulse oximetry. *From Podszus T, Greenberg H, Scharf S: Influence of sleep state and sleep disordered breathing on cardiovascular function. In Sanders NA, Sullivan CE (eds): Sleep and Breathing. New York: Marcel Decker, 1994, pp. 257–310.*

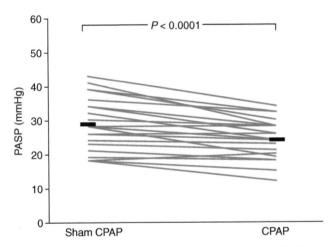

FIGURE 17–8 A reduction in pulmonary arterial systolic pressure (PASP) (Doppler Echo) after 3 months of continuous positive airway pressure (CPAP) treatment in CPAP versus sham CPAP. This was a **randomized cross-over trial**. *From Arias MA, García-Río F, Alonso-Fernández A, et al: Pulmonary hypertension in obstructive sleep apnoea: effects of continuous positive airway pressure: a randomized, controlled cross-over study. Eur Heart J 2006;27:1106–1113.*

responsible. One long-term case series showed that patients with OSA and pulmonary hypertension had stable pulmonary pressures over 5 years when treated with CPAP.[63] Another study found that CPAP improved pulmonary arterial pressure and vascular reactivity in OSA.[64] Alchanatis and colleagues[65] found mild daytime pulmonary hypertension in a group of OSA patients without lung disease that reversed after 6 months of CPAP. Arias and associates[66] performed a randomized cross-over trial (sham or effective CPAP) for 12 weeks. CPAP resulted in lower pulmonary arterial systolic pressure compared with sham (Fig. 17–8).

ARRHYTHMIAS

In normal individuals, the heart rate is lower during NREM sleep than during wakefulness. This is thought to be due to parasympathetic predominance during sleep.[5] In patients with OSA, the heart rate varies in cycles: slowing with apnea onset; increasing slightly, staying the same, or decreasing during apnea; and increasing dramatically in the postapneic period[67-69] (Fig. 17–9). Early studies attributed the slowing of heart rate during apnea to increased vagal tone and hypoxia.[67] The slowing was diminished by atropine and supplemental oxygen. Later studies have not consistently found a reduction in heart rate in the last part of apnea.[68,69] The increased vagal tone during apnea is the result of hypoxic stimulation of the carotid body **during absent ventilation.** With resumption of respiration, inflation of the lungs decreases vagal tone and the hypoxic influences on sympathetic tone are unmasked (tachycardia). Bonsignore and coworkers[68] found that the heart rate during apnea could increase, stay the same, or decrease depending on relative amounts of parasympathetic and sympathetic tone. One investigation suggested that the individual differences in the effect of apnea on heart rate may be secondary to differences in the response of the carotid body to hypoxia.[70] Although the cyclic changes in heart rate are sometimes referred to as *brady-tachycardia*, the heart rate often remains between 60 and 90 bpm in most patients.

Guilleminault and colleagues[71] reported on 400 patients with sleep apnea. Forty-eight percent had some type of arrhythmia. Twenty percent had more than two premature ventricular contractions (PVCs)/min during sleep, 7% had severe bradycardia to less than 30 bpm, 3% had nonsustained ventricular tachycardia, and 5% and 3% had Mobitz type I and type II second-degree block, respectively. Sinus

FIGURE 17–9 Changes in heart rate associated with obstructive apnea. ECG = electrocardiogram; SaO$_2$ = arterial oxygen saturation. *From Berry RB: Sleep Medicine Pearls, 2nd ed. Philadelphia: Hanley & Belfus, 2003, p. 195.*

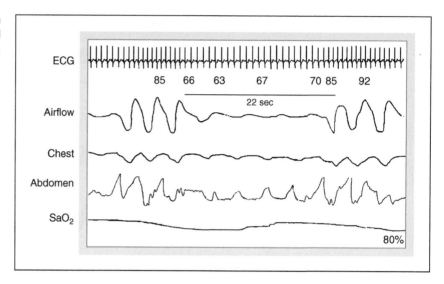

arrest from 2.5 to 13 seconds was noted in 11%. A prospective study of 45 recently diagnosed OSA patients used Holter monitoring for 18 hours after diagnosis and again after 2 to 3 days of CPAP.[72] Only 8 of the 45 had significant rhythm disturbances including ventricular tachycardia, atrial fibrillation (Afib), supraventricular tachycardia, and second- or third-degree heart block. In 7 of these 8 patients, CPAP resulted in the abolition of rhythm disturbances.

The parasympathetic predominance during apnea in some patients may have little significance, except in cases of significant bradycardia or heart block. One study documented a reversal of atrioventricular conduction block on CPAP treatment.[73] The periods of tachycardia and elevated blood pressure postapnea increase myocardial oxygen demand at the same time that hypoxemia exists, predisposing to ischemia and possibly tachyarrhythmias. In normal individuals, sleep usually is a time of reduced tachyarrhythmias and ischemia. Patients with OSA may not enjoy the same protection. PVCs are not uncommon in patients with OSA. However, in some patients, the PVC frequency is actually lower during sleep. Shepard and associates[74] found no correlation between the SaO$_2$ at desaturation and PVC frequency during sleep unless the SaO$_2$ was less than 60%.

Heart rate variability has been used as a tool to study the balance of parasympathetic and sympathetic tone in patients with OSA. During wakefulness, OSA patients show less heart rate variability than normal individuals. This is thought secondary to an increase in sympathetic tone that is still present during the day. After successful treatment with CPAP, the heart rate variability may increase suggesting a drop in sympathetic activity. Khoo and coworkers[75] found that CPAP treatment of OSA improved vagal heart rate control and that the degree of improvement varied directly with the amount of CPAP adherence.

Gami and colleagues[76] found that the risk of developing Afib was more associated with obesity and the degree of arterial oxygen desaturation than the AHI. Untreated OSA appears to worsen arrhythmia control. Kanagala and

associates[77] found that patients with untreated OSA had a higher recurrence of Afib after cardioversion than patients without a polysomnographic diagnosis of sleep apnea. Appropriate treatment with CPAP in OSA was associated with a lower recurrence of Afib. Mehra and coworkers[78] evaluated a cohort of older men and found that sleep-disordered breathing was associated with Afib and complex ventricular events (CVEs). The prevalence of CVE was associated with OSA and hypoxemia whereas Afib was associated with central sleep apnea (CSA). An evaluation of the Sleep Heart Health cohort found that, although the rate of arrhythmias was low, the relative risk of Afib or nonsustained ventricular tachycardia was much higher following respiratory events.[79] In Figure 17–10, a patient with OSA changes from sinus rhythm to Afib after apnea termination. Ryan and coworkers[80] performed a randomized, controlled trial of CPAP in heart failure patients to determine whether ventricular premature beats (VPBs) would decrease. The study found that CPAP did reduce VPB frequency (58% reduction) during sleep. The urinary norepinephrine concentration also decreased. No changes were noted in the control group.[80]

CORONARY ARTERY DISEASE

The Sleep Heart Health Study of a large prospective cohort of patients found evidence of a slight increase in risk of having self-reported coronary artery disease (CAD) at even low levels of sleep apnea (prevalence) (see Table 17–2).[81] Peker and colleagues[82] found an increase in mortality in patients with CAD who had untreated OSA. Gottlieb and associates[83] evaluated the Sleep Heart Health cohort data and found an increased risk of **incident** CAD was associated with the presence of OSA in men younger than 70 years of age. The association was strongest for severe OSA. Milleron and coworkers[84] found CPAP treatment of patients with OSA and CAD improved event-free survival (Fig. 17–11). The end point was a composite of cardiovascular death, acute coronary syndrome, hospitalization for CHF, or need for

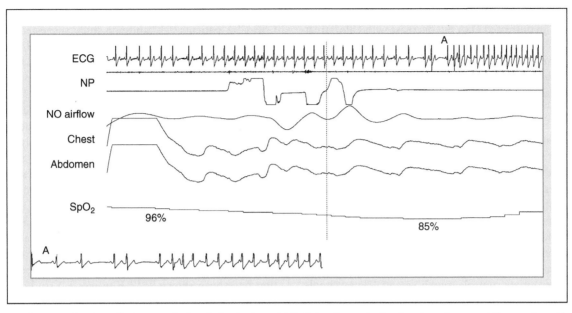

FIGURE 17–10 A patient with sleep apnea in sinus rhythm develops atrial fibrillation after termination of an obstructive apnea. A blow-up of area *A* is shown in the lower left corner. NO airflow = nasal oral thermal flow; NP = nasal pressure; SpO$_2$ = pulse oximetry. The tracing is 60 seconds in duration.

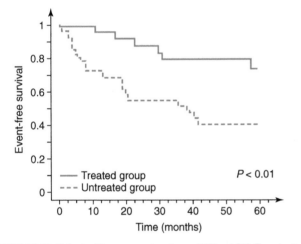

FIGURE 17–11 Patients with coronary artery disease (CAD) and OSA. Those treated with CPAP had improved survival compared with untreated patients. *From Milleron O, Pillière R, Foucher A, et al: Benefits of obstructive sleep apnoea treatment in coronary artery disease: a long-term follow-up study. Eur Heart J 2004;25:728–734.*

coronary revascularization. The control group was patients who declined CPAP (not a randomized trial). The mean follow-up was 86 months.

ATHEROSCLEROSIS AND THROMBOSIS

There have also been a growing number of studies showing changes in blood components or indicators of inflammation in OSA that may be associated with an increased risk of atherosclerosis or thrombosis (Table 17–4). In OSA, there is an increase in the early morning hematocrit[85] and fibrinogen levels[86] that decrease after CPAP treatment. The levels of vascular endothelial growth factor (VEGF),[87] extent of neutrophil,[88,89] and platelet activation[90] are also reduced with

TABLE 17–4	
Effect of Obstructive Sleep Apnea on Factors Contributing to Atherosclerosis and Thrombosis	
UNTREATED OSA	**IMPROVED WITH CPAP**
Increased am hematocrit—Kreiger, 1990[85]	Less natriuresis
Increased fibrinogen—Chin, 1996[86]	Yes[86]
Neutrophil activation[89]	Yes[89]
Increased visceral fat[97]	Decreased visceral fat[97]
Platelet activation—Bokinsky, 1995[90]	Yes[90]
VEGF—Lavie, 2002[87]	Yes[87]
Reactive oxygen species—Dyugovskaya, 2002[88]	Yes[88]
Superoxide release—Schulz, 2000[89]	Yes[89]
Elevated C-reactive protein[91–93]	Yes[93]
Elevated IL-6[91]	Yes[91]
Elevated TNF-alpha, IL-8[94]	Yes[94]
CPAP = continuous positive airway pressure; IL = interleukin; OSA = obstructive sleep apnea; TNF-alpha = tumor necrosis factor-alpha; VEGF = vascular endothelial growth factor.	

CPAP treatment of patients with OSA. Inflammation is now believed to play a role in atherosclerosis or plaque rupture. The level of C-reactive protein (a marker of inflammation) is reduced with CPAP treatment.[91–93] Intermittent hypoxia (hypoxia-reoxygenation) is believed to selectively activate several inflammatory pathways.[94] For example, tumor necrosis factor-alpha (TNF-alpha) and interleukin-8 (IL-8) are elevated in untreated OSA but decrease with CPAP treatment.[95] TNF-alpha can also cause daytime sleepiness. In this study, higher TNF-alpha levels were associated with higher Epworth Sleepiness Scale scores and worsened arterial oxygen desaturation. Other studies found a reduction in leptin[96] (a hormone secreted by adipose tissue) and a reduction in visceral fat[97] on CPAP treatment. Increased visceral fat is associated with an increased risk of cardiac disease. Of note, not all studies have found an association between OSA and leptin that is independent of the degree of obesity. In some studies, increased leptin levels were associated with the degree of obesity rather than with the AHI.[98] Endothelial function is impaired (specifically NO-dependent flow-mediated dilatation) in patients with OSA, and studies suggest improvement after CPAP.[99]

In studies comparing OSA patients with normal subjects, using an appropriate control group is essential. For example, it is often difficult to match groups for obesity. Trials of the effects of CPAP do not require a normal control group. However, many of the previously discussed studies of effects of CPAP on inflammatory changes in OSA patients were not randomized, controlled trials. Therefore, the results need to be confirmed by controlled trials. For example, a recent randomized, controlled trial of CPAP found no change in several inflammatory mediators following 4 weeks of CPAP.[100] Another study found decreases in C-reactive protein after CPAP treatment only in those patients with good CPAP compliance and with elevated C-reactive protein levels at baseline.[93] Therefore, results may vary depending on the characteristics of the patients at baseline and the compliance with CPAP treatment.

CONGESTIVE HEART FAILURE

The Sleep Heart Health study found that the presence of OSA increases the risk of having CHF (see Table 17–2).[81] Conversely, studies have suggested that sleep-disordered breathing is common in patients with CHF.[101,102] One should not assume that complaints of disturbed nocturnal sleep are simply secondary to heart failure. Sin and colleagues[103] retrospectively evaluated a group of patients with significant LV failure referred to the sleep laboratory and found that risk factors for OSA included an increased BMI for men and increased age for women. In patients with CHF and OSA, negative intrathoracic pressure, hypoxemia, and increased sympathetic tone associated with the apneas are believed to negatively affect ventricular function.[5,103] Treatment of OSA with nasal CPAP in patients with CHF has been found to improve the ejection fraction and symptoms in a number of studies.[104–106] This appears to occur because of a reduction in sympathetic tone and a decrease in ventricular afterload.[103] However, all studies have not shown a significant benefit.[107] To date, no study has confirmed a reduction in mortality with CPAP treatment.

Patients with CHF may manifest Cheyne-Stokes breathing (CSB) type of CSA (see Chapter 21). Short-term studies showed that CPAP improved the ejection fraction in CSB-CSA patients,[108,109] and one study suggested that there may be a survival advantage if patients with CHF and CSB-CSA were treated with CPAP.[109] However, a large randomized trial of CPAP versus standard care in patients with CSB-CSA was unable to show a survival benefit.[110] However, only roughly 50% of the patients in this study responded to CPAP. An analysis of the subgroup that responded to CPAP did have a survival advantage (a post-hoc analysis).[111] The reasons CPAP treatment improves CSA[102] are unclear but could include beneficial effects on hemodynamics (decreased afterload), reduction in pulmonary wedge pressure (may reduce ventilatory drive), or induction of mild increases in PCO_2. The latter two possibilities might stabilize ventilatory control (see Chaper 21). Adaptive servoventilation (ASV) has been more successful than CPAP in **acutely** reducing the AHI in patients with CSB-CSA and benefits in cardiac function have been shown.[112–115] However, no study has shown that ASV treatment improves survival.

CEREBROVASCULAR ACCIDENTS AND OSA

A number of studies have shown a high prevalence of sleep-disordered breathing in patients soon after a cerebrovascular accident (CVA).[116,117] Although the predominant form of sleep-disordered breathing is OSA, CSA with CSB can also occur.[11,118] The CSB-CSA is believed to occur early in the post-CVA period and then usually resolves. In contrast, OSA seems to persist after a CVA. However, the temporal relationship between OSA and stroke is not well defined. It is not known whether brain damage from CVA causes sleep apnea or if sleep apnea preceded the stroke. If so, is the presence of sleep apnea an independent risk factor for the development of a CVA? The Sleep Heart Health Study showed an increased risk of having a self-reported CVA (prevalence) if OSA is present (see Table 17–2).[81] In a recently published study, Redline and associates[119] evaluated the Sleep Heart Health data and found an increased risk for **incident** ischemic stroke in men with mild to moderate OSA. In this study, data were adjusted for a number of confounders that complicated the analysis including obesity. If there is a causal role for OSA in stroke, what are the mechanisms? As noted previously, OSA may predispose to atherosclerosis, hypertension, and early morning hemoconcentration. These factors increase the risk of stroke. During sleep apnea, there are increases in intracranial pressure (ICP)[120] and decreases in cerebral blood flow.[121] There is an increase in ICP with each apneic event and the rise tends to be correlated with the length of apnea. The increase in ICP is thought to be secondary to increases in central venous pressure, systemic pressure, and cerebral vasodilatation from increases in $PaCO_2$ during respiratory events. Because cerebral perfusion is proportional to the mean arterial pressure (MAP) – ICP, increases in ICP may reduce perfusion pressure even if MAP also rises. Studies of cerebral blood flow velocity using Doppler monitoring have shown that flow velocity increases in early apnea, then has approximately a 25% fall below baseline at end apnea.[121]

There is some evidence that the presence of OSA in patients who have suffered a CVA is a bad prognostic sign regardless of whether OSA precedes or follows the CVA. Good and coworkers[122] found that the Barthel index (a multifaced scale measuring mobility and activities of daily living that is used to assess patients after stroke) was significantly lower in patients with OSA and CVA compared with those with no evidence of OSA after CVA. The presence of OSA was determined at discharge and the Barthel index was lower at 3 and 12 months in the OSA-CVA group. Martinez-Garcia and colleagues[123] found that CPAP treatment reduced the mortality after ischemic stroke in patients with concomitant OSA. However, adherence to CPAP in patients with a recent CVA tends to be low.

ERECTILE DYSFUNCTION

An association between erectile dysfunction and sleep disorders appears to exist in survey studies relying on self-report and in small case series.[124] Hormonal, neural, and endothelial mechanisms have been implicated in linking sleep disorders with erectile dysfunction. Treatment of sleep disorders, specifically sleep apnea with CPAP, has been shown to improve patient erectile function.[125]

DIABETES

Obesity is a major confounding factor in the analysis of the association between diabetes mellitus (DM) and OSA because both are worsened with increased BMI. Studies have found that obese and nonobese patients have abnormal glucose metabolism related to OSA. Punjabi and Beamer[126] found that independent of adiposity, sleep-disordered breathing was associated with impairment of insulin sensitivity, glucose effectiveness, and pancreatic beta cell function. Harsch and associates[127] found that CPAP rapidly improved insulin sensitivity, although the greatest results were in nonobese patients. Babu and coworkers[128] found that in diabetic OSA patients with a hemoglobin A1c greater than 7%, CPAP treatment reduced the A1c. Lam and colleagues[129] compared sham CPAP and effective CPAP in patients with OSA and found that 1 week of CPAP improved insulin sensitivity in nondiabetic males, and the improvement was maintained for 12 weeks of treatment in those with moderate obesity. Conversely, West and associates[130] were not able to show an improvement in insulin resistance with CPAP treatment. Although these studies do suggest that OSA independent of obesity impairs glucose metabolism, the effect may be more pronounced in nonobese patients. The impact of treatment of OSA on long-term diabetes and the diabetic complications remains to be determined.

NOCTURIA

It has been a common clinical observation that many patients with OSA who start CPAP treatment report fewer awakenings to urinate. Hajduk and coworkers[131] found a high incidence of pathologic nocturia (PN; defined as ≥2 urination events/night) in OSA patients. The percentage of PN was 47.8% and age, arousal index, AHI, and measures of oxygenation were predictors of the presence of PN. Some of the reported effect of CPAP treatment could be due to better sleep. However, studies have shown a reduced sodium excretion in OSA patients treated with CPAP. Krieger and colleagues[132] found that OSA patients had greater urinary flows and greater urinary sodium excretion compared with controls. Nasal CPAP resulted in a reduction in urinary flow and sodium and chloride excretion. A second study by the same group found evidence of increased guanosine 3'5'-cyclic monophosphate excretion in untreated OSA patients, which reflects atrial natriuretic peptide (ANP) release. The authors hypothesized that atrial stretch during sleep apnea induced release of ANP, which caused increased sodium excretion.[133] Umlauf and associates[134] also found increased nocturia and elevated urinary ANP when the AHI was greater than or equal to 15/hr. Fitzgerald and coworkers[135] found that CPAP decreased nocturia in OSA patients.

CONSEQUENCES OF CHILDHOOD OSA

Many of the important consequences of untreated pediatric OSA are listed in Table 17–5.[136] They are divided into neurobehavioral, metabolic, and cardiovascular groups.

TABLE 17–5
Sequelae of Pediatric Obstructive Sleep Apnea
NEUROCOGNITIVE
Decreased quality of life
Aggressive behavior
Poor school performance
Depression
Attention deficit
Hyperactivity
Moodiness
METABOLIC
Elevated C-reactive protein
Insulin resistance
Hypercholesterolemia
Elevated transaminases
Decreased insulin-like growth factor
Decreased/altered growth hormone secretion
Increased leptin
CARDIOVASCULAR
Autonomic dysfunction
Systemic hypertension
Absent blood pressure "dipping" during sleep
Left ventricular dysfunction
Pulmonary hypertension
Abnormal heart rate variability
Elevated vascular endothelial growth factor
From Katz E, Ambrosio CM: Pediatric obstructive sleep apnea. Clin Chest Med 2010;31:221.

Neurobehavioral

Studies have suggested that both habitual snoring and childhood OSA are associated with behavioral problems, particularly hyperactivity and inattentive behaviors.[136-139] These may improve after effective treatment (usually with tonsillectomy and adenoidectomy). Sometimes, a diagnosis of attention-deficit disorder is made when a patient actually has OSA. Conversely, one should not assume every child with attention deficit disorder and hyperactivity (ADHD) has OSA. Children with OSA often have poor school performance and performance on tests of intelligence that improve with treatment. Both hypoxia and sleep fragmentation may cause neurocognitive changes. Although studies suggest that most impairment is reversible with treatment, it is still not known whether an irreversible component of central nervous system damage occurs with untreated OSA. Although excessive daytime sleepiness is less prominent in childhood OSA compared with OSA in adults, it does occur and may be unrecognized. Using the MSLT, daytime sleepiness is thought to occur in between 13% and 40% of patients.[136,140] Daytime sleepiness is often more prominent in obese children with pediatric OSA.

Metabolic and Inflammatory Consequences

Untreated pediatric OSA has been associated with a failure to thrive.[136,141,142] The possible origin is a reduction in insulin-like growth factor (IGF) and growth hormone secretion. IGF-binding protein (IGF-3) correlates with growth hormone secretion and is decreased in some children with OSA. These changes are reversible and catch-up growth occurs with adequate treatment. Today with the obesity epidemic, obesity is more often noted than failure to thrive. Up to one half of childhood OSA patients have obesity.[143] Leptin, an adipocyte-secreted hormone, is increased in children with OSA and decreases after treatment.[144,145]

Leukotrienes and their receptors are increased in adenotonsillar tissue and exhaled condensates of children with OSA.[146,147] The combination of nasal inhaled steroid and the leukotriene inhibitors (montelukast) was found to have benefit in a study of patients with residual sleepiness after tonsillectomy and adenoidectomy.[148] However, long-term success with anti-inflammatory therapy has not been established. Children with OSA may also have elevated serum levels of TNF-alpha, C-reactive protein, IL-6 and IL-8, and interferon-gamma levels.[136] These changes can occur independent of obesity.

Cardiovascular Consequences

Children with OSA have similar cardiovascular consequences as adults but changes occur at the much lower AHI values typical in children.[136] Children with "severe" OSA (AHI > 10/hr) may have lack of nocturnal blood pressure dipping and high AM blood pressure. In severe cases, RV and LV hypertrophy have been described.

CLINICAL REVIEW QUESTIONS

1. OSA is associated with all of the following EXCEPT:
   A. Increased daytime sympathetic tone.
   B. Increased heart rate variability.
   C. Endothelial dysfunction.
   D. Increased nocturnal sodium excretion.

2. During sleep, patients with OSA experience:
   A. Decreased venous return.
   B. Negative intrathoracic pressure.
   C. Decreased systemic afterload.
   D. Parasympathetic predominance.

3. All of the following are associated with increased mortality in OSA EXCEPT:
   A. Severe arterial oxygen desaturation.
   B. Age > 70 years.
   C. Severe versus mild OSA.
   D. Co-morbid conditions (DM, CHF, COPD).

4. All of the following are true concerning patients with a recent stroke who are found to have sleep apnea EXCEPT:
   A. CSA is more common than OSA.
   B. Worse prognosis.
   C. Improved prognosis with CPAP treatment.
   D. Low adherence to CPAP treatment.

5. Untreated OSA is associated with all of the following EXCEPT:
   A. Decreased leptin.
   B. Increased C-reactive protein.
   C. Increased AM hematocrit.
   D. Increased VEGF.

Answers

1. **B.** Untreated OSA is associated with decreased heart rate variability. This is thought to be due to higher sympathetic compared with parasympathetic tone.

2. **B.** Due to negative intrathoracic pressure there is increased venous return and increased systemic afterload. Sympathetic tone is increased during sleep compared to normal individuals.

3. **B.** Most of the available evidence suggests an increased risk for middle-aged rather than older (age > 70 years) patients.

4. **A.** Although both OSA and CSA can occurs after stroke, OSA is much more common. Studies suggest that the presence of sleep apnea is associated with a worse prognosis and that CPAP treatment improves outcome. However, adherence with CPAP treatment is problematic.

5. **A.** Some studies have shown an increase in leptin with untreated OSA, whereas other studies have suggested this finding is more related to obesity than to OSA.

REFERENCES

1. Platt AB, Kuna ST, Field SH, et al: Adherence to sleep apnea therapy and use of lipid-lowering drugs: a study of the healthy-user effect. Chest 2010;137:102–108.
2. Villar I, Izuel M, Carrizo S, et al: Medication adherence and persistence in severe obstructive sleep apnea. Sleep 2009; 32:623–628.
3. Brown DL, Anderson CS, Chervin RD, et al: Ethical issues in the conduct of clinical trials in obstructive sleep apnea. J Clin Sleep Med 2011;7:103–108.
4. Dempsey JA, Veasey SC, Morgan BJ, O'Donnell CP: Pathophysiology of sleep apnea. Physiol Rev 2010;90:47–112.
5. Bradley TD, Floras JS: Obstructive sleep apnea and its cardiovascular consequences. Lancet 2009;373:82–93.
6. Somers VK, Dyken ME, Clary MP, Abboud FM: Sympathetic neural mechanisms in obstructive sleep apnea. J Clin Invest 1995;96:1897–1904.
7. He J, Kryger MH, Zorick FJ, et al: Mortality and apnea index in obstructive sleep apnea. Chest 1988;94:9–14.
8. Lavie P, Herer P, Peled R, et al: Mortality in sleep apnea patients: a multivariate analysis of risk factors. Sleep 1995; 18:149–157.
9. Lavie P, Lavie L, Herer P: All-cause mortality in males with sleep apnea syndrome: declining mortality rates with age. Eur Respir J 2005;25:514–520.
10. Lavie P, Herer P, Lavie L: Mortality risk factors in sleep apnoea: a matched case-control study. J Sleep Res 2007;16:128–134.
11. Lavie P, Lavie L: Unexpected survival advantage in elderly people with moderate sleep apnoea. J Sleep Res 2009;18: 397–403.
12. Marshall NS, Wong KK, Liu PY, et al: Sleep apnea as an independent risk factor for all-cause mortality: the Busselton Health Study. Sleep 2008;31:1079–1085.
13. Marin JM, Carrizo S, Vicente E, Agusti AGN: Long-term cardiovascular outcomes in men with obstructive sleep apnea-hypopnea with or without treatment with continuous positive airway pressure an observational study. Lancet 2005;365: 1046–1053.
14. Yaggi HK, Concato J, Kernan WN, et al: Obstructive sleep apnea as a risk factor for stroke and death. N Engl J Med 2005;353:2034–2041.
15. Young T, Finn L, Peppard PE, et al: Sleep disordered breathing and mortality: eighteen-year follow-up of the Wisconsin Sleep Cohort. Sleep 2008;31:1071–1078.
16. Punjabi N, Caffo BS, Goodwin JL, et al: Sleep-disordered breathing and mortality: a prospective cohort study. PLOSMed 2009;6:e1000132.
17. Gami AS, Howard DE, Olson EJ, Somers VK: Day-night pattern of sudden death in obstructive sleep apnea. N Engl J Med 2005;352:1206–1214.
18. Bonnet MH: Performance and sleepiness as a function of frequency and placement of sleep disruption. Psychophysiology 1986;3:263–271.
19. Roehrs T, Merlotti L, Petrucelli N, et al: Experimental sleep fragmentation. Sleep 1994;17:438–443.
20. Johns MW: Daytime sleepiness, snoring, and obstructive sleep apnea. The Epworth Sleepiness Scale. Chest 1993;103:30–36.
21. Guilleminault C, Partinen M, Quera-Salva A, et al: Determinants of daytime sleepiness in obstructive sleep apnea. Chest 1988;94:32–37.
22. Cheshire K, Engleman H, Deary I, et al: Factors impairing daytime performance in patients with sleep apnea/hypopnea syndrome. Arch Intern Med 1992;152:538–541.
23. Bennett LS, Langford BA, Stradling JR: Sleep fragmentation indices as predictors of daytime sleepiness and nCPAP response in obstructive sleep apnea. Am J Respir Crit Care Med 1998;158:778–786.
24. Martin SE, Wraith PK, Deary IJ, Douglas NJ: The effect of nonvisible sleep fragmentation on daytime function. Am J Respir Crit Care Med 1997;155:1596–1601.
25. Marcus CL: Sleep-disordered breathing in children. Am J Respir Crit Care Med 2001;164:16–30.
26. Capdevila OS, Kheirandish-Gozal L, Gozal D: Pediatric obstructive sleep apnea. Proc Am Thorac Soc 2008;5: 274–282.
27. Gottlieb DJ, Whitney CW, Bonekat WH, et al: Relation of sleepiness to respiratory disturbance index. Am J Respir Crit Care Med 1999;159:502–507.
28. Findley LJ, Barth JT, Powers DC, et al: Cognitive impairment in patients with obstructive sleep apnea and associated hypoxemia. Chest 1986;90:686–690.
29. Arzt M, Young T, Finn L, et al: Sleepiness and sleep in patients with both systolic heart failure and obstructive sleep apnea. Arch Intern Med 2006;166:1716–1722.
30. Findley LJ, Unverzagt ME, Suratt PM: Automobile accidents involving patients with obstructive sleep apnea. Am Rev Respir Dis 1988;138:337–340.
31. Cassel W, Ploch C, Becker D, et al: Risk of traffic accidents in patients with sleep disordered breathing: reduction with nasal CPAP. Eur Respir J 1996;9:2602–2611.
32. Tregear S, Reston J, Schoelles K, Phillips B: Obstructive sleep apnea and risk of motor vehicle crash: systematic review and meta-analysis. J Clin Sleep Med 2009;5:573–581.
33. American Thoracic Society Official Statement: Sleep apnea, sleepiness, and driving risk. Am J Respir Crit Care Med 1994; 150:1463–1473.
34. Hartenbaum N, Collop N, Rosen IM, et al: Sleep apnea and commercial motor vehicle operators: statement from the joint task force of the American College of Chest Physicians, the American College of Occupational and Environmental Medicine, and the National Sleep Foundation. Chest 2006; 130:902–905.
35. George CFP, Boudreau AC, Smiley A: Simulated driving performance in patients with obstructive sleep apnea. Am J Respir Crit Care Med 1996;154:175–181.
36. Sagaspe P, Taillard J, Chaumet G, et al: Maintenance of wakefulness test as a predictor of driving performance in patients with untreated obstructive sleep apnea. Sleep 2007; 30:327–330.
37. Philip P, Sagaspe P, Taillard J, et al: Maintenance of wakefulness test, obstructive sleep apnea syndrome and driving risk. Ann Neurol 2008;64:410–416.
38. Hack M, Davies RJ, Mullins R, et al: Randomised prospective parallel trial of therapeutic versus subtherapeutic nasal continuous positive airway pressure on simulated steering performance in patients with obstructive sleep apnoea. Thorax 2000;55:224–231.
39. George CF: Reduction in motor-vehicle collisions following treatment of sleep apnea with nasal CPAP. Thorax 2001;56: 508–512.
40. Tregear S, Reston J, Schoelles K, Phillips B: Continuous positive airway pressure reduces risk of motor vehicle crash among drivers with obstructive sleep apnea: systematic review and meta-analysis. Sleep 2010;33:1373–1380.
41. Suzuki M, Guilleminault G, Otsuka K, Shimomi T: Blood pressure "dipping" and "non-dipping" in obstructive sleep apnea syndrome patients. Sleep 1996;19:382–387.
42. Brooks D, Horner RL, Kozar LF, et al: Obstructive sleep apnea as a cause of systemic hypertension. Evidence from a canine model. J Clin Invest 1997;99:106–109.
43. Kales A, Bixler EO, Cadieux RJ, et al: Sleep apnea in a hypertensive population. Lancet 1984;3:1005–1008.
44. Carlson JT, Hedner JA, Ejnell H, Peterson LE: High prevalence of hypertension in sleep apnea patients independent of obesity. Am J Respir Crit Care Med 1994;150:72–77.

45. Nieto FJ, Young TB, Lind BK, et al: Association of sleep-disordered breathing, sleep apnea, and hypertension in a large community-based study. Sleep Heart Health Study. JAMA 2000;283:1829–1836.

46. Peppard PE, Young T, Palta M, Skatrud J: Prospective study of the association between sleep-disordered breathing and hypertension. N Engl J Med 2000;342:1378–1384.

47. O'Connor GT, Caffo B, Newman AB, et al. Prospective study of sleep disordered breathing and hypertension. Am J Respir Crit Care Med 2009;179:1159–1164.

48. Verdecchia P, Schillaci G, Guerrieri M, et al: Circadian blood pressure changes and left ventricular hypertrophy in essential hypertension. Circulation 1990;81:528–536.

49. Brotman DJ, Davidson MB, Boumitri M, Vidt DG: Impaired diurnal blood pressure variation and all-cause mortality. Am J Hypertens 2008;21:92–97.

50. Gonzaga CC, Gaddam KK, Ahmed MI, et al: Severity of obstructive sleep apnea is related to aldosterone status in subjects with resistant hypertension. J Clin Sleep Med 2010; 6:363–368.

51. Lozano L, Tovar JL, Sampol G, et al: Continuous positive airway pressure treatment in sleep apnea patients with resistant hypertension: a randomized, controlled trial. J Hypertens 2010;28:2161–2168.

52. Becker HF, Jerrentrup A, Ploch T, et al: Effect of nasal continuous positive airway pressure treatment on blood pressure in patients with obstructive sleep apnea. Circulation 2003; 107:68–73.

53. Pepperell JCT, Ramdassingh-Dow S, Crosthwaite N, et al: Ambulatory blood pressure after therapeutic and subtherapeutic nasal continuous positive airway pressure for obstructive sleep apnea: a randomized parallel trial. Lancet 2002; 359:204–210.

54. Faccendia J, Mackay TW, Bood NA, Douglas NJ: Randomized placebo-controlled trial of continuous positive airway pressure on blood pressure in the sleep apnea-hypopnea syndrome. Am J Respir Crit Care Med 2001;163:344–348.

55. Engleman HM, Gough K, Martin SE, et al: Ambulatory blood pressure on and off continuous positive airway pressure therapy for the sleep apnea-hypopnea syndrome: Effects in "non-dippers." Sleep 1996;19:378–381.

56. Dimsdale JE, Loredo JS, Profant J: Effect of continuous positive pressure on blood pressure placebo trial. Hypertension 2000;35:144–147.

57. Haentjens P, Meerhaeghe AV, Moscariello A, et al: The impact of continuous positive airway pressure on blood pressure in patients with obstructive sleep apnea syndrome. Arch Intern Med 2007;167:757–765.

58. Heude E, Bourgin P, Feigel P, et al: Ambulatory monitoring of blood pressure disturbs sleep and raises systolic pressure at night in patients suspected of suffering from sleep-disordered breathing. Clin Sci (Colch) 1996;91:45–50.

59. Podszus T, Greenberg H, Scharf S: Influence of sleep state and sleep disordered breathing on cardiovascular function. In Sanders NA, Sullivan CE (eds): Sleep and Breathing. New York: Marcel Decker, 1994, pp. 257–310.

60. Sajkov D, McEvoy RD: Obstructive sleep apnea and pulmonary hypertension. Progr Cardiovasc Dis 2009;51:363–370.

61. Weitzenblum E, Krieger J, Apprill M, et al: Daytime pulmonary hypertension in patients with obstructive sleep apnea syndrome. Am Rev Respir Dis 1988;138:345–349.

62. Sajkov D, Cowie RJ, Thornton AT, et al: Pulmonary hypertension and hypoxemia in obstructive sleep apnea syndrome. Am J Respir Crit Care Med 1994;149:416–422.

63. Chaouat A, Weitzenblum E, Kessler R, et al: Five-year effects of nasal continuous positive airway pressure in obstructive sleep apnoea syndrome. Eur Respir J 1997;10:2578–2582.

64. Sajkov D, Wang T, Saunders NA, et al: Continuous positive airway pressure treatment improves pulmonary hemodynamics in patients with obstructive sleep apnea. Am J Respir Crit Care Med 2002;165:152–158.

65. Alchanatis M, Tourkohoriti G, Kakouros S, et al: Daytime pulmonary hypertension in patients with obstructive sleep apnea: the effect of continuous positive airway pressure on pulmonary hemodynamics. Respiration 2001;68:566–572.

66. Arias MA, García-Río F, Alonso-Fernández A, et al: Pulmonary hypertension in obstructive sleep apnoea: effects of continuous positive airway pressure: a randomized, controlled cross-over study. Eur Heart J 2006;27:1106–1113.

67. Zwillich C, Devlin T, White D, et al: Bradycardia during sleep apnea. Characteristics and mechanisms. J Clin Invest 1982; 69:1286–1292.

68. Bonsignore MR, Romano S, Marrone O, et al: Different heart rate patterns in obstructive sleep apnea during NREM sleep. Sleep 1997;20:1167–1174.

69. Weiss JW, Remsburg S, Garpestad E, et al: Hemodynamic consequences of obstructive sleep apnea. Sleep 1996;19: 388–397.

70. Sato F, Nishimura M, Sinano H, et al: Heart rate during obstructive sleep apnea depends on individual hypoxic chemosensitivity of the carotid body. Circulation 1997;96: 274–281.

71. Guilleminault C, Connoly SJ, Winkle RA: Cardiac arrhythmia and conduction disturbances during sleep in 400 patients with sleep apnea syndrome. Am J Cardiol 1983;52:490–494.

72. Harbison J, O'Reilly P, McNicholas WT: Cardiac rhythm disturbances in obstructive sleep apnea syndrome: effects of nasal continuous positive airway pressure therapy. Chest 2000;118:591–595.

73. Becker H, Brandenburg U, Peter JH, et al: Reversal of sinus arrest and atrioventricular conduction block in sleep apnea during nasal continuous positive airway pressure. Am J Respir Crit Care Med 1995;151:215–218.

74. Shepard JW Jr, Garrison MW, Grither DA, et al: Relationship of ventricular ectopy to oxyhemoglobin desaturation in patients with obstructive sleep apnea. Chest 1985;88:335–340.

75. Khoo MC, Belozeroff V, Berry RB, Sassoon CSH: Cardiac autonomic control in obstructive sleep apnea: effects of long term CPAP therapy. Am J Respir Crit Care Med 2001;164: 807–812.

76. Gami AS, Hodge DO, Herges RM, et al: Obstructive sleep apnea, obesity, and the risk of incident atrial fibrillation. J Am Coll Cardiol 2007;49:565–571.

77. Kanagala R, Murali NS, Friedman PA, et al: Obstructive sleep apnea and the recurrence of atrial fibrillation. Circulation 2003;107:2589–2594.

78. Mehra R, Stone KL, Varosy PD, et al: Nocturnal arrhythmias across a spectrum of obstructive and central sleep-disordered breathing in older men: outcomes of sleep disorders in older men (MrOS sleep) study. Arch Intern Med 2009;169: 1147–1155.

79. Monahan K, Storfer-Isser A, Mehra R, et al: Triggering of nocturnal arrhythmias by sleep-disordered breathing events. J Am Coll Cardiol 2009;54:1797–1804.

80. Ryan CM, Usui K, Floras JS, Bradley TD: Effect of continuous positive airway pressure on ventricular ectopy in heart failure patients with obstructive sleep apnea. Thorax 2005;60: 781–785.

81. Shahar E, Whitney CW, Redline S, et al: Sleep-disordered breathing and cardiovascular disease: cross-sectional results of the Sleep Heart Health Study. Am J Respir Crit Care Med 2001;163:19–25.

82. Peker Y, Hender J, Kraiczi H, Loth S: Respiratory disturbance index: an independent predictor of mortality in coronary artery disease. Am J Respir Crit Care Med 2000;162:81–86.

83. Gottlieb DJ, Yenokyan G, Newman AB, et al: Prospective study of obstructive sleep apnea and incident coronary heart disease and heart failure: the Sleep Heart Health Study. Circulation 2010;122:352–360.

84. Milleron O, Pillière R, Foucher A, et al: Benefits of obstructive sleep apnoea treatment in coronary artery disease: a long-term follow-up study. Eur Heart J 2004;25:728–734.

85. Kreiger J, Sforza E, Barthelmebs M, et al: Overnight decreases in hematocrit after nasal CPAP with patients with OSA. Chest 1990;97:729–730.

86. Chin K, Ohi M, Kita H, et al: Effects of NCPAP therapy on fibrinogen levels in obstructive sleep apnea syndrome. Am J Respir Crit Care Med 1996;153:1972–1976.

87. Lavie L, Kraiczi H, Hefetz A, et al: Plasma vascular endothelial growth factor in sleep apnea syndrome: effects of nasal continuous positive air pressure treatment. Am J Respir Crit Care Med 2002;165:1624–1628.

88. Dyugovskaya L, Lavie P, Lavie L: Increased adhesion molecules expression and production of reactive oxygen species in leukocytes of sleep apnea patients. Am J Respir Crit Care Med 2002;165:934–939.

89. Schulz R, Mahmoudi S, Hattar K, et al: Enhanced release of superoxide from polymorphonuclear neutrophils in obstructive sleep apnea. Impact of continuous positive airway pressure therapy. Am J Respir Crit Care Med 2000;162:566–570.

90. Bokinsky G, Miller M, Ault K, et al: Spontaneous platelet activation and aggregation during obstructive sleep apnea and its response to therapy with nasal continuous positive airway pressure. A preliminary investigation. Chest 1995; 108:625–630.

91. Yokoe T, Minoguchi K, Matsuo H, et al: Elevated levels of C-reactive protein and interleukin-6 in patients with obstructive sleep apnea syndrome are decreased by nasal continuous positive airway pressure. Circulation 2003;107:1129–1134.

92. Shamsuzzaman AS, Winnicki M, Lanfranchi P, et al: Elevated C-reactive protein in patients with obstructive sleep apnea. Circulation 2002;105:2462–2464.

93. Ishida K, Kato M, Kato Y, et al: Appropriate use of nasal continuous positive airway pressure decreases elevated C reactive protein in patients with obstructive sleep apnea. Chest 2009;136:125–129.

94. Ryan S, Taylor CT, McNicholas WT: Selective activation of inflammatory pathways by intermittent hypoxia in obstructive sleep apnea syndrome. Circulation 2005;112: 2660–2667.

95. Ryan S, Taylor CT, McNicholas WT: Predictors of elevated nuclear factor-kappaB-dependent genes in obstructive sleep apnea syndrome. Am J Respir Crit Care Med 2006;174: 824–830.

96. Shimizu K, Chin K, Nakamura T, et al: Plasma leptin levels and cardiac sympathetic function in patients with obstructive sleep apnoea-hypopnoea syndrome. Thorax 2002; 57:429–434.

97. Chin K, Shimizu K, Nakamura T, et al: Changes in intra-abdominal visceral fat and serum leptin levels in patients with obstructive sleep apnea syndrome following nasal continuous positive airway pressure therapy. Circulation 1999; 100:706–712.

98. Ursavas A, Ilcol YO, Nalci N, et al: Ghrelin, leptin, adiponectin, and resistin levels in sleep apnea syndrome: role of obesity. Ann Thorac Med 2010;5:161–165.

99. Bayram NA, Ciftci B, Keles T, et al: Endothelial function in normotensive men with obstructive sleep apnea before and 6 months after CPAP treatment. Sleep 2009;32:1257–1263.

100. Kohler M, Ayers L, Pepperell JC, et al: Effects of continuous positive airway pressure on systemic inflammation in patients with moderate to severe obstructive sleep apnoea: a randomized controlled trial. Thorax 2009;64:67–73.

101. Oldenburg O, Lamp B, Faber L, et al: Sleep-disordered breathing in patients with symptomatic heart failure: a contemporary study of prevalence in and characteristics of 700 patients. Eur J Heart Fail 2007;9:251–257.

102. Leung RST, Bradley TD: Sleep apnea and cardiovascular disease. Am J Respir Crit Care Med 2001;164:2147–2165.

103. Sin D, Fitzgerald F, Parker J: Risk factors for central and obstructive sleep apnea in 450 men and women with congestive heart failure. Am J Respir Crit Care Med 1999;160: 1101–1106.

104. Malone S, Liu PP, Holloway R, et al: Obstructive sleep apnea in patients with dilated cardiomyopathy: effects of continuous positive airway pressure. Lancet 1991;33:1480–1484.

105. Kaneko Y, Floras JS, Usui K, et al: Cardiovascular effects of continuous positive airway pressure in patients with heart failure and obstructive sleep apnea. N Engl J Med 2003; 348:1233–1241.

106. Mansfield DR, Gollogly NC, Kaye DM, et al: Controlled trial of continuous positive airway pressure in obstructive sleep apnea and heart failure. Am J Respir Crit Care Med 2004; 169:361–366.

107. Egea CJ, Aizpuru F, Pinto JA, et al: Cardiac function after CPAP therapy in patients with chronic heart failure and sleep apnea: a multicenter study. Sleep Med 2008;9:660–666.

108. Naughton MT, Liu PP, Bernard DC, et al: Treatment of congestive heart failure and Cheyne-Stokes respiration during sleep by continuous positive airway pressure. Am J Respir Crit Care Med 1995;151:92–97.

109. Sin DD, Logan AG, Fitzgerald FS, et al: Effects of continuous positive airway pressure on cardiovascular outcomes in heart failure patients with and without Cheyne-Stokes respiration. Circulation 2000;102:61–66.

110. Bradley TD, Logan AG, Kimoff RJ, et al, and the CANPAP Investigators: Continuous positive airway pressure for central sleep apnea and heart failure. N Engl J Med 2005;353: 2025–2033.

111. Arzt M, Floras JS, Logan AG, et al: Suppression of central sleep apnea by continuous positive airway pressure and transplant-free survival in heart failure: a post hoc analysis of the Canadian Continuous Positive Airway Pressure for Patients with Central Sleep Apnea and Heart Failure Trial (CANPAP). Circulation 2007;115:3173–3180.

112. Teschler H, Döhring J, Wang YM, Berthon-Jones M: Adaptive pressure support servoventilation: a novel treatment for Cheyne-Stokes respiration in heart failure. Am J Respir Crit Care Med 2001;164:614–619.

113. Oldenburg O, Schmidt A, Lamp B, et al: Adaptive servoventilation improves cardiac function in patients with chronic heart failure and Cheyne-Stokes respiration. Eur J Heart Fail 2008;10:581–586.

114. Philippe C, Stoïca-Herman M, Drouot X, et al: Compliance with and effectiveness of adaptive servoventilation versus continuous positive airway pressure in the treatment of Cheyne-Stokes respiration in heart failure over a six-month period. Heart 2006;92:337–342.

115. Pepperell JC, Maskell NA, Jones DR, et al: A randomized controlled trial of adaptive ventilation for Cheyne-Stokes breathing in heart failure. Am J Respir Crit Care Med 2008; 168:1109–1114.

116. Turkington P, Bamfor J, Wanklyn P, et al: Prevalence and predictors of upper airway obstruction in the first 24 hours after acute stroke. Stroke 2002;33:2037–2041.

117. Para O, Arboix A, Bechichi S, et al: Time course of sleep-related breathing disorders in first-ever stroke or transient ischemic attack. Am J Respir Crit Care Med 2000;161: 375–380.

118. Siccoli MM, Valko PO, Hermann DM, Bassetti CL: Central periodic breathing during sleep in 7 patients with acute

ischemic stroke—neurogenic and cardiogenic factors. J Neurol 2008;255:1687–1692.

119. Redline S, Yenokyan G, Gottlieb DJ, et al: Obstructive sleep apnea-hypopnea and incident stroke: the Sleep Heart Health study. Am J Respir Crit Care Med 2010;182:269–277.

120. Sugita Y, Susami I, Yoshio T, et al: Marked episodic elevation of cerebral spinal fluid pressure during nocturnal sleep in patients with sleep apnea hypersomnia syndrome. Electroencephalgr Clin Neurophysiol 1985;60:214–219.

121. Balfors EM: Impairment of cerebral perfusion during obstructive sleep apneas. Am J Respir Crit Care Med 1994;150:1587–1591.

122. Good DC, Henkle JQ, Gelber D, et al: Sleep disordered breathing and poor functional outcome after stroke. Stroke 1996;27:252–259.

123. Martinez-Garcia MA, Soler-Cataluna JJ, Ejarque-Martinez L, et al: Continuous positive airway pressure treatment reduces mortality in patients with ischemic stroke and obstructive sleep apnea: a five-year follow-up. Am J Respir Crit Care Med 2008;180:36–41.

124. Jankowski JT, Seftel AD, Strohl KP: Erectile dysfunction and sleep related disorders. J Urol 2008;179:837–841.

125. Gonçalves MA, Guilleminault C, Ramos E, et al: Erectile dysfunction, obstructive sleep apnea syndrome and nasal CPAP treatment. Sleep Med 2005;6:333–339.

126. Punjabi N, Beamer BA: Alterations in glucose disposal in sleep-disordered breathing. Am J Respir Crit Care Med 2009;179:235–240.

127. Harsch IA, Schahin SP, Radespiel-Troger M, et al: Continuous positive airway pressure treatment rapidly improves insulin sensitivity in patients with obstructive sleep apnea syndrome. Am J Respir Crit Care Med 2004;169:156–162.

128. Babu AR, Herdegen J, Fogelfeld L, et al: Type 2 diabetes, glycemic control, and continuous positive airway pressure in obstructive sleep apnea. Arch Intern Med 2005;165:447–452.

129. Lam JC, Lam B, Yao TJ, et al: A randomized controlled trial of nasal positive airway pressure on insulin sensitivity in obstructive sleep apnea. Eur Respir J 2010;35:138–145.

130. West SD, Nicoll DJ, Wallace DM, et al: Effect of CPAP on insulin resistance and HbA1c in men with obstructive sleep apnea and type 2 diabetes. Thorax 2007;62:969–974.

131. Hajduk IA, Strollo PJ, Jasani RR, et al: Prevalence and predictors of nocturia in obstructive sleep apnea hypopnea syndrome—a retrospective study. Sleep 2003;26:61–64.

132. Krieger J, Imbs JL, Schmidt M, Kurtz D: Renal function in patients with obstructive sleep apnea. Effects of nasal continuous positive airway pressure. Arch Intern Med 1988;148:1337–1340.

133. Krieger J, Schmidt M, Sforza E, et al: Urinary excretion of guanosine 3':5'-cyclic monophosphate during sleep in obstructive sleep apnea patients with and without nasal continuous positive airway pressure. Clin Sci (Lond) 1989;76:31–37.

134. Umlauf MG, Chasens ER, Greevy RA, et al: Obstructive sleep apnea, nocturia and polyuria in older adults. Sleep 2004;27:139–144.

135. Fitzgerald MP, Mulligan M, Parthasarathy S: Nocturic frequency is related to severity of obstructive sleep apnea, improves with continuous positive airways treatment. Am J Obstet Gynecol 2006;194:1399–1403.

136. Katz E, Ambrosio CM: Pediatric obstructive sleep apnea. Clin Chest Med 2010;31:221–234.

137. Owens JA: Neurocognitive and behavioral impact of sleep disordered breathing in children. Pediatr Pulmonol 2009;44:417–422.

138. Gozal D: Obstructive sleep apnea in children: implications for the developing central nervous system. Semin Pediatr Neurol 2008;15:100–106.

139. Capdevila OS, Kheirandish-Gozal L, Dayyat E, Gozal D: Pediatric obstructive sleep apnea: complications, management, and long-term outcomes. Proc Am Thorac Soc 2008;5:274–282.

140. Gozal D, Kheirandish-Gozal L: Obesity and excessive daytime sleepiness in prepubertal children with obstructive sleep apnea. Pediatrics 2009;123:13–18.

141. Guilleminault C, Eldridge FL, Simmons FB, et al: Sleep apnea in eight children. Pediatrics 1976;58:23–30.

142. Brouillette RT, Fernbach SK, Hunt CE: Obstructive sleep apnea in infants and children. J Pediatr 1982;100:31–40.

143. Gozal D, Simakajornboon N, Holbrook CR, et al: Secular trends in obesity and parentally-reported daytime sleepiness among children referred to a pediatric sleep center for snoring and suspected sleep-disordered breathing (SDB). Sleep 2006;29:A74.

144. Tauman R, Serpero LD, Capdevila OS, et al: Adipokines in children with sleep disordered breathing. Sleep 2007;30:443–449.

145. Nakra N, Bhargava S, Dzuira J, et al: Sleep-disordered breathing in children with metabolic syndrome: the role of leptin and sympathetic nervous system activity and the effect of continuous positive airway pressure. Pediatrics 2008;122:e634–e642.

146. Goldbart AD, Goldman JL, Li RC, et al: Differential expression of cysteinyl leukotriene receptors 1 and 2 in tonsils of children with obstructive sleep apnea syndrome or recurrent infection. Chest 2004;12:613–618.

147. Goldbart AD, Krishna J, Li RC, et al: Inflammatory mediators in exhaled condensate of children with obstructive sleep apnea syndrome. Chest 2006;130:143–148.

148. Kheirandish L, Goldbart AD, Gozal D: Intranasal steroids and oral leukotriene modifier therapy in residual sleep-disordered breathing after tonsillectomy and adenoidectomy in children. Pediatrics 2006;117:e61–e66.

Chapter 18

Obstructive Sleep Apnea Treatment Overview and Medical Treatments

Chapter Points

- The choice of treatment for OSA depends on OSA severity, symptoms, co-morbid medical conditions, patient preference, and sometimes economic issues.
- Treatment options for snoring included the side sleep position, treatment of nasal congestion, weight loss (adjunctive), an OA, or upper airway surgery.
- Treatment options for mild OSA include the side sleep position, treatment of nasal congestion, weight loss (adjunctive), an OA, or upper airway surgery. If the patient is symptomatic, PAP treatment can also be effective if the patient is motivated.
- Treatment options for moderate OSA include PAP (treatment of choice), an OA, or upper airway surgery. Weight loss or the side sleep position is adjunctive.
- Treatment options for severe OSA include PAP (treatment of choice), upper airway surgery such as the MMA (if anatomy is favorable and the patient is a good surgical candidate), or an OA (third option).
- Mild to moderate weight loss can reduce the AHI, but weight loss takes time and is considered adjunctive therapy.
- Bariatric surgery resulting in weight loss can reduce the AHI. However, a substantial fraction of patients with presurgery OSA continue to need treatment after weight loss stabilizes. In some patients, the required level of CPAP is lower. OSA can return even in the absence of weight gain.
- Positional therapy can be effective in patients with positional OSA, but long-term studies of effectiveness are lacking. Sleep in the lateral position or with the head elevated can reduce the level of CPAP required to keep the airway open.
- Modafinil (armodafinil) is indicated for treatment of residual excessive daytime sleepiness in patients with OSA on effective CPAP treatment (good adherence and effective pressure) when other sleep disorders have been ruled out. Continued monitoring of PAP adherence is essential.
- The AASM practice parameters state that supplemental oxygen treatment is not indicated for treatment of OSA. However, individual patients may benefit if they do not tolerate or do refuse more effective treatment. Oxygen treatment can increase event duration. Significant worsening of nocturnal and daytime hypercapnia can occur in some patients with the use of supplemental oxygen.

INTRODUCTION

The severity of obstructive sleep apnea (OSA), co-morbid conditions, patient preference, and financial considerations may all factor into the choice of treatment modality[1-6] (Table 18–1). The American Academy of Sleep Medicine (AASM) has published practice parameters for medical,[3] surgical,[4] oral appliance (OA),[5] and positive airway pressure (PAP)[6] treatments for sleep apnea. Medical treatments for OSA are discussed in this chapter. Treatment of OSA with PAP is discussed in detail in Chapter 19 and OA and surgical treatment of OSA are covered in Chapter 20. Although treatment options for OSA are usually classified by apnea-hypopnea index (AHI) severity, symptoms do not correlate well with the AHI. Therefore, the goal should be "treat the patient, not the AHI." Another concept to consider is efficacy versus effectiveness. For example, continuous positive airway pressure (CPAP) is very efficacious, often lowering the AHI to less than 5 to 10/hr. However, the effectiveness of CPAP depends on adherence to treatment. If CPAP reduces the AHI from 55 to 5/hr but is used only 50% of the time during sleep, the effective average AHI is really 30/hr. The ideal OSA treatment goals include normalization of the AHI and nocturnal oxygenation and resolution of symptoms associated with OSA.

TABLE 18-1

Treatment Alternatives for Obstructive Sleep Apnea (Adults)[4-6]

	SNORING	MILD	MODERATE	SEVERE
Primary	Treat nasal congestion Lateral positioning	Oral appliance or Upper airway surgery	PAP	PAP
Secondary	Oral appliance or Upper airway surgery	PAP (if symptomatic)	Oral appliance or Upper airway surgery	Upper airway surgery or Oral appliance
Adjunctive	Weight loss	Weight loss Lateral positioning	Weight loss Lateral positioning	Weight loss Lateral positioning

PAP = positive airway pressure.

SHOULD MILD OSA PATIENTS BE TREATED?

Whereas most clinicians recommend treatment of patients with an AHI of 15/hr or greater even if not symptomatic, treatment of mild OSA remains controversial.[7,8] However, there can be night-to-night variability in the AHI and even patients with mild OSA can be symptomatic. In the Sleep Heart Health Study, 28% of individuals with an AHI greater than 5 but less than 15 had subjective sleepiness (Epworth Sleepiness Scale [ESS] ≥ 11).[9] The Wisconsin cohort study found a 2.03 greater risk of incident hypertension in patients with an AHI in the range of 5 to 14.9 compared with individuals without sleep apnea (AHI = 0/hr).[10] The fact that even mild OSA could have adverse consequences is supported by a recent finding that snoring alone can cause carotid atherosclerosis.[11] Effective treatment of patients with mild OSA can improve symptoms. A meta-analysis of treatment studies of mild to moderate OSA found that CPAP significantly reduced subjective sleepiness (the ESS decreased by 1.2 points) and improved objective wakefulness (measure of wakefulness test [MWT] sleep latency increased by 2.1 min).[12] Conversely, Barbé and coworkers[13] found no benefit to CPAP treatment in a group of nonsleepy patients with mild to moderate OSA. Whereas suboptimal CPAP adherence has often been reported in studies of patients with mild OSA, several studies found 40% to 60% of patients had greater than 4 hours use for 70% of nights.[7]

WHOM TO TREAT

At least four treatment considerations affect the decision to treat a patient with OSA. The first category is the severity of OSA as based on the AHI or extent of arterial oxygen desaturation. The second consideration is presence or absence of symptoms. Symptomatic OSA should always be treated but the choice of treatment may vary, as noted later. The third consideration is the impact of OSA on the sleep of the patient's bed partner. Loud snoring and apnea may cause marital discord and impair the sleep of the patient's bed partner.[14] In some cases, sleeping in separate bedrooms is the most acceptable solution. However, if this is not acceptable,

treatment of the OSA patient can significantly improve the sleep of the bed partner.[14] The fourth category is the increased risk of adverse cardiovascular morbidity and mortality associated with untreated sleep apnea. The evidence that untreated sleep apnea is associated with an increased risk of death or adverse cardiovascular event is strongest for severe OSA (AHI > 30/hr) and in men who are 40 to 70 years of age.[15,16] The evidence is less clear for moderate OSA and for women. However, the presence of certain co-morbid conditions such as coronary artery disease, cerebrovascular disease, arrhythmias, or congestive heart failure may increase the risk even for milder degrees of sleep apnea.[17] Given that PAP treatment is safe and effective, treatment of patients with moderate OSA is recommended even if patients are asymptomatic.

Table 18-2 illustrates an approach to the decision of whom to treat. Symptomatic patients with all severities of OSA should be treated with an effective therapy. Asymptomatic patients with moderate to severe OSA should also be treated. For asymptomatic patients with mild OSA and no obvious significant medical co-morbidities, either observation or conservative treatment (weight loss/lateral positioning) is reasonable. The patient should be informed that even mild OSA carries some increased risk of cardiovascular morbidity. For asymptomatic patients with mild OSA and **significant medical co-morbidities,** treatment decisions should be individualized based on the patient's motivation to undergo treatment. Treatment success in asymptomatic patients with mild OSA requires them to be motivated.

TREATMENT SELECTION

Treatment options for snoring, mild, moderate, and severe OSA are discussed in detail in the following sections. The options by category of AHI severity are listed in Table 18-1.

Snoring

For snoring patients for whom treatment is felt necessary, a number of therapies are available including weight loss,

TABLE 18-2

Consideration—Whom to Treat?

	SYMPTOMATIC	ASYMPTOMATIC	ASYMPTOMATIC
AHI		No significant medical morbidities	Significant medical morbidities
Mild	Treat	Observation or conservative treatment	? Treat
Moderate	Treat	Treat	Treat
Severe	Treat	Treat	Treat
Conservative treatment: weight loss, side sleep position, treat nasal congestion, avoid alcohol.			
AHI = apnea-hypopnea index.			

medical treatment of nasal congestion, the side (lateral) sleeping position, and avoidance of alcohol. If medical treatment does not improve nasal congestion, nasal surgery may address this problem, although improvement in snoring is variable.[18,19] OAs or upper airway surgery involving the palate may improve snoring in many patients.[6,20-25] The surgical procedures commonly used for snoring include laser-assisted uvulopalatoplasty (LAUP), radiofrequency palatoplasty, and uvulopalatopharyngoplasty (UPPP).[21-23] The Pillar procedure involves insertion of Teflon strips into the palate. The success of this procedure is variable, and sometimes additional strip insertion is needed.[22] A controlled study comparing the Pillar procedure with a sham surgery found modest improvement in snoring without a significant improvement in the AHI.[23] The LAUP procedure is not recommended for treatment of sleep apnea.[24] The recently published American Academy of Sleep Medicine (AASM) practice parameters for surgical treatment of OSA[4] state "palatal implants may be effective in some patients with mild OSA who cannot tolerate or are unwilling to adhere to PAP therapy, or in whom oral appliances have been considered and found ineffective or undesirable." However, the evidence to support this recommendation is not very convincing and it is not clear that palatal implants are any more effective for sleep apnea than the LAUP procedure.

Mild OSA

For mild OSA, one may again begin with conservative measures in (especially in asymptomatic patients) including treatment of nasal congestion, weight loss, or the lateral sleeping position. Weight loss takes time, and if the patient is symptomatic, weight loss should be considered a secondary (adjunctive) treatment.[3] Both OAs and upper airway surgery are reasonably effective for mild OSA.[4,5,20-25] PAP is very efficacious at reducing the AHI,[1,2,6] but acceptance and adherence are typically lower than with more severe OSA. PAP treatment is not indicated in mild OSA if patients are asymptomatic and have no co-morbid cardiovascular disorders.[2] In symptomatic patients with mild OSA, some patients may prefer a trial of PAP rather than an OA or upper airway surgery. PAP treatment is safe and it is often difficult to predict who will benefit. If the patient is motivated to try

PAP, the dictum "when in doubt, pressurize the snout" should be considered.[26] If PAP is not an acceptable option, the choice between upper airway surgery or an OA to treat mild OSA often depends upon financial considerations and patient preference. At the present time, many insurance plans will not pay for OA treatment for sleep apnea. However, OA treatment is now reimbursed by Medicare if certain conditions are met (see Chapter 20). Reimbursement by insurance or Medicare requires that patients with mild OSA be symptomatic.

Moderate OSA

For moderate OSA, the treatment of choice is some form of PAP.[1,2,5] For moderate OSA, OA treatment and upper airway surgery are less reliable than PAP at reducing the AHI to less than 10/hr. However, they may be more acceptable to some patients and more "effective" if patients do not have reasonable PAP adherence.[1,5,20,21] Upper airway surgery obviates the need for treatment adherence. Treatment adherence is still an issue with OA treatment, and currently, there is no method to objectively monitor adherence to OA treatment. A recent AASM task force review concluded that OA was about 50% effective for moderate OSA (defined as a treatment AHI < 10/hr).[20] A meta-analysis of surgery in OSA patients concluded that palatal surgery with or without genioglossus advancement was approximately 30% effective, using a strict outcome measure of reduction in the AHI to less than 10/hr.[25] Therefore, for moderate OSA, PAP is the most reliably efficacious treatment. It is very effective if adherence is adequate. Most clinicians would recommend a trial of PAP therapy for patients with moderate OSA. If this treatment is not acceptable or the patient is not adherent to PAP treatment, upper airway surgery or an OA would be alternatives.

The AASM practice parameters for the surgical treatment of OSA[4] state "Uvulopalatopharyngoplasty (UPPP) as a sole procedure, with or without tonsillectomy, does not reliably normalize the AHI when treating moderate to severe OSA. Therefore, patients with severe OSA should initially be offered PAP therapy, while those with moderate OSA should initially be offered either PAP therapy or oral appliances." However, economics or patient preference may favor surgery over OA treatment in some settings. If patients with moderate OSA pursue weight loss with bariatric surgery, an effective immediate treatment for OSA is indicated because weight loss takes time.

Severe OSA

For severe OSA, PAP is the treatment of choice because of its effectiveness and safety.[1,2,6] Unfortunately, acceptance and adherence can be as low as 50% depending on the definition of adherence. The maxillary mandibular advancement (MMA) operation can result in acceptable residual AHIs in many patients with severe OSA.[4,21] A recent meta-analysis found that up to 90% of patients undergoing MMA had improvement in symptoms and a postoperative AHI less than 20/hr (only 30% had a reduction in AHI to < 10/hr)[25] (Table 18–3). Some surgeons perform MMA only after other surgical procedures have failed. However, in very obese patients with retrognathia, performing MMA as the first surgical procedure is recommended by some clinicians. Tracheostomy is effective when life-threatening OSA and respiratory failure are present and the patient is not compliant with PAP treatment.[4] Surgical treatment options are discussed in more detail in Chapter 20. If neither PAP nor surgery is an acceptable treatment option, some patients with severe OSA will have significant improvement in the AHI with OA treatment. Although the AHI is usually not reduced below 10/hr, one could argue that a drop from 80/hr to 20/hr is worthwhile, especially if there is symptomatic improvement and an improvement in oxygenation.

PATIENT EDUCATION BEFORE TREATMENT

Following polysomnography (PSG) or portable monitoring (home sleep testing, limited-channel sleep testing), the physician ordering the study should discuss the findings and the consequences of untreated sleep apnea with the patient (Table 18–4).[1] The factors that can exacerbate OSA, including weight gain, insufficient sleep, medications, and alcohol consumption, should also be addressed. The available treatment options and the pros and cons of each option should be discussed. Whereas most patients look to the physician

for ultimate recommendations, involving the patient and spouse in decision making is essential to improve treatment outcomes. Drowsy driving counseling should be performed and documented. Many patients have co-morbid conditions such as depression, insomnia, restless legs syndrome (RLS), or chronic pain that will make compliance with PAP or other treatments more difficult. These should be evaluated and treated.

FOLLOW-UP AND OUTCOMES ASSESSMENT

Following treatment initiation, careful follow-up is essential because OSA is a chronic disease. Table 18–5 lists some

---

TABLE 18–4

Patient Education and Co-morbid Disorders

PATIENT EDUCATION

- Testing results—discuss with the patient without excessive medical jargon, answer questions
- Pathophysiology of OSA
- Consequences of untreated OSA
- Treatment options—pros and cons
- Drowsy driving counseling

EVALUATION AND TREATMENT OF CO-MORBID DISORDERS

- RLS
- Depression
- Insomnia
- Insufficient sleep
- Chronic pain
- Narcolepsy

OSA = obstructive sleep apnea; RLS = restless legs syndrome.

TABLE 18–3

Meta-Analysis Results for Upper Airway Surgery (% Success Rates)

CRITERIA	50% REDUCTION IN AHI TO ≤ 20/HR	AHI < 10/HR	AHI < 5/HR
Phase I	55%	31.5%	13%
Phase II	86%	45%	43%

Phase I = uvulopalatoplasty with or without genioglossus advancement and hyoid advancement; Phase II = MMA.
AHI = apnea-hypopnea index; MMA = maxillary-mandibular advancement.
From Elshaug AG, Moss JR, Southcott A, et al: Redefining success in airway surgery for obstructive sleep apnea: a meta-analysis and synthesis of the evidence. Sleep 2007;30:461–467.

TABLE 18–5

Assessments for Treatment Follow-up

ASSESSMENTS

- Objective adherence
- Epworth Sleepiness Scale, resolution of sleepiness
- Quality of life
- Patient and spousal satisfaction

COUNSELING

- Increased adherence
- Proper maintenance of equipment
- Avoidance of factors worsening disease
- Weight loss
- Adequate amount of sleep

TABLE 18-6
American Academy of Sleep Medicine Practice Parameter Recommendations for Medical Treatment of Obstructive Sleep Apnea
WEIGHT REDUCTION
• Successful dietary weight loss may improve the AHI in obese OSA patients. (Guideline)
• Dietary weight loss should be combined with primary treatment of OSA. (Option)
• Bariatric surgery may be **adjunctive** in treatment of OSA in obese patients. (Option)
POSITIONAL THERAPIES
• Positional therapy, consisting of a method that keeps the patient in a nonsupine position, is an effective secondary therapy or can be a supplement to primary therapies for OSA in patients who have a low AHI in the nonsupine versus the supine position. (Guideline)
OXYGEN SUPPLEMENTATION
• Oxygen supplementation is not recommended as a primary treatment for OSA. (Option)
NASAL CORTICOSTEROIDS
• Topical nasal corticosteroids may improve the AHI in patients with OSA and concurrent rhinitis and, thus, may be a useful adjunct to primary therapies for OSA. (Guideline)
MODAFINIL, ARMODAFINIL
• Modafinil is recommended for treatment of residual excessive sleepiness in OSA patients who have sleepiness despite effective PAP treatment and who are lacking any other identifiable cause for their sleepiness. (Standard)
OTHER TREATMENTS (NOT RECOMMENDED)
• Protriptyline, SSRIs, aminophylline, estrogen preparations with or without progesterone, and short-acting decongestants.
AHI = apnea-hypopnea index; OSA = obstructive sleep apnea; PAP = positive airway pressure; SSRIs = selective serotonin reuptake inhibitors.

outcome assessments that were suggested in recent clinical guidelines.[1] A follow-up sleep study is recommended after upper airway surgery for moderate to severe OSA[1,4,5,27] and after final adjustment of an OA as treatment for all severities of OSA.[5]

MEDICAL TREATMENTS FOR OSA

Practice parameters have been published for use of "medical" treatments for OSA[3] including weight loss, positioning, medications, oxygen, and alerting agents (Table 18–6). Documentation of the effectiveness of treatment and continued monitoring of adherence are important.

Weight Loss

Obesity is a major risk factor for the development of OSA. In some studies, approximately 70% of patients with OSA were obese (body weight > 120% of predicted). In the Wisconsin cohort study, for every standard deviation increase in the body mass index (BMI), there was a fourfold increase in the prevalence of OSA.[28] A BMI of 25.0 to 29.9 kg/m² is considered overweight, greater than 30 is obesity, and greater than 40 is severe obesity. Many studies have documented that weight loss of modest proportions (5–10%) can produce significant improvement in sleep apnea[29–34] as well as decrease upper airway collapsibility.[35]

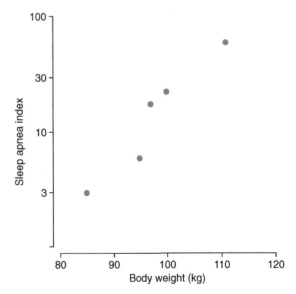

FIGURE 18-1 Decrease in apnea-hypopnea index (AHI) with weight loss. The y axis is a logarithmic scale. The weight loss was due to medication. *From Browman CP, Sampson MG, Yolles SF, et al: Obstructive sleep apnea and body weight. Chest 1984;85:435–436.*

Figure 18–1 illustrates the AHI versus weight of a patient undergoing weight loss.[29] Even patients with mild obesity (110–115% of ideal body weight) can benefit from weight reduction.[30] Peppard and colleagues[34] followed the effects of weight change on AHI. A 10% weight gain predicted an approximate 32% increase in the AHI. A 10% weight loss predicted a 26% reduction in the AHI. A 10% increase in weight was associated with a sixfold increase in the risk of developing moderate to severe OSA.

The effectiveness in reducing the AHI with weight loss varies among patients. This may be due to the fact that a given amount of weight loss may have more effect on upper body obesity or upper airway anatomy in one individual than in another. One study found that neck fat was the best predictor of a high AHI in women whereas central obesity was a better predictor in men.[36] Weight loss may also be less effective in reducing the AHI if skeletal abnormalities play a more prominent role in the pathogenesis of OSA in a given patient. The level of nasal CPAP required to maintain upper airway patency may decrease after weight reduction. Lettieri and associates[37] reported a reduction in required CPAP from 11.5 to 8.4 cm H_2O after weight loss (BMI dropped from 51 to 32 kg/m²) in a group of patients undergoing bariatric surgery. However, the magnitude of this effect can vary significantly between patients.

Behavioral, surgical, and pharmacologic approaches to weight loss have all been successful in selected groups of patients. The major problem to date has been maintenance of weight loss. Johansson and coworkers[31] (Table 18–7) studied the effects of a very low energy diet on OSA in patients on CPAP (intervention vs. control group) with moderate to severe OSA. At 9 weeks, the intervention group had lost weight (–18.8 kg) with a drop in AHI of 23/hr. Tuomilehtol and colleagues[32] reported on use of lifestyle intervention and weight reduction in mild OSA. Although both the weight and the AHI decreases were small, a significant number of the intervention group dropped their AHI below 5/hr. In the AHEAD (Action for Health in Diabetes) study, weight loss also resulted in a drop in the AHI.[33] Grunstein and associates[38] reported on a 2-year reduction in sleep apnea symptoms following surgically induced weight loss. Another study of the effect of the weight reduction with subitramine found a reduction of 7.9 kg was associated with a 30% reduction in the AHI (change in AHI 16/hr).[39]

Today, bariatric surgery is performed as a treatment for morbid obesity.[40,41] However, it could be considered as an adjunctive treatment for OSA. The most common bariatric operation is a Roux-en-Y procedure, although other surgery such as laparoscopic gastric banding may be tried for less obese patients. The mortality of the Roux-en-Y procedure is less than 2%.[40,41] Greenburg and coworkers[42] performed a meta-analysis of bariatric surgery and the effects on OSA in morbidly obese patients. Twelve studies including 342 patients were analyzed. The mean BMI was reduced by 17.9 kg/m² (baseline 55.3 kg/m²) and the AHI was reduced from 54.7 to 15.8/hr. The authors concluded that bariatric surgery does result in both dramatic weight loss and improvement of the AHI, but not always to normal levels. Many patients will still likely require treatment of OSA (CPAP and others). In another series of 24 consecutive patients undergoing bariatric surgery, only 4% were cured of OSA.[40] Pillar and colleagues[43] reported on a patient who had recurrence

TABLE 18–7
Selected Studies of Weight Loss in Obstructive Sleep Apnea

WEIGHT REDUCTION AT 1 YR IN MILD OSA WITH VERY LOW CALORIE DIET*	CONTROL	INTERVENTION
Weight (kg)	92.3	101.2
AHI (#/hr)	9.3	10.0
AHI supine	21.3	20.1
Change in AHI	0.3	–4.0
Change in weight (kg)	–2.4	–10.7

EFFECTS OF A VERY LOW ENERGY DIET (9 WK)†	CONTROL	INTERVENTION
Weight (kg)—Baseline	111.7	113.4
Change in weight (kg)	1.1	–18.7
AHI (#/hr)—Baseline	37	37
Change in AHI	–2	–25

EFFECTS OF MILD TO MODERATE WEIGHT LOSS‡	BASELINE	WEIGHT LOSS
Weight (kg)	106	96.9
Apnea index	55	29.2

AHI = apnea-hypopnea index; OSA = obstructive sleep apnea.
*Adapted from Tuomilehto HPI, Seppa JM, Partine MM, et al: Lifestyle intervention with weight reduction: first-line treatment in mild obstructive sleep apnea. Am J Respir Crit Care Med 2009;179:320–327.
†From Johansson K, Neovius M, Lagerros YT, et al. Effect of a very low energy diet on moderate and severe sleep apnea in obese men: a randomised controlled trial. BMJ 2009;339:b4609.
‡From Smith PL, Gold AR, Meyers DA, et al: Weight loss in mildly to moderately obese patients with obstructive sleep apnea. Ann Intern Med 1985;103:850–855.

of OSA after previous weight loss **without concomitant weight gain**. This illustrates the need for continued clinical follow-up. Sampol and associates[44] followed 24 patients "cured" by weight loss for a mean of 94 months. Six of the 13 patients who maintained weight loss had recurrence of OSA (AHI = 40.5/hr).

The AASM practice parameters for use of medical treatments for OSA recommended that weight loss be combined with a primary treatment for OSA[3] (see Table 18–6). This recommendation is based on the fact that weight loss takes time, results vary between patients, and OSA can recur even if initially improved by weight loss. It was stated that bariatric surgery "may" be adjunctive in treatment of OSA in obese patients. This recommendation falls short of recommendation of bariatric surgery as a primary treatment for OSA treatment given the variable improvement in the AHI. Patients with OSA undergoing bariatric surgery should be treated with an effective treatment (usually CPAP) in the postoperative period and during weight loss. If a sleep study after significant weight loss documents a "cure," stopping primary treatment could be considered. If significant OSA is still present, a lower level of CPAP may be effective.[37] If CPAP or other treatment for OSA is stopped, patients should be followed closely for signs and symptoms of recurrence (Table 18–8).

Posture and Positional Treatment

Many patients with OSA have a significant worsening of apnea in the supine position.[45] Some but not all studies have found an increase in upper airway size in the lateral position. Walsh and coworkers,[46] using optical coherence tomography in awake normal subjects and patients with sleep apnea, found airway size not to change (supine to lateral) but airway shape was more circular (Fig. 18–2A). A circular shape may be more resistant to closure. In contrast, Isono and colleagues[47] found a larger airway in the lateral position in anesthetized normal subjects. Walsh and coworkers[46] did not find a difference in shape between OSA patients and normal

individuals. However, other studies have found OSA patients to have an upper airway with narrower lateral dimensions (see Fig. 18–2B).[48,49] Changes in airway shape or size with changes in posture could be due to an effect of gravity on the tissue surrounding the upper airway or to posterior movement of the tongue. Reductions in lung volume in the supine position may also reduce upper airway size. A limitation of many studies of the upper airway in OSA patients is that the patients were evaluated either awake or under anesthesia. Neither of these circumstances may accurately represent what happens during sleep.

Neill and associates[50] found that elevation of the head by 30° improved airway stability (compared with the supine position) in OSA patients as measured by airway occlusion during sleep. In this study, lateral sleep positioning had less of a stabilizing effect compared with elevation of the head. This suggests that sleeping with the head elevated may reduce the AHI more in some patients than sleeping in the lateral position. In the same study, CPAP was also progressively elevated until apneas and hypopneas were abolished. The mean effective pressure was 10.4 cm H_2O in the supine position, 5.3 cm H_2O with the head-elevated position, and 5.5 cm H_2O in the lateral position.

A considerable number of patients with a significant overall AHI will have minimal sleep apnea in the lateral position. In fact, many of these patients have chronically favored this position at home. In one study, approximately 55% of a large group of patients with sleep apnea had positional sleep apnea, defined as an AHI at least two times higher in the supine than in the nonsupine position.[45] Because the amount of supine sleep can dramatically affect the overall AHI, **one must always note the amount of supine sleep when interpreting a sleep study or comparing the results of different sleep studies.**

Avoiding the supine posture has been proposed as a treatment for sleep apnea. To maintain the lateral posture during

TABLE 18–8
Weight Loss Treatment for Obstructive Sleep Apnea
• Weight loss is considered a secondary or adjunctive treatment.
• Modest weight loss can be helpful (10% weight loss is associated with a 26% reduction in the AHI).
• Recurrence of OSA can occur after previous weight loss despite maintenance of lower weight.
• Bariatric surgery rarely cures patients of OSA but may reduce the required level of CPAP.
AHI = apnea-hypopnea index; CPAP = continuous positive airway pressure; OSA = obstructive sleep apnea.

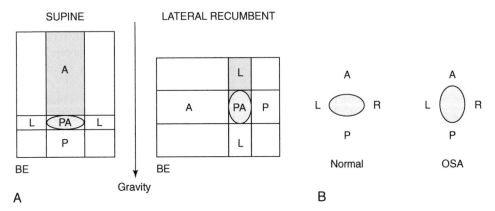

FIGURE 18–2 A, Schematic of changes in upper airway shape. In the lateral position the pharyngeal airway (PA) has a rounder shape. A = anterior; BE = bony enclosure; L = lateral; P = posterior. **B,** Schematic of upper airway shape found in normal and obstructive sleep apnea (OSA) patients with the supine position in other studies. R = right. **A,** *From Walsh JH, Leigh MS, Paduch A, et al: Effect of body posture on pharyngeal shape and size in adults with and without obstructive sleep apnea. Sleep 2008;31:1543–1549.* **B,** *From Schwab RJ, Gefter WB, Hoffman EA, Pack AI: Dynamic upper airway imaging during awake respiration in normal subjects and patients with sleep disordered breathing. Am Rev Respir Dis 1993;148:1385.*

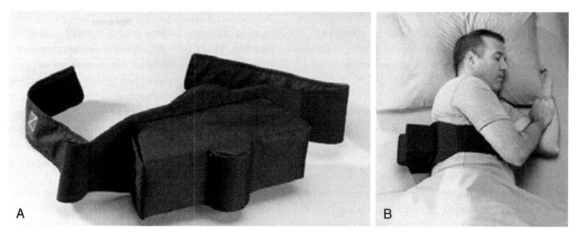

FIGURE 18–3 A, and B, A lateral positioning device. The ZZsoma Positional Sleeper. *From Permut I, Diaz-Abad M, Eissam C, et al: Comparison of positional therapy to CPAP in patients with positional obstructive sleep apnea. J Clin Sleep Med 2010;6:238–243.*

sleep, a number of night shirts or straps with foam balls or cushions are available that prevent comfortable supine sleep[51,52] (Fig. 18–3). Another approach was "training" with an auditory alarm when patients turn supine.[53] Jokic and coworkers[52] performed a randomized cross-over trial of position therapy and CPAP in a group of patients with positional OSA. The positional device consisted of a backpack with a foam ball (10 × 5.5 inches). Positional treatment was slightly less effective than CPAP but there was no difference in improvement in the ESS, sleep architecture, or subjective sleep quality. There have been no long-term studies of positional therapy. Permut and colleagues[51] found positional treatment (see Fig. 18–3) to be as effective as CPAP as assessed by one night of PSG in a group of patients with mild and positional OSA. McEvoy and associates[54] also found a lower AHI, better oxygen saturation, and better sleep quality in the seated sleeping posture (60°) compared with the supine position. Skinner and coworkers[55] studied the effect of a shoulder-head elevation pillow in mild to moderate OSA. In 7 of 14 patients, the AHI dropped to less than 10/hr. In contrast with CPAP, the AHI was less than 5/hr in all patients. There seems little doubt that positional treatment would work in a number of patients with positional OSA. However, a recent study found poor adherence to the "tennis ball technique."[56] Studies of long-term outcomes with more comfortable positioner devices are needed.

An increase in the required CPAP pressure to maintain upper airway patency is commonly required in the supine compared with the lateral body position.[57,58] Oksenberg and colleagues[57] documented about a 3-cm H_2O difference between supine and nonsupine postures. As noted previously, Neill and associates[50] noted a significantly lower PAP was needed in the lateral position or with the head elevated. In pressure-intolerant patients undergoing CPAP treatment, one approach might be to lower the pressure to one effective in the lateral position and encourage patients to sleep in that position (or use a device to discourage supine sleep), at least during an adaptation period. Nocturnal oximetry at home and/or observation of the residual AHI recorded on the

TABLE 18–9
Treatment of Nasal Congestion/Rhinitis[3]
• Short-acting nasal decongestants are not recommended for treatment of OSA. (Option)
• Topical nasal corticosteroids may improve the AHI in patients with OSA and concurrent rhinitis and, thus, be useful adjuncts to primary therapies for OSA. (Guideline)
AHI = apnea-hypopnea index; OSA = obstructive sleep apnea.

CPAP device are methods to document the efficacy of this approach.

Medical Therapies to Improve Nasal Patency

The AASM practice parameters for medical treatment[3] did not recommend use of short-acting nasal decongestants (Table 18–9). The major consideration is the development of rhinitis medicamentosa.[59] A study by Kiely and associates,[60] using a placebo-controlled, randomized, cross-over design, found a modest reduction in the AHI in a group of apneic snorers with intranasal fluticasone but no reduction in snoring noise in nonapneic snorers. There was no improvement in objective sleep quality. Of interest, the improvement in the AHI was correlated with a reduction in the nasal resistance. A treatment effect is likely only if intranasal steroids improve nasal resistance, and this change may not occur in all patients.

Supplemental Oxygen

Supplemental oxygen can improve nocturnal oxygenation in patients with OSA. In a study by Smith and coworkers,[61] nocturnal supplemental oxygen did not improve objective daytime sleepiness but did improve nocturnal oxygenation in a group of patients with OSA. In general, oxygen does not significantly reduce the AHI or improve daytime sleepiness.[61–63] Caution is advised in hypercapnic OSA

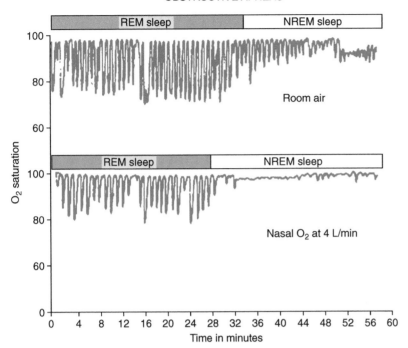

OXYGEN SATURATION DURING REPETITIVE OBSTRUCTIVE APNEAS

FIGURE 18-4 Effects of supplemental oxygen on oxygen desaturation during repetitive obstructive apneas. Supplemental oxygen at 4 L/min did not completely eliminate events (which appear slightly longer during rapid eye movement [REM] sleep). NREM = non–rapid eye movement. *From Alford NJ, Fletcher EC, Nickeson D: Acute oxygen in patients with sleep apnea and COPD. Chest 1986;89:30–38.*

patients, because some may develop worsening hypercapnia, especially on high flow rates of oxygen.[65] In some studies, acute administration of oxygen caused prolongation of apneas.[62-65] Supplemental oxygen tends to convert central and mixed apneas to obstructive apneas.[66] Loredo and colleagues[67] compared oxygen with CPAP treatment in OSA. CPAP improved sleep quality but supplemental oxygen improved only nocturnal oxygenation. It should also be noted that supplemental oxygen often improves but does not normalize nocturnal oxygen saturation in patients with severe drops in the arterial oxygen saturation[65] (Fig. 18–4). Norman and associates[68] compared supplemental oxygen with CPAP with respect to changes in blood pressure in a group of patients with OSA. CPAP reduced daytime and nighttime blood pressure whereas supplemental oxygen had no effect. Supplemental oxygen did improve nocturnal oxygenation. In summary, supplemental nocturnal oxygen is not the treatment of choice for OSA, but individual patients may benefit from this treatment if all other treatment options fail. The AASM practice parameters for medical treatment of OSA state that supplemental oxygen is not indicated for treatment of OSA.[3]

Persistent Daytime Sleepiness on CPAP

A substantial number of patients with OSA continue to have daytime sleepiness despite adequate PAP treatment.[69,70] In such patients, the first steps are to document adequate objective PAP adherence, document effective treatment, and to try sleep extension if indicated. Other causes of persistent daytime sleepiness despite PAP treatment include medications and other sleep disorders (narcolepsy, periodic limb movement disorder, idiopathic hypersomnia, depression). Other sleep disorders should be ruled out if clinically indicated. Of note, although some might assume 6 to 7 hours of nightly CPAP adherence to be "good adherence," in patients with continued daytime sleepiness, the first step would be an attempt at **sleep extension**. This includes using CPAP during naps. Another option would be an empirically small increase in CPAP pressure. Adequacy of pressure should also be documented because a surprisingly high percentage of patients remain inadequately treated.[71] Many PAP devices today give an estimate of the residual AHI. Finally, one might consider a repeat PAP titration if there is any suspicion that the current level of CPAP is not effective.

Modafinil, Armodafinil, and Stimulants

If daytime sleepiness persists on optimized CPAP treatment and there is no identifiable additional sleep disorder/cause of sleepiness, treatment with an alerting agent (modafinil [Provigil] or armodafinil [Nuvigil]) is indicated.[3] These medications have been shown to improve daytime alertness (subjective and objective) using randomized, placebo-controlled studies in OSA patients with residual sleepiness despite adequate PAP treatment.[69,70,72-76] Figure 18–5 illustrates improvement in the ESS in patients taking modafinil compared with placebo. Figure 18–6 displays results documenting an improvement in objective daytime sleepiness (longer sleep latency) with modafinil compared with placebo. The side effects of modafinil and use of this medication are discussed in more detail in Chapter 24. Headache is the most common side effect of modafinil. The Stevens-Johnson syndrome is a very rare but severe complication of modafinil treatment.

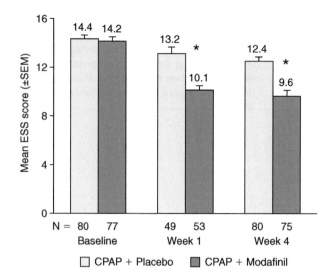

FIGURE 18–5 Modafinil decreased the Epworth Sleepiness Scale (ESS) compared with placebo at week 1 and week 4. *$P = .001$ placebo versus modafinil. Modafinil decreased the ESS compared with placebo. CPAP = continuous positive airway pressure; SEM = standard error of the mean. *From Pack AI, Black JE, Schwartz JR, Matheson JK: Modafinil as adjunct therapy for daytime sleepiness in obstructive sleep apnea. Am J Respir Crit Care Med 2001;164:1675–1681.*

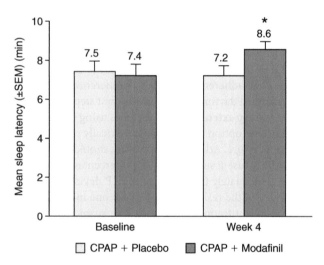

FIGURE 18–6 Mean multiple sleep latency test (MSLT) sleep latency at baseline and after treatment with nasal continuous positive airway pressure (nCPAP) and modafinil or nCPAP plus placebo. *$P = .021$. Modafinil increased the sleep latency. SEM = standard error of the mean. *From Pack AI, Black JE, Schwartz JR, Matheson JK: Modafinil as adjunct therapy for daytime sleepiness in obstructive sleep apnea. Am J Respir Crit Care Med 2001;164:1675–1681.*

During treatment of OSA patients with modafinil, it is essential to document continued adequate adherence to PAP treatment. In one study evaluating the addition of modafinil to CPAP treatment, poorer CPAP use was noted with modafinil than with placebo.[70] The usual modafinil dose is 200 to 400 mg in the morning. Some patients will benefit from a split dose if they have an increase in sleepiness in the late afternoon (modafinil 200 mg q AM and 100–200 mg q 2 PM). Patients with OSA who are adherent to PAP treatment will sometimes not be able to use CPAP for various reasons

(e.g., upper respiratory tract infection). A recent study by Williams and coworkers[77] documented that use of modafinil did help the ability of the patients to function in this circumstance.

Armodafinil (Nu-vigil) is the R enantiomer of modafinil and has a longer half-life than the L enantiomer. The dose of armodafinil is 150 to 250 mg daily. One would expect armodafinil to be as effective for daytime sleepiness as modafinil, but fewer studies have been published.[78,79] Armodafinil has also been shown to be effective in treatment of wakefulness in CPAP-adherent patients with OSA with co-morbid depression.[78] This is an important issue because a significant proportion of patients with OSA do suffer from depression.

Unfortunately, the addition of modafinil has minimal or modest benefits in a significant number of OSA patients who are still sleepy on PAP treatment. Kingshott and colleagues[70] found no improvement in ESS or multiple sleep latency test (MSLT) with modafinil but did find an improvement in the MWT sleep latency. Although stimulants are not U.S. Food and Drug Administration (FDA) or AASM practice parameter approved for treatment of persistent sleepiness, there are individual OSA patients with persistent daytime sleepiness despite adequate PAP treatment who will respond better to stimulants (methylphenidate, amphetamine) than to modafinil. Treatment with stimulants in addition to PAP could be tried if patients continue to have disabling sleepiness despite other measures. If clinically indicated, the possibility of coexistent narcolepsy should be ruled out. (This situation is discussed in Chapter 24). Performing an overnight sleep study on CPAP followed by an MSLT on CPAP can help document coexistent narcolepsy. If the MSLT is positive for narcolepsy, stimulants could certainly be used if modafinil was not effective. If the MSLT is negative or not possible (current treatment with an antidepressant), one could still try the addition of a stimulant to PAP treatment as a last resort (an "off-label" treatment).

Overview of Treatment of Pediatric OSA

Pediatric OSA is diagnosed if the apnea index >1/hr or the obstructive AHI (OAHI) >1–2/hr. OAHI values of 1 to <5, 5–10, and >10/hr are considered to characterize mild, moderate, and severe pediatric OSA.[80] These classifications are arbitrary and fail to account for different susceptibility in children to sleep disruption or hypoxemia. Patients with an OAHI <5/hr are treated based on the presence of significant symptoms. The treatment of choice for most patients with pediatric OSA is tonsillectomy and adenoidectomy (TNA) (see Chapter 21). Even if patients are obese or the AHI is elevated to the severe range, TNA is usually recommended unless minimal tonsillar and adenoidal tissues are present. PSG after surgical healing is recommended in all patients by some clinicians. Certainly, patients with residual symptoms on a pre-treatment OAHI in the moderate to severe range should be studied. If a significant residual OAHI is present after TNA, possible treatments include weight loss, positive airway pressure (see Chapter 20), dental procedures such as rapid maxillary expansion (see Chapter 21), or medications to reduce adenoidal and tonsillar inflammation.

Medications for Pediatric OSA

Leukotrienes and their receptors are increased in adenotonsillar tissue and exhaled condensates of children with OSA.[81,82] The combination of nasal inhaled steroid and the leukotriene inhibitors (montelukast) was found to have benefit in a study of patients with residual sleepiness after tonsillectomy and adenoidectomy.[83]

CLINICAL REVIEW QUESTIONS

1. A 40-year-old man without daytime sleepiness undergoes a PSG. The AHI = 50/hr with a low arterial oxygen saturation (SaO_2) of 80%. On physical examination, a very long uvula and a mild tonsillar enlargement is present. Which treatment do you recommend?
   A. UPPP.
   B. CPAP.
   C. OA.
   D. MMA.

2. A 50-year-old woman with a BMI of 35, AHI of 40/hr cannot tolerate CPAP. She does not want surgery. What do you recommend?
   A. Bariatric surgery.
   B. Nocturnal oxygen.
   C. Structured medical weight loss (diet modification).
   D. Protriptyline.
   E. OA.

3. A 35-year-old woman with previously documented OSA stopped CPAP of 10 cm H_2O after weight loss of 50 pounds following bariatric surgery was documented to reduce the AHI to less than 5/hr (study performed without CPAP). Over the last 6 months, daytime sleepiness has returned, although snoring is described only as mild. The patient's body weight has not changed since the last sleep study. What do you recommend?
   A. PSG.
   B. Thyroid function studies.
   C. Modafinil.
   D. CPAP of 10 cm H_2O

4. A 40-year-old man has persistent severe daytime sleepiness (ESS 15/24) despite good adherence to CPAP of 10 cm H_2O (average nightly use of 6 hr). A recent sleep study showed an AHI of 2/hr on CPAP of 10 cm H_2O during supine REM sleep. The patient's wife reports no snoring or apnea on treatment. He is taking fluoxetine for depression and denies symptoms of cataplexy. What do you recommend?

   A. Sleep extension and, if not successful, modafinil.
   B. PSG on CPAP followed by MSLT.
   C. Addition of methylphenidate.
   D. A repeat PAP PSG titration.

5. A 30-year-old man with a BMI of 19 denies sleepiness but is a very loud snorer. This is worse when he drinks alcohol or has worsening of nasal congestion. A sleep study revealed an overall AHI of 15/hr. He has declined CPAP or uvuloplasty and cannot afford an OA. An overnight summary of the sleep study is shown in Figure 18–7. What treatment do you recommend?
   A. Pillar procedure (palatal implants).
   B. Supplemental oxygen.
   C. Nasal corticosteroid and positional therapy.
   D. Mirtazapine.

Answers

1. **B.** The treatment of choice for severe OSA is CPAP (or other PAP treatment) even if some potentially surgically correctable anatomic changes are present.

2. **E.** Protriptyline and supplemental oxygen are not recommended treatments for OSA. Weight loss with either a dietary or a surgical intervention takes time and is considered a secondary treatment. Although an OA is not the treatment of choice for severe OSA, it can be effective in a significant proportion of patients. If severe arterial oxygen desaturation is present and no other treatments are acceptable, one might use supplemental oxygen, although the benefit of oxygen treatment for OSA is unproven. A sleep study on OA treatment should be performed to document efficacy.

3. **A.** A PSG is indicated to determine whether significant OSA has returned. This can occur after bariatric surgery even if weight loss has been maintained. Restarting CPAP is not indicated without documentation of the need for treatment and lower pressure may be effective. If a PSG documents significant OSA, a PSG PAP titration can be performed to determine an effective pressure level at the new lower weight.

4. **A.** Of the answers presented, this is the best option. An MSLT is often of limited value if a patient is taking a selective serotonin reuptake inhibitor. Methylphenidate is not FDA approved for treatment of residual daytime sleepiness on CPAP treatment. A repeat PSG CPAP titration is not unreasonable, but a recent study showed good control at the current treatment pressure.

5. **C.** The figure reveals postural OSA with few respiratory events in nonsupine positions. Nasal corticosteroids and positional therapy are the best answer, although the long-term effectiveness of positional therapy is unproved.

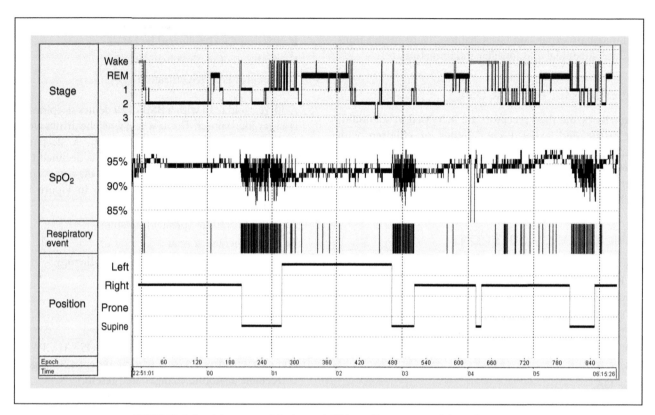

FIGURE 18–7 Overnight summary of the sleep study. REM = rapid eye movement; SpO$_2$ = pulse oximetry.

REFERENCES

1. Epstein LJ, Kristo D, Strollo PJ Jr, et al, Adult Obstructive Sleep Apnea Task Force of the American Academy of Sleep Medicine: Clinical guideline for the evaluation, management and long-term care of obstructive sleep apnea in adults. J Clin Sleep Med 2009;5:263–276.
2. Loube DI, Gay PC, Strohl KP, et al: Indications for positive airway pressure treatment of adult sleep apnea patients. A consensus statement. Chest 1999;115:863–866.
3. Morgenthaler TI, Kapen S, Lee-Chiong T, et al: Practice parameters for the medical therapy of obstructive sleep apnea. Sleep 2006;29:1031–1035.
4. Aurora RN, Casey KR, Kristo D, et al: Practice parameters for the surgical modifications of the upper airway for obstructive sleep apnea in adults. Sleep 2010;33:1408–1413.
5. Kushida CA, Morgenthaler TI, Littner MR, et al: American Academy of Sleep Medicine practice parameters for the treatment of snoring and obstructive sleep apnea with oral appliances: an update for 2005. Sleep 2006;29:240–243.
6. Kushida CA, Littner MR, Hirshkowitz M, et al: American Academy of Sleep Medicine Practice parameters for the use of continuous and bilevel positive airway pressure devices to treat adult patients with sleep-related breathing disorders. Sleep 2006;29:375–380.
7. Brown LK: Mild obstructive sleep apnea should be treated. J Clin Sleep Med 2007;3:259–261.
8. Littner MR: Mild obstructive sleep apnea should not be treated. J Clin Sleep Med 2007;3:262–264.
9. Gottlieb DJ, Whitney CW, Bonekat WH, et al: Relation of sleepiness to respiratory disturbance index. Am J Respir Crit Care Med 1999;159:502–507.
10. Peppard PE, Young T, Palta M, Skatrud J: Prospective study of the association between sleep disordered breathing and hypertension. N Engl J Med 2000;342:1378–1384.
11. Lee SA, Amis TC, Byth K, et al: Heavy snoring as a cause of carotid artery atherosclerosis. Sleep 2008;31:1207–1213.
12. Marshall NS, Barnes M, Travier N, et al: Continuous positive airway pressure reduces daytime sleepiness in mild to moderate obstructive sleep apnea: a meta-analysis. Thorax 2006;61:430–434.
13. Barbé F, Mayoralas LR, Duran J, et al: Treatment with continuous positive airway pressure is not effective in patients with sleep apnea but no daytime sleepiness: a randomized, controlled trial. Ann Intern Med 2001;134:1015–1023.
14. Beninati W, Harris CD, Herold DL, Shepard JW Jr: The effect of snoring and obstructive sleep apnea on the sleep quality of bed partners. Mayo Clin Proc 1999;74:955–958.
15. Punjabi NM, Caffo BS, Goodwin JL, et al: Sleep-disordered breathing and mortality: a prospective cohort study. PLoS Med 2009;6:e1000132.
16. Marin JM, Carrizo S, Vicente E, Agusti AGN: Long-term cardiovascular outcomes in men with obstructive sleep apnea-hypopnea with or without treatment with continuous positive airway pressure: an observational study. Lancet 2005;365:1046–1053.
17. Lavie P, Herer P, Lavie L: Mortality risk factors in sleep apnoea: a matched case-control study. J Sleep Res 2007;16:128–134.
18. Kohler M, Bloch KE, Stradling JR: The role of the nose in the pathogenesis of obstructive sleep apnea and snoring. Eur Respir J 2007;30:1208–1215.
19. Koutsourelakis I, Georgoulopoulos G, Perraki E, et al: Randomized trial of nasal surgery for fixed nasal obstruction in obstructive sleep apnea. Eur Respir J 2008;31:110–117.
20. Ferguson KA, Cartwright R, Rogers R, et al: Oral appliances for snoring and obstructive sleep apnea: a review. Sleep 2006;29:244–262.
21. Caples SM, Rowley JA, Prinsell JR, et al: Surgical modifications of the upper airway for obstructive sleep apnea in adults: a systematic review and meta-analysis. Sleep 2010;33:1396–1407.

22. Friedman M, Schalch P, Lin HC, et al: Palatal implants for the treatment of snoring and obstructive sleep apnea/hypopnea syndrome. Otolaryngol Head Neck Surg 2008;138:209–216.

23. Steward DL, Huntley TC, Woodson BT, Surdulescu V: Palate implants for obstructive sleep apnea: multi-institution, randomized, placebo-controlled study. Otolaryngol Head Neck Surg 2008;139:506–510.

24. Littner M, Kushida CA, Hartse K, et al: Practice parameters for the use of laser-assisted uvulopalatoplasty. Sleep 2001; 245:603–619.

25. Elshaug AG, Moss JR, Southcott A, et al: Redefining success in airway surgery for obstructive sleep apnea: a meta-analysis and synthesis of the evidence. Sleep 2007;30:461–467.

26. Personal communication from Philip Westbrook, MD, 1983.

27. Kushida CA, Littner MR, Morgenthaler T, Alessi CA: Practice parameters for the indications for polysomnography and related procedures: an update for 2005. Sleep 2005;28:499–521.

28. Young T, Pelta M, Dempsey J, et al: The occurrence of sleep disordered breathing among middle aged adults. N Engl J Med 1993;328:1230–1235.

29. Browman CP, Sampson MG, Yolles SF, et al: Obstructive sleep apnea and body weight. Chest 1984;85:435–436.

30. Smith PL, Gold AR, Meyers DA, et al: Weight loss in mildly to moderately obese patients with obstructive sleep apnea. Ann Intern Med 1985;103:850–855.

31. Johansson K, Neovius M, Lagerros YT, et al: Effect of a very low energy diet on moderate and severe sleep apnea in obese men: a randomised controlled trial. BMJ 2009;339:b4609.

32. Tuomilehto HPI, Seppa JM, Partine MM, et al: Lifestyle intervention with weight reduction: first-line treatment in mild obstructive sleep apnea. Am J Respir Crit Care Med 2009; 179:320–327.

33. Foster GD, Borradaile KE, Sanders MH, et al: A randomized study on the effect of weight loss on obstructive sleep apnea among obese patients with type 2 diabetes: the Sleep AHEAD study. Arch Intern Med 2009;169:1619–1626.

34. Peppard PE, Young T, Palta M, et al: Longitudinal study of moderate weight change and sleep disordered breathing. JAMA 2000;284:3015–3021.

35. Schwartz AR, Gold AR, Schubert N, et al: Effect of weight loss on upper airway collapsibility in obstructive sleep apnea. Am Rev Respir Dis 1991;144:494–498.

36. Simpson L, Mukherjee S, Cooper MN, et al: Sex differences in the association of regional fat distribution with the severity of obstructive sleep apnea. Sleep 2009;33:467–474.

37. Lettieri CJ, Eliasson AH, Greenburg DL: Persistence of obstructive sleep apnea after surgical weight loss. J Clin Sleep Med 2008;4:333–338.

38. Grunstein RR, Stenlöf KS, Hedner JA, et al: Two year reduction in sleep apnea symptoms and associated diabetes incidence after weight loss in severe obesity. Sleep 2007;30:703–710.

39. Phillips CL, Yee B, Trenell MI, et al: Changes in regional adiposity and cardiometabolic function following a weight loss program with sibutramine in obese men with obstructive sleep apnea. J Clin Sleep Med 2009;5:416–421.

40. Fritscher LG, Canani S, Mottin CC, et al: Bariatric surgery in the treatment of obstructive sleep apnea in morbidly obese patients. Respiration 2007;74:647–652.

41. Flancbaum L, Belsley S: Factors affecting morbidity and mortality of Roux-en-Y gastric bypass for clinically severe obesity: an analysis of 1000 consecutive patients by a single surgeon. Gastrointest Surg 2007;11:500–507.

42. Greenburg DL, Lettieri CJ, Eliasson AH: Effects of surgical weight loss on measures of obstructive sleep apnea: a meta-analysis. Am J Med 2009;122:535–542.

43. Pillar G, Peled R, Lavie P: Recurrence of sleep apnea without concomitant weight increase 7.5 years after weight reduction surgery. Chest 1994;106:1702–1704.

44. Sampol G, Sagales MT, Marti S, et al: Long-term efficacy of dietary weight loss in sleep apnea/hypopnea syndrome. Eur Respir J 1998;12:1156–1159.

45. Oksenberg A, Silverberg DS, Arons E, Radwan H: Positional vs nonpositional obstructive sleep apnea patients. Chest 1997;112: 629–639.

46. Walsh JH, Leigh MS, Paduch A, et al: Effect of body posture on pharyngeal shape and size in adults with and without obstructive sleep apnea. Sleep 2008;31:1543–1549.

47. Isono S, Tanaka A, Nishino T: Lateral position decreases collapsibility of the passive pharynx in patients with obstructive sleep apnea. Anesthesiology 2002;97:780–785.

48. Schwab RJ, Gefter WB, Hoffman EA, Pack AI: Dynamic upper airway imaging during awake respiration in normal subjects and patients with sleep disordered breathing. Am Rev Respir Dis 1993;148:1385.

49. Fogel RB, Malhotra A, Dialagiorgou G, et al: Anatomic and physiologic predictors of apnea severity in morbidly obese subjects. Sleep 2003;26:150–155.

50. Neill AM, Angus SM, Sajkov D, McEvoy RD: Effects of sleep posture on upper airway stability in patients with obstructive sleep apnea. Am J Respir Crit Care Med 1997;155: 199–204.

51. Permut I, Diaz-Abad M, Eissam C, et al: Comparison of positional therapy to CPAP in patients with positional obstructive sleep apnea. J Clin Sleep Med 2010;6:238–243.

52. Jokic R, Klimaszewski A, Crossley M, et al: Positional treatment vs continuous positive airway pressure in patients with positional obstructive sleep apnea syndrome. Chest 1999;115: 771–781.

53. Cartwright RD, Lloyd S, Lilie J, Kravitz H: Sleep position training for sleep apnea syndrome: a preliminary study. Sleep 1985; 8:87–94.

54. McEvoy RD, Sharp DJ, Thornton AT: The effects of posture on obstructive sleep apnea. Am Rev Respir Dis 1986;133: 662–666.

55. Skinner MA, Kingshott RN, Jones DR, et al: Elevated posture for the management of obstructive sleep apnea. Sleep Breath 2004;8:193–200.

56. Bignold JJ, Deans-Costi G, Goldsworthy MR, et al: Poor long-term patient compliance with the tennis ball technique for treating positional obstructive sleep apnea. J Clin Sleep Med 2009;5:428–430.

57. Oksenberg A, Silverberg DS, Arons E, et al: The sleep supine position has a major effect on optimal nasal CPAP. Chest 1999; 116:1000–1006.

58. Pevernagie DA, Shepard JW Jr: Relations between sleep stage, posture and effective nasal CPAP levels in OSA. Sleep 1992; 15:162–167.

59. Doshi J: Rhinitis medicamentosa: what an otolaryngologist needs to know. Eur Arch Otolaryngol 2009;266:623–625.

60. Kiely JL, Nolan P, McNicholas WT: Intranasal corticosteroid therapy for obstructive sleep apnea in patients with co-existing rhinitis. Thorax 2004;59:35–55.

61. Smith PL, Haponik EF, Bleecker ER: The effects of oxygen in patients with sleep apnea. Am Rev Respir Dis 1984;130: 958–963.

62. Martin RJ, Sander MH, Gray BA, Pennock BE: Acute and long term ventilatory effects in adult sleep apnea. Am Rev Respir Dis 1982;125:175–180.

63. Gold AR, Schwartz AR, Bleecker ER, Smith PL: The effect of chronic nocturnal oxygen administration upon sleep apnea. Am Rev Respir Dis 1986;134:925–929.

64. Fletcher E, Munafo DA: Role of nocturnal oxygen therapy in obstructive sleep apnea. Should it be used? Chest 1990; 98:1497–1504.

65. Alford NJ, Fletcher EC, Nickeson D: Acute oxygen in patients with sleep apnea and COPD. Chest 1986;89:30–38.

66. Gold AR, Bleecker ER, Smith PL: A shift from central and mixed sleep apnea to obstructive sleep apnea resulting from low flow oxygen. Am Rev Respir Dis 1985;132:220–223.

67. Loredo JS, Ancoli-Israel S, Kim E, et al: Effect of continuous positive airway pressure versus supplemental oxygen on sleep quality in obstructive sleep apnea: a placebo-CPAP-controlled study. Sleep 2006;29:564–571.

68. Norman D, Loredo JS, Nelesen RA, et al: Effects of continuous positive airway pressure versus supplemental oxygen on 24 hour ambulatory blood pressure. Hypertension 2006;47: 840–845.

69. Pack AI, Black JE, Schwartz JR, Matheson JK: Modafinil as adjunct therapy for daytime sleepiness in obstructive sleep apnea. Am J Respir Crit Care Med 2001;164:1675–1681.

70. Kingshott RN, Vennelle M, Coleman EL, et al: Randomized, double-blind, placebo-controlled crossover trial of modafinil in the treatment of residual excessive daytime sleepiness in the sleep apnea/hypopnea syndrome. Am J Respir Crit Care Med 2001;163:918–923.

71. Pittman SD, Pillar G, Berry RB, et al: Follow-up assessment of CPAP efficacy in patients with obstructive sleep apnea using an ambulatory device based on peripheral arterial tonometry. Sleep Breath 2006;10:123–131.

72. Dinges DF, Weaver TE: Effects of modafinil on sustained attention performance and quality of life in OSA patients with residual sleepiness while being treated with nCPAP. Sleep Med 2003;4:393–402.

73. Schwartz JR, Hirshkowitz M, Erman MK, Schmidt-Nowara W: Modafinil as adjunct therapy for daytime sleepiness in obstructive sleep apnea: a 12-week, open-label study. Chest 2003;124: 2192–2199.

74. Black JE, Hirshkowitz M: Modafinil for treatment of residual excessive sleepiness in nasal continuous positive airway pressure–treated obstructive sleep apnea/hypopnea syndrome. Sleep 2005;28:464–471.

75. Weaver TE, Chasens ER, Arora S: Modafinil improves functional outcomes in patients with residual excessive sleepiness associated with CPAP treatment. J Clin Sleep Med 2009; 5:499–505.

76. Roth T, Rippon GA, Arora S: Armodafinil improves wakefulness and long-term episodic memory in nCPAP-adherent patients with excessive sleepiness associated with obstructive sleep apnea. Sleep Breath 2008;12:53–62.

77. Williams SC, Marshall NS, Kennerson M, et al: Modafinil effects during acute continuous positive airway pressure withdrawal: a randomized crossover double-blind placebo-controlled trial. Am J Respir Crit Care Med 2010;181: 825–831.

78. Krystal AD, Harsh JR, Yang RR, et al: A double-blind, placebo-controlled study of armodafinil for excessive sleepiness in patients with treated obstructive sleep apnea and comorbid depression. J Clin Psychiatry 2010;71:32–40.

79. Roth T, Schwartz JR, Hirshkowitz M, et al: Evaluation of the safety of modafinil for treatment of excessive sleepiness. J Clin Sleep Med 2007;3:595–602.

80. Katz ES, D'Ambrosio CM: Pediatric obstructive sleep apnea syndrome. Clin Chest Med 2010;31:221–234.

81. Goldbart AD, Goldman JL, Li RC, et al: Differential expression of cysteinyl leukotriene receptors 1 and 2 in tonsils of children with obstructive sleep apnea syndrome or recurrent infection. Chest 2004;12:613–618.

82. Goldbart AD, Krishna J, Li RC, et al: Inflammatory mediators in exhaled condensate of children with obstructive sleep apnea syndrome. Chest 2006;130:143–148.

83. Kheirandish L, Goldbart AD, Gozal D: Intranasal steroids and oral leukotriene modifier therapy in residual sleep-disordered breathing after tonsillectomy and adenoidectomy in children. Pediatrics 2006;117:e61–e66.

Chapter 19

Positive Airway Pressure Treatment

Chapter Points

- PAP is the treatment of choice for patients with moderate to severe OSA and is an option in symptomatic patients with mild OSA.
- Although many variants of PAP have been developed, CPAP remains the treatment of choice for most OSA patients.
- BPAP devices deliver separately adjustable IPAP and EPAP with IPAP > EPAP.
- APAP devices provide the lowest effective pressure for a given posture and sleep stage.
- BPAP, APAP, or flexible PAP devices have not significantly improved adherence to PAP treatment for unselected patients. However, individual patients may benefit from these treatment modes.
- BPAP in the spontaneous mode is used for pressure intolerant OSA patients and to deliver pressure support (PS = IPAP − EPAP).
- BPAP in the ST mode (backup rate) is used for NPPV treatment of patients who have central apneas or central ventilatory control disorders.
- BPAP-ST is also used for patients who may not reliably trigger a transition for EPAP to IPAP due to neuromuscular or chest wall disorders.
- ASV is used for patients with an instability in ventilatory control manifested by CSB-central apneas, central apneas from narcotics, or CompSA of unknown etiology that does not improve with chronic CPAP treatment.
- PAP treatment is very effective at reversing or improving many manifestations of OSA. However, acceptance and adherence are major problems.
- There is a dose response to CPAP usage with the Epworth Sleepiness Scale improving with as little as 4 hours of use but objective improvement in sleepiness and quality of life measures usually require longer CPAP use for maximal benefit.
- Objective monitoring of adherence is essential for successful PAP treatment. This should be performed early after treatment initiation and at continuous intervals.
- Documentation of adequate objective adherence is the first step to evaluate persistent sleepiness despite PAP treatment.
- A PSG PAP titration is the standard approach for choosing an effective pressure.
- Higher CPAP is needed in the supine position and during REM sleep.
- Unattended APAP titration can be used to determine an effective level of CPAP (90th or 95th percentile pressure).
- Chronic treatment with APAP devices in properly selected patients eliminates the need for a PSG titration but does not significantly improve adherence.

Since the original description of continuous positive airway pressure (CPAP) treatment for obstructive sleep apnea (OSA) by Sullivan, Issa, and Berthon-Jones in 1981,[1] positive airway pressure (PAP) remains the mainstay of treatment for moderate to severe OSA in adults.[2-5] Despite many advances in technology, the major challenge facing clinicians is improving adherence to PAP treatment.[6]

MECHANISM OF ACTION

PAP works by splinting the upper airway open during sleep.[7-9] Studies have shown CPAP to increase upper airway size, especially in the lateral dimension (Fig. 19–1). Positive intraluminal pressure expands the upper airway (pneumatic splint). This is a passive process because upper airway muscle activity is reduced by CPAP.[10] Although the pneumatic splint is the main mechanism of action, an increase in lung volume due to CPAP may also increase upper airway size and/or stiffen the upper airway walls, making them less collapsible. In general, upper airway size increases as lung volume increases.[11] This is thought due to a downward pull on upper

FIGURE 19–1 Change in the upper airway of a normal individual after application of continuous positive airway pressure (CPAP) of 0 cm H₂O **(A)** and CPAP of 15 cm H₂O **(B).** The airway increases in size mainly in the lateral dimension. *From Schwab RJ: Upper airway imaging. Clin Chest Med 1998;19:33–54.*

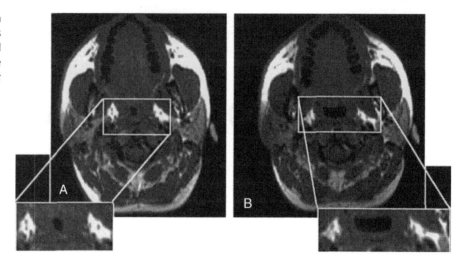

TABLE 19–1	
Modes of Positive Airway Pressure Devices	
CPAP	• Continuous pressure during inhalation and exhalation.
BPAP (S mode)	• IPAP. • EPAP. • IPAP − EPAP = PS. • BPAP may be better tolerated in patients complaining of difficulty exhaling on CPAP.
Flexible PAP, expiratory pressure relief (Cflex, EPR)	• Pressure falls in early exhalation. • Returns to set pressure at end-exhalation.
APAP autotitrating, autoadjusting PAP (autoCPAP)	• Titrates between maximum and minimum pressure limits to prevent apnea, hypopnea, airflow flattening, and airway vibration (snoring).
Auto-BPAP	• Titrates IPAP and EPAP between EPAPmin and IPAPmax with PSmin = 3 and PSmax set by the clinician. PSmax constrained by IPAPmax.
BPAP with backup rate (NPPV)	BPAP modes • ST. • T.
ASV	PS varies to stabilize breathing. EPAP set to eliminate airway obstruction. Backup rate AVAILABLE (see Table 19–2).
APAP = autoadjusting positive airway pressure; ASV = adaptive servoventilation; BPAP = bilevel positive airway pressure; CPAP = continuous positive airway pressure; EPAP = expiratory positive airway pressure; EPR = expiratory pressure relief; IPAP = inspiratory positive airway pressure; NPPV = noninvasive positive pressure ventilation; PAP = positive airway pressure; PS = pressure support; S mode = spontaneous mode; ST = spontaneous timed mode; T = timed mode.	

airway structures during lung expansion ("tracheal tug").[12] Whereas CPAP maintains a positive intraluminal pressure during both inspiration and expiration, one study using only expiratory positive airway pressure (EPAP) showed a reduction in respiratory events.[13] Another study was not able to reproduce a beneficial effect of EPAP.[14] This could be due to differences in study design or the method of delivery of EPAP (threshold valve vs. expiratory resistance).

EFFECTIVENESS

Numerous studies have shown that PAP can bring the apnea-hypopnea index (AHI) down to below 5 to 10/hr in the majority of patients.[2] The virtual elimination of apnea and hypopnea improves arterial oxygen saturation and decreases respiratory arousals. In some patients, PAP treatment can also increase the amount of stage N3 and stage R (rapid eye movement [REM] sleep). An occasional patient with very severe apnea will have a large REM or stage N3 sleep rebound on the first night of PAP treatment. This is most commonly seen when an entire night of polysomnography (PSG) is available for PAP titration. The most difficult problem with PAP treatment is that adherence is suboptimal in a large percentage of patients.[6] Many of the benefits of PAP treatment are discussed in Chapter 17.

MODES OF PAP

A number of modes of delivering PAP exist (Table 19–1). CPAP delivers a predetermined constant pressure during

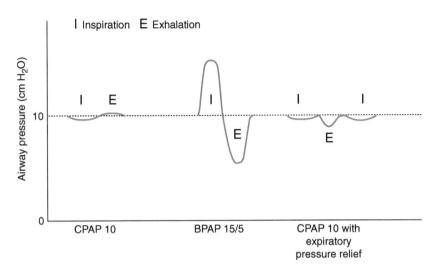

I Inspiration E Exhalation

both inspiration and exhalation (Fig. 19–2). Bilevel positive airway pressure (BPAP) delivers separately adjustable higher inspiratory positive airway pressure (IPAP) and lower EPAP (see Fig. 19–2).[15] Of note, in unselected patients, BPAP treatment does not result in higher rates of adherence than CPAP.[16] A Cochrane database analysis of six studies and 285 participants found no significant difference in usage with BPAP compared with CPAP.[17] However, some patients failing CPAP will tolerate BPAP.[18,19] This is especially true of patients having difficulty exhaling or with complaints of bloating. The IPAP-EPAP differential (pressure support [PS]) is useful for augmenting ventilation in patients with OSA and concomitant hypoventilation. These groups include the obesity hypoventilation syndrome (OHS) and the "overlap syndrome" (OSA + chronic obstructive pulmonary disease [COPD]). Some patients with the OHS or the overlap syndrome can be adequately treated with CPAP alone.[20,21] However, other patients in this group require BPAP, especially if significant hypoventilation is present.

BPAP is also used for noninvasive positive pressure ventilation (NPPV) in chronic alveolar hypoventilation syndromes.[22] In patients with OSA and OHS, BPAP is usually used in the spontaneous (S) mode. In this mode, the patient cycles the device from EPAP to IPAP and sets the respiratory rate. BPAP is also available with a backup rate (spontaneous-time [ST] mode) or a set respiratory rate (timed [T] mode). These modes are used to provide NPPV to patients who unreliably cycle the device between IPAP and EPAP due to muscle weakness or abnormal central ventilatory control (central apnea). In the ST mode, the device will provide a machine-triggered breath with the specified IPAPtime (inspiratory time) if no spontaneous breath occurs within a time window. For example, if the backup rate is 12 breaths/min, there is a 5-second window following the start of the last breath. If no spontaneous breath occurs during the time window, the machine will deliver a machine-triggered breath (Fig. 19–3). In the T mode, the device delivers IPAP/EPAP cycles with a set IPAPtime at a specified respiratory rate. For example, with a rate of 20, the cycle time is 3 seconds. If IPAPtime = 1 sec, then EPAP time = 2 sec. The

IPAP time is usually set at 1.2 to 1.6 seconds depending on the backup rate.

Autoadjusting (autotitrating) positive airway pressure (autoCPAP, autoPAP, APAP) devices were developed with two potential uses: (1) autotitrating PAP to select an effective level of CPAP without the need for an attended titration and (2) autoadjusting PAP for chronic treatment with the advantage of delivering the lowest effective pressure in any circumstance.[23–26] Chronic treatment with APAP would also eliminate the requirement for a CPAP titration. When APAP was first developed, improvement in PAP adherence was a goal. Although there are conflicting data, one meta-analysis showed that APAP does not improve adherence compared with CPAP.[27] A more recent larger meta-analysis of 30 studies and 1136 participants found a statistically significant difference in machine usage of 0.21 hour (12 min), which is not clinically significant.[17] However, individual patients may tolerate APAP better than CPAP.

The APAP algorithms vary between different devices, but in most instances, the pressure changes in response to variations in airflow magnitude (apnea or hypopnea), airflow limitation (flattening of the airflow contour), snoring (vibration), and/or airway impedance.[23] The pressure changes gradually between the preset lower and upper pressure limits (Pmax, Pmin) to avoid inducing arousal. If none of the monitored variables is detected, the device slowly lowers the pressure to a minimum effective setting. The pressure varies during the night in response to changes in body position or sleep stage that may alter the pressure required to maintain an open upper airway (Fig. 19–4). The **average** pressure is typically only 2 to 3 cm H_2O lower than the fixed pressure that would be effective during the entire night but can be up to 6 cm H_2O lower.[28] Of note, different brands of devices may respond very differently to changes in airflow.[29] High air leak (mask or mouth leak), which simulates physiologic events, and inability to differentiate between central and obstructive apnea by these devices can result in errors in APAP titration.[23,30] The APAP devices have no method of determining whether inspiratory effort is present during an apnea. In the past, some autotitration algorithms would not titrate above

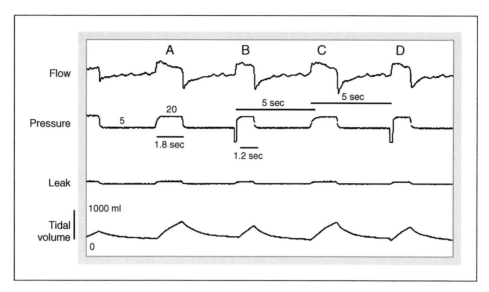

FIGURE 19–3 Tracings of flow, pressure, leak, and tidal volume signals provided by the positive airway pressure device while a patient is breathing on BPAP spontaneous timed (ST) mode with a backup rate of 12 breaths/min. Breaths *A* and *C* are patient-initiated and breaths *B* and *D* are machine-cycled breaths. If the device does not cycle from expiratory positive airway pressure (EPAP) to inspiratory positive airway pressure (IPAP) within a 5-second window, a machine breath (IPAPcycle) for the chosen inspiratory time (IPAPtime) occurs (breath *B*). The particular noninvasive positive airway pressure (NPPV) device illustrated supplies a negative-pressure spike signifying a machine-triggered breath. Note the shorter inspiratory time in breath *B* compared with breath *A*. Although the peak flow rates are similar, the tidal volume differs between breaths *A* and *B* due to a different IPAPtime. This illustrates the utility of recording tidal volume as well as flow.

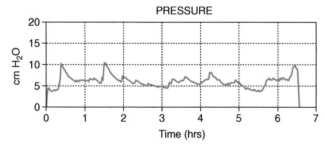

FIGURE 19–4 A single-night tracing of a patient using autoadjusting positive airway pressure (APAP) to determine an effective level of CPAP. The pressure limits were Pmax = 18 and Pmin = 4. The 95th percentile pressure was 9.8 cm H_2O. A CPAP of 10 cm H_2O was chosen for chronic treatment.

10 cm H_2O unless snoring or airflow limitation was present. Other algorithms would not continue to increase pressure if this did not reduce apnea (nonresponsive apnea). New technology used by Philips-Respironics attempts to differentiate "clear airway apneas" versus obstructive apneas by delivering a small pressure pulse (1–2 cm H_2O pressure pulse) after approximately 6 seconds of a reduction in airflow (Fig. 19–5). If the pressure pulse does produce an increase in flow, this is compatible with an open airway (clear airway). If the pressure pulse does not increase flow, the airway is closed. An APAP device using this technology does not increase pressure for "clear airway" apneas. Note that a closed airway

FIGURE 19–5 Method of determining whether an apnea is associated with an open airway (clear airway apnea) or a closed airway (obstructive apnea). The method cannot tell whether there is inspiratory effort, so a closed airway central apnea is labeled as an obstructive apnea. CPAP = continuous positive airway pressure.

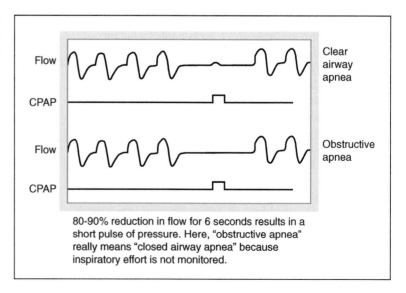

80-90% reduction in flow for 6 seconds results in a short pulse of pressure. Here, "obstructive apnea" really means "closed airway apnea" because inspiratory effort is not monitored.

can occur with some central apneas.[31] Thus, using this approach, some apneas classified as obstructive could actually be closed airway central apneas. The use of APAP devices for autotitration is discussed in more detail in later sections.

An autoBPAP device is also available (Fig. 19–6). The physician sets the minimum EPAP, and the minimum and maximum pressure support (IPAP-EPAP), as well as the maximum IPAP. The minimum PS is 3 cm H_2O by default. The machine then adjusts both the EPAP and the IPAP to maintain an open airway. The advantages of autoBPAP over other PAP modes remain to be demonstrated. A recent study found autoBPAP to be useful as "rescue" therapy in patients not compliant to CPAP treatment in spite of the usual interventions.[32] Thus, autoBPAP could potentially be useful in very pressure-intolerant patients who find BPAP alone unacceptable or in patients for whom an effective bilevel pressure is not known.

Adaptive servoventilation (ASV)[33-38] is a variant of BPAP that was developed to treat Cheyne-Stokes central apnea in patients with congestive heart failure.[33,37,38] Both ASV and BPAP devices with a backup rate are approved for use with patients with central apnea and complex sleep apnea (CompSA; central apnea that persists or appears during a PAP titration). ASV devices attempt to stabilize ventilation in patients with ventilatory instability such as Cheyne-Stokes breathing (CSB),[33,37,38] narcotic-induced central apnea,[36] and CompSA of unknown etiology.[34,35] During an ASV titration, a level of EPAP is chosen to keep the upper airway open (preventing obstructive apnea) and the IPAP-EPAP difference (PS) automatically adapts between minimum and maximum levels to stabilize ventilation (Fig. 19–7).

ASV devices from two manufacturers are available in the United States (Table 19–2). They both adjust pressures with a goal of stabilizing ventilation. The ResMed device (VPAP Adapt SV) uses a goal of providing 90% of the recent average

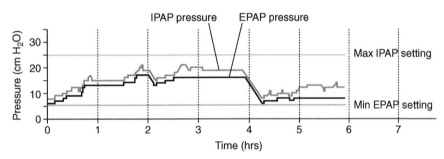

FIGURE 19–6 An overnight pressure-versus-time tracing is shown for a patient using autobilevel positive airway pressure (PAP) with a minimum expiratory positive airway pressure (EPAP) of 6 cm H_2O and a maximum inspiratory airway pressure (IPAP) of 25 cm H_2O. The 90th percentile IPAP and EPAP pressures were 19.2 cm H_2O and 16.2 cm H_2O, respectively. The average IPAP and EPAP values were 14.6 cm H_2O and 11.8 cm H_2O, respectively. *From Kakkar RK, Berry RB: Positive airway pressure treatment for obstructive sleep apnea. Chest 2007;132:1057–1072.*

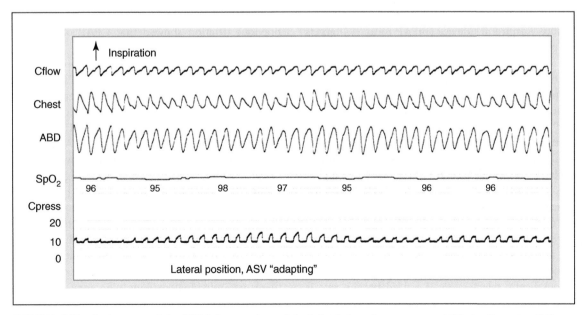

FIGURE 19–7 The adaptive servoventilation (ASV) device responds to variation in flow by increasing pressure support (PS) when flow and ventilation are low and decreasing PS when flow is high. ABD = abdomen; Cflow = flow signal from the PAP device; Cpress = delivered pressure; SpO₂ = pulse oximetry.

TABLE 19-2

Adaptive Servoventilation Devices

BRAND NAME	RESMED ADAPT SV	PHILIPS-RESPIRONICS AUTO BIPAP SV ADVANCED
Target	90% of previous average ventilation (moving time window)	90% of average peak flow (moving time window)
EPAP	• EPP titrated manually • To prevent upper airway obstruction	EPAP automatically adjusted between EPAPmin and EPAPmax
IPAP	• Max available 25 cm H_2O • Varies to deliver optimal PS • Limits: PSmin to PSmax depending on EPP and maximum machine pressure • PSmin ≥ 3 cm H_2O	• Max pressure up to 30 cm H_2O • IPAP varies to deliver PS between PSmin (can be 0) to PSmax • PSmax constrained by maximum pressure and current level of EPAP
Backup rate	• Automatic Approximately 15 breaths/min	• Auto rate • Fixed rate
Inspiratory time	• Automatic	• Automatic in auto rate mode • Set in manual rate mode (default 1.5 sec)
Recommended initial settings	EPP = 4 cm H_2O • PSmin ≥ 3 cm H_2O • PSmax ≥ 10 cm H_2O	EPAPmin = 4 cm H_2O EPAPmax = 15 cm H_2O PSmin = 0 PSmax = 20 Max pressure = 25 cm H_2O Rate: auto If rate set, use IPAPtime (I-time) = 1.5 sec

BiPAP = bilevel positive airway pressure; EPAP = expiratory positive airway pressure; EPP = EPAP; IPAP = inspiratory positive airway pressure; PS = pressure support; SV = servoventilation.

ventilation (moving time window). With low tidal volume, the PS increases, and with high tidal volume, the PS decreases. An automatic backup rate triggers an IPAP/EPAP cycle if central apnea is present (default 15 breaths/min). The technologist can only adjust the EPAP (termed "EPP" for this brand of ASV). The PS is constrained by PSmax (≥10 cm H_2O is recommended) and the maximum IPAP is constrained by maximum pressure of 25 cm H_2O.

The Philips-Respironics device (BiPAP Auto SV) targets 90% of the previous average peak flow (moving time average) and has a within-breath adjustment capability. The IPAP increases to provide PS between the limits of **PSmin and PSmax** as needed to augment flow. The EPAP is adjusted to maintain an open upper airway. The BiPAP Auto SV provides CPAP = EPAP if ventilation is stable and if PSmin = 0 (default setting). The backup rate can be set at a fixed rate (or rate = 0) but usually the autorate is used. The autorate provides a background rate of 8 to 10 breaths/min or higher depending on previous percentage of patient-triggered breaths. The rate is increased based on current cycle time and EPAPtime (time since start of the EPAP cycle). If a fixed backup rate is specified, an IPAPtime (or inspiratory time [Ti]) must also be specified. The Ti is usually 1.2 to 1.6 sec (recommended 1.5 sec). However, in the autorate mode, the device automatically selects a Ti. If a fixed backup rate is used, the manufacturer suggests starting at 2 breaths/min below the spontaneous rate (minimum 8–10). The latest version of the BiPAP Auto SV device, called *BiPAP Auto SV*

advanced, can automatically titrate EPAP with algorithms similar to the one used for APAP devices to overcome any obstructive component of breathing. The clinician specifies EPAPmin and EPAPmax and the device titrates EPAP between those settings. The initial EPAPmin = 4 cm H_2O unless it is known or suspected that CPAP higher than 10 cm H_2O is needed to maintain an open upper airway. In that case, EPAPmin of 6 to 8 cm H_2O is used. For example, a previous titration showed that CPAP of 12 cm H_2O was needed during REM sleep.

Of note, patients with CSB-central apnea and CompSA (including patients on narcotics) can also be treated with BPAP in the ST mode. One study comparing BPAP-ST with ASV in patients with central apnea and CompSA found ASV to result in only a slightly lower AHI than BPAP-ST.[34] However, stabilizing ventilation with BPAP-ST in this situation often requires a high backup rate (with a high proportion of machine-triggered breaths). Higher PS is usually needed to deliver a machine-triggered breath because the patient does not assist with inspiration. It is preferable to have the patient trigger the majority of breaths because timing and effective ventilation are usually better. Thus, ASV is generally preferable because, if ventilation is stabilized, a majority of the breaths will be patient-triggered. However, there are individual patients who may respond better to BPAP-ST.

An important concept when using ASV is that of closed airway central apnea. As noted previously, during

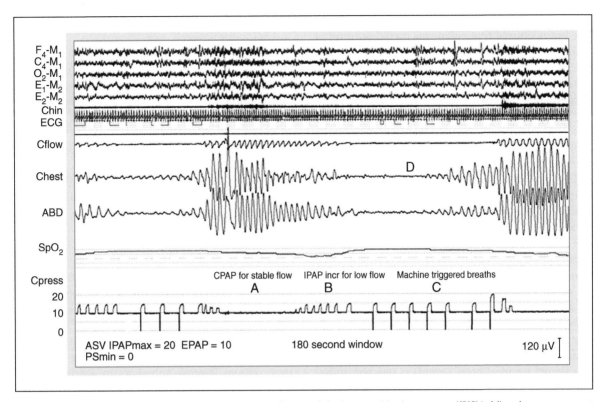

FIGURE 19–8 A patient with Cheyne-Stokes breathing on a BPAP Auto SV device. *A,* Continuous positive airway pressure (CPAP) is delivered as pressure support (PS) equals PSmin (here = 0) and flow is high. *B,* PS increases as flow is low. *C,* Machine-triggered breaths during a central apnea. *D,* The machine-triggered PS was not effective due to a closed upper airway. An increase in expiratory positive airway pressure (EPAP) is needed. ABD = abdomen; ASV = adaptive servoventilation; Cpress = delivered pressure; ECG = electrocardiogram; IPAP = inspiratory positive airway pressure; SpO_2 = pulse oximetry. *From Brown LK: Adaptive servoventilation for sleep apnea: technology, titration protocols, and treatment efficacy. Sleep Med Clin 2010;5:433.*

central apnea, the upper airway may close.[31] For example, during a mixed apnea, the airway has closed during the central portion. If a closed airway central apnea occurs, the machine-triggered PS will not effectively deliver flow (or tidal volume). In this case, higher EPAP is needed (Fig. 19–8). ASV was not specifically designed for patients with nocturnal hypoventilation. However, some patients with CompSA due to narcotics have both hypoventilation and instability in breathing. A higher PSmin ($\geq$4 cm H_2O) may be needed if the arterial oxygen saturation (SaO_2) remains low but breathing is regular. Another situation in which PSmin greater than 0 is useful is the pressure-intolerant patient. Rather than using EPAP of 16, one could use an EPAP of 14 and a PSmin of 4. Thus, the device would deliver a basal pressure of 18/14 cm H_2O with higher IPAP as needed to stabilize ventilation. This example also illustrates that if a patient requires high EPAP, quite high IPAP values may be needed to deliver an adequate PS.

VOLUME-TARGETED BPAP

Recently, volume-targeted bilevel positive airway pressure (VT-BPAP) has been developed in which the IPAP-EPAP difference is automatically adjusted to deliver a target tidal volume.[39–42] VT-BPAP has the potential advantage of automatically varying the PS to deliver a targeted tidal volume if the condition of the patient changes. For example, if respiratory muscle strength declined and the tidal volume decreased, the device would deliver higher PS to return the delivered tidal volume to the targeted level. VT-BPAP can be used in the S, ST, or T mode. Relatively few studies on VT-BPAP devices have been published. To date, only one VT-BPAP device is available in the United States (Average Volume Assured Pressure Support [AVAPS], Philips-Respironics). Storre and colleagues[39] compared BPAP and AVAPS (both in the ST mode) using a randomized, crossover trial in patients with OHS. AVAPS resulted in a slightly higher ventilation and lower arterial partial pressure of carbon dioxide ($PaCO_2$) without any better sleep quality or quality of life measures compared with BPAP-ST. Using the same device, Ambrogio and associates[40] studied an assortment of patients with chronic alveolar hypoventilation who were stable on BPAP support. A validation night preceded the study nights to ensure the BPAP settings were adequate and to provide guidance for the AVAPS settings. Patients then were studied on BPAP or AVAPS in random order. On AVAPS, the minute ventilation was greater than on BPAP but sleep quality was comparable between the two NPPV modes. Using a different VT-BPAP device, Janssens and coworkers[41] monitored patients with the OHS using either BPAP or

VT-BPAP for one night each in random order. Sleep quality was worse but nocturnal transcutaneous partial pressure of carbon dioxide (TcPCO$_2$) was slightly lower on VT-BPAP. It is possible that patients might have exhibited better sleep quality after a longer period of adaptation to the VT-BPAP. Jaye and colleagues[42] compared BPAP-ST with an autotitrating bilevel ventilator (autoVPAP) in patients with stable neuromuscular and chest wall disease with nocturnal hypoventilation and found autoVPAP to produce comparable control of nocturnal oxygenation without compromising sleep quality. The mean nocturnal TcPCO$_2$ was higher with autoVPAP, although the difference was unlikely to be clinically significant. AutoVPAP (ResMed, Poway, CA) is not currently available in the United States. These studies suggest VT-BPAP can be effective, but the role of VT-BPAP in the NPPV treatment of patients with chronic alveolar hypoventilation syndromes remains to be determined.

When VT-BPAP is used, the purpose of a PSG PAP titration is to select a level of EPAP that eliminates obstructive events (obstructive apnea and hypopnea) and document that the device does deliver adequate tidal volumes. According to the manufacturer's recommendations, a target tidal volume of 8 cc/kg (based on ideal body weight) is selected. Initial settings are EPAP = 4 cm H$_2$O, IPAPmin = EPAP + 4 cm H$_2$O, and IPAPmax = 25 to 30 cm H$_2$O. If VT-BPAP is used in the ST or T mode, the backup rate and Ti must also be specified. A default Ti (IPAPtime) of 1.5 seconds is recommended by the manufacturer.

COMFORT MEASURES

Ramp

Most PAP devices, with the exception of certain APAP devices, allow the patient to trigger the ramp option. In the ramp option, the pressure starts at a preset level—usually a low level of CPAP—and then slowly increases to the treatment pressure (CPAP) over the set ramp time. Some APAP devices have a "settling time" at a low pressure before the device starts autoadjusting pressure. The ramp option is appealing and can be used during midnight awakenings to help patients return to sleep. However, no study has shown that the ramp option increased adherence.

Flexible Pressure

Two manufacturers of PAP devices have developed flexible PAP in an attempt to improve patient comfort and adherence. Some PAP devices manufactured by Philips-Respironics provide several comfort options (Cflex, Cflex+, and Aflex) (Fig. 19–9). ResMed devices offer expiratory pressure relief (EPR). However, there are no convincing data that any of these options improve adherence in unselected patients. In Cflex, expiratory pressure drops at the start of exhalation but returns to the set CPAP at end-exhalation. The amount of drop (Cflex 1, 2, 3) is determined by a proprietary algorithm. In general, there is a greater pressure drop for greater flow during exhalation. Cflex is available on APAP devices as well

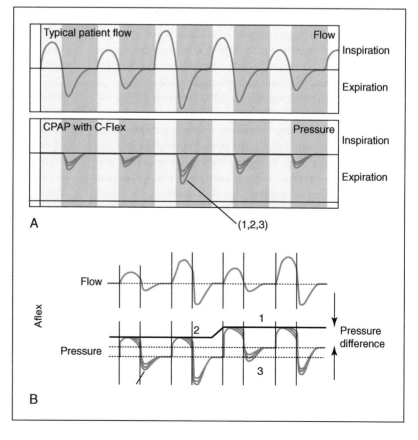

FIGURE 19–9 A, C-Flex. The pressure drops at the start of exhalation (the amount depends on expiratory flow and the C-Flex setting, 1, 2, or 3) but returns to the set continuous positive airway pressure (CPAP) pressure at end-exhalation. **B,** Aflex. *(1)* The inspiratory pressure autoadjusts as per autoadjusting positive airway pressure (APAP), *(2)* smoothing of transition from inspiration to exhalation, *(3)* expiratory pressure relief similar to C-Flex. The end-expiratory pressure is 2 cm H$_2$O below the inspiratory pressure (pressure difference). *A,* From Mulgrew AT, Cheema R, Fleetham J, et al: Efficacy and patient satisfaction with autoadjusting CPAP with variable expiratory pressure vs standard CPAP: a two-night randomized crossover trial. Sleep Breath 2007;11:31–37.

as CPAP. Cflex+ adds a smoothing of the transition from inhalation to exhalation. Aflex is a form of APAP that provides a 2 cm H_2O lower end-expiratory pressure than the inspiratory pressure (in addition to the features of Cflex+). For both BPAP and autoBPAP devices, a form of expiratory pressure relief is available (Biflex). The technology provides a smoothing of transition from IPAP to EPAP as well as expiratory pressure relief during the EPAP cycle (Biflex 1, 2, 3).

ResMed devices provide EPR and drop the pressure during the start of exhalation pressure by 1, 2, or 3 cm H_2O (EPR 1, 2, 3). The EPR can be used full time or only during the ramp period. EPR is not available with ResMed APAP devices.

An initial study found that flexible PAP improved adherence by about $\frac{1}{2}$ hour using a cross-over design.[43] A number of subsequent studies in patients on CPAP[44-48] or APAP[49] have not found an increase in adherence. The mode can still be useful for individual patients who find CPAP difficult to tolerate. Conversely, some patients actually prefer CPAP to flexible PAP.

Humidification

Today, most PAP devices come with the option of an integrated heated humidification system. They can be used in the cool humidity mode if desired. Heated humidity (HH) can deliver a greater level of moisture than cool humidification and may be especially useful in patients with mouth leak or nasal congestion. Mouth leak can cause a dramatic fall in relative humidity[50] (Fig. 19–10) and a loss of humidity from the upper airway/CPAP system, thus drying the nasal or oral mucosa. Drying of the nasal mucosa increases nasal resistance and this is minimized by use of HH.[51,52] HH is more effective than cool at delivering moisture. The level of humidity can be adjusted by the patient to meet variable needs. An occasional patient will prefer cool humidity (heat turned off) or no humidity at all. Adequate cleaning of the humidifier chamber and hoses does require extra patient effort. A number of technologic advances for adjusting humidity to prevent rain-out in the tubing and mask have recently been introduced. One study suggested that use of humidity is associated with an increase in risk of infectious complications[53] that can be reduced with use of a filter.[54] There is an occasional patient with recurrent sinus infections who seems to do better without humidification—but the etiology of this improvement is unclear.

Studies determining whether HH improves either acceptance of CPAP after titration or long-term adherence to CPAP treatment have found conflicting results. Massie and associates[55] studied patients who received either HH or cool humidity for 3 weeks (random order), a 2-week washout period of no humidity, and 3 weeks of the alternative humidity. Patients on HH had about $\frac{1}{2}$ hour greater objective adherence than those on no humidity (Table 19–3). However, several other studies have not found an improvement in adherence[56-61] with the use of HH for PAP treatment. Other

TABLE 19–3			
Effect of Humidity on Outcomes			
	HEATED HUMIDITY	**COLD PASSOVER HUMIDITY**	**NO HUMIDITY**
Usage (hr/night)	5.52 ± 2.1*	5.15 ± 1.9	4.93 ± 2.2
Epworth Sleepiness Scale	6.2 ± 3.8	7.2 ± 4.8	6.7 ± 3.9
Feeling on awakening	74 ± 15.9†	68.9 ± 23.4	62.0 ± 23.4
Satisfaction with CPAP	73.9 ± 19.1†	72.9 ± 22.6‡	62.3 ± 27.6
Adverse side effects score	4.9 ± 3.3	6.2 ± 3.8	6.5 ± 4.9

*P < .008.
†P < .05. Heated humidity versus no humidity.
‡P < .05. Cool humidity versus no humidity.[54]
Data from Massie CA, Hart RW: Clinical outcomes related to interface type in patients with obstructive sleep apnea/hypopnea syndrome who are using continuous positive airway pressure. Chest 2003;123:1112–1118.

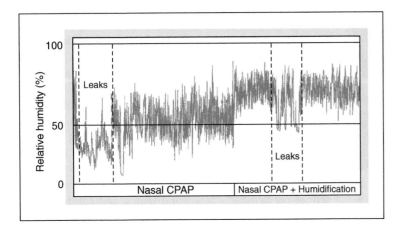

FIGURE 19–10 This tracing shows a fall in the relative humidity at the nasal mask during mouth leaks (leak detected by an oral thermistor). Heated humidification minimized but did not eliminate the fall in relative humidity. CPAP = continuous positive airway pressure. *From Martins de Araujo MT, Vieira SB, Vasquez EC, Fleury B: Heated humidification or face mask to prevent upper airway dryness during continuous positive airway pressure therapy. Chest 2000;117:142–147.*

investigations could not document a benefit from the "pro-phylactic" use of HH for titration. A criticism of these studies is that patients with baseline nasal congestion or dryness were not targeted. It seems reasonable to use humidity in patients with complaints of nasal congestion or mouth breathing at baseline. Certainly, in some patients, use of HH is crucial, and in others, it may improve satisfaction. Rainout in the tubing and the mask is a significant problem for some patients. Lowering the CPAP unit to a level below the bed (water flows back into the humidifier chamber by gravity), reducing the humidity setting, or using a tube insulator may help. New technology recently available adjusts the humidifier setting based on room temperature and relative humidity. However, it is not clear that this technology will improve adherence. In the practice parameters for PAP treatment (Appendix 19–1), use of HH is recommended to improve CPAP utilization.[3] In the clinical guidelines for titration, having HH available for titration was recommended.[62]

Interfaces

When CPAP devices became available commercially, the first interfaces were nasal masks. Today, a large variety of interfaces is available (Fig. 19–11), but it may still be difficult to obtain a good mask fit. Nasal pillow masks are often better tolerated than traditional nasal masks by patients with claustrophobia and are useful in patients with a mustache or edentulous patients who have no dental support for the upper lip.[63] It is essential to use a size of pillow large enough to provide a good seal. A wide variety of nasal masks with gel or air cushion interfaces is available. For patients who

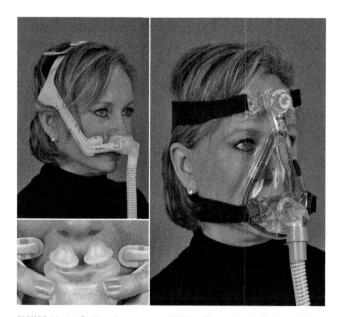

FIGURE 19–11 Positive airway pressure (PAP) interface options. **Left,** A nasal pillows mask (Swift LT for her by ResMed, Poway, CA). **Right,** A full face mask (Quattro by ResMed, Poway, CA).

have severe nasal congestion or open their mouths during PAP treatment, oronasal (full face masks)[64,65] and oral interfaces[66,67] are available. Oronasal masks have to seal over a large area, and this makes finding a good fit very difficult in some patients. In edentulous patients, oronasal masks may also compress the soft tissues. Patients tend to overtighten masks, and this can cause damage to the nasal bridge or actually impair the ability of the mask to seal. Often, a trial of several masks is needed to find one that patients can use comfortably. This is a challenge because insurance providers typically will pay for only one mask every 3 to 6 months. This is one situation in which trying several different types of mask in the sleep center before the titration can be very useful. Adequate care and replacement of masks are also essential to maximize their ability to seal. If the patient gets up to use the bathroom during the night, we encourage disconnection of the hose from mask rather than taking off the mask. Masks that are removed in the middle of the night are often not replaced.

INDICATIONS FOR PAP TREATMENT

Important elements of the AASM practice parameters for the use of PAP and APAP are listed in Appendix 19–1. Treatment with PAP is indicated for patients with moderate to severe OSA (with or without symptoms).[2,3] PAP treatment is an option for patients with mild OSA who are symptomatic and choose PAP over other treatment options (upper airway surgery or an oral appliance). The Centers for Medicare and Medicaid Services (CMS) requirements for PAP reimbursement are specified in the National Carrier Determination 240.4.[68] Patients must be diagnosed with either a PSG or a home sleep test (HST) that follows Medicare requirements for those evaluations (discussed in Chapter 13). CPAP treatment is reimbursed for an initial 12-week period if the AHI is 15/hr or greater with or without symptoms or if the AHI is 5/hr or greater but less than 14/hr if certain symptoms (excessive daytime sleepiness, impaired cognition, mood disorders, or insomnia) or certain disorders (hypertension, ischemic heart disease, or history of stroke) are present. For continued payment after that period, adequate objective adherence must be documented. For at least 1 month during the qualifying period, CPAP must be ≥4 hours for ≥70% of nights. A face-to-face evaluation of the patient by the physician ordering CPAP and documentation of a benefit from treatment are also required. The exact requirements vary with different local carrier determinations (LCDs) (Appendix 19–2). Most other health insurance providers follow similar guidelines.

As noted in Chapters 18 and 20, the initial treatment for most children with OSA is tonsillectomy and adenoidectomy. However, residual sleep apnea is present in a significant portion of patients.[69] The clinician must then decide on further treatment recommendations based on the residual AHI and symptoms. Excessive daytime sleepiness, poor school performance, behavioral issues, and cardiovascular consequences should all be considered. PAP is an effective option provided that both the parents and the patient accept this treatment. The exact AHI cutoff is not well defined, but many pediatricians consider a residual greater than 5/hr as indicating significant OSA in children and an indication for CPAP treatment. Those less symptomatic patients with an AHI between 1 and 5 are in a gray zone and treatment must be individualized. Starting CPAP in children often requires periods of adaptation to a mask before a titration can be attempted.[62,70] Other options include weight loss, dental procedures, or intranasal steroids and leukotriene modifier therapy.[71]

ADHERENCE—DEFINITIONS AND MEASUREMENT

Despite the excellent efficacy of PAP devices for reducing the AHI, the actual effectiveness is much lower. For example, if CPAP reduces the AHI from 40 to 5/hr but is used only 50% of nights, the mean AHI has only been reduced to 25/hr. Monitoring PAP adherence at one time involved looking at the run time meter on devices. Then the devices began to record both blower hours and time at pressure (actual use). Today, PAP machines have both internal memory and removal memory (smart cards, memory sticks, or disks). The removable media can store extensive information on adherence and patterns of use. The recorded device information can be assessed by direct machine interrogation (internal memory) or transferring of information on removable media to a computer. Some devices when attached to a modem can send information to a central location and physicians can obtain ongoing data on a patient. Other devices can communicate with a central location using wireless technology. The data obtained from PAP devices often includes useful information on leak as well as an estimate of the residual AHI. Detailed daily information can show important patterns, for example, consistent mask removal at 5 AM. As discussed later, it has been shown that the pattern of use is established early and that objective adherence (not patient report) is essential to guide treatment. Data via modem or wireless communication can provide information during the critical first weeks of use without requiring the patient to come to a clinic or a durable medical equipment office.

Adherence rates are defined in many ways. Most devices compute the percentage of days used, the average use all days (averaging in 0s for days not used), average nightly use (days used), and the percentage of nights used ≥4 hours. An early paper reporting measurement of objective adherence by Kribbs and coworkers[72] defined regular users as those who used CPAP at least 4 hr/day on at least 70% of nights. In their study, only 46% of patients met this criterion.

PAP Adherence in Large Studies

There has been a tremendous variability in the reported rates of PAP adherence. This is due to a number of factors including different populations (moderate to severe OSA vs. all

patients), different definitions of adherence, different length of follow-up, and different algorithms of initiating PAP treatment and following patients. One of the largest studies of long-term adherence with nasal CPAP reported only 68% of patients were still using CPAP at 5 years.[73] Pépin and colleagues[74] found 79% of patients using CPAP for longer than 4 hours on 70% of nights at 3 months. Sin and coworkers[75] followed patients with an AHI greater than 20/hr and found greater than 85% were using the device longer than 3.5 hr/night at 6 months. Kohler and associates[76] found that 81% of patients were using CPAP at 5 years.

Factors Influencing Adherence and Importance of Early Adherence

Several studies have addressed the factors associated with good versus poor PAP adherence (Table 19–4). In general, the factors identified to date explain relatively little of the large variance in CPAP acceptance and adherence.[73,74,76,77] The level of pressure does not seem to be important. Finding an acceptable interface is often the biggest challenge in getting patients to adhere to PAP treatment. However, there is no evidence for the superiority of any type of interface. Although a great deal of effort is spent in intervening for side effects, the presence or absence of side effects does not seem to be a major determinant of PAP use.[77] Patients may be willing to tolerate side effects if there is a significant improvement in pretreatment symptoms. Factors favoring better adherence include symptomatic daytime sleepiness, good response in sleepiness to treatment, and to a lesser extent disease severity (AHI). In one study a high arterial oxygen desaturation index predicted good adherence.[76] Poor prognostic factors include spouse referral and high nasal resistance.[75,78] Whether CPAP treatment follows a split night (diagnostic/PAP titration) or separate diagnostic and PAP titration studies does not seem to affect PAP adherence. Early adherence is a good predictor of long term PAP use. In a study of 32 patients followed for 9 weeks, the nightly duration of use differed between compliant and noncompliant patients by the fourth night of use.[79] Budhiraja and colleagues[80] found that long-term adherence to CPAP can be predicted as early as 3 days after CPAP initiation.

TABLE 19–4		
Factors Predicting Good or Worse Adherence		
GOOD ADHERENCE	**WORSE ADHERENCE**	**NO EFFECT**
• More sleepy • Higher AHI • Greater perception of benefit • Good early adherence	• Spouse referred • Not sleepy • High nasal resistance • Poor early adherence	• Level of pressure • Pressure technology—minimal if any effect
AHI = apnea-hypopnea index.		

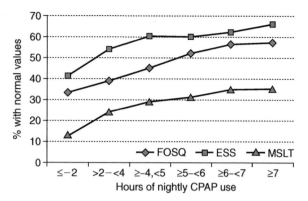

FIGURE 19–12 Cumulative proportion of participants obtaining normal threshold values on the Epworth Sleepiness Scale (ESS), multiple sleep latency test (MSLT), and Functional Outcomes of Sleep Questionnaire (FOSQ). CPAP = continuous positive airway pressure. *From Weaver TE, Maislin G, Dinges DF, et al: Relationship between hours of CPAP use and achieving normal levels of sleepiness and daily functioning. Sleep 2007;30:711–719.*

TABLE 19–5
Methods to Improve Positive Airway Pressure Adherence
• Education about OSA and PAP by staff, video, printed information
• Involvement of significant other/spouse
• Subsequent mask and headgear adjustment or change as needed
• PAP help line
• Unsolicited telephone follow-up
• Early interventions for side effects and concerns
• Objective monitoring of adherence
• Early and regular clinic visits
OSA = obstructive sleep apnea; PAP = positive airway pressure.

How Much Adherence Is Enough?

Weaver and associates[81] studied patients before and after 3 months of therapy and correlated objective adherence with improvement in functioning (Fig. 19–12). Thresholds above which further improvements were less likely relative to nightly duration of CPAP use were identified for Epworth Sleepiness Scale score (4 hr), multiple sleep latency test (6 hr), and Functional Outcomes Associated with Sleepiness Questionnaire (7.5 hr). Thus, as usage increases, subjective sleepiness, then objective sleepiness, and last, quality of life measures improve. The amount of necessary usage depends on what outcome is being evaluated. As noted above, the current Medicare guidelines state that devices will be reimbursed after 12 weeks only if objective adherence for a period of 1 month shows ≥4 hours of use for ≥70% of nights and the treating physician documents in a face-to-face meeting that the patient is benefiting from PAP treatment (see Appendix 19–2). However, many patients require much greater than 4 hours nightly use to experience a resolution of excessive sleepiness. Campos-Rodriguez and coworkers[82] followed a historical cohort of 871 patients with OSA for a mean of 48 months. Five-year cumulative survival was highest in the group of patients who used PAP therapy more than 6 hours per night on average (96.4% survival) compared with patients who used PAP from 1 to 6 hours per night (91.3% survival) and patients who used PAP less than 1 hour per night (85.5%). The same group conducted a prospective cohort study of 55 patients with hypertension.[83] Patients with average use greater than 5.3 hr/day and hypertension at entry to the study had a drop in mean arterial blood pressure of about 4 mm Hg.

Interventions to Improve Adherence

The literature on this subject is somewhat difficult to interpret because most programs use a number of interventions to try to improve adherence[6] (Table 19–5). Although education about OSA and PAP treatment is recommended, there is no evidence that this dramatically improves adherence.[84] Comprehensive programs of education (patient and bed partner), early contact, and interventions,[85] a simple CPAP help line,[86] or group education[87] have improved adherence in some studies. Cognitive behavioral interventions have shown promise.[88,89] Timely interventions for side effects and discomforts would also seem reasonable, although not proved to improve adherence. Table 19–6 presents common problems and possible solutions. Finding a comfortable and well-fitting mask interface is one of the biggest challenges in PAP treatment. Proper sizing and mask adjustment are essential and should be checked at every visit to the physician or respiratory therapist providing PAP support. If necessary, a different mask type could be tried. For mouth leaks, the addition of a chin strap, higher humidity, or a full face mask is an option. Sometimes, a leak will respond to slight lowering of pressure or switch from CPAP to BPAP if all else fails. Nasal pillows may help deal with claustrophobia. Unintentional mask removal may indicate a leak or inadequate pressure. Nasal congestion can be addressed with nasal steroids, antihistamines, increased humidity, or reduced mask leak. Rhinitis/rhinorrhea may respond to nasal ipratropium bromide. For pressure intolerance, use of a lower pressure, addition of flexible CPAP, a change to APAP or BPAP, and education about using the ramp are all options.

Hypnotics, Alcohol, and CPAP

Patients with both insomnia and OSA pose a difficult problem. In addition, some patients who normally have no problems with insomnia will have problems falling asleep or staying asleep on CPAP. Some clinicians have been hesitant to prescribe hypnotics, believing that this may reduce the effectiveness of CPAP. There has also been a concern that the use of alcohol could increase the required level of CPAP above that demonstrated to be effective in the sleep center.

TABLE 19–6

Interventions for Common Positive Airway Pressure Treatment Side Effects

POSITIVE PRESSURE SIDE EFFECTS	INTERVENTIONS
MASK SIDE EFFECTS	
Air leaks • Conjunctivitis • Discomfort • Noise	Proper mask fitting Proper mask application (education) Different brand/type of mask
Skin breakdown	Avoid overtightening—intervene as above for leaks Alternate between different mask types Nasal prongs/pillows Tape barrier for skin protection
Mouth leaks Mouth dryness	Treat nasal congestion if present (see below) Chin strap Heated humidity Full face (oronasal) mask Consider BPAP, flexible PAP, lower pressure, APAP
Mask claustrophobia	Nasal pillows/prongs interface Desensitization
Unintentional mask removal	Low-pressure alarm Consider increase in pressure
NASAL SYMPTOMS	
Congestion/obstruction	Nasal steroid inhaler Antihistamines (if allergic component) Nasal saline Humidification (heated) Full face (oronasal) mask Nighttime topical decongestants (oxymetazoline) as a last resort
Epistaxis Pain	Nasal saline Humidification (heated)
Rhinorrhea	Nasal ipratropium bromide
OTHER PROBLEMS	
Pressure intolerance	Ramp Flexible PAP BPAP APAP Lower prescription pressure temporarily—accept higher AHI Lower pressure + adjunctive measures (elevated head of bed, side sleeping position, weight loss)
Aerophagia/bloating	BPAP, flexible PAP, reduce pressure

AHI = apnea-hypopnea index; APAP = autoadjusting positive airway pressure; BPAP = bilevel positive airway pressure; PAP = positive airway pressure.

However, one study found that moderate alcohol consumption near bedtime did not impair the efficacy of CPAP.[90] Another study found that zolpidem, a commonly used hypnotic, did not impair efficacy of a given level of CPAP.[91] Conversely, it has been hypothesized that using a hypnotic might improve adherence to PAP in some patients. A study by Bradshaw and colleagues[92] using zolpidem did not find an improvement. In contrast, Lettieri and associates[93,94] found improvement during CPAP titration (sleep quality) and long-term adherence with eszopiclone (a hypnotic with a longer duration of action that zolpidem). It is possible that a longer-acting medication is needed to improve CPAP adherence. Although routine use of a hypnotic cannot currently be recommended, at least temporary use of a hypnotic should be considered if insomnia is a major obstacle to CPAP use.

CPAP/BPAP TITRATION FOR OSA

A PSG is the standard method PAP for titration and is usually accomplished either as the second part of a split study or during an entire night after a previous diagnostic study. The American Academy of Sleep Medicine (AASM) practice parameters for the use of PSG provide guidance about when a split study is acceptable.[95] A split study is recommended only if the AHI is greater than 40/hr and 2 hours of monitoring have occurred. In addition, 3 hours of PAP titration is the minimum acceptable duration. If an adequate titration is not obtained, a repeat PSG titration is indicated. Of note, these recommendations for a split study are based on limited data and some sleep centers have more lenient criteria for use of a split study. CMS guidelines for qualifying a patient for PAP formerly required at least 2 hours of recorded sleep in the diagnostic portion of a split study. This requirement has been dropped. If less than 2 hours of sleep are recorded, the minimum number of apneas and hypopneas must equal the number that would have been required if 2 hours of sleep had been recorded[68] (see also Appendix 19–2). For example, to meet a cutoff of an AHI of 15/hr, a total of 30 apneas and hypopneas must be recorded. Recently, Clinical Guidelines for the Titration of BPAP and CPAP for Obstructive Sleep Apnea were written by a task force of the AASM and approved by the board of directors.[62] Excerpts from the titration guidelines are discussed later. The reader is referred to this informative document.

General Titration Considerations

A number of general recommendations for PAP titration are listed in Table 19–7. Before PAP titration, the patient should be educated about OSA, PAP treatment, and the PAP titration process.[3,62] They should be given mask interface options. They should try on one or more interfaces while breathing on low pressure (CPAP practice). If a split study has been ordered, these events should take place before any diagnostic monitoring begins. A number of interfaces should be available (nasal, oronasal, oral, pillows) including masks in sizes suitable for children if a child is being studied. HH should be available as well as a source of supplemental oxygen.

Pediatric Considerations

PAP titrations in children require some extra considerations. Children are often given a mask to play with and try on during the day for a week before scheduled studies. The child should be desensitized to the mask during the day by wearing it for increasing periods of time while engaging in a fun activity (e.g., watching a favorite video). Split-night studies are not recommended for children. If the child without previous mask desensitization undergoes a split-night study, you may frighten the child and this will make subsequent CPAP use unlikely. Pediatric size masks should be available. Durable medical equipment providers and sleep technologists skilled and willing to provide care for pediatric-age patients should be utilized.[62,96] Studies have shown that structured behavioral interventions help with compliance (graduated exposure, positive reinforcement, dealing with escape and avoidance behavior, and praising distracting activities that allow the child to wear a mask).[70,97,98]

Monitoring during Positive-Pressure Titration

Most positive-pressure devices used in the sleep disorders center provide several analog or digital outputs that can be

---

TABLE 19–7

Positive Airway Pressure Titration (Equipment, Patient Preparation, and General Recommendations)

All potential PAP candidates (PAP titration and potential split titration)	• PAP education. • Mask fitting, try several interfaces. • Acclimatization period with low pressure.
Monitoring	• Airflow monitored from machine flow signal. • RERAs identified by flattening of the machine flow signal associated with arousal. • Leak, machine pressure recorded if possible.
Interfaces	• Nasal, full face (oronasal), nasal pillows, oral should be available. • Interfaces in pediatric sizes if children are studied.
High leak—one higher than expected for a given interface and pressure	• Mask adjustment, refit, change.
Heated humidity available	Used for nasal congestion or dryness
Treatment emergent central apneas	Let the patient settle down—if they reach stage N3, central apneas may stop. Try lowering CPAP or IPAP. Do not switch from CPAP to BPAP as a response to central apneas unless a backup rate is used.
Repeat PAP titration	Less than 3 hours during PAP titration of split study. Good or acceptable titration results **NOT** obtained.

BPAP = bilevel positive airway pressure; CPAP = continuous positive airway pressure; IPAP = inspiratory positive airway pressure; PAP = positive airway pressure; RERAs = respiratory effort–related arousals.

TABLE 19–8

Monitoring during Positive Airway Pressure or Noninvasive Positive Pressure Ventilation Titration

PARAMETER	SENSOR	REASON
Airflow	PAP/NPPV device output (accurate internal flow sensor).	Detection of apnea, hypopnea, and RERAs.
Leak	Leak estimate by PAP or NPPV device from accurate flow measurement.	Total leak = intentional + unintentional leak (some device output an estimate of unintentional leak rather than total leak).
Snoring	Piezoelectric sensor or microphone.	Detection of snoring.
Pressure	External pressure transducer or NPPV device signal (internal pressure sensor).	Documentation of amount and pattern of pressure delivery.
Chest and abdominal movement	Respiratory inductance plethysmography.	Differentiating central and obstructive events, detection of paradox.
NPPV		
Tidal volume	NPPV device output (from integration of flow signal).	Estimate of tidal volume.
Respiratory muscle EMG	Bipolar monitoring: use surface electrodes over the diaphragm or intercostal muscles.	Absence or reduction in respiratory muscle EMG suggests adequate respiratory muscle rest has been achieved.
$P_{ET}CO_2$	Side stream via nasal cannula in nares under the mask.	Breath-by-breath estimate of $PaCO_2$.
$TcPCO_2$	Transcutaneous sensor.	Estimate of trends in $PaCO_2$.

EMG = electromyogram; NPPV = noninvasive positive pressure ventilation; PAP = positive airway pressure; $PaCO_2$ = arterial partial pressure of carbon dioxide; $P_{ET}CO_2$ = end-tidal carbon dioxide pressure; RERAs = respiratory effort–related arousals; $TcPCO_2$ = transcutaneous carbon dioxide pressure.

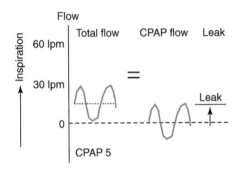

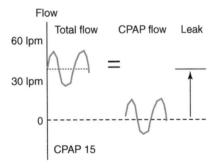

FIGURE 19–13 Total flow increases with pressure but is separated into a variable component (continuous positive airway pressure [CPAP] flow) and a more constant component (leak). The leak includes intentional (mask orifice) and unintentional leak. Note that CPAP flow is also called machine flow, CFlow, or PAP flow. Note that on higher CPAP, the total flow increases (see Figure 19–14) as the intentional flow increases (even if unintentional leak does not increase).

recorded (Table 19–8).[62] The total flow delivered by the machine is measured by an accurate flow sensor in the PAP device. Use of a thermal device under the mask to monitor flow is not recommended. The total flow is then divided by the device into two components (Equation 19–1) that are supplied for monitoring: (1) the PAP flow (also known as CPAP flow, Cflow, or machine flow), which varies with inspiration and expiration, and (2) the leak (bias flow), which is a fairly constant portion due to system leak (Fig. 19–13). The CPAP flow signal is used to score respiratory events (apneas, hypopneas, or respiratory event–related arousals [RERAs]). The same respiratory scoring rules defined by the AASM scoring manual are utilized with the exception that there is one flow signal rather than the usual two (oronasal thermal flow and nasal pressure).[99] The total leak is due to the intentional leak (to prevent rebreathing) and unintentional leak (Equation 19–2). All CPAP mask interfaces have a built-in orifice system consisting of small holes to provide an intentional leak that washes out exhaled CO_2 from the mask and prevents rebreathing. This intentional leak increases with the amount of pressure and varies between different masks (Fig. 19–14). The unintentional leak is due to mask or mouth leak (in the case of a nasal mask). Leak is seen by the machine as bias or constant baseline inspiratory flow onto which the variations in patient flow is superimposed. The leak signal provided by some devices is the total leak whereas others provide an estimate of unintentional leak by subtracting the expected leak given the mask and pressure (mask type must be specified). Absolute values are less useful than relative increases in leak.

$$\text{Total flow} = \text{PAP flow} + \text{Leak} \qquad \text{Equation 19–1}$$

$$\text{Leak} = \text{Intentional leak} + \text{Unintentional leak} \qquad \text{Equation 19–2}$$

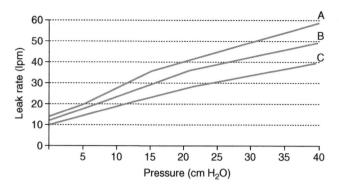

FIGURE 19-14 Intentional leak increases with pressure and depends on the mask type (*A*, *B*, or *C*). Information is available with each mask.

The PAP flow signal provides not only an estimate of the magnitude of flow but also information from the inspiratory flow contour. High upper airway resistance is manifested by a flattened profile[100] (Fig. 19-15). The normal profile is a rounded one. Figure 19-16 shows that the CPAP flow signal is flat at a pressure of 7 cm H_2O and snoring is present. These findings suggest significant upper airway narrowing is still present. An increase in CPAP results in a round signal shape and cessation of snoring.

CPAP flow signals are usually either filtered or insufficiently sampled to show snoring. Snoring can be detected by a snoring sensor placed on the neck or from pressure vibrations in mask pressure. Nearly all sleep center PAP units will also provide a signal of the "machine pressure." This is the pressure at the machine outlet and can differ slightly from the set pressure (value entered by technologist). The actual

FIGURE 19-15 The shape of the PAP device flow signal changes with increased upper airway resistance, becoming flattened consistent with airflow limitation. Here, a drop in continuous positive airway pressure (CPAP; *arrow*) results in change of flow signal and increased pressure gradient across the upper airway (increased resistance). *From Condos R, Norman RG, Krishnasamy I, et al: Flow limitation as a noninvasive assessment of residual upper-airway resistance during continuous positive airway pressure therapy of obstructive sleep apnea. Am J Respir Crit Care Med 1994;150:475–480.*

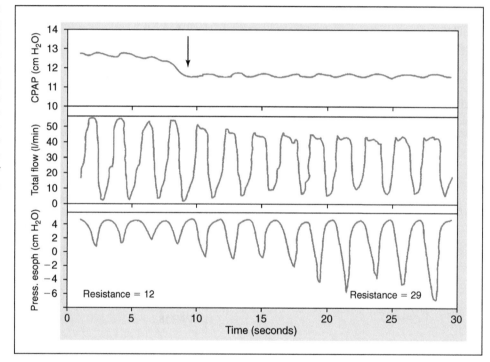

FIGURE 19-16 Flattening in the continuous positive airway pressure (CPAP) flow signal (*arrow*) suggests high upper airway resistance, and this is consistent with the appearance of snoring. Here, inspiration is associated with an upward deflection in flow. After only 1 cm H_2O increase in pressure, the CPAP flow signal is now round and the snoring has stopped.

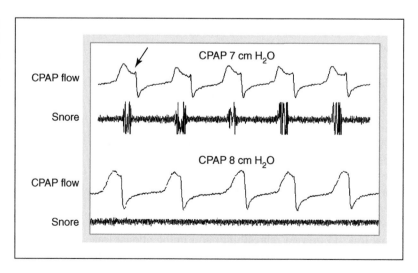

mask pressure may be somewhat lower during inhalation and sometimes slightly higher during exhalation. Mask pressure can also be directly measured by connecting the mask to a pressure transducer. Actual mask pressure can then be recorded.

PAP units also provide a leak signal that can be monitored and recorded. Recording of the leak signal is useful for the physician reviewing a PAP titration. The trend in the leak is more useful than the absolute number. If the patient has not moved and leak suddenly increases, this could be a hint that mouth leak is occurring (assuming the patient is wearing a nasal mask). Sometimes, an increase in leak can occur with the onset of REM sleep. Relaxation in the facial musculature can sometimes produce mask or mouth leaks. In Figure 19–17, there is a sudden increase in leak in a patient wearing

a nasal mask and chin strap when there is a transition to REM sleep. Because there was no change in pressure or body movement, this suggests that mouth leak was present (confirmed by video monitoring). Observation using video (zooming in) can show an open mouth or fluttering of the lips during mouth leak. If the flow signal becomes truncated during expiration, this means that part or all of flow during exhalation is not sensed by the machine flow sensor (no flow returning to the hose/device system) consistent with an expiratory leak from either the mask or the mouth. If the patient is wearing a nasal mask (which has not moved), the sudden appearance of truncated expiratory flow (often associated with vibration in the snoring sensor) is suggestive of expiratory mouth leak (Fig. 19–18). The technician does not necessarily have to intervene unless mouth leak is arousing the

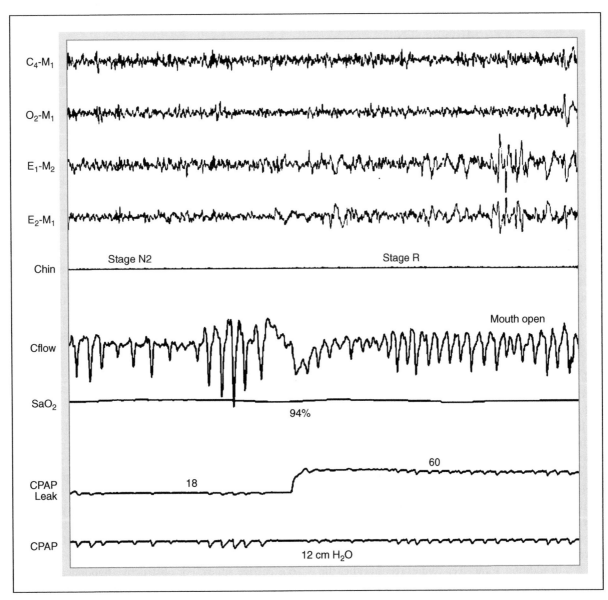

FIGURE 19–17 A 120-second tracing shows flow from the continuous positive airway pressure device (Cflow), leak, and the delivered pressure at the device outlet (CPAP). The patient was wearing a nasal mask and chin strap. At the transition to stage R, a large increase in leak was noted. The patient was not noted to move but video observation showed that one corner of his mouth had opened slightly. Note that the increase in leak signal lags behind the obvious change in flow that occurs a few seconds earlier. Stage R is associated with muscle hypotonia. SaO$_2$ = arterial oxygen saturation.

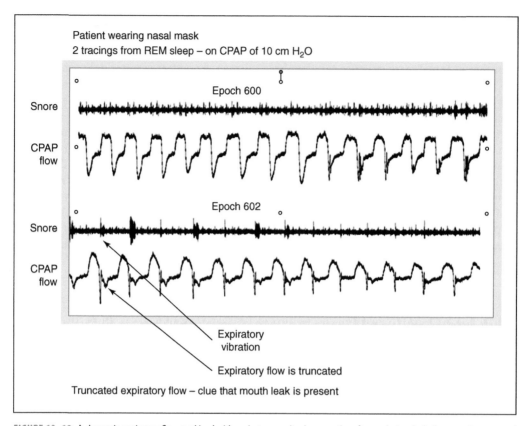

FIGURE 19–18 A change in expiratory flow combined with expiratory snoring is suggestive of an expiratory leak. Compare the truncated expiratory flow in epoch 602 with the normal expiratory flow in epoch 602. This is due to expiratory mask or mouth leak (if a nasal mask is being used). This patient was using a nasal mask and subtle lip fluttering was noted on video. The expiratory flow is truncated because part of the expiratory flow does not pass into the tubing ("escapes" from the system) and is not sensed by the device flow sensor. Inspiration is upward. CPAP = continuous positive airway pressure; REM = rapid eye movement.

patient or preventing PAP from maintaining a patent airway. If mouth leak is a problem, either using a chin strap or an oronasal mask or lowering the pressure could be considered.

Additional Monitoring for NPPV Titration

For NPPV titration, it is useful to record the tidal volume signal from the PAP device that is derived from integration of the flow signal (see Fig. 19–3).[22] Tidal volume depends both on flow and inspiratory time. Therefore, monitoring the flow signal alone may not provide an accurate estimate of ventilation. Some sleep centers that perform NPPV in patients with neuromuscular disorders also record an intercostal electromyogram (EMG) or surface diaphragmatic EMG with techniques similar to those for leg EMG. If the signal decreases, tidal volume increases and respiratory rate decreases; these changes suggest that adequate respiratory muscle rest is being delivered by the current level of PS (Fig. 19–19).[101,102] In addition, some sleep centers record either the end-tidal partial carbon dioxide pressure ($P_{ET}CO_2$) or $TcPCO_2$.[103,104] However, the exhaled gas sampled for the $P_{ET}CO_2$ measurement can be diluted by NPPV flow. A common method is to use a small nasal cannula under the mask that suctions exhaled air at the nares before it can be

diluted. A downside is that this can cause problems with the mask seal. Another option is to record is the $TcPCO_2$. These surrogate measures of PCO_2 are useful only if calibrated and validated (ideally with an arterial or capillary blood gas).[22,99] As mentioned in Chapter 8, a $P_{ET}CO_2$ tracing should show a plateau.

Titration Protocol

The recommended PAP titration protocol for adults and children is shown in Tables 19–9 and 19–10.[62] CPAP is usually started at 4 to 5 cm H_2O and then increased for obstructive apneas, hypopneas, RERAs, and snoring. Usually, as pressure is increased, the apneas → hypopneas → RERAs → snoring resolve in that order.[105] CPAP is increased in adults after two obstructive apneas, three hypopneas, or five RERAs and no more often than every 5 minutes. When titrating BPAP, starting pressures of 8/4 cm H_2O are typically used. Both IPAP and EPAP are increased together for obstructive apnea. For obstructive hypopneas, RERAs, and snoring, the IPAP alone is increased. The clinical guidelines suggest that the IPAP-EPAP difference should be at least 4 but not greater than 10 cm H_2O. Note that, when NPPV titration is discussed later, a wider IPAP-EPAP difference can be used. In general, if the IPAP-EPAP difference widens,

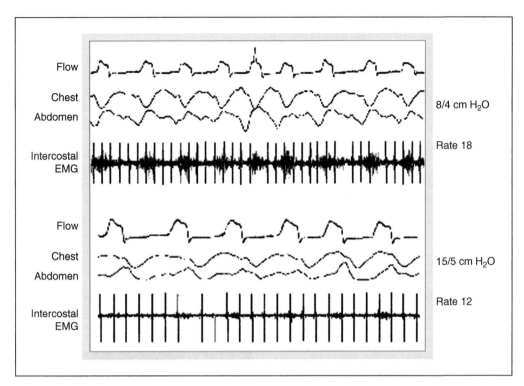

FIGURE 19-19 A patient with neuromuscular disease underwent an NPPV titration. When the level of pressure support was increased, there was a decrease in the respiratory rate and in the intercostal electromyogram (EMG). *From Berry RB: Initiating NPPV treatment with patients with chronic hypoventilation. Sleep Med Clin 2010;5:485–505.*

TABLE 19-9

Continuous Positive Airway Pressure Titration Guidelines[62]

	ADULTS AND CHILDREN > 12 YR	CHILDREN < 12 YR
Beginning pressure (cm H_2O; minimum)	4	4
Maximum pressure (cm H_2O)	20	15
Increase CPAP in at least 1 cm H_2O increments no more frequently than every 5 min	Increase pressure for: ≥2 obstructive apneas ≥3 hypopneas ≥5 RERAs ≥3 min loud snoring	Increase pressure for: ≥1 obstructive apnea ≥1 hypopnea ≥3 RERAs ≥1 min loud snoring
Switch to BPAP	Intolerant to CPAP Events still present on CPAP of 15 cm H_2O (option)	

Snoring guidelines state that pressure "may" be increased.
BPAP = bilevel positive airway pressure; CPAP = continuous positive airway pressure; RERAs = respiratory effort–related arousals.

an increase in EPAP is often needed to maintain upper airway patency. **Higher PAP is needed for the supine position and during REM sleep.**[106,107] For this reason, an effective pressure during **supine REM sleep** should be determined if possible during the titration.[62] Note that the recommended maximum CPAP and number of events triggering pressure changes are lower in children.

If the patient awakens and complains of excessive pressure, pressure should be lowered. If this does not work, a switch from CPAP to BPAP or use of flexible PAP may be tried. When switching from CPAP to BPAP, one approach is to use IPAP 2 cm H_2O higher than CPAP and EPAP 2 cm H_2O lower. Thus, with a change from CPAP of 16, one would

use BPAP 18/14 cm H_2O. Another approach is to use EPAP = CPAP, and IPAP = EPAP + 4 cm H_2O and titrate pressure upward if needed. Of note, in pressure-intolerant patients, sleep in the lateral position or with the head elevated can be tried to reduce the required level of pressure.[108] If mouth leak is a problem, a chin strap can be tried followed by an oronasal mask. In patients with allergic rhinitis or nasal congestion, use of HH from the start of the study is suggested. Although studies have not shown a benefit from using "prophylactic" HH in all patients, many sleep centers find it to be very useful. Once the nose is congested, this problem is not easily reversed. If there is excessive mask leak, a readjustment of the mask, change in mask size, or change in mask

TABLE 19-10
Bilevel Positive Airway Pressure Titration Guidelines[62]

	ADULTS	CHILDREN < 12 YR
Beginning pressure (cm H_2O) IPAP/EPAP	8/4	8/4
Maximum IPAP (cm H_2O)	30	20
Minimum PS (cm H_2O)	4	4
Maximum PS (cm H_2O)	10	10
Increase BOTH **IPAP AND EPAP** in at least 1 cm H_2O increments no more frequently than every 5 min	Increase pressure for: ≥2 obstructive apneas	Increase pressure for: ≥1 obstructive apnea
Increase **IPAP** in at least 1 cm H_2O increments no more frequently than every 5 min	Increase pressure for: ≥3 hypopneas ≥5 RERAs ≥3 min loud snoring	Increase pressure for: ≥1 hypopnea ≥3 RERAs ≥1 min loud snoring

Snoring guidelines state that pressure "may" be increased.
EPAP = expiratory positive airway pressure; IPAP = inspiratory positive airway pressure; PS = pressure support = IPAP − EPAP; RERAs = respiratory effort–related arousals.

---

type is indicated. Overtightening of the mask straps is strongly discouraged. It is also worth mentioning that some patients with severe upper airway narrowing may tolerate a higher initial pressure (8–10 cm H_2O) better than the usual low starting pressure. This is also true of patients already using CPAP at home. If the patient is not falling asleep on PAP, he or she should be asked what is bothering him or her.

PAP and Supplemental Oxygen

The addition of supplemental oxygen during PAP titration is sometimes needed[62] (Table 19–11). Some patients will exhibit significant arterial oxygen desaturation despite adequate airflow, especially during REM sleep. Persistent hypoxemia in these conditions may be due to hypoventilation or ventilation-perfusion mismatch (often due to chronic lung disease). In some studies of titration in patients with OHS, a substantial number of patients required the addition of supplemental oxygen. If the awake supine patient has an SaO_2 of 88% or lower or is already on supplemental oxygen to maintain an acceptable awake SaO_2, the addition of supplemental oxygen will definitely be needed. Recall that even in normal subjects, the arterial partial pressure of oxygen (PaO_2) falls on the order of 5 to 10 mm Hg during sleep.

Before adding supplemental oxygen, one can attempt to adjust the PAP pressure settings to prevent the need for this additional treatment. If the patient is requiring high oxygen flows, optimizing PAP may allow reduction in the required oxygen flow rate. First, an increase in CPAP can be tried to eliminate unrecognized high upper airway resistance. If this is not successful or not tolerated, CPAP can be changed to BPAP (Fig. 19–20). If the patient is already on BPAP, the level of PS can be increased. If these interventions do not increase the SaO_2 to an acceptable level or if higher pressure is not tolerated, supplemental oxygen can be added to PAP. One can start at 1 L/min flow and titrate up every 10 to 15 minutes

TABLE 19-11
Addition of Supplemental Oxygen during Positive Airway Pressure Titration

Addition of supplemental oxygen
- Awake supine SaO_2 while breathing room air ≤ 88%.
- During PAP titration when SaO_2 ≤ 88% for ≥ 5 min **in the absence of obstructive respiratory events.**
- Goal of addition of supplemental oxygen SaO_2 between 88% and 94%.

Minimum starting rate of oxygen is 1 L/min.

O_2 rate increased by 1 L/min with an interval no shorter than 15 min until SaO_2 is between 88% and 94%.

Attach supplemental oxygen at PAP device outlet.

Weaning down of oxygen flow may be attempted by change from CPAP to BPAP or increased in IPAP if already on BPAP.

BPAP = bilevel positive airway pressure; CPAP = continuous positive airway pressure; IPAP = inspiratory positive airway pressure; PAP = positive airway pressure; SaO_2 = arterial oxygen saturation.
Adapted from Kushida CA, Chediak A, Berry RB, et al: Positive Airway Pressure Titration Task Force, American Academy of Sleep Medicine: Clinical guidelines for the manual titration of positive airway pressure in patients with obstructive sleep apnea. J Clin Sleep Med 2008;4:157–171.

---

with a goal of attaining an acceptable SaO_2 (88–94%). Most clinicians would use a target 92% to 94% to allow for variability and a margin of safety.

It is important to recognize that the **effective oxygen concentration** will depend on both the supplemental oxygen flow (L/min) and the machine flow[109,110] (Fig. 19–21). Increases in machine flow associated with higher pressure or mask/mouth leak can dilute a given flow of supplemental oxygen. For example, if a patient with chronic lung disease requires supplemental oxygen at 2 L/min to maintain an SaO_2 of 94% while awake without CPAP, on CPAP the

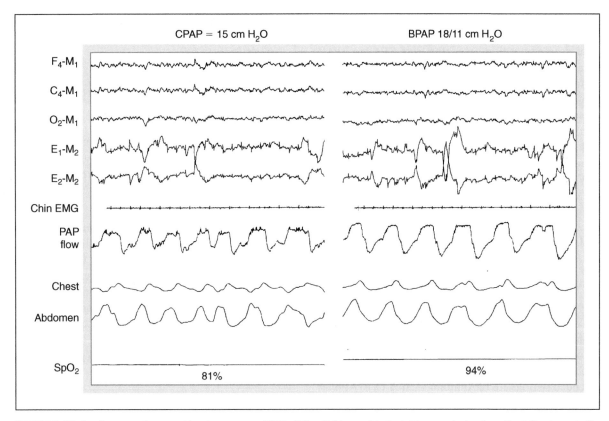

FIGURE 19–20 A patient on continuous positive airway pressure (CPAP) of 15 cm H_2O has persistent arterial oxygen desaturation without discrete events. The options are to add supplemental oxygen, try an increase in CPAP, or switch to bilevel positive airway pressure (BPAP). A switch to BPAP was effective in this patient. EMG = electromyogram; PAP = positive airway pressure; SpO_2 = pulse oximetry.

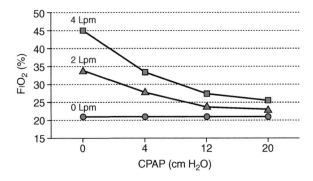

FIGURE 19–21 Approximate change in effective fractional concentration of oxygen in inspired gas (FiO_2) with supplemental oxygen and various continuous positive airway pressure (CPAP) levels in a model system. *Plotted from data from Yoder EA, Klann K, Strohl KP: Inspired oxygen concentrations during positive pressure therapy. Sleep Breath 2004;8:1–5.*

required supplemental oxygen flow will likely be much higher (assuming the same fractional concentration of oxygen on CPAP treatment is still required).

Complex Sleep Apnea

CompSA is defined as a form of central apnea specifically identified by the persistence or emergence of central apneas or hypopneas upon exposure to CPAP or a BPAP without a backup rate when obstructive events have disappeared. Patient with CompSA have predominantly obstructive or mixed apneas during the diagnostic sleep study (or diagnostic portion of a split study) occurring at 5/hr or greater. The CMS definition of CompSA requires that greater than 50% of the residual respiratory events on PAP are central apneas or central hypopneas, the central AHI is 5/hr or greater, and the total AHI is 5 or greater (Appendix 19-3). Patients with a combination of OSA and CSB may manifest CSB-central apneas when CPAP eliminates obstructive events. These patients meet the definition of CompSA. Other patients taking potent opiates develop central apneas on CPAP (treatment emergent central apneas) or central apneas persist on CPAP. Other patients may manifest CompSA without an obvious cause (idiopathic CompSA). The treatment of CompSA is discussed in detail in Chapter 21.

Patients with Cheyne-Stokes central apnea or idiopathic CompSA tend to have high ventilatory drives or difficulty maintaining sleep. Central apnea occurs because the $PaCO_2$ drops below the apneic threshold. The approach to CompSA and PAP titration protocol for handling central apneas varies between sleep centers.[111-113] One approach is to increase CPAP only until the obstructive apneas and hypopneas are eliminated. CPAP is increased further only if RERAs are believed to be causing central apneas (after the arousals). Many patients will stabilize if they enter stage N3 sleep (i.e., patience rather than increasing the CPAP). A small reduction in pressure to one not associated with central apneas can also be tried. Some patients will also improve in the lateral sleeping position. Switching from CPAP to BPAP without a backup rate is NOT indicated and may actually contribute to ventilatory instability. Many patients with CompSA when treated with CPAP on a chronic basis will have a resolution of the central apneas.[111,112] Others with CSB or narcotics as a cause for ventilatory instability may continue to have frequent central events on chronic CPAP treatment. These patients should undergo another PAP titration with ASV or BPAP with a backup rate.[113,114] Unless there are financial constraints, it is better to utilize an entire night to perform an ASV titration. As discussed in Chapter 21 some patients with CompSA are more easily treated in REM than NREM sleep.

ASV Titration Protocol

The protocol for ASV titration varies with the type of device (Adapt SV vs. BiPAP AutoSV). For the Adapt SV, EPP = 4 cm H_2O, PSmax of 10 cm H_2O or greater is recommended. EPAP should be increased slowly to allow the unstable ventilatory pattern to stabilize. For the BiPAP auto SV advanced, recommended settings are EPAPmin = 4 cm H_2O, EPAPmax = 15 cm H_2O, PSmin = 0 cm H_2O, PSmax = 20 cm H_2O, Max pressure = 25 cm H_2O, rate = auto. If it is known that CPAP greater than 10 cm H_2O is needed to prevent obstructive apnea, EPAPmin of 6 to 8 cm H_2O could be tried. For pressure-intolerant patients or those with a component of hypoventilation (narcotics), PSmin of 4 cm H_2O could be used. Of note, most insurance providers have definite criteria for reimbursement for ASV or BPAP with a backup rate (Appendix 19-3). Usually more than 50% of the events on CPAP must be either central apneas or central hypopneas. Although most sleep centers do not report central hypopneas, this may be one case in which it is necessary to meet reimbursement guidelines. In the AASM scoring manual, identifying hypopneas as central or obstructive was recommended only if a quantitative measure of respiratory effort was recorded (esophageal pressure, calibrated respiratory inductance plethysmography [RIP] belts, or diaphragmatic/intercostal EMG).[99]

Adequacy of PAP Titration

According to the AASM clinical guidelines for the titration of CPAP and BPAP,[62] an optimal titration is one that reduces the AHI to less than 5/hr for at least 15 minutes and should include supine REM sleep at the final pressure without repeated arousals. A good titration results in an AHI < 10/hr or at least a 50% reduction in the AHI if the baseline AHI is less than 15/hr. A good titration should include supine REM sleep at the selected pressure that is not continually interrupted by arousals. An adequate titration is one that does not reduce the AHI < 10/hr but does reduce the AHI by 75% from baseline, or one in which criteria for optimal or good titration is met with the exception that supine REM sleep did

TABLE 19-12
Alternative Methods of Starting Positive Airway Pressure
• PSG titration → CPAP treatment.
• Autotitration → CPAP treatment.
• APAP treatment.
• CPAP treatment with empirical pressure then adjustments based on symptoms, oximetry, or machine-residual AHI.
AHI = apnea-hypopnea index; APAP = autoadjusting positive airway pressure; CPAP = continuous positive airway pressure; PSG = polysomnography.

not occur at the selected pressure. An unacceptable titration does not meet any of these criteria. If clinically indicated, a repeat titration should be ordered. In optimal, good, and acceptable titrations, the SaO_2 should remain above 90% at the treatment pressure selected for chronic use. If a titration shows borderline oxygenation, it is then prudent to check nocturnal oximetry while the patient uses PAP at home.

ALTERNATIVE METHODS OF STARTING PAP TREATMENT

A number of options are available for starting PAP after a diagnosis of OSA has been made **without** the use of a PSG PAP titration.[26,115-120] These options are especially relevant if the diagnosis of OSA is based on a portable monitoring (PM) study. The titration alternatives can also be used for patients who are unwilling or unable to have a standard PSG titration. The alternatives are listed in Table 19-12 and include treating the patient with an APAP device (titration not needed), performing autotitration at home for several days to a week (at least 3 days optimum) with subsequent CPAP treatment based on the results, and starting PAP treatment based on a prediction equation with subsequent adjustment based on symptoms, machine readings, and nocturnal oximetry. Equations to predict the optimal CPAP level have been developed (Equation 19-3).[116] The prediction equation can provide an empirical treatment level or a reasonable starting point for a PAP titration. However, the optimal treatment pressure may differ substantially from the predicted pressure. In our experience the formula considerably underestimates the required pressure, especially in men.

$$CPAP\ predicted = (0.16 \times BMI) + (0.13 \times NC) + (0.04 \times AHI) - 5.12$$

$$Equation\ 19-3$$

where BMI = body mass index and NC = neck circumference in centimeters.

Example: BMI = 30, NC = 16 inches (40.6 cm), AHI = 30/hr

$$CPAP\ pred = (0.16 \times 30) + (0.13 \times 40.6) + (0.04 \times 30) - 5.12$$
$$= 4.8 + 5.3 + 1.2 - 5.12 = 7\ cm\ H_2O$$

Most PAP devices provide an estimate of the residual AHI. Some devices also separate apneas into "clear airway apneas" and "obstructive apneas." Desia and coworkers[121] recently compared the PAP device residual AHI with PSG and found that using a PAP AHI of 8/hr had a sensitivity and specificity of 0.94 and 0.90, respectively, for detecting a PSG AHI greater than 10/hr.

Masa and coworkers[115] compared three clinical pathways including standard PSG titration, autotitration for one night followed by CPAP treatment based on the results, and CPAP based on a prediction formula with subsequent adjustments based on symptoms. At the end of a 12-week period, all patients were studied on their current CPAP pressure. All three methods resulted in equivalent CPAP adherence, control of the AHI, and improvement in subjective sleepiness. Of note, 23% of the eligible patients were excluded. Other studies comparing algorithms using alternative modes of initiating PAP treatment with PSG found similar results.[117-120] If a patient is diagnosed as having sleep apnea by PM, one of the three alternative methods or traditional PSG titration is needed if PAP treatment is indicated. Using PM followed by a PSG titration would seem to have little advantage compared with a split PSG study (if available). However, sometimes the results of PM uncover an unexpected problem (central apneas, low baseline SaO_2, or CSB). If these are present, a PSG titration is definitely indicated.

Patient Selection for Alternative Titrations

Patients with a number of conditions are not suitable for APAP titration or treatment.[23-25,115] These include patients who require or are likely to require supplemental oxygen (low baseline SaO_2), patients with hypoventilation, patients likely to have central apneas (narcotics, congestive heart failure), and patients who may require very high pressures. Patients with severe pressure intolerance or moderate to severe COPD who may require BPAP should also undergo a PSG titration if possible.

Technique of Autotitration

The patient is educated about OSA and PAP treatment and has mask fitting and instructions on use of an APAP device. It is often useful for the patient to take a brief practice nap during which she or he applies the interface, activates the APAP device, and "naps" for about 15 or 20 minutes.[115,119] This allows identification of interface problems and allows for adjustment or change of interface. The patient then sleeps on the APAP device at home for several nights. Usually, the pressure limits of the device are set from 4 to 20 cm H_2O. In large patients likely to require high CPAP, starting with pressure of 4 cm H_2O may be uncomfortable, so a higher low-pressure limit is chosen (8–10 cm H_2O). For the pressure-intolerant patient, a lower upper limit of pressure can be chosen. A telephone hotline is available for interventions similar to PAP treatment. The device is then returned and the information transferred to a computer. The quality of the autotitration can be noted including amount of use (adherence), residual AHI, and amount of leak. Typically,

TABLE 19–13

Examples of Autoadjusting Positive Airway Pressure Titration

	PATIENT 1	PATIENT 2	PATIENT 3
Min pressure limit (cm H_2O)	4	4	4
Max pressure limit (cm H_2O)	20	20	20
Days used	14/14	3/6	11/12
Average use	6 hr 31 min	2 hr 2 min	5 hr 5 min
90th percentile pressure (cm H_2O)	11.8	9.5	12.0
Average pressure (cm H_2O)	9.2	8	8.0
AHI	4.0	3	15
Large leak*	5 min	1 hr	12 min

*Large leak defined as leak > twice the average leak of interfaces at a given pressure.
AHI = apnea-hypopnea index.

either the 95th percentile pressure or the 90th percentile pressure (depending on device) is chosen for chronic PAP treatment. If the APAP titration is suboptimal owing to poor adherence, high leak, or high residual AHI, another attempt can be made using a different mask, HH, or other interventions. If two attempts at an APAP titration are unsuccessful, the patient can be referred for a PSG titration. Table 19–13 shows three examples of typical APAP titrations. Patient 1 is ideal with good adherence, low leak, a 90th percentile pressure well within pressure limits, and a good residual AHI. Based on this study, CPAP of 12 cm H_2O could be used for chronic treatment. Patient 2 is an example of a poor titration. There is poor adherence and very high leak. The patient complained of being dry despite using a high humidity setting. The patient could be changed from a nasal to a full face mask and the study repeated. Patient 3 shows good adherence but the residual AHI is very high. The apnea index was 13/hr and the hypopnea index 2/hr. The patient was taking methadone. The high residual AHI was believed to be due to central apneas. The patient was referred for a PSG PAP titration. In retrospect, the patient was not a good candidate for an APAP titration.

Follow-up of Patients on PAP Treatment

Because the pattern of adherence is set early, obtaining a download within the first week and having a face-to-face visit at or soon after 4 weeks of use is recommended. As noted previously, CMS rules require at least 1 month of 70% of nights with greater than 4 hours of use. This month of adherence must occur within the first 3 months of CPAP use for treatment to continue to be reimbursed. In addition to

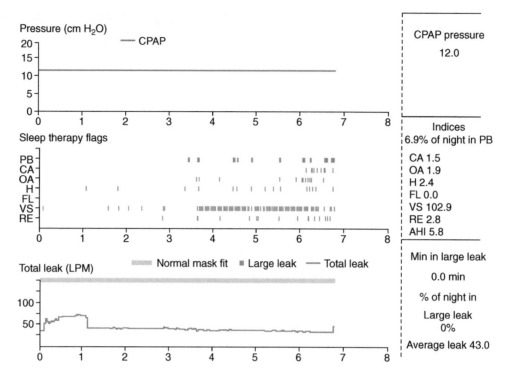

FIGURE 19–22 Sample PAP device download on a patient using continuous positive airway pressure (CPAP) of 12 cm H$_2$O. The residual apnea-hypopnea index (AHI) is 5.8 (adequate) but snoring is very prominent in the second half of the night. Leak is not increased. On the basis of this information CPAP was increased to 13 cm H$_2$O. Large leak is defined as a leak greater than twice the intentional leak from interfaces at that pressure. CA = clear airway apnea; FL = flow limitation; H = hypopnea; OA = obstructive airway apnea; PB = periodic breathing; RE = respiratory effort–related arousal; VS = vibratory snore.

the adherence data, most PAP machines give information on leak and residual AHI. Some can give detailed information about residual events including clear airway events (central apneas). Three studies found a surprisingly high proportion of patients "well treated" with CPAP who had elevated AHI values on their current treatment pressures.[122–124] A high residual AHI found on CPAP machine download would suggest that the current pressure was inadequate (unless the events were central apneas) or that an inadequate mask seal significantly reduced the delivered pressure. Some CPAP and APAP devices present the residual AHI, AHI, hypopnea index (HI), and a snoring index. If the residual apnea index exceeds the HI, this is a clue that central apnea may be present. Recall that as pressure increased, first obstructive apnea then hypopnea resolve. However, false elevations of the AHI can occur. Recently, CPAP and APAP devices can separate apneas into obstructive apneas and "clear airway apneas." In Figure 19–22, a sample report from a patient on CPAP shows a reasonable residual AHI and no evidence of excessive leak. However, there is evidence of considerable snoring and slightly higher pressure is indicated. A high residual AHI in a patient with congestive heart failure or potent narcotic use would suggest the possibility of central apneas. High leak would suggest need for better interface fit. The interface could be adjusted or changed to a different size or interface type. **We have found it very useful to pressurize the mask in the office before the patient leaves to check the seal.** If extreme dryness is present and a reasonable humidity

setting has been used, the function of the humidifier should be checked, the possibility of mouth leak considered (if the patient has a nasal mask), or the fit of the mask should be evaluated. If a mouth leak is suspected, one could try a full face mask or chin strap. The patient's bed partner often provides important clues as to persistent snoring or apnea, pulling the mask off during the night, noisy mask, or mouth leak. Most clinicians have the patient fill out an Epworth Sleepiness Scale each visit; this is used along with questions about the quality of sleep to assess effectiveness of CPAP treatment. In patients with significant insomnia, use of a hypnotic could be considered once sleep hygiene and medication side effects are optimized.

NPPV Titration and Treatment

The titration of NPPV focuses on providing ventilatory support in addition to maintaining an open airway.[22,124] Patients with neuromuscular disorders, thoracic cage disorders, or disorders of inadequate ventilatory control may not be obese and may not require as high an EPAP as patients with OSA or OHS.[22,125,126] IPAP and EPAP are titrated as per the protocol discussed previously to eliminate obstructive events. However, the goal is to provide adequate PS without using excessive pressure. Therefore, BPAP of 16/4 or 20/5 cm H$_2$O might be typical pressures. The ST mode is used for treatment of all patients with central ventilatory control disorders and is also recommended for patients with neuromuscular disorders and thoracic cage disorders. These patients may not reliably cycle the BPAP device from EPAP to IPAP. The ST mode is also needed if central apneas are noted during the NPPV titration. The backup rate is usually set 1 to 2 breaths below the sleeping spontaneous breathing rate (8–10 breaths/min minimum). The cycle time in seconds is equal to 60 divided by the respiratory rate in breaths per minute. The Ti is chosen between 30% and 40% of the cycle time. When expressed as a fraction of the cycle time, this is also known as the *%IPAP time*.

> Example: If the respiratory rate = 15,
>   cycle time = 60/15 = 4 sec.

> If the %IPAP time is 30%, the Ti would be 1.2 sec.

In general, patients with airflow obstruction (COPD) are best treated with 30% %IPAP time and those with restrictive disorders may do better with 40% %IPAP time. One manufacturer recommends using 1.5 seconds as the default inspiratory time for BPAP-ST. The rise time is the time from start of the IPAP cycle until IPAP pressure is reached. It is typically around 200 msec (200–600 msec) but can be varied for patient comfort.

Goals of NPPV Titration and Treatment

The goals of the NPPV treatment vary between patients[22,125,126] but generally include (1) improving sleep quality and preventing nocturnal dyspnea, (2) preventing nocturnal hypoventilation (or worsening of hypoventilation during sleep if daytime hypoventilation is present), and (3) providing respiratory muscle rest. For patients with daytime hypoventilation, use of NPPV can improve the quality of life and delay or prevent the progression of respiratory failure.[125,126] The indications for NPPV[127] are discussed in

Chapter 21. The nocturnal $PaCO_2$ goal is a value equal to or less than the daytime $PaCO_2$. However, sufficient PS may not be tolerated initially. NPPV can be started on an outpatient basis at low pressure (BPAP 8/4) and increased as tolerated based on patient symptoms and oximetry, daytime $P_{ET}CO_2$ measurements, or daytime arterial blood gas measurements.[128] However, an NPPV PSG titration is recommended and allows a treatment to be chosen (IPAP, EPAP, backup rate) that will eliminate obstructive apnea/hypopnea and deliver optimal PS. Some patients will also require the addition of supplemental oxygen. Close follow-up is needed because the given level of pressure support may prove inadequate if respiratory muscles weaken.

Titration using VT-BPAP is performed to determine an effective EPAP. The ST mode is commonly used. The device will automatically adjust PS to provide a desired tidal volume. If pressure intolerance is a problem, a lower tidal volume target with a higher respiratory rate (spontaneous or machine-triggered) may be better tolerated.

NPPV Titration Protocol

Before the titration, the patient should be educated about the process and be able to try different interfaces with low pressure. Monitoring during a NPPV titration uses methods similar to those for a PAP titration.[22,125] A BPAP device with capability to function in the ST or T mode is needed. Most NPPV devices provide an analog output of tidal volume that can be recorded. As shown in Figure 19-3, monitoring and recording tidal volume in addition to flow is useful because tidal volume depends on both flow and Ti. A Best Clinical Practices NPPV titration protocol has recently been published by the AASM and is a useful guide to NPPV titration.[22] Some of the titration recommendations are listed in Table 19-14. Generally, a starting pressure

TABLE 19-14			
Recommendations for Adjustment of Pressure Support during Noninvasive Positive Pressure Ventilation Titration			
PRESSURE CHANGE	**TRIGGER**	**DURATION BETWEEN CHANGES**	**GOAL**
IPAP/EPAP increased	Eliminate apnea, hypopnea RERA (see Table 19-10)	≥5 min	Prevent apnea, hypopnea, RERAs, snoring.
PS increased 1–2 cm H_2O	Low tidal volume (<6–8 cc/kg IBW)	≥5 min	Adequate tidal volume.
PS increased 1–2 cm H_2O	$PaCO_2$ > 10 mm Hg above goal	≥10 min	Adequate ventilation and $PaCO_2$
PS increased 1–2 cm H_2O	Respiratory muscle rest not achieved	≥10 min	Adequate respiratory muscle rest. Reduction of respiratory rate with higher tidal volumes and/or reduction in inspiratory respiratory EMG activity.
PS increased 1–2 cm H_2O	SaO_2 < 90% with tidal volume < 8 cc/kg (assumes discrete apnea, hypopnea, RERAs not present)	≥5 min	Adequate oxygenation.

EMG = electromyogram; EPAP = expiratory positive airway pressure; IBW = ideal body weight; IPAP = inspiratory positive airway pressure; $PaCO_2$ = arterial carbon dioxide pressure; PS = pressure support; RERA = respiratory effort–related arousal; SaO_2 = arterial oxygen saturation.

BPAP of 8/4 cm H_2O is used. The IPAP and EPAP are both increased if obstructive apneas are noted. IPAP is increased for obstructive hypopneas. Otherwise, the IPAP is adjusted to deliver adequate PS. The adequacy of PS can be assessed by monitoring the delivered tidal volume (goal $\geq$ 6–8 mL/kg ideal body weight) and the SaO_2. If the sleep center has the ability to monitor $P_{ET}CO_2$ or $TcPCO_2$, these measurements can help guide the titration (if devices are calibrated and validated). Monitoring of $P_{ET}CO_2$ requires using a nasal cannula under the mask to avoid dilution of the sampled gas. If there is continued arterial oxygen desaturation, PS can be increased to reach a slightly higher tidal volume goal. If further increases in ventilation are desired but the patient does not tolerate high PS, use of a higher backup rate can be tried.

As PS is increased, the finding of a higher tidal volume and lower respiratory rate is compatible with a level of support providing respiratory muscle rest. However, use of surface EMG recordings of respiratory muscle activity can also be useful. A reduction in respiratory muscle EMG activity as PS increases would be evidence that a level of support was providing muscle rest. Supplemental oxygen can be added if desaturation persists despite optimization of NPPV. The same considerations for supplemental oxygen apply as for CPAP/BPAP titrations for sleep apnea.

Reimbursement for NPPV Devices

NPPV devices are called RADs (respiratory-assist devices) and these are of two types: E0470 (BPAP) and E0471 (BPAP-ST). RADs have specific criteria for reimbursement depending on the type of patient (see Appendix 19–3). The different categories include neuromuscular disease/chest wall disorders, hypoventilation, central apnea/CompSA, and COPD. A summary of the major CMS criteria is listed in Appendix 19–3. The criteria may vary with the local carrier determination and/or private health providers.

CLINICAL REVIEW QUESTIONS

1. Which of the following is most predictive of good PAP adherence?
   A. Epworth Sleepiness Scale 16.
   B. Treatment prescription CPAP = 8 cm H_2O vs. 16 cm H_2O.
   C. Spouse referral.
   D. Entire night for PAP titration.

2. A patient with amyotrophic lateral sclerosis (ALS) who weighs 70 kg is started on empirical BPAP-ST with pressure of 8/4 cm H_2O and a backup rate of 12 breaths/min. The patient reports improved sleep and his wife notes no snoring. On the basis of the following 6-week download what do you recommend?

Apnea-hypopnea index (AHI)	Hypopnea index (HI)
Adherence (all nights)	7.5/hr
AHI	4.0/hr Apnea index 0.5/hr HI 3.5/hr
Large leak	10 min
Average tidal volume	400 mL
Average rate	20
Patient-triggered breaths	99%

   A. Continue present treatment.
   B. BPAP 12/4 cm H_2O.
   C. BPAP 10/6 cm H_2O.
   D. Increase backup rate to 18 breaths/min.

3. Which of the following is most likely to be an effective treatment for a patient with the OHS (BMI = 40 kg/m^2), neck circumference (NC) of 19 inches, and daytime PCO_2 of 60 mm Hg?
   A. BPAP 19/16 cm H_2O.
   B. BPAP 22/14 cm H_2O.
   C. BPAP 16/8 cm H_2O.
   D. BPAP 16/6 cm H_2O.

4. A patient treated with CPAP of 12 cm H_2O complains of severe bloating. Pressure is reduced to 10 cm H_2O but bloating continues and the patient's wife notes mild snoring. What do you recommend?
   A. CPAP 8 cm H_2O.
   B. APAP range 4–16 cm H_2O.
   C. BPAP 12/8 cm H_2O.
   D. BPAP 10/6 cm H_2O.

5. A patient with severe COPD requiring supplemental oxygen at 2 L/min during the day is found to have severe OSA with an AHI of 40/hr. BPAP of 16/12 cm H_2O is the optimal treatment pressure. The patient is started on the combination of BPAP and oxygen. Which of the following is likely true about the required oxygen flow on BPAP treatment?
   A. 2.5 L/min should be adequate.
   B. Higher BPAP would require higher supplemental oxygen flow.
   C. The required supplemental oxygen flow would increase with high mouth leak.
   D. A and B.
   E. B and C.

6. A patient with OSA undergoes an attended PAP titration. The CPAP treatment table follows. What pressure do you recommend? (CA = central apnea; H = hypopnea; MA = mixed apnea; OA = obstructive apnea; TST = total sleep time). Assume all sleep is in the supine position.

CPAP	TST	REM SLEEP	AHI	AHI REM	OA	MA	CA	H
7	30	0	20	0	10	0	0	0
8	30	10	10	30	0	0	0	5
9	30	20	4	6	0	0	0	2
10	30	10	10	0	0	0	5	0
11	30	10	20	0	0	0	10	0

A. 7.

B. 8.

C. 9.

D. 10.

E. 11.

Answers

1. A. Patients with daytime sleepiness are more likely to experience a symptomatic benefit and adhere to PAP treatment. The level of pressure does not seem to be a factor in unselected patients. Individual patients may benefit from interventions such as BPAP, APAP, autoB-PAP, or flexible PAP. Use of a split-night study versus an entire night of titration does not seem to be a major factor in most studies.

2. B. The tidal volume is low and respiratory rate high. For a 70-kg individual, the ideal tidal volume is around 500 to 600 mL (6–8 mL/kg). An increase in PS is indicated. Because the AHI is low, there is no need to increase the EPAP. If tidal volume increases, one would expect the respiratory rate to decrease (e.g., 20–15 breaths/min). At this point, there is no indication to use a higher respiratory rate.

3. B. In patients with OSA or OHS and a large neck circumference, a relatively high CPAP or EPAP is needed to prevent obstructive apnea. BPAP with a PS of 4 cm H_2O might be used in a patient with OSA and pressure intolerance to keep the upper airway open. Some patients with OHS who will respond to CPAP alone experience a reduction in daytime PCO_2 with chronic treatment. However, given the significant hypercapnia, a higher PS (if tolerated) is indicated. EPAP of 8 would be unlikely to prevent obstructive apnea (at least during supine REM sleep). If the patient did not tolerate BPAP of 22/14, one could try 20/14 cm H_2O.

4. C. One could argue that any of the answers might be reasonable. However, patients with bloating often require a change to BPAP. A BPAP of 12/8 should provide similar treatment to CPAP of 10. At this level, there was only mild snoring. If bloating persists, one could try lower pressure. CPAP of 8 cm H_2O would also likely provide relief from bloating but would likely result in an increased AHI. In some situations, this might be acceptable. On APAP, the mean pressure is often 2 to 6 cm H_2O below the 90th percentile pressure (commonly selected for CPAP). In most individuals, the difference is in the 2 cm H_2O range. This may not provide enough pressure reduction but would not be an unreasonable approach.

5. E. The patient likely requires fairly high BPAP and, therefore, 2.5 L/min will likely not be adequate given that 2 L/min provides a daytime SaO_2 of only 94%. The required supplemental oxygen flow increases with increasing levels of PAP due to the higher delivered flow rate. The supplemental oxygen flow can be adjusted during a PSG PAP titration. However, checking nocturnal oximetry on treatment is suggested to determine oxygen requirements in the home setting.

6. C. On CPAP of 9 cm H_2O, the AHI = 4/hr and supine REM sleep was recorded. Higher pressure was associated with central apneas.

REFERENCES

1. Sullivan CE, Issa FG, Berthon-Jones M, et al: Reversal of obstructive sleep apnoea by continuous positive airway pressure applied through the nares. Lancet 1981;1:862–865.
2. Gay P, Weaver T, Loube D, et al: Evaluation of positive airway pressure treatment for sleep related breathing disorders in adults. Sleep 2006;29:381–401.
3. Kushida CA, Littner MR, Hirshkowitz M, et al: Practice parameters for the use of continuous and bilevel positive airway pressure devices to treat adult patients with sleep related breathing disorders. Sleep 2006;29:375–380.
4. Loube DI, Gay PC, Strohl KP, et al: Indications for positive airway pressure treatment of adult sleep apnea patients. A consensus statement. Chest 1999;115:863–866.
5. Kakkar RK, Berry RB: Positive airway pressure treatment for obstructive sleep apnea. Chest 2007;132:1057–1072.
6. Weaver TE, Grunstein RR: Adherence to continuous positive airway pressure therapy: the challenge to effective treatment. Proc Am Thorac Soc 2008;5:173–178.
7. Schwab RJ: Upper airway imaging. Clin Chest Med 1998; 19:33–54.
8. Kuna ST, Bedi DG, Ryckman C: Effect of nasal airway positive pressure on upper airway size and configuration. Am Rev Respir Dis 1988;138:969–975.
9. Schwab RJ, Pack AI, Gupta KB, et al: Upper airway and soft tissue structural changes influences by CPAP in normal subjects. Am J Respir Crit Care Med 1996;154:1106–1116.
10. Alex CG, Aronson RM, Onal E, Lopata M: Effects of continuous positive airway pressure on upper airway and respiratory muscle activity. J Appl Physiol 1987;62:2026–2030.
11. Heinzer RC, Stanchina ML, Malhotra A, et al: Lung volume and continuous positive airway pressure requirements in obstructive sleep apnea. Am J Respir Crit Care Med 2005; 172:114–117.
12. Van de Graaff WB: Thoracic influences on upper airway patency. J Appl Physiol 1988;65:2124–2131.
13. Mahadevia AK, Onal E, Lopata M: Effects of expiratory positive airway pressure on sleep-induced respiratory abnormalities in patients with hypersomnia-sleep apnea syndrome. Am Rev Respir Dis 1983;128:708–711.
14. Heinzer R, White DP, Malhotra A, et al: Effect of expiratory positive airway pressure on sleep disordered breathing. Sleep 2008;31:429–432.
15. Sanders MH, Kern N: Obstructive sleep apnea treated by independently adjusted inspiratory and expiratory positive airway pressures via nasal mask. Chest 1990;98:317–324.

16. Reeves-Hoché MK, Hudgel DW, Meck R, et al: Continuous versus bilevel positive airway pressure for obstructive sleep apnea. Am J Respir Crit Care Med 1995;151:443–449.

17. Smith I, Lasserson TJ: Pressure modification for improving usage of continuous positive airway pressure machines in adults with obstructive sleep apnoea. Update of Cochrane Database Syst Rev 2004;4:CD003531. Cochrane Database Syst Rev 2009;4:CD003531.

18. Ballard RD, Gay PC, Strollo PJ: Interventions to improve compliance in sleep apnea patients previously non-compliant with continuous positive airway pressure. J Clin Sleep Med 2007; 3:706–712.

19. Schafer H, Ewig S, Hasper E, et al: Failure of CPAP therapy in obstructive sleep apnea syndrome: predictive factors and treatment with bilevel positive airway pressure. Respir Med 1998;92:208–215.

20. Berger KI, Ayappa I, Chatr-Amontri B, et al: Obesity hypoventilation syndrome as a spectrum of respiratory disturbances during sleep. Chest 2001;120:1231–1238.

21. Piper AJ, Wang D, Yee BJ, et al: Randomized trial of CPAP vs bilevel support in the treatment of obesity hypoventilation syndrome without severe nocturnal desaturation. Thorax 2008;63:395–401.

22. Berry RB, Chediak A, Brown LK, et al: Best clinical practices for the sleep center adjustment of noninvasive positive pressure ventilation (NPPV) in stable chronic alveolar hypoventilation syndromes. J Clin Sleep Med 2010;6:491–509.

23. Berry RB, Parish JM, Hartse KM: The use of auto-titrating continuous positive airway pressure for treatment of adult obstructive sleep apnea. An American Academy of Sleep Medicine Review. Sleep 2002;25:148–173.

24. Littner M, Hirshkowitz M, Davila D, et al: Practice parameters for the use of auto-titrating continuous positive airway pressure devices for titrating pressures and treating adult patients with obstructive sleep apnea syndrome. An American Academy of Sleep Medicine report. Sleep 2002;25:143–147.

25. Morgenthaler TI, Aurora RN, Brown T, et al: Standards of Practice Committee of the AASM: Practice parameters for the use of autotitrating continuous positive airway pressure devices for titrating pressures and treating adult patients with obstructive sleep apnea syndrome: an update for 2007. Sleep 2008;31:141–147.

26. Masa JF, Jimenez A, Duran J, et al: Alternative methods of titrating continuous positive airway pressure. Am J Respir Crit Care Med 2004;170:1218–1224.

27. Ayas NT, Patel SR, Malhotra A, et al: Auto-titrating versus standard continuous positive airway pressure for the treatment of obstructive sleep apnea: results of a meta-analysis. Sleep 2004;27:249–253.

28. Randerath WJ, Schraeder O, Galetke W, et al: Autoadjusting CPAP therapy based on impedance efficacy, compliance and acceptance. Am J Respir Crit Care Med 2001;163:652–657.

29. Farre R, Montserrat JM, Rigau J, et al: Response of automatic continuous positive airway pressure devices to different sleep breathing patterns: a bench study. Am J Respir Crit Care Med 2002;166:469–473.

30. Coller D, Stanley D, Parthasarathy S: Effect of air leak on the performance of auto-PAP devices: a bench study. Sleep Breath 2005;9:167–175.

31. Badr MS, Toiber F, Skatrud JB, et al: Pharyngeal narrowing/occlusion during central apnea. J Appl Physiol 1995;78:1806–1815.

32. Gentina T, Fortin F, Douay B, et al: Auto bi-level with pressure relief during exhalation as a rescue therapy for optimally treated obstructive sleep apnoea patients with poor compliance to continuous positive airways pressure therapy—a pilot study. Sleep Breath Epub ahead of print 2010;March 4.

33. Teschler H, Döhring J, Wang YM, Berthon-Jones M: Adaptive pressure support servo-ventilation: a novel treatment for Cheyne-Stokes respiration in heart failure. Am J Respir Crit Care Med 2001;164:614–619.

34. Morgenthaler TI, Gay PC, Gordon N, Brown LK: Adaptive servoventilation versus noninvasive positive pressure ventilation for central, mixed, and complex sleep apnea syndromes. Sleep 2007;30:468–475.

35. Allam JS, Olson EJ, Gay PC, Morgenthaler TI: Efficacy of adaptive servoventilation in treatment of complex and central sleep apnea syndromes. Chest 2007;132:1839–1846.

36. Javaheri S, Malik A, Smith J, Chung E: Adaptive pressure support servoventilation: a novel treatment for sleep apnea associated with use of opioids. J Clin Sleep Med 2008; 4:305–310.

37. Philippe C, Stoïca-Herman M, Drouot X, et al: Compliance with and effectiveness of adaptive servoventilation versus continuous positive airway pressure in the treatment of Cheyne-Stokes respiration in heart failure over a six-month period. Heart 2006;92:337–342.

38. Pepperell JC, Maskell NA, Jones DR, et al: A randomized controlled trial of adaptive ventilation for Cheyne-Stokes breathing in heart failure. Am J Respir Crit Care Med 2003;168:1109–1114; Epub 2003;August 19.

39. Storre JH, Seuthe B, Fiechter R, et al: Average volume-assured pressure support in obesity hypoventilation: a randomized crossover trial. Chest 2006;130:815–821.

40. Ambrogio C, Lowman X, Kuo M, et al: Sleep and non-invasive ventilation in patients with chronic respiratory failure. Intensive Care Med 2009;35:306–313.

41. Janssens JP, Metzger M, Sforza E: Impact of volume targeting on efficacy of bi-level non-invasive ventilation and sleep in obesity hypoventilation syndrome. Respir Med 2009;103: 165–172.

42. Jaye J, Chatwin M, Dayer M, et al: Autotitration versus standard noninvasive ventilation: a randomized crossover trial. Eur Respir J 2009;33:566–573.

43. Aloia MS, Stanchina M, Arnedt JT, et al: Treatment adherence and outcomes in flexible vs standard continuous positive airway pressure therapy. Chest 2005;172:2085–2093.

44. Bakker J, Campbell A, Neill A: Randomized controlled trial comparing flexible and continuous positive airway pressure delivery: effects on compliance, objective and subjective sleepiness and vigilance. Sleep 2010;33:523–529.

45. Dolan DC, Okonkwo R, Gfullner F, et al: Longitudinal comparison study of pressure relief (C-Flex) vs. CPAP in OSA patients. Sleep Breath 2009;13:73–77.

46. Marshall NS, Neill AM, Campbell AJ: Randomised trial of compliance with flexible (C-Flex) and standard continuous positive airway pressure for severe obstructive sleep apnea. Sleep Breath 2008;12:393–396.

47. Pépin JL, Muir JF, Gentina T, et al: Pressure reduction during exhalation in sleep apnea patients treated by continuous positive airway pressure. Chest 2009;136:490–497.

48. Nilius G, Happel A, Domanski U, Ruhle KH: Pressure-relief continuous positive airway pressure vs constant continuous positive airway pressure: a comparison of efficacy and compliance. Chest 2006;130:1018–1024.

49. Mulgrew AT, Cheema R, Fleetham J, et al: Efficacy and patient satisfaction with autoadjusting CPAP with variable expiratory pressure vs standard CPAP: a two-night randomized crossover trial. Sleep Breath 2007;11:31–37.

50. Martins de Araujo MT, Vieira SB, Vasquez EC, Fleury B: Heated humidification or face mask to prevent upper airway dryness during continuous positive airway pressure therapy. Chest 2000;117:142–147.

51. Hayes MJ, McGregor FB, Roberts DN, et al: Continuous positive airway pressure with a mouth leak: effect on nasal mucosal blood flow and nasal geometry. Thorax 1995;50:1179–1182.

52. Richards GN, Cistulli PA, Ungar RG, et al: Mouth leak with nasal continuous positive airway pressure increases nasal

airway resistance. Am J Respir Crit Care Med 1996;154: 182–186.

53. Sanner BM, Fluerenbrock N, Kleiber-Imbeck A, et al: Effect of continuous positive airway pressure therapy on infectious complications in patients with obstructive sleep apnea syndrome. Respiration 2001;68:483–487.

54. Ortolano GA, Schaffer J, McAlister MB, et al: Filters reduce the risk of bacterial transmission from contaminated heated humidifiers used with CPAP for obstructive sleep apnea. J Clin Sleep Med 2007;3:700–705.

55. Massie CA, Hart RW, Peralez K, Richards GN: Effects of humidification on nasal symptoms and compliance in sleep apnea patients using continuous positive airway pressure. Chest 1999;116:403–408.

56. Ryan S, Doherty LS, Nolan GM, et al: Effects of heated humidification and topical steroids on compliance, nasal symptoms, and quality of life in patients with obstructive sleep apnea syndrome using nasal continuous positive airway pressure. J Clin Sleep Med 2009;5:422–427.

57. Worsnop CJ, Miseski S, Rochford PD: The routine use of humidification with nasal continuous positive airway pressure. Int Med J 2009;40:650–656.

58. Nilius G, Domanski U, Franke KJ, Ruhle KH: Impact of a controlled heated breathing tube humidifier on sleep quality during CPAP therapy in a cool sleeping environment. Eur Respir J 2008;31:830–836.

59. Duong M, Jayaram L, Camfferman D, et al: Use of heated humidification during nasal CPAP titration in obstructive sleep apnoea syndrome. Eur Respir J 2005;26: 679–685.

60. Mador MJ, Krauza M, Pervez A, et al: Effect of heated humidification on compliance and quality of life in patients with sleep apnea using nasal continuous positive airway pressure. Chest 2005;28:2151–2158.

61. Wiest GH, Harsch IA, Fuchs FS, et al: Initiation of CPAP therapy for OSA: does prophylactic humidification during CPAP pressure titration improve initial patient acceptance and comfort? Respiration 2002;69:406–412.

62. Kushida CA, Chediak A, Berry RB, et al: Positive Airway Pressure Titration Task Force, American Academy of Sleep Medicine: Clinical guidelines for the manual titration of positive airway pressure in patients with obstructive sleep apnea. J Clin Sleep Med 2008;4:157–171.

63. Massie CA, Hart RW: Clinical outcomes related to interface type in patients with obstructive sleep apnea/hypopnea syndrome who are using continuous positive airway pressure. Chest 2003;123:1112–1118.

64. Prosise GL, Berry RB: Oral-nasal continuous positive airway pressure as a treatment for obstructive sleep apnea. Chest 1994;106:180–186.

65. Sanders MH, Kern NB, Stiller RA, et al: CPAP therapy via oronasal mask for obstructive sleep apnea. Chest 1994;106: 774–779.

66. Anderson FE, Kingshott RN, Taylor DR, et al: A randomized crossover efficacy trial of oral CPAP (Oracle) compared with nasal CPAP in the management of obstructive sleep apnea. Sleep 2003;26:721–726.

67. Beecroft J, Zanon S, Lukic D, Hanley P: Oral continuous positive airway pressure for sleep apnea. Chest 2003;124: 2200–2208.

68. Department of Health and Human Services Centers for Medicare and Medicaid Services: National Carrier Determination (NCD) for Continuous Positive Airway Pressure (CPAP) Therapy For Obstructive Sleep Apnea (OSA) (240.4). Available at http://www.cms.gov/medicare-coverage-database/details/ncd-etails.aspx?NCDId=226&ncdver=3&DocID=240.4&bc=gAAAABAAAAAA& See also recent transmittal R96 at http://www.cms.gov/transmittals/downloads/R96NCD.pdf.

69. Capdevila OS, Kheirandish-Gozal L, Dayat E, Gozal D: Pediatric obstructive sleep apnea. Proc Am Thorac Soc 2008;5: 274–282.

70. Rains JC: Treatment of obstructive sleep apnea in pediatric patients. Behavioral intervention for compliance with nasal continuous positive airway pressure. Clin Pediatr (Phila) 1995;34:535–541.

71. Kheirandish L, Goldbart D, Gozal D: Intranasal steroids and oral leukotriene modifier therapy in residual sleep disordered breathing after tonsillectomy and adenoidectomy in children. Pediatrics 2006;117:e61–e66.

72. Kribbs NB, Pack AI, Kline LR, et al: Objective measurement of patterns of nasal CPAP use by patients with obstructive sleep apnea. Am Rev Respir Dis 1993;147:887–895.

73. McArdle N, Devereux G, Heidarnejad H, et al: Long-term use of CPAP therapy for sleep apnea/hypopnea syndrome. Am J Respir Crit Care Med 1999;159:1108–1114.

74. Pépin JL, Krieger J, Rodenstein D, et al: Effective compliance during the first 3 months of continuous positive airway pressure. A European prospective study of 121 patients. Am J Respir Crit Care Med 1999;160:1124–1129.

75. Sin DD, Mayers I, Man GC, Pawluk L: Long-term compliance rates to continuous positive airway pressure in obstructive sleep apnea: a population-based study. Chest 2002;121:430–435.

76. Kohler M, Smith D, Tippett V, Stradling JR: Predictors of long-term compliance with continuous positive airway pressure. Thorax 2010;65:829–832.

77. Engleman HM, Wild MR: Improving CPAP use by patients with the sleep apnoea/hypopnoea syndrome (SAHS). Sleep Med Rev 2003;7:81–99.

78. Sugiura T, Noda A, Nakata S, et al: Influence of nasal resistance on initial acceptance of continuous positive airway pressure in treatment for obstructive sleep apnea syndrome. Respiration 2007;74:56–60.

79. Weaver TE, Kribbs NB, Pack AI, et al: Night-to-night variability in CPAP use over the first three months of treatment. Sleep 1997;20:278–283.

80. Budhiraja R, Parthasarathy S, Drake CL, et al: Early CPAP use identified subsequent adherence to CPAP therapy. Sleep 2007;30:320–324.

81. Weaver TE, Maislin G, Dinges DF, et al: Relationship between hours of CPAP use and achieving normal levels of sleepiness and daily functioning. Sleep 2007;30:711–719.

82. Campos-Rodriguez F, Pena-Grinan N, Reyes-Nunez N, et al: Mortality in obstructive sleep apnea-hypopnea patients treated with positive airway pressure. Chest 2005;128:624–633.

83. Campos-Rodriguez F, Perez-Ronchel J, Grilo-Reina A, et al: Long-term effect of continuous positive airway pressure on BP in patients with hypertension and sleep apnea. Chest 2007;132:1847–1852.

84. Smith I, Nadig V, Lasserson TJ: Educational, supportive and behavioural interventions to improve usage of continuous positive airway pressure machines for adults with obstructive sleep apnoea. Cochrane Database Syst Rev 2009;2:CD007736.

85. Hoy CJ, Vennelle M, Kingshott RN, et al: Can intensive support improve continuous positive airway pressure use in patients with the sleep apnea/hypopnea syndrome? Am J Respir Crit Care Med 1999;159:1096–1100.

86. Chervin RD, Theut S, Bassetti C, Aldrich MS: Compliance of nasal CPAP can be improved by simple interventions. Sleep 1997;20:284–289.

87. Likar LL, Panciera TM, Erickson AD, et al: Group education sessions and compliance with nasal CPAP therapy. Chest 1997;111:1273–1277.

88. Richard D, Bartlett DJ, Wong K, et al: Increased adherence to CPAP with a group cognitive behavioral treatment intervention: a randomized trial. Sleep 2007;30:635–640.

89. Aloia MS, Smith K, Arndt JT, et al: Brief behavioral therapies reduce early positive airway pressure discontinuation rates in sleep apnea syndrome: preliminary findings. Behav Sleep Med 2007;5:89–104.

90. Berry RB, Desa MM, Light RW: Effect of ethanol on the efficacy of nasal continuous positive airway pressure as a treatment for obstructive sleep apnea. Chest 1991;99:339–343.

91. Berry RB, Patel PB: Effect of zolpidem on the efficacy of continuous positive airway pressure as treatment for obstructive sleep apnea. Sleep 2006;29:1052–1056.

92. Bradshaw DA, Ruff GA, Murphy DP: An oral hypnotic medication does not improve continuous positive airway pressure compliance in men with obstructive sleep apnea. Chest 2006;130:1369–1376.

93. Lettieri CJ, Shah AA, Holley AB, et al: CPAP promotion and prognosis—the Army Sleep Apnea Program Trial. Effects of a short course of eszopiclone on continuous positive airway pressure adherence: a randomized trial. Ann Intern Med 2009;151:696–702.

94. Lettieri CJ, Quast TN, Eliasson AH, Andrada T: Eszopiclone improves overnight polysomnography and continuous positive airway pressure titration: a prospective, randomized, placebo-controlled trial. Sleep 2008;31:1310–1316.

95. Kushida CA, Littner M, Morgenthaler T, et al: Practice parameters for the indications for polysomnography and related procedures: an update for 2005. Sleep 2005;28:499–521.

96. Marcus CL, Rosen G, Davidson-Ward S, et al: Adherence to and effectiveness of positive airway pressure therapy in children with obstructive sleep apnea. Pediatrics 2006;117:e442–e451.

97. Koontz KL, Slifer KJ, Cataldo MD, Marcus CL: Improving pediatric compliance with positive airway pressure therapy: the impact of behavioral intervention. Sleep 2003;26:1010–1015.

98. Kirk VG, O'Donnell AR: Continuous positive airway pressure for children: a discussion on how to maximize compliance. Sleep Med Rev 2006;10:119–127.

99. Iber C, Ancoli-Israel S, Chesson A, Quan SF for the American Academy of Sleep Medicine: The AASM Manual for the Scoring of Sleep and Associated Events: Rules, Terminology and Technical Specifications, 1st ed. Westchester, IL: American Academy of Sleep Medicine, 2007.

100. Condos R, Norman RG, Krishnasamy I, et al: Flow limitation as a noninvasive assessment of residual upper-airway resistance during continuous positive airway pressure therapy of obstructive sleep apnea. Am J Respir Crit Care Med 1994;150:475–480.

101. Bennett JR, Dunroy HMA, Corfield DR, et al: Respiratory muscle activity during REM sleep in patients with diaphragm paralysis. Neurology 2004;61:134–137.

102. White JES, Drinnan MJ, Smithson AJ, et al: Respiratory muscle activity and oxygenation during sleep in patients with muscle weakness. Eur Respir J 1995;8:808–814.

103. Paiva R, Krivec U, Aubertin G, et al: Carbon dioxide monitoring during noninvasive respiratory support in children. Intensive Care Med 2009;35:1068–1074.

104. Kirk VG, Batuyong ED, Bohn SG: Transcutaneous carbon dioxide monitoring and capnography during pediatric polysomnography. Sleep 2006;29:1601–1608.

105. Montserrat JM, Ballester E, Olivi H, et al: Time-course of stepwise CPAP titration. Behavior of respiratory and neurological variables. Am J Respir Crit Care Med 1995;152:1854–1859.

106. Oksenberg A, Silverberg DS, Arons E, et al: The sleep supine position has a major effect on optimal nasal CPAP. Chest 1999;116:1000–1006.

107. Pevernagie DA, Shepard JW Jr: Relations between sleep stage, posture and effective nasal CPAP levels in OSA. Sleep 1992;15:162–167.

108. Neill AM, Angus SM, Sajkov D, McEvoy RD: Effects of sleep posture on upper airway stability in patients with obstructive sleep apnea. Am J Respir Crit Care Med 1997;155:199–204.

109. Yoder EA, Klann K, Strohl KP: Inspired oxygen concentrations during positive pressure therapy. Sleep Breath 2004;8:1–5.

110. Schwartz AR, Kacmarek RM, Hess DR: Factors affecting oxygen delivery with bilevel positive airway pressure. Respir Care 2004;49:270–275.

111. Dernaika T, Tawk M, Nazir S, et al: The significance and outcome of continuous positive airway pressure–related central sleep apnea during split-night sleep studies. Chest 2007;132:81–87.

112. Javaheri S, Smith J, Chung E: The prevalence and natural history of complex sleep apnea. J Clin Sleep Med 2009;5:205–211.

113. Pusalavidyasagar SS, Olson EJ, Gay PC, Morgenthaler TI: Treatment of complex sleep apnea syndrome: a retrospective comparative review. Sleep Med 2006;7:474–479.

114. Javaheri S: Positive airway pressure treatment of central sleep apnea with emphasis on heart failure, opioids, and complex sleep apnea. Sleep Med Clin 2010;5:407–418.

115. Skomro RP, Gjevre J, Reid J, et al: Outcomes of home-based diagnosis and treatment of obstructive sleep apnea. Chest 2010;138:257–263.

116. Oliver Z, Hoffstein V: Predicting effective continuous positive airway pressure. Chest 2000;117:1061–1064.

117. Fitzpatrick MF, Alloway CED, Wakeford TM, et al: Can patients with obstructive sleep apnea titrate their own continuous positive airway pressure? Am J Respir Crit Care Med 2003;167:716–722.

118. Mulgrew AT, Fox N, Ayas NT, Ryan CF: Diagnosis and initial management of obstructive sleep apnea without polysomnography: a randomized validation study. Ann Intern Med 2007;146:157–166.

119. Berry RB, Hill G, Thompson L, McLaurin V: Portable monitoring and autotitration versus polysomnography for the diagnosis and treatment of sleep apnea. Sleep 2008;31:1423–1431.

120. Antic NA, Buchan C, Esterman A, et al: A randomized controlled trial of nurse-led care for symptomatic moderate-severe obstructive sleep apnea. Am J Respir Crit Care Med 2009;179:501–508.

121. Desai H, Patel A, Patel P, et al: Accuracy of auto-titration CPAP to estimate the residual apnea-hypopnea index in patients with obstructive sleep apnea on treatment with auto-titration CPAP. Sleep Breath 2009;13:383–390.

122. Pittman SD, Pillar G, Berry RB, et al: Follow-up assessment of CPAP efficacy in patients with obstructive sleep apnea using an ambulatory device based on peripheral arterial tonometry. Sleep Breath 2006;10:123–131.

123. Baltzan MA, Kassissia I, Elkholi O, et al: Prevalence of persistent sleep apnea in patients treated with continuous positive airway pressure. Sleep 2006;29:557–563.

124. Mulgrew AT, Lawati NA, Ayas NT, et al: Residual sleep apnea on polysomnograpy after 3 months of CPAP therapy. Clinical implications and patterns. Sleep Med 2010;11:119–125.

125. Berry RB: Initiating NPPV treatment with patients with chronic hypoventilation. Sleep Med Clin 2010;5:485–505.

126. Perrin C, D'Ambrosio C, White A, Hill NS: Sleep in restrictive and neuromuscular respiratory disorders. Semin Respir Crit Care Med 2005;26:117–130.

127. American College of Chest Physicians: Clinical indications for noninvasive positive pressure ventilation in chronic respiratory failure due to restrictive lung disease, COPD, and nocturnal hypoventilation—a consensus conference report. Chest 1999;116:521–534.

128. Gruis KL, Brown DL, Lisabeth LD, et al: Longitudinal assessment of noninvasive positive pressure ventilation adjustments in ALS patients. J Neurol Sci 2006;247:59–63.

Practice Parameters for APAP and CPAP/BPAP (Selected Recommendations)

CPAP/BPAP Recommendations*

4.1.1 Treatment with CPAP must be based on a prior diagnosis of OSA established using an acceptable method. (Standard)

4.1.2 CPAP is indicated for the treatment of moderate to severe OSA. (Standard)

4.1.3 CPAP is recommended for the treatment of mild OSA. (Option)

4.1.4 CPAP is indicated for improving self-reported sleepiness in patients with OSA. (Standard)

4.1.5 CPAP is recommended for improving quality of life in patients with OSA. (Option)

4.2.1 Full-night, attended polysomnography performed in the laboratory is the preferred approach for titration to determine optimal PAP; however, split-night, diagnostic-titration studies are usually adequate. (Guideline)

4.3.1 CPAP usage should be objectively monitored to help ensure utilization. (Standard)

4.3.2 Close follow-up for PAP usage and problems in patients with OSA by appropriately trained health care providers is indicated to establish effective utilization patterns and remediate problems, if needed. This is especially important during the first few weeks of PAP use. (Standard)

4.3.3 The addition of heated humidification is indicated to improve CPAP utilization. (Standard)

4.3.4 The addition of a systematic educational program is indicated to improve PAP utilization. (Standard)

4.4.1 After initial CPAP setup, long-term follow-up for CPAP-treated patients with OSA by appropriately trained health care providers is indicated yearly and as needed to troubleshoot PAP mask, machine, or usage problems. (Option)

4.4.2 CPAP and BPAP therapy are safe; side effects and adverse events are mainly minor and reversible. (Standard)

4.5.1 While the literature mainly supports CPAP therapy, BPAP is an optional therapy in some cases in which high pressure is needed and the patient experiences difficulty exhaling against a fixed pressure or coexisting central hypoventilation is present. (Guideline)

4.5.2 BPAP may be useful in treating some forms of restrictive lung disease or hypoventilation syndromes associated with daytime hypercapnia. (Option)

APAP Recommendations†

3.1. APAP is not recommended to diagnose OSA. (Standard)

3.2. Patients with CHF, significant lung disease such as COPD, patients expected to have nocturnal arterial oxyhemoglobin desaturation due to conditions other than OSA (e.g., obesity hypoventilation syndrome), patients who do not snore (either naturally or as a result of palate surgery), and patients who have central sleep apnea syndromes are not currently candidates for APAP titration or treatment. (Standard)

3.3. APAP devices are not currently recommended for split-night titration. (Standard)

3.4. Certain APAP devices may be used during attended titration with polysomnography to identify a single pressure for use with standard CPAP for treatment of moderate to severe OSA. (Guideline)

3.5. Certain APAP devices may be initiated and used in the self-adjusting mode for unattended treatment of patients with moderate to severe OSA without significant co-morbidities (CHF, COPD, central sleep apnea syndromes, or hypoventilation syndromes). (Option)

3.6. Certain APAP devices may be used in an unattended way to determine a fixed CPAP treatment pressure for patients with moderate to severe OSA without significant co-morbidities (CHF, COPD, central sleep apnea syndromes, or hypoventilation syndromes). (Option)

*From Kushida CA, Littner MR, Hirshkowitz M, et al: Practice parameters for the use of continuous and bilevel positive airway pressure devices to treat adult patients with sleep related breathing disorders. Sleep 2006;29:375–380.

†From Morgenthaler TI, Aurora RN, Brown T, et al: Standards of Practice Committee of the AASM: Practice parameters for the use of autotitrating continuous positive airway pressure devices for titrating pressures and treating adult patients with obstructive sleep apnea syndrome: an update for 2007. Sleep 2008;31:141–147.

3.7. Patients being treated with fixed CPAP on the basis of APAP titration or being treated with APAP must have close clinical follow-up to determine treatment effectiveness and safety. This is especially important during the first few weeks of PAP use. (Standard)

3.8. A re-evaluation and, if necessary, a standard attended CPAP titration should be performed if symptoms do not resolve or if the APAP treatment otherwise appears to lack efficacy. (Standard)

APAP = autotitrating positive airway pressure; BPAP = bilevel positive airway pressure; CHF = congestive heart failure; COPD = chronic obstructive airway pressure; CPAP = continuous positive airway pressure; OSA = obstructive sleep apnea; PAP = positive airway pressure.

The details of local carrier determinations can vary by region and are frequently updated.

Excerpts from the Local Carrier Determination (LCD) for Positive Airway Pressure (PAP) devices for the treatment of Obstructive Sleep Apnea (L11518) CIGNA-DMAC.

Initial Coverage

A single level continuous positive airway pressure (CPAP) device (E0601) is covered for the treatment of obstructive sleep apnea (OSA) if criteria A–C are met:

A. The patient has a face-to-face clinical evaluation by the treating physician prior to the sleep test to assess the patient for OSA.
B. The patient has a Medicare-covered sleep test that meets either of the following criteria (1 or 2):
  1. The apnea-hypopnea index (AHI) or Respiratory Disturbance Index (RDI)* is greater than or equal to 15 events per hour with a minimum of 30 events; **or**
  2. The AHI or RDI is greater than or equal to 5 and less than or equal to 14 events per hour with a minimum of 10 events and documentation of:
    a. Excessive daytime sleepiness, impaired cognition, mood disorders, or insomnia; **or**
    b. Hypertension, ischemic heart disease, or history of stroke.
C. The patient and/or their caregiver have received instruction from the supplier of the CPAP device and accessories in the proper use and care of the equipment.

If a claim for a CPAP (E0601) is submitted and all of the criteria above have not been met, it will be denied as not medically necessary.

Sleep Tests

Coverage of a PAP device for the treatment of OSA is limited to claims where the diagnosis of OSA is based upon a Medicare-covered sleep test (Type I, II, III, IV, Other). A Medicare-covered sleep test must be either a polysomnogram performed in a facility-based laboratory (Type I study) or a home sleep test (HST) (Types II, III, IV, or Other). The test must be ordered by the beneficiary's treating physician and conducted by an entity that qualifies as a Medicare provider of sleep tests and is in compliance with all applicable state regulatory requirements.

---

*Here RDI is used for Home Sleep Testing as # apneas + hypopneas/hr of monitoring time; respiratory event–related arousals (RERAs) are not included in either the AHI or the RDI.

A Type I sleep test is the continuous and simultaneous monitoring and recording of various physiological and pathophysiological parameters of sleep with physician review, interpretation, and report. It is facility-based and must include sleep staging, which is defined to include a 1–4 lead electroencephalogram (EEG), electro-oculogram (EOG), submental electromyogram (EMG) and electrocardiogram (ECG). It must also include at least the following additional parameters of sleep: airflow, respiratory effort, and oxygen saturation by oximetry. It may be performed either as a whole night study for diagnosis only or as a split night study to diagnose and initially evaluate treatment.

An HST is performed unattended in the beneficiary's home using a portable monitoring device. A portable monitoring device for conducting an HST must meet one of the following criteria:

Type II device—Monitors and records a minimum of seven (7) channels: EEG, EOG, EMG, ECG/heart rate, airflow, respiratory movement/effort and oxygen saturation; **or**
Type III device—Monitors and records a minimum of four (4) channels: respiratory movement/effort, airflow, ECG/heart rate and oxygen saturation; **or**
Type IV device—Monitors and records a minimum of three (3) channels, one of which is airflow that allows direct calculation of an AHI or RDI; **or**
Other—Devices that monitor and record a minimum of three (3) channels that include actigraphy, oximetry, and peripheral arterial tone that allow calculation of an AHI or RDI.

Continued Coverage beyond the First 3 Months of Therapy

Continued coverage of a PAP device (E0470 or E0601) beyond the first three months of therapy requires that no sooner than the 31st day but no later than the 91st day after initiating therapy, the treating physician must

1. Face-to-face a clinical re-evaluation by the treating physician with documentation that the symptoms of OSA have improved; and
2. Objective evidence of adherence to use of the PAP device, reviewed by the treating physician

Adherence to therapy is defined as use of PAP ≥ 4 hours per night on 70% of nights during a consecutive thirty (30) day period anytime during the first three (3) months of initial usage.

If the above criteria are not met, continued coverage of a PAP device and related accessories will be denied as not medically necessary.

Beneficiaries who fail the initial 12-week trial are eligible to re-qualify for a PAP device but must have both:

1. Face-to-face clinical re-evaluation by the treating physician to determine the etiology of the failure to respond to PAP therapy; **and**
2. Repeat sleep test in a facility-based setting (Type 1 study).

Available at http://www.cms.gov/medicare-coverage-database/details/lcd-details.aspx?ContrNum=18003&ContrTypeId=10&LCDId=11518&ver=55&Date =01%2f01%2f2011&DocID=L11518&bc=iAAAABAAQAAA&

Medicare Criteria for Reimbursement for Respiratory-Assist Devices

Device terminology: E0470 = BPAP no backup rate; E0471 = BPAP with backup rate

Requirements for Initial Coverage for 3 Months

A. Restrictive thoracic and neuromuscular disorders (Table 19–15)
B. Hypoventilation syndrome (Table 19–16)
C. Central apnea/CompSA (Table 19–17)
D. Severe COPD (Table 19–18)

Coverage beyond 3 Months

Coverage beyond 3 months requires a physician evaluation no sooner than the 61st day after starting the RAD. The medical record should document relevant symptoms and usage of the device up to that time. Failure of the patient to be consistently using the device for an average of 4 hours per 24-hour period by the time of re-evaluation would represent noncompliant utilization for the intended purpose and expectations of benefit. This would constitute reason for Medicare to deny continued coverage as not medically necessary. A signed and dated statement by the treating physician no sooner than 61 days after initiating device use, declaring that the patient is compliantly using the device (an average of 4 hours per 24-hour period) and that the patient is benefiting from its use, must be obtained by the supplier of the device before continued coverage beyond 3 months.

TABLE 19–15

Medicare Guidelines for Reimbursement for Respiratory Assist Device Restrictive Thoracic and Neuromuscular Disorders

Criterion A: There is documentation in the patient's medical record of a neuromuscular disease (ALS) or severe thoracic cage abnormality
AND
Criterion B1: $PaCO_2 \geq 45$ mmHg while **awake** and breathing patient's prescribed FiO_2.
AND Criterion B2 OR B3
Criterion B2: Sleep oximetry shows $SaO_2 \leq 88\%$ for at least 5 min of nocturnal recording time while breathing prescribed FiO_2 (2 hr minimum recording time).
OR
Criterion B3 (NMD only): Maximal inspiratory pressure < 60 cm H_2O or FVC < 50% predicted.
AND
Criterion C: COPD does not contribute significantly to the patient's pulmonary limitation.

Either E0470 or E0471 (backup rate) will be covered for first 3 mo of treatment.

ALS = amyotrophic lateral sclerosis; COPD = chronic obstructive pulmonary disease; FiO_2 = fractional concentration of oxygen in inspired gas; FVC = forced vital capacity; NMD = neuromuscular disease; $PaCO_2$ = arterial partial pressure of carbon dioxide; SaO_2 = arterial oxygen saturation.

BPAP = bilevel positive airway pressure; COPD = chronic obstructive pulmonary disease; CompSA = complex sleep apnea; RAD = respiratory-assist device.
Available at http://www.cms.gov/mcd/viewlcd.asp?lcd_id=5023&lcd_version=56&show=all

TABLE 19-16

Medicare Guidelines for Reimbursement for Respiratory Assist Device Hypoventilation Syndrome

HYPOVENTILATION SYNDROME (E0470 DEVICE, BPAP WITHOUT A BACKUP RATE)
An E0470 will be covered for first 3 mo of treatment if Criteria A and B and either C or D is met. **Criterion A:** Arterial blood gas $PaCO_2 \geq 45$ mm Hg while **awake** and breathing patient's prescribed FIO_2. **AND** **Criterion B:** Spirometry shows an $FEV_1/FVC \geq 70\%$ and $FEV_1 \geq 50\%$ of predicted. **AND either Criterion C or D** **Criterion C:** An arterial blood gas $PaCO_2$, done during sleep or immediately on awakening, and breathing the patient's prescribed FIO_2, show the beneficiary's $PaCO_2$ worsened 7 mm Hg compared with original result in Criterion A. **Criterion D:** A facility-based PSG demonstrates oxygen saturation < 88% for 5 min of nocturnal recording time (minimal recording time of 2 hr) that is not caused by obstructive upper airway events.
HYPOVENTILATION SYNDROME (E0471 DEVICE, BPAP WITH A BACKUP RATE)
An E0471 will be covered for first 3 mo of treatment if criterion A and B and either C or D is met. **Criterion A:** A covered E0470 device is being used **AND** **Criterion B:** Spirometry shows an $FEV_1/FVC \geq 70\%$ and $FEV_1 \geq 50\%$ of predicted. **AND either Criterion C or D** **Criterion C:** An arterial blood gas $PaCO_2$, done while **awake,** and breathing the patient's prescribed FIO_2, show the beneficiary's $PaCO_2$ worsened 7 mm Hg compared with the arterial blood gas result used to qualify the patient for the E0470 device. **Criterion D:** A facility-based PSG demonstrates SaO_2 < 88% for 5 min of nocturnal recording time (minimal recording time of 2 hr) that is not caused by obstructive upper airway events (AHI < 5/hr) **while using** an E0470 device.

AHI = apnea-hypopnea index; BPAP = bilevel positive airway pressure; FEV_1 = forced expiratory volume in 1 second; FVC = forced vital capacity; $PaCO_2$ = arterial partial pressure of carbon dioxide; PSG = polysomnography; SaO_2 = arterial oxygen saturation.

TABLE 19-17

Medicare Guidelines for Reimbursement for Respiratory-Assist Device Central Apnea and Complex Sleep Apnea (E0470 or E0471)

Before initiating therapy, a complete facility-based attended PSG must be performed documenting the following criteria: **Criterion A:** Diagnosis of central sleep apnea or complex sleep apnea. **AND** **Criterion B:** Significant improvement of the sleep-associated hypoventilation with the use of E0470 or E0471 device on settings that will be prescribed for initial use at home, while breathing the patient's usual prescribed FIO_2.
Central sleep apnea is defined as 1. AHI > 5/hr. 2. Central apnea/hypopnea > 50% of the total apneas and hypopneas. 3. Central apneas or hypopneas $\geq$ 5/hr. 4. Symptoms of excessive sleepiness or disturbed sleep. Complex sleep apnea is a form of central apnea specifically identified by the persistence or emergence of central apneas or hypopneas upon exposure to CPAP or an E0470 when obstructive events have disappeared. These patients have predominantly obstructive or mixed apneas during the diagnostic sleep study occurring at $\geq$ 5/hr. With use of a CPAP or E0470, they show a pattern of apneas and hypopneas that meet the definition of central sleep apnea described previously.

AHI = apnea-hypopnea index; CPAP = continuous positive airway pressure; FIO_2 = fractional concentration of oxygen in inspired gas; PSG = polysomnography.

TABLE 19-18

Medicare Guidelines for Reimbursement for Respiratory-Assist Device Severe Chronic Obstructive Pulmonary Disease (E0470*)

Criterion A: An arterial blood gas $PaCO_2 \geq 52$ mm Hg, done while awake and breathing the patient's prescribed FIO_2. **AND** **Criterion B:** Sleep oximetry demonstrates oxygen saturations < 88% for at least 5 min nocturnal recording time, done while breathing oxygen at 2 L/min or the patient's prescribed FIO_2 (whichever is higher), 2-hr minimum recording time. **AND** **Criterion C:** Before initiating therapy, OSA (and treatment with CPAP) has been considered and ruled out. If all above criteria are met, an E0470 with be covered for the first 3 mo of therapy.

*E0470 = BPAP with no backup rate.
CPAP = continuous positive airway pressure; FIO_2 = fractional concentration of oxygen in inspired gas; OSA = obstructive sleep apnea; $PaCO_2$ = arterial partial pressure of carbon dioxide.

Chapter 20

Oral Appliance and Surgical Treatment for Obstructive Sleep Apnea

Chapter Points

- Before treatment of snoring with an OA, the presence or absence of OSA should be determined. If OSA is present, treatment plans may change based on severity. In addition, the presence of OSA mandates different follow-up.
- Treatment with an OA is indicated for patients with primary snoring (when patients do not respond to weight loss or the side sleep position).
- Although not as efficacious as CPAP, OAs are indicated for use in patients with **mild to moderate OSA** who prefer OAs to CPAP, do not respond to CPAP, are not appropriate candidates for CPAP, or fail treatment attempts with CPAP or treatment with behavioral measures such as weight loss or sleep position change.
- OAs are **not** indicated for initial treatment of **severe OSA**. Positive airway pressure is the treatment of choice for patients with severe OSA. Upper airway surgery may also supersede use of OA in patients for whom surgery is predicted to be highly effective.
- OA devices include MRAs and tongue retaining/stabilizing devices. The effectiveness of MRAs is better documented and, at least some studies suggest, better tolerated by patients.
- Adjustable custom-fitted MRAs are preferred over monobloc (boil and bite appliances).
- A qualified dentist should evaluate potential OA treatment candidates for suitability of OA treatment from the dental standpoint, supervise appliance fitting and adjustment, and see patients for long-term follow-up to determine whether adverse changes in dentition have occurred due to OA treatment.
- Follow-up sleep testing after optimal OA adjustment is NOT indicated for treatment of **primary snoring** but is indicated for treatment of **all severities of OSA**. Sleep testing may include a PSG, an attended type 3 home sleep test, or unattended type 3 home sleep test (airflow, effort, saturation, pulse, or electrocardiogram).
- Follow-up with the treating clinician is needed to assess the patient for signs and symptoms of worsening OSA. If worsening is suspected, repeat sleep testing with the OA in place is indicated.
- The presence and severity of OSA must be determined before initiating any type of upper airway surgical treatment for presumed snoring.
- Before undergoing surgery, patients should be advised of potential success rates and complications as well as treatment alternatives.
- Tracheostomy is the only surgery uniformly effective for severe OSA, although some series suggest MMA may be 45% to 85% effective depending on how surgical success is defined.
- MMA is indicated for initial treatment of severe OSA in patients who cannot tolerate or are unwilling to adhere to PAP therapy and in whom OAs have been considered and found ineffective or undesirable.
- UPPP does not reliably normalize the AHI in patients with moderate to severe OSA. Patients with severe OSA should be offered PAP treatment. Patients with moderate OSA should initially be offered PAP therapy or an OA.
- A PSG is recommended before TNA in children to determine whether OSA is present and to determine the severity. A PSG after TNA is recommended for patients with persistent symptoms of OSA. Many clinicians recommended a post-treatment PSG in children with moderate to severe OSA before TNA (AHI 5–10 or > 10/hr, respectively).

ORAL APPLIANCE TREATMENT FOR OSA

ORAL APPLIANCES

An oral appliance (OA) can be defined as a device inserted into the mouth for treatment of snoring or obstructive sleep apnea (OSA).[1-5] There are two main types, the tongue retaining (stabilizing) device (TRD/TSD)[6-9] (Fig. 20–1) and the mandibular repositioning appliances (MRAs) (Figs. 20–2 to 20–4). The TSD/TRDs hold the tongue in a forward position by retaining the tongue in a suction bulb.[6-9] The MRAs are attached to the dental arches and provide variable degrees of bite opening and mandibular advancement. The MRAs are also called *mandibular advancing devices (MADs)* or *mandibular repositioning devices (MRDs)*. MRAs can come in monobloc (boil and bit) fixed configurations or custom-fitted appliances that can be adjusted to change the amount of mandibular protrusion (advancement).

Evaluation of the Patient

Each candidate for an OA should be examined by a qualified dentist to determine whether an OA is feasible and safe from a dental standpoint. The dental examination should focus on

FIGURE 20–1 **Left,** Tongue retaining device (TRD). **Right,** Tongue stabilizing device (TSD). The TRD is fabricated for each patient whereas the TSD comes in three standard sizes (small, medium, and large).

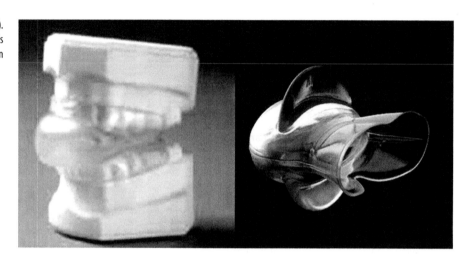

FIGURE 20–2 A Herbst appliance. The side arms allow adjustment of the amount of mandibular protrusion. *From Berry RB: Sleep Medicine Pearls. 2nd ed. Philadelphia: Hanley & Belfus, 2003, p. 175.*

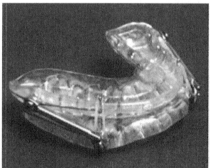
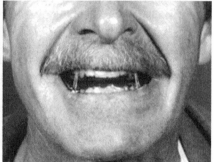

Herbst appliance

FIGURE 20–3 The patient is shown with and without the Herbst appliance. The appliance moves the chin noticeably forward.

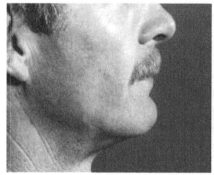
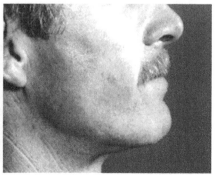

Before   Herbst appliance

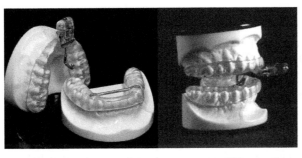
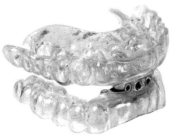

FIGURE 20–4 Versions of the Thornton anterior positioner (TAP) oral appliance, which consists of two separate arches connected by an advancing mechanism. **Left two panels,** The adjustment apparatus extends outward from the maxillary arch. This is turned to change the amount of protrusion of the mandible by moving the hook which pulls the bar forward. **Right,** TAP-3 appliance; key is used to advance the mandibular arch.

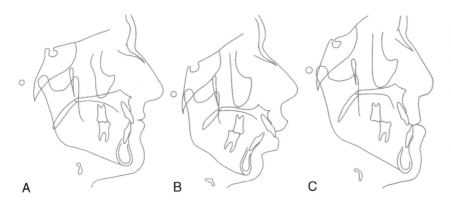

A   B   C

FIGURE 20–5 Lateral cephalometric views of three distinct skeletal occlusions. **A,** A skeletal class I occlusion. There is nearly ideal and dental balance. **B,** A skeletal class II malocclusion (overjet, or retrognathia). There is mandibular deficiency. Note the everted lower lip and distance between the upper and the lower incisors. **C,** A skeletal class III occlusion with mandibular hyperplasia and maxillary hypoplasia (or prognathia). The upper incisor is behind the lower incisor. *A–C, From Conely RS: Orthodontic considerations related to sleep disordered breathing. Sleep Med Clin 2009;5:80.*

the temporomandibular joint (TMJ), evidence or history of bruxism, quality of dental occlusion, the presence of significant periodontal disease, overall dental health, and protrusive ability. Cephalometrics or dental radiographs may be indicated.[10] The patient's occlusion type should be noted. Three classes (types) of skeletal occlusions are illustrated in Figure 20–5. One might expect that patients with mandibular deficiency (retrognathia) would benefit the most from an OA but the amount of improvement is somewhat unpredictable. The location of airway occlusion during sleep might also be expected to predict the response to OA treatment. Patients with occlusion mainly in the retroglossal area rather than the retropalatal area might be expected to improve the most with a MRA. However, in one study, some patients with upper airway occlusion mainly in the velopharynx also improved with MRA treatment.[11]

Exclusions and Contraindications

Patients must have a minimal amount of healthy teeth for an MRA. A minimum of 6 to 10 teeth in each arch is needed.[1,5] However, treatment with dental implants can permit future MRA treatment in patients with insufficient dentition at the time of evaluation. Patients must be able to open the jaw adequately for OA insertion and must have the ability to voluntarily protrude the mandible. Moderate to severe TMJ disease or inadequate protrusive ability are contraindications. Mild TMJ dysfunction may actually improve with the

jaw positioned anteriorly during sleep. Moderate to severe bruxism is also a contraindication in most cases. Bruxism during sleep can actually damage some types of OAs. However, bruxism in some patients improves with adequate treatment of OSA. An experienced dental practitioner should evaluate patients with bruxism for suitability for an OA. A history of bruxism may also alter the choice of the type of OA used. Of note, edentulous patients can be treated with a TRD/TSD.

Mechanism of Action of OAs

OAs are believed to work by increasing upper airway size. TRDs/TSDs move the tongue forward. MRAs move the tongue and mandible forward, increasing the posterior airspace. By stabilizing the mandibular position, MRAs resist the downward rotation of the mandible with sleep and the accompanying retrusion of the mandible. They may also tense palatal muscles. Some studies have found an increase in upper airway muscle tone with an MRA in place.[12] As noted previously, patients with airway closure mainly in the velopharynx may also respond to OA treatment. In agreement with this finding, a study of the effect of an MRA on upper airway size during wakefulness using fiberoptic endoscopy found the most significant increase in airway size was at the velopharynx.[13] Another study of videofluoroscopy during sleep found increases in both the retroglossal and the retropalatal airway size during sleep with an MRA in place.[14]

Effectiveness

A number of studies (some controlled) have demonstrated that OA devices are effective in reducing the apnea-hypopnea index (AHI) in mild, moderate, and severe OSA.[1,2] However, because OAs are less effective than continuous positive airway pressure (CPAP) in reducing the AHI to less than 10/hr, CPAP is considered the treatment of choice for moderate to severe OSA. American Academy of Sleep Medicine (AASM) practice parameters[2] state that OAs are indicated for treatment of mild and moderate OSA as well as snoring. The practice parameters also state that OAs can be used in severe OSA, although generally considered a third-line treatment after positive airway pressure (PAP) and surgery. A summary of effectiveness in a systematic review of OAs published in 2006 is listed in Table 20–1. Although results differed considerably between studies, OA treatment was found to be successful in about 50% of patients with mild to moderate OSA (using an AHI < 10/hr as the definition of success).[1] Of note, some patients with severe OSA can have an impressive reduction in the AHI, although rarely to a value less than 10/hr (Fig. 20–6).

Studies have also documented that OA treatment improves both subjective and objective sleepiness. Using a controlled cross-over design (OA without protrusion as control), Gotsopoulos and coworkers[15] found significant improvement in the subjective sleepiness (Epworth Sleepiness Scale decreased from 9 to 7) and objective sleepiness as assessed by the multiple sleep latency test (mean sleep latency increased from 9.1 to 10.3 min).

Factors Predicting Effectiveness

Four variables appear to contribute to the degree of effectiveness of OA treatment of OSA.[1,16,17] These include (1) the severity of the OSA, (2) amount of protrusion by the MRA, (3) the presence or absence of positional sleep apnea, and (4) the body mass index (BMI).[1] The degree of protrusion of the mandible with MRAs varies typically from 6 to 10 mm or from 50% to 75% of the maximum the patient can voluntarily protrude the mandible on request. One study using the same OA with different protrusions found a reduced AHI with greater protrusion.[16] Positional OSA defined as a supine AHI > 2 × lateral AHI predicts that OA will be more effective[1,17] (Fig. 20–7). OA treatment also is more effective in mild to moderate OSA (better chance of treatment AHI falling in acceptable range). They also appear to be more effective in the less obese patient.

Devices

The TSD is manufactured in three prefabricated sizes (small, medium, and large), whereas TRDs are custom-fitted to each patient. The patient inserts the tongue into the device and gently pumps the bulb to apply suction. Once the tongue is inserted, the bulb is released and the tongue is held forward by suction. One study found the TSD to significantly reduce the AHI, although not quite as well as an MRA.[9] In addition, the TSD had a lower compliance rate and was more likely to

TABLE 20–1		
Range of Effectiveness of Oral Appliances*		
	MILD TO MODERATE OSA	**SEVERE OSA**
OA success	57–81%	14–61%

*Success is defined as a reduction of the AHI to < 10/hr.
AHI = apnea-hypopnea index; OA = oral appliance; OSA = obstructive sleep apnea.
From Ferguson KA, Cartwright R, Rogers R, et al: Oral appliances for snoring and obstructive sleep apnea: a review. Sleep 2006;29:244–262.

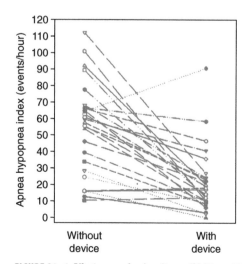
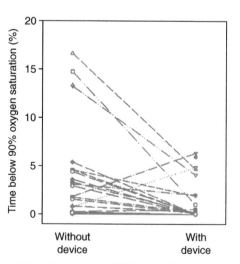

FIGURE 20–6　Effectiveness of oral appliances (OAs) in a wide range of obstructive sleep apnea (OSA) patients. Note that some patients with severe OSA had dramatic falls in the apnea-hypopnea index (AHI) and improvement in the arterial oxygen saturation (SaO_2). *From Henke KG, Frantz DE, Kuna ST: An oral mandibular advancement device for obstructive sleep apnea. Am J Respir Crit Care Med 2000;161:423.*

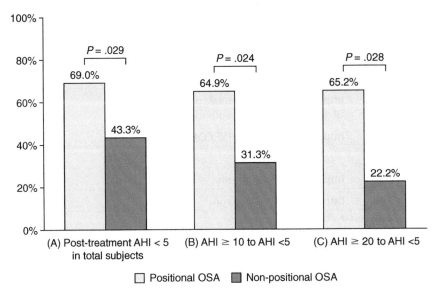

☐ Positional OSA ■ Non-positional OSA

FIGURE 20-7 Effectiveness of OAs on positional and nonpositional obstructive sleep apnea (OSA). Positional OSA was defined as patients with an apnea-hypopnea index [AHI] supine > 2 × AHI nonsupine. **A,** Percentage of ALL positional and nonpositional patients with a post-treatment AHI < 5/hr. **B,** Considering only patients with a pretreatment AHI ≥ 10/hr, the percentage of positional and nonpositional patients with a post-treatment AHI < 5/hr. That is, "AHI ≥ 10 to < 5/hr." **C,** Considering only patients with a pretreatment AHI ≥ 20/hr, the percentage of positional and nonpositional patients with a post-treatment AHI < 5/hr is shown. For the entire group and those with moderate and severe OSA, the OA was more effective in positional than in nonpositional OSA. Note that the presence or absence of positional OSA was most important in patients with a high pretreatment AHI **(C)**. *From Chung JW, Enciso R, Levendowski DJ, et al: Treatment outcomes of mandibular advancement devices in positional and nonpositional OSA patients. Oral Surg Oral Med Oral Pathol Oral Radiol Endod 2010;109:724–731.*

TABLE 20-2	
Attributes of an Ideal Oral Appliance	
ATTRIBUTE	**COMMENT**
Adjustable	Allows for modification if dental work is needed.
Titratable	Ability to modify vertical opening or advancement of mandible.
Full tooth coverage	Makes certain upper and lower teeth are fully engaged to prevent tooth movement.
Posterior support	The upper and lower components should have contact in the posterior area for stabilization of TMJ.
Mandibular mobility	Allows free movement of mandible during sleep—beneficial in patients with bruxism.
Adequate lip seal	Improves nasal breathing, prevents drying of teeth.
Adequate tongue space	Prevents collapse of tongue into oropharyngeal airway.

TMJ = temporomandibular joint.
Adapted from Bailey DR, Hoekema A: Oral appliance therapy in sleep medicine. Sleep Med Clin 2010;5:91–98.

come out during the night. However, the TSD (see Fig. 20–1) may be an affordable alternative for some patients. Purchase of a TSD requires a prescription from a doctor or dentist (approximate price range is $125–$180).

Some ideal attributes for an MRA are listed in Table 20–2. The ideal device has coverage of both arches and is adjustable (protrusion can be changed). A recent study compared a custom-made and thermoplastic OA for the treatment of mild OSA. The custom-made device was more effective.[18] However, custom-made devices are typically much more expensive. OAs are now viewed by the U.S. Food and Drug Administration (FDA) as class 2 medical devices and, as such, must adhere to more detailed standards with special controls.[19] A short list of commonly used devices is presented in Table 20–3. A more extensive list is available in Reference 5. A list of FDA-approved devices can be found at http://www.accessdata.fda.gov/scripts/cdrh/cfdocs/cfPMN/pmn.cfm

Titration/Adjustment of OAs

After OAs are fabricated, they are usually adjusted by the dentist taking care of the patient for fit and comfort. Patients are then instructed to slowly increase mandibular protrusion until symptoms improve (cessation of snoring and improvement in sleep quality) or until either the maximum protrusion is reached or further advances are not tolerated. In one study, patients were studied during polysomnography (PSG) and a remotely controlled mandibular appliance was advanced until respiratory events were controlled or until further advances were not tolerated.[20] The results of the PSG OA titration were highly predictive of the effectiveness of chronic OA treatment with a permanent device. In another study, patients were allowed to adjust their devices at home.[21] During a PSG if persistent events were noted, further adjustment during the PSG was performed by protocol (increased protrusion in 1-mm increments). Of the patients completing the protocol, 55% were successfully treated (AHI < 10/hr) after home titration. A total of 64.9% of patients were successfully treated overall. **Thus, some patients will likely need further adjustments either during or after a PSG documenting the efficacy of OA treatment.**

Adherence to OA Treatment

Studies of adherence to OA treatment have almost always relied on patient report. There is a single report of the use

TABLE 20-3

Selected Oral Appliances

DEVICE	TELEPHONE NUMBER	WEBSITE
Tongue retaining device	800-828-7626	
Tongue stabilizing device	800-854-7256 (United States)	http://www.glidewelldental.com Glidewell Dental is the authorized U.S. dealer.
TAP	866-AMI-SNOR	http://www.TAPINTOSLEEP.COM
SUAD Herbst	888-447-6673	
Klearway	800-828-7626	http://www.klearway.com
OASYS	888-866-2727	http://www.oasyssleep.com

FDA = U.S. Food and Drug Administration; OASYS = oral/nasal airway system; TAP = Thornton anterior positioner.
After Bailey DR, Hoekema A: Oral appliance therapy in sleep medicine. Sleep Med Clin 2010;5:91–98.
See complete list on FDA website: **http://www.accessdata.fda.gov/scripts/cdrh/cfdocs/cfPMN/pmn.cfm**

TABLE 20-4

Comparison of Oral Appliance and Continuous Positive Airway Pressure

AUTHOR	TOTAL NO. N	AHI BASELINE	AHI CPAP	AHI MRA	ESS BASELINE	ESS CPAP	ESS MRA	RX SUCCESS CPAP	RX SUCCESS MRA	CRITERION (AHI#/hr)
Barnes, 2004[27]	104	21.3 ± 12.8	4.8 ± 4.7	14.0 ± 10.1	10.2 ± 4.7	9.2 ± 3.8	9.2 ± 3.7	Not stated	49%	<10
Clark, 1996[28]	23	33.9 ± 14.3	11.2 ± 3.9	19.9 ± 12.8				52%	19%	<10
Engleman, 2002[29]	51	31 ± 26	8 ± 6	15 ± 16	14 ± 4	8 ± 5	12 ± 5	66%	47%	<10
Ferguson, 1997[25]	24	26.8 ± 11.9	4.2 ± 2.2	13.6 ± 14.5	10.7 ± 3.4	5.1 ± 3.3	4.7 ± 2.6	70%	55%	<10 + SI
Ferguson, 1996[26]	25	24.5 ± 8.8	3.6 ± 1.7	9.7 ± 7.3				62%	48%	<10 + SI
Randerath, 2002[30]	20	17.5 ± 7.7	3.2 ± 2.9	13.8 ± 11.1				100%	30%	<10
Tan, 2002[31]	24	22.2 ± 9.6	31. ± 2.8	8.0 ± 10.9	13.4 ± 4.6	8.1 ± 4.1	9.2 ± 1	Not stated	67%	<10

AHI = apnea-hypopnea index; CPAP = continuous positive airway pressure; ESS = Epworth Sleepiness Scale; MRA = mandibular repositioning appliance; SI = symptoms improved.
From Ferguson KA, Cartwright R, Rogers R, et al: Oral appliances for snoring and obstructive sleep apnea: a review. Sleep 2006;29:244–262.

of a temperature-sensitive embedded monitor to objectively determine OA use.[13] OA adherence rates tend to decrease with the duration of use. One study reported 60% adherence at 1 year and 48% at 2 years.[22] Another study reported adherence dropped from 82% to 62% over 4 years.[23] The reasons for discontinuing OA included side effects, complications, and lack of efficacy. In a questionnaire study of OA patients 5 years after starting treatment, 64% of respondents were using the OA. Of these, 93% were using the OA more than 4 nights/wk. Of those stopping OA treatment, the causes were discomfort (44%), little or no effect (34%), and the patient changing to CPAP treatment (23%).[24] In two crossover studies of CPAP, adherence to OA was equal to or better than to CPAP.[25,26]

Effectiveness Compared with Other Treatments

A number of studies have compared OA and CPAP (Table 20-4).[25-31] They show that OAs are not as effective as CPAP but are effective in a significant proportion of patients

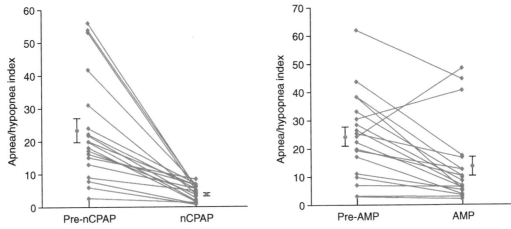

FIGURE 20–8   The AHI as determined by home monitoring before and after treatment with nasal continuous positive airway pressure (nCPAP; **left**) and an anterior mandibular positioner (AMP; **right**). The AHI was significantly reduced (P < .05) by both devices, although the posttreatment AHI was lower with nCPAP. *From Ferguson KA, Ono T, Lowe AA, et al: A short-term controlled trial of an adjustable oral appliance for the treatment of mild to moderate obstructive sleep apnoea. Thorax 1997;52:362–368.*

(19–67%) (Fig. 20–8).[1] In some studies listed in Table 20–4, a significant proportion of patients preferred the OA to CPAP. In some studies, improvement in daytime sleepiness was similar with both OA and CPAP treatment even if the AHI was higher with OA than with CPAP. In the study by Barnes and colleagues[27] using a cross-over design, 28% preferred CPAP, 41% preferred the OA, and 31% preferred placebo (a tablet). In a study by Ferguson and associates,[25] the compliance to an OA and CPAP were similar but patient satisfaction was better with an OA.

OA Treatment Guidelines

The AASM practice parameters for the OA treatment of patients with snoring and OSA[2] are listed in Appendix 20–1. The guidelines are summarized in Boxes 20–1 and 20–2. The presence or absence of OSA must be determined before OA treatment. It is important to determine whether OSA or snoring is being treated. If OSA is present, the severity has implications for treatment selection and the probability of success with OA. The OA should be fitted by a qualified dental professional. The treatment goals for snoring are to reduce noise to an acceptable level. For OSA, treatment goals are to reduce the AHI, improve oxygenation, and improve sleep quality. OAs are indicated for primary snoring that does not respond to simple measures such as weight loss, lateral position, and treatment of nasal congestion. OAs are also indicated for mild to moderate OSA. It is acknowledged that CPAP may be more effective. CPAP rather than OA should be the first treatment for severe OSA. If CPAP is not accepted, upper airway surgery or an OA should be considered. Upper airway surgery may also supersede use of OA in patients for whom surgery is predicted to be highly effective. In patients with severe OSA who decline CPAP or surgery, a trial of OA may be reasonable. Another indication for OA would be patients who had failed surgery and do not want CPAP or further surgery.

BOX 20–1

OA Treatment Guidelines

1. **Initial diagnosis:** Presence or absence of OSA must be determined before OA treatment.
2. **Appliance fitting:** OA treatment should be managed by dental practitioners with training in sleep medicine and sleep-related breathing disorders.
3. Cephalometrics are not always needed, but if used, qualified professionals should perform and evaluate.
4. **Primary snoring**—Goal of OA is to reduce snoring to a subjectively acceptable level.
5. **OSA**—Goals of treatment are resolution of clinical signs and symptoms of OSA, and normalization of the AHI and arterial oxygen saturation.
6. OAs are indicated for treatment of **primary snoring** in patients who do not respond to or are not appropriate candidates for weight loss or sleep position change.
7. OA treatment is indicated for **mild to moderate OSA**
   a. OA is not as efficacious as CPAP but is preferred by some patients.
   b. OA is indicated with CPAP failures.
   c. OA treatment is indicated when there is failure of weight loss or side sleep position treatments for mild OSA.
8. OAs are not indicated for **initial** treatment of severe OSA. Upper airway surgery may also supersede use of OA in patients for whom surgery is predicted to be highly effective.

AHI = apnea-hypopnea index; CPAP = continuous positive airway pressure; OA = oral appliance; OSA = obstructive sleep apnea.

Adjustment of OA is usually preformed over days to weeks with progressive protrusion until obvious apnea and snoring have ceased or the limit of the device or patient tolerance is reached. A study can then be performed to assess efficacy. As noted in a later section, documentation of efficacy with some type of sleep study is indicated for **any level**

BOX 20–2

Follow-up after Oral Appliance Treatment
1. Follow-up sleep testing is **not** indicated after OA treatment of primary snoring. 2. Follow-up sleep testing with the OA in place **is indicated** after final adjustments of fit have been performed. • All OSA severities. • PSG or *attended* type III cardiopulmonary test (PM) (recent PM guidelines stated unattended portable monitoring PM "may be indicated" for this purpose). 3. Follow-up visits with dental specialist until optimal fit and efficacy are shown. 4. Follow-up dental visits every 6 months for first year, and annually thereafter. 5. Regular visits with clinician supervising treatment of OSA. 6. Repeat sleep study with OA in place if signs or symptoms of OSA worsen or recur.
OA = oral appliance; OSA = obstructive sleep apnea; PM = portable monitoring; PSG = polysomnography.

of OSA severity. For snoring alone, subjective improvement may suffice.

Follow-up

The practice parameters do not mandate repeat sleep testing for OA treatment of snoring. For **all severities of OSA,** repeat sleep testing with the patient wearing the OA is indicated to document effectiveness (see Box 20–2).[2] The practice parameters state either PSG or an attended type 3 cardiopulmonary test is acceptable to assess the efficacy of OA treatment. Recent clinical guidelines for portable monitoring (PM) also state that unattended PM "may be indicated" to determine the adequacy of non-PAP treatment.[32] In fact, either unattended cardiopulmonary monitoring or attended PSG is usually used to determine the effectiveness of OA treatment. Follow-up visits with the dentist who fabricated the OA device are also indicated every 6 months, then yearly. This is to ensure side effects are not significant and the amount of protrusion is optimized. Follow-up with the clinician directing sleep apnea treatment is also indicated to be certain OSA symptoms are controlled and do not recur. **If symptoms return while the patient is using the OA, repeat sleep testing with OA in place is indicated.**

Centers for Medicaid and Medicare Services Coverage of OA Treatment

The Centers for Medicaid and Medicare Services (CMS) has recognized certain types of OAs as reasonable and necessary for treatment of OSA. The criteria for reimbursement have been published in the form of local carrier determinations (LCDs) by Durable Medical Administrative Contractors (DMACs). An excerpt from one LCD is listed in Appendix

BOX 20–3

Side Effects of Oral Appliance
1. Minor and temporary a. Excessive salivation b. Tooth pain c. TMJ tenderness d. Tongue pain (TSD/TRD) 2. Chronic and more severe a. Tooth movement b. TMJ dysfunction/pain c. Gum disease d. Dry mouth
TMJ = temporomandibular joint; TRD = tongue retaining device; TSD = tongue stabilizing device.

20–2. Only custom-fabricated mandibular advancement OA (E0486) devices are covered. Coverage requires a face-to-face clinical evaluation prior to a Medicare-covered sleep test. The patient must meet one of the following criteria: (1) AHI ≥ 15/hr or respiratory disturbance index (RDI; events/hr of monitoring time using a home sleep test) ≥ 15/hr or a minimum of 30 events, (2) AHI (RDI) values 5 to ≤ 14 with certain symptoms or disorders (see Appendix 20–2), AHI > 30 or RDI > 30 if the patient cannot tolerate a PAP device or if the treating physician feels PAP treatment is contraindicated. Note that testing for diagnosis cannot be performed by the person or organization supplying the OA. The OA device must be ordered by the treating physician following review of the report of the sleep test. The device is provided and billed for/by a licensed dentist (DDS or DMD). Custom-fabricated devices that work by positioning of the tongue (E1399) or a prefabricated OA (E0485) are not covered.

Side Effects and Complications

The available research suggests that side effects and complications (Box 20–3) may be grouped as follows: (1) minor and temporary side effects and (2) moderate to severe and continuous side effects.

1. Minor and temporary side effects: These can occur at any stage during treatment, are minor in severity, tend to resolve in a short period of time, or are easily tolerated if they do not resolve and they do not prevent regular use of the appliance. Commonly reported minor and temporary side effects included TMJ pain, myofascial pain, tooth pain, excessive salivation, TMJ sounds, dry mouth, gum irritation, and morning-after occlusal changes. These phenomena were observed in a wide range of frequencies from 6% to 86% of patients.[1] Patients undergoing TRD and TSD treatments may report a sore tongue or difficulty with the device slipping off during the night.
2. Moderate to severe and continuous side effects: These can occur at any stage during treatment, are moderate to severe in intensity, tend not to resolve over time, and may

result in discontinuation of appliance use. More severe and continuous side effects included TMJ pain, myofascial pain, tongue pain (tongue devices only), gagging (soft palate lifter mostly), tooth pain, gum pain, dry mouth, and salivation.[1] Occasionally, these phenomena prevent continued use of the appliance. Several studies have found long-term changes in dental occlusion but the results vary between studies. The changes are relatively mild in most patients. One study found occlusal changes after a mean treatment duration of about 30 months.[33] The anteroposterior position of the molars and the inclination of upper and lower incisors changed with MRA treatment. No skeletal changes in mandibular position were noted.

Combinations of OA with Other Treatments

Use of OA in patients with persistent sleep apnea after uvulopalatopharyngoplasty (UPPP) was reported by Millman and coworkers[34] in 18 patients. The post UPPP AHI was 37.2/hr and the arterial oxygen saturation (SaO₂) nadir was 84%. With OA treatment, the AHI fell to 15.3/hr and the SaO₂ nadir was 87.9%. With the addition of a Herbst device, 10 of the patients had a fall in the AHI to less than 10/hr.

Effects of OA Treatment on Consequences of OSA

There have been few studies of the effects of OA treatment of OSA on the cardiovascular consequences of OSA. Gotsopoulos and colleagues[35] found that OAs reduced blood pressure in a randomized, controlled trial. Another study found an improvement (normalization) of heart rate variability after 3 months of OA treatment.[36] More studies of the impact of OAs are expected in the future.

SURGICAL TREATMENTS FOR OSA

Tracheostomy was the first treatment available for OSA.[37] Since that time, a number of surgical options have become available (Box 20–4).[38–41] These are more acceptable than tracheostomy but none is more effective. Recently, a systematic review of surgical treatment options for treatment of OSA in adults and practice parameters have been published by the AASM (Appendix 20–3).[40,41]

Evaluation for Possible Surgical Treatment

The typical evaluation of patients with snoring or OSA for possible upper airway surgery includes fiberoptic examination of the nose, pharynx, and hypopharynx.[42] Fiberoptic pharyngoscopy while the patient performs a Müller maneuver (inspiration with the nose occluded) is performed to help identify the most prominent site of collapse (retropalatal or retroglossal/hypopharyngeal area). A limitation of this technique, which is typically performed during wakefulness and often in an upright posture, is that the results may not correspond to what happens during supine sleep. Lateral cephalometric radiographs are also standard and can help visualize bony abnormalities and the posterior airspace. On cephalometrics, OSA patients tend to have long soft palates, small posterior air spaces (<10 mm behind the tongue), mandibular deficiency, and a long distance to the hyoid. **The AASM practice parameters for surgical treatment of OSA mandate that all patients scheduled for surgery to correct snoring or OSA should undergo PSG for diagnosis and to assess severity.**[39,41]

Indications for Surgical Treatment

The AASM practice parameters for surgical treatment of OSA have recently been updated[40,41] (see Appendix 20–3). The practice parameters state that the presence and severity of OSA must be determined before initiating surgical therapy. The patient should be advised about the success of surgical procedures and side effects as well as the success rate of alternative treatments. The practice parameters state that PAP should first be offered to patients with severe OSA and either PAP or an OA for patients with moderate OSA.[41] For those requiring the stepped procedure approach, patients should be informed that multiple surgical procedures may be needed.[39]

Surgical Options

A number of surgical options are available (see Box 20–4).[38–48] Each is briefly discussed and then an overall approach is presented.

Tracheostomy

This procedure bypasses all obstructions and is uniformly effective at preventing upper airway obstruction.[37–41] Some patients will still require supplemental oxygen, and some patients with the obesity hypoventilation syndrome may continue to hypoventilate during sleep or require oxygen for persistent nocturnal desaturation. The main use of tracheostomy is for patients who have life-threatening OSA (often the obesity hypoventilation syndrome with recurrent hypercapnic respiratory failure) and are poorly adherent to PAP treatment. Another use is as a temporary measure while patients

BOX 20–4

Surgical Options
BYPASSES ALL OBSTRUCTION
Tracheostomy
SELECTIVELY IMPROVES UPPER AIRWAY OBSTRUCTION
Nasal reconstruction UPPP and LAUP Genioglossus advancement Hyoid advancement MMA Temperature-controlled RF tongue base reduction
LAUP = laser-assisted uvuloplasty; MMA = maxillomandibular advancement; RF = radiofrequency; UPPP = uvulopalatopharyngoplasty.

recover from other upper airway surgery. Tracheostomy is cosmetically unacceptable to most patients. The indications used in one large series included (1) disabling sleepiness with severe consequences, (2) cardiac arrhythmias with sleep apnea, (3) cor pulmonale, (4) AHI > 40/hr, (5) frequent desaturations below 40%, and (6) no improvement after other therapy.[37] Recent AASM practice parameters state that tracheostomy has been found to be an effective single intervention.[41] However, this "operation should be considered only when other options do not exist, have failed, are refused, or when this operation is deemed necessary by clinical urgency." Tracheostomy has significant complications in patients with OSA.[37,43] For example, anesthesia and intubation tend to be more difficult in patients with large necks and narrow upper airways. Postoperative complications include stoma infection/granulation tissue, accidental decannulation, obstruction of the tube when the head is turned or hyperextended, recurrent purulent bronchitis, and psychosocial difficulties (depression).[37-39,43] Noncuffed, size 6 French tubes usually suffice. A longer-than-usual tracheostomy tube may be needed for very obese patients with thick necks. The end of the tracheostomy tube typically is plugged during the day and, because of its small size, air flows around it between the lungs and the upper airway. If resistance to flow around the tube is a problem, a fenestrated tube (hole at bend of the superior end of the tube) may be used. During sleep, the tracheostomy tube is unplugged to bypass the upper airway obstruction. However, one must not forget that very obese patients can still occlude the tracheostomy opening with "triple chins."

Nasal Obstruction

Nasal obstruction can lead to mouth breathing during sleep. This causes rotation of the mandible and retrodisplacement of the tongue base back into the pharynx. The major areas of focus include the nasal valve/alar cartilage area, septum, and turbinates (mostly inferior turbinates). One study found that radiofrequency ablation (RFA) of turbinate hypertrophy can improve nasal CPAP adherence in selected patients.[49] Long-term studies are needed to better define the indications for this procedure. A randomized, controlled trial of nasal surgery (vs. placebo surgery) found improvement in the amount of nasal breathing during sleep (less mouth breathing) but minimal effects on the AHI. The surgeries include resection of the deviated nasal septum and submucous

resection of the inferior turbinates.[50] A review of the role of the nose in the pathogenesis of OSA and snoring found no published evidence to support the use of nasal surgery (correction of septal deviation or external valve collapse) as a treatment of OSA.[51] Thus, whereas nasal surgery can improve the quality of life for some patients, it is considered as an adjunctive rather than a primary treatment for OSA.

Palatal Implants

The Pillar procedure involves insertion of Teflon strips into the palate and can be done in the office or outpatient surgery center. The purpose of the strips is to stiffen the palate (reduced snoring). The success is variable and sometimes additional strip insertion is needed.[40,54-56] A randomized, placebo-controlled study (sham implant procedure as control) of palatal implants (PIs) in mild OSA found that the AHI in both placebo and PI groups actually increased![53] Although the increase in the AHI was significantly less with PI compared with control, this can hardly be seen as documentation of PI effectiveness. Snoring was slightly but significantly improved more with PI than with control. Although the evidence that palatal implant surgery is effective in patients with OSA is very marginal, recent practice parameters stated "Palatal implants may be effective in some patients with mild OSA who cannot tolerate or are unwilling to adhere to PAP therapy, or in whom oral appliances have been considered and found ineffective or undesirable (Option)."[41] Thus, PIs may be effective in some patients with mild OSA but results are variable at best.

Laser-Assisted Uvuloplasty

Laser-assisted palatoplasty or uvuloplasty (LAP or LAUP) was introduced recently as a treatment for snoring.[46,54-56] In this procedure, only a small portion of the uvula/soft palate is removed (Fig. 20–9). Usually two trenches on either side of the uvula are cut. Some also remove the end of the uvula. With time and scarring, the palate stiffens and elevates. This procedure can be done on an outpatient basis using local anesthesia. It is generally considered a treatment for snoring but has been used for very mild sleep apnea when suitable upper airway anatomy exists. The long-term efficacy of LAP remains to be established. The standard of practice committee of the AASM was unable to recommend this procedure for sleep apnea based on the current published evidence in

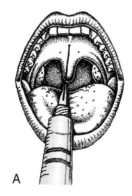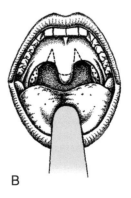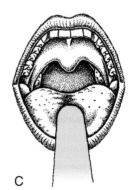

FIGURE 20–9 Laser uvulopalatoplasty. **A,** Local anesthetic is injected. **B,** The CO$_2$ laser is used to excise vertical trenches of the soft palate on either aspect of the uvula up to the muscular sling. Thirty percent to 90% of the uvula is excised or vaporized. **C,** The postoperative result necessitates 4 to 5 weeks for complete healing and scarring to production traction forces to improve airway patency. *A–C, From Li KK, Powell NB, Riley RW: Surgical management of OSA. In Lee-Chiong TL, Sateia MJ, Carskadon MA (eds): Sleep Medicine. Philadelphia: Hanley & Belfus, 2002, p. 439, reproduced with permission.*

A   B   C

2001.[54] Recent practice parameters for surgical treatment of OSA state "LAUP is not routinely recommended as a treatment for obstructive sleep apnea syndrome (Standard)."[41]

Radiofrequency Ablation

Radiofrequency has been used in the upper airway with and without temperature control of the probe tip. RFA has been used for treatment of the soft palate, base of the tongue, and treatment of multiple levels.[40,46,47,56] Somnoplasty (a variant of RFA) is a method of palatoplasty for treatment of snoring, appears to be well tolerated (possibly less pain), but is no more effective than traditional UPPP.[40,56] It can be performed as an outpatient procedure. Repeated treatments may be needed. Several other procedures that utilize cautery or injection of sclerotic agents to stiffen the palate have also been used.[46] The recent practice parameters for surgical treatment of OSA state "RFA can be considered as a treatment in patients with mild to moderate OSA who cannot tolerate or who are unwilling to adhere to PAP, or in whom oral appliances have been considered and have been found ineffective or undesirable (Option)." RFA of the palate is not more effective than traditional UPPP.

Uvulopalatopharyngoplasty

UPPP is an operation that removes residual tonsillar tissue, the uvula, a portion of the soft palate, and redundant tissue from the pharyngeal area (Fig. 20–10).[46–48,57] Its disadvantages include the need for general anesthesia and considerable postoperative pain. The most frequent complication (Box 20–5) is velopharyngeal insufficiency, which is manifested as some degree of nasal reflux when drinking fluids.[58–60] This usually resolves within a month of surgery. Other potential complications include voice change, postoperative bleeding, nasopharyngeal stenosis (secondary to scarring), or a persistent globus sensation. A few cases of severe postsurgical bleeding or upper airway obstruction requiring reintubation have been reported. It is prudent to admit patients to the intensive care unit after surgery for close observation if significant OSA is present. Significant apnea and desaturation

can occur during the recovery period in patients with severe OSA. These problems often can be managed with nasal CPAP.

However, the major problem with UPPP is less-than-perfect efficacy as a treatment for OSA.[40,41,61] UPPP does not address airway narrowing behind the tongue or in the hypopharynx; therefore, it is not universally effective in preventing sleep apnea. UPPP is generally reasonably effective in decreasing the incidence or loudness of snoring (vibration of the soft palate). In general, 40% to 50% of all patients undergoing UPPP have about a 50% decrease in their AHI, to less than 20/hr, or about a 30% chance of a postoperative AHI dropping below 10/hr.[38,40,60,61] The results will, of course, depend on the presurgery AHI and the locations of upper airway obstruction. Frequently, the number of apneas decreases and the number of hypopneas increases after UPPP. Of interest, one study of UPPP failures found the site of upper airway obstruction to still occur at the retropalatal area.[62] Sasse and associates[63] reported on a group of patients in whom the AHI was actually higher after UPPP. Another study reported that a significant number of initial responders

BOX 20–5

Complications from Uvulopalatopharyngoplasty
IMMEDIATE
Pain—can be severe
Velopharyngeal incompetence (fluid out the nose during swallowing)
Voice change
Globus sensation—"mucus in the back of the throat"
Worsening of apnea in the postoperative period
DELAYED
Return of snoring
Worsening of OSA
Nasopharyngeal stenosis
Increased probability of mouth leak during CPAP treatment
CPAP = continuous positive airway pressure; OSA = obstructive sleep apnea.

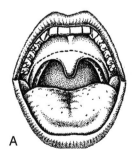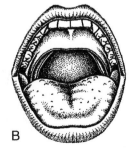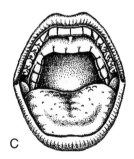

A   B   C

FIGURE 20–10 Technique of uvulopalatopharyngoplasty. **A,** Redundant soft palate and tonsillar pillar mucosa are outlined. **B,** Tonsils, tonsil pillar mucosa, and posterior soft palate are excised. The extent of the soft palate excision is determined by placing traction on the uvula and noting the position of the mucosal crease. **C,** Mucosal flaps of the lateral pharyngeal wall and nasal palatal muscle are advanced to the anterior pillar and/or mucosa of the soft palate. The wound is closed with 3-0 polyglactin braided suture. **A–C,** *From Li KK, Powell NB, Riley RW: Surgical management of OSA. In Lee-Chiong TL, Sateia MJ, Carskadon MA (eds): Sleep Medicine. Philadelphia: Hanley & Belfus, 2002, p. 439, reproduced with permission.*

to UPPP may later relapse, especially if there is weight gain.[64] **Thus, patients treated with UPPP should be restudied if symptoms or signs of sleep apnea return.**

Recent practice parameters for surgical treatment of OSA state "UPPP as a sole procedure, with or without tonsillectomy, does not reliably normalize the AHI when treating moderate to severe OSA. Therefore, patients with severe OSA should initially be offered positive airway pressure therapy, while those with moderate OSA should initially be offered either PAP therapy or oral appliances (Option)."[41]

Several methods have been studied to determine whether UPPP responders can be identified preoperatively. These methods include cephalometric radiographs, computed axial tomography, fluoroscopy, fiberoptic endoscopy of the upper airway during Müller maneuvers (precipitating airway collapse), and upper airway pressure monitoring during sleep.[42,62,64] In some of these methods, the patient is upright, and in most, the patient is awake. Therefore, it is not surprising that predictions of what happens during sleep are less than perfect. In general, patients with obstruction only in the retropalatal area are the most likely to respond to UPPP. However, no method can predict with certainty which patients will benefit from this surgery. As previously noted, a few studies have determined that the site of upper airway obstruction in UPPP failures is the retropalatal area. Presumably, postsurgical changes secondary to either palatal edema or scarring are to blame.[62]

UPPP is considered less effective than nasal CPAP because it is less likely to eliminate apnea and normalize sleep. However, when nasal CPAP is refused or not tolerated, UPPP can be a treatment alternative—especially in mild to moderate apnea. With disease of this severity, there usually is a reasonable chance of obtaining a postoperative AHI less than 15/hr. If UPPP fails, there is always the option of trying nasal CPAP. However, one study suggested that when nasal CPAP is used after UPPP, air leak via the mouth may be more likely.[65] Of interest, a retrospective study of a Veterans Administration (VA) population found better survival in patients after UPPP than treatment with CPAP.[66] The study was not adjusted for OSA severity or for the amount of CPAP use. However, it does point out the need for prospective long-term evaluation of relative UPPP efficacy compared with CPAP.

Uvulopalatal Flap

This surgery is a modification of the UPPP and, instead of removing the uvula and soft palate, the uvula is retracted and tucked superiorly under the soft palate. The pharyngeal pillars are sutured back and tonsils are removed in this procedure as well. The advantages are less postoperative pain and perhaps less nasopharyngeal reflux. The results are similar to UPPP. The procedure cannot be done if the palate is very long or bulky.[45,47]

Genioglossus Advancement/Hyoid Advancement

In the genioglossus advancement (GA) (Fig. 20–11), the attachment of the genioglossus at the genoid tubercle of the mandible is advanced by making a limited rectangular mandibular osteotomy to include the genial tubercle (site of attachment of genioglossus and geniohyoid on the mandible).[38,40,44,45,48] The rectangular piece of bone with muscular attachments is advanced and rotated to prevent retraction of the piece of bone back into the mandible. A screw is then placed for stabilization.

When initially introduced, the second component of the surgery, hyoid advancement (HA) (Fig. 20–12) was called "hyoid myotomy with suspension." The original surgery consisted of release of the hyoid from its inferior muscular attachments and suspension from the anterior mandible with suture or ligament. Today, the hyoid is often attached to the superior border of the thyroid cartilage. This modification has increased the response rate to approximately 80%. Some surgeons perform only the GA at the first surgery with the HA performed only if needed at a subsequent operation. The GAHA does not require any change in dental occlusion. Complications of GAHA include transient anesthesia of the lower anterior teeth (all) and, rarely, tooth injury. Indications for GAHA include a small posterior airspace by lateral cephalometrics (<10 mm), an increased mandible-to-thyroid distance (>20 mm) by cephalometrics, mandibular deficiency, tongue base prominence on nasopharyngoscopy, or macroglossia.[44]

FIGURE 20–11 Technique of genioglossus advancement. A rectangular window of symphyseal bone consisting of the geniotubercle is advanced anteriorly, rotated to allow body overlap, and immobilized with a titanium screw. **Left,** Anterior view. **Right,** Lateral view. *From Li KK: Hypoglossal airway surgery. Otolaryngol Clin North Am 2007; 40:845–853.*

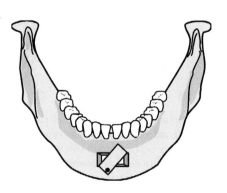
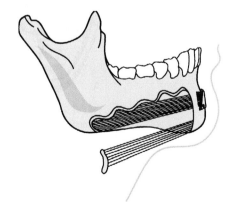

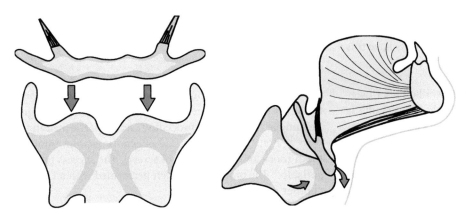

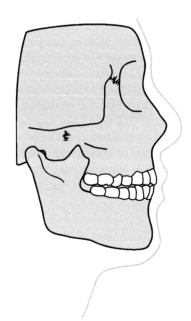

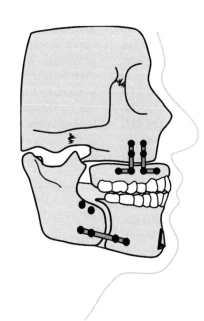

FIGURE 20–12 Technique of hyoid advancement (HA). The hyoid bone is isolated, the inferior body is dissected clean, and the majority of the suprahyoid musculature remains intact. The hyoid is advanced over the thyroid lamina and immobilized with sutures placed through the superior aspect of the thyroid cartilage. **Left,** Anterior view. **Right,** Lateral view. *From Li KK: Hypoglossal airway surgery. Otolaryngol Clin North Am 2007;40:845–853.*

FIGURE 20–13 Technique of maxillomandibular advancement osteotomy procedure (lateral view). Le Fort I maxillary osteotomy with rigid plate fixation and a bilateral sagittal split mandibular osteotomy with bicortical screw fixation. The advancement is at least 10 mm. *From Li KK: Hypoglossal airway surgery. Otolaryngol Clin North Am 2007;40:845–853.*

The recent AASM practice parameters for surgical treatment of OSA did not provide a specific statement about the GA or HA procedures. The practice parameters state "multilevel or stepwise surgery (MLS), as a combined procedure or stepwise operations, is acceptable in patients with narrowing of multiple sites in the upper airway, particularly if they have failed UPPP as a sole treatment (Option)."[41]

Maxillomandibular Advancement

Maxillomandibular advancement (MMA) is a complex upper airway surgery, but excluding tracheostomy, this procedure has the best record of success as a treatment for OSA (Fig. 20-13). The maxilla and mandible are advanced together and both upper and lower teeth are moved to maintain adequate occlusion.[44,45,48,67] The procedure increases the retrolingual and, to a small extent, the retropalatal segments of the upper airway. The maxilla is moved by a Le Fort I osteotomy and the mandible by a sagittal split osteotomy. Numbness of the chin and cheek areas is an expected complication that resolves in 6 to 12 months in most patients. The indications for MMA are listed in Box 20-6. In some

BOX 20–6

Indications for Maxillomandibular Advancement
FIRST SURGICAL OPTION
Severe OSA (especially with minimally redundant palate)
Retrognathia or facial skeletal deficiency
Morbid obesity
Adequate health to undergo surgery
SECOND SURGERY
Failed previous surgical procedures
OSA = obstructive sleep apnea.

institutions, MMA is performed only after UPPP and GAHA. For patients with severe OSA and/or mandibular deficiency, MMA can also be offered as the initial surgery. If the palate is long, doing a UPPP at the same time as the MMA is also an option.

The MMA enlarges the pharyngeal and hypopharyngeal areas by moving the skeletal framework and tensions the suprahyoid and velopharyngeal musculature. Whereas patients with retrognathia may be especially good candidates, this procedure does not require that patients have this problem.

MMA Procedure The maxillary procedure is a Le Fort I osteotomy above the apices of the upper teeth. The maxilla is advanced 10 to 12 mm and stabilized with plates. The mandibular procedure involves a sagittal split osteotomy. The medial and lateral cortex of the mandible is separated at the ramus region with care to preserve the inferior alveolar nerve. The dentated mandibular segment is then advanced to align with the maxilla and rigid fixation is performed with screws or plates.

Outcomes of MMA Response rates up to 90% have been published—depending on the definition of surgical success. Li and coworkers[67] reported 95% "cure" rate defined as an AHI < 20/hr and at least a 50% reduction. In a group of patients who responded to MMA (36 of 40 studied), the AHI dropped from 69.6/hr preoperatively to 7.7/hr postoperatively. A recent meta-analysis found MMA to reduce the AHI to less than 20/hr in 80% to 90%.[61] This procedure is usually offered only at large tertiary hospitals by experienced maxillofacial surgeons. The recent AASM practice parameters for surgical treatment of OSA state "MMA is indicated for surgical treatment of severe OSA in patients who cannot tolerate or are unwilling to adhere to positive airway pressure therapy, or in whom oral appliances, which are often more appropriate in mild and moderate OSA patients, have been considered and found ineffective or undesirable (Option)."[41] The reason for the grade of Option rather than a higher grade of Guideline is that the published studies were considered "low quality of evidence" because they were small and not controlled. Other than tracheostomy, the procedure is most likely to significantly improve the AHI in patients with severe OSA, although the AHI is often not normalized. Of note, there are individual patients with severe OSA in whom OA treatment may be equally effective.

Tongue Procedures

In an attempt to avoid surgery involving the mandible or maxilla, procedures directed at the tongue have also been developed.[45,46,68] Laser midline glossectomy (LMG) and lingualplasty (LP) increase the retroglossal airway by removing tongue tissue. When combined with UPPP, the procedures are known collectively as UPPGP or UPPLP. Due to a number of side effects including postoperative bleeding, odynophagia, and alterations in speech, these are rarely performed today. Temperature-controlled radiofrequency tongue base reduction has also been used to reduce the retroglossal obstruction. Serial treatments are usually required. Side effects have included a single report of a tongue abscess and temporary pain on swallowing or local ulceration. An initial study showed the AHI improved from 39.6/hr to 17.9/hr.[68] However, long-term follow-up showed relapse (AHI = 28.7/hr) without major weight gain. This procedure is usually

used as an adjunctive measure with other procedures. After the first procedure, subsequent procedures are often done in an outpatient surgery center.

Tongue Base Suspension Suture A suspension suture is looped from an anchor screw on the inner surface of the mandible to the base of the tongue. The suture is tensioned, bringing the tongue forward. The procedure can be performed in less than ½ hour and has few side effects (infection, injury to tooth roots, and detachment of screw). The success rates are variable.[69] The procedure is often performed with a UPPP or another procedure.

Overall Surgical Approach

The overall surgical approach depends on OSA severity, upper airway anatomy, prior treatment failures, and patient preference. Box 20–7 presents a summary of recommendations from recent surgical practice parameters. One approach to treatment is to classify patients as type 1 to 3. Obstruction can be classified as type 1 to 3 based on the predominant level of upper airway obstruction.[44,46] A type 1 obstruction is at the retropalatal area. Type 3 obstruction is at the hypopharyngeal area (behind the tongue or lower), and type 2 is a combined obstruction (palate + hypopharynx). Type 1 patients are considered favorable candidates for palatal

BOX 20–7

Surgical Practice Parameter Recommendations	
PROCEDURE	INDICATIONS/CONDITIONS
Tracheostomy	• Other options do not exist or have failed. • Clinical urgency (e.g., repeated bouts of hypercapnic respiratory failure).
MMA	• Severe OSA. • Unwilling or unable to tolerate PAP. • OA considered and undesirable or ineffective.
UPPP	• Snoring, mild OSA. • Moderate OSA—only after offering PAP treatment and OAs.
Palatal implants	• May be effective in some patients with mild OSA. • Indicated for OSA treatment IF patients cannot tolerate/adhere to PAP therapy and OA treatment is considered and found ineffective and undesirable.
Multilevel or stepwise surgery	• Upper airway narrowing at multiple sites. • Have failed UPPP as sole treatment.

MMA = maxillomandibular advancement; OA = oral appliance; OSA = obstructive sleep apnea; PAP = positive airway pressure; UPPP = uvulopalatopharyngoplasty.
From Caples SM, Rowley JA, Prinsell JR, et al: Surgical modifications of the upper airway for obstructive sleep apnea in adults: a systematic review and meta-analysis. Sleep 2010;33:1396–1407.

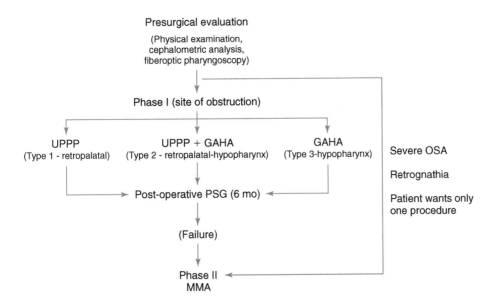

Presurgical evaluation

(Physical examination,
cephalometric analysis,
fiberoptic pharyngoscopy)

Phase I (site of obstruction)

UPPP
(Type 1 - retropalatal)

UPPP + GAHA
(Type 2 - retropalatal-hypopharynx)

GAHA
(Type 3-hypopharynx)

Severe OSA

Retrognathia

Patient wants only
one procedure

Post-operative PSG (6 mo)

(Failure)

Phase II
MMA

FIGURE 20–14 Stepped surgical approach to treatment of obstructive sleep apnea (OSA) based on the site of upper airway obstruction. GAHA = genioglossal advancement/hyoid advancement; MMA = maxillomandibular advancement; PSG = polysomnography; UPPP = uvulopalatopharyngoplasty. *Adapted from Li KK, Powell NB, Riley RW: Surgical management of obstructive sleep apnea. In Lee-Chiong TL, Sateia MJ, Caraskadon MA (eds): Sleep Medicine. Philadelphia: Hanley & Belfus, 2002, pp. 435–446.*

procedures (UPPP). Type 3 are candidates for procedures addressing the retroglossal space (GA, with or without HA [also called *hypoid myotomy*], or MMA). Type 2 patients are candidates for combined UPPP and GAHA or MMA. A systematic stepped surgical approach has been advocated such as the one used at Stanford (Fig. 20–14).[44,46] A postoperative PSG is performed in 6 months and treatment failures can then be offered MMA. Because an occasional patient with type 2 obstruction will improve with UPPP, in some centers, a retrolingual procedure is added only after UPPP fails. In some other centers, patients with severe OSA, severe mandibular deficiency, or very small posterior air spaces are offered MMA with or without UPPP as the first procedure. Some patients also want to avoid multiple procedures and this more aggressive approach may be more acceptable to them.

Success Rates of Upper Airway Surgery

A recent meta-analysis and synthesis of evidence for success in upper airway surgery was reported by Elshaug and colleagues[61] (Table 20–5). A traditional metric of success has been a 50% reduction in the AHI and/or 20/hr or less. These authors suggested a more rigorous approach with reduction less than 10 or 5/hr being the goal of success. Phase I surgery included palatal surgery with or without other procedures such as GA or GAHA. Phase II surgery was the MMA with or without additional procedures. Of course, the percentage termed successful will depend on the initial severity.

SURGERY FOR PEDIATRIC OSA

Tonsillectomy and Adenoidectomy

Tonsillectomy and adenoidectomy (TNA) has been the standard treatment for OSA in pediatric patients for many years

TABLE 20–5			
Meta-analysis Results for Upper Airway Surgery (% Success Rates)			
CRITERIA	50% REDUCTION IN AHI AND/OR TO ≤ 20/HR	AHI < 10/HR	AHI < 5/HR
Phase I*	55%	31.5%	13%
Phase II†	86%	45%	43%

*Phase I (UPPP, GA, HA, or combination).
†Phase II (MMA).
GA = genioglossus advancement; HA = hyoid advancement; MMA = maxillomandibular advancement; UPPP = uvulopalatopharyngoplasty.
From Elshaug AG, Moss JR, Southcott A, et al: Redefining success in airway surgery for obstructive sleep apnea: a meta-analysis and synthesis of the evidence. Sleep 2007;30:461–467.

(Fig. 20–15). There are over 400,000 surgeries per year. It is estimated that PSG is performed in only about 10% of patients undergoing TNA.[70] Studies have shown that history and physical examination are **not** accurate in predicting the presence or absence of OSA. The size of tonsils is not predictive of OSA. However, the need for routine PSG before TNA for childhood sleep apnea is still debated.[70,71] Both the American Academy of Pediatrics[72] and the American Thoracic Society[73] recommend preoperative PSG.

Earlier studies found that TNA successfully eliminated OSA in 75% to 100% of patients. Recent prospective studies using postoperative PSG have found lower cure rates (depending on the definition of success).[74-77] A prospective study of 199 children with OSA found 46% continued to have elevated AHI (AHI > 1/hr) on follow-up PSG performed 3 to 5 months later.[74] A high Mallampati score (3 or 4), turbinate hypertrophy, retroposition of the mandible, and

FIGURE 20–15 Tonsillectomy and adenoidectomy. The adenoid and tonsillar tissues are removed and the lateral pharyngeal walls are sutured to prevent collapse. *From Won CHJ, Li KK, Guilleminault C: Surgical treatment of obstructive sleep apnea. Proc Am Thorac Soc 2008;5:193–199.*

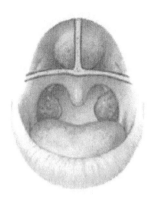
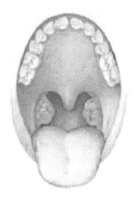
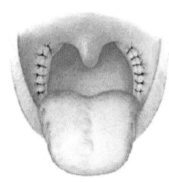

a deviated septum were predictive of an elevated postoperative AHI.[74] Another study of a cohort of 110 children found complete normalization of AHI was present in only 25% of patients.[75] A meta-analysis by Brietzke and Gallagher[76] found 82% of patients to be successfully treated for OSA. In the studies analyzed, treatment success varied between studies (AHI < 1–5/hr). Another meta-analysis of the efficacy of TNA by Friedman and associates[77] found "cure," defined as an AHI < 1/hr, to occur in about 60% of patients. Most patients undergoing TNA do improve symptomatically, but frequently significant residual OSA is still present. **TNA is still considered the initial treatment of choice in pediatric patients with OSA.** A postsurgery PSG is recommended and other treatments (including weight reduction or CPAP) may be needed. Complications from the TNA include bleeding, pain, infection, and weight loss.[72,73,78]

Performing a PSG before TNA has a number of advantages: (1) accurate diagnosis and avoiding unnecessary surgery, (2) PSG results provide parents with an estimate of chance of success; patients with an elevated AHI may require additional treatment beyond TNA, and (3) the PSG and clinical evaluation may reveal factors indicating increased risk for postoperative complications. These patients require overnight or at least extended monitoring of the SaO_2. Proposed risk factors for TNA requiring overnight hospitalization or more long-term recovery room monitoring are listed in Box 20–8.[72,78] Nasal CPAP can be used to manage postoperative complications in very severely affected individuals. The need for routine postoperative PSG in patients who have undergone TNA (after surgical healing) is also a subject of controversy.[70,71] A PSG is definitely indicated if signs or symptoms of OSA continue or return after a period of improvement. One can also make a case for a postoperative PSG in patients with moderate or severe OSA (AHI of 5–10 or > 10/hr, respectively) or significant obesity.

Rapid Maxillary Expansion

Rapid maxillary expansion (RME) in conjunction with TNA has been shown to be successful in treating children with OSA and maxillary contraction (high arched palate

BOX 20–8

Criteria for Increased Risk of Tonsillectomy and Adenoidectomy

CLINICAL CRITERIA

Age < 2 yr
Craniofacial abnormalities affecting the pharyngeal airway (especially midface hypoplasia or micro-/retrognathia)
Failure to thrive
Hypotonia
Cor pulmonale
Morbid obesity or daytime hypercapnia
Previous upper airway trauma
Undergoing a UPPP in addition to TNA

PSG CRITERIA

AHI > 40/hr
SaO_2 nadir < 70%

SaO_2 = arterial oxygen saturation; TNA = tonsillectomy and adenoidectomy; UPPP = uvulopalatopharyngoplasty.
From Rosen GM, Muckle RP, Mahowald MW, et al: Postoperative respiratory compromise in children with obstructive sleep apnea syndrome: can it be anticipated? Pediatrics 1994;93:784–788.

and unilateral or bilateral cross-bite).[79–81] RME requires an orthodontic device (Fig. 20–16) anchored to two upper molars on each side of the jaw that applies daily pressure causing each half of the maxilla to grow apart. This technique aims to expand the hard palate laterally, raise the soft palate, and widen the nasal passages. RME needs to occur before cartilage becomes bone (5–16 yr of age). Distraction osteogenesis is defined as the mechanical induction of new bone between two bony surfaces that are gradually distracted (separated). If RMD is not successful or deemed insufficient, mandibular distraction osteogenesis is performed surgically. A surgeon uses a saw to create osteotomies in the mandible and then either an internal or an external device is used to expand the bones. Mandibular distraction osteogenesis is often used to treat sleep apnea in patients with severe congenital abnormalities of the mandible (micrognathia) as in the Treacher Collins syndrome or Pierre Robin syndrome.[82]

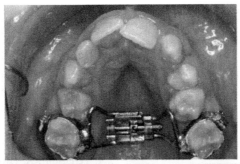

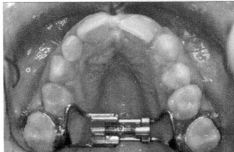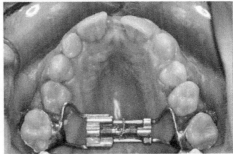

FIGURE 20–16 Occlusal sequence of treatment with rapid maxillary expansion from crowding in the upper central incisors **(top)** to a wide space **(bottom).** Note how the palatal vault has changed. *From Pirelli P, Saponara M, Guilleminault C: Rapid maxillary expansion in children with obstructive sleep apnea syndrome. Sleep 2004;27:764.*

CLINICAL REVIEW QUESTIONS

1. A 53-year-old man was diagnosed with moderate OSA with an AHI of 20/hr about 4 years ago. He underwent a UPPP and a postoperative PSG showed an AHI of 8/hr. He noted resolution of snoring and daytime sleepiness. Recently, he began to have return of his daytime sleepiness, although minimal snoring is present. No weight gain has been noted. What do you recommend?

   A. An OA.

   B. PSG.

   C. Modafinil.

   D. Weight loss.

2. An 11-year-old male has a history of snoring and daytime sleepiness. On physical examination, he is obese (BMI = 30) and has 4+ enlarged tonsils. A sleep study shows an AHI of 20/hr with all events being obstructive apneas or hypopneas. What treatment do you recommend?

   A. TNA.

   B. CPAP.

   C. Weight loss.

   D. UPPP.

3. A 40-year-old man with loud snoring but no witnessed apnea or daytime sleepiness is considering the palatal implant surgery for snoring. He is seeking a second opinion. What do you recommend?

   A. PSG; if OSA is present, PI surgery not indicated.

   B. Proceed with palatal surgery but obtain postprocedure PSG.

   C. Palatal surgery, PSG only if symptoms appear.

   D. OA rather than PI treatment, PSG if symptoms appear.

4. A 35-year-old man has moderate OSA with an AHI of 20/hr. Fiberoptic examination of the upper airway with the Müller maneuver demonstrates obstruction at both the retropalatal and the retroglossal areas. What surgery do your recommend?

   A. UPPP + GAHA.

   B. UPPP.

   C. GAHA.

   D. MMA.

5. Of the following factors, which is predictive of a good response to an OA?

   A. Higher BMI.

   B. Mild retrognathia.

   C. Presence of postural OSA.

   D. Rapid eye movement–related OSA.

6. A 40-year-old woman has loud snoring and mild OSA (AHI 10/hr). She also has nasal congestion with septal deviation and hypertrophy of the inferior turbinates. She has good dentition and no TMJ problems. Her oropharynx is a Mallampati 2, and she has a long uvula. Which of the following treatment options do you recommend?

   A. LAUP.

   B. Nasal surgery.

   C. OA.

   D. OA or UPPP

7. A 40-year-old man has severe daytime sleepiness and an AHI of 40/hr with moderate arterial oxygen desaturation. The patient's only medical problems are obesity and hypertension. Multiple attempts at PAP treatment have been unsuccessful. Which treatment alternatives do you recommend?

   A. UPPP.

   B. UPPP + GAHA.

   C. MMA.

   D. OA.

Answers

1. **B.** Recurrence of OSA following initial success after UPPP has been reported even without weight gain. In this patient, a PSG is indicated to determine whether OSA has returned and, if so, the severity. The cause of the daytime sleepiness should be determined before treatment.

2. **A.** Although this patient is at risk of having considerable postoperative OSA, a TNA is still the first-line treatment in pediatric patients unless minimal tonsillar tissue is present. A postoperative PSG is essential to rule out significant residual OSA (even if symptoms improve).

3. **A.** A PSG is indicated to determine whether primary snoring or OSA is present. This is true whether the patient undergoes upper airway surgery or treatment with an OA. If moderate OSA is present, PI surgery is not indicated. If mild OSA is present, PI is indicated with reservations. The surgical practice parameters state "palatal implants may be effective in some patients with mild OSA who cannot tolerate or are unwilling to adhere to PAP therapy, or in whom oral appliances have been considered and found ineffective or undesirable." If mild OSA is present, an OA will likely be more effective for both snoring and OSA. If PI or OA treatment is used to treat OSA, a post-treatment PSG (after surgical healing or with the OA in place after adjustment) is indicated. The type of treatment that is indicated will depend on the severity of OSA and the patient's preference.

4. **A.** The combined surgery is indicated in patients with obstruction in both retropalatal and retroglossal areas. The MMA might be effective but, because the patient is not severe, this would not usually be the first surgical option. In the step approach, this would be considered only if phase I surgery was not successful.

5. **C.** Patients with postural OSA usually have a better response to OA therapy.

6. **D.** An LAUP is not indicated for OSA. Nasal surgery would be considered adjunctive. Either an OA or a UPPP would be a reasonable treatment alternative.

7. **C.** In patients with severe OSA in whom PAP treatment has failed (or not tolerated), the treatment options include OA and MMA. Given the severity of symptoms and desaturation, MMA is indicated. OA can be effective in some patients with severe OSA. If the patient declines surgery or is not a good surgical candidate, then OA treatment may be the best option.

REFERENCES

1. Ferguson KA, Cartwright R, Rogers R, et al: Oral appliances for snoring and obstructive sleep apnea: a review. Sleep 2006;29:244–262.
2. Kushida CA, Morgenthaler TI, Littner MR, et al: American Academy of Sleep Medicine. Practice parameters for the treatment of snoring and obstructive sleep apnea with oral appliances: an update for 2005. Sleep 2006;29:240–243.
3. Thorpy M, Chesson A, Derderian S, et al: Practice parameters for the treatment of snoring and obstructive sleep apnea with oral appliances. Sleep 1995;18:511–513.
4. Schmidt-Nowara W, Lowe A, Wiegand L, et al: Oral appliances for treatment of snoring and obstructive sleep apnea. Sleep 1995;18:501–510.
5. Bailey DR, Hoekema A: Oral appliance therapy in sleep medicine. Sleep Med Clin 2010;5:91–98.
6. Cartwright R: Return of the TRD. J Clin Sleep Med 2009; 5:439–440.
7. Lazard DS, Blumen M, Lévy P, et al: The tongue-retaining device: efficacy and side effects in obstructive sleep apnea syndrome. J Clin Sleep Med 2009;5:431–438.
8. Dort L, Brant R: A randomized, controlled, crossover study of a noncustomized tongue retaining device for sleep disordered breathing. Sleep Breath 2008;12:369–373.
9. Deane SA, Cistulli PA, Ng AT, et al: Comparison of mandibular advancement splint and tongue stabilizing device in obstructive sleep apnea: a randomized controlled trial. Sleep 2009;32: 648–653.
10. Conely RS: Orthodontic considerations related to sleep disordered breathing. Sleep Med Clin 2009;5:71–89.
11. Henke KG, Fratnz DE, Kuna ST: An oral mandibular advancement device for obstructive sleep apnea. Am J Respir Crit Care Med 2000;161:420–425.
12. Tsuiki S, Ono T, Kuroda T: Mandibular advancement modulates respiratory-related genioglossus electromyographic activity. Sleep Breath 2000;4:53–57.
13. Lowe AA, Sjoholm TT, Ryan CF, et al: Treatment, airway, and compliance effects of a titratable oral appliance. Sleep 2000; 23(Suppl 4):S172–S178.
14. Lee CH, Kin JW, Lee HJ, et al: An investigation of upper airway changes associated with mandibular advancement device using sleep videofluoroscopy in patients with obstructive sleep apnea. Arch Otolaryngol Head Neck Surg 2009;135:910–914.
15. Gotsopoulos H, Chen C, Qian J, Cistulli PA: Oral appliance therapy improves symptoms in obstructive sleep apnea. Am J Respir Crit Care Med 2002;166:743–748.
16. Walker-Engström ML, Rinquiest K, Vestling O, et al: A prospective randomized study comparing two different degrees of mandibular advancement with a dental appliance in treatment of obstructive sleep apnea. Sleep Breath 2003;7:119–130.
17. Chung JW, Enciso R, Levendowski DJ, et al: Treatment outcomes of mandibular advancement devices in positional and nonpositional OSA patients. Oral Surg Oral Med Oral Pathol Oral Radiol Endod 2010;109:724–731.
18. Vanderveken OM, Devolder A, Marklund M, et al: Comparison of a custom-made and a thermoplastic oral appliance for the treatment of mild sleep apnea. Am J Respir Crit Care Med 2008:178:197–202.

19. Center for Devices and Radiologic Health, U.S. Food and Drug Administration: Class II special controls guidance document: intraoral devices for snoring and/or obstructive sleep apnea: guidance for industry. FDA Bull November 12, 2002.

20. Tsai WH, Vazquez J, Oshima T, et al: Remotely controlled mandibular positioner predicts efficacy of an oral appliance in sleep apnea. Am J Respir Crit Care Med 2004;170:366–370.

21. Krishnan V, Collop N, Scherr S: An evaluation of a titration strategy for prescription of an oral appliance for obstructive sleep apnea. Chest 2008;133:1135–1141.

22. Clark GT, Sohn JW, Hong CN: Treating obstructive sleep apnea and snoring: assessment of an anterior mandibular positioning device. J Am Dent Assoc 2000;131:765–771.

23. Walker-Engström ML, Tegelberg Å, Wilhelmsson B, Ringqvist I: 4-year follow-up of treatment with dental appliance or uvulopalatopharyngoplasty in patients with obstructive sleep apnea: a randomized study. Chest 2002;121:739–746.

24. de Almeida FR, Lowe AA, Tsuiki S, et al: Long-term compliance and side effects of oral appliances used for the treatment of snoring and obstructive sleep apnea syndrome. J Clin Sleep Med 2005;1:143–152.

25. Ferguson KA, Ono T, Lowe AA, et al: A randomized crossover study of an oral appliance vs nasal-continuous positive airway pressure in the treatment of mild-moderate obstructive sleep apnea. Chest 1996;109:1269–1275.

26. Ferguson KA, Ono T, Lowe AA, et al: A short-term controlled trial of an adjustable oral appliance for the treatment of mild to moderate obstructive sleep apnoea. Thorax 1997;52: 362–368.

27. Barnes M, McEvoy RD, Banks S, et al: Efficacy of positive airway pressure and oral appliance in mild to moderate obstructive sleep apnea. Am J Respir Crit Care Med 2004;170:656–664.

28. Clark GT, Blumenfeld I, Yoffe N, et al: A crossover study comparing the efficacy of continuous positive airway pressure with anterior mandibular positioning devices on patients with obstructive sleep apnea. Chest 1996;109:1477–1483.

29. Engleman HM, McDonald JP, Graham D, et al: Randomized crossover trial of two treatments for sleep apnea/hypopnea syndrome: continuous positive airway pressure and mandibular repositioning splint. Am J Respir Crit Care Med 2002;166: 855–859.

30. Randerath WJ, Heise M, Hinz R, Ruehle KH: An individually adjustable oral appliance vs continuous positive airway pressure in mild to moderate obstructive sleep apnea. Chest 2002;122:569–575.

31. Tan YK, L'Estrange PR, Luo YK, et al: Mandibular advancement splints and continuous positive airway pressure in patients with obstructive sleep apnea: a randomized cross-over trial. Eur J Orthod 2002;24:239–249.

32. Collop NA, McDowell W, Boehlecke B, et al: Clinical guidelines for the use of unattended portable monitors in the diagnosis of obstructive sleep apnea in adult patients. J Clin Sleep Med 2007;3:737–747.

33. Rose E, Statts R, Virchow C, Jonas IE: Occlusal and skeletal effects of an oral appliance in treatment of obstructive sleep apnea. Chest 2002;122:871–877.

34. Millman RP, Rosenberg CL, Carlisle CC, et al: The efficacy of oral appliances in the treatment of persistent sleep apnea after uvulopalatopharyngoplasty. Chest 1998;113:992–996.

35. Gotsopoulos H, Kelly JJ, Cistulli PA: Oral appliance therapy reduces blood pressure in obstructive sleep apnea: a randomized, controlled trial. Sleep 2004;27:934–941.

36. Coruzzi P, Gualerzi M, Bernkopf E, et al: Effects of an oral appliance on autonomic cardiac modulation in obstructive sleep apnea. Chest 2006;130:1362–1368.

37. Guilleminault C, Simmons B, Motta J, et al: Obstructive sleep apnea syndrome and tracheostomy. Arch Intern Med 1981; 141:985–988.

38. Sher AE, Schechtman KB, Piccirillo JF: The efficacy of surgical modifications of the upper airway in adults with obstructive sleep apnea syndrome. Sleep 1996;19:156–177.

39. American Sleep Disorders Association, Standards of Practice Committee: Practice parameters for the treatment of obstructive sleep apnea in adults: the efficacy of surgical modifications of the upper airway. Sleep 1996;19:152–155.

40. Caples SM, Rowley JA, Prinsell JR, et al: Surgical modifications of the upper airway for obstructive sleep apnea in adults: a systematic review and meta-analysis. Sleep 2010;33:1396–1407.

41. Aurora RN, Casey KR, Kristo D, et al: Practice parameters for the surgical modifications of the upper airway for obstructive sleep apnea in adults. Sleep 2010;33:1408–1413.

42. Sher AE, Thorpy MJ, Spielman AJ, et al: Predictive values of Müller maneuver in selection of patients for uvulopalatopharyngoplasty. Laryngoscope 1985;95:1483–1487.

43. Conway WA, Victor L, Magilligan DJ, et al: Adverse effects of tracheostomy for sleep apnea. JAMA 1981;246:347–350.

44. Li KK, Powell NB, Riley RW: Surgical management of obstructive sleep apnea. In Lee-Chiong TL, Sateia MJ, Caraskadon MA (eds): Sleep Medicine. Philadelphia: Hanley & Belfus, 2002, pp. 435–446.

45. Won CHJ, Li KK, Guilleminault C: Surgical treatment of obstructive sleep apnea. Proc Am Thorac Soc 2008;5:193–199.

46. Powell NB: Contemporary surgery for obstructive sleep apnea. Clin Exp Otolaryngol 2009;2:107–114.

47. Friedman M, Schalch P: Surgery of the palate and oropharynx. Otolaryngol Clin North Am 2007;40:829–843.

48. Li KK: Hypopharyngeal airway surgery. Otolaryngol Clin North Am 2007;40:845–853.

49. Powell NB, Zonato AI, Weaver EM, et al: Radiofrequency treatment of turbinate hypertrophy in subjects using continuous positive airway pressure: a randomized, double-blind, placebo-controlled clinical pilot trial. Laryngoscope 2001; 111:1783–1790.

50. Koutsourelakis I, Georgoulopoulos G, Perraki E, et al: Randomized trial of nasal surgery for fixed nasal obstruction in obstructive sleep apnea. Eur Respir J 2008;31:110–117.

51. Kohler M, Bloch KE, Stradling JR: The role of the nose in the pathogenesis of obstructive sleep apnea and snoring. Eur Respir J 2007;30:1208–1215.

52. Friedman M, Schalch P, Lin HC, et al: Palatal implants for the treatment of snoring and obstructive sleep apnea/hypopnea syndrome. Otolaryngol Head Neck Surg 2008;138:209–216.

53. Steward DL, Huntley TC, Woodson BT, Surdulescu V: Palate implants for obstructive sleep apnea: multi-institution, randomized, placebo-controlled study. Otolaryngol Head Neck Surg 2008;139:506–510.

54. Littner M, Kushida CA, Hartse K, et al: Practice parameters for the use of laser-assisted uvulopalatoplasty. Sleep 2001; 245:603–619.

55. Ryan CF, Love LL: Unpredictable results of laser assisted uvulopalatoplasty in the treatment of obstructive sleep apnea. Thorax 2000;55:399–404.

56. Powell NB, Riley RW, Troell RJ, et al: Radiofrequency volumetric tissue reduction of the palate in subjects with sleep-disordered breathing. Chest 1998;113:1163–1174.

57. Fujita S, Conway W, Zorick F, Roth T: Surgical correction of anatomic abnormalities in obstructive sleep apnea. Uvulopalatopharyngoplasty. Otolaryngol Head Neck Surg 1981; 89:923–934.

58. Larsson LH, Carlsson-Norlander B, Svanborg E: Four year follow-up after uvulopalatopharyngoplasty in 50 unselected patients with obstructive sleep apnea syndrome. Laryngoscope 1994;104:1362–1368.

59. Fairbanks DNF: Uvulopalatopharyngoplasty complications and avoidance strategies. Otolaryngol Head Neck Surg 1990; 102:239–245.

60. Franklin KA, Anttla H, Axelsson S, et al: Effects and side-effects of surgery for snoring and OSA: a systematic review. Sleep 2009;32:27–36.

61. Elshaug AG, Moss JR, Southcott A, et al: Redefining success in airway surgery for obstructive sleep apnea: a meta-analysis and synthesis of the evidence. Sleep 2007;30:461–467.

62. Hudgel DW, Harasick T, Katz RL, et al: Uvulopalatopharyngo-plasty in obstructive apnea: value of preoperative localization of site of upper airway narrowing during sleep. Am Rev Respir Dis 1991;143:942–946.

63. Sasse SA, Mahutte CK, Dickel M, Berry RB: The characteristics of five patients with obstructive sleep apnea whose apnea-hypopnea index deteriorated after uvulopalatopharygoplasty. Sleep Breath 2002;6:77–84.

64. Launois SH, Feroah TR, Campbell WN, et al: Site of pharyngeal narrowing predicts outcome of surgery for obstructive sleep apnea. Am Rev Respir Dis 1993;147:182–189.

65. Mortimore IL, Bradley PA, Murray JAM, Douglas NJ: Uvulo-palatoplasty may compromise nasal CPAP therapy in sleep apnea syndrome. Am J Respir Crit Care Med 1996;154:1759–1762.

66. Weaver EM, Maynard C, Yueth B: Survival of veterans with sleep apnea: continuous positive airway pressure versus surgery. Otolaryngol Head Neck Surg 2004;130:659–665.

67. Li KK, Powell NB, Riley RW, et al: Long term results of maxillomandibular advancement surgery. Sleep Breath 2000; 3:137–139.

68. Li K, Powell NB, Riley RW, Guilleminault C: Temperature controlled radiofrequency tongue base reduction for sleep disordered breathing: long term outcomes. Otolaryngol Head Neck Surg 2002;127:230–234.

69. Miller FR, Watson D, Malis D: Role of tongue base suspension suture with the repose system bone screw in the multilevel surgical management of obstructive sleep apnea. Otolaryngol Head Neck Surg 2002;126:392–398.

70. Hoban TF: Polysomnography should be required both before and after adenotonsillectomy for childhood sleep disordered breathing. J Clin Sleep Med 2007;3:675–677.

71. Friedman N: Polysomnography should not be required before and after adenotonsillectomy for childhood sleep disordered breathing. J Clin Sleep Med 2007;3:678–680.

72. American Academy of Pediatrics: Clinical practice guideline. Diagnosis and management of childhood obstructive sleep apnea syndrome. Pediatrics 2002;109:704–712.

73. American Thoracic Society: Standards and indications for cardiopulmonary sleep studies in children. Am J Respir Crit Care Med 1996;153:866–878.

74. Guilleminault C, Huang YS, Glamann C, Chan A: Adenotonsillectomy and obstructive sleep apnea in children: a prospective survey. Otolaryngol Head Neck Surg 2007;136:169–175.

75. Tauman R, Gulliver TE, Krishna J, et al: Persistence of obstructive sleep apnea syndrome in children after adenotonsillectomy. J Pediatr 2006;121:803–808.

76. Brietzke SE, Gallagher D: The effectiveness of tonsillectomy and adenoidectomy in the treatment of pediatric obstructive sleep apnea/hypopnea syndrome: a meta-analysis. Otolaryngol Head Neck Surg 2006;134:979–984.

77. Friedman M, Wilson M, Chang HW: Updated systematic review of tonsillectomy and adenoidectomy for treatment of pediatric obstructive sleep apnea/hypopnea syndrome. Otolaryngol Head Neck Surg 2009;140:800–808.

78. Rosen GM, Muckle RP, Mahowald MW, et al: Postoperative respiratory compromise in children with obstructive sleep apnea syndrome: can it be anticipated? Pediatrics 1994;93:784–788.

79. Pirelli P, Saponara M, Guilleminault C: Rapid maxillary expansion in children with obstructive sleep apnea syndrome. Sleep 2004;27:761–766.

80. Cistulli PA, Palmisano RG, Poole MD: Treatment of obstructive sleep apnea syndrome by rapid maxillary expansion. Sleep 1998;21:831–835.

81. Villa MP, Malagola C, Pagani J, et al: Rapid maxillary expansion in children with obstructive sleep apnea syndrome: 12-month follow-up. Sleep Med 2007;8:128–134.

82. Cohen SR, Simms C, Burstein F: Mandibular distraction osteogenesis in the treatment of upper airway obstruction in children with craniofacial deformities. Plast Reconstr Surg 1998; 101:312–318.

Summary of AASM Practice Parameters for the Use of Oral Appliances for Treatment of Snoring and Obstructive Sleep Apnea

3.1 Diagnosis

3.1.1 The presence or absence of OSA must be determined before initiating treatment with OAs to identify those patients at risk due to complications of sleep apnea and to provide a baseline to establish the effectiveness of subsequent treatment. Detailed diagnostic criteria for OSA are available and include clinical signs, symptoms, and the findings identified by polysomnography. The severity of sleep-related respiratory problems must be established in order to make an appropriate treatment decision. (Standard)

3.2 Appliance Fitting

3.2.1 OAs should be fitted by qualified dental personnel who are trained and experienced in the overall care of oral health, the temporomandibular joint, dental occlusion, and associated oral structures. Dental management of patients with OAs should be overseen by practitioners who have undertaken serious training in sleep medicine and/or sleep-related breathing disorders with focused emphasis on the proper protocol for diagnosis, treatment, and follow-up. (Option)

3.2.2 Although cephalometric evaluation is not always required for patients who will use an OA, appropriately trained professionals should perform these examinations when they are deemed necessary. (Option)

3.3.1 Treatment Objectives

3.3.1.1 For patients with primary snoring without features of OSA or upper airway resistance syndrome, the treatment objective is to reduce the snoring to a subjectively acceptable level. (Standard)

3.3.1.2 For patients with OSA, the desired outcome of treatment includes the resolution of the clinical signs and symptoms of OSA and the normalization of the apnea-hypopnea index and oxyhemoglobin saturation. (Standard)

3.3.2 OAs are appropriate for use in patients with primary snoring who do not respond to or are not appropriate candidates for treatment with behavioral measures such as weight loss or sleep position change. (Guideline)

3.3.3 Although not as efficacious as CPAP, OAs are indicated for use in patients with mild to moderate OSA who prefer OAs to CPAP, or who do not respond to CPAP, are not appropriate candidates for CPAP, or who fail treatment attempts with CPAP or treatment with behavioral measures such as weight loss or sleep position change. (Guideline)

3.3.4 Patients with severe OSA should have an initial trial of nasal CPAP because greater effectiveness has been shown with this intervention than with the use of OAs. Upper airway surgery (including tonsillectomy and adenoidectomy, craniofacial operations, and tracheostomy) may also supersede use of OAs in patients for whom these operations are predicted to be highly effective in treating sleep apnea. (Guideline)

3.4 Follow-up

3.4.1 Follow-up sleep testing is not indicated for patients with primary snoring. (Guideline)

3.4.2 To ensure satisfactory therapeutic benefit from OAs, patients with OSA should undergo polysomnography or an attended cardiorespiratory (type 3) sleep study with the OA in place after final adjustments of fit have been performed. (Guideline)

3.4.3 Patients with OSA who are treated with OAs should return for follow-up office visits with the dental specialist. Once optimal fit is obtained and efficacy shown, dental specialist follow-up at every 6 months is recommended for the first year, and at least annually thereafter. The purpose of follow-up is to monitor patient adherence, evaluate device deterioration or maladjustment, evaluate the health of the oral structures and integrity of the occlusion, and assess the patient for signs and symptoms of worsening OSA. Intolerance and improper use of the device are potential problems for patients using OAs, which require patient effort to use properly. OAs may aggravate temporomandibular joint disease and may cause dental misalignment and discomfort that are unique to each device. In addition, OAs can be rendered ineffective by patient alteration of the device. (Option)

3.4.4 Patients with OSA who are treated with OAs should return for periodic follow-up office visits with the referring clinician. The purpose of follow-up is to assess the patient for signs and symptoms of worsening OSA. Close communication with the dental specialist is most conducive to good patient care. An objective re-evaluation of respiration during sleep is indicated if signs or symptoms of OSA worsen or recur. (Option)

CPAP = continuous positive airway pressure; OA = oral appliance; OSA = obstructive sleep apnea.
From Kushida CA, Morgenthaler TI, Littner MR, et al: American Academy of Sleep Medicine. Practice parameters for the treatment of snoring and obstructive sleep apnea with oral appliances: an update for 2005. Sleep 2006;29:240–243.

Excerpts from Local Coverage Determination for Oral Appliances for Obstructive Sleep Apnea (L28606)

A custom-fabricated mandibular advancement oral appliance (E0486) used to treat obstructive sleep apnea (OSA) is covered if criteria A–D are met.

A. The patient has a face-to-face clinical evaluation by the treating physician prior to the sleep test to assess the patient for OSA testing.
B. The patient has a Medicare-covered sleep test that meets one of the following criteria (1–3):
1. The apnea-hypopnea index (AHI) or respiratory disturbance index (RDI) ≥ 15 events/hr with a minimum of 30 events; or
2. The AHI or RDI ≥ 5 and ≤ 14 events/hr with a minimum of 10 events and documentation of
   a. Excessive daytime sleepiness, impaired cognition, mood disorders, or insomnia; or
   b. Hypertension, ischemic heart disease, or history of stroke, or
3. If the AHI > 30 or the RDI > 30 and meets either of the following (a or b):
   a. The patient is not able to tolerate a positive airway pressure (PAP) device, or
   b. The treating physician determines that the use of a PAP device is contraindicated.

C. The device is ordered by the treating physician following review of the report of the sleep test. (The physician who provides the order for the oral appliance could be different from the one who performed the clinical evaluation in criterion A.)
D. The device is provided and billed for by a licensed dentist (DDS or DMD).

If all of these criteria (A–D) are not met, the custom-fabricated oral appliance (E0486) will be denied as not reasonable and necessary.

Custom-fabricated appliances that achieve their effect through positioning of the tongue (E1399) will be denied as not reasonable and necessary. There is insufficient evidence to show that these items are effective therapy for OSA.

A prefabricated OA (E0485) will be denied as not reasonable and necessary. There is insufficient evidence to show that these items are effective therapy for OSA.

Custom-fabricated mandibular advancement devices that do not meet the requirements in the Coding Guidelines section of the Related Policy Article (E1399) will be denied as not reasonable and necessary.

Note: Here AHI = apnea + hypopnea index (hypopnea = 30% drop in flow + ≥ 4% desaturation).
RDI is determined by a type 3 or type 4 home sleep test (RDI = apneas + hypopneas/hour of monitoring time).
Available at Noridian https://www.noridianmedicare.com/dme/coverage/docs/lcds/current_lcds/oral_appliances.htm%3f

Summary of Practice Parameters for Surgical Treatment of Obstructive Sleep Apnea in Adults

4.1 Diagnosis

4.1.1 The presence and severity of OSA must be determined before initiating surgical therapy. (Standard)

4.1.2 The patient should be advised about potential surgical success rates and complications, availability of alternative treatment options such as nasal PAP and oral appliances, and the levels of effectiveness and success rates of these alternative treatments. (Standard)

4.2 Treatment objective: The desired outcomes of treatment include resolution of the clinical signs and symptoms of OSA and the normalization of sleep quality, the AHI, and oxyhemoglobin levels. (Standard)

4.3 Surgical Procedures

4.3.1 Tracheostomy: Tracheostomy has been shown to be an effective single intervention to treat OSA. This operation should be considered only when other options do not exist, have failed, are refused, or when this operation is deemed necessary by clinical urgency. (Option)

4.3.2 Maxillomandibular advancement: MMA is indicated for surgical treatment of severe OSA in patients who cannot tolerate or are unwilling to adhere to PAP therapy, or in whom oral appliances, which are often more appropriate in mild and moderate OSA patients, have been considered and found ineffective or undesirable. (Option)

4.3.3 Uvulopalatopharyngoplasty as a single surgical procedure: UPPP as a sole procedure, with or without tonsillectomy, does not reliably normalize the AHI when treating moderate to severe OSA. Therefore, patients with severe OSA should initially be offered PAP therapy, while those

with moderate OSA should initially be offered either PAP therapy or oral appliances. (Option)

4.3.4 Multilevel or stepwise surgery. Use of MLS, as a combined procedure or stepwise operations, is acceptable in patients with narrowing of multiple sites in the upper airway, particularly if they have failed UPPP as a sole treatment. (Option)

4.3.5 Laser-assisted uvulopalatoplasy: LAUP is not routinely recommended as a treatment for OSA syndrome. (Standard)

4.3.6 Radiofrequency ablation: RFA can be considered as a treatment in patients with mild to moderate OSA who cannot tolerate or who are unwilling to adhere to PAP, or in whom oral appliances have been considered and have been found ineffective or undesirable.

4.3.7 Palatal implants: Palatal implants may be effective in some patients with mild OSA who cannot tolerate or are unwilling to adhere to PAP therapy, or in whom oral appliances have been considered and found ineffective or undesirable. (Option)

5.0 Follow-up

Postoperatively after an appropriate period of healing, patients should undergo follow-up evaluation including an objective measure of the presence and severity of sleep-disordered breathing and oxygen saturation, as well as clinical assessment for residual symptoms. In addition, patients should be followed over time to detect recurrent of disease. (Standard)

AHI = apnea-hypopnea index; LAUP = laser-assisted uvuloplasty; MMA = maxillomandibular advancement; MLS = multilevel or stepwise surgery; OSA = obstructive sleep apnea; PAP = positive airway pressure; RFA = radiofrequency ablation; UPPP = uvulopalatopharyngoplasty.

From Aurora RN, Casey KR, Kristo D, et al: Practice parameters for the surgical modifications of the upper airway for obstructive sleep apnea in adults. Sleep 2010;33:1408–1413.

Chapter 21

Central Sleep Apnea and Hypoventilation Syndromes

Chapter Points

- Hypocapnic CSA occurs because the $PaCO_2$ falls below the AT. The propensity for this type of central apnea to occur is increased when there is a small difference between the sleeping $PaCO_2$ during sleep and the AT.
- Hypocapnic CSA disorders include primary CSA (idiopathic CSA), CSB-CSA, HAPB, and some types of CompSA.
- Hypocapnic CSA is often less severe during REM sleep because this sleep stage is associated with lower ventilatory responses to $PaCO_2$ and PaO_2, and ventilation varies with the phasic changes of this sleep stage.
- CompSA is defined as the persistence or emergence of central apneas during a PAP titration in a patient with predominantly obstructive or mixed respiratory events during the diagnostic portion.
- CompSA can occur in patients with a combination of OSA and CSB, patients taking opiates, or patients without an obvious etiology (idiopathic).
- CompSA patients without CSB or opiate medication usually experience a resolution of CSA with chronic CPAP treatment. Patients with persistent CSA on CPAP require adaptive servo-ventilation or BPAP with a backup rate for effective treatment.
- Hypercapnic CSA syndromes are characterized by sleep-related hypoventilation with variable amounts of CSA. Some patients may have a normal daytime $PaCO_2$.
- The CCHS is a rare disorder usually present from birth and is characterized by alveolar hypoventilation without evidence of lung, neuromuscular, or structural brainstem abnormalities. The disorder is due to mutations in the *PHOX2b* gene.
- Opiate (narcotic)-associated sleep-disordered breathing can be manifested by long obstructive apneas, a slow respiratory rate, ataxic breathing, periodic breathing-central apneas or CompSA. Some patients have daytime hypoventilation.

- Patients with RTCD or NMD may manifest daytime hypoventilation that worsens during sleep or exhibit hypoventilation only during sleep early in the disease course. Although classified under the hypercapnic CSA subgroup, many patients have relatively few discrete central apneas.
- In RTCD/NMD patients, nocturnal gas exchange is usually the most abnormal during REM sleep.
- Nocturnal oximetry may reveal significant desaturation even if the forced vital capacity is not severely reduced. If OSA is suspected PSG is indicated.
- The treatment of choice for CSA/nocturnal hypoventilation in RTCD/NMD patients is NPPV.
- In RTCD/NMD patients a daytime $PaCO_2 \geq 45$ mm Hg or nocturnal oximetry showing ≥ 5 minutes with an $SaO_2 \leq 88\%$ is considered an indication for nocturnal NPPV.
- In patients with an NMD, an FVC < 50% of predicted or a maximal inspiratory force less than 60 cm H_2O is also considered an indication for NPPV.
- Patients with restrictive chest wall disorders may require relatively high pressure support.
- Most clinicians would treat RTCD/NMD patients with BPAP using a backup rate (BPAP-ST).

The central sleep apnea (CSA) syndromes include a diverse group of disorders associated with the presence of central apnea during sleep (Fig. 21–1).[1-3] In some of the disorders discussed in this chapter, the patients have primarily nocturnal hypoventilation (increased arterial partial pressure of carbon dioxide [$PaCO_2$]) due to inadequate tidal volume and/or respiratory rate with relatively few discrete central apneas. However, discussion of patients with central apnea and hypoventilation syndromes together is useful clinically because they have many similar aspects of pathophysiology and treatment.

FIGURE 21–1 A central sleep apnea event in a patient with the idiopathic central sleep apnea syndrome (primary central sleep apnea). Note that the central apnea followed a large breath. EMG = electromyogram; SpO$_2$ = pulse oximetry. *Adapted from Berry RB: Sleep Medicine Pearls, 2nd ed. Philadelphia: Hanley & Belfus, 2003, p. 237.*

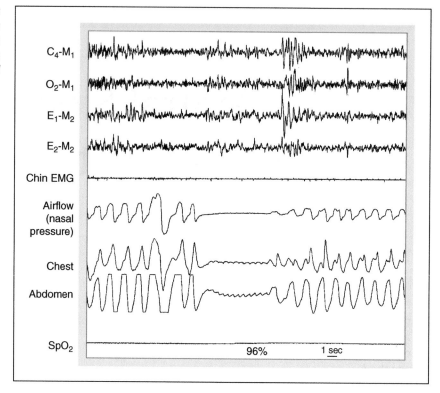

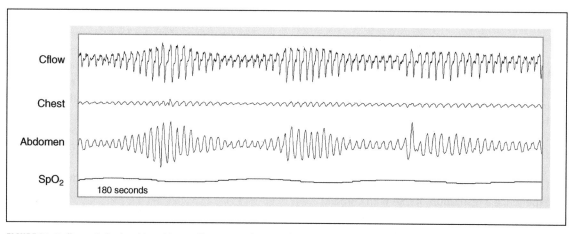

FIGURE 21–2 Cheyne-Stokes breathing with central hypopnea at the nadir of ventilatory effort. This patient had obstructive and mixed apneas during the diagnostic portion of a sleep study. When placed on continuous positive airway pressure (CPAP), the underlying ventilatory instability was uncovered. Here, Cflow is the signal from the accurate flow transducer in the positive airway pressure (PAP) device. SpO$_2$ = pulse oximetry.

Central apnea in adults is defined as a cessation in airflow of 10 seconds or longer that is associated with an absence of respiratory effort.[4] During diagnostic studies oronasal thermal sensor signal is used to detect apnea. During a positive airway pressure (PAP) titration the PAP flow signal is used. The diagnosis of a CSA *syndrome* requires that the majority of apneic events be central in nature. The exact proportion of central events required is not clear, with various authors diagnosing the CSA syndromes when 50% to 80% of the events are central. Traditionally, patients with

CSA have accounted for less than 5% to 15% of patients with sleep apnea evaluated at most sleep centers. However, two factors have increased the number of CSA patients being evaluated. First, there has been an increased recognition of sleep-disordered breathing in congestive heart failure (CHF) and a substantial number of patients with systolic heart failure have Cheyne-Stokes breathing central sleep apnea (CSB-CSA) (Fig. 21–2). Second, recently, there has been more aggressive use of opiates to control pain. As discussed in this chapter, many patients develop central apnea as a

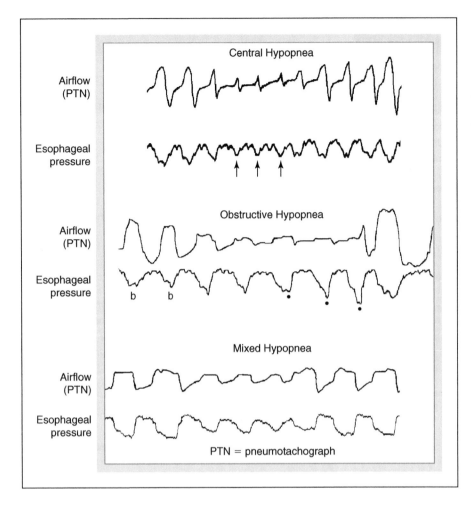

FIGURE 21-3 Central, obstructive, and mixed hypopneas. In central hypopnea, the flow falls in proportion to the respiratory effort. The airflow profile using an accurate measure of airflow (including nasal pressure or CPAP flow) shows a round contour. In obstructive hypopnea, there is evidence of airflow limitation (flat airflow shape) and flow falls even though respiratory effort stays the same or increases. In mixed hypopnea, there is a fall in respiratory effort but the fall in flow is proportionately greater and there is evidence of airflow limitation. *Adapted from Berry RB: Sleep Medicine Pearls, 2nd ed. Philadelphia: Hanley & Belfus, 2003, p. 83.*

result of the use of potent narcotics. Central apnea may occur either at baseline or once patients are exposed to PAP treatment. Thus, sleep centers can expect to see more patients with CSA.

Many patients who exhibit central apneas also exhibit central hypopneas (see Fig. 21-2). The challenges in defining central hypopnea were discussed in earlier chapters. The American Academy of Sleep Medicine (AASM) scoring manual discourages identification of central hypopnea unless an accurate method to quantify respiratory effort is being used (esophageal pressure or respiratory inductance plethysmography).[4] In general, central hypopneas are characterized by a proportionate decrease in both airflow and respiratory effort (Fig. 21-3).[5] Usually, there is no snoring or chest-abdominal paradox and the nasal pressure or PAP device flow signal is fairly rounded (minimal or no signs of airflow limitation).

CLASSIFICATION OF CSA SYNDROMES

There is a number of classifications of CSA and the hypoventilation syndrome but none of these classifications is entirely satisfactory.[1,6] The International Classification of Sleep Disorders, 2nd edition (ICSD-2) lists five CSA syndromes (Box

BOX 21-1

Central Sleep Apnea Syndromes

1. Primary central sleep apnea
2. Cheyne-Stokes breathing pattern
3. High-altitude periodic breathing
4. Central sleep apnea due to drug or substance
5. Primary sleep apnea of infancy

From American Academy of Sleep Medicine: ICSD-2 International Classification of Sleep Disorders, 2nd ed. Diagnostic and Coding Manual. Westchester, IL: American Academy of Sleep Medicine, 2005.

21-1).[6] Primary CSA is termed *idiopathic central sleep apnea (ICSA)* in this chapter, in keeping with much of the literature. Primary CSA, CSB-CSA, and high-altitude periodic breathing (HAPB) are hypocapnic forms of CSA. Patients with these syndromes have a **normal or low PaCO_2** during wakefulness. During sleep, these patients do not develop hypercapnia. In contrast, patients with CSA due to drug or substance and primary sleep apnea of infancy have normal or increased daytime $PaCO_2$ and may develop or have worsening hypercapnia during sleep. The ICSD-2 lists five

BOX 21–2

Hypoventilation Syndromes

1. Sleep-related nonobstructive alveolar hypoventilation, idiopathic
   Comment: Rare, usually case reports
2. Congenital central alveolar hypoventilation syndrome
   Example: Central congenital hypoventilation syndrome
3. Sleep-related hypoventilation due to medical condition
   A. Sleep-related hypoventilaton/hypoxemia due to lower airways obstruction
      Examples: Hypercapnic COPD, bronchiectasis, or cystic fibrosis
   B. Sleep-related hypoxemia due to pulmonary parenchymal or vascular pathology
      Example: Sleep-related hypoventilation with idiopathic pulmonary fibrosis or other interstitial lung diseases or pulmonary vascular disease associated with end-stage lung disease
   C. Sleep-related hypoventilation/hypoxemia due to neuromuscular and chest wall disorders
      Examples: Obesity hypoventilation syndrome, neuromuscular disease, kyphoscoliosis

See Appendix 21–1 for diagnostic criteria.
COPD = chronic obstructive pulmonary disease.
From American Academy of Sleep Medicine: ICSD-2 International Classification of Sleep Disorders, 2nd ed. Diagnostic and Coding Manual. American Academy of Sleep Medicine. Westchester, IL: American Academy of Sleep Medicine, 2005.

BOX 21–3

Central Sleep Apnea Syndromes

HYPOCAPNIC (normal or low daytime PCO_2)

1. Idiopathic central sleep apnea
2. Cheyne-Stokes breathing—central sleep apnea
   Associated with congestive heart failure
   Associated with neurologic disease
3. Periodic breathing at high altitude
4. Complex sleep apnea (treatment emergent or persistent sleep apnea)
   - Idiopathic complex sleep apnea*
   - Combined OSA and CSB (CPAP eliminates obstruction and unmasks CSB–CSA)

HYPERCAPNIC†

1. Won't breathe
   A. Central hypoventilation
      - Congenital central hypoventilation syndrome
      - Idiopathic central hypoventilation syndrome
      - Brain tumors, cerebrovascular disease
      - Structural brain disorders—Chiari's syndrome
      - Apnea of infancy
   B. Medication-induced central sleep apnea (narcotics/opiates)
      - Central sleep apnea with normal or increased daytime PCO_2
      - Complex sleep apnea (treatment emergent or persistent central sleep apnea)
   C. Obesity hypoventilation syndrome
2. "Can't Breathe"
   A. Restrictive thoracic cage disorders
   B. Neuromuscular disorders
      i. Motor neuron disease including poliomyelitis
      ii. Neuropathy
      iii. Neuromuscular junction disorders (myasthenia gravis)
      iv. Myopathy (muscular dystrophy)

*Idiopathic complex sleep apnea refers to patients with CompSA who do not have Cheyne-Stokes breathing or are not taking narcotics or other medications altering ventilatory drive.
†Some patients with these disorders may have normal daytime $PaCO_2$.
CompSA = complex sleep apnea; CPAP = continuous positive airway pressure; CSA = central sleep apnea; CSB = Cheyne-Stokes breathing; OSA = obstructive sleep apnea; $PaCO_2$ = arterial partial pressure of carbon dioxide; PCO_2 = partial pressure of carbon dioxide.

categories of hypoventilation syndromes (Box 21–2). Idiopathic nonobstructive hypoventilation is due to an abnormality of ventilatory control of unknown etiology. Congenital hypoventilation syndrome is due to abnormal ventilatory control due to a genetic abnormality. Three groups of disorders with hypoxemia or hypercapnia during sleep are listed. The first is due to lower airways obstruction (e.g., chronic obstructive pulmonary disease), the second is due to pulmonary parenchymal or vascular disorders (e.g., pulmonary fibrosis, interstitial lung disease), and the third is due to abnormality of the chest wall or neuromuscular disorders (e.g., kyphoscoliosis, amyotrophic lateral sclerosis [ALS], obesity hypoventilation syndrome [OHS]). Patients with the OHS are discussed in Chapter 15. The effects of chronic obstructive pulmonary disease on sleep (including hypercapnia) are discussed in Chapter 22.

This chapter utilizes a classification of the CSA syndromes adapted from one proposed by Bradley and coworkers[1] (Box 21–3) that subdivides patients into hypocapnic and hypercapnic groups. Patients with hypocapnic CSA tend to have low to normal daytime $PaCO_2$ values. The disorders in this group include ICSA, CSB-CSA, HAPB, and treatment-persistent/-emergent CSA.

The term *complex sleep apnea (CompSA)* has been used to identify patients who have primarily obstructive or mixed events during diagnostic studies but develop central apneas on PAP treatment (treatment-emergent central apneas) or have significant persistent central apneas on PAP treatment (treatment-persistent central sleep apnea).[7] It is not unusual for patients with obstructive sleep apnea (OSA; predominantly obstructive apneas and hypopneas) to have some mixed or central apneas during diagnostic studies.[8,9] PAP will eliminate central and mixed as well as obstructive apneas in many of these patients on the first treatment night (or during the initial PAP treatment).[9] In other patients, central apneas will persist after airway obstruction is eliminated. In the early studies of the effect of treatment of OSA patients

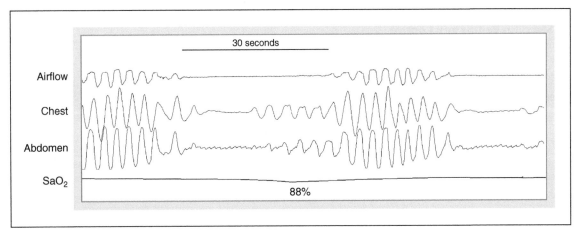

FIGURE 21-4 A mixed apnea. Note the crescendo-decrescendo pattern of ventilatory effort. When the patient was placed on CPAP, the mixed apneas were converted to central apneas of the Cheyne-Stokes type. Another hint that the patient has congestive heart failure is the delay in the arterial oxygen saturation (SaO₂) nadir. The 88% occurs before the termination of the event pictured. In fact, this desaturation is not due to the event pictured but to the previous event. Airflow = nasal pressure. *From Malhotra A, Berry RB, White DP: Central sleep apnea. In Carney P, Berry RB, Geyer JW (eds): Clinical Sleep Medicine. Philadelphia: Lippincott Williams & Wilkins, 2005, p. 341.*

with tracheostomy (elimination of obstruction), patients were found to have residual central apneas that tended to resolve with chronic treatment.[8] The term *CompSA* is also sometimes used to include patients with narcotic-associated sleep-disordered breathing who have persistent or emergent central apneas on PAP. Patients with this condition usually have high normal or mildly increased PaCO₂ during wakefulness. In this chapter, this group is discussed under the hypercapnic CSA group. It is also not uncommon for patients with CHF to have a combination of obstructive or mixed apnea and CSB-CSA (Fig. 21-4).[10] In some of these patients, application of PAP will eliminate obstruction but frequent central apneas of the Cheyne-Stokes type may persist or emerge. For this reason, the term *CompSA* is sometimes applied. These patients are discussed with the nonhypercapnic CSA disorders. Patients with CompSA without an obvious etiology (no narcotics or heart failure) are termed *idiopathic CompSA* for lack of a better terminology. These patients have an instability in ventilatory control either at baseline or due to PAP treatment. Because they have normal or low daytime PaCO₂, they are discussed in the hypocapnic CSA sections.

The hypercapnic CSA syndromes associated with hypoventilation include those with a defect in ventilatory control (congenital central alveolar hypoventilation, acquired central alveolar hypoventilation, CSA due to medication/substance), patients with the OHS, thoracic cage disorders, and neuromuscular disorders. The hypercapnic CSA group can be divided into a "won't breathe" group (can reduce their PaCO₂ with voluntary increases in ventilation) and a "can't breathe" group due to an abnormal thoracic cage or neuromuscular weakness. This classification is not entirely satisfactory because patients with OHS have various combinations of OSA, abnormal ventilatory control, and respiratory pump abnormality (mass loading due to obesity). Of note, early in

the disease course, **some patients with chronic hypoventilation syndromes will have an increased PaCO₂ only during sleep.** They may present with complaints of disturbed sleep or nocturnal dyspnea, morning headaches, daytime sleepiness, or insomnia. Later in the disease course, these may present with hypercapnic respiratory failure and cor pulmonale.

PATHOPHYSIOLOGY OF CSA

Effects of Normal Physiologic Changes

In normal individuals, there is a 2 to 8 mm Hg rise in PaCO₂ during non–rapid eye movement (NREM) sleep. This is thought due to loss of the wakefulness drive, reduction of the hypercapnic and hypoxic ventilatory drives, and increased upper airway resistance (Table 21-1).[11] The wakefulness drive is a poorly understood generalized augmentation of ventilation associated with the wakefulness state. During NREM sleep, ventilation is totally under metabolic control (chemoreceptors). Ventilatory control centers respond to information from the peripheral chemoreceptors including the carotid body (arterial partial pressure of oxygen [PaO₂] and PaCO₂) and medullary chemoreceptors (H⁺ due to changes in PaCO₂).[11] During rapid eye movement (REM) sleep, ventilation is irregular and nonmetabolic factors also affect ventilation. The hypercapnic and hypoxic ventilatory drives are lower during REM than during NREM sleep. In addition, during REM sleep, there is generalized skeletal muscle hypotonia.[11-13] The contribution of accessory muscles of ventilation is either reduced or absent and ventilation depends entirely on the diaphragm. The loss of accessory inspiratory muscles can compromise the ability to maintain adequate ventilation, especially in patients with muscle weakness or a high work of breathing. During the phasic changes of REM sleep (associated with bursts of eye

TABLE 21–1

Effect of Sleep on Ventilatory Control

	WAKE	NREM	REM
Wakefulness drive	Present	Absent	Absent
Central chemoreceptors (H$^+$, PCO$_2$)	Intact	Reduced	Very reduced
Peripheral chemoreceptors (PO$_2$, PCO$_2$ [H$^+$])	Intact	Reduced	Very reduced
Apneic threshold	Not present	Present	N/A
Behavioral and other nonventilatory control center influences	Present	Absent	Periods of reduced tidal volume during phasic REM sleep often associated with bursts of eye movements

N/A = not applicable; NREM = non-rapid eye movement; PCO$_2$ = partial pressure of carbon dioxide; PO$_2$ = partial pressure of oxygen; REM = rapid eye movement.

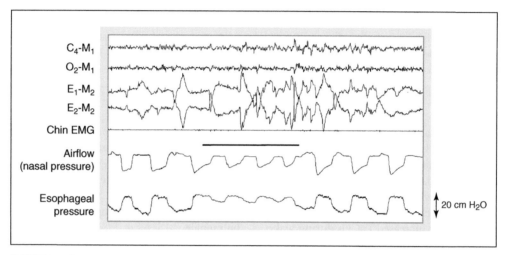

FIGURE 21–5 Respiration during rapid eye movement (REM) sleep. Periods of diminished diaphragmatic activity (reflected in decreased esophageal pressure excursions) and tidal volume associated with the phasic changes of REM sleep (associated with bursts of eye movements). EMG = electromyogram. *From Berry RB: Sleep Medicine Pearls, 2nd ed. Philadelphia: Hanley & Belfus, 2003, p. 31.*

movements), there is often additional inhibition of upper airway muscles and diaphragmatic activity resulting in episodes of central apnea or reduced tidal volume (Fig. 21–5).[12,13] Patients with hypercapnic CSA/hypoventilation syndromes usually have worse oxygenation and highest PaCO$_2$ during REM sleep. It is of interest that some patients with hypocapnic CSA due to ventilatory control instability may actually have better oxygen saturation during REM than during NREM sleep. For example, in the ICSA or CSB-CSA syndromes, central apneas generally do not occur during REM sleep. Some patients with CompSA will also have a much better response to CPAP during REM sleep than during NREM sleep.

Ventilatory Control in Hypocapnic CSA

A number of factors contribute to the occurrence of hypocapnic CSA (Table 21–2). Patients with hypocapnic CSA have a normal or low daytime PaCO$_2$ and high ventilatory responses to hypercapnia. They develop central apnea because the PaCO$_2$ falls below the apneic threshold (AT) to be discussed in the following section.[14,15] From a ventilatory

TABLE 21–2

Mechanisms Inducing Central Apnea

IDIOPATHIC CENTRAL SLEEP APNEA	CHEYNE-STOKES BREATHING
High hypercapnic ventilatory drive (high controller gain)	• High hypercapnic ventilatory response (high controller gain)
Small sleeping PCO$_2$—AT difference	• High sympathetic activity
Sleep state instability (arousals)	• Pulmonary congestion—high PCWP (J receptor stimulation)
	• Delay in arterial blood reaching chemoreceptors
	• Small sleeping PCO$_2$—AT difference

AT = apneic threshold; PCO$_2$ = partial pressure of carbon dioxide; PCWP = pulmonary capillary wedge pressure.

control model standpoint, they have high system loop gain and ventilatory instability.[16,17] Central apneas are more common in stage N1 and N2 rather than stage N3 sleep because ventilation is less stable on transition from wakefulness to sleep. Sleep stage changes and arousal predispose to

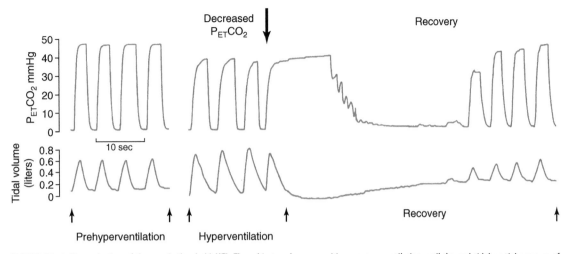

FIGURE 21-6 Determination of the apneic threshold (AT). The subject undergoes positive-pressure ventilation until the end-tidal partial pressure of carbon dioxide ($P_{ET}CO_2$) drops and the ventilator is turned off. If $P_{ET}CO_2$ is below the AT, central apnea ensues. *From Skatrud JB, Dempsey JA: Interaction of sleep state and chemical stimuli in sustaining rhythmic ventilation. J Appl Physiol 1983;55:813–822.*

the occurrence of central apneas in patients with hypocapnic CSA.[18] Hypocapnic central apneas are uncommon during REM sleep because ventilation is not totally under metabolic control and the ventilatory response to hypercapnia is lower than during NREM sleep, making ventilatory instability less likely. Short central apneas can occur during REM sleep during bursts of eye movements but these are likely not due to a lowering of $PaCO_2$ below the AT.

Apneic Threshold

During wakefulness, hypocapnia does not cause cessation of breathing due to the presence of the wakefulness stimulus to breathing. During NREM sleep, ventilation depends completely on metabolic control. If the $PaCO_2$ falls below a characteristic value (AT) for each individual, a central apnea occurs[14,15] (Fig. 21-6). Ventilation does not resume until the $PaCO_2$ climbs above (and actually slightly higher than) the AT. The AT can be experimentally determined by serial runs of hyperventilation with positive-pressure ventilation that progressively drop the $PaCO_2$ to various levels below the eucapnic $PaCO_2$ level during sleep. The positive-pressure ventilation is terminated suddenly, and if the $PaCO_2$ has dropped below the AT, a central apnea occurs. For example, suppose the spontaneous sleeping $PaCO_2$ is 42 mm Hg, then trials could progressively induce $PaCO_2$ values of 41, 40, 39, 38, 37, and so on. The level at which a central apnea occurs when the positive-pressure device is turned off is the AT. As noted previously, the sleeping $PaCO_2$ is normally about 2 to 8 mm Hg above waking value. The typical AT is usually **at or 1 to 2 mm Hg lower than the waking $PaCO_2$.** In Figure 21-7, during normoxia, an individual end-tidal partial pressure of carbon dioxide ($P_{ET}CO_2$) increases with sleep from 40 to 44 mm Hg. Hyperventilation trials with positive-pressure ventilation resulted in central apnea (apnea duration > 0 sec) in a range of $P_{ET}CO_2$ values from about 38 to 42 mm Hg.

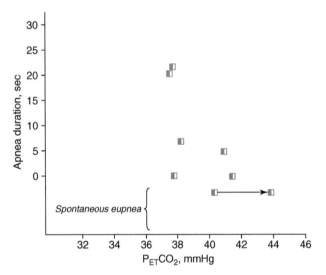

FIGURE 21-7 The results of determination of the apneic threshold (AT) in an individual who spontaneously increases the end-tidal partial pressure of carbon dioxide ($P_{ET}CO_2$) from slightly above 40 mm Hg when awake to 44 mm Hg during sleep (spontaneous eupnea shown by *arrow*). The AT varied but was usually at or slightly below the awake arterial carbon dioxide pressure ($PaCO_2$) value. $P_{ET}CO_2$ values from 38 mm Hg to slightly above 40 mm Hg resulted in central apnea (apnea duration > 0 sec). Note that there was some variability with one trial resulting in a $P_{ET}CO_2$ of 38 mm Hg that did not result in central apnea. *From Skatrud JB, Dempsey JA: Interaction of sleep state and chemical stimuli in sustaining rhythmic ventilation. J Appl Physiol 1983;55:813–822.*

Of note, it is the **difference** between the sleeping $PaCO_2$ and the AT rather than the position of the AT that is the critical determinant of the propensity to develop central apnea. The smaller the $PaCO_2$-AT difference the more likely CSA is to occur. Figure 21-8 shows awake and sleeping $PaCO_2$ values for CHF patients with and without periodic breathing. Those with periodic breathing have a small difference between the sleeping $PaCO_2$ and the AT. This is because the $PaCO_2$ increased relatively little with transition from

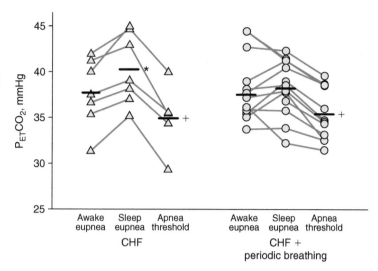

FIGURE 21–8 The awake eupnea end-tidal partial pressure of carbon dioxide ($PaCO_2$), sleeping $P_{ET}CO_2$, and apneic threshold (AT) for patients with congestive heart failure (CHF) with and without periodic breathing. The patients with periodic breathing had a small sleeping $P_{ET}CO_2$—AT difference. *From Xie A, Skatrud JG, Puelo DS, et al: Apnea-hypopnea threshold for CO_2 in patients with congestive heart failure. Am Respir Crit Care Med 2002;165:1245–1250.*

wake to sleep but the AT did not show a corresponding decrease.[19]

Studies have shown that the $PaCO_2$-AT difference can vary with changes in ventilatory drive.[20] Specifically, the $PaCO_2$-AT difference increases with the induction of metabolic acidosis (acetazolamide) and decreases with metabolic alkalosis. This is somewhat counterintuitive because one might expect that further increases in ventilatory drive due to metabolic acidosis would increase the propensity for central apnea. In contrast to metabolic acidosis, hypocapnic hypoxia decreases the $PaCO_2$-AT difference. Thus, hypoxemia can increase the likelihood of central apnea. A detailed description of the factors that affect the $PaCO_2$-AT difference is found in references 15 and 20.

Loop Gain

Ventilatory control stability has also been analyzed using feedback control theory focusing on the loop gain (LG) of the respiratory system.[2,16,17] The LG is determined by the plant gain (ability of increases in ventilation by the lungs/respiratory muscles to reduce the $PaCO_2$) and the controller gain (change in ventilation induced by a change in $PaCO_2$) (Fig. 21–9). High plant gain ($\Delta PaCO_2/\Delta$ ventilation) is associated with hypercapnia and low physiologic dead space. Owing to the hyperbolic relationship between ventilation and $PaCO_2$, small changes in ventilation induce larger changes in $PaCO_2$ if hypercapnia is present (Fig. 21–10A). Controller gain depends on the sensitivity of the ventilatory control centers to changes in $PaCO_2$. Controller gain can be expressed as Δ Ventilation/Δ $PaCO_2$. The LG = plant gain × controller gain. A system with a high LG (LG > 1) is unstable (see Fig. 21–10B). High controller gain or high plant gain can destabilize the system. In hypocapnic CSA, the major factors causing instability are the high controller gain and the effect of wake-to-sleep transitions.

Upper Airway and Posture Effects

Both ICSA and CSB-CSA tend to be worse in the supine position.[21,22] In ICSA patients, Issa and Sullivan[21] found

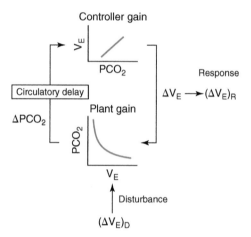

Loop gain (LG) = plant gain × controller gain

FIGURE 21–9 The interaction between controller gain and plant gain for the respiratory system. High controller gain or high plant gain results in a large response to a small disturbance (change in ventilation). D = disturbance; PCO_2 = partial pressure of carbon dioxide; R = response; V_E = volume of expired gas. *From White DP: Central sleep apnea. In Kryger MH, Roth T, Dement WC (eds): Principles and Practice of Sleep Medicine. Philadelphia: Elsevier, 2005, pp. 969–981.*

central apnea to be more frequent in the supine position. They hypothesized that upper airway reflexes may trigger central apnea because upper airway anesthesia abolished central apnea in two patients. In addition, high levels of continuous positive airway pressure (CPAP) abolished central apnea. CSB-CSA has also been noted to be more prominent in the supine position.[22] It is not known whether this is due to upper airway factors or to changes in oxygenation or pulmonary congestion.

HYPOCAPNIC CSA SYNDROMES

Patterns of Ventilation in ICSA and CSB

The patterns of ventilation differ between patients with CSB-CSA and patients with ICSA. In both groups, the

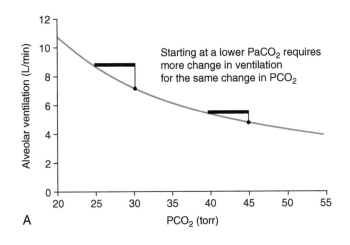

FIGURE 21–10   **A,** Starting at a lower arterial partial pressure of carbon dioxide ($PaCO_2$) means that to induce a given change in partial pressure of carbon dioxide (PCO_2) requires a large change in ventilation (smaller plant gain). **B,** A system with a loop gain (LG) of 1 or greater is unstable and tends to oscillate after a disturbance. **A** and **B,** From White DP: Pathogenesis of obstructive and central sleep apnea. Am J Respir Crit Care Med 2005;172:1363–1370.

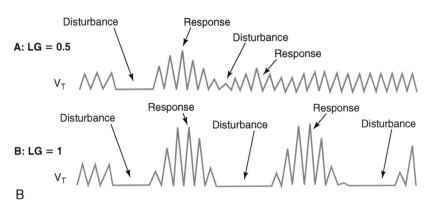

TABLE 21–3

Differences in Respiration between Patients with Idiopathic Central Sleep Apnea and Cheyne-Stokes Breathing

	CENTRAL APNEA DURATION (SEC)	CYCLE LENGTH (SEC)	VENTILATORY PHASE (BETWEEN APNEAS) (SEC)	DELAY IN SaO_2 NADIR (SEC)
ICSA	20.9	37.3	16.7	10.3
CSB-CSA (CHF)	22.3	59.0	36.7	24.3

CHF = congestive heart failure; CSA = central sleep apnea; CSB = Cheyne-Stokes breathing; ICSA = idiopathic central sleep apnea; SaO_2 = arterial oxygen saturation. From Hall MJ, Xie A, Rutherford R, Bradley TD: Cycle length of periodic breathing with and without heart failure. Am J Respir Crit Care Med 1996;154:376–381.

central apneas typically are 20 to 40 seconds in duration. In ICSA, there is typically a short ventilatory phase of 2 to 4 breaths between central apneas, and arousals tend to occur at apnea termination (Fig. 21–11). Patients with CSB have a longer ventilatory phase between consecutive apneas, and the ventilatory phase has a characteristic crescendo-decrescendo morphology. Hall and colleagues[23] compared cycle length between patients with ICSA and CSB-CSA due to heart failure (Table 21–3). The apnea durations were similar but cycle length was longer in CSB-CSA due to a long ventilatory phase. The CSA-CSB patients also had a longer delay in the arterial oxygen saturation (SaO_2) nadir. The lower the cardiac output, the longer the ventilatory phase and the delay in SaO_2 nadir. This is believed due

to a long circulation time. The patterns of ventilation in treatment-emergent CSA (nonhypercapnic, non-CSB CompSA) resembles that of ICSA.

Idiopathic CSA (Primary CSA)

These patients have central apneas of unknown etiology. CHF, neurologic disorders, or medications suppressing ventilation are not present. The prevalence varies but is thought to be 5% to 10% of patients being studied in sleep centers. Patients may present with symptoms similar to those of patients with OSA. These may include daytime sleepiness or insomnia, snoring, witnessed breathing pauses, and disturbed sleep. They tend to be thinner than patients with OSA

CSA-CSB has longer cycle length due to a longer ventilatory phase

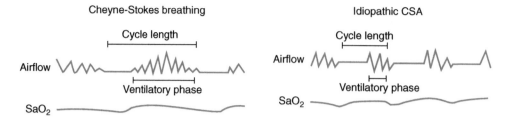

CSA-CSB often has arousal at the zenith of ventilatory effort and the nadir in the SaO₂ is delayed

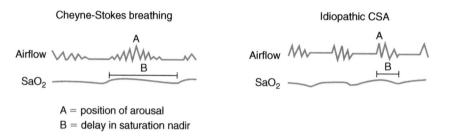

A = position of arousal
B = delay in saturation nadir

FIGURE 21–11 Schematic illustrations of the difference between idiopathic central sleep apnea (CSA) and Cheyne-Stokes breathing (CSB) central apnea associated with heart failure. The ventilatory phase is longer in CSB-CSA, arousal occurs at the zenith of ventilation, and the nadir in the arterial oxygen saturation (SaO₂) is delayed.

BOX 21–4

Primary Central Sleep Apnea—Diagnostic Criteria

A. The patient reports at least one of the following:
  i. Excessive daytime sleepiness.
  ii. Frequent arousals and awakenings during sleep or insomnia complaints.
  iii. Awakening short of breath.
B. Polysomnography shows five or more central apneas per hour of sleep.
C. The disorder is not better explained by another current sleep disorder, medical or neurologic disorder, medication use, or substance use disorder.

From American Academy of Sleep Medicine: ICSD-2 International Classification of Sleep Disorders, 2nd ed. Diagnostic and Coding Manual. Westchester, IL: American Academy of Sleep Medicine, 2005.

and have less prominent snoring. In the ICSD-2, the terminology for this patient group is *primary CSA* (Box 21–4).

Pathophysiology of Idiopathic CSA

As reflected in the term "idiopathic," the etiology of primary CSA is unknown. However, the patients have ventilatory instability due to a high hypercapnic ventilatory response[24] or sleep state instability.[18] These patients tend to have decreased PaCO₂ values during wakefulness. Often, central apnea can be triggered by only one or two large breaths (see Fig. 21–1). The periods of increased ventilation triggering central apneas often are associated with arousal. Arousal may

trigger a transient increase in ventilation and a fall in PaCO₂. This transient fall in PaCO₂ is then associated with a central apnea as the patient returns to sleep. As discussed previously, in some patients with ICSA, central apnea occurs mainly in the supine position.[21] Studies have documented a response to CPAP in some ICSA patients.[21,25] In research studies, the addition of **dead space or inhalation of PaCO₂** with the goal of increasing and/or stabilizing the PaCO₂ has been shown to reduce central apnea in ICSA patients.[26] However, these interventions have not been tried for long-term treatment nor are they practical.

Polysomnography

Sleep studies in patients with ICSA typically reveal frequent, isolated central apneas or runs of central apneas (a form of periodic breathing). A run of central apneas may follow arousal from a nonrespiratory stimulus. Central apneas in ICSA patients occur during NREM sleep, most commonly in stage 1 or 2 sleep. Central apnea in these patients is much less common during stage N3 and REM sleep. The percentage of total respiratory events that must be central is not well defined but is usually taken as greater than 50%.

Treatment of ICSA

Because idiopathic CSA is rare, most treatment information comes from small case series (no randomized, controlled studies) and no long-term studies of the effectiveness of any treatment have been published. There is no uniform consensus about the best treatment for patients with ICSA. This group is heterogeneous, and treatment must be

BOX 21–5

Possible Treatments for Idiopathic Central Sleep Apnea

CPAP
Hypnotics
Respiratory stimulants (acetazolamide)
Oxygen therapy??

CPAP = continuous positive airway pressure.

individualized (Box 21–5). Various respiratory stimulants have been tried as treatments for idiopathic CSA, with variable amounts of success.[27–29] The best evidence is for use of acetazolamide (Diamox), which is a carbonic anhydrase inhibitor. Acetazolamide induces a metabolic acidosis and reduces the pH even if the $PaCO_2$ also decreases slightly. DeBacker and associates[27] studied the effects of acetazolamide 250 mg 1 hour before sleep after 1 month of treatment in ICSA patients. The apnea-hypopnea index (AHI) was reduced by about 50% and symptoms improved, although sleep efficiency was not significantly better.[27]

Another treatment approach is to decrease arousals and promote stage N3 sleep where ventilation is more stable and the $PaCO_2$ likely slightly higher. Hypnotics including triazolam and zolpidem have been tried.[30–32] A recent trial of zolpidem 10 mg in ICSA was reported by Quadri and coworkers.[31] The central AHI decreased from 30 to 13.5/hr and subjective sleepiness as measured by the Epworth Sleepiness Scale improved (from 13 to 8). However, in some patients, obstructive events increased with hypnotic treatment. Of note, hypnotics are relatively contraindicated in hypercapnic CSA.

As noted previously, CPAP also appears to be effective treatment in some patients with ICSA.[21,25] The mechanisms by which CPAP works are unknown. Four possibilities are that nasal CPAP minimizes overshoots in $PaCO_2$ after arousal, slightly increases the sleeping $PaCO_2$ in patients who are hypocapnic at baseline, prevents high upper airway resistance from inducing arousals, or prevents significant negative upper airway pressure (which may trigger reflex central apnea). Patients who snore or have central apnea mainly in the supine position might be assumed to be the best candidates for CPAP treatment. Of note, one case report found that CPAP helped but bilevel positive airway pressure (BPAP) worsened CSA.[33] BPAP may destabilize the system by augmenting ventilation. No study evaluating the effect of adaptive servo-ventilation (ASV), a mode designed to stabilize ventilation, in ICSA has been published but a trial of that treatment might be reasonable. Supplemental oxygen has been shown to improve CSA in patients with CSB.[34,35] However, an evaluation of supplemental oxygen in ICSA patients has not been published. Supplemental oxygen might work by decreasing ventilatory instability by blunting the hypercapnic ventilatory response. The hypercapnic ventilatory response is increased by hypoxia and decreased by hyperoxia.

CSB WITH CSA

CSB occurs most commonly in patients with left ventricular systolic dysfunction[36–38] but also can occur in patients with diastolic CHF or neurologic disorders.[39,40] The neurologic disorders associated with CSB include a prior cerebrovascular accident (CVA) and neurodegenerative disorders. CSB may be present in up to 30% of patients in the first few days after stroke.[39,41] Central apnea tends to resolve and is less commonly seen in studies of patients studied several months after stroke. OSA is the predominant form of sleep apnea present in patients after CVA. Of interest, a recent study suggested that a significant proportion of CSB-CSA in stroke patients was due to occult cardiovascular disease.[42] CSA-CSB has also recently been reported in patients with heart failure with normal systolic function (diastolic heart failure).[40]

CSB-CSA due to systolic CHF is probably the most common cause of CSA seen today. Javaheri and colleagues[36] found occult sleep-disordered breathing in 45% of a group with stable heart failure and an ejection fraction less than 45% and CSA was common in the affected individuals. MacDonald and associates[37] studied a group of patients in stable CHF with maximal modern medical management and found 61% to have some form of sleep-disordered breathing (31% central apnea and 30% OSA). Oldenberg and coworkers[38] studied 700 patients with CHF and found similar results. It should be noted that many patients in these studies had various amounts of both central and obstructive apneas. Defining what percentage of events qualified the patient for the central apnea group was somewhat arbitrary. In addition, **patients can vary in the percentage of central events overnight**[43] **or from night to night.**[44] In any case, the prevalence of CSB-CSA is very high in patients with significant systolic heart failure.

Patients with CSA-CSB may complain of the typical symptoms of sleep apnea including disturbed sleep or daytime sleepiness. However, in most studies, the majority of patients do not complain of subjective excessive daytime sleepiness. Thus, a high index of suspicion is needed to suspect the presence of CSB. Nocturnal sleep complaints are often assumed to be secondary to CHF rather than to co-morbid sleep apnea. Despite the lack of subjective sleepiness complaints in CSB-CSA patients, studies have documented improvement in sleep quality and objective daytime sleepiness with successful treatment.[45]

Polysomnography in CSB-CSA

The crescendo-decrescendo morphology of CSB-CSA has previously been discussed (see Figs. 21–2, 21–4, and 21–11). Another characteristic to appreciate is the long delay in the nadir in the SaO_2 tracing after event termination due to a prolonged circulation time (low cardiac output) (Fig. 21–12). The distinctive pattern of CSB may not be recognized during a diagnostic study in a patient who has **both OSA and underlying CSB.**[10] However, during a subsequent PAP titration, pure CSB-CSA may emerge when upper airway

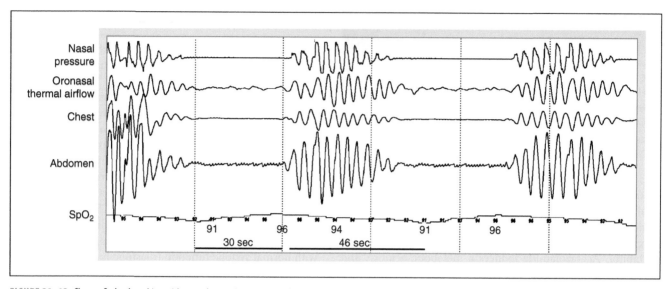

FIGURE 21–12 Cheyne-Stokes breathing with central apnea in a patient with systolic heart failure central apnea. Note the long delay in the nadir in the pulse oximetry (SpO_2). The tracing is 180 seconds and the *vertical lines* denote 30-second epochs.

obstruction is eliminated (Fig. 21–13). The possibility of underlying CSB should be considered if mixed apneas during the diagnostic study have a long central component or if the nadir in the SaO_2 following obstructive event termination is delayed. If central hypopneas rather than central apneas are present, this may also make CSB more difficult to recognize. As noted previously, central hypopneas rather than apneas can occur at the nadirs in ventilatory effort (see Fig. 21–2). The typical CSB cycle time is relatively long at 60 to 90 seconds and may be missed if a short time window is used to monitor sleep during a PAP titration. Figure 21–13 also illustrates the typical cessation of CSB-CSA when a patient transitions from NREM to REM sleep.

Pathophysiology of CSB-CSA

The factors contributing to CSB include high ventilatory drive (high sympathetic tone, pulmonary congestion), long circulation time, and a small difference between the sleeping $PaCO_2$ and the AT. Patients with CSB have low daytime $PaCO_2$ compared with CHF patients without CSB[46,47] due to increased ventilatory drive. High drive is thought to be due to increased sympathetic tone and pulmonary congestion stimulation of lung J receptors. In one study of patients with CHF, the higher the pulmonary capillary wedge pressure, the lower the awake $PaCO_2$ (Fig. 21–14A).[48] In another study, the higher the pulmonary capillary wedge pressure, the higher the AHI (see Fig. 21–14B).[49] As noted previously, CHF patients with CSB also have a small difference between the sleeping $PaCO_2$ and the AT.[19]

One might expect CHF patients with CSA to have lower cardiac output or ejection fraction compared with those that do not have periodic breathing. However, one study comparing groups with CHF with and without CSB found the two groups had similar ejection fractions but the CSB patients

had a lower daytime $PaCO_2$.[47] Other studies have found lower ejection fractions in patients with CSB.[37] A study by Sin and colleagues[50] of 450 men and women with CHF identified risk factors for the presence of OSA and CSA. Risk factors for CSA included male sex, atrial fibrillation, age older than 60, and hypocapnia ($PaCO_2 < 38$ mm Hg) during wakefulness. Risk factors for OSA included a high body mass index (BMI) in men and an increase in age in women. The presence of CSB-CSA also has prognostic implications. **Studies have suggested that the presence of CSA in patients with CHF is associated with a worse prognosis** (Fig. 21–15).[51,52]

Treatment of CSB-CSA

CSB-CSA in patients with CHF may improve with improved medical treatment of heart failure.[53] Transplantation may also cure CSB-CSA.[54] A number of treatments have been tried including aminophylline,[55] acetazolamide,[56] hypnotics,[57] oxygen,[34,35,58,59] and PAP[52,60,61] (Box 21–6). Neither aminophylline (can increase arrhythmias) nor acetazolamide has been widely used. One study found temazepam reduced the arousal index without worsening oxygenation but the amount of CSB was not improved.[57] In contrast, a number of studies of 1 to 3 months' duration have documented improvement with CPAP in a substantial number of patients showing an improvement in sleep quality and ejection fraction and reduced sympathetic activity.[52,60,61] Titration of CPAP in CSB-CSA patients differs from that in OSA patients. On a given titration night, a pressure that eliminates CSA cannot usually be found. Typically, pressure is increased until obstructive events are eliminated and then increased to 8 to 10 cm H_2O (if pressure is not already above that level). In some studies of CPAP treatment for CSB-CSA, CPAP was started on an outpatient basis and increased

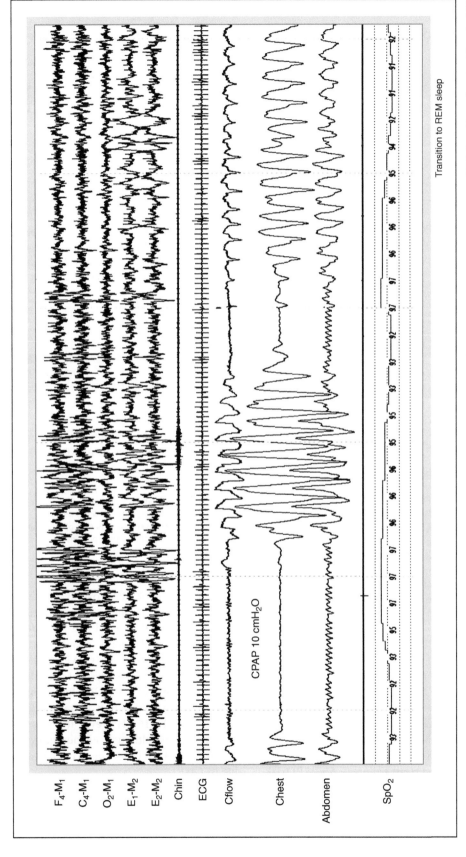

FIGURE 21–13　Note the presence of CSB-CSA on continuous positive airway pressure (CPAP). Also note the sudden cessation of CSB-CSA on transition to rapid eye movement (REM) sleep. Cflow = flow signal from the CPAP device; ECG = electrocardiogram; SpO₂ = pulse oximetry.

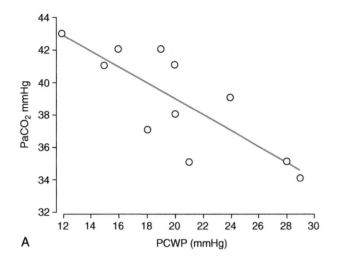

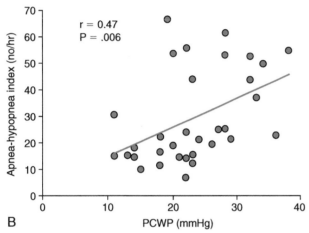

FIGURE 21-14 **A,** The higher the pulmonary capillary wedge pressure (PCWP), the lower the daytime arterial partial pressure of carbon dioxide ($PaCO_2$) in a group of patients with congestive heart failure. **B,** The higher the PCWP, the higher the apnea-hypopnea index (AHI; central events) in a patient with congestive heart failure and CSB-CSA. **A,** From Lorenzi-Filho G, Azevedo ER, Parker JD, Bradley TD: Relationship of carbon dioxide tension in arterial blood to pulmonary wedge pressure in heart failure. Eur Respir J 2002;19:37–40. **B,** From Solin P, Bergin P, Richardson M, et al: Influence of pulmonary capillary wedge pressure on central apnea in heart failure. Circulation 1999;99:1574–1579.

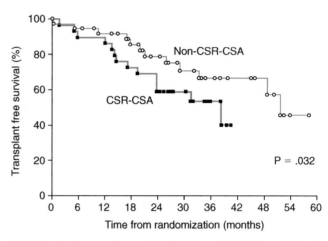

FIGURE 21-15 Transplant-free survival in CHF patients with CSR-CSA was significantly worse than in those with Cheyne-Stokes respiration (CSR)-CSA independent of the use of CPAP. *From Sin DD, Fitzgerald F, Parker JD, et al: Risk factors for central and obstructive sleep apnea in 450 men and women with congestive heart failure. Am J Respir Crit Care Med 1999;160:64.*

BOX 21–6

Treatments for Cheyne-Stokes Breathing–Central Sleep Apnea Associated with Heart Failure

- Optimize medical management (lower PCWP)
- Supplemental oxygen
- CPAP (effective in ~40–50%)
- BPAP with backup rate (BPAP-ST)
- ASV
- Transplant

Note: Theophylline and acetazolamide (case report) have been reported to be effective but are not used in clinical practice.
ASV = adaptive servo-ventilation; BPAP = bilevel positive airway pressure; CPAP = continuous positive airway pressure; PCWP = pulmonary capillary wedge pressure; ST = spontaneous-timed mode.

slowly with a goal of 8 to 10 cm H_2O commonly recommended.[62] One randomized trial of CPAP provided preliminary evidence of prolonged survival in patients with CSB-CSA treated with CPAP.[52] The ability of CPAP to improve mortality was subsequently investigated by the Canadian Continuous Positive Airway Pressure for Patients with Central Sleep Apnea and Heart Failure (CANPAP) trial. This large, multicenter, randomized, controlled trial compared CPAP and standard treatment for patients with CHF and CSB-CSA.[62] Unfortunately, the trial failed to show a survival benefit with CPAP treatment and there was a trend for higher early mortality in the CPAP group. The results of the study were disappointing, but analysis showed that only about 50% of patients responded to CPAP (defined as an AHI < 15/hr on a sleep study after 3 mo of treatment).

The average level of CPAP over 3 months was around 9 cm H_2O. Of interest, Javaheri and associates[63] during a single night of titration also found that 57% of patients responded to CPAP. Given that only about 50% of patients in the CANPAP trial responded to CPAP (AHI < 15/hr), the results are not surprising. An analysis of the subgroups responding and not responding to CPAP[64] showed improvement in survival and ejection fraction in responders compared with controls (Fig. 21–16). However, this was a post-hoc analysis and the results, although encouraging, do not prove the effectiveness of CPAP for unselected patients with CSB-CSA due to CHF.

Because only about 50% of patients with CSB-CSA improve with CPAP treatment, ASV was developed to stabilize breathing in CSB-CSA patients. A study by Teschler and coworkers[65] compared CPAP, oxygen, BPAP with a backup rate (BPAP-ST [spontaneous-timed mode]), and ASV each used for a single night (Fig. 21–17). This study showed a modest improvement in the AHI with oxygen and CPAP. BPAP-ST was more effective. ASV reduced the AHI to very

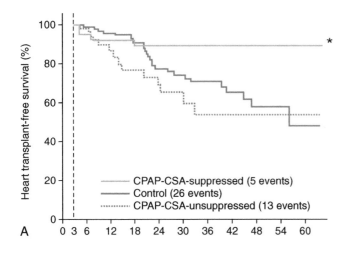

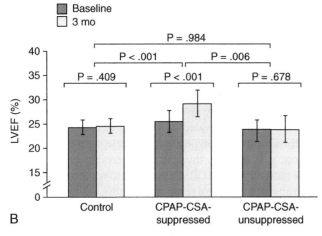

FIGURE 21-16 Results from an analysis of the data from the Canadian Continuous Positive Airway Pressure for Patients with Central Sleep Apnea and Heart Failure (CANPAP) study. **A,** The patients who responded to continuous positive airway pressure (CPAP; *) had better survival than the controls or the nonresponders. CSA = central sleep apnea. **B,** The responders had an improvement in the left ventricular ejection fraction (LVEF). **A and B,** From Naughton M, Bernard D, Tam A, et al: Role of hyperventilation in the pathogenesis of central sleep apnea in patients with congestive heart failure. Am Rev Respir Dis 1993;148:330–338.

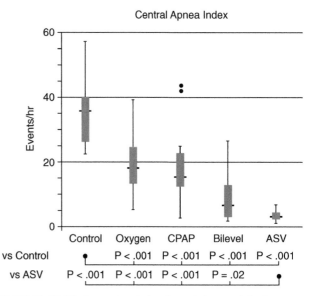

FIGURE 21-17 Effectiveness in reducing the central apnea index by oxygen, continuous positive airway pressure (CPAP), bilevel positive airway pressure (BPAP) with a backup rate, and adaptive servoventilation (ASV). ASV was the most successful at lowering the central apnea index. The figure shows box plots: *horizontal bar* (median); *thick vertical bars* (interquartile range); *thin bars* (range excluding outliers); *dots* (outliers). From Teschler H, Döhring J, Wang YM, Berthon-Jones M: Adaptive pressure support servo-ventilation: a novel treatment for Cheyne-Stokes respiration in heart failure. Am J Respir Crit Care Med 2001;164:614–619.

low levels typical of CPAP titrations in OSA patients. Another study found BPAP-ST to improve breathing in CSB-CSA patients.[66] A number of studies have documented that ASV is well tolerated and effective in CSB-CSA patients.[45,67,68] In general, sleep quality improves with ASV treatment and some studies have shown an improvement in ejection fraction.[67] Details of the use of ASV are discussed in Chapter 19. At the present time, a randomized trial of ASV is in progress to determine whether this treatment can improve mortality in patients with CHF and CSB-CSA.

If a patient with CHF has predominantly OSA on a diagnostic study, then a CPAP titration is certainly indicated. If underlying CSB is suspected in a patient with predominantly obstructive events, a CPAP titration would still be indicated because a study must demonstrate that the patient has CompSA (emergence of frequent central apneas on CPAP) before a device with a backup rate (ASV) is reimbursed by

most insurance carriers. Conversely, if a patient has predominantly CSB-CSA on the diagnostic study, one may proceed directly with an ASV titration unless reimbursement issues mandate an initial trial of CPAP. The Centers for Medicare and Medicaid Services (http://www.cms.gov/mcd/viewlcd.asp?lcd_id=5023&lcd_version=56&show=all) and many insurance carriers no longer require an attempt at CPAP if a patient meets criteria for CSA on the diagnostic study. A PSG must demonstrate the effectiveness of BPAP-ST or ASV for treatment of CSA.

CMS criteria for CSA include:

1. AHI ≥ 5/hr,
2. Central apneas/hypopneas > 50% of the total apneas and hypopneas, and
3. Central apneas/hypopneas ≥ 5/hr, and
4. Symptoms of excessive daytime sleepiness or disrupted sleep.

Of note, some clinicians would still order a titration with CPAP (at least during the initial part of the titration). Failure of CPAP would then trigger an ASV titration during the rest of the study. A problem with this approach is that there may be insufficient time for an optimal ASV titration.

In summary, while the best treatment for patients with CSB-CSA remains controversial, most clinicians would use ASV unless a patient has a satisfactory response to CPAP. Of note, BPAP **without** a backup rate is unlikely to be effective if CPAP is not effective. Attempts to optimize treatment of CHF are an essential component of treatment in patients with CSB-CSA associated with heart failure. In fact, optimization of medical treatment of CHF should be the first treatment intervention in patients with CSB-CSA due to heart failure.

COMPLEX SLEEP APNEA

CompSA has been defined in many ways[7,68,69] but the CMS definition is one of the most widely used. *CompSA* is defined as a form of CSA identified by the persistence or emergence of central sleep **apneas or hypopneas** upon exposure to CPAP or BPAP without a backup rate when obstructive events have disappeared. These patients have predominantly obstructive or mixed apneas during the diagnostic portion of the study occurring 5/hr or more. With use of CPAP or BPAP without a backup rate, they show a pattern of apneas and hypopneas that meets the definition of CSA (see previous section).

CompSA includes patients with no obvious cause for treatment-emergent central apneas (idiopathic) as well as some patients with a combination of OSA and CSB-CSA or medication-induced central sleep apnea. However, these last two groups are discussed in separate sections due to their unique features. This section discusses mainly the "idiopathic" CompSA group, which is composed of patients who develop treatment-emergent CSA without an obvious cause.

Pathophysiology

Patients with CompSA are thought to have an instability in ventilatory control or a sleep state instability.[69] The underlying instability is believed to be exacerbated by CPAP or BPAP. CPAP or BPAP could result in a lower sleeping $PaCO_2$ by decreasing upper airway resistance. CompSA patients probably also have low ATs and difficulty reaching stable sleep. Some studies show a male predominance.[70,71]

Incidence and Natural History

The incidence of CompSA varies between studies.[7,70-74] Javaheri and colleagues[72] published a large retrospective analysis of 1286 patients with a diagnosis of OSA who underwent a CPAP titration and 6.5% of the patients had treatment-emergent CSA. These patients had the most severe OSA and had a central apnea index (CAI) of 5/hr or greater at baseline. Of the 84 patients with CompSA, 42 returned for a second titration. In 33 patients (78%), CSA was eliminated by CPAP. Of note, most patients in this study had diagnostic and titration sleep studies on separate nights (no split studies). In split studies, rapid titration could predispose to CompSA. Dernaika and associates[73] reported on a population of 116 patients who met criteria for a split-night study. Twenty-three (19.8%) had CSA during a CPAP titration. Fourteen of these patients underwent chronic CPAP treatment. Repeat PSG with CPAP was performed an average of 9 weeks after treatment. Objective adherence was documented. CSA resolved in 12 of the 14 (92%). Lehman and coworkers[74] reported on 100 patients with a retrospective analysis; 13 subjects (13%) had CSA-CPAP. Risk factors included male sex, cardiac disease, and CSA on baseline PSG.[74] In a referral sleep clinic setting, Morganthaler and colleagues[7] found that 15% of 223 consecutive patients referred for a sleep study had CompSA.

Thus, the incidence of CompSA will depend on the clinical setting and whether patients taking opioids and those with CSB are included. The published studies suggest that CSA will resolve in a large proportion of patients with chronic CPAP treatment or with ASV treatment if indicated.[70,74] However, if patients with CompSA do not have improvement in control of sleep apnea, they tend to have poor sleep quality and are at risk for poor adherence. In one study, patients with CompSA had more mask issues and more complaints of removal of the mask.[74]

Polysomnography

CompSA patients have primarily obstructive or mixed apneas and obstructive hypopneas during the diagnostic study (or diagnostic portion of a split study). A small number of central apneas may also occur. During the PAP titration, the AHI remains elevated due to persistence or emergence of central apneas or hypopneas. Because central hypopneas are not well defined, this can be a problem in identifying these patients. Often, CPAP is titrated to very high pressures in an attempt to control respiratory events. Of interest, CPAP may be more effective in CompSA patients during REM sleep or in the lateral body position. Often an effective level of CPAP appears to have been found, only to have the patient change to the supine position with a subsequent return of frequent central apneas. Figures 21–18 and 21–19 show tracings on CPAP of a typical CompSA patient. In REM sleep, respiration on CPAP is relatively stable on CPAP of 10 cm H_2O (see Fig. 21–18, top panel). In stage N2, periodic breathing with central apneas and hypopneas developed on the same level of CPAP (see Fig. 21–18, bottom panel). Subsequently, the pressure was raised to 12 cm H_2O without benefit. After repeated arousals, the patient attained stage N3 and respiration on CPAP of 12 cm H_2O stabilized (see Fig. 21–19, top panel). However, after a subsequent arousal, the periodic breathing returned (see Fig. 21–19, bottom panel). These tracings emphasize that patients with "idiopathic" CompSA often are better controlled during REM sleep and, if they can attain stage N3, respiration may stabilize.

Treatment of CompSA

The best treatment for CompSA remains controversial. In the absence of CSB-CSA or opioids, it appears that a significant portion will improve with chronic CPAP alone.[72,73] The only problem with watchful waiting is that if the AHI remains high, sleep quality will be impaired and adherence may decrease. Therefore, it is prudent to assess patients soon after starting CPAP. Many CPAP devices provide the ability to estimate residual events. It is also important to remember

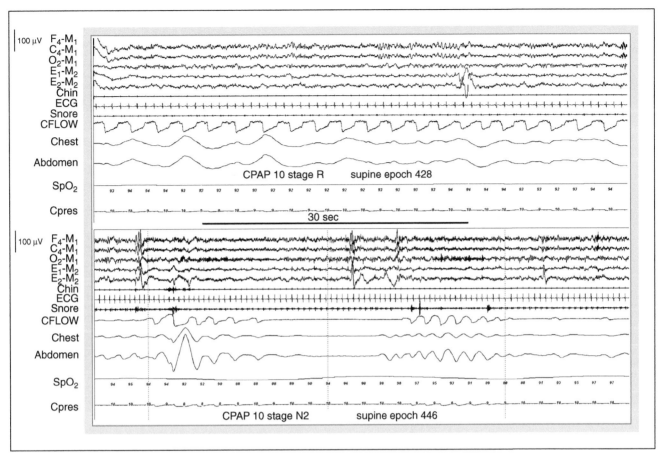

FIGURE 21–18 A patient with complex sleep apnea (CompSA). **Top,** The patient is in stage R on continuous positive airway pressure (CPAP) of 10 cm H_2O with stable breathing. Cflow = flow from PAP device; Cpres = pressure from PAP device; ECG = electrocardiogram; SpO_2 = pulse oximetry. **Bottom,** A few epochs later in stage N1 or N2 on the same pressure, recurrent central apneas are noted.

that the patient is being treated, not the AHI. Therefore, if a patient reports good sleep and objective adherence is good, intervention may not be necessary if the residual AHI remains mildly elevated (5–10/hr). If patients do not improve or if the residual AHI is high, most clinicians would order a titration with ASV. Studies have documented that ASV is effective in the majority of CompSA patients.[75,76] A higher minimal amount of pressure support may be needed if there is significant nocturnal hypoventilation. Another option would be treatment with BPAP-ST (backup rate) if ASV is not effective. In one study comparing BPAP-ST with ASV, both reduced the central apnea index, although ASV was slightly more effective.[75] ASV may be able to treat CompSA patients using lower average pressures and a decreased number of machine-triggered breaths compared with BPAP-ST. The main adjustment required during ASV titration is titration of expiratory positive airway pressure (EPAP). In general, the EPAP will need to be at or close to the level of CPAP needed to prevent obstructive apnea. This is often the pressure that was effective during supine REM sleep. However, if high EPAP is needed, this means that a fairly high inspiratory positive airway pressure (IPAP) is required

to provide a reasonable amount of pressure support (IPAP-EPAP). As discussed in Chapter 19, an ASV device that automatically adjusts the EPAP during the night (between EPAPmin and EPAPmax) is now available from one manufacturer. This option could be useful in a pressure-intolerant patient or in one in whom the ASV titration does not document an effective EPAP setting.

HIGH-ALTITUDE PERIODIC BREATHING

The ICSD-2 diagnostic criteria for HAPB are listed in Box 21–7. Periodic breathing is actually a normal adaptation to high altitude. Some individuals develop mainly central hypopnea whereas others have frank central apnea.[77] As in all hypocapnic CSA syndromes, the disorder is worse in NREM than in REM sleep.

HAPB occurs in nearly everyone at 7600 m and is associated with fragmented sleep (decreased stage N3) from arousals. There are repeated cycling periods of hyperpnea and apnea/hypopnea (periodic breathing). Patients complain of poor sleep quality or suffocation. There is no association between HAPB and the other altitude syndromes including

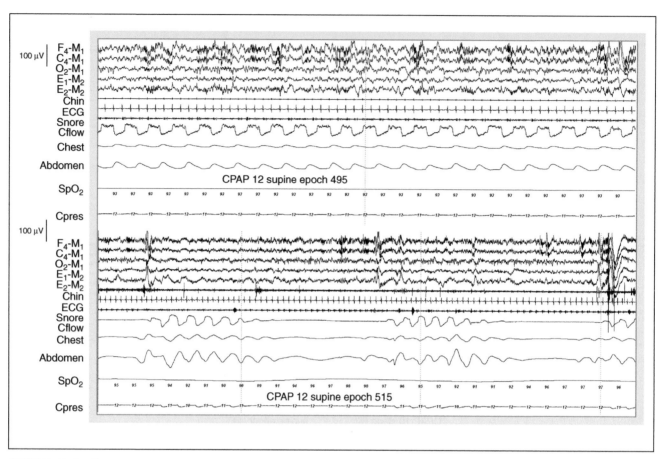

FIGURE 21–19 **Top,** The same patient in Figure 21–18 attained stage N3 sleep and respiration stabilized on the same continuous positive airway pressure (CPAP) of 12 cm H_2O. Cflow = flow signal from the CPAP device; Cpres = delivered pressure by the CPAP device; ECG = electrocardiogram; SpO_2 = pulse oximetry. **Bottom,** After an arousal, the pattern of periodic breathing returned on the same level of CPAP.

BOX 21–7

High-Altitude Periodic Breathing—Diagnostic Criteria

A. Recent ascent to altitude of at least 4000 m.

B. Polysomnography demonstrates recurrent central apneas primarily during NREM sleep at a frequency of > 5/hr. The cycle length should be 12–34 sec.

Note: This is a normal adaptation to altitude. An AHI cutoff separating normal and abnormal is not defined. Symptoms of recurrent awakenings or fatigue may occur.

AHI = apnea-hypopnea index; NREM = non–rapid eye movement.
From American Academy of Sleep Medicine: ICSD-2 International Classification of Sleep Disorders, 2nd ed. Diagnostic and Coding Manual. American Academy of Sleep Medicine. Westchester, IL: American Academy of Sleep Medicine, 2005.

high-altitude pulmonary edema, high-altitude cerebral edema, and acute mountain sickness, although patients with acute mountain sickness will usually have HAPB.

Pathophysiology

Hypoxemia at altitude increases ventilatory drive, and this results in periodic breathing. Individuals with a high hypercapnic ventilatory drive are more likely to develop HAPB.

Treatment

Most patients gradually adapt to altitude. Benzodiazepines have been used for the sleep disturbance and acetazolamide has been used for acute mountain sickness including sleep disturbance. For an in-depth discussion of high-altitude illness, the reader is referred to reference 77.

HYPERCAPNIC CSA AND HYPOVENTILATION SYNDROMES NOT DUE TO LUNG DISEASE

These disorders have in common sleep-related hypoventilation with variable amounts of central apnea and a normal or increased awake $PaCO_2$. Recall that sleep-related hypoventilation is defined as an increase in the $PaCO_2 \geq 10$ mm Hg compared to an awake value. Daytime hypoventilation is defined as a $PaCO_2 \geq 45$ mm Hg. In some patients, early in the disease course only nocturnal hypoventilation is present (see Box 21–3). This section does not discuss patients with nocturnal hypoventilation due to lung disease (see Chapter 22). In patients with hypoventilation not primarily due to lung disease, the etiology is either the control of ventilation (won't breathe) or the respiratory pump (thoracic cage or respiratory muscles) (can't breathe). The won't breath group can, with voluntary effort, lower their $PaCO_2$ values. The hypercapnic CSA syndromes are classified in the ICSD-2 under the hypoventilation syndromes. The hypoventilation syndromes included in the ICSD-2 are listed in Box 21–2. Detailed diagnostic criteria are listed in Appendix 21–1. The ICSD-2 classification of hypoventilation syndromes is not completely satisfactory because the OHS is probably better classified with OSA syndromes rather than with neuromuscular disorders and disorders of the thoracic cage. In addition, some causes of central hypoventilation (brain tumor) are neither idiopathic nor congenital.

Mechanisms of Hypercapnic CSA and/or Hypoventilation

The mechanisms of CSA and/or hypoventilation in the group of patients with hypercapnic CSA include alterations in chemoreceptors, central ventilatory control centers, central nervous system (CNS) respiratory pattern generators, lesions of CNS or spinal cord motor pathways (trauma, tumor), motor neuron disease (ALS), dysfunction of motor nerves, neuromuscular junction disorders (myasthenia gravis), myopathies (muscular dystrophy), or disorders of the thoracic cage (Fig. 21–20).

Evaluation of Patients with Suspected Hypoventilation

The diagnosis of hypoventilation (daytime or nocturnal) should be considered in all patients with the disorders listed in Box 21–3 or Figure 21–20 who complain of nocturnal symptoms including insomnia, dyspnea, disturbed sleep, or frequent awakenings. However, lack of symptoms does not rule out hypoventilation. The development of right heart failure should also trigger suspicion but is often a late sign (Fig. 21–21). A reduced daytime SaO_2 (≤92%) or an elevated serum HCO_3 (possible compensation for chronic respiratory acidosis) should also increase suspicion of hypoventilation.[78] In patients with normal lungs (normal alveolar-arterial [A-a] gradient), significant hypoventilation can be present and the SaO_2 remains in the low-normal range (Box 21–8). An arterial blood gas with a $PaCO_2$ of 45 mm Hg or greater during the day is the most definite method to diagnose daytime hypoventilation. Depending on the clinical setting, a careful neurologic examination, pulmonary function testing, chest radiography, CNS imaging (ventilatory control dysfunction suspected), genetic testing (if congenital central hypoventilation syndrome [CCHS] is a possibility), and PSG may be useful.[78] Early in the disease course, some patients have only

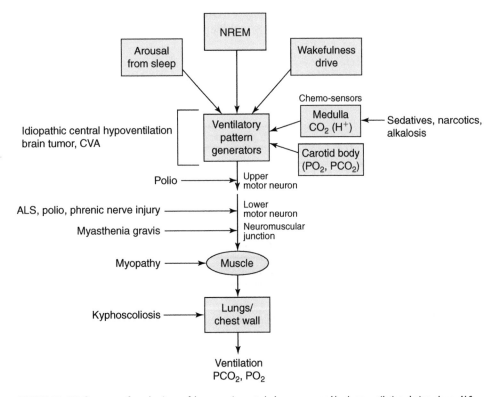

MECHANISMS OF HYPERCAPNIC CENTRAL SLEEP APNEA AND/OR HYPOVENTILATION DURING SLEEP

FIGURE 21–20 Summary of mechanisms of hypercapnic central sleep apnea and/or hypoventilation during sleep. ALS = amyotrophic lateral sclerosis; CVA = cerebrovascular accident; NREM = non–rapid eye movement; PCO_2 = partial pressure of carbon dioxide; PO_2 = partial pressure of oxygen. *From Malhotra A, Berry RB, White DP: Central sleep apnea. In Carney P, Berry RB, Geyer JW (eds): Clinical Sleep Medicine. Philadelphia: Lippincott Williams & Wilkins, 2005, p. 338.*

nocturnal hypoventilation (see Fig. 21–21). An arterial blood gas drawn immediately on awakening can confirm nocturnal hypoventilation. Noninvasive methods such as $P_{ET}CO_2$ monitoring or transcutaneous carbon dioxide ($TcPCO_2$) monitoring can also be used if their accuracy can be documented. Figure 21–22 shows PSG in a patient with muscular dystrophy with hypoventilation documented by $P_{ET}CO_2$. Nocturnal oximetry in patients with suspected hypoventilation may detect unexpected arterial oxygen desaturation. Whereas this does not document nocturnal hypoventilation, it would indicate the need for further diagnostic and therapeutic interventions. Further comments on diagnostic evaluation are included in specific disorders.

BOX 21–8

Example of a Patient with Daytime Hypoventilation Due to Neuromuscular Disease*
Room air arterial blood gas: pH 7.36; PCO_2 60 mm Hg; PaO_2 70 mm Hg, SaO_2 = 93% PAO_2 = 150 − 60/0.8 = 150 − 75 = 75 A-a gradient = PAO_2 − PaO_2 = 75 − 70 = 5 (Normal)

FEV_1	1.5 L (50% of predicted)
FVC	2.0 L (52% of predicted)
FEV_1/FVC	0.80

*See Chapter 10 for discussion or respiratory physiology and pulmonary function testing.
A-a gradient = alveolar-arterial gradient; FEV_1 = forced expiratory volume in 1 second; FVC = forced vital capacity; PAO_2 = alveolar partial pressure of oxygen; PaO_2 = arterial partial pressure of oxygen; PCO_2 = partial pressure of carbon dioxide; SaO_2 = arterial oxygen saturation.

Congenital Central Hypoventilation Syndrome

CCHS is a rare disorder affecting approximately 1 per 200,000 live births.[79] CCHS is usually present from birth and is characterized by alveolar hypoventilation without evidence of lung, neuromuscular, or structural brainstem abnormalities. During wakefulness, many patients have normal ventilation, although ventilatory responses to hypercapnia or hypoxemia by the rebreathing method are absent or blunted and a perception of dyspnea is absent. The most severely affected CCHS patients also have hypoventilation during wakefulness. Those patients with normal awake ventilation do have peripheral chemoreceptor responses to hypoxemia or hypercapnia.[80] It has been hypothesized that the central integration of chemoreceptor information rather than the chemoreceptors themselves is the abnormality in patients with CCHS. One study found that CCHS patients did have intact arousal responses to hypercapnia.[81] However, such arousals do not reliably result in an appropriate ventilatory response and rapid reversal of hypoxemia.

During sleep, all CCHS patients have worsening of ventilation with profound hypoventilation exhibited by normal respiratory rates and diminished tidal volumes associated with severe falls in the SaO_2.[79,82] The abnormalities are often worse during NREM than REM sleep because the control of breathing is entirely metabolic during NREM sleep. In any case, the arousal responses are significantly impaired because long periods of hypercapnic hypoxemia without arousal are not unusual.

Other forms of autonomic dysregulation may be seen in these patients. These abnormalities can include Hirschsprung's

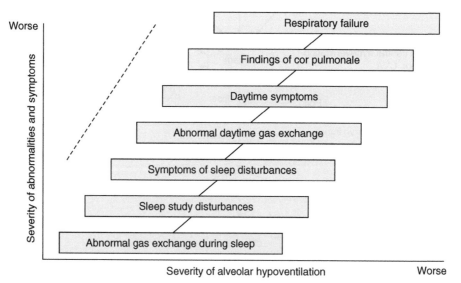

FIGURE 21–21 The severity of symptoms of alveolar hypoventilation are related to the degree of alveolar hypoventilation. As hypoventilation increases in severity, symptoms increase from only abnormalities during sleep to daytime symptoms and finally to symptoms of overt respiratory failure. In patients with reduced cardiopulmonary reserve from co-morbid conditions, this relationship is shifted upward and to the left as shown by the *dashed line*. From American College of Chest Physicians: *Clinical indications for noninvasive positive pressure ventilation in chronic respiratory failure due to restrictive lung disease, COPD, and nocturnal hypoventilation—a consensus conference report. Chest 1999;116:530.*

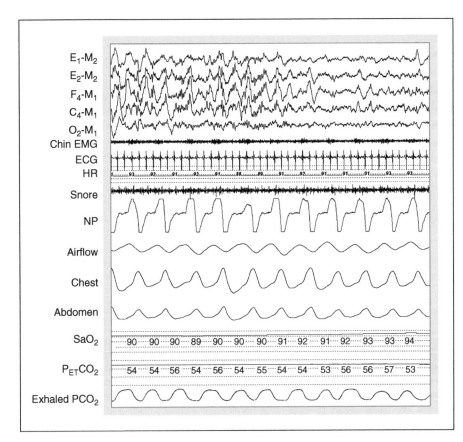

FIGURE 21-22 A 30-second tracing of NREM sleep in a patient with muscular dystrophy shows nocturnal hypoventilation with minimal drop in the arterial oxygen saturation (SaO$_2$). ECG = electrocardiogram; EMG = electromyogram; Exhaled PCO$_2$ = partial pressure of carbon dioxide (capnography tracing); HR = heart rate; NP = nasal pressure; P$_{ET}$CO$_2$ = end-tidal partial pressure of carbon dioxide. *From Wagner MH, Berry RB: Disturbed sleep in a patient with Duchenne muscular dystrophy. J Clin Sleep Med 2008;4:173–175.*

disease (20%) usually presenting with constipation, esophageal dysmotility presenting with feeding difficulty, tumors of neural crest origin (6%) such as neuroblastoma or ganglioneuroma, decreased heart rate variability, decreased heart rate response to exercise, decreased papillary light response, intermittent profuse sweating, and dysregulation of body temperature with decreased baseline body temperature.[78,82,83] CCHS patients are at risk for adverse outcomes from respiratory infections because they may not exhibit a fever or complain of dyspnea even if severely hypoxemic.

The diagnosis of CCHS should be considered if apneic or cyanotic spells are noted in infants, especially if associated with sleep. The most severe cases occur in patients who do not breathe adequately during wakefulness after birth and require immediate ventilatory support. In others, the abnormalities are noted when the infants sleep. Milder cases may present later with signs of cor pulmonale or hypoxic damage to CNS structures. Some cases may not present until late childhood and a few present in adulthood.[84,85] The diagnosis of CCHS depends on exclusion of other causes of hypoventilation such as brainstem malformation, inborn errors of metabolism, myopathy, diaphragmatic paralysis, lung or respiratory pump abnormalities. PSG with P$_{ET}$CO$_2$ monitoring usually reveals high P$_{ET}$CO$_2$ and low tidal volume (Fig. 21–23).[82]

A suspected diagnosis is confirmed by genetic testing for mutations in the *PHOX2b* gene.[79,82,86,87] Most persons with CCHS are heterozygous for polyalanine repeat expansion mutations in exon 3 of *PHOX2b*. The expansion results in lengthening the normal 20-repeat polyalanine tract to 25–33 repeats. Longer expansions are associated with more severe phenotypes. Most mutations occur de novo, but in families with CCHS, it is inherited as an autosomal dominant trait.

Treatment includes lifelong ventilatory support for all patients during sleep. Some patients will require ventilatory support while awake as well. Ventilatory support for severe cases is usually provided by a volume-cycled ventilator via a tracheostomy. In older and milder patients, noninvasive mask ventilation may suffice.[79,83,87] Diaphragmatic pacing has also been used during the day. Diaphragmatic pacing at night requires the presence of a tracheostomy, because obstructive events usually occur when the upper airway muscles do not contract in synchrony with the diaphragm. Infants in CCHS must be closely monitored because they are at risk for hypoventilation or apnea at sleep onset. These children are also at increased risk during chest infections owing to their abnormal temperature control, lack of perception of dyspnea, and nonappearance of respiratory distress. Noninvasive positive-pressure ventilation (NPPV) with BPAP with a backup rate has been successfully used in infants when parents have refused tracheostomy.[88,89] Appropriate alarms are essential. Older children may be transitioned to NPPV if their symptoms are milder and they are adherent to treatment.

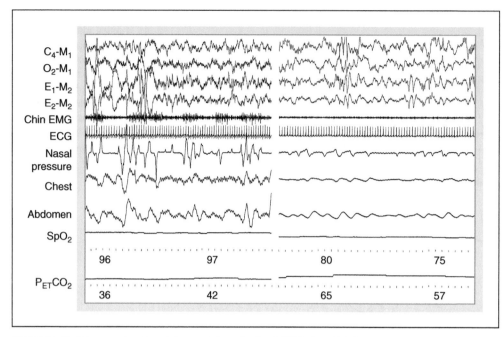

FIGURE 21–23 Thirty-second tracings during wakefulness **(left)** and NREM sleep **(right)** in a patient with congenital central hypoventilation syndrome. Right central and occipital electroencephalographic (C_4-M_1, O_2-M_1) and right and left electro-oculographic derivations (E_1-M_2, E_2-M_2) as well as a chin electromyogram (EMG) tracing are shown. During sleep, there is a dramatic reduction in tidal volume, increase in end-tidal partial pressure of carbon dioxide $P_{ET}CO_2$, and decrease in pulse oximetry (SpO_2). ECG = electrocardiogram. *From Wagner MH, Berry RB: A full term infant with cyanotic episodes. Congenital central hypoventilation syndrome. J Clin Sleep Med 2007;3:425–426.*

Other Neural Disorders Causing Central Hypoventilation

CSA and hypoventilation due to abnormalities in the control of ventilation have been noted in a wide variety of disorders but most are relatively uncommon. These include idiopathic central hypoventilation, neurodegenerative disorders with autonomic dysfunction[90] such as multiple system atrophy, paraneoplastic encephalitis,[91] and tumors of the medulla.[92,93] CSA and OSA can occur late in the course in patients with prior polio infection (postpolio syndrome).[94] The Chiari syndrome is discussed in the next section.

Chiari's Malformation

Sleep-related breathing disorders are common in both children and adults with Chiari's malformation (CM).[95,96] With the increased use of magnetic resonance imaging (MRI), cases are often detected before symptoms begin. *CM type I* is defined as herniation of the cerebellar tonsils through the foramen magnum. CM II includes caudal displacement of the vermis and is usually associated with myelodysplasia and meningomyelocele. In CM I, obstructive apneas, central apneas, or a combination can occur. Nocturnal hypoventilation without discrete apneas can also occur. A minority of CM I patients have daytime hypercapnia, but the disorder is included in this section because central apnea is believed to be secondary to alterations in brainstem control of respiration. Presenting symptoms of CM include worsening of

snoring, breathing pauses, headaches, neck pain, ataxia, oculomotor disturbances, scoliosis, and lower cranial nerve palsies. Although CM I can present in infancy and childhood, the most common presentation is in **young adulthood between 20 and 40 years.** Sleep apnea is believed due to pressure on the medullary structures controlling ventilation and upper airway muscles. Surgical decompression (posterior fossa decompression, duraplasty, and cervical laminectomy) often improves the degree of sleep apnea, although significant apnea can be present in the postoperative period. There have been reports of patients treated for obstructive hydrocephalus with shunts who experienced an acute worsening of sleep apnea as the only manifestation of shunt failure.

CSA Due to Medication (Opiate/Narcotic-Induced CSA)

The opiate-induced sleep-related breathing disorder (OSRBD) is increasingly common with more aggressive treatment of chronic pain with potent narcotics including morphine, fentanyl, and methadone, often in very high doses. Affected patients may manifest obstructive apneas—often of long duration, ataxic breathing, low sleeping respiratory rates, and central apneas either intermittent or in the form of periodic breathing.[97,98] They also tend to have either persistent or treatment-emergent central apneas on CPAP (a form of CompSA). The etiology of the disorder is believed to be depression of central drive by opiate medications. Although opiate-induced CSA is placed in the hypercapnic

CSA group, patients often have either normal or only mildly increased daytime $PaCO_2$ values (45–50 mm Hg). However, patients with OSRBD more often exhibit significant worsening of hypoventilation during sleep. The many breathing abnormalities noted in OSRBDs are listed in Box 21–9. An unusual characteristic noted during sleep studies is the ataxic breathing pattern—variation in tidal volume and respiratory rate (Fig. 21–24). Some patients actually have central apneas during stage N3 sleep (uncommon in other types of central sleep apnea) and others have a low respiratory rate during sleep (see Fig. 21–24) or periodic breathing with repetitive central apneas that are typically short in duration (Fig.

21–25). Individual patients may have long obstructive apneas during REM sleep or mixed apneas with a long central component. Patients may also exhibit relatively few central apneas until placed on CPAP (Fig. 21–26). As in CSB-CSA, patients with opiates are often more effectively treated with CPAP during REM sleep (Fig. 21–27).

Treatment

Some patients will improve with a reduction in narcotic dose,[2] but this is rarely acceptable to the patient. Other patients with mainly obstructive events may respond to CPAP. However, central apneas either persist or emerge on CPAP in a significant number of patients (see Figs. 21–25 and 21–26). There is a single case report of use of acetazolamide[99] as an adjunct to CPAP treatment in patients with narcotic-induced CompSA. Treatment with either BPAP with a backup rate or ASV can be successful in narcotic-induced CompSA.[100-102] Relatively few studies using ASV in patients with opiate-induced CSA have been published. One study found ASV less effective but the EPAP probably was not adequately increased to eliminate obstruction.[101] When using ASV, it is essential to increase EPAP sufficiently to prevent upper airway closure.[100,102] Javaheri and associates[102] found ASV to be an effective treatment for both central and obstructive apnea in narcotic-induced CompSA.

Primary Sleep Apnea of Infancy

This syndrome was formerly termed "primary sleep apnea of the newborn." As the name implies, this syndrome is characterized by CSA due to an immature respiratory control

---

BOX 21–9

Important Facts about Opiates and Sleep-Related Breathing Disorders

- Ataxic breathing—variation in respiratory rate and tidal volume.
- Slow respiratory rate during sleep.
- Intermittent central apneas (even during stage N3) or periodic breathing with central apneas.
- Long obstructive apneas.
- Relatively few arousals, amount of stage N3 can be increased.
- In some patients, NREM AHI » REM AHI.
- Treatment-emergent central apneas are common even if diagnostic study shows mainly obstructive events.

AHI = apnea-hypopnea index; NREM = non–rapid eye movement; REM = rapid eye movement.

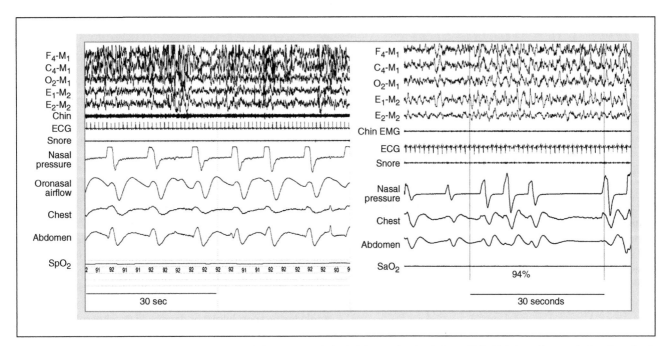

FIGURE 21–24 **Left,** Low respiratory rate in a patient on methadone (6–7 breaths/min). A 60-second tracing is shown. **Right,** Variation in flow amplitude and rate (ataxic breathing) in another patient on methadone. ECG = electrocardiogram; EMG = electromyogram; SaO_2 = arterial oxygen saturation; SpO_2 = pulse oximetry.

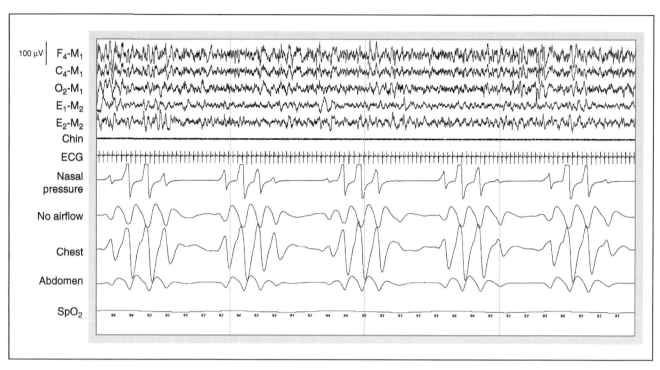

FIGURE 21–25 Periodic breathing during a diagnostic study in a patient on a fentanyl patch. Repeated central apneas are noted without any arousals. Respiratory events without arousals is common in opiate-induced central sleep apnea. ECG = electrocardiogram; SpO_2 = pulse oximetry.

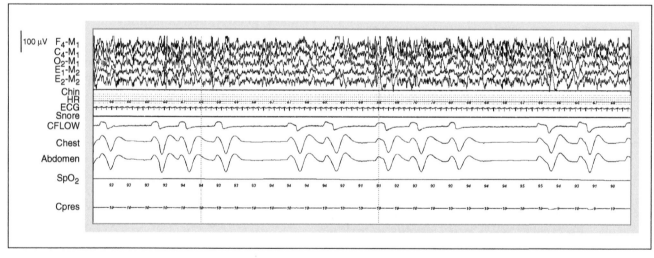

FIGURE 21–26 Periodic breathing with central apneas on CPAP of 10 cm H_2O during NREM sleep. The patient was taking methadone. Cflow = flow signal from the CPAP device; Cpres = pressure from PAP device; ECG = electrocardiogram; HR = heart rate; SpO_2 = pulse oximetry.

system.[6,103] **Periodic breathing is a normal finding in premature infants** but is deemed pathologic only if the duration of apnea is greater than 20 seconds or if the events are associated with desaturation or other physiologic compromise. The disorder may be treated with caffeine or low-dose theophylline[104] (Box 21–10).

Restrictive Thoracic Cage Disorders

Disorders causing restriction of the thoracic cage due to disease of the spine, chest wall, or pleura can result in

hypoventilation. Causes include thoracoplasty, fibrothorax, kyphoscoliosis, and ankylosing spondylitis.[6,105] In general, isolated nocturnal hypoventilation precedes daytime hypoventilation. These disorders result in extrinsic restrictive ventilatory dysfunction[78] (Fig. 21–28). In patients with chest wall disease, the total lung capacity is decreased and the functional residual capacity is either normal to increased (ankylosing spondylitis) or decreased (kyphoscoliosis).[78] The chest wall has decreased compliance, so there is an increased work of breathing. Patients tend to take rapid shallow breaths. The severity of impairment may be roughly gauged by the

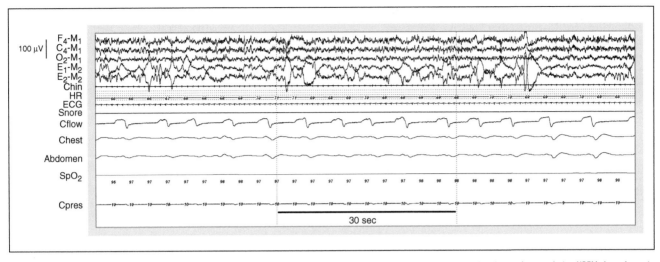

FIGURE 21–27 Good control of respiratory events with CPAP of 10 cm H_2O during REM sleep in the patient with methadone-induced central apnea during NREM sleep shown in Figure 21-26. Cflow = flow signal from the CPAP device; ECG = electrocardiogram; HR = heart rate; SpO_2 = pulse oximetry.

BOX 21–10

Primary Sleep Apnea of Infancy—Diagnostic Criteria

APNEA OF PREMATURITY

A. One of the following is recorded in an infant < 37 wk conceptional age:

1. Prolonged central respiratory pauses of ≥ 20 sec in duration.
2. Shorter-duration events include obstructive or mixed respiratory patterns and are associated with a significant physiologic compromise, including decrease in heart rate, hypoxemia, clinical symptoms, or the need for nursing intervention.

APNEA OF INFANCY

A. One of the following is recorded in an infant of conceptual age ≥ 37 wk:

1. Prolonged central respiratory pauses of ≥ 20 sec in duration.
2. Shorter duration events including obstructive or mixed respiratory patterns and are associated with bradycardia, cyanosis, pallor, or marked hypotonia.

B. For either diagnosis, the disorder is not better explained by another current sleep disorder, medical or neurologic disorder, or medication.

From American Academy of Sleep Medicine: ICSD-2 International Classification of Sleep Disorders, 2nd ed. Diagnostic and Coding Manual. American Academy of Sleep Medicine. Westchester, IL: American Academy of Sleep Medicine, 2005.

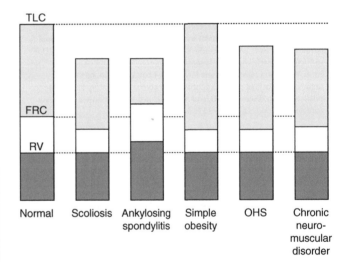

FIGURE 21–28 Changes in lung volumes in patients with extrinsic restrictive ventilatory dysfunction. In patients with obesity, scoliosis, and the obesity hypoventilation syndrome (OHS), the functional residual capacity (FRC) is decreased. In chronic neuromuscular disorders, both the total lung capacity (TLC) and the FRC are reduced. In patients with neuromuscular disorders, the residual volume (RV) is usually unchanged unless significant expiratory muscle weakness is present (quadriplegia). *From Berry RB, Sriram P: Evaluation of hypoventilation. Semin Respir Crit Care Med 2009;30:303–314.*

forced vital capacity (FVC). An FVC less than 50% of predicted is considered severe.[106] However, patients with FVCs higher than 50% may hypoventilate and desaturate at night. Nocturnal oximetry is a useful tool in this setting. A daytime $PaCO_2$ documenting hypoventilation or nocturnal oximetry documenting 5 minutes or longer with an SaO_2 of 88% or lower is considered an indication for nocturnal NPPV (Table 21–4).[106] However, PSG is the most sensitive test to determine nocturnal hypoventilation and rule out coexistent OSA. Hypoventilation is often inferred from documenting arterial oxygen desaturation without discrete events. This practice has been discouraged by the AASM scoring manual.[4] However, many sleep centers do not have the ability to monitor $PaCO_2$ noninvasively. An arterial blood gas on awakening is one approach. The most severe desaturation usually occurs during REM sleep (Fig. 21–29).

TABLE 21–4

Indications for Noninvasive Positive-Pressure Ventilation Treatment in Restrictive Thoracic Chest Wall Disease and Neuromuscular Disease

RTCD	Symptoms of hypoventilation (morning headache, daytime somnolence) AND one of the following: Physiologic criteria • $PaCO_2 > 45$ mm Hg (daytime) • Nocturnal oximetry demonstrating $SaO_2 < 88\%$ for ≥ 5 min*
NMD	Symptoms of hypoventilation (morning headache, daytime somnolence) AND one of the following: Physiologic criteria • $PaCO_2 > 45$ mm Hg (daytime) • Nocturnal oximetry demonstrating $SaO_2 < 88\%$ for ≥ 5 min* • FVC < 50% of predicted • Maximal inspiratory pressure < 60 cm H_2O

*The ACCP conference used at least 5 "consecutive" minutes. However, the Centers for Medicare and Medicaid Services indications for respiratory assist devices does not include "consecutive" but only ≥5 min with an $SaO_2 \leq 88\%$. FVC = forced vital capacity; NMD = neuromuscular disease; $PaCO_2$ = arterial partial pressure of carbon dioxide; SaO_2 = arterial oxygen saturation; RTCD = restrictive thoracic chest wall disease.
From American College of Chest Physicians: Clinical indications for noninvasive positive pressure ventilation in chronic respiratory failure due to restrictive lung disease, COPD, and nocturnal hypoventilation—a consensus conference report. Chest 1999;116:521–534.

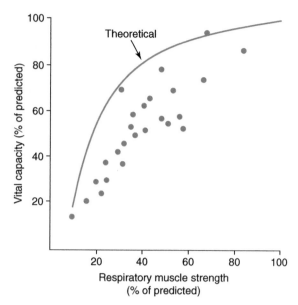

FIGURE 21–30 The vital capacity in patients with neuromuscular disease is decreased out of proportion to the degree of muscle weakness. This implies a change in the chest wall or lungs that decreases the respiratory system compliance. *From De Troyer A, Borenstein S, Cordier R: Analysis of lung volume restriction in patients with respiratory muscle weakness. Thorax 1980;35:603–610.*

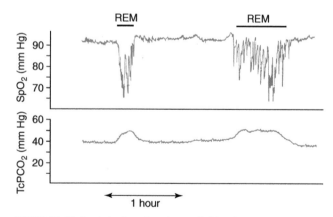

FIGURE 21–29 Trends in the pulse oximetry (SpO_2) and transcutaneous partial pressure of carbon dioxide ($TcPCO_2$) during the night in a patient with neuromuscular disease. Note the simultaneous increase in $TcPCO_2$ and decrease in the SpO_2 during episodes of rapid eye movement (REM) sleep. PCO_2 = partial pressure of carbon dioxide.

Treatment of Restrictive Thoracic Cage Disorders

Early intervention may prevent the onset of cor pulmonale and improve sleep quality. Most clinicians would start treatment after documentation of nocturnal desaturation or hypoventilation. Nocturnal ventilatory support rather than supplemental oxygen is the treatment of choice. A number of studies have evaluated the use of NPPV in these patients.[107-110] NPPV is usually provided using BPAP in the ST mode with a mask interface. NPPV can be started on an outpatient basis, but NPPV titration with PSG is the ideal method to select appropriate treatment. Due to the low compliance of the respiratory system, high pressure support (IPAP-EPAP) up to 20 cm H_2O may be needed to deliver an adequate tidal volume. Some patients may be ventilated with lower pressure support and higher than spontaneous respiratory rates. NPPV is discussed in more detail in Chapter 19.

Neuromuscular Weakness

Hypoventilation can occur with disorders that impair function at any point from premotor neuron to muscle. These sites include disorders of the premotor neurons, neural pathways to lower motor neurons, peripheral nerve disorders, disorders of the neuromuscular junction (myasthenia gravis), or myopathies (muscular dystrophy).

These disorders result in extrinsic restrictive ventilatory dysfunction. Later in the disease course, abnormalities of the lung can also occur. Although it is often said that testing respiratory muscle strength (maximum inspiratory force, expiratory force) is the most sensitive method to detect respiratory weakness, these tests require special expertise to avoid erroneous measurements and normative values for strength vary considerably.[78] The FVC is a very useful measurement in neuromuscular disease (NMD). Studies have shown that the FVC is reduced out of proportion to the degree of muscle weakness, making it a fairly sensitive means of documenting the significance of suspected respiratory muscle weakness[111] (Fig. 21–30). The American College of

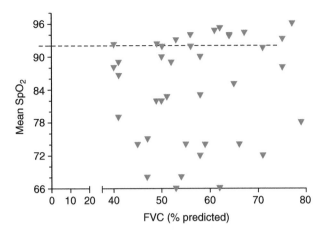

FIGURE 21–31 The mean arterial oxygen saturation (SpO$_2$) determined by nocturnal oximetry is plotted against the forced vital capacity (FVC; % predicted) for a group of patients with ALS. Note that many patients with an FVC greater than 50% of predicted had substantial nocturnal desaturation (and presumably nocturnal hypoventilation). *From Morgan RS, McNally S, Alexander M, et al: Use of sniff nasal inspiratory force to predict survival in amyotrophic lateral sclerosis. Am J Respir Crit Care Med 2005;171:101.*

Chest Physicians (ACCP) consensus guidelines[106] recommended an FVC less than 50% of predicted or a maximal inspiratory pressure less than 60 cm H$_2$O as indications for NPPV treatment (see Table 21–4). However, this degree of FVC impairment is not sensitive for detection of nocturnal desaturation (Fig. 21–31). Therefore, nocturnal oximetry or PSG is recommended if the patient complains of poor sleep quality, frequent awakenings, or nocturnal dyspnea. Of interest, some patients with NMD cannot make a good mouth seal to allow estimate of inspiratory force. One study found using nasal inspiratory pressure was useful in assessing prognosis.[112] Nocturnal oximetry showing more than 5 minutes of continuous desaturation less than 88% is considered an indication for beginning NPPV treatment.[106] Patients with NMD typically have the lowest SaO$_2$ and high PaCO$_2$ during REM sleep.

Treatment of Nocturnal Hypoventilation Due to NMD

In the past, volume ventilation via a tracheostomy was the usual mode of ventilatory support in NMD patients. Today, NPPV using BPAP-ST with a mask interface is the most widely used treatment.[105,106,113–115] NPPV can be started at low levels and increased based on nocturnal oximetry, daytime PaCO$_2$ measurements, or symptoms.[114] For example, using BPAP-ST at 8/4 cm H$_2$O with backup rate of 1 to 2 breaths/min below the spontaneous rate. A more precise approach is NPPV titration with PSG. Not all patients will tolerate an optimal degree of pressure support on the first night of treatment. BPAP with a backup rate is recommended because patients may **not** consistently trigger IPAP-EPAP cycles due to muscle weakness. NPPV treatment initiation is discussed in more detail in Chapter 19.

The goals of NPPV treatment should be individualized but include improved sleep quality and quality of life,

prevention of worsening of hypoventilation, and avoiding cor pulmonale. A randomized study in ALS patients found increased survival with NPPV in the group of patients with less severe bulbar dysfunction.[115] The average IPAP and EPAP settings were 15 and 6 cm H$_2$O, respectively. This and other studies reported improvement in quality of life with NPPV. Patients with bulbar involvement may have more difficulty tolerating NPPV and mask ventilation. These patients may also have a greater risk of aspiration than those without upper airway dysfunction.

CLINICAL REVIEW QUESTIONS

1. All of the following are true about CCHS **EXCEPT**
   A. It is associated with Hirschsprung's disease.
   B. It is due to mutations in the *PHOX2b* gene.
   C. Hypoventilation is manifested by low tidal volume.
   D. Patients develop dyspnea when hypoxic.
   E. Patients may require 24-hour ventilatory support from birth.

2. Which of the following does **NOT** predispose a patient to hypocapnic CSA?
   A. Large PCO$_2$-AT gradient.
   B. Increased hypercapnic ventilatory drive.
   C. Frequent arousals.
   D. NREM > REM sleep.
   E. Supine > nonsupine sleep.

3. Which of the following patients with CSB-CSA likely has the lowest cardiac output and the longest delay in the SaO$_2$ nadir?

PATIENT	CYCLE LENGTH (START OF ONE CENTRAL APNEA UNTIL THE NEXT)	APNEA LENGTH
A	40	20
B	75	25
C	50	25
D	50	20

4. A patient with suspected sleep apnea undergoes a split sleep study. During the diagnostic portion, the AHI is 50/hr with 40 obstructive apneas, 10 mixed apneas, 0 central apneas, and 30 hypopneas. During the CPAP titration on CPAP of 10 cm H$_2$O, obstructive apneas are abolished but frequent central apneas of the Cheyne-Stokes type are noted. The AHI on 10 cm H$_2$O is 40/hr. Higher pressure is no more effective. What do you recommend?
   A. Optimize cardiac function.
   B. Treatment with CPAP of 10 cm H$_2$O.
   C. Titration with ASV.
   D. A and B.
   E. A and C.

5. Which of the following is likely present in a patient with CSB-CSA associated with heart failure?
   A. High wedge pressure (left ventricular end-diastolic pressure).
   B. Low hypercapnic ventilatory response.
   C. Daytime $PaCO_2$ = 44 mm Hg.
   D. Normal left atrial size.

6. A 50-year-old man undergoes a split sleep study. The results are shown below. The central apneas were not of the Cheyne-Stokes type. What do you recommend?

	DIAGNOSTIC	TITRATION
Total sleep time (min)	120	150
REM sleep (min)	10	40
AHI (#/hr)	45	22
Obstructive apneas (no.)	40	15
Central apneas (no.)	5	30
Mixed apneas (no.)	5	0
Hypopneas (no.)	40	10

CPAP	TST	REM SLEEP	AHI	AHI REM	OA	MA	CA	H
6	15	0	40	0	10	0	0	0
7	15	0	40	0	5	0	0	5
8	30	10	10	30	0	0	0	5
9	30	20	0	0	0	0	0	0
10	30	10	10	0	0	0	5	0
11	30	10	40	0	0	0	20	0

   A. CPAP of 8 cm H_2O.
   B. CPAP of 9 cm H_2O.
   C. CPAP of 10 cm H_2O.
   D. ASV titration.
   E. BPAP-ST titration.

7. A patient with a progressive neuromuscular disorder reports mild snoring and has a daytime $PaCO_2$ of 42 mm Hg. However, nocturnal oximetry reveals an $SaO_2 \leq 88\%$ for 15 min. The FVC is 60% of predicted and the maximum inspiratory force is 70 cm H_2O. What do you recommend?
   A. Nocturnal supplemental oxygen.
   B. Diagnostic PSG and PSG for titration with CPAP.
   C. Diagnostic PSG and PSG for titration with BPAP.
   D. Diagnostic PSG and PSG for titration with BPAP-ST.
   E. Empirical treatment with BPAP-ST 8/4 cm H_2O and backup rate of 12 breaths/min.

Answers

1. **D.** Patients with CCHS do not experience dyspnea when hypoxemic and are at risk from death due to respiratory infections.

2. **A.** A small $PaCO_2$-AT gradient predisposes to hypocapnic CSA.

3. **B.** A longer ventilatory phase between events is associated with a longer circulation time, lower cardiac output, and a longer delay in the SaO_2 nadir. The ventilatory phase = cycle length − apnea duration = A (20 sec), B (50 sec), C (25 sec), D (30 sec).

4. **E.** CSB may improve with improvement in cardiac function. CPAP was not effective at reducing the AHI. The patient may receive some benefit from CPAP, which did eliminate OSA, but the residual AHI due to central apnea is quite high. ASV can often reduce the AHI to less than 5/hr. Whereas ASV is more effective at acutely reducing the AHI, no direct long-term comparisons have been performed with CPAP treatment of patients with CSB-CSA. However, short-term studies of ASV do report improvement in symptoms and some report improvement in cardiac function.

5. **A.** Patients with CSB-CSA are more likely to have a large left atrium, atrial fibrillation, a low daytime PCO_2, and an elevated wedge pressure.

6. **B.** The patient has treatment-emergent CSA. CPAP of 9 cm H_2O was effective at eliminating obstructive events. Higher pressure was associated with central apneas. In other patients, treatment-emergent central apneas may occur on pressures needed to prevent obstructive apneas during REM sleep. The treatment-emergent central apneas may resolve with chronic CPAP treatment (especially if the patient does not have CSB or is taking potent narcotics).

7. **D.** The patient may have nocturnal hypoventilation, and NPPV rather than supplemental oxygen is indicated for treatment of nocturnal hypoventilation. Some clinicians would begin empirical BPAP 8/4 cm H_2O with upward titration as indicated. However, a diagnostic PSG is indicated to determine if OSA, nocturnal hypoventilation, or both are present. If the nocturnal arterial oxygen desaturation is due to OSA alone, one might consider treatment with CPAP. However, given the likely need for NPPV in the future, treatment with BPAP rather than CPAP is probably the best answer. A titration with NPPV (BPAP-ST) can eliminate OSA events and treat nocturnal hypoventilation as well as provide respiratory muscle rest. BPAP with a backup rate is recommended for patients with neuromuscular disorders because they may not trigger IPAP/EPAP cycles due to weak muscles (especially during REM sleep). A backup rate will also provide intervention for central apneas. Of note, a saw-tooth pattern in the oximetry tracings used to screen a neuromuscular disorder patient for abnormal nocturnal gas exchange would suggest that sleep apnea is present (discrete events).

REFERENCES

1. Bradley TD, McNicholas WT, Rutherford R, et al: Clinical and physiologic heterogeneity of the central sleep apnea syndrome. Am Rev Respir Dis 1986;134:217–221.
2. Eckert DJ, Jordan AS, Merchia P, Malhotra A: Central sleep apnea. Chest 2007;131:595–607.
3. Malhotra A, Berry RB, White DP: Central sleep apnea. In Carney P, Berry RB, Geyer JW (eds): Clinical Sleep Medicine. Philadelphia: Lippincott Williams & Wilkins, 2005, pp. 331–334.
4. Iber C, Ancoli-Israel S, Chesson A, Quan SF for the American Academy of Sleep Medicine: The AASM Manual for the Scoring of Sleep and Associated Events: Rules, Terminology and Technical Specification, 1st ed. Westchester, IL: American Academy of Sleep Medicine, 2007.
5. Berry RB: Esophageal and nasal pressure monitoring during sleep. In Lee-Chiong TL, Sateia MJ, Carskadon MA (eds): Sleep Medicine. Philadelphia: Hanley & Belfus, 2002, pp. 661–679.
6. American Academy of Sleep Medicine: ICSD-2 International Classification of Sleep Disorders, 2nd ed. Diagnostic and Coding Manual. Westchester, IL: American Academy of Sleep Medicine, 2005.
7. Morgenthaler TI, Kagramanov V, Hanak V, Decker PA: Complex sleep apnea syndrome: is it a unique clinical syndrome? Sleep 2006;29:1203–1209.
8. Guilleminault C, Cummisky J: Progressive improvement of apnea index and ventilatory response to CO_2 after tracheostomy in obstructive sleep apnea syndrome. Am Rev Respir Dis 1982;126:14–20.
9. Iber C, Davies SF, Chapman RC, Mahowald MM: A possible mechanism for mixed apnea in obstructive sleep apnea. Chest 1986;89:800–805.
10. Dowdell WT, Javaheri S, McGinnis W: Cheyne-Stokes respiration presenting as a sleep apnea syndrome. Am Rev Respir Dis 1990;141:874.
11. Douglas NJ: Respiratory physiology: control of ventilation. In Kryger MH, Roth T, Dement WC (eds): Principles and Practice of Sleep Medicine, 5th ed. Philadelphia: Elsevier, 2005, pp. 224–243.
12. Gould GA, Gugger M, Molloy J, et al: Breathing pattern and eye movement density during REM sleep in humans. Am Rev Respir Dis 1988;138:874–877.
13. Kline LR, Hendricks JC, Davies RO, Pack AI: Control of activity of the diaphragm in rapid-eye-movement sleep. J Appl Physiol 1986;61:1293–1300.
14. Skatrud JB, Dempsey JA: Interaction of sleep state and chemical stimuli in sustaining rhythmic ventilation. J Appl Physiol 1983:55:813–822.
15. Dempsey J: Crossing the apneic threshold. Causes and consequences. Exp Physiol 2004;90:13–24.
16. White DP: Pathogenesis of obstructive and central sleep apnea. Am J Respir Crit Care Med 2005;172:1363–1370.
17. White DP: Central sleep apnea. In Kryger MH, Roth T, Dement WC (eds): Principles and Practice of Sleep Medicine. Philadelphia: Elsevier, 2005, pp. 969–981.
18. Xie A, Wong B, Phillipson EA, et al: Interaction of hyperventilation and arousal in pathogenesis of idiopathic central sleep apnea. Am J Respir Crit Care Med 1994; 150:489–495.
19. Xie A, Skatrud JG, Puelo DS, et al: Apnea-hypopnea threshold for CO_2 in patients with congestive heart failure. Am Respir Crit Care Med 2002;165:1245–1250.
20. Nakayama H, Smith CA, Rodman JR, et al: Effect of ventilatory drive on carbon dioxide sensitivity below eupnea during sleep. Am J Respir Crit Care Med 2002;165: 1251–1260.
21. Issa FG, Sullivan CE: Reversal of central sleep apnea using nasal CPAP. Chest 1986;90:165–171.
22. Szollosi I, Roebuck T, Thompson B, Naughton MT: Lateral sleeping position reduces severity of central sleep apnea/Cheyne-Stokes respiration. Sleep 2006;29:1045–1051.
23. Hall MJ, Xie A, Rutherford R, Bradley TD: Cycle length of periodic breathing with and without heart failure. Am J Respir Crit Care Med 1996;154:376–381.
24. Xie A, Rutherford R, Rankin F, et al: Hypocapnia and increased ventilatory responsiveness in patients with idiopathic central sleep apnea. Am J Respir Crit Care Med 1995; 152:1950–1955.
25. Hoffstein V, Slutsky AS: Central sleep apnea reversed by continuous positive airway pressure. Am Rev Respir Dis 1987; 135:1210–1212.
26. Xie A, Rankin F, Rutherford R, et al: Effects of inhaled CO_2 and added dead space on idiopathic central sleep apnea. Am Rev Respir Dis 1997;82:918–926.
27. DeBacker WA, Verbacken J, Willemen M, et al: Central apnea index decreases after prolonged treatment with acetazolamide. Am J Respir Crit Care Med 1995;151:87–91.
28. Shore ET, Millman RP: Central sleep apnea and acetazolamide therapy. Arch Intern Med 1983;143:1278–1280.
29. White DP, Zwillich CW, Pickett CK, et al: Central sleep apnea. Improvement with acetazolamide therapy. Arch Intern Med 1982;142:1816–1819.
30. Bonnet MH, Dexter JR, Arand DL: The effect of triazolam on arousal and respiration in central sleep apnea patients. Sleep 1990;13:31–41.
31. Quadri S, Drake C, Hudgel DW: Improvement of idiopathic central sleep apnea with zolpidem. J Clin Sleep Med 2009; 15:122–129.
32. Grimaldi D, Provini F, Vertrugno R, et al: Idiopathic central sleep apnea syndrome treated with zolpidem. Neurol Sci 2008;29:255–257.
33. Hommura F, Nishimura M, Oguri M, et al: Continuous versus bilevel positive airway pressure in a patient with idiopathic central sleep apnea. Am J Respir Crit Care Med 1997;155: 1482–1485.
34. Franklin KA, Eriksson P, Sahlin C, et al: Reversal of central sleep apnea with oxygen. Chest 1997;111:163–169.
35. Hanly PJ, Millar TW, Steljes DG, et al: The effect of oxygen on respiration and sleep in patients with congestive heart failure. Ann Intern Med 1989;111:777–782.
36. Javaheri S, Parker TJ, Wexler L, et al: Occult sleep-disordered breathing in stable congestion heart failure. Ann Intern Med 1995;122:487–492.
37. MacDonald M, Fang J, Pittman SD, et al: The current prevalence of sleep disordered breathing in congestive heart failure patients treated with beta-blockers. J Clin Sleep Med 2008; 4:38–42.
38. Oldenburg O, Lamp B, Faber L, et al: Sleep-disordered breathing in patients with symptomatic heart failure: a contemporary study of prevalence in and characteristics of 700 patients. Eur J Heart Fail 2007;9:251–257.
39. Siccoli MM, Valko PO, Herman DM, Bassetti CL: Central periodic breathing during sleep in 74 patients with acute ischemic stroke. J Neurol 2008;255:1687–1692.
40. Bitter T, Faber L, Hering D, et al: Sleep-disordered breathing in heart failure with normal left ventricular ejection fraction. Eur J Heart Fail 2009;11:602–608.
41. Hermann DM, Siccoli M, Kirov P, et al: Central periodic breathing during sleep in ischemic stroke. Stroke 2007;38: 1082–1084.
42. Nopmaneejumruslers C, Kaneko Y, Hajek V, et al: Cheyne-Stokes respiration in stroke: relationship to hypocapnia and occult cardiac dysfunction. Am J Respir Crit Care Med 2005; 171:1048–1052.

43. Tkacova R, Niroumand M, Lorenzi-Filho G, Bradley TD: Overnight shift from obstructive to central apneas in patients with heart failure: role of PCO_2 and circulatory delay. Circulation 2001;103:238–243.

44. Tkacova R, Wang H, Bradley TD: Night-to-night alterations in sleep apnea type in patients with heart failure. J Sleep Res 2006;15:321–328.

45. Pepperell JC, Maskell NA, Jones DR, et al: A randomized controlled trial of adaptive ventilation for Cheyne-Stokes breathing in heart failure. Am J Respir Crit Care Med 2003; 168:1109–1114.

46. Javaheri S, Corbett WS: Association of low $PaCO_2$ with ventral sleep apnea and ventricular arrhythmias in ambulatory patients with stable heart failure. Ann Intern Med 1998;128: 204–207.

47. Naughton M, Bernard D, Tam A, et al: Role of hyperventilation in the pathogenesis of central sleep apnea in patients with congestive heart failure. Am Rev Respir Dis 1993;148: 330–338.

48. Lorenzi-Filho G, Azevedo ER, Parker JD, Bradley TD: Relationship of carbon dioxide tension in arterial blood to pulmonary wedge pressure in heart failure. Eur Respir J 2002;19: 37–40.

49. Solin P, Bergin P, Richardson M, et al: Influence of pulmonary capillary wedge pressure on central apnea in heart failure. Circulation 1999;99:1574–1579

50. Sin DD, Fitzgerald F, Parker JD, et al: Risk factors for central and obstructive sleep apnea in 450 men and women with congestive heart failure. Am J Respir Crit Care Med 1999;160: 1101–1106.

51. Hanly PJ, Zuberi-Khokhar NS: Increased mortality associated with Cheyne-Stokes respiration in patients with congestive heart failure. Am J Respir Crit Care Med 1996;153: 272–276.

52. Sin DD, Logan AG, Fitzgerald FS, et al: Effects of continuous positive airway pressure on cardiovascular outcomes in heart failure patients with and without Cheyne-Stokes respiration. Circulation 2000;102:61–66.

53. Dark DS, Pingleton SK, Kerby GR, et al: Breathing pattern abnormalities and arterial oxygen desaturation during sleep in the congestive heart failure syndrome: improvement following medical therapy. Chest 1987;91:833–836.

54. Braver HM, Brandes WC, Kubiet MA, et al: Effect of cardiac transplantation on Cheyne-Stokes respiration occurring during sleep. Am J Cardiol 1995;76:632–634.

55. Javaheri S, Parker TJ, Wexler L, et al: Effect of theophylline on sleep-disordered breathing in heart failure. N Engl J Med 1996;335:562–567.

56. Javaheri S: Acetazolamide improves central sleep apnea in heart failure: a double-blind, prospective study. Am J Respir Crit Care Med 2006;173:234–237.

57. Biberdorf DJ, Steens R, Millar TW, Kryger MH: Benzodiazepines in congestive heart failure: effects of temazepam on arousability and Cheyne-Stokes respiration. Sleep 1993;16: 529–538.

58. Javaheri S, Ahmend M, Parker TJ: Effects of nasal O_2 on sleep-related disordered breathing in ambulatory patients with stable heart failure. Sleep 1999;22:1101–1106.

59. Staniforth AD, Kinnera WJM, Straling R, et al: Effect of oxygen on sleep quality, cognitive function and sympathetic activity in patients with chronic heart failure and Cheyne-Stokes respiration. Eur Heart J 1998;19:922–928.

60. Naughton MT, Liu PP, Bernard DC, et al: Treatment of congestive heart failure and Cheyne-Stokes respiration during sleep by continuous positive airway pressure. Am J Respir Crit Care Med 1995;151:92–97.

61. Naughton MT, Benard DC, Liu PP, et al: Effects of nasal CPAP on sympathetic activity in patients with heart failure and central sleep apnea. Am J Respir Crit Care Med 1995;152: 473–479.

62. Bradley TD, Logan AG, Kimoff RJ, et al, CANPAP Investigators: Continuous positive airway pressure for central sleep apnea and heart failure. N Engl J Med 2005;353:2025–2033.

63. Javaheri S: Effects of continuous positive airway pressure on sleep apnea and ventricular irritability in patients with heart failure. Circulation 2000;101:392–397.

64. Arzt M, Floras JS, Logan AG, et al, CANPAP Investigators: Suppression of central sleep apnea by continuous positive airway pressure and transplant-free survival in heart failure: a post hoc analysis of the Canadian Continuous Positive Airway Pressure for Patients with Central Sleep Apnea and Heart Failure Trial (CANPAP). Circulation 2007;115:3173–3180.

65. Teschler H, Döhring J, Wang YM, Berthon-Jones M: Adaptive pressure support servo-ventilation: a novel treatment for Cheyne-Stokes respiration in heart failure. Am J Respir Crit Care Med 2001;164:614–619.

66. Wilson GN, Wilcox I, Piper AJ, et al: Noninvasive pressure preset ventilation for the treatment of Cheyne-Stokes respiration during sleep. Eur Respir J 2001;17:1250–1257.

67. Oldenburg O, Schmidt A, Lamp B, et al: Adaptive servoventilation improves cardiac function in patients with chronic heart failure and Cheyne-Stokes respiration. Eur J Heart Fail 2008;10:581–586.

68. Philippe C, Stoïca-Herman M, Drouot X, et al: Compliance with and effectiveness of adaptive servoventilation versus continuous positive airway pressure in the treatment of Cheyne-Stokes respiration in heart failure over a six-month period. Heart 2006;92:337–342.

69. Thomas RJ, Terzano MG, Parrino L, Weiss JW: Obstructive sleep-disordered breathing with a dominant cyclic alternating pattern—a recognizable polysomnographic variant with practical clinical implications. Sleep 2004;27:229–234.

70. Kuzniar TJ, Pusalavidyasagar S, Gay PC, Morgenthaler TI: Natural course of complex sleep apnea—a retrospective study. Sleep Breath 2008;12:135–139.

71. Pusalavidyasagar SS, Olson EJ, Gay PC, Morgenthaler TI: Treatment of complex sleep apnea syndrome: a retrospective comparative review. Sleep Med 2006;7:474–479.

72. Javaheri S, Smith J, Chung E: The prevalence and natural history of complex sleep apnea. J Clin Sleep Med 2009;5: 205–211.

73. Dernaika T, Tawk M, Nazir S, et al: The significance and outcome of continuous positive airway pressure–related central sleep apnea during split-night sleep studies. Chest 2007;132:81–87.

74. Lehman S, Antic NA, Thompson C, et al: Central sleep apnea on commencement of continuous positive airway pressure in patients with a primary diagnosis of obstructive sleep apnea-hypopnea. J Clin Sleep Med 2007;3:462–466.

75. Morgenthaler TI, Gay PC, Gordon N, Brown LK: Adaptive servoventilation versus noninvasive positive pressure ventilation for central, mixed, and complex sleep apnea syndromes. Sleep 2007;30:468–475.

76. Allam JS, Olson EJ, Gay PC, Morgenthaler TI: Efficacy of adaptive servoventilation in treatment of complex and central sleep apnea syndromes. Chest 2007;132:1839–1846.

77. Hackett PH, Roach RC: High altitude illness. N Engl J Med 2001;345:107–113.

78. Berry RB, Sriram P: Evaluation of hypoventilation. Semin Respir Crit Care Med 2009;30:303–314.

79. Weese-Mayer DE, Berry-Kravis EM, Ceccherini I, et al: ATS Congenital Central Hypoventilation Syndrome Subcommittee. An official ATS clinical policy statement: congenital central hypoventilation syndrome: genetic basis, diagnosis, and management. Am J Respir Crit Care Med 2010;181:626–644.

80. Gozal D, Marcus CL, Shoseyov D, Keens TB: Peripheral chemoreceptor function in children with the congenital hypoventilation syndrome. J Appl Physiol 1993;74:379–387.

81. Marcus CL, Bautista DB, Amihyia A, et al: Hypercapnic arousal responses in children with congenital central hypoventilation syndrome. Pediatrics 1991;88:993–998.

82. Wagner MH, Berry RB: A full term infant with cyanotic episodes. Congenital central hypoventilation syndrome. J Clin Sleep Med 2007;3:425–426.

83. Grigg-Damberger M, Wells A: Central congenital hypoventilation syndrome: changing face of a less mysterious but more complex genetic disorder. Semin Respir Crit Care Med 2009; 30:262–274.

84. Weese-Mayer DE, Berry-Kravis EM, Zhou L: Adult identified with congenital central hypoventilation syndrome—mutation in PHOX2b gene and late-onset CHS. Am J Respir Crit Care Med 2005;171:88.

85. Katz ES, McGrath S, Marcus CL: Late-onset central hypoventilation with hypothalamic dysfunction: a distinct clinical syndrome. Pediatr Pulmonol 2000;29:62–88.

86. Weese-Mayer DE, Berry-Kravis EM: Genetics of congenital central hypoventilation syndrome: lessons from a seemingly orphan disease. Am J Respir Crit Care Med 2004;170:16–21.

87. Berry-Kravis EM, Zhou L, Rand CM, Weese-Mayer DE: Congenital central hypoventilation syndrome *PHOX2b* mutations and phenotype. Am J Respir Crit Care Med 2006;174: 1139–1144.

88. Tibballs J, Henning RD: Noninvasive ventilatory strategies in the management of a newborn infant and three children with congenital central hypoventilation syndrome. Pediatr Pulmonol 2003;36:544–548.

89. Ramesh P, Boit P, Samuels M: Mask ventilation in the early management of congenital central hypoventilation syndrome. Arch Dis Child Fetal Neonatal Ed 2008;93:F400–F403.

90. McNicholas W, Rutherford R, Grossman R, et al: Abnormal respiratory pattern generation in patients with autonomic dysfunction. Am Rev Respir Dis 1938;128:429–433.

91. Gómez-Choco MJ, Zarranz JJ, Saiz A, et al: Central hypoventilation as the presenting symptom in Hu associated paraneoplastic encephalomyelitis. J Neurol Neurosurg Psychiatry 2007;78:1143–1145.

92. Matsuyama M, Nakazawa K, Katou M, et al: Central alveolar hypoventilation syndrome due to surgical resection for bulbar hemangioblastoma. Intern Med 2009;48:925–930.

93. Ramar K: Central alveolar hypoventilation and failure to wean from the ventilator. J Clin Sleep Med 2009;5:583–585.

94. Steljes DG, Kryger MH, Kirk BW, Millar TW: Sleep in post-polio syndrome. Chest 1990;98:52–57.

95. Dauvilleriers Y, Stal V, Coubes P, et al: Chiari malformation and sleep related breathing disorders. J Neurol Neurosurg Psychiatry 2007;78:1344–1348.

96. Herschberger ML, Chidekel A: Arnold-Chiari malformation type I and sleep disordered breathing. J Pediatr Health Care 2003;17:190–197.

97. Farney RJ, Walker JM, Cloward TV, Rhondeau S: Sleep-disordered breathing associated with long-term opioid therapy. Chest 2003;123:632–639.

98. Wang D, Teichtahl H, Drummer O, et al: Central sleep apnea in stable methadone maintenance treatment patients. Chest 2005;1238:1348–1356.

99. Glidewell RN, Orr WC, Imes N: Acetazolamide as an adjunct to CPAP treatment: a case of complex sleep apnea in a patient on long-acting opioid therapy. J Clin Sleep Med 2009;5: 63–64.

100. Morgenthaler TI: The quest for stability in an unstable world: adaptive servoventilation in opioid induced complex sleep apnea syndrome. J Clin Sleep Med 2008;4:321–323.

101. Farney RJ, Walker JM, Boyle KM, et al: Adaptive servoventilation (ASV) in patients with sleep disordered breathing associated with chronic opioid medications for non-malignant pain. J Clin Sleep Med 2008;4:311–319.

102. Javaheri S, Malik A, Smith J, Chung E: Adaptive pressure support servoventilation: a novel treatment for sleep apnea associated with use of opioids. J Clin Sleep Med 2008;4: 305–310.

103. Melichar PK, Miletin J, Dittrichova J: Differential diagnosis of apneas in preterm infancy. Primary apnea of infancy. Eur J Pediatr 2009;168:195–201.

104. Henderson-Smart DJ, Steer PA: Caffeine versus theophylline for apnea in preterm infants. Cochrane Database Syst Rev 2010;1:CD000273.

105. Perrin C, D'Ambrosio C, White A, Hill NS: Sleep in restrictive and neuromuscular respiratory disorders. Semin Respir Crit Care Med 2005;26:117–130.

106. American College of Chest Physicians: Clinical indications for noninvasive positive pressure ventilation in chronic respiratory failure due to restrictive lung disease, COPD, and nocturnal hypoventilation—a consensus conference report. Chest 1999;116:521–534.

107. Ellis ER, Grunstein RR, Chan S, et al: Noninvasive ventilatory support during sleep improves respiratory failure in kyphoscoliosis. Chest 1988;94:811–815.

108. Gonzalez C, Ferris G, Diaz J, et al: Kyphoscoliotic ventilatory insufficiency: effects of long-term intermittent positive-pressure ventilation. Chest 2003;124:857–862.

109. Budweiser S, Heinemann F, Fischer W, et al: Impact of ventilation parameters and duration of ventilator use on non-invasive home ventilation in restrictive thoracic disorders. Respiration 2006;73:488–494.

110. Piper AJ, Sullivan CE: Effects of long-term nocturnal ventilation on spontaneous breathing during sleep in neuromuscular and chest wall disorders. Eur Respir J 1996;9:151.

111. De Troyer A, Borenstein S, Cordier R: Analysis of lung volume restriction in patients with respiratory muscle weakness. Thorax 1980;35:603–610.

112. Morgan RS, McNally S, Alexander M, et al: Use of sniff nasal inspiratory force to predict survival in amyotrophic lateral sclerosis. Am J Respir Crit Care Med 2005;171:269–274.

113. Simonds AK, Ward S, Heather S, et al: Outcome of pediatric domiciliary mask ventilation in neuromuscular and skeletal disease. Eur Respir J 2000;16:476–481.

114. Gruis KL, Brown DL, Lisabeth LD, et al: Longitudinal assessment of noninvasive positive pressure ventilation adjustments in ALS patients. J Neurol Sci 2006;247:59–63.

115. Bourke SC, Tomlinson M, Williams TL, et al: Effects of non-invasive ventilation on survival and quality of life in patients with amyotrophic lateral sclerosis: a randomized controlled trial. Lancet Neurol 2006;5:140–147.

Sleep-Related Hypoventilation Syndromes— Diagnostic Criteria

1. Sleep-Related Nonobstructive Alveolar Hypoventilation, Idiopathic
   A. Polysomnographic monitoring demonstrates episodes of shallow breathing longer than 10 seconds in duration associated with arterial oxygen desaturation and frequent arousals from sleep associated with the breathing disturbances or brady-tachycardia.
   Note: Although symptoms are not mandatory to make this diagnosis, patients often report excessive daytime sleepiness, frequent arousals and awakenings during sleep, or insomnia complaints.
   B. No primary lung diseases, skeletal malformations, or peripheral neuromuscular disorders that affect ventilation are present.
   C. The disorder is not better explained by another current sleep disorder, medical or neurologic disorder, mental disorder, medication use, or substance use disorder.
   Key features: No obvious cause such as a medical disorder or structural problems with the lung or chest wall. These patients do not have a congenital form of alveolar hypoventilation. However, late-onset congenital central hypoventilation has been described.
2. Congenital Central Alveolar Hypoventilation Syndrome
   A. The patient exhibits shallow breathing, or cyanosis and apnea, of perinatal onset during sleep.
   Note: In severely affected infants, consequences of hypoxia, including pulmonary hypertension and cor pulmonale, may also be present.
   B. Hypoventilation is worse during sleep than during wakefulness.
   C. The rebreathing ventilatory response to hypoxia and hypercapnia is absent or diminished.
   D. Polysomnographic monitoring during sleep demonstrates severe hypercapnia and hypoxia predominantly without apnea.
   E. The disorder is not explained by another current sleep disorder, medical or neurologic disorder, medication use, or substance use disorder.
3. Sleep-Related Hypoventilation Due to Medical Condition
   I. Sleep-Related Hypoventilaton/Hypoxemia Due to Lower Airways Obstruction

   A. Lower airways obstructive disease is present (as evidenced by a forced expiratory volume exhaled in one second/forced vital capacity ratio less than 70% on pulmonary function testing) and is believed to be the primary cause of hypoxemia.
   B. Polysomnography or sleeping arterial blood gas determination shows at least one of the following:
      i. An SpO_2, during sleep of less than 90% for more than 5 minutes with a nadir of at least 85%.
      ii. More than 30% of total sleep time with an SpO_2 of less than 90%.
      iii. Sleeping arterial blood gas with $PaCO_2$ that is abnormally high or disproportionately increased relative to levels during wakefulness.
   C. The disorder is not better explained by another current sleep disorder, another medical or neurologic disorder, medication use, or substance use disorder.
   II. Sleep-Related Hypoxemia Due to Pulmonary Parenchymal or Vascular Pathology
   A. Lung parenchymal disease or pulmonary vascular disease is present and believed to be the primary cause of hypoxemia.
   B. Polysomnography or sleeping arterial blood gas determination shows at least one of the following:
      i. An SpO_2 during sleep of less than 90% for more than 5 minutes with a nadir of at least 85%.
      ii. More than 30% of total sleep time at an SpO_2 of less than 90.
      iii. Sleeping arterial blood gas with $PaCO_2$ that is abnormally high or disproportionately increased relative to levels during wakefulness.
   C. The disorder is not better explained by another current sleep disorder, another medical or neurologic disorder, medication use, or substance use disorder.
   III. Sleep-Related Hypoventilation/Hypoxemia Due to Neuromuscular and Chest Wall Disorders

A. A neuromuscular or chest wall disorder is present and believed to be the primary cause of hypoventilation/hypoxemia.

B. Polysomnography or sleeping arterial blood gas determination shows at least one of the following:

   i. An SpO_2 during sleep of less than 90% for more than 5 minutes with a nadir of at least 85%.

   ii. More than 30% of the total sleep time at an SpO_2 of less than 90%.

   iii. Sleeping arterial blood gas with $PaCO_2$ that is abnormally high or disproportionately increased relative to levels during wakefulness.

C. The disorder is not better explained by another current sleep disorder, another medical or neurologic disorder, medication use, or substance use disorder.

Examples: Obesity hypoventilation syndrome, neuromuscular disease, kyphoscoliosis.

$PaCO_2$ = arterial partial pressure of carbon dioxide; SpO_2 = pulse oximetry.

From American Academy of Sleep Medicine: ICSD-2 International Classification of Sleep Disorders, 2nd ed. Diagnostic and Coding Manual. American Academy of Sleep Medicine. Westchester, IL: American Academy of Sleep Medicine, 2005.

Chapter 22

Sleep and Obstructive Lung Disease

Chapter Points

- Patients with COPD may experience NOD without discrete apneas and hypopneas.
- In COPD, the NOD is worse during REM sleep.
- NOD during REM sleep is often characterized by long periods of irregular and reduced tidal volume.
- A saw-tooth pattern on a nocturnal oximetry tracing in a COPD patient suggests the possibility of coexisting sleep apnea.
- If the awake SaO_2 is low, even the normal fall in PO_2 with sleep will result in greater desaturation (drop in SaO_2) due to the initial position on the steep portion of the oxyhemoglobin dissociation curve.
- Mechanisms of NOD in COPD patients include a low baseline SaO_2 as well as hypopneic breathing during REM sleep characterized by a low tidal volume (hypoventilation) and a reduction in the FRC (greater V̇/Q̇ mismatch).
- Nocturnal oxygen supplementation has not been proven to improve sleep quality in patients with COPD.
- Long-term oxygen treatment (24 hr/day) improves survival in COPD patients with daytime hypoxemia ($PaO_2 \leq 55$ mm Hg, $SaO_2 \leq 88\%$ OR PaO_2 55–59 mm Hg and evidence of cor pulmonale; see Box 22-2).
- The benefit of nocturnal oxygen supplementation in patients with a daytime $PaO_2 \geq 60$ mm Hg is unproven. However, nocturnal supplemental oxygen is usually provided if significant nocturnal hypoxemia is documented (>5 min with $SaO_2 \leq 88\%$; see Box 22-2).
- Poor sleep quality in COPD patients is believed due to medication side effects, nocturnal cough, and dyspnea.
- Bronchodilator therapy improves nocturnal gas exchange in COPD, but only a few studies have documented an improvement in sleep quality. If bronchodilators are used, medications with a long duration of action are preferred.
- Benzodiazepine receptor agonists can be used with caution to treat insomnia in stable COPD patients **without** hypercapnic respiratory failure. A melatonin receptor agonist (ramelteon) was demonstrated not to worsen gas exchange and did improve sleep quality in

one study. Sedating antidepressants are another option, but their efficacy as a hypnotic in COPD patients is unproven.
- Patients with a combination of COPD and OSA (OLS) often require treatment with a combination of PAP and supplemental oxygen. Bronchodilator therapy may improve nocturnal gas exchange and smoking cessation should be encouraged.
- BPAP may be better tolerated than CPAP in some patients with the combination of COPD and OSA.
- Nocturnal oxygen therapy in hypercapnic COPD patients without OSA generally results in only mild increases in the $PaCO_2$. A greater increase in nocturnal $PaCO_2$ may occur in patients with a combination of OSA and COPD when supplemental oxygen is administered.
- Studies suggest that OLS patients on long-term oxygen therapy have better outcomes if OSA is effectively treated with PAP.
- Patients with nocturnal asthma experience a greater than normal fall in the FEV_1 (morning dippers). This can be documented by peak flow measurements at bedtime and on awakening.
- Frequent awakening from nocturnal asthma is one of the defining characteristics of moderate to severe asthma. The presence of nocturnal asthma symptoms means asthma is suboptimally controlled.
- An inhaled corticosteroid is the first step in treating patients with nocturnal asthma. The next option is addition of a long-acting inhaled beta agonist.

OBSTRUCTIVE VENTILATORY DYSFUNCTION

Obstructive ventilatory dysfunction (OVD) describes a pattern of pulmonary dysfunction characterized by a reduced ratio of the forced expiratory volume in 1 second (FEV_1) to the forced vital capacity (FVC) on spirometry. In addition to the reduced FEV_1/FVC ratio there is a reduction in flow manifested by a reduction in the FEV_1 (Fig. 22–1).[1-4] Patients with very mild OVD may have a normal FEV_1 but a reduced

FEV$_1$/FVC ratio. For convenience, the lower limit of normal for the FEV$_1$ is assumed to be 80% of predicted and the lower limit of normal for the FEV$_1$/FVC ratio is assumed to be 0.70. However, using a slightly higher value of the FEV$_1$/FVC ratio for the lower limit of normal is appropriate in younger

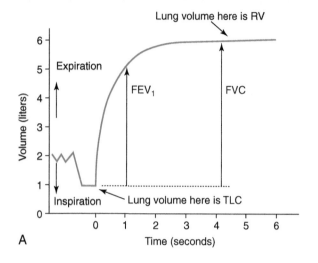

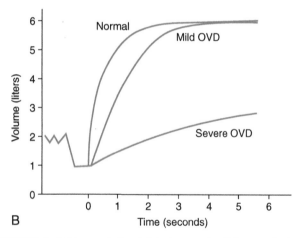

FIGURE 22–1 **A,** Spirometry is the exhaled volume per time. **B,** Patterns of patients with mild and severe obstructive ventilatory dysfunction (OVD). The hallmark of obstruction is a reduced forced expiratory volume in 1 second–to–forced vital capacity (FEV$_1$/FVC) ratio. RV = residual volume; TLC = total lung capacity.

patients. For example, using 90% of predicted as the lower limit of normal for the FEV$_1$/FVC ratio may be more sensitive for identification of OVD. Patients with OVD have normal or increased lung volumes (residual volume [RV], function residual capacity [FRC], and total lung capacity [TLC]) (Fig. 22–2). The first lung volume to be affected is the RV. Most patients with OVD have an elevated RV due to airtrapping from small airway narrowing and closure. With more severe disease, the FRC and then the TLC may also be increased (hyperinflation). However, the relative increase in the RV is greater than any increase in the FRC or TLC. In moderate to severe OVD, the increase in RV is large enough (compared with any increase in the TLC) to cause a reduction in the FVC (see Fig. 22–2). The increase in the FRC and TLC is due to loss of lung elastic recoil (emphysema) or airway disease (asthma).

A significant acute response to inhaled bronchodilator is defined by a 12% or greater increase in the FEV$_1$ or FVC with a minimum of 200 mL absolute increase. Lack of an acute bronchodilator response does not rule out a benefit from chronic bronchodilator therapy.

The common OVD disorders are listed in Table 22–1. These include asthma (bronchospasm = reversible airway obstruction), chronic bronchitis (productive cough/sputum production usually with OVD), and emphysema (destruction of alveoli and increased size of terminal airspaces). Patients often have a mixture of these manifestations and are said to have chronic obstructive pulmonary disease (COPD). Patients with asthma may have normal pulmonary function between exacerbations that can occur after upper respiratory tract infections, exposure to allergens, or exercise. They typically demonstrate a large improvement in the FEV$_1$ or FVC after inhaled bronchodilator. Asthmatics have bronchial hyperresponsiveness to methacholine challenge (>20% fall in FEV$_1$ after inhaling low concentrations), allergen, or exercise challenge (>20% fall in FEV$_1$ after exercise). A diagnosis of asthma can be made in a patient with normal pulmonary function by demonstration of bronchial hyperresponsiveness. Some asthma patients have persistent airflow obstruction and require inhaled or even oral corticosteroids for improvement. Patients with severe asthma can have

FIGURE 22–2 Lung volumes including total lung capacity (TLC), functional residual capacity (FRC), and residual volume (RV). In obstructive ventilatory dysfunction (OVD), the RV increases more than the FRC and TLC. In moderate to severe OVD, the RV increase may be enough to decrease the vital capacity (VC). ERV = expiratory reserve volume; IC = inspiratory capacity; Vt = tidal volume.

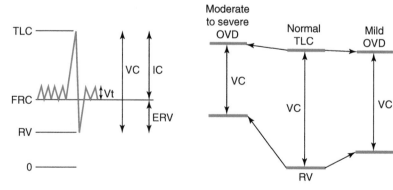

RV = residual volume
FRC = function residual capacity
TLC = total lung capacity

TABLE 22–1

Spectrum of Obstructive Ventilatory Dysfunction

	DIAGNOSIS	DIFFUSING CAPACITY	BRONCHODILATOR RESPONSE	AIRTRAPPING AND HYPERINFLATION
Asthma	Reversible airflow obstruction (physiologic diagnosis)	Normal	Yes >12% often 25%	May be present
Chronic bronchitis	Productive sputum for ≥ 3 mo for 2 consecutive yr (clinical diagnosis)	Normal	Sometimes 10–15%	Air trapping (high RV)
Emphysema	Destruction of gas-exchanging units and enlargement of terminal airspaces (pathologic diagnosis)	Decreased	Rarely	Yes
Mixed chronic bronchitis and emphysema (COPD)	Combination	Decreased	None or small	Yes

In OVD the increase in RV > increase in FRC > increase in TLC.
Air trapping manifested by an increased RV and hyperinflation manifested by an increased FRC and TLC.
COPD = chronic obstructive pulmonary disease; FRC = functional residual capacity; OVD = obstructive ventilatory dysfunction; RV = residual volume; TLC = total lung capacity.

TABLE 22–2

GOLD Criteria for Chronic Obstructive Pulmonary Disease Severity

STAGE	DESCRIPTION	FINDINGS (BASED ON POSTBRONCHODILATOR FEV_1)
0	At risk	Risk factors and chronic symptoms but normal spirometry
I	Mild	$FEV_1/FVC \leq 70\%$ FEV_1 at least 80% of predicted value May have symptoms
II	Moderate	$FEV_1/FVC \leq 70\%$ FEV_1 50% to < 80% of predicted value May have chronic symptoms
III	Severe	$FEV_1/FVC \leq 70\%$ FEV_1 30% to < 50% of predicted value May have chronic symptoms
IV	Very severe	$FEV_1/FVC \leq 70\%$ $FEV_1 < 30\%$ of predicted value or $FEV_1 < 50\%$ of predicted value + chronic respiratory failure Respiratory failure: $PaO_2 < 60$ mm Hg with or without $PaCO_2 > 50$ mm Hg while breathing room air at sea level

FEV_1 = postbronchodilator forced expiratory volume in 1 second; FVC = forced vital capacity; $PaCO_2$ = arterial partial pressure of carbon dioxide; PaO_2 = arterial partial pressure of oxygen.
From Rabe KF, Hurd S, Anzueto A, et al: Global Initiative for Chronic Obstructive Lung Disease. Global strategy for the diagnosis, management, and prevention of chronic obstructive pulmonary disease: GOLD executive summary. Am J Respir Crit Care Med 2007;176:532–555.

hyperinflation and even hypercapnic respiratory failure. Patients with COPD and predominantly chronic bronchitis typically have recurrent exacerbations and tend to have lower arterial partial pressure of oxygen (PaO_2) values earlier in the disease course. Some may develop hypercapnia and cor pulmonale (blue bloaters). Other OVD patients have predominantly emphysema with severe hyperinflation (due to loss of lung elastic recoil) and relative preservation of PaO_2 levels until late in the disease course. They present with dyspnea and, because of the relatively spared PaO_2, are called "pink puffers."

CHRONIC OBSTRUCTIVE PULMONARY DISEASE

COPD is the fourth leading cause of death in the United States.[4] The major cause of COPD is cigarette smoking. Patients with COPD may die from respiratory failure or lung cancer. Although they typically present to physicians with complaints of bronchitis or dyspnea, they also frequently complain of poor-quality sleep. The Global Initiative for Chronic Obstructive Lung Disease (GOLD) has defined severity criteria (Table 22–2).[4] In general, an FEV_1 less than 30% to 40% of predicted or 1.0 L for a normal-sized

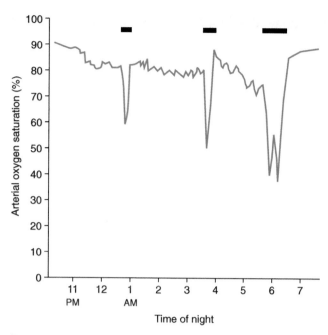

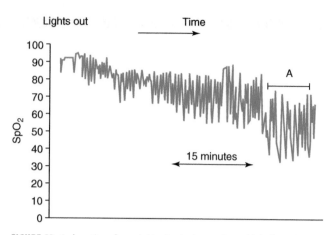

FIGURE 22–4 A portion of overnight oximetry in a patient with both snoring and moderate COPD. The baseline is reduced during sleep but the saw-tooth pattern is suggestive of obstructive sleep apnea. A = period of REM sleep. *From Berry RB: Sleep Medicine Pearls 2nd ed. Philadelphia: Hanley & Belfus, 2003, p. 227.*

FIGURE 22–3 Nocturnal oximetry in a patient with severe chronic obstructive pulmonary disease (COPD). The awake arterial oxygen saturation (SaO$_2$) is mildly reduced at 92% but falls to the low 80s with sleep. Further severe falls in the SaO$_2$ occur during rapid eye movement (REM) sleep (*dark bars*). Note that the worst period of desaturation was noted in the early morning hours. *From Berry RB: Sleep Medicine Pearls, 2nd ed. Philadelphia: Hanley & Belfus, 2003, p. 216.*

individual indicates very severe disease. Daytime hypercapnia is usually associated with an FEV$_1$ of 30% to 40% of predicted or less. Patients with the overlap syndrome (COPD + obstructive sleep apnea [OSA]) can develop hypercapnia with higher FEV$_1$ values.

Sleep in COPD

Sleep in patients with COPD is often impaired in both duration and quality.[5–7] Many patients also have significant hypercapnia and hypoxemia at night. Ten percent to 15% of patients may also have concomitant OSA that worsens nocturnal gas exchange (overlap syndrome). The typical pattern of nocturnal oxygen desaturation (NOD) in a patient with COPD is shown in Figure 22–3. The baseline sleeping arterial oxygen saturation (SaO$_2$) falls 2% to 4% from the awake baseline with minor fluctuations until much larger drops are noted during rapid eye movement (REM; stage R) sleep. In contrast, a typical oximetry of a patient with the overlap syndrome is shown in Figure 22–4. There is a low baseline sleeping SaO$_2$ and a saw-tooth pattern consistent with repeated discrete events. Whereas central sleep apnea could cause a saw-tooth pattern, this is most likely to represent OSA.

Etiology of Abnormal Nocturnal Gas Exchange

Patients with COPD often experience exaggerations of normal sleep-related changes in ventilation. The most severe desaturation occurs during REM sleep. The major

BOX 22–1

Major Mechanisms of Nocturnal Oxygen Desaturation in Chronic Obstructive Pulmonary Disease

- Hypoventilation—believed by most to be the most important factor
  - Decreased chemosensitivity (REM < NREM < wake)
  - Reliance on accessory respiratory muscles and loss of this assistance during REM atonia
  - Increased upper airway resistance
  - Lower alveolar ventilation per minute ventilation (high dead space–to–tidal volume ratio—due to high dead space and low tidal volume)
- Ventilation-perfusion mismatching (drop in PaO$_2$ exceeds the increase in PaCO$_2$)
  - High closing volume and decreases in FRC—especially during REM-associated hypopnea
- Coexisting sleep apnea (12–15%)—especially blue bloaters
- Low awake SaO$_2$—starting position on the steep portion of the oxygen-hemoglobin saturation curve (larger fall in SaO$_2$ for a given fall in PaO$_2$)

FRC = functional residual capacity; NREM = non–rapid eye movement; PaCO$_2$ = arterial partial pressure of carbon dioxide; PaO$_2$ = arterial partial pressure of oxygen; REM = rapid eye movement; SaO$_2$ = arterial oxygen saturation.

mechanisms of nocturnal arterial oxygen desaturation are listed in Box 22–1. The relative importance of hypoventilation and ventilation-perfusion ($\dot{V}/\dot{Q}$) mismatch is still debated.

Normal Individuals

During non–rapid eye movement (NREM) sleep, CO$_2$ production falls but alveolar ventilation falls proportionately more and arterial pressure of carbon dioxide (PaCO$_2$)

increases slightly (Fig. 22–5). Recall that $PaCO_2$ = constant × (CO_2 production)/(alveolar ventilation); see Chapter 10. The fall in ventilation is due to a loss of the wakefulness stimulus to breathe, decreased ventilatory responses (chemosensitivity) to hypoxia and hypercapnia, and increased upper airway resistance.[5,7] The increase in $PaCO_2$ results in a mild decrease in the PaO_2. However, because the awake PaO_2 value is on the flat portion of the oxygen-hemoglobin saturation curve (Fig. 22–6), minimal drops in the SaO_2 are noted (e.g., from 97% to 95%). The FRC may decrease slightly from wake to NREM sleep (Fig. 22–7).[8,9]

During REM sleep in normal individuals, ventilation is irregular and periods of reduced tidal volume occur, often during bursts of REMs. Skeletal muscle hypotonia reduces the contribution from the accessory respiratory muscles and respiration depends on the diaphragm.[8,9] Two studies did not find a lower FRC during REM compared with NREM sleep

in normal individuals (see Fig. 22–7).[8,10] During REM sleep, there is typically a decrease in chest wall movement,[9] likely due to chest wall hypotonia. These REM-associated physiologic changes result in a slight increase in $PaCO_2$ and decreases in PaO_2 during REM compared with NREM sleep. The slight fall in PaO_2 results in minimal changes in the SaO_2 due to the position of the oxygen-hemoglobin saturation curve (see Fig. 22–6).

Sleep-Related Changes in Respiration in COPD

Koo and colleagues[11] studied 15 patients with severe COPD (FEV_1 of 0.96 L) with a mean daytime PaO_2 greater than

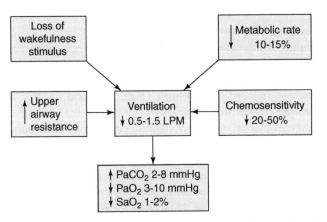

FIGURE 22–5 Normal changes in gas exchange during sleep. $PaCO_2$ = arterial partial pressure of carbon dioxide; PaO_2 = arterial partial pressure of oxygen; SaO_2 = arterial oxygen saturation. *Adapted from Mohsenin V: Sleep in chronic obstructive pulmonary disease. Semin Respir Crit Care Med 2005;26:109–115.*

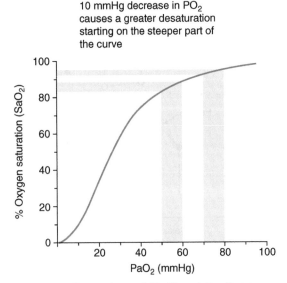

FIGURE 22–6 The same drop in the arterial partial pressure of oxygen (PaO_2) is associated with a greater drop in the arterial oxygen saturation (SaO_2) when the initial partial pressure of oxygen (PO_2) is 60 rather than 80 mm Hg.

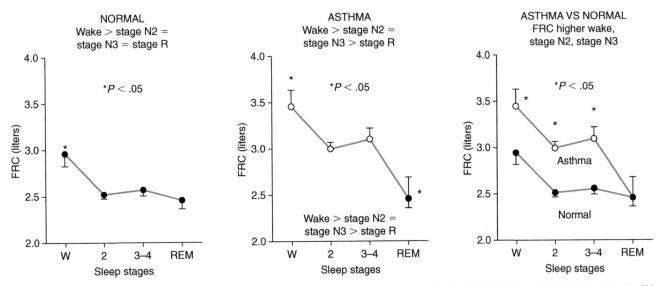

FIGURE 22–7 **(Left)** In normal subjects the FRC is lower during sleep but the FRC does not differ between stages 2, 3–4, and REM (N2, N3, and R). **(Middle)** In asthma the FRC decreases from wake to stage N2–N3 and then further decreases during REM sleep. **(Right)** FRC during wake and stages N2 and N3 is higher in asthmatics compared to normal individuals. In this study the FRC during REM sleep was similar in asthmatics and normal individuals. FRC = functional residual capacity; REM = rapid eye movement. *Adapted from Ballard RD, Irvin CG, Martin RJ, et al: Influence of sleep on lung volume in asthmatic patients and normal subjects. J Appl Physiol 1990;68:2034–2041.*

60 mm Hg and found a mean decrease in PaO_2 of 13.5 mm Hg and a mean increase in $PaCO_2$ of 8.3 mm Hg during REM sleep (Fig. 22–8). Although patients with daytime hypercapnia or a low awake PaO_2 or SaO_2 are more likely to have worse gas exchange during sleep, up to 25% of patients with

COPD exhibit REM-related hypoventilation and NOD, despite having a daytime PaO_2 above 60 mm Hg.[12]

Non–Rapid Eye Movement During supine wakefulness, patients with COPD often start with low-normal or slightly decreased SaO_2 values. Therefore, even the normal fall in PaO_2 with sleep will cause a greater decrease in the SaO_2. Koo and colleagues[11] documented a fall in PaO_2 of approximately 8 mm Hg from wake to NREM sleep and an increase in $PaCO_2$ of about 5 mm Hg. In patients with COPD, the onset of NREM sleep is associated with mild falls in the SaO_2 (4–8%) and $PaCO_2$ increases. If obstructive apneas or hypopneas are present, the degree of desaturation is worsened. Due to hyperinflation, the diaphragm is at a mechanical disadvantage and there is more dependence on the accessory muscles of respiration. In a study by Becker and coworkers[13] of a group of hypercapnic patients with COPD, the minute ventilation fell by 16% from wake to NREM.

Rapid Eye Movement During REM sleep, there are more profound periods of arterial oxygen desaturation compared with NREM sleep in patients with COPD. These episodes of desaturation are characterized by long periods of irregular breathing and reduced tidal volume (Figs. 22–9 and 22–10). In contrast to obstructive hypopnea in OSA patients, the onset and termination of these nonapneic periods of REM desaturation are less well defined. As noted previously, it is believed that REM-associated hypotonia reduces the contribution for the intercostal muscles so that ventilation depends on the diaphragm. Hyperinflation in patients with COPD reduces the effectiveness of the diaphragm. During the periods of REM-associated diaphragmatic inhibition (often during bursts of eye movements),[13–15] the tidal volume and minute ventilation often decrease dramatically (see Figs. 22–9 and

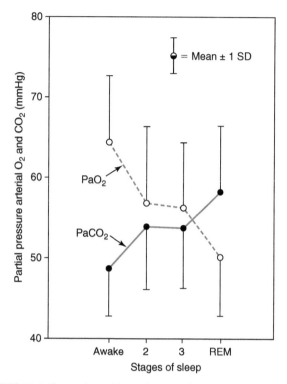

FIGURE 22–8 Changes in arterial partial pressure of carbon dioxide ($PaCO_2$) and arterial partial pressure of oxygen (PaO_2) during sleep in a group of patients with severe COPD. Here stages 2, 3, and REM represent stages N2, N3, and R. REM = rapid eye movement; SD = standard deviation. *From Koo KW, Sax DS, Snider GL: Arterial blood gases and pH during sleep in chronic obstructive pulmonary disease. Am J Med 1975;58:663–670.*

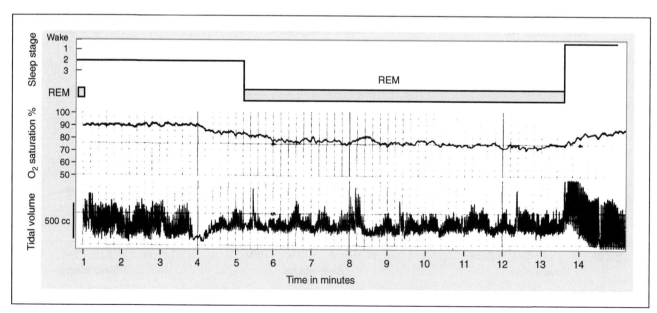

FIGURE 22–9 An episode of hypopneic breathing during rapid eye movement (REM) sleep in a patient with COPD. The episode lasted over 10 minutes. *From Fletcher EC, Gray BA, Levin DC: Nonapneic mechanisms of arterial oxygen desaturation during rapid-eye-movement sleep. J Appl Physiol 1983;54:632–639.*

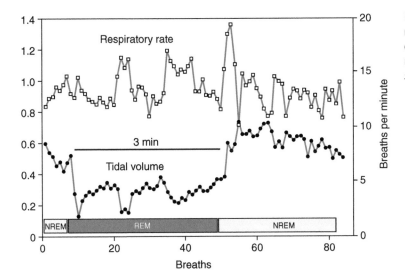

FIGURE 22-10 Fall in tidal volume during a period of rapid eye movement (REM)−associated hypoventilation. Note that there is no overall significant change in the respiratory rate. NREM = non−rapid eye movement. *From Becker HF, Piper AJ, Flynn WE, et al: Breathing during sleep in patients with nocturnal desaturation. Am J Respir Crit Care Med 1999;159:112−118.*

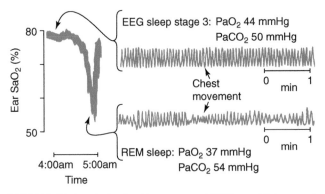

FIGURE 22-11 An episode of rapid eye movement (REM)−associated nonapneic desaturation in a patient with COPD. The decrease in arterial partial pressure of oxygen (PaO_2) was greater than the increase in the arterial partial pressure of carbon dioxide ($PaCO_2$). Stage 3 and REM denote stages N3 and R. EEG = electroencephalogram; SaO_2 = arterial oxygen saturation. *From Catterall JR, Calverley PMA, MacNee W, et al: Mechanism of transient nocturnal hypoxemia in hypoxic chronic bronchitis and emphysema. J Appl Physiol 1985;59:1698−1703.*

22-10). The drop in alveolar ventilation is even larger than the change in minute ventilation due to an increase in the dead space–to–tidal volume ratio (see Chapter 10). In one study of a group of hypercapnic patients with COPD, the minute ventilation fell by 32% from wake to REM sleep (compared with 16% from wake to NREM).[13] Studies have documented increases in $PaCO_2$ during these episodes.[11,15,16] Figure 22-10 illustrates a nonapneic period of REM-associated fall in tidal volume.

V̇/Q̇ Mismatch Whereas hypoventilation definitely occurs during periods of nonapneic desaturation (also called hypopneic breathing), Catterall and associates[16,17] directly measured arterial blood gases and found the PaO_2 dropped more than the $PaCO_2$ increased (Fig. 22-11). Therefore, increased V̇/Q̇ mismatch is believed to play a role in REM-associated desaturation (in addition to hypoventilation).[15,16] However, as Catterall and associates[16,17] and others have pointed out,

the usual blood gas analysis of the relationship between PaO_2 and $PaCO_2$ depends on an assumption of steady state. This condition does not exist during the transient periods of hypopneic breathing. Because oxygen stores in the body are much smaller than carbon dioxide stores, a change in ventilation may affect PaO_2 more than $PaCO_2$.

Many patients with COPD have an increase in FRC in the upright position (hyperinflation). In the supine position, the FRC may be slightly lower during wakefulness. Ballard and coworkers[10] found similar FRC values during wake, NREM, and REM sleep in patients with emphysema. However, in asthmatics, another study found that the FRC does decrease from wake to NREM and from NREM to REM (see Fig. 22-7).[10] COPD patients with a significant component of airways disease could experience a drop in FRC during REM sleep. In a given patient with COPD, the FRC may also be affected by the degree of obesity. Furthermore, assigning a single FRC value to stage R sleep is problematic because breathing during REM sleep is very inhomogeneous. Hudgel and coworkers[14] found no decrease in FRC during transition from stage N2 to stage R sleep in a group of five patients with COPD. However, **during episodes of hypopneic breathing in REM sleep, there was a fall in FRC.** The same study found that those COPD patients who desaturated during REM sleep had longer periods of hypopneic breathing (Fig. 22-12). Thus, it seems likely that the FRC during hypopneic breathing in COPD is lower than during NREM sleep. Whether the absolute value is below normal may vary between patients.

A fall in the FRC during hypopneic breathing in COPD patients may have greater consequences than in normal individuals. In COPD, the closing volume (CV), the volume at which small airway closure is significant, is closer to the FRC than in normal individuals. During the hypopneic breathing of REM sleep, the FRC falls below the CV (Fig. 22-13). This means that during tidal breathing, more alveoli are either not ventilated or underventilated. This results in worsening of V̇/Q̇ mismatch (already abnormal awake) and worsening

FIGURE 22-12 Hypopnea and hyperpnea in REM sleep in a COPD patient. Raw intercostal and diaphragmatic electromyogram (EMG), esophageal pressure, and arterial oxygen saturation (SaO₂) are shown. This is the end of an episode of REM hypopneic breathing. Note the increase in end-expiratory volume (*) at the end of the episode. The *solid bar* shows that the end-expiratory volume after the hypopnea ends is higher than during the hypopneic breathing. Also note the decreased intercostal EMG and greater reduction in chest wall movement. *From Hudgel DW, Martin RJ, Capehart M, et al: Contribution of hypoventilation to sleep oxygen desaturation in chronic obstructive pulmonary disease. J Appl Physiol 1983; 55:669–677.*

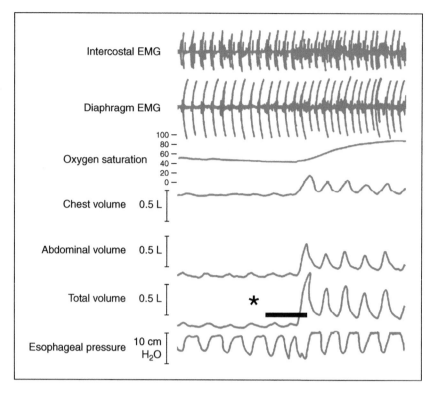

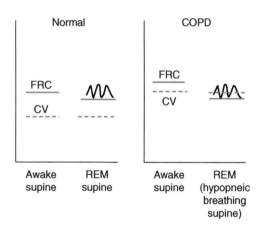

FIGURE 22-13 In patients with chronic obstructive pulmonary disease (COPD), the closing volume (CV) is nearer the functional residual capacity (FRC) than in normal individuals. The fall in FRC associated with hypopneic breathing during rapid eye movement (REM) sleep results in tidal breathing below the CV. This worsens ventilation-perfusion mismatch. Note that, in this figure, the FRC for COPD during hypopneic breathing in REM sleep is shown as approximately equal to that of a normal individual during REM sleep. The actual FRC in COPD patients may depend on other factors such as obesity and vary between individuals.

hypoxemia. Hudgel and coworkers[14] concluded that hypoventilation, and to a lesser extent $\dot{V}/\dot{Q}$ mismatch, causes REM-associated desaturation. Fletcher and associates[15] found an increase in venous admixture during REM hypopnea episodes and concluded that $\dot{V}/\dot{Q}$ mismatch was a significant cause of hypoxemia. The relative roles of hypoventilation and $\dot{V}/\dot{Q}$ mismatch in inducing nocturnal desaturation during hypopneic breathing during REM sleep are still debated. The analysis is complicated by the non–steady-state condition of transient hypopneic breathing.

Time of Night and Circadian Variation in Lung Function
REM episodes in the early morning have greatest REM density and the greatest variation in ventilation even in normal individuals.[19] These REM periods also are typically longer. In the early morning hours, there is greater lower airway resistance due to circadian changes in bronchomotor tone that are exaggerated in many patients with COPD.[5,6] Ballard and colleagues[18] found an increase in upper airway resistance but not lower airway resistance during the night in a group of patients with emphysema. Conversely, lower airway resistance does increase in asthmatics[20] and likely in some COPD patients with a significant component of airway disease. These factors help explain **why the most severe and longest REM-associated desaturation typically occurs in the early morning hours**.

COPD Types and Respiration during Sleep
Several studies have tried to find factors predicting more severe desaturation during sleep in COPD. As might be expected, a **lower awake PaO₂ and higher PaCO₂** predict more dramatic changes in gas exchange during sleep. One study compared blue bloaters and pink puffers and found the former were more likely to desaturate during sleep (Table 22–3).[21] Analysis of the Sleep Heart Health data suggested that the odds of having desaturation more than 5% of total sleep time was minimally increased until the FEV₁/FVC ratio was less than 60% (Table 22–4).[22] A plot of awake SaO₂ versus

TABLE 22-3 Arterial Oxygen Saturation during Wake and Sleep—Variation with Chronic Obstructive Pulmonary Disease Type		
	PINK PUFFER (%)	**BLUE BLOATER (%)**
SaO_2 awake and sitting	93	88.4
SaO_2 awake and supine	92.3	80.5
SaO_2 sleep	92.3	77.3
Maximal fall in SaO_2	4.7	29.5
Episodes of arterial oxygen desaturation	3.5	22.7
$SaO_2 < 80\%$ (min)	0.08	120.0

From DeMarco FJ Jr, Wynne JW, Block AJ, et al: Oxygen desaturation during sleep as a determinant of the "blue and bloated" syndrome. Chest 1981;79:621–625.

TABLE 22-4 Adjusted Odds of Desaturation > 5% of Total Sleep Time*	
FEV$_1$/FVC	**ADJUSTED ODDS RATIO**
>80	1.0
75.9–79.9	0.92
70.0–74.9	1.01
65.0–69.9	1.32
60–64.9	1.92
<60	3.36

*Excludes subjects with AHI > 15/hr.
AHI = apnea-hypopnea index; FEV_1 = forced expiratory volume in 1 second; FVC = forced vital capacity.
From Sanders MH, Newman AB, Haggerty CL, et al: Sleep and sleep-disordered breathing in adults with predominantly mild obstructive airway disease. Am J Respir Crit Care Med 2003;167:7–14.

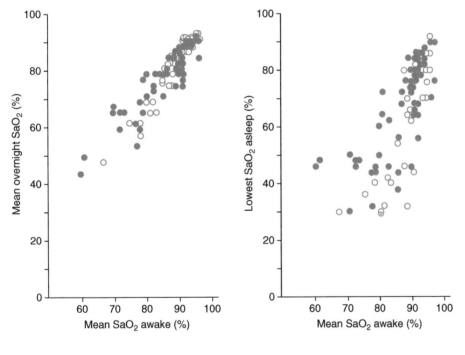

FIGURE 22–14 The relationship between mean arterial oxygen saturation (SaO_2) during wakefulness and the mean overnight SaO_2 during sleep **(left)** or lowest SaO_2 asleep **(right)**. The *closed* and *open circles* represent patients from different centers. *From Connaughton JJ, Catterall JR, Elton RA, et al: Do sleep studies contribute to the management of patients with severe chronic obstructive pulmonary disease? Am Rev Respir Dis 1988;138:341–344.*

minimum sleeping value is shown in Figure 22–14. Patients with lower awake SaO_2 or PaO_2 values tend to have lower values at night.[23] However, there is considerable variability and oximetry or polysomnography (PSG) is needed to reliably exclude NOD.

Sleep Quality in COPD
Sleep quality is impaired with reductions in total sleep time, stage N3 sleep, and REM sleep. In contrast, the wake after sleep onset (WASO) and stage N1 sleep are increased as is the total arousal index. Patients often complain of insomnia but can also complain of daytime sleepiness if OSA is also present. A study of NOD in COPD patients not on 24-hour oxygen found no difference in quality of life, subjective sleepiness, or subjective sleep quality in COPD patients who had NOD compared with those who did not.[24] It is likely that other factors such as cough, nocturnal dyspnea, and medication side effects have greater effect than transient hypoxemia on sleep quality. In many patients, the NOD is less than 15 minutes and confined to the last few REM periods of the night.

Treatment of Sleep-Related Hypoxemia in COPD
Studies have shown that long-term oxygen therapy (LTOT) will improve survival in patients with COPD with daytime hypoxemia.[25-27] The standard indication for 24-hour

BOX 22–2

Indications for Supplemental Oxygen

Local Carrier Determination (LCD) 11446 (Cigna) for CMS 240.2 National Carrier Determination

GROUP I (INITIAL COVERAGE LIMITED TO 12 MO)

1. $PO_2 \leq 55$ mm Hg or $SaO_2 \leq 88\%$ at rest awake (breathing room air, stable medical condition).
2. $PO_2 \leq 55$ mm Hg or $SaO_2 \leq 88\%$ for at least 5 min while asleep. Oxygen is provided during sleep only.
3. Decrease in $PO_2 > 10$ mm Hg or a decrease in $SaO_2 \geq 5\%$ for at least 5 min during sleep associated with symptoms.*
4. $PO_2 < 55$ mm Hg or $SaO_2 \leq 88\%$ during exercise in a patient with a PaO_2 at $\geq 56\%$ or $SaO_2 \geq 89\%$ at rest. Oxygen provided during exercise.

GROUP II (INITIAL COVERAGE LIMITED TO 3 MO)

The presence of (a) an arterial PO_2 of 56–59 mm Hg or an arterial oxygen saturation of 89% at rest (awake), during sleep for at least 5 min, or during exercise (as described in Group 1 criteria) and (b) any one of the following:

1. Dependent edema suggesting CHF.
2. Pulmonary HTN or cor pulmonale determined by measurement of pulmonary artery pressure, gated blood pool scan, echocardiogram, or "P" pulmonale on ECG (P wave ≥ 3 mm in standard leads II, III, or aVF) or
3. Erythrocythemia with Hct > 56%.
4. $PaO_2 \leq 55$ mm Hg or $SaO_2 \leq 88\%$ during exercise, O_2 supplied only for exercise.

See also CMS 240.2 NCD for Home Oxygen
  L11446 can be found at https://www.virtuox.net/dyndocs/Documents/LCDforOxygen.pdf

*Symptoms: impairment of consciousness, nocturnal restlessness, insomnia or signs of cor pulmonale, P pulmonale on ECG, documented pulmonary HTN, erythrocytosis.
CHF = congestive heart failure; CMS = Centers for Medicare and Medicaid Services; ECG = electrocardiogram; Hct = hematocrit; HTN = hypertension; PaO_2 = arterial partial pressure of oxygen; PO_2 = partial pressure of oxygen; SaO_2 = arterial oxygen saturation.

TABLE 22–5

Studies of Effects of Supplemental Oxygen on Sleep Quality in Chronic Obstructive Pulmonary Disease

	CALVERLY[29] (N = 6)	FLEETHAM[30] (N = 15)
Total sleep time	Increased	No change
Stage N3	Increased	No change
REM sleep	Increased	No change
Arousals	Decreased	No change

REM = rapid eye movement.

supplemental oxygen is a daytime $PaO_2 \leq 55$ mm Hg at rest when the patient is in stable condition. PaO_2 values from 56 to 59 mm Hg are also an indication of a need for oxygen therapy if signs of dysfunction (right heart failure) are present. Typical requirements for Medicare reimbursement for supplemental oxygen are listed in Box 22–2. The criteria vary between regions (Local Carrier Determinations). Patients qualifying for 24-hour supplemental oxygen will obviously be using nocturnal oxygen. However, one study found that at least 50% of patients on LTOT needed increased oxygen flow during sleep.[28] The utility of treating isolated NOD (daytime $PaO_2 > 60$ mm Hg) is unproven. However, most clinicians would treat patients who have a nocturnal SaO_2 less than 88% for a substantial period of time. Most insurance providers require at least 5 minutes less than or equal to 88% (see Box 22–2).

One study found an improvement in sleep quality with supplemental oxygen,[29] and another did not.[30] Both were relatively small studies and this question remains to be answered (Table 22–5). A randomized trial of supplemental oxygen in patients with isolated NOD (daytime $PaO_2 > 60$ mm Hg) did not find a survival benefit (although there were only a small number of deaths) but nocturnal oxygen did improve the pulmonary artery pressure.[31] Chaouat and coworkers[32] also performed a randomized trial of nocturnal oxygen in a similar patient group. They found no benefit of oxygen treatment with respect to mortality, the increase in pulmonary artery pressure, or the subsequent need for daytime oxygen. Connaughton and colleagues[23] found that those patients with a worse NOD than expected based on daytime gas exchange did not have a worse prognosis and argued against the use of routine sleep studies or nocturnal oximetry in COPD patients. On the other hand nocturnal oximetry is indicated if the patient complains of nocturnal symptoms or has evidence of cor pulmonale. In acute respiratory failure, administration of high-flow oxygen can significantly worsen hypercapnia but low-flow supplemental oxygen produces only mild to moderate increases in nocturnal $PaCO_2$ unless patients have sleep apnea[33] (Fig. 22–15). Another study found that increasing the nocturnal oxygen flow rate by even 1 L/min resulted in a lower pH and higher $PaCO_2$ in the morning.[34] It seems prudent to use the lowest oxygen flow required to maintain adequate nocturnal oxygenation, especially in hypercapnic patients.

Bronchodilators Treatment with bronchodilators, especially long-acting inhaled bronchodilators, does improve nocturnal oxygenation in COPD patients. Most studies of the effects of bronchodilators on sleep have **not** shown improvement in **sleep quality**. Conversely, quality was usually not worsened. One study compared the combination of sustained-action theophylline and a short-acting inhaled beta agonist bronchodilator at bedtime versus the inhaled bronchodilator + placebo.[35] The addition of theophylline did not worsen sleep quality but improved the morning FEV_1

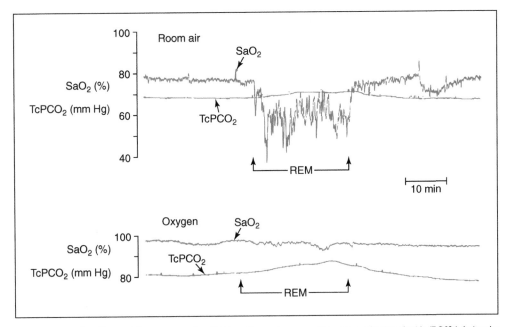

FIGURE 22–15 **Top,** The arterial oxygen saturation (SaO$_2$) and transcutaneous partial pressure of carbon dioxide (TcPCO$_2$) during the night with an impressive drop in the SaO$_2$ during rapid eye movement (REM) sleep associated with a mild increase in the TcPCO$_2$. The TcPCO$_2$ is approximately 70 mm Hg during NREM sleep. **Bottom,** The same patient on supplemental oxygen with a TcPCO$_2$ now approximately 80 mm Hg. There is improved SaO$_2$, although the TcPCO$_2$ increases during REM sleep. *From Goldstein RS, Ramcharan V, Bowes G, et al: Effect of supplemental nocturnal oxygen on gas exchange in patients with severe obstructive lung disease. N Engl J Med 1984;310:425–429.*

and SaO$_2$ during NREM sleep.[35] Martin and associates[36] found that inhaled ipratropium bromide (a short-acting anticholinergic) given by nebulizer improved subjective sleep quality, NOD, and the amount of REM sleep. This study used 4 nights of sleep monitoring, allowing patients to acclimate to the monitoring equipment. McNicholas and coworkers[37] found that tiotropium (a long-acting inhaled anticholinergic) given either in the morning or in the evening improved the SaO$_2$ during REM sleep compared with placebo but did not improve sleep quality. Ryan and colleagues[38] found that salmeterol, a long-acting inhaled beta agonist, improved nocturnal oxygenation without impairing sleep quality. Donahue and associates[39] compared fluticasone propionate/salmeterol with ipratropium bromide/albuterol during an 8-week period. The former treatment combination was more effective at reducing nocturnal and sleep symptoms. The use of inhaled corticosteroids in patients with COPD remains somewhat controversial and the controversy was reviewed by Sin and Man.[40] The use of inhaled corticosteroids does not improve mortality but, in some studies, improved the quality of life, reduced exacerbations, and improved lung function when added to a long-acting bronchodilator. Based on the previously mentioned studies, most clinicians would use a long-acting beta agonist or anticholinergic in patients with significant COPD who complain of nocturnal dyspnea, cough, or poor sleep quality. Inhaled corticosteroids are also a reasonable addition especially if the patient has repeated COPD exacerbations, a significant component of bronchospasm, or do not respond to other treatments.

Hypnotics in COPD Patients Hypnotics have been used with some caution in patients with COPD. In general, in nonhypercapnic patients, clinically significant worsening of gas exchange does not occur with benzodiazepine receptor agonists.[41] Girault and coworkers[42] studied 10 patients with severe COPD before and after 10 days of zolpidem 10 mg and could find no worsening in performance or gas exchange. Of interest, the only objective improvement in sleep was an increase in stage N2. Subjective sleep quality was also improved (not placebo-controlled). Another study found no detrimental effects from temazepam 10 mg.[43] Steens and colleagues[44] studied the effects of zolpidem and triazolam in mild to moderate COPD. Total sleep time was increased as well as sleep efficiency without an adverse effect on gas exchange. This was a randomized, double-blind, placebo-controlled study. A double-blind, placebo-controlled crossover study of patients with moderate to severe COPD evaluated the effects of 8 mg of ramelteon, a melatonin agonist with no respiratory depressant properties. This study found no worsening of nocturnal gas exchange.[45] However, there was an improvement in total sleep time, sleep efficiency, and the latency to persistent sleep on ramelteon compared to placebo. This medication has a short duration of action and is generally used for sleep-onset insomnia. However, the duration of action may vary between individuals. In summary, the benzodiazepine receptor agonists are probably safe in nonhypercapnic nonhypoxemic patients. However, caution is still required. Ramelteon is a safe hypnotic that may be effective in some patients with COPD. Many clinicians use sedating antidepressants as hypnotics (e.g., trazodone), believing that this is safer. However, the utility of the use of sedating antidepressants to improve sleep quality in COPD patients has never been documented.

Nocturnal Noninvasive Positive-Pressure Ventilation For patients with COPD who present with hypercapnic respiratory failure, noninvasive positive-pressure ventilation (NPPV) has proved to be an effective treatment, often avoiding the need for intubation and mechanical ventilation. The results for long-term use are much less clear. Those COPD patients most likely to benefit are individuals with substantial daytime CO_2 retention and NOD who are highly motivated. A consensus conference recommended the following indications for NPPV in patients with COPD[46]:

1. Symptoms criteria (e.g., fatigue, dyspnea, or morning headache),
2. Physiologic criteria daytime $PaCO_2 > 55$ or $50-54$ mm Hg with NOD, or
3. $PaCO_2$ $50-54$ mm Hg with recurrent hospitalization related to episodes of hypercapnic respiratory failure.

Patients with severe swallowing dysfunction or those who cannot protect their airway are not candidates for NPPV.

Overlap Syndrome

The overlap syndrome (OLS) consists of patients with both OSA and COPD (Box 22-3). One study found that OSA is no more frequent in COPD patients than in the general population.[22] That is, the prevalence of OSA in COPD patients is the same as in the general population. However, because both are common, the combination is also fairly common. The two groups of OSA patients with daytime hypercapnia include patients with the obesity hypoventilation syndrome and some patients with OLS.[47-49] Patients with OLS tend to have severe NOD even if they do not have daytime hypercapnia. Patients with COPD usually become hypercapnic when the FEV_1 is around 1.0 liters (or 40% of predicted). OLS patients can be hypercapnic with milder reductions in the FEV_1 (Table 22-6, Study #2). However, OLS patients can also maintain a normal daytime PCO_2 even when their FEV_1 is quite reduced (Table 22-6, Study #1). In clinical practice, one often treats patients with a combination of COPD, OSA, and severe obesity who have significant hypoventilation. It is difficult to know how to label them because they likely have components of both OHS and OLS.

Treatment of OLS

Treatment of patients with OLS with supplemental oxygen alone can result in significant increases in nocturnal $PaCO_2$. In Figure 22-16, on room air, there is a saw-tooth pattern in the SaO_2 tracing. As mentioned previously, this is a clue that OSA as well as COPD is present. On the bottom, the patient is on supplemental oxygen and the transcutaneous partial pressure of carbon dioxide ($TcPCO_2$) has climbed from approximately 60 mm Hg (top tracing) to just below

BOX 22–3

Overlap Syndrome

- Combination of OSA and COPD.
- Prevalence of OSA in COPD is the same as the general population.
- Predisposes OSA patients to more severe arterial oxygen desaturation.
- Hypercapnia may occur in OLS at FEV_1 values greater than typically associated with hypercapnia in patients with COPD without OSA.
- Optimal treatment of OLS
  - PAP (CPAP or BPAP), BPAP may be better tolerated.
  - Supplemental oxygen if needed (low awake or baseline sleeping SaO_2).
  - Bronchodilator treatment and smoking cessation.
- Nocturnal supplemental oxygen alone is not adequate treatment, may be associated with significant hypercapnia during sleep and worse outcomes.
- OLS patients who adhere to CPAP (in addition to oxygen if needed) have a better outcome.*
- OLS patients have an increased risk of death and hospitalization due to severe COPD exacerbations.†
- Treatment with CPAP may improve survival of OLS patients and decrease hospitalizations.†

*From Machado MCL, Vollmer WM, Togeiro SM, et al: CPAP and survival in moderate to severe obstructive sleep apnea syndrome and hypoxemic COPD. Eur Respir J 2010;35:132–137.
†From Marin JM, Soriano JB, Carrizo SJ, et al: Outcomes in patients with chronic obstructive pulmonary disease and obstructive sleep apnea. Am J Respir Crit Care Med 2010;182:325–331.
BPAP = bilevel positive airway pressure; COPD = chronic obstructive pulmonary disease; CPAP = continuous positive airway pressure; FEV_1 = forced expiratory volume in 1 second; OLS = overlap syndrome; OSA = obstructive sleep apnea; PAP = positive airway pressure; SaO_2 = arterial oxygen saturation.

90 mm Hg. Therefore, use of supplemental oxygen in patients with OLS and significant daytime hypercapnia may worsen nocturnal hypercapnia. Fletcher and associates[50] followed patients with chronic lung disease and OSA including a group treated with oxygen but no effective treatment for sleep apnea. They found that patients who did not have adequate treatment for OSA had no improvement in their pulmonary hemodynamics whereas those who had effective treatment improved. A recent observational study of patients with OSA and hypoxemic COPD receiving LTOT found that those who accepted continuous positive airway pressure (CPAP; in addition to oxygen) and adhered to treatment had a better survival than those who did not.[51] Another study by Marin and coworkers[52] of patients with OLS found an increased risk of death and hospitalization due to COPD exacerbations. CPAP treatment was associated with improved survival and decreased hospitalizations. The treatment of patients with OLS includes treatment of their COPD and CPAP or bilevel positive airway pressure (BPAP) with supplemental oxygen if needed. If significant CO_2 retention is present, most clinicians would use BPAP. Some patients with COPD have difficulty exhaling on CPAP and may be more adherent to treatment with BPAP.

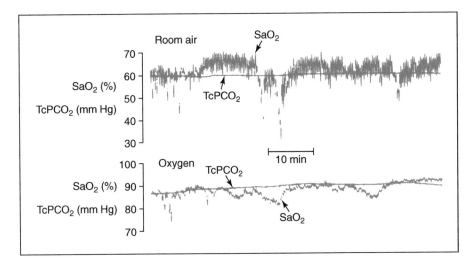

FIGURE 22–16 A patient with obstructive sleep apnea (OSA) and COPD. **Top,** A saw-tooth pattern in the arterial oxygen saturation (SaO_2) is noted while the patient breathes room air. The transcutaneous partial pressure of carbon dioxide ($TcPCO_2$) is approximately 60 mm Hg and the SaO_2 is severely reduced. **Bottom,** The patient is breathing supplemental oxygen. The SaO_2 is improved but the $TcPCO_2$ has increased dramatically to just below 90 mm Hg. *From Goldstein RS, Ramcharan V, Bowes G, et al: Effect of supplemental nocturnal oxygen on gas exchange in patients with severe obstructive lung disease. N Engl J Med 1984;310:425–429.*

TABLE 22–6			
Eucapnic and Hypercapnic Patients with Overlap Syndrome			
	STUDY #1 OLS EUCAPNIC (N = 14)	**STUDY #1 OLS HYPERCAPNIC (N = 14)**	**STUDY #2 OLS HYPERCAPNIC (N = 7)**
FEV₁ (liters)	1.01	1.12	2.03 (61% pred)
FEV₁/FVC	0.44	0.47	0.61
PaO₂ (mm Hg)	71	60	52
PaCO₂ (mm Hg)	40	50	51
NREM AHI	AHI 40	51	57 (AHI NREM + REM)
Lowest SaO₂	85	77	no data

AHI = apnea-hypopnea index; FEV₁ = forced expiratory volume in 1 second; FVC = forced vital capacity; NREM = non-rapid eye movement; OLS = overlap syndrome; PaCO₂ = arterial partial pressure of carbon dioxide; PaO₂ = arterial partial pressure of oxygen; REM = rapid eye movement; SaO₂ = arterial oxygen saturation.
Study #1 Chan CS, Grunstein RR, Bye PT, et al: Obstructive sleep apnea with severe chronic airflow limitation. Am Rev Respir Dis 1989;140:1274–1278.
Study #2 Bradley TD, Rutherford R, Lue F, et al: Role of diffuse airway obstruction in the hypercapnia of obstructive sleep apnea. Am Rev Respir Dis 1986;134:920–924.

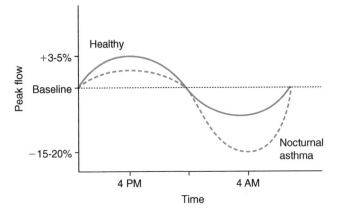

FIGURE 22–17 Both healthy individuals (*solid line*) and subjects with nocturnal asthma (*dotted line*) have circadian alterations in lung function with nadirs occurring at approximately 4 AM. The circadian variation in lung function is increased in subjects with nocturnal asthma and might exceed 20% over the course of the 24-hour period. *From Sutherland ER: Nocturnal asthma. J Allergy Clin Immunol 2005;116:1179–1186.*

BOX 22–4

Manifestations of Nocturnal Asthma
Morning drop in FEV₁ > 15% (often 15–50%) Increased circadian variation in FEV₁ Decreased response to bronchodilators during early AM Increased bronchial hyperresponsiveness to methacholine Nocturnal awakenings with symptoms of asthma
FEV₁ = forced expiratory volume in 1 second.

ASTHMA

Nocturnal asthma is usually defined as occurring in patients with a 15% or greater drop in the peak flow (or FEV₁) between bedtime and morning awakening.[53,54] Even normal persons have a circadian variation in lung function with the best function around 4 PM and the worst at 4 AM. However, the variation is much greater in patients with asthma. Asthmatic patients can experience a 20% to 50% drop in the FEV₁ from bedtime until morning ("morning dippers") (Fig. 22–17). The overnight drop in lung function is also associated with airway hyperresponsiveness, increasing airway inflammation, and a decreased response to inhaled bronchodilators.[54-57] Some of the manifestations of nocturnal asthma are listed in Box 22–4.

Important considerations for the diagnosis and treatment of nocturnal asthma are listed in Box 22–5.

Epidemiology

The largest study of the prevalence of nocturnal asthma was reported by Turner-Warwick in 1988[58] and surveyed 7729

BOX 22–5

Diagnosis and Treatment of Nocturnal Asthma

1. The degree of diurnal variation in airflow can most easily be documented by peak flow measurements at bedtime and on awakening.
2. When OSA is present in asthmatic patients, adequate treatment of OSA may improve the asthma.
3. The addition of a long-acting bronchodilator is indicated if patients with nocturnal asthma do not respond to inhaled steroids or if the required dose of inhaled steroids is higher than desired.
4. Long-acting inhaled beta agonists taken at bedtime have been shown to improve morning flow rates as well as, if not better than, theophylline and may improve perceptions of sleep quality more than theophylline in some patients.
5. If theophylline is used for nocturnal asthma, dosing should be such that the highest levels are during the night or the early morning hours.
6. Treatment of GER does not appear to improve asthma in patients who do not complain of GER symptoms. Treatment of GER is indicated in symptomatic patients (complain of GER symptoms).

GER = gastroesophageal reflux; OSA = obstructive sleep apnea.

BOX 22–6

Possible Causes of Circadian Variation in Asthma

- Increased nocturnal parasympathetic (vagal) tone
- Decreased circulating cortisol and epinephrine
- Influx of inflammatory cells into the lung
- Nocturnal gastroesophageal reflux
- Allergen exposure (bed mites, dust)
- Obstructive sleep apnea (snoring)
- Adverse effect of sleep (controlling for time of day and body position)

asthmatics. The study revealed that 74% woke up at least once each week with asthma symptoms and 65% woke up with symptoms at least 3 times/wk. In those who considered their asthma "mild," 26% woke up every night with symptoms of asthma. The majority of respiratory arrests or sudden death occurred from midnight to 8 AM.[59] **The presence and frequency of nocturnal asthma (nocturnal awakening) is one of the criteria for determining the severity of asthma.** Persistent mild, moderate, and severe asthma are characterized by nocturnal awakenings 3 to 4 times/mo, more than once weekly but not nightly, and usually 7 times/wk, respectively (Expert Panel Report 3, National Heart, Lung, and Blood Institute PR3, http://www.nhlbi.nih.gov/guidelines/asthma/asthgdln.pdf).

Etiology of Nocturnal Asthma

The etiology of this circadian variation is likely multifactorial with a number of proposed mechanisms (Box 22–6). These include circadian changes in the amounts of circulating steroids, catecholamines, and inflammatory mediators in the lungs as well as a nocturnal increase in cholinergic tone.[56,60] Studies of infusions of adrenaline[61] or administration of high-dose steroids[62] were not able to eliminate the circadian variation in bronchomotor tone. The relative role of other circadian rhythms and sleep in causing nocturnal worsening of asthma has been controversial. One study found the dip in peak flow moved to the daytime sleep period in shift workers.[63]

Sleep also appears to have an adverse effect on asthma, independent of other factors. Ballard and colleagues[20] found that sleep increased lower airway resistance by comparing supine nighttime changes between asthmatics and normal individuals who either slept in the supine position or were kept awake while supine. In asthmatics, there was a progressive increase in lower airway resistance over the night (both wake and sleep) but the increase in resistance was greater during sleep (Fig. 22–18). In another study, Ballard and associates[10] found that despite elevated lung volumes during wakefulness, the FRC of asthmatics had a larger than normal drop during sleep with the lowest levels during REM. The FRC was lower during REM compared to NREM sleep (see Fig. 22–7).

Airway Inflammation

Kraft and coworkers[64] found the biopsy of the small airway at 4 AM showed differences in the number of eosinophils per unit volume in asthmatics with nocturnal asthma compared with patients with non-nocturnal asthma. No differences in eosinophils were found in the large airways. In nocturnal asthma patients, there were more alveolar eosinophils at 4 AM than at 4 PM. A later study by the same group found that CD4+ lymphocytes (important for eosinophil recruitment) were increased in alveolar tissue at night in nocturnal asthma but not in asthmatic patients without nocturnal asthma.[65] Kelly and colleagues[66] investigated circadian changes in airway inflammation in patients with mild atopic asthma (mean FEV_1 93% of predicted). In this patient population, bronchoalveolar lavage (BAL) fluid contained increased numbers of macrophages, neutrophils, and CD4+ T lymphocytes at 4 AM versus 4 PM. In addition, the percentage of CD4+ T lymphocytes in the 4 AM lavage fluid was inversely correlated with the 4 AM FEV_1.

Melatonin

Melatonin, a hormone secreted by the pineal gland at night (in darkness), has proinflammatory effects. The addition of melatonin to zymosan stimulation of peripheral blood monocytes increased the production of interleukin-1 (IL-1), IL-6, and tumor necrosis factor-alpha (TNF-alpha) when compared with zymosan stimulation alone in normal controls and asthmatic patients.[67] The cytokine production was higher in patients with asthma than in normal subjects.

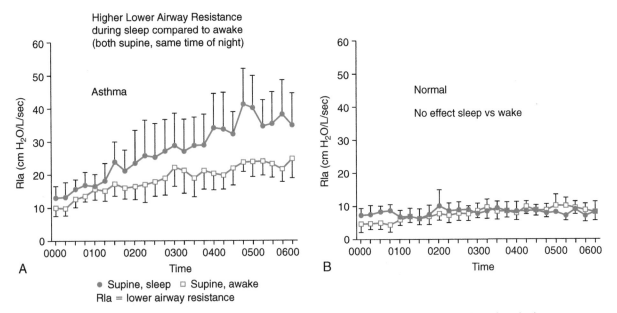

FIGURE 22–18 A, In asthmatics, lower airway resistance (Rla) increased overnight during supine wake and sleep. However, during sleep, the change was greater. **B,** In normal subjects, there was minimal change overnight and no difference between wake and sleep. **A and B,** From Ballard RD, Saathoff MC, Patel DK, et al: Effect of sleep on nocturnal bronchoconstriction and ventilatory patterns in asthmatics. J Appl Physiol 1989;67:243–249.

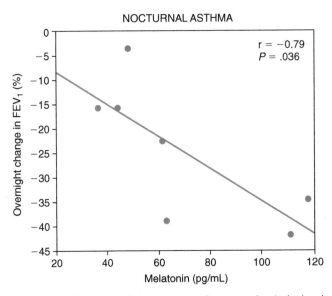

FIGURE 22–19 Inverse correlation between peak serum melatonin level and percentage overnight change in forced expiratory volume in 1 second (FEV₁) in subjects with nocturnal asthma. *From Sutherland ER, Ellison MC, Kraft M, et al: Elevated serum melatonin is associated with the nocturnal worsening of asthma. J Allergy Clin Immunol 2003;112:513–517.*

Another study found that melatonin levels are higher in patients with nocturnal asthma than in both asthmatic patients without nocturnal asthma and healthy control subjects.[68] In subjects with nocturnal asthma, there was an inverse correlation between melatonin level and overnight decrease in lung function (Fig. 22–19). The clinical importance of the effects of melatonin on asthma remains to be determined. Other studies are needed to confirm these results.

Factors Worsening Nocturnal Asthma

Allergens in the Bedroom

The importance of allergens in the bedroom is controversial. Woodcock and associates[69] were not able to find a benefit from having patients use allergen-impermeable bed covers. It still seems prudent to minimize exposure to allergens if possible.

Gastroesophageal Reflux

Several studies have supported the idea that gastroesophageal reflux (GER) may worsen asthma. Studies have shown that GER as defined by abnormal esophageal pH monitoring can occur in 62% of patients without GER symptoms.[70] Harding and coworkers[71] treated 22 patients with both asthma and GER (documented by 24-hr pH monitoring) for 3 months with doses of omperazole documented to normalize 24-hour pH monitoring. Seventy-three percent of the patients had improvement in either asthma symptoms (67%) or peak expiratory flow (20%). Cuttitta and colleagues[72] investigated the relationship of reduced esophageal pH (evidence of GER) and lower airway resistance. The most important predictor of an increase in lower airway resistance was the duration of esophageal acid contact. However, studies have not conclusively shown that treatment of GER will improve asthma. A systematic review published in 2001 concluded that treatment of GER does not improve asthma.[73] A parallel-group, randomized, double-blind study of esomperazole for treatment of poorly controlled asthma (patient did not complain of GER) found no difference in episodes of asthma exacerbations between placebo and esomperazole groups.[74] GER was found in 40% of patients using pH monitoring (asymptomatic). No subgroup of patients could be identified in which treatment of GER improved asthma. The investigators concluded the GER is unlikely to be a major factor in uncontrolled asthma. However, this group of patients **did not** have GER symptoms. Treatment of patients with asthma and GER could be considered (for GER alone) but may also help asthma in individual patients. However, there is no evidence that treatment of GER in patients with intractable asthma without symptomatic GER is of benefit.

OSA/Obesity

If OSA is present in patients with asthma, treatment with nasal CPAP can improve the asthma. Chan and associates[75] treated patients with both OSA and asthma and found that the peak expiratory flow rate improved in the morning and night after 2 weeks of treatment. In another study, weight loss in a group of obese asthmatics improved pulmonary function.[76]

Diagnosis of Nocturnal Asthma

The easiest way to diagnose severe nocturnal worsening of asthma is to have the patient record peak flow measurements at bedtime and upon awakening. Although there is not a widely accepted criteria, a fall in the peak flow of greater than 15% (evening to awakening) supports the diagnosis of nocturnal asthma.

Chronotherapy

Chronotherapy is the design of treatment to respond to circadian changes in disease. If theophylline is used, dosing so that the peak level will occur in the early morning may improve effectiveness. Martin and coworkers[77] compared twice-daily sustained-release theophylline versus once-daily sustained-release theophylline in subjects with nocturnal

asthma and demonstrated that administration of the once-daily preparation at 7 PM resulted in a higher serum theophylline concentration at night than did an equivalent dose of the twice-daily preparation given at 7 PM and 7 AM. The 7 AM FEV_1 was higher in subjects who received the once-daily preparation. The dosing of oral[78] or inhaled steroids[79] at 3 to 4 PM appears to have a greater effect on nocturnal asthma. A double-blind, placebo-controlled study evaluated the effects of a 50-mg oral dose of prednisone given at 8:00 AM, 3:00 PM, or 8:00 PM on overnight spirometry, blood eosinophil counts, and BAL cytology in seven individuals who had asthma.[79] A single prednisone dose at 3:00 PM resulted in a reduction in the overnight percentage decrease in FEV_1 and improvement in the FEV_1 measured at 4:00 AM. In contrast, neither the 8:00 AM nor the 8:00 PM prednisone dose resulted in overnight spirometric improvement. After the 3:00 PM prednisone dose, blood eosinophil counts were also significantly reduced at both 8:00 PM and 4:00 AM. These findings have not altered the usual clinical practice of administering oral steroids in the morning.

Treatment of Nocturnal Asthma

Important treatment considerations for nocturnal asthma are listed in Box 22–5, and general asthma guidelines (Step treatment) are listed in Table 22–7. Reducing the burden of allergen exposure by keeping the bedroom free of dust may help. The foundation of treatment of chronic persistent asthma is inhaled corticosteroids. Weersink and colleagues[80] studied a group with nocturnal asthma and patients were treated with inhaled fluticasone, salmeterol (a long-acting beta agonist [LABA]), or the combination. The three treatments all reduced the circadian variation in peak flow to less than 10% (Fig. 22–20), improved the bronchial

---

TABLE 22–7

Guidelines for Asthma Management

INTERMITTENT ASTHMA	PERSISTENT ASTHMA				
STEP 1	**STEP 2**	**STEP 3**	**STEP 4**	**STEP 5**	**STEP 6**
Preferred: SABA prn	**Preferred:** Low-dose ICS **Alternatives:** Cromolyn, LTRA, nedcromil, or theophylline	**Preferred:** Low-dose ICS + LABA **Or** Medium-dose ICS **Alternatives:** ICS + either LTRA, theophylline, or zileuton	**Preferred:** Medium-dose ICS + LABA **Alternatives:** Medium-dose ICS + either LTRA, theophylline, or zileuton	**Preferred:** High-dose ICS + LABA **And** Consider omalizumab for patients who have allergies	**Preferred:** High-dose ICS + LABA + oral corticosteroid **And** Consider omalizumab for patients who have allergies

ICS = inhaled corticosteroid; LABA = long-acting beta agonist; LTRA = leukotriene receptor antagonist; SABA = short-acting beta agonist.
Adapted from Expert Panel Report 3: Guidelines for the Diagnosis and Management of Asthma. National Heart, Lung, and Blood Institute—National Asthma Education and Prevention Program. Available at http://www.nhlbi.nih.gov/guidelines/asthma/asthgdln.pdf

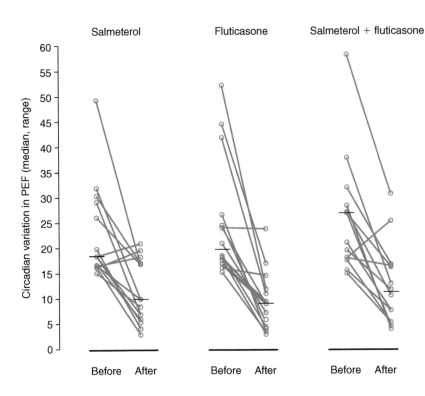

FIGURE 22–20 Effects of three treatment regimens on the variability in peak expiratory flow (PEF) over the night. All three were effective. *From Weersink EJM, Douma RR, Postma DS, et al: Fluticasone propionate, salmeterol xinafoate, and their combination in the treatment of nocturnal asthma. Am J Respir Crit Care Med 1997;155:1241–1246.*

hyperresponsiveness to methacholine both day and night, and improved cognitive performance during daytime testing. Thus, the usual practice is to start with inhaled steroids and add a long-acting inhaled beta agonist if symptoms persist (see Table 22-7).

Both inhaled long-acting beta agonists and sustained-action theophylline preparations have been effective in treatment of nocturnal asthma.[77,81–84] Selby and associates[82] found only a slight advantage for salmeterol compared with theophylline in sleep quality (fewer arousals). The falls in morning flow rates were similar but awakenings were less frequent on salmeterol. Weigand and coworkers[83] found salmeterol to be more effective than theophylline at preventing the morning drop in flow rates. The drugs did not differ in PSG findings, but patients perceived better sleep with salmeterol than with theophylline. In any case, the long-acting beta agonists require less attention to dosing than theophylline. Whereas asthmatics generally have a greater response to beta agonists than anticholinergic medications, vagal tone is increased at night. Therefore, one might expect that inhaled anticholinergics might be helpful. There is evidence that the addition of an inhaled anticholinergic to standard treatment may be helpful in some patients with moderate to severe asthma.[84] A recent study[85] documented the effectiveness of the addition of tiotropium (long-acting anticholinergic) to patients still not well controlled with an inhaled steroid. This approach may provide an alternative to long-acting beta agonists or an additional treatment if the combination of inhaled steroids and a long-acting beta agonist is unable to control nocturnal symptoms.

Although theophylline could have stimulatory effects and impair sleep, this possible side effect is probably outweighed by benefit from bronchodilator effects in some patients. As noted previously, if theophylline is used, the dosing should be altered so levels are relatively high at night. Because of the need to follow theophylline levels and adjust the dose to both obtain optimal treatment and avoid serious toxicity, long-acting beta agonists are favored by most clinicians. If there are symptoms of nocturnal GER, treatment with a proton pump inhibitor may improve asthma in some patients. The evening proton pump inhibitor should be given before the evening meal rather than at bedtime. If sleep apnea is present, treatment with CPAP may improve asthma in some patients.[75]

CLINICAL REVIEW QUESTIONS

1. A 50-year-old man with moderate COPD has a room air blood gas showing a PaO$_2$ of 60 mm Hg. He undergoes nocturnal oximetry that reveals 200 minutes with an SaO$_2$ less than 88%. There are long periods in which the average SaO$_2$ is around 85%. A saw-tooth pattern is seen in about half of the tracing. The patient reports snoring but no daytime sleepiness. What do you recommend?

A. Treatment with supplemental oxygen at 2 L/min.

B. Treatment with supplemental oxygen at 2 L/min and repeat the oximetry.

C. PSG.

D. Addition of an inhaled long-acting beta agonist and repeat the oximetry.

2. Which of the following is (are) mechanisms of nonapneic (hypopneic) NOD during REM sleep?

A. Low baseline SaO$_2$.

B. Intercostal muscle hypotonia.

C. Hypoventilation.

D. $\dot{V}/\dot{Q}$ mismatch.

E. All of the above.

3. Which of the following is thought to play a role in the morning fall in the FEV_1 in asthma patients?

A. High cortisol levels at night.

B. High circulating catecholamines.

C. Increased inflammatory cells in the lung.

D. Low parasympathetic tone.

4. Which of the following are predictive of significant arterial oxygen desaturation during sleep in a patient with COPD?

A. Daytime $PaCO_2$ = 55 mm Hg.

B. Pink puffer COPD type.

C. Blue bloater clinical type.

D. Daytime PaO_2 = 70 mm Hg.

E. A and C.

F. B and D.

5. In spirometry, which of the following is used to assess the severity of COPD (GOLD criteria)?

A. FEV_1 (% predicted).

B. FVC (% predicted).

C. FEV_1/FVC (% predicted).

D. Postbronchodilator FEV_1 (% predicted).

E. Postbronchodilator FVC (% predicted).

6. A 30-year-old patient with known intermittent asthma has begun to develop awakenings with dyspnea and cough twice weekly. The evening peak flow is 450 L/min and that on awakening in the morning is 350 L/min. The patient has been using a short-acting beta agonist intermittently. What do you recommend?

A. Short-acting beta agonist at bedtime.

B. Long-acting beta agonist at bedtime.

C. Inhaled corticosteroids.

D. Inhaled corticosteroids and long-acting beta agonist at bedtime.

Answers

1. **C.** Although the patient may well require supplemental oxygen as a component of therapy, the presence or absence of OSA must be determined. The saw-tooth pattern suggests sleep apnea is present and that the patient has OLS. Optimal therapy includes treatment of both OSA and COPD.

2. **E.**

3. **C.** Increased inflammatory cells appear to enter the airways and lung. Cortisol and circulating catecholamine levels are lower during the night and parasympathetic tone is higher during sleep.

4. **E.** Worse nocturnal SaO_2 is predicted by a lower daytime SaO_2/PaO_2, hypercapnia, and the blue bloater clinical type.

5. **D.**

6. **C.** The patient has nocturnal asthma evidenced by a 22% fall in the peak flow as well as symptoms. The treatment of choice is inhaled corticosteroids. If this is not effective, the addition of a long-acting beta agonist is the next step. However, the patient may improve with inhaled corticosteroids alone.

REFERENCES

1. Lung function testing: selection of reference values and interpretative strategies. Am Rev Respir Dis 1991;144:1202–1218.
2. Crapo RO: Pulmonary function testing. N Engl J Med 1994;331:25.
3. Pellegrino R, Viegi G, Brusasco V, et al: Interpretative strategies for lung function tests. Eur Respir J 2005;26:948–968.
4. Rabe KF, Hurd S, Anzueto A, et al: Global Initiative for Chronic Obstructive Lung Disease. Global strategy for the diagnosis, management, and prevention of chronic obstructive pulmonary disease: GOLD executive summary. Am J Respir Crit Care Med 2007;176:532–555.
5. Mohsenin V: Sleep in chronic obstructive pulmonary disease. Semin Respir Crit Care Med 2005;26:109–115.
6. Collop N: Sleep and sleep disorders in chronic obstructive pulmonary disease. Respiration 2010;80:78–86.
7. Douglas NJ, Flenley DC: Breathing during sleep in patients with obstructive lung disease. Am Rev Respir Dis 1990; 141:1055–1070.
8. Hudgel DW, Devodatta P: Decrease in functional residual capacity during sleep in normal humans. J Appl Physiol 1984;57:1319–1325.
9. Tabachnik E, Muller NL, Bryan C, et al: Changes in ventilation and chest wall mechanics during sleep in normal adolescents. J Appl Physiol 1981;51:557–564.
10. Ballard RD, Irvin CG, Martin RJ, et al: Influence of sleep on lung volume in asthmatic patients and normal subjects. J Appl Physiol 1990;68:2034–2041.
11. Koo KW, Sax DS, Snider GL: Arterial blood gases and pH during sleep in chronic obstructive pulmonary disease. Am J Med 1975;58:663–670.
12. Fletcher EC, Miller J, Divine GW, et al: Nocturnal oxyhemoglobin desaturation in COPD patients with arterial oxygen tensions above 60 mm Hg. Chest 1987;92:604–608.
13. Becker HF, Piper AJ, Flynn WE, et al: Breathing during sleep in patients with nocturnal desaturation. Am J Respir Crit Care Med 1999;159:112–118.
14. Hudgel DW, Martin RJ, Capehart M, et al: Contribution of hypoventilation to sleep oxygen desaturation in chronic obstructive pulmonary disease. J Appl Physiol 1983;55:669–677.
15. Fletcher EC, Gray BA, Levin DC: Nonapneic mechanisms of arterial oxygen desaturation during rapid-eye-movement sleep. J Appl Physiol 1983;54:632–639.
16. Catterall JR, Calverley PMA, MacNee W, et al: Mechanism of transient nocturnal hypoxemia in hypoxic chronic bronchitis and emphysema. J Appl Physiol 1985;59:1698–1703.
17. Catterall JR, Douglas NJ, Calverley PM, et al: Transient hypoxemia during sleep in chronic obstructive pulmonary disease is not a sleep apnea syndrome. Am Rev Respir Dis 1983; 128:24–29.
18. Ballard RD, Clover CW, Suh BY: Influence of sleep on respiratory function in emphysema. Am J Respir Crit Care Med 1995;151:945–951.

19. Gould GA, Gugger M, Molloy J, et al: Breathing pattern and eye movement density during REM sleep in humans. Am Rev Respir Dis 1988;138:874–877.
20. Ballard RD, Saathoff MC, Patel DK, et al: Effect of sleep on nocturnal bronchoconstriction and ventilatory patterns in asthmatics. J Appl Physiol 1989;67:243–249.
21. DeMarco FJ Jr, Wynne JW, Block AJ, et al: Oxygen desaturation during sleep as a determinant of the "blue and bloated" syndrome. Chest 1981;79:621–625.
22. Sanders MH, Newman AB, Haggerty CL, et al: Sleep and sleep-disordered breathing in adults with predominantly mild obstructive airway disease. Am J Respir Crit Care Med 2003;167:7–14.
23. Connaughton JJ, Catterall JR, Elton RA, et al: Do sleep studies contribute to the management of patients with severe chronic obstructive pulmonary disease? Am Rev Respir Dis 1988;138:341–344.
24. Lewis CA, Fergusson W, Eaton T, et al: Isolated nocturnal desaturation in COPD: prevalence and impact on quality of life and sleep. Thorax 2009;64:133–138.
25. Nocturnal Oxygen Therapy Trial Group: Continuous or nocturnal oxygen therapy in hypoxemic chronic obstructive lung disease. Ann Intern Med 1980;93:391–398.
26. Medical Research Council Working Party: Long-term domiciliary oxygen therapy in chronic hypoxic cor pulmonale complicating chronic bronchitis and emphysema: report of the Medical Research Council Working Party. Lancet 1981;1:681–686.
27. Kim V, Benditt JO, Wise RA, Sharafkhaneh A: Oxygen therapy in chronic obstructive pulmonary disease [review]. Proc Am Thorac Soc 2008;5:513–518.
28. Plywaczewski R, Sliwinski P, Nowinski A, et al: Incidence of nocturnal desaturation while breathing oxygen in COPD patients undergoing long-term oxygen therapy. Chest 2000;117:679–683.
29. Calverley PM, Brezinova V, Douglas NJ, et al: The effect of oxygenation on sleep quality in chronic bronchitis and emphysema. Am Rev Respir Dis 1982;126:206–210.
30. Fleetham J, West P, Mezon B, et al: Sleep, arousals, and oxygen desaturation in chronic obstructive pulmonary disease: the effect of oxygen therapy. Am Rev Respir Dis 1982;126:429–433.
31. Fletcher EC, Luckett RA, Goodnight-White S, et al: A double-blind trial of nocturnal supplemental oxygen for sleep desaturation in patients with chronic obstructive pulmonary disease and a daytime PO_2 above 60 mm Hg. Am Rev Respir Dis 1992;145:1070–1076.
32. Chaouat A, Weitzenblum E, Kessler R, et al: A randomized trial of oxygen therapy in chronic obstructive pulmonary disease. Eur Respir J 1999;14:1002–1008.
33. Goldstein RS, Ramcharan V, Bowes G, et al: Effect of supplemental nocturnal oxygen on gas exchange in patients with severe obstructive lung disease. N Engl J Med 1984;310:425–429.
34. Samolski D, Tárrega J, Antón A, et al: Sleep hypoventilation due to increased nocturnal oxygen flow in hypercapnic COPD patients. Respirology 2010;15:283–288.
35. Berry RB, Desa MM, Branum JP, et al: Effect of theophylline on sleep and sleep-disordered breathing in patients with chronic obstructive pulmonary disease. Am Rev Respir Dis 1991;143:245–250.
36. Martin RJ, Bartelson BL, Smith P, et al: Effect of ipratropium bromide treatment on oxygen saturation and sleep quality in COPD. Chest 1999;115:1338–1345.
37. McNicholas WT, Calverly PMA, Edward JC: Long-acting inhaled anticholinergic therapy improves sleeping oxygen saturation in COPD. Eur Respir J 2004;23:825–831.
38. Ryan S, Doherty LS, Rock C, et al: Effects of salmeterol on sleeping oxygen saturation in chronic obstructive pulmonary disease. Respiration 2010;79:475–481.
39. Donohue JF, Kalberg C, Emmett A, et al: A short-term comparison of fluticasone propionate/salmeterol with ipratropium bromide/albuterol for the treatment of COPD. Treat Respir Med 2004;3:173–181.
40. Sin DD, Man SFP: Steroids in COPD: still up in the air? Eur Respir J 2010;35:949–951.
41. Roth T: Hypnotic use for insomnia management in chronic obstructive pulmonary disease. Sleep Med 2009;10:19–25.
42. Girault C, Muir JF, Mihaltan F, et al: Effects of repeated administration of zolpidem on sleep, diurnal and nocturnal respiratory function, vigilance, and physical performance in patients with COPD. Chest 1996;110:1203–1211.
43. Stege G, Heijdra YF, van den Elshout FJ, et al: Temazepam 10 mg does not affect breathing and gas exchange in patients with severe normocapnic COPD. Respir Med 2010;104:518–524.
44. Steens RD, Pouliot Z, Millar TW, et al: Effects of zolpidem and triazolam on sleep and respiration in mild to moderate chronic obstructive pulmonary disease. Sleep 1993;16:318–326.
45. Kryger M, Roth T, Wang-Weigand S, et al: The effects of ramelteon on respiration during sleep in subjects with moderate to severe chronic obstructive pulmonary disease. Sleep Breath 2009;13:79–84.
46. Clinical indications for noninvasive positive pressure ventilation in chronic respiratory failure due to restrictive lung disease, COPD, and nocturnal hypoventilation—a consensus conference report. Chest 1999;116:521–534.
47. Weitzenblum E, Chaouat A, Kessler R, Canuet M: Overlap syndrome. Obstructive sleep apnea syndrome in patients with chronic obstructive pulmonary disease. Proc Thorac Soc 2008;5:237–241.
48. Kessler R, Chaouat A, Schinkewitch PH, et al:. The obesity-hypoventilation syndrome revisited: a prospective study of 34 consecutive cases. Chest 2001;120:369–376.
49. Bradley TD, Rutherford R, Lue F, et al: Role of diffuse airway obstruction in the hypercapnia of obstructive sleep apnea. Am Rev Respir Dis 1986;134:920–924.
50. Fletcher EC, Schaaf JW, Miller J, Fletcher JG: Long-term cardiopulmonary sequelae in patients with sleep apnea and chronic lung disease. Am Rev Respir Dis 1987;135:525–533.
51. Machado MCL, Vollmer WM, Togeiro SM, et al: CPAP and survival in moderate to severe obstructive sleep apnea syndrome and hypoxemic COPD. Eur Respir J 2010;35:132–137.
52. Marin JM, Soriano JB, Carrizo SJ, et al: Outcomes in patients with chronic obstructive pulmonary disease and obstructive sleep apnea. Am J Respir Crit Care Med 2010;182:325–331.
53. Martin RJ: Nocturnal asthma: circadian rhythms and therapeutic interventions. Am Rev Respir Dis 1993;147:525–528.
54. Atanasov ST, Calhoun WJ: The relationship between sleep and asthma. Sleep Med Clin 2007;2:9–18.
55. Sutherland ER: Nocturnal asthma. J Allergy Clin Immunol 2005;116:1179–1186.
56. Martin RJ, Cicutto LC, Ballard RD: Factors related to the nocturnal worsening of asthma. Am Rev Respir Dis 1990;141:33–38.
57. Hendeles L, Beaty R, Ahrens R, et al: Response to inhaled albuterol during nocturnal asthma. J Allergy Clin Immunol 2004;113:1058–1062.
58. Turner-Warwick M: Epidemiology of nocturnal asthma. Am J Med 1988;85:6–8.
59. Cochrane GM, Clark JH: A survey of asthma mortality in patients between ages 35 and 64 in the Greater London hospitals in 1971. Thorax 1975;30:300–305.
60. Martin RJ, Banks-Schlegel S: Chronobiology of asthma. Am J Respir Crit Care Med 1998;158:1002–1007.
61. Morrison JF, Teale C, Pearson SB, et al: Adrenaline and nocturnal asthma. BMJ 1990;301:473–476.

62. Clark TJ, Hetzel MR: Diurnal variation of asthma. Br J Dis Chest 1977;71:87–92.
63. Hetzel MR, Clark TJ: Does sleep cause nocturnal asthma? Thorax 1979;34:749–754.
64. Kraft M, Djukanovic R, Wilson S, et al: Alveolar tissue inflammation in asthma. Am J Respir Crit Care Med 1996;154:1505–1510.
65. Kraft M, Martin RJ, Wilson S, et al: Lymphocyte and eosinophil influx into alveolar tissue in nocturnal asthma. Am J Respir Crit Care Med 1999;159:228–234.
66. Kelly EA, Houtman JJ, Jarjour NN: Inflammatory changes associated with circadian variation in pulmonary function in subjects with mild asthma. Clin Exp Allergy 2004;34:227–233.
67. Sutherland ER, Martin RJ, Ellison MC, et al: Immunomodulatory effects of melatonin in asthma. Am J Respir Crit Care Med 2002;166:1055–1061.
68. Sutherland ER, Ellison MC, Kraft M, et al: Elevated serum melatonin is associated with the nocturnal worsening of asthma. J Allergy Clin Immunol 2003;112:513–517.
69. Woodcock A, Forster L, Matthews E, et al: Control of exposure to mite allergen and allergen impermeable bed covers for adults with asthma. N Engl J Med 2003;349:225–257.
70. Harding SM, Guzzo MR, Richter JE: The prevalence of gastroesophageal reflux in asthma patients with reflux symptoms. Am J Respir Crit Care Med 2000;162:34–39.
71. Harding SM, Richter JE, Guzzo MR, et al: Asthma and gastroesophageal reflux: acid suppressive therapy improves asthma outcomes. Am J Med 1996;100:395–405.
72. Cuttitta G, Cibella F, Visconti A, et al: Spontaneous gastroesophageal reflux and airway patency during the night in adult asthmatics. Am J Respir Crit Care Med 2000;161:177–181.
73. Coughlan JL, Gibson PG, Henry RL: Medical treatment for reflux oesophagitis does not consistently improve asthma control: a systematic review. Thorax 2001;56:198–204.
74. ALA Asthma Clinical Research Centers: Efficacy of esomeprazole for treatment of poorly controlled asthma. N Engl J Med 2009;360:1487–1499.
75. Chan CS, Woolcock AJ, Sullivan CE: Nocturnal asthma: role of snoring and obstructive sleep apnea. Am Rev Respir Dis 1988;137:1502–1504.
76. Hakala K, Stenius-Aarniala B, Sovijarvi A: Effects of weight loss on peak flow variability, airways obstruction, and lung volumes in obese patients with asthma. Chest 2000;118:1315–1321.
77. Martin RJ, Cicutto LC, Ballard RD, et al: Circadian variations in theophylline concentrations and the treatment of nocturnal asthma. Am Rev Respir Dis 1989;139:475–478.
78. Pincus DJ, Humeston TR, Martin RJ: Further studies on the chronotherapy of asthma with inhaled steroids: the effect of dosage timing on drug efficacy. J Allergy Clin Immunol 1997;100:771–777.
79. Beam WR, Weiner DE, Martin RJ: Timing of prednisone and alterations of airways inflammation in nocturnal asthma. Am Rev Respir Dis 1992;146:1524–1530.
80. Weersink EJM, Douma RR, Postma DS, et al: Fluticasone propionate, salmeterol xinafoate, and their combination in the treatment of nocturnal asthma. Am J Respir Crit Care Med 1997;155:1241–1246.
81. Kraft M, Wenzel SE, Bettinger CM, et al: The effect of salmeterol on nocturnal symptoms, airway function, and inflammation in asthma. Chest 1997;111:1249–1254.
82. Selby C, Engleman HM, Fitzpatrick MF, et al: Inhaled salmeterol or oral theophylline in nocturnal asthma? Am J Respir Crit Care Med 1997;155:104–108.
83. Weigand L, Mende CN, Zaidel G, et al: Salmeterol vs theophylline. Sleep and efficacy outcomes in patients with nocturnal asthma. Chest 1999;115:1525–1532.
84. Gelb AF, Karpel J, Wise RA, et al: Bronchodilator efficacy of the fixed combination of ipratropium and albuterol compared to albuterol alone in moderate-to-severe persistent asthma. Pulm Pharmacol Ther 2008;21:630–636.
85. Peters SP, Kunselman SJ, Icitovic N, et al, National Heart, Lung, and Blood Institute Asthma Clinical Research Network: Tiotropium bromide step-up therapy for adults with uncontrolled asthma. N Engl J Med 2010;363:1715–1726.

Chapter 23

The Restless Leg Syndrome, Periodic Limb Movements in Sleep, and the Periodic Limb Movement Disorder

Chapter Points

- A diagnosis of the RLS is based on **clinical history.** The essential elements include **URGE** (**U**rge to move, **R**est makes symptoms worse, **G**ets better with movement—temporary improvement in symptoms with movement, and **E**vening is worse [symptoms worse in the evening, at least at the onset of the syndrome]).
- Supportive clinical features for the diagnosis of RLS include a family history, improvement with dopaminergic treatment, and the presence of PLMS on PSG.
- **Secondary causes of RLS** included renal failure, pregnancy, iron deficiency, and medications. Medications frequently worsening RLS include first-generation antihistamines, antidepressants (except bupropion), and dopamine blockers (phenothiazines, metochlopramide).
- A diagnosis of PLMD is based on both history and PSG findings: (1) A complaint of sleep disturbance or daytime fatigue, (2) PSG findings PLMSI > 5/hr (children) and > 15/hr in adults, (3) Symptoms are not better explained by another sleep, medical, or neurologic disorder, or medication use (e.g., OSA). **A diagnosis of RLS excludes a diagnosis of PLMD.** A complaint of sleep disturbance must be made by the patient (in contrast to the bedmate).
- **PLMS is a PSG finding.** PLMS is very common in older adults and is most often asymptomatic. PLMS can be associated with OSA, narcolepsy, and RBD.
- About 80% of patients with RLS will have a PLMS index ≥ 5/hr on PSG.
- The PLMD may precede a diagnosis of RLS in children. A diagnosis of RLS is difficult in children because they

may not report traditional symptoms. They may present with "growing pains."
- Treatment options for RLS include conservative measures, dopaminergic medications (LD/CD and DAs), anticonvulsants, opiates and opioid agonists, and sedative hypnotics.
- LD/CD is a rapidly absorbed dopaminergic medication (LD is a precursor of dopamine) that is effective treatment of RLS. It is a good option for intermittent RLS. However, the medication has a short duration of action and continued use results in augmentation in up to 80% of cases (especially with doses of LD > 200 mg daily).
- The **DAs ropinirole and pramipexole** are FDA approved for treatment of RLS in adults and are considered the **treatment of choice for daily RLS.** They must be given 2 hours before symptoms to be most effective.
- Anticonvulsants are also effective for RLS/PLMD. Due to a good safety profile, gabapentin is the anticonvulsant recommended for RLS treatment. Doses of 900 to 1500 mg of gabapentin may be needed to be effective. A slow upward titration of the dose starting at 300 mg may improve tolerance to use. Gabapentin is considered a first-line medication by some clinicians if RLS is associated with pain.
- Narcotics are effective treatment for RLS. They may be especially useful in patients who develop augmentation or do not tolerate DAs. If given only at bedtime, they usually do not result in dependence. For milder cases, codeine, propoxyphene, or tramadol may be effective. For moderate RLS, hydrocodone (combined with acetaminophen in the United States)

or oxycodone is often used. For severe RLS, oxycodone or methadone has been used with success.

- Sedative hypnotics may be useful in milder RLS associated with insomnia or can be combined with other classes of medications. Most of the published treatment trials used clonazepam (long half-life), but other BZRAs may also be effective.
- **Augmentation** describes a phenomenon that is characterized by one or more of the following: (1) earlier symptom onset, (2) greater severity of symptoms at the same dose/or escalating dose, (3) reduced latency to onset of symptoms with rest, and (4) spread of symptoms to involve new body parts (arms as well as legs).
- **Low serum ferritin** (<45 to 50 μg/mL) is a risk factor for development of augmentation.
- RLS patients with a ferritin less than 45 to 50 μg/mL may improve with iron supplementation. The usual dose is ferrous sulfate 325 mg tid with each dose given with 100 to 200 mg of ascorbic acid to improve absorption. Patients with augmentation may improve with iron supplementation.

The restless legs syndrome (RLS), periodic limb movements in sleep (PLMS), and the periodic limb movement disorder (PLMD) are three distinct but related entities[1-6] (Table 23–1). A diagnosis of RLS is based on clinical history. PLMS is a polysomnography (PSG) finding that may or may not be clinically important. The PLMD is diagnosed in patients with PLMS on PSG who have a sleep complaint (sleep-onset or maintenance insomnia or, less commonly, daytime sleepiness) not better explained by another sleep disorder.[6] PLMS is a very common finding especially in older patients (Fig. 23–1) and is often asymptomatic.[5,7-11] Approximately 80 to 90% of patients with RLS will have findings of PLMS on

PSG.[12] The percentage of patients with PLMS who have RLS has not been well-defined, but the vast majority of patients with PLMS do not have RLS. PLMS has been associated with narcolepsy, the REM sleep behavior disorder, and obstructive sleep apnea (OSA). A diagnosis of RLS excludes PLMD. PLMS is very common, RLS is common, and PLMD is thought to be rare. Chapter 12 outlines the scoring criteria for PLMS in detail with examples of illustrative tracings. This chapter emphasizes the clinical significance of PLMS.

RESTLESS LEGS SYNDROME

The RLS is a common disorder often underdiagnosed and improperly treated. In 1995, the International Restless Legs Syndrome Study Group (IRLSSG)[11] published a statement on

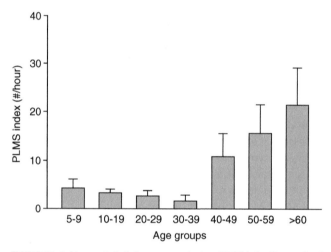

FIGURE 23–1 Mean periodic limb movements in sleep (PLMS) index (# events/hr of sleep) at different ages for normal healthy individuals. The average PLMS index increases in older individuals. Error bars are SEM. *From Pennestri M, Whittom S, Adam B, et al: PLMS and PLMW in healthy subjects as a function of age: prevalence and interval distribution. Sleep 2006;29:1183–1187.*

TABLE 23–1			
Different Leg Movement Conditions			
	RLS	**PLMS**	**PLMD**
Diagnosis	History	PSG	PSG + History
Prevalence	Common	Very common • Asymptomatic individuals • Narcolepsy • REM sleep behavior disorder • OSA	Rare
Associated findings	• ~80% have PLMS	• Usually asymptomatic or symptoms are not due to PLMS • A minority of patients have RLS	• Must exclude other causes of insomnia or daytime sleepiness
Relationship with other leg movement conditions	A diagnosis of RLS excludes a diagnosis of PLMD	A PSG finding not a disorder	Not diagnosed if RLS is present
OSA = obstructive sleep disorder; PLMD = periodic limb movement disorder; PLMS = periodic limb movement in sleep; PSG = polysomnography; REM = rapid eye movement; RLS = restless leg syndrome.			

BOX 23–1

Diagnostic Criteria for Restless Legs Syndrome

A. The patient reports **an urge to move the legs,** usually accompanied or caused by uncomfortable and unpleasant sensations in the legs.

B. The urge to move or unpleasant sensations **begin or worsen during periods of rest** or inactivity such as lying or sitting.

C. The urge to move or unpleasant sensations are partially or totally relieved by movement, such as walking or stretching, as long as the activity continues.

D. The urge to move or sensations are worse, or only occur, in the evening or night.

E. The condition is not better explained by another current sleep disorder, medical or neurologic disorder, medication use, or substance use disorder.

From American Academy of Sleep Medicine: ICSD-2 International Classification of Sleep Disorders, 2nd ed. Diagnostic and Coding Manual. Westchester, IL: American Academy of Sleep Medicine, 2005.

BOX 23–2

Abnormal Sensations in Restless Legs Syndrome

COMMON PATIENT DESCRIPTIONS OF SENSATIONS

- Creepy, crawly.
- Ants crawling under the skin.
- Worms crawling in the veins.
- Pepsi-Cola in the veins.
- Nervous feet "gotta move."
- Itching under the skin, itchy bones.
- Crazy legs/Elvis legs.
- Toothache feeling—can't leave it alone.
- Excited nerves, electric-like shocks.

CHARACTERISTICS OF SENSATIONS

- Daytime symptoms if RLS is severe.
- If RLS very severe, symptoms may not be worse at night.
- Usually bilateral but can be unilateral.
- Arms may be involved in 30–50%.
- Sensations are painful in 20%.
- May be absent—simply urge to move.

RLS = restless legs syndrome.

the primary and associated features of the syndrome. The criteria were refined during a workshop at the National Institutes of Health (NIH).[13] The criteria form the basis for the International Classification of Sleep Disorders, 2nd edition (ICSD-2) diagnostic criteria for RLS[6] (Box 23–1). There are four essential diagnostic criteria for RLS (**URGE = urge to move, rest induced, gets better with activity, evening and night worse**).

The Essential RLS Diagnostic Criteria[6,13]

1. The patient reports *an urge to move the legs*, usually accompanied or caused by uncomfortable and unpleasant sensations in the legs. Of note, the urge to move can be present without associated symptoms. Commonly reported RLS sensations are listed in Box 23–2. Although called the "restless legs syndrome," symptoms can occur in the arms as well as the legs in 30% to 50% of the patients.[12,13] Although RLS symptoms are usually bilateral, some patients report symptoms mainly in one extremity.[12] About 20% of RLS patients report the leg sensations to be painful. Involuntary leg movements may also be reported without an urge to move ("the legs just move on their own"). As discussed later, this is a manifestation of periodic limb movements during wake (PLMW).

2. RLS symptoms begin or worsen during periods of inactivity such as lying or sitting. Being stationary and having decreased mental activity appear to both worsen symptoms.

3. The urge to move or unpleasant sensations are totally or partially relieved by movements such as walking or stretching as long as the activity continues (temporary relief). Rubbing the legs or taking hot or cold baths may improve symptoms in some patients. Of note, increased

mental activity or eating can improve the symptoms ("popcorn therapy" while watching a movie).

4. The urge to move or unpleasant sensations are worse in the evening or night. **If RLS has become very severe, nocturnal worsening may not be reported but should have been present earlier in the disease course.** When RLS is severe, daytime symptoms can occur especially during periods of inactivity.

Supportive Clinical Features

Some patients will report atypical symptoms.[13] The supportive clinical features of RLS (Box 23–3) may help resolve diagnostic uncertainty. They are not required for a diagnosis of RLS. In studies of groups of patients with RLS, a familial history is reported in 50% to 60% of the cases. A family history of RLS is supportive of the diagnosis. An improvement with a trial of dopaminergic treatment is also evidence that symptoms represent the RLS. However, one must be aware of the placebo effect. Placebo-controlled studies in RLS report considerable improvement in symptoms with inactive medication. The periodic limb movements in sleep index (PLMSI) is defined as the number of periodic limb movements (PLMs) per hour of sleep. The criteria for scoring a leg movement as a periodic leg movement are discussed in Chapter 12. It is difficult to define a normal PLMSI (see Fig. 23–1). In the past, some sleep centers considered a PLMSI of 5/hr or greater to be abnormal. However, many asymptomatic individuals have much higher PLMSI values,[7-9] The presence of PLMS can provide supporting evidence for the presence of the RLS. One study employing a PLMSI cutoff of 5/hr reported that 80.2% of patients with RLS had PLMS (87% if 2 nights were monitored).[12] Patients with RLS often

BOX 23–3

Supportive Clinical Features of Restless Legs Syndrome

FAMILY HISTORY

- The prevalence of RLS among first-degree relatives of patients with RLS is 3 to 5 times greater than in people without RLS.
- 50–60% of patients with RLS report a family member with RLS.

RESPONSE TO DOPAMINERGIC THERAPY

- Nearly all patients with RLS show at least an initial positive therapeutic response to either L-dopa or a dopamine receptor agonist at doses considered low compared with those used to treat Parkinson's disease.

PERIODIC LIMB MOVEMENTS (DURING WAKEFULNESS OR SLEEP)

- Involuntary movements during wake or sleep.
- PLMS occur in at least 80% of patients with RLS—however, PLMS commonly occur in other disorders and in the elderly.
- PLMW is a manifestation of RLS.

PLMS = periodic leg movements in sleep; PLMW = periodic leg movements during wake; RLS = restless legs syndrome.
Adapted from Allen RP, Picchietti D, Hening W, et al. Restless legs syndrome: diagnostic criteria, special considerations, and epidemiology. A report from the Restless Legs Syndrome Diagnosis and Epidemiology Workshop at the National Institutes of Health. Sleep Med 2003;4:101–119.

report repetitive involuntary leg movements during wakefulness when at rest especially at night. This is a manifestation of PLMW (periodic limb movements during wake).

Differential Diagnosis of RLS/PLMS

The differential diagnosis of RLS/PLMS includes a number of mimics[13–16] (Table 23–2 and Box 23–4). Most of these are not associated with an urge to move. Often, the movements are not worse at night and symptoms are not temporarily improved by movement.

Hypnic jerks are usually single, whole body jerks that occur at sleep onset. They are not associated with abnormal sensations.

Neuropathy may present as pain and/or burning in the legs or feet but is usually associated with an abnormal neurologic examination and is not associated with an urge to move. Neuropathic pain is usually not improved with movement or rubbing. The pain may be worse at night but is usually present during the day. **RLS and neuropathy can exist together.**

Positional discomfort is associated with a need to move in bed to relieve pressure that compresses nerves, limits blood flow, or stretches tissue. The sensations may be painful but are improved with change in position rather than with movement.

Neuroleptic akathisia is characterized by involuntary movement of the face or extremities (such as body rocking,

TABLE 23–2

Characteristics of Restless Legs Syndrome Mimics

	URGE TO MOVE	ABNORMAL SENSATIONS	WORSE IN THE EVENING/NIGHT	IMPROVED BY MOVEMENT	NEUROLOGIC STUDIES	NEUROLEPTIC USE
RLS	Yes	Usually	Always	Temporary improvement	Neurologic examination usually normal, EMG often normal	No
Hypnic jerk	No	No	Sleep onset	Single whole body jerk	Normal	No
Neuropathy	No	Yes, can be painful	Sometimes	No	Decreased sensation, abnormal EMG/nerve conduction	No
Positional discomfort	Yes	Usually	Usually	Change in position not movement	Variable	No
Neuroleptic akathisia	Inner restlessness	No	Not usually	Not usually	Variable	**YES**
Leg cramps	No	**Pain localized to muscle**	Sometimes	Stretching not movement	Normal	No
Claudication	No	Pain	Not usually	Walking may worsen	Decreased pulses	No
Painful legs, moving toes syndrome	No	**Pain, burning**	Not usually	No	Abnormal EMG, MRI may show lumbosacral nerve compression	No

EMG = electromyogram; MRI = magnetic resonance imaging; RLS = restless legs syndrome.

BOX 23–4

Differential Diagnosis of Restless Legs Syndrome and Periodic Limb Movements in Sleep
Hypnic jerks—whole body jerks at sleep onset, involuntary, no urge to move.
Positional discomfort—need to move in bed to relieve pressure that compresses nerves, limits blood flow, or stretches tissue.
Sleep-related leg cramps—muscle hardening and pain of specific muscle groups, tenderness and sensitivity remain after cramping subsides, stretching more than movement provides relief.
Neuroleptic akathisia—generalized nature of need to move the body and the occurrence in association with use of dopamine receptor antagonists (phenothiazines, metaclopramide).
Painful legs–moving toes syndrome—pain in the lower limbs with spontaneous movements of the toes or feet. The pain is most often burning and the movements consist of flexion/extension, abduction/adduction, fanning, or clawing of the toes, fingers, foot, or hand. Painless variants exist. Causes include nerve root lesions, herpes zoster, HIV, neuroleptics, chemotherapeutic agents, peripheral trauma, and polyneuropathy for alcoholism.
HIV = human immunodeficiency virus.

BOX 23–5

Causes of Restless Legs Syndrome		
PRIMARY RLS		
• Familial		
• Idiopathic		
• Characteristics		
• Earlier age of onset and slower progression		
• Familial occurrence more likely		
SECONDARY RLS		
• Iron deficiency		
• Low normal ferritin level (<45–50 µg/L) is related to increasing severity of RLS even if hemoglobin is normal		
• Pregnancy		
• Neuropathy—diabetic and others		
• Multiple sclerosis		
• Renal failure (transplant but NOT dialysis cures RLS)		
• Parkinson's disease		
• Medications		
• First-generation (sedating) antihistamines (diphenhydramine)		
• Antinausea medication—prochlorperazine		
• Dopamine receptor blockers—metoclopramide		
• Antidepressants (SSRIs, SNRIs)—exception is bupropion		
RLS = restless legs syndrome; SNRIs = selective serotonin and norepinephrine reuptake inhibitors; SSRIs = selective serotonin reuptake inhibitors.		

marching in place, or movement of the extremities) and is NOT worse during the night or at rest. There is invariably a **history of use of neuroleptics** (phenothiazines) and other dopamine blockers (metoclopramide). The movements are associated with inner restlessness but not abnormal sensations.

The **painful legs–moving toes (PLMT) syndrome**[13,16] is characterized by pain in the lower limbs with spontaneous movements of the toes or feet. Variants of PLMT that are painless or involve the arms and hands also exist. The pain is most often burning in nature and commonly precedes spontaneous movements consisting of flexion/extension, abduction/adduction, fanning, or clawing of the toes, fingers, foot, or hand. Causes of PLMT include nerve root lesions, herpes zoster, human immunodeficiency virus (HIV), neuroleptics, chemotherapeutic agents, peripheral trauma, and polyneuropathy from alcoholism.

Nocturnal leg cramps are associated with localized severe pain and tightness in a muscle. These are improved with stretching but not just movement.

Claudication may be associated with pain even at rest, if severe, but is usually NOT improved with movement. Usually, claudication symptoms are worse with exertion.

Causes of RLS

Common causes of RLS are listed in Box 23–5. RLS is often divided into *primary RLS* (independent of other disorders) and *secondary RLS* (due to an identifiable cause such as a

medical disorder, condition, or medication). The cause of primary RLS is not known. There may be an abnormality in iron transport into the central nervous system or utilization of iron as it relates to dopaminergic neurons. Causes of secondary RLS include renal failure, pregnancy, iron deficiency (with or without anemia), and certain medications. Medications associated with RLS include tricyclic antidepressants, serotonin reuptake inhibitors, dopamine blockers (phenothiazines, haloperidol, metoclopramide), sedating antihistamines (diphenhydramine), and antinausea medications (prochlorperazine). RLS associated with renal failure is not helped by dialysis but is cured by renal transplantation. The RLS of pregnancy commonly vanishes or improves with delivery. It is prudent to check a serum iron, total iron-binding capacity (TIBC), and ferritin in patients with RLS. It is recommended that RLS patients have a ferritin above 45 to 50 µg/mL.[17] The RLS of iron deficiency may improve with iron supplementation. If the onset of RLS can be linked to the start of a given medication, a switch to an alternate medication can be tried. For example, bupropion is an antidepressant that does not worsen RLS.[18] In one study, selective serotonin reuptake inhibitor (SSRI) medications and venlafaxine were more likely to be associated with PLMS than either a control group or a group taking bupropion.[19] Thus, bupropion might be less likely to cause or worsen RLS.

Familial Patterns and Genetics

In 50% to 60% of cases of RLS, a family history of RLS can be found.[13,20] Twin studies show a high concordance rate. Most pedigrees suggest an autosomal dominant pattern; however, a recessive pattern with a carrier phenotype is also possible. Familial RLS has onset of symptoms at a younger age and is more slowly progressive. The genetics of RLS, as in many medical conditions, is complex[21-30] (Table 23-3). Linkage studies have found RLS loci but no related disease-causing sequence variants have been found. More recent genome-wide association studies have identified three genomic regions *MEIS1*, *BTBD9*, and *MAP2K5/LBXCOR1*. In one study, the presence of a genetic risk for the **presence of PLMS** was found whether or not RLS symptoms were present.[29]

Pathophysiology of RLS

The pathophysiology of RLS is not well understood.[21,31-34] Central nervous system iron homeostatic dysregulation is thought to be the basic mechanism. Cerebrospinal fluid (CSF) ferritin is lower (and transferrin is higher) in RLS patients. Magnetic resonance imaging (MRI) using special sequencing techniques can provide measures of iron concentration in specific brain regions. Using this technique, imaging showed **reduced iron stores** in the striatum and red nucleus.[34] The dopaminergic system is also believed to be involved in RLS. Iron is a cofactor for the enzyme tyrosine-hydroxylase, which is a rate-limiting step in the formation of dopamine. RLS patients show a greater circadian variation in dopamine metabolites than controls. This would be consistent with the circadian component of RLS. The current theory of the causation of RLS is sometimes called the *iron-dopamine hypothesis.*

Clinical Features of RLS

A number of features of RLS have clinical utility (Box 23-6). These include information about the prevalence of RLS as well as variations in the presentation of RLS and symptoms associated with RLS.

Prevalence of RLS

A number of studies have attempted to define the prevalence of RLS. The results vary considerably due to the use of

BOX 23-6

Clinical Features of Restless Legs Syndrome
PREVALENCE OF RLS
• 5–10% in general population
• Women > men
NATURAL CLINICAL COURSE
• Can begin at any age
• RLS can be intermittent
• Variable course
• Early onset (<50 yr)—onset is insidious
• Late onset—abrupt and more severe
REASONS RLS PATIENTS SEEK MEDICAL ATTENTION
• Leg discomfort
• Sleep disturbance—the primary reason most patients seek medical attention
• Sleep-onset and -maintenance insomnia
• Daytime sleepiness much less common
RLS = restless legs syndrome.

TABLE 23-3

Genetic Linkages and Associations in Restless Legs Syndrome

LINKAGES			
AUTHOR	**POPULATION**	**CHROMOSOME**	**MODEL**
RLS-1—Desautels, 2001[22]	French Canadian	12q	Recessive
RLS-2—Bonati, 2003[23]	Italian	14q	Dominant
RLS-3—Chen, 2004[24]	United States	9p	Dominant
RLS-4—Levchenko, 2006,[25] 2009[26]	French Canadian	20p	Dominant
RLS-5—Pichler, 2006[27]	Italian	2q	Dominant
ASSOCIATIONS			
AUTHOR	**POPULATION**	**CHROMOSOME**	**GENE**
Winkelmann, 2007[28]	French Canadian/ European	2p	*MEIS1*, exon 9
		6p	*BTBD9*, intron 5
		15q	*MAP2K5, LBXCOR1*
Stefannson, 2007[29]	Icelandic/US	6p	*BTBD9*
Winklemann, 2007[30]	European	12q	*BTBDR*, intron 5

Adapted from Hening WA, Buchfuhrer MJ, Lee HB: Clinical Management of Restless Legs Syndrome. West Islip, NY: Professional Communications, 2008, pp. 56–57.

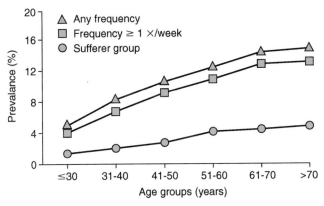

FIGURE 23-2 Prevalence of restless legs syndrome (RLS) at different age groups for patients reporting any frequency of RLS symptoms, those reporting frequency greater than 1/wk, and sufferers (reporting RLS symptoms ≥2/wk and some impact from the symptoms when they occurred). *From Hening WA, Buchfuhrer MJ, Lee HB: Clinical management of restless legs syndrome. West Islip, NY: Professional Communications, 2008; and Hening W, Walters AS, Allen RP, et al: Impact, diagnosis and management of restless legs syndrome in a primary care population: the REST (RLS Epidemiology, Symptoms, and Treatment) Primary Care Study. Sleep Med 2004;5:237–246.*

TABLE 23-4	
Manifestation of Restless Legs Syndrome in Restless Legs Syndrome "Sufferers" (N = 551)	
At least one sleep-related symptom	43.4%
Consulted MD about symptoms	64.8%
Given RLS diagnosis	24.9%
ON NIGHTS WHEN RLS SYMPTOMS PRESENT	
>30 min to fall asleep	68.6%
≥3 awakenings	60.1%

RLS = restless legs syndrome.
Data from Hening W, Walters AS, Allen RP, et al: Impact, diagnosis and management of restless legs syndrome in a primary care population: the REST (RLS Epidemiology, Symptoms, and Treatment) Primary Care Study. Sleep Med 2004;5:237–246.

different RLS diagnostic criteria and different methods (survey vs. direct patient interview).[1,2,13,35,36] Approximately 5% to 10% of adults in Northern European countries report RLS symptoms. RLS is approximately **1.5 to 2 times more common in women** than in men. However, much of the difference in RLS prevalence between men and women is likely due to the association of RLS with pregnancy. The Restless Legs Epidemiology, Symptoms, and Treatment Study (REST)[35] was a large questionnaire evaluation of 23,052 primary care patients. The study found that the overall prevalence of weekly RLS symptoms was 9.6% and that the prevalence increased with age (Fig. 23-2). A large international study of a general population (REST general population study) found that 5% of the respondents experience RLS symptoms weekly and 2.7% reported symptoms at least twice weekly and that the symptoms had a negative impact on their life.[36]

Onset and Clinical Course of RLS

RLS can begin at any age and the clinical course is variable. Two patterns are commonly seen (see Box 23-6).[13] An early onset (age < 50 yr) characterized by insidious onset, less severity, and higher familial association. A late onset RLS (age > 50 yr) is characterized by a more abrupt onset and more severe manifestations. Late-onset RLS patients also tend to have lower ferritin levels compared with early-onset RLS patients.

Sleep Disturbance Associated with RLS

The two most common complaints that cause RLS patients to seek medical attention are the uncomfortable leg sensations and the disturbance of sleep. Beyond the significant discomfort caused by RLS symptoms, the disorder can cause difficulty with sleep initiation and maintenance A recent large questionnaire study of 23,052 primary care patients identified a group of "RLS sufferers" (N = 551) with RLS symptoms twice or more weekly and a negative impact from RLS symptoms.[35] In this group, 43.4% complained of sleep-related symptoms but only 6% complained of daytime sleepiness. On nights that RLS symptoms were present, 69% complained of taking over 30 minutes to fall asleep and 60% complained of three or more awakenings per night (Table 23-4). Daytime sleepiness is a less common symptom than insomnia but can occur. In a general population study, the prevalence of RLS of any frequency was 7.2%, weekly RLS symptoms was 5%, and twice-weekly symptoms with distressing symptoms was 2.7%.[36] Of the group with RLS twice weekly or more, 81% had reported symptoms to primary physicians but only 6.2% were given a diagnosis of RLS.

The etiology of sleep disturbance from RLS includes a delay in sleep onset due to RLS symptoms. If the patient awakens, the return to sleep may also be delayed by RLS symptoms. Because the majority of RLS patients have PLMS, it might be assumed that arousals associated with PLMS contribute to sleep disturbance. However, the PLMSI (number of PLMs/hr of sleep) is not highly correlated with any measure of sleep disturbance in most studies of RLS patients.[12] In a study of unmedicated RLS patients, Hornyak and coworkers[37] found that the IRLSSG rating scale (IRLS) score[38,39] (RLS symptoms severity) correlated with the PLMS arousal index but not the PLMSI. However, even the relationship between the IRLSSG rating scale (IRLS) and the PLMS arousal index was very weak (r = 0.22, P = .03).

Medical Evaluation in RLS

The diagnostic evaluation (Box 23-7) should include a history to elicit the essential and associated features of RLS. A detailed medication history including over-the-counter (OTC) medications (sedating antihistamines) is very important. The IRLSSG developed a rating scale for RLS symptoms called the *IRLSSG rating scale (IRLS)*.[38,39] A slight revision of

BOX 23–7

Medical Evaluation of Restless Legs Syndrome Patients

HISTORY

- Presence of essential RLS criteria
- RLS in family members
- Neuroleptic use?
- Detailed medication history (including OTC medications)

PHYSICAL EXAMINATION

- Neurologic—signs of neuropathy

LABORATORY

- Ferritin, TIBC, % iron saturation
- Renal function

OTC = over the counter; RLS = restless legs syndrome; TIBC = total iron-binding capacity.

BOX 23–8

International Restless Legs Syndrome Study Group Rating Scale (IRLS)—Version 2.1

In the past week …

1. Overall, how would you rate the RLS discomfort in your legs or arms?
   (4) Very severe (3) Severe (2) Moderate (1) Mild (0) None
2. Overall, how would you rate the need to move around because of your RLS symptoms?
   (4) Very severe (3) Severe (2) Moderate (1) Mild (0) None
3. Overall, how much relief of your RLS arm or leg discomfort did you get from moving around?
   (4) No relief (3) Slight relief (2) Moderate relief (1) Either complete or almost complete relief (0) No RLS symptoms to be relieved
4. Overall, how severe was your **sleep disturbance** due to your RLS symptoms?
   (4) Very severe (3) Severe (2) Moderate (1) Mild (0) None
5. How severe was your **tiredness or sleepiness** due to your RLS symptoms?
   (4) Very severe (3) Severe (2) Moderate (1) Mild (0) None
6. How severe was your RLS as a whole?
   (4) Very severe (3) Severe (2) Moderate (1) Mild (0) None
7. How often did you get RLS symptoms?
   (4) Very often [6–7 days/wk] (3) Often [4–5 days/wk] (2) Sometimes [2–3 days/wk] (1) Occasionally [≤1 day/wk] (0) Never
8. When you had RLS symptoms, how severe were they on average?
   (4) Very severe [≥8 hr/24 hr] (3) Severe [3–8 hr/24 hr] (2) Moderate [1–3 hr/24 hr] (1) Mild [<1 hr/24 hr] (0) None
9. Overall, how severe was the impact of your RLS symptoms on your ability to carry out your daily affairs—for example, carrying out a satisfactory family, home, social, or work life?
   (4) Very severe (3) Severe (2) Moderate (1) Mild (0) None
10. How severe was your mood disturbance due to your RLS symptoms—for example, angry, depressed, sad, anxious, or irritable?
    (4) Very severe (3) Severe (2) Moderate (1) Mild (0) None

RLS = restless legs syndrome.
From International Restless Legs Syndrome Study Group. Validation of the International restless legs syndrome rating scale for the restless legs syndrome. Sleep Med 2003;4:121–122.

the validated scale[38] was published as an appendix to an editorial.[39] The IRLS is useful to quantify RLS symptom severity and the effects of treatment (Box 23–8). The scale is used in research studies but also has clinical utility in following patients on treatment.

Physical examination should look for signs of neuropathy. Laboratory studies should check renal and thyroid function. A serum iron level, TIBC, % iron saturation, and ferritin levels should be checked. The ferritin is the most useful single test. However, ferritin can be elevated by inflammatory processes. If the ferritin level is less than 45 to 50 μg, iron supplementation may improve symptoms.[17] An iron saturation less than 20% or an elevated TIBC may be useful if the ferritin is elevated due to inflammation. PSG is NOT required in most cases of RLS unless sleep apnea or another sleep disorder is suspected. Of note, abnormal movements during sleep including leg kicks can occur with OSA. If there is a suspicion of other causes of abnormal nocturnal movements such as OSA, epilepsy, sleep-related rhythmic movement disorder, or the rapid eye movement (REM) sleep behavior disorder (RBD), a sleep study is indicated. As noted previously, daytime sleepiness is NOT a common symptom of RLS and the presence of this symptom should prompt consideration of disorders other than RLS. In addition, a combination of sleep disorders, for example, RLS and sleep apnea, is not uncommon.

PSG Findings in RLS Patients

In a study of 133 patients with RLS, it was found that the PLMSI was greater than 5/hr in 80.2% of RLS patients.[12] The PLMSI did increase with RLS severity. There was also a significant correlation between the PLMSI and the periodic limb movement in wake index (PLMWI). However, there was no correlation between PLMSI and measures of sleep disturbance such as sleep efficiency and nocturnal awakenings. Another study found a weak correlation between the PLMS arousal index and RLS severity.[37] Therefore, PLMS does not appear to be a major cause of sleep disturbance in most patients with RLS. The PSG is more likely to be abnormal if patients with RLS complain of sleep problems (Table 23–5).[12] In looking at the classification of RLS severity in this table, note that the classification was influenced by sleep complaints as well as RLS symptoms. Whereas the finding of PLMS should always alert the clinician to the possibility of RLS, PLMS is also common in patients with sleep apnea, narcolepsy, and the RBD.

TABLE 23-5

Polysomnography Findings in Groups with Mild, Moderate, and Severe Restless Legs Syndrome

SEVERITY*	MILD	MODERATE	SEVERE	P
N	11	38	82	
Age (yr)	46.7	49.0	52.7	NS
Sleep latency (min)	11.7	20.2	20.2	NS
Sleep efficiency (%)	82.2	80.1	72.7	.01
PLMSI (#/hr)	10.6	24.7	33.2	<.05
PLMWI	29.1	25.8	31.0	NS

*Patients were rated as mild, moderate, or severe based on frequency and severity of RLS complaints, severity of sleep-onset insomnia, and frequency and duration of nocturnal awakenings.
NS = not significant; PLMSI = periodic limb movements in sleep index; PLMWI = periodic limb movements during wake index.
From Montplasir J, Boucher S, Poirer G, et al: Clinical, polysomnographic, and genetic characteristics of restless legs syndrome: a study of 133 patients diagnosed with new standard criteria. Mov Disord 1997;12:61–65.

BOX 23-9

Criteria for Diagnosis of Restless Legs Syndrome in Children (Age 2–12 yr)

A alone or B + C

A. The child meets all four essential adult criteria for RLS and relates a description in his or her own words that is consistent with leg discomfort.

OR

B. The child meets all adult criteria for RLS but does NOT relate a description in his or her own words that is consistent with leg discomfort.

AND

C. The child has at least two of the following three findings:
  i. Sleep disturbance for age.
  ii. A biologic parent or sibling with definite RLS.
  iii. A PSG documented PLM index of ≥ 5/hr (≥5/hr of sleep)

PLM = periodic limb movement; PSG = polysomnography; RLS = restless legs syndrome.
From American Academy of Sleep Medicine: ICSD-2 International Classification of Sleep Disorders, 2nd ed. Diagnostic and Coding Manual. Westchester, IL: American Academy of Sleep Medicine, 2005.

RLS in Children

RLS can be difficult to diagnose in children.[6,13,40-43] Some complain of typical RLS symptoms while others complain of "growing pains" or simply have difficulty "sitting still." The ICSD-2 diagnostic criteria for RLS in children are shown in Box 23–9. These criteria are based on the NIH workshop on RLS, which listed criteria for probable and possible RLS for research purposes.[13] The Peds REST study found criteria for definite RLS in 1.9% of children aged 8 to 11 years and 2% in adolescents age 12 to 17 years.[40] Of note, PLMS is less common in children and a PLMSI of 5/hr or greater is considered abnormal. Some children with attention deficit hyperactivity disorder (ADHD) have PLMS and possible RLS and vice versa.[44] The relationship of RLS and ADHD remains to be determined.

PERIODIC LIMB MOVEMENTS IN SLEEP

In the earlier descriptions of PLMS, the phenomenon was referred to as "nocturnal myoclonus," but this terminology is no longer used. As discussed in detail in Chapter 12, the limb movements (LMs) composing PLMS are characterized by the rhythmic repetitive stereotypic dorsiflexion/extension of the big toe, dorsiflexion at the ankle, and sometimes flexion at the knee and hip joints. Individual LMs that meet criteria for being a component of a PLM series are called PLMs. Criteria for identifying LMs qualifying as PLMs were first proposed by Coleman[3] and later revised by a task force of the American Academy of Sleep Medicine (AASM) in 1993.[45] A revised scoring system was published in 2006 by the World Association of Sleep Medicine in association with the IRLSSG.[46] Criteria for scoring PLMs during both sleep (PLMS) and wake (PLMW) were published. The major

change was that the maximum duration of PLM events was extended from 5 to 10 seconds and voltage amplitude criteria were used to define a significant LM. Similar scoring criteria for PLMS were published in the AASM scoring manual.[47] The AASM manual did not provide criteria for scoring PLMW. As reviewed in Chapter 12, for LMs to be counted as part of a PLM series (to be PLMs), they must be 0.5 to 10 seconds in duration and have an amplitude greater than 8 μV above the resting baseline anterior tibial electromyogram (EMG) level. The time of onset of successive LMs must be between 5 and 90 seconds. If two leg EMG bursts are separated by less than 5 seconds from onset to onset, they are considered a single LM if they occur on the same or different legs. LMs must occur in groups of four or more to be considered PLMs (part of a PLM sequence). An LM is not scored as a PLM if it occurs during a period starting 0.5 second before the start of the apnea/hypopnea to 0.5 second after an apnea and hypopnea. How to handle PLMs associated with RERAs was not mentioned, but many clinicians would consider these as associated with respiratory events.

PLMSI and PSG Findings

The PLMSI is the number of PLM events per hour of sleep. The ICSD, first edition,[48] listed the following grading of the severity of PLMs: PLMSI < 5 normal, 5–24 mild, 25–49 moderate, and ≥ 50/hr severe. However, these cutoffs are entirely arbitrary and are not based on any outcome data. Given the high prevalence of PLMS in asymptomatic individuals, there is unlikely to be a value separating asymptomatic from symptomatic populations. The ICSD-2 chose a PLMSI **greater than 15/hr in adults and greater than 5/hr in children as part of the diagnostic criteria for the PLMD.**[6] However, asymptomatic individuals can have quite high PLMSI values.

PLMs occur most commonly in stage N1 and N2 but can also occur in stage N3 or, less commonly, during stage R sleep.[49,50] The PLMSI is often higher during the first part of the night. Culpepper and colleagues[50] described two patterns of PLMS. In one pattern, PLMS was much more common in the first part of the night. In the second pattern, PLMS was more evenly distributed across the night. The interval between individual PLMs increases from stage N1 to stage N3. PLMs are less likely to cause arousal from stage N3 sleep. Frequent PLMs have been described during REM sleep in patients with spinal cord injury[51] and the RBD.[52,53] The AASM scoring manual did not define criteria for PLMW, but others have used criteria similar to those used for PLMS[54] (except that patients are awake). In PLMW, the periodicity is less regular and shorter than typical of PLMS. It was found that PLMW events tend to be longer (5–10 sec in duration) compared with typical PLMS events.

PLMS and Arousals

An individual PLM and an arousal are considered to be associated with each other when there is 0.5 second or less from the end of one event to the onset of the other event regardless of which is first.[47] Overlapping events are considered to be associated. The **PLMS arousal index** is the number of PLMS arousals per hour of sleep. There are no widely accepted normal values for the PLMS arousal index. The ICSD-1[48] listed a PLMS arousal index of 25/hr or greater as severe. One study looking at the association of PLMs and arousals found that 49% of electroencephalogram (EEG) arousals occurred before PLMs, 30.6% simultaneously, and 23.2% occurred just after the LMs.[55] PLMs can often be associated with K complexes or delta bursts that do not meet criteria for cortical arousal. Of note, autonomic changes (increase in heart rate, increase in blood pressure, change in pulse transit time) can occur in association with the PLMs **with and without cortical arousals**[56,57] and these "autonomic arousals" are more common than cortical arousals. Figure 23–3 shows the change in heart rate before and after PLM events with and without cortical arousal. Of note, some have hypothesized that PLMs and arousals are both secondary to a periodic central activation leading to both arousals and PLMS.[58,59] In one study of RLS patients, treatment with L-dopa (LD) did not change the frequency of K-alpha complexes, although the PLMSI decreased.[58]

Differential Diagnosis of PLMS

The differential of other periodic movements includes hypnogogic foot tremor (HFT), alternating leg movement activities (ALMAs), excessive fragmentary myoclonus, and rhythmic movement disorder.[6,47] The reader is referred to

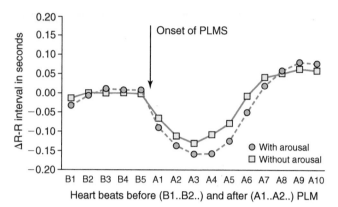

FIGURE 23–3 Change in heart rate after periodic limb movements in sleep (PLMS). The heart rate increased (R-R interval decreased) whether or not the PLM is associated with a cortical arousal. The increase in heart rate is **higher for a few beats after the periodic leg movement (PLM) if an arousal is present.** *From Sforza E, Nicolas A, Lavigne G, et al: EEG and cardiac activation during periodic leg movements in sleep. Neurology 1999;52:786–792.*

Chapter 12 on movement monitoring for more details on these entities.

Clinical Significance of the PLMSI and PLMS Arousal Index

The clinical significance of PLMS and the utility of monitoring LMs have been the subject of controversy[59,60] and Pro-Con debates.[61,62] The utility of counting PLMS arousals has also been questioned because the index does not appear to correlate with subjective measures of disturbed sleep, daytime sleepiness, or the sense of nonrestorative sleep.[60] Clearly, PLMs are very common in asymptomatic patient populations. For example, a PLMSI greater than 5/hr is seen in 30% to 86% of adults aged 60 or older. Claman and associates[9] studied 455 older community-dwelling women and found that 66% had a PLMSI greater than 5/hr and 52% greater than 15/hr. The associations between the PLMSI and the PLMS arousal index with measures of sleep quality were determined. The associations were adjusted for age, body mass index (BMI), apnea-hypopnea index, and antidepressant medication use. An increased **PLMSI** was associated with a statistically significant higher total arousal index (but the difference was very small) but not impairment of other indices of sleep quality. A higher **PLMS arousal index** was associated with lower total sleep time, less stage N3, and a higher total arousal index. However, neither a higher PLMSI nor a higher PLMS arousal index was associated with worse subjective daytime sleepiness by Epworth Sleepiness Scale. Carrier and coworkers[63] found a PLMSI of greater than 10/hr in 43/70 healthy middle-aged subjects without sleep complaints. Sleep quality was not worse in those with a higher PLMSI. The Pittsburgh Sleep Quality Index was slightly worse in men with higher PLMSI. The difference was statistically significant but not clinically significant. It remains to be determined whether determination of the PLMS arousal

TABLE 23–6

Syndromes in which Periodic Limb Movements in Sleep Are Common

DISORDER	PREVALENCE OF PLMS
RLS	80–90% with PLMSI > 5/hr
Narcolepsy	45–65%[5,59]
REM sleep behavior disorder	PLMS > 4/hr 70%[52,53] Unlike most other disorders, PLMs commonly continue during stage R
OSA	24%[65]

OSA = obstructive sleep apnea; PLMs = periodic limb movements; PLMS = periodic limb movements in sleep; PLMSI = periodic limb movement in sleep index; REM = rapid eye movement; RLS = restless legs syndrome.

index really adds anything of clinical significance to other measures of sleep quality.

PLMS and Other Disorders

PLMS is common in a number of disorders other than RLS (Table 23–6) including narcolepsy, the RBD, neuropathies of diverse etiology, and OSA.[5,52,53,64–66] An increase in PLMSI (compared to a diagnostic study) was noted during a continuous positive airway pressure (CPAP) titration and a repeat study on CPAP (2 weeks to 7 months later).[64] Chervin and colleagues[65] evaluated 1124 patients with suspected or confirmed OSA and found that a higher PLMS arousal index was associated with **decreased** objective sleepiness by multiple sleep latency test (MSLT). In this study, 24% of the OSA patients had a PLMSI greater than 5/hr. **In most patients diagnosed with OSA on a sleep study, the incidental finding of PLMS is usually of no or limited clinical significance. It should prompt the clinician to check for symptoms of the RLS.** PLMS can be associated with respiratory event–related arousals (RERAs), and indeed, patients once diagnosed with PLMD on the basis of PSG using thermal airflow sensors can now be noted to have LMs associated with RERAs[66] due to more sensitive detection of subtle respiratory events using nasal pressure monitoring of airflow. As noted previously, LMs associated with apneas and hypopneas are not considered PLMs. Baran and associates[67] found PLMs tended to increase during the CPAP titration in severe OSA patients but to decrease in milder OSA patients. They hypothesized that CPAP unmasked PLMs in some severe patients, but in the milder patients, prevented RERAs and, therefore, decreased PLMs.

PERIODIC LIMB MOVEMENT DISORDER

In this disorder, PLMs, as described previously, result in clinical sleep disturbance (sleep maintenance insomnia, daytime sleepiness, or fatigue). The clinical symptoms are not better explained by another primary sleep disorder. Thus, the diagnosis depends on PSG to demonstrate PLMS and exclusion of other causes of the symptoms by a clinical

BOX 23–10

Periodic Limb Movement Disorder Diagnostic Criteria (ICSD-2)*

A. PLMS present—LMs meet criteria to be PLMs
   i. 0.5–10 sec in duration.
   ii. Amplitude > 8 μV above baseline.
   iii. In a sequence of four or more movements.
   iv. Onset of consecutive LMs >5 and <90 sec.
B. PLMS index >15/hr in adults, >5/hr in children.
C. There is a clinical sleep disturbance or complaint of daytime fatigue.
D. The PLMS and clinical sleep disturbance are not better explained by another current sleep disorder, medical or neurologic, or psychiatric disorder.

Notes:
1. A diagnosis of RLS excludes PLMD.
2. If PLMs are present without sleep complaint, they can simply be noted as a PSG finding.
3. If only the bed partner's sleep is disturbed, this is not sufficient to make a diagnosis of PLMD.
*Updated according to the AASM scoring manual.
LMs = limb movements; PLMs = periodic limb movements; PLMS = periodic limb movements in sleep.

history and PSG (Box 23–10). Recall that a diagnosis of RLS excludes a diagnosis of PLMD. ICSD-1 stated "The patient has a complaint of insomnia or excessive sleepiness. The patient occasionally will be asymptomatic, and the movements are noticed by an observer." In ICSD-2,[6] a complaint of sleep disturbance **by the patient** is required for a diagnosis of PLMD.

Prevalence and Manifestations of PLMD

Although PLMS is common, PLMD is thought to be rare. The exact prevalence of the PLMD is unknown. Patients rarely are aware that they have PLMS until informed by their bed partner. The disturbance of the bed partner's sleep by PLMS is thought to be more common than PLMD. Some of the patients previously thought to have PLMD on the basis of sleep studies that monitored airflow with a thermal device rather than nasal pressure may have actually had RERA or hypopnea-associated PLMS. In these patients, the symptoms of daytime sleepiness may have been due to mild OSA rather than PLMD.[66] Other patients with PLMD may have had somewhat atypical symptoms of RLS without prominent sensations. **The finding of PLMS in children can be especially helpful because RLS symptoms are often difficult to elicit.** It has also been proposed that in children, **PLMD (PLMS with sleep disturbance) may precede the development of symptoms of RLS.**[41]

PSG and Objective Findings

The PLMSI in asymptomatic patients and patients with PLMD overlap. The ICSD-2 criteria for PLMS include the requirement of a PLMSI of 15/hr or greater in adults and

5/hr or greater in children (see Box 23–10). However, many asymptomatic individuals have a PLMSI greater than 15/hr. Mendelson[60] evaluated a group of 67 patients felt to have the PLMD. The patients had both a PSG and MSLT. The overall sleep latency was around 10 minutes (near normal). There was no significant correlation between the PLM arousal index and the sleep latency on a MSLT or a measure of subjective sleepiness.

TREATMENT OF RLS AND PLMD

Nonpharmacologic treatments of RLS may be appropriate in mild or intermittent cases of RLS. Iron supplementation may improve RLS symptoms if iron stores are low. A number of medications (Table 23–7) can be used to treat RLS.[68–76] The major medication groups include the dopaminergic medications (the **dopamine precursor LD and dopamine agonists [DAs]), opiates, anticonvulsant medications, and sedative-hypnotic medications** (usually benzodiazepine receptor agonists [BZRAs]). Similar medications have been used to treat the PLMD with the exception that opiates have not been well studied for this indication. Of note, two DAs, ropinirole and pramipexole, are the only two medications that are U.S. Food and Drug Administration (FDA) approved for RLS treatment.

Nonpharmacologic Treatments

In mild and intermittent RLS, nonpharmacologic treatments may be useful. These include stretching, heating or cooling of the extremities (warm bath), and a trial of avoidance of alcohol and caffeine. Antidepressant treatment can sometimes be associated with initiation or worsening of RLS. However, if antidepressant treatment is deemed necessary, RLS can be treated as if primary RLS was present. Studies have suggested that bupropion either improves[18] or does not worsen PLMS,[19] so use of this medication could be considered. However, concerns about RLS should not limit effective treatment of depression. Iron deficiency can cause or worsen RLS. A ferritin level is recommended in RLS patients because this disorder may be the only indication that low iron stores are present. Most clinicians recommend that a ferritin level above 45 to 50 µg/mL be achieved in RLS patients.[17,70] Patients should also be evaluated for occult gastrointestinal blood loss if clinically indicated. Typical iron supplementation is ferrous sulfate 325 mg tid with the addition of 100 to 200 mg of ascorbic acid with each dose (to improve absorption). Iron absorption is better when ingested with an empty stomach. However, some patients must take iron with food to avoid severe gastrointestinal upset. Monitoring of ferritin levels is recommended to ensure adequate replenishment of iron stores and to avoid inducing iron overload. When ferritin levels exceed the goal, iron supplementation can be stopped. It is important to note that iron supplementation alone does not always improve RLS. However, many patients will have better results with treatment with standard RLS medications.

Dopaminergic Medications

LD is a precursor that is converted to dopamine by dopa decarboxylase (DDC). Carbidopa (CD) does not penetrate the blood-brain barrier but acts as an inhibitor of DDC outside the central nervous system. Therefore, there is less peripheral conversion of LD to dopamine. This results in fewer side effects and an increased amount of LD reaching the brain. LD/CD is very effective in RLS and has a quick onset of action.[68–71] There are two problems with use of LD/CD in treating RLS. First, the drug has a short duration of action and there may be a rebound in symptoms in the early morning hours. The patient can take another dose at that time. There are longer-acting forms of LD/CD but they have a slower onset of action. The second problem is that continued use of LD/CD, especially at high doses (LD > 200 mg/day), commonly results in augmentation (a change in the effectiveness of dopaminergic medications, discussed later). In some studies, up to 80% of patients taking LD/CD for RLS develop augmentation.[72]

The ergotamine-related DA pergolide is effective but rarely used for RLS treatment due to the severe associated nausea and the rare potential for retroperitoneal fibrosis.[68,69,72] The nonergotamine DAs pramipexole and ropinirole are considered the treatments of choice for moderate to severe RLS.[69,70] Randomized, controlled studies have documented the efficacy of these medications for treating RLS and PLMD.[73–77] They have a sufficiently long duration of action such that rebound usually does not occur. Augmentation, discussed in detail later, can occur in up to 30% of patients but is usually mild and can be controlled by taking a portion of the dose at an earlier time (split dose).[70,78] Both augmentation and side effects from the DAs can be minimized by starting at a low dose (0.125 for pramipexole and 0.25 mg for ropiniriole) with a slow upward titration every 3 to 5 days as needed. It is important to note that both drugs have a long time of onset of 1 to 3 hours and, ideally, should be taken at least 2 hours before symptoms are expected. If patients have symptoms in the morning, one can try treatment with twice or three times a day dosing. Of note, some patients will respond better to pramipexole than to ropinirole and vice versa. Switching DAs is also an intervention that can be tried if augmentation develops.

Few studies have been published concerning treatment of PLMD and RLS in children. **No medication is FDA approved for treatment of PLMD or RLS in children.** However, it appears that dopaminergic therapy is effective treatment for PLMD or RLS in children.[41–43]

All dopaminergic medications share similar side effects (Box 23–11). Nausea is the most common side effect, but headache, light-headedness, somnolence, and insomnia can occur. Less frequent side effects include peripheral edema and sleep attacks. The **dopamine dysregulation syndrome** is a dysfunction of the rewards system in subjects taking dopamine treatment. The most common symptom is craving for dopaminergic medication sometimes associated with taking extra doses even in the absence of symptoms that

TABLE 23-7

Medications Used to Treat the Restless Leg Syndrome

	DOSE FORMS (MG)	INITIAL DOSE (MG)	USUAL EFFECTIVE DOSE (MG)	MAX DOSE (24 HR)	TIME TO ONSET OF ACTION	HALF-LIFE (HR)/ ELIMINATION (H, R)
DOPAMINE PRECURSORS						
CD/LD (Sinemet)	25/100	½–1 tablet of 25/100	100–200 of LD	200 LD hs	30 min	1.5–3 H
CD/LD CR (Sinemet CR)	25/100 50/200	½–1 tablet of 25/100	100–200 of LD	200 LD hs	120 min	6–8 H
DOPAMINE AGONISTS						
Pramipexole (Mirapex)	0.125 0.25	0.125	0.25–0.75	1.5 mg	120 min 2–3 hr max effect	8–12 R
Ropinirole (Requip)	0.25 0.5	0.25	0.5–2.0	4.0 mg 2 or 3 divided doses	60–120 min 1–3 hr max effect	6 H
OPIOIDS						
Propoxyphene napsylate (Darvon) Propoxyphene HCl	100 32, 65	100 65	100 65	100 mg q4h 600/24 hr 65 mg q4h 390/24 hr	15–60 min, peak level 2–2.5 hr	4–6 H, R
HC/APAP (Lortab, Vicoden)	5, 7.5, 10/325 5, 7.5, 10/500	5	5–15 HC	20–30 mg/day in 2 or 3 divided doses	1.3 hr peak level	3–4 (hydrocodone)
Oxycodone	5, 10, 15	5	5–15	5–30 q4h	10–15 min, peak level 30–60 min	3–6 H, R
Methadone	5, 10	2.5–5	5–15	15	30–60 min	8–59 H
Tramadol	50	50	50–100	50–100 q4h 400 mg/24 hr	1 hr, peak level 2–3 hr	6–7 H
BENZODIAZEPINE RECEPTOR AGONISTS						
Clonazepam (Klonopin)	0.5	0.25	0.25–1.0	2 mg	60–120 min peak level	19–39 H
Temazepam (Restoril)	15, 30	30 (15 elderly)	15–30	30 mg	45–60 min, peak level 90–120 min	8–9 H
Zolpidem Zolpidem-CR (Ambien CR)	5, 10 6.25, 12.5	10 (5 elderly) 12.5 (6.25 elderly)	5–10 6.25–12.5	10 mg 12.5 mg	30 min, peak level 90 min	2.5–3 H
Eszopiclone (Lunesta)	1, 2, 3	2 (1 elderly)	2–3	3 mg	<30 min, peak level 60 min	6 H
Zalpelon (Sonata)	5, 10, 20	10	10–20	20 mg	15–30 min, peak level 30–90 min	1–2 H
ANTICONVULSANTS						
Gabapentin (Neurontin)	100, 300	300	600–1800 200–300 after HD	2400 mg	Peak level 2–4 hr Slow upward titration recommended	5–7 R

APAP = acetaminophen; CD = carbidopa; CR = controlled release; H = hepatic metabolism; HC = hydrocodone; HD = hemodialysis; LD = l-dopa; R = renal metabolism.

BOX 23–11

Side Effects from Dopaminergic Medications

COMMON ACUTE EFFECTS

- Nausea, less commonly vomiting
- Light-headedness, rarely syncope
- Headache
- Somnolence
- Insomnia

LESS COMMON ADVERSE EFFECTS

- Peripheral edema
- Sleep attacks
- Dopamine dysregulation syndrome
  - Craving for dopaminergic medications including taking extra doses without clinical symptoms
  - Impulse control disorders
    - Hypersexuality
    - Pathologic gambling
    - Excessive shopping

SUBACUTE TO LATE-ONSET ADVERSE EFFECTS

- Augmentation
  - Advance in time of onset of symptoms
  - Greater severity of symptoms when present
  - Reduced latency to onset of symptoms at rest
  - Spread of symptoms to involve new body parts

ADVERSE EFFECTS PRIMARILY NOTED IN PARKINSON'S DISEASE

- Dyskinesias
- Hallucinations
- Psychosis

SIDE EFFECTS ASSOCIATED WITH ERGOTAMINE DOPAMINE AGONISTS

- Severe nausea
- Fibrotic syndromes
  - Retroperitoneal fibrosis
  - Pleural-pulmonary fibrosis
  - Fibrotic cardiomyopathy
  - Valvular disease

Adapted from Hening WA, Buchfuhrer MJ, Lee HB: Clinical Management of Restless Legs Syndrome. West Islip, NY: Professional Communications, 2008.

BOX 23–12

Approaches to Augmentation

1. If on LD/CD, stop and change to a DA (avoid LD/CD in daily RLS, avoid dose > 200 mg LD).
2. If on a DA and earlier symptom onset is the problem, split the dose and give half of the dose earlier.
3. If patient is taking a DA, try changing to the other DA.
4. If patient is taking a DA and morning symptoms are a problem, try an evening and morning dose of medication.
5. If very severe augmentation, stop the DA or LD/CD and add high-potency opiate.
6. Avoid high doses of DAs, use combination therapy (add opiate, gabapentin, or BZRA).
7. Low iron stores may predispose to augmentation.

BZRA = benzodiazepine receptor agonist; CD = carbidopa; DA = dopamine agonist; LD = L-dopa; RLS = restless legs syndrome.

Augmentation

Augmentation is defined as a change in the efficacy of RLS treatment with dopaminergic medications[70,78] (see Box 23–11). It is characterized by one or more of the following: (1) earlier symptom onset, (2) greater severity of symptoms at the same dose, (3) reduced latency to onset of symptoms with rest, and (4) spread of symptoms to involve new body parts (arms as well as legs). The greater severity of symptoms is often noted even though medication dose has been increased. Patients with severe augmentation are usually on LD/CD or a very high dose of a DA. As noted previously, augmentation is common on daily LD/CD (80%) but can occur in patients taking a DA (≤30%)—although it is usually milder. When using a DA, it is imperative to be certain the patient is taking the DA **early enough** before increasing the dose. Using the lowest effective dose of DA is prudent to minimize augmentation.

Approaches to augmentation are listed in Box 23–12. Low iron stores appear to increase the frequency or severity of augmentation so this problem should be treated if dopaminergic medications are being used.[80] If the patient is on LD/CD, the first approach would be to change to a DA. If the patient is on a DA and symptoms occur earlier in the evening, the medication dose could be split or another dose added earlier (e.g., pramipexole 0.125 mg at 6 PM and 9 PM). If the problem is morning symptoms, a morning dose could be added (bid to tid dosing). Sometimes a midday dose is not needed due to the "RLS protected time period" in the middle of the day. If RLS symptoms become more intense on the current dose of DA, approaches include an increase in dose (unless already on a high dose) or a switch to the other DA. Sometimes patients respond better to one DA than to the other. Many physicians would rather add another class of medication (an opiate or gabapentin) rather than increase the DA dose above a moderate level. If augmentation is severe or the current DA dose is high, the best approach is probably stopping the DA (although severe exacerbation of RLS can occur) and adding a high-potency opiate with or

indicate the need for additional medication. It can also be associated with defects in impulse control (compulsive gambling, hypersexuality, or compulsive shopping). While the dopamine dysregulation appears to be more common in Parkinson's disease than in RLS, the problem is increasingly reported as complication of DA treatment of RLS.[79] When the DAs are used to treat Parkinson's disease in much higher doses than those used to treat RLS, they can be associated with dyskinesias, hallucinations, or psychosis. The ergotamine-derived DAs (pergolide) are rarely used today. They are associated with severe nausea and, rarely, fibrotic syndromes.

without another class of medication. Clearly, the best approach is to not use LD/CD for daily RLS, use the lowest dose possible of the DA with slow upward titration, and correction of low iron stores (goal ferritin > 45–50 µg/L).

Opioids/Opiates

Opiates and opioid receptor agonists (tramadol) can be effective treatment for RLS.[70,81,82] They are fairly rapidly acting and can be used either singly or in combination with other medication groups such as DAs. Milder RLS may respond to low-potency opiates (propoxyphene, codeine) or opioid agonists (tramadol). Moderate to severe RLS may respond to high-potency opiates (hydrocodone, oxycodone, methadone). Hydrocodone is available in the United States in combination with acetaminophen (APAP). One must be cautious not to prescribe an excessive dose of APAP. For example, it is preferable to use hydrocodone/APAP 10/325 rather than 2 tablets of 5/325 mg. A maximum of 2 g of APAP/day can be used, although lower doses can be harmful if liver disease is present. Side effects of opiates include nausea and constipation. These medications should not be used with alcohol and should be used with caution in patients with OSA. Due to the potential of abuse and dependence, opiates are not the drugs of choice for daily RLS. However, studies and clinical experience suggest that dependence is not a problem if patients do not have a history of opiate dependence and take medication only at night. Typical doses of opiates/opioid agonists to treat RLS include tramadol 50 to 100 mg, propoxyphene napsylate 100 mg, hydrocodone 5 to 15 mg, oxycodone 5 to 15 mg, and methadone 5 to 15 mg (see Table 23–7).[70]

Anticonvulsant Medications

Although a number of these medications have been used (including carbamazepine, valproic acid, and gabapentin), gabapentin is preferred because of its better safety profile. Some consider gabapentin the drug of choice for patients with RLS associated with pain.[70] The efficacy of gabapentin has been demonstrated by uncontrolled[83] and controlled[84] trials in patients with RLS. One of these studies also reported a decrease in the PLMSI compared with placebo.[84] Patients reporting the symptoms of pain received the most benefit from gabapentin. The usual starting dose of gabapentin is 300 mg administered at night ½ to 1 hour before symptoms. The average effective dose is quite high (900–1500 mg) (Fig. 23–4). Side effects include sedation, fatigue, ataxia, nausea, and peripheral edema. Serious reactions include leukopenia, thrombocytopenia, and depression. A slow upward titration has been used in studies of gabapentin with an increase of 300 to 600 mg every 1 to 2 weeks. This may improve tolerance to relatively high doses of gabapentin. A controlled cross-over study demonstrated that gabapentin was effective treatment of RLS in renal failure patients on hemodialysis.[85] In this study, a dose of 200 to 300 mg was given after each dialysis session. Gabapentin is **cleared by the kidney so a**

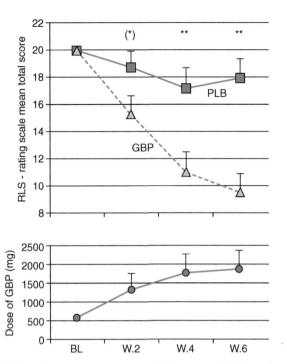

FIGURE 23–4 Change in restless legs syndrome (RLS) symptoms (RLS rating scale, see Box 23–8) on gabapentin (GBP) and placebo (PLB) during dose escalation. *P = NS; ** P < .05 GBP vs. PLB. Note that fairly high doses of GBP were needed to be effective. BL = baseline; W.2, W.4, W.6 after 2, 4, and 6 weeks of treatment. *From Garcia-Borreguero D, Larrosa O, de la Llave Y, et al: Treatment of restless legs syndrome with gabapentin. Neurology 2002;59:1573–1579.*

reduced dose is needed in patients with renal insufficiency. One problem with gabapentin is that there is large interpatient variability in absorption and plasma levels due to saturable absorption in the upper intestine. The prodrug gabapentin enacarbil (GEn, XP13512) is rapidly absorbed throughout the gastrointestinal tract and, once absorbed, is converted to gabapentin. This drug delays the time to peak gabapentin plasma levels and provides dose-proportional exposure. A placebo-controlled study demonstrated efficacy of GEn for RLS treatment.[86] This medication may be a treatment alternative in the future. A recent double-blind, placebo-controlled study found that pregabalin (Lyrica) in a mean dose of 333 mg was an effective treatment for RLS.[87] Treatment was started at 150 mg and increased as needed. Pregabalin (like gabapentin) is a ligand that binds to the α2δ (alpha2delta) subunit of the voltage-dependent calcium channel in the central nervous system. Pregabalin was developed as an anticonvulsant but is approved for treatment of neuropathic pain and fibromyalgia. Side effects include dizziness and drowsiness, blurred vision, and ataxia. It is more expensive than gabapentin but could be considered if a patient does not tolerate or improve with a DA and does not tolerate gabapentin.

Sedative Hypnotics

The BZRAs including both benzodiazepines (triazolam, temazepam, clonazepam) and nonbenzodiazepines

TABLE 23-8

Benzodiazepine Receptor Agonists and Periodic Limb Movement in Sleep/Periodic Limb Movement Disorder

MEDICATION/ STUDY	STUDY DESIGN	DISORDER	DECREASED PLMSI	SLEEP IMPROVED	IMPROVED SYMPTOMS
Clonazepam and temazepam Mitler, 1986[88]	Case series	PLMS	No	Sleep efficiency improved	Improved subjective sleep quality but not alertness
Clonazepam Peled, 1987[89]	Placebo-controlled	PLMS	Yes	Sleep latency decreased Sleep efficiency improved	N/A
Triazolam Bonnet, 1990[90]	Double-blind, placebo-controlled cross-over	PLMS with sleep fragmentation	No	Sleep efficiency increased Total sleep time increased	Objective daytime alertness improved
Triazolam Doghramji, 1991[91]	Cross-over, placebo-controlled	PLMS	No	Decreased PLM arousal index	Less daytime sleepiness MSLT
Clonazepam Saletu, 2001[92]	Placebo-controlled, single-blind with cross-over with clonazepam given first	PLMD and RLS	No	Yes	Improved subjective sleep quality

MSLT = multiple sleep latency test; N/A = not applicable; PLM = periodic limb movement; PLMD = periodic limb movement disorder; PLMS = periodic limb movement in sleep; PLMSI = periodic limb movement in sleep index; RLS = restless leg syndrome.

(zolpidem, zaleplon, eszopiclone) can be used for treatment of RLS or PLMD.[70,88–92] Clonazepam, a potent and long-acting BZRA, has been the most studied[88,89,92] (Table 23-8). The BZRAs work mainly by reducing the sleep latency, increasing sleep efficiency, and reducing the arousals due to PLMS. Most studies have NOT found a decrease in the PLMSI. Unfortunately, clonazepam can cause profound morning grogginess due to its long half-life. The BZRAs with a short duration of action (triazolam,[90,91] zaleplon, or zolpidem) or an intermediate duration of action (zolpidem-CR, eszopiclone, temazepam) are likely to be as effective and better tolerated. In patients with early morning awakening, a change from the shorter-acting to the medium-duration medications may be helpful. This class of medications should be used with caution in patients with OSA or severe lung disease. Side effects include hallucinations, sleep-related eating disorder, confusion, falls, morning grogginess, and unpleasant taste (eszopiclone).

RLS Treatment Algorithm

In choosing treatment, it is useful to classify the patient using the approach of Silber and coworkers[70] into the following groups: (1) mild/intermittent RLS symptoms, (2) daily RLS symptoms, and (3) refractory RLS symptoms (Table 23-9). The mild/intermittent group may be treated with conservative measures such as avoiding precipitating medications (sedating antihistamines) and substances (alcohol, caffeine), warm baths, and iron supplementation if there are low iron stores. If a RLS medication is used, it should be rapidly acting because the patient can often not predict that symptoms will

occur. LD/CD in the short-acting form is active within ½ hour and, therefore, is a good choice for treatment with intermittent RLS (that may not be predictable). A DA will be effective, although the time to onset is delayed for 1 to 3 hours. Ropinirole may have a more rapid effect than pramipexole. Other choices are low-potency opiates such as propoxyphene or codeine. Sedative-hypnotics may also be effective.

Daily RLS

Daily RLS of moderate severity requires a different approach from milder disease. Although LD/CD may be effective, it is associated with augmentation in 80% of the cases. In addition, due to the short duration of action, patients may have rebound (return of symptoms in the middle of the night or morning). The options are taking an additional short-acting LD/CD in the middle of the night or using a continuous-release LD/CD preparation. The longer-acting preparation has a slow onset. **One of the nonergotamine DAs (ropinirole or pramipexole) is considered the treatment of choice for daily/moderate to severe RLS.**[70]

The initial dose should be low (0.125 pramipexole 0.25 ropinirole) and given 2 hours before symptom onset. The dose can be slowly increased every 3 to 5 days. The usual effective dose ranges are 0.25 to 0.75 mg for pramipexole and 0.5 to 1.5 mg for ropinirole (higher doses have been used by some clinicians). If a given DA is not effective, the other should be tried because some patients respond better to either pramipexole or ropinirole. If the clinical response is inadequate or side effects prevent the use of the DA, a low- to moderate-potency opiate, gabapentin, or a sedative-hypnotic

TABLE 23–9

Treatment Algorithm for Restless Leg Syndrome

Mild/intermittent RLS	Nonpharmacologic	Abstain from caffeine, nicotine, alcohol. Iron replacement. Discontinue drugs (find alternate) that may worsen or cause RLS. Alerting activities.	
	Pharmacologic	Levodopa/carbidopa—rapid onset. DA—slow onset (2 hr). Low-potency opiates/opioid agonist (propoxyphene, tramadol). Sedative-hypnotic BZRA.	
Daily RLS	First choice	DA	• Ropinirole or pramipexole • If side effects or not effective, change to the other DA. • If side effects on both DAs, use second or third choice.
	Second choice	Opiates—low to high potency	• Low potency: propoxyphene, tramadol. • High potency: hydrocodone/APAP, oxycodone, methadone. • Use DA if unsuccessful.
	Third choice (unless pain or history of addiction)	Gabapentin Sedative-hypnotic	• Gabapentin may be first choice in patients with painful sensations. • Use DA if unsuccessful.
Refractory RLS RLS treated with DA then 1. Inadequate initial response 2. Response inadequate with time 3. Intolerable side effects 4. Augmentation	If DA is initially effective but augmentation develops.	• Split DA dose • Change to another DA	Ropinirole (0.25–1.5 mg) Pramipexole (0.125–0.75 mg)
	Moderate to severe augmentation or DA not tolerated	• Change to high-potency opiate	Oxycodone (5–15 mg), methadone (5–10 mg).
	Moderate to severe augmentation or DA not tolerated Pain prominent Addiction concerns	• Change to gabapentin	Start gabapentin 300–600 mg, lower in elderly, or renal failure. May require 1300–1800 mg
	Inadequate initial response DA only partially effective at moderate dose or highest tolerated dose.	• Add BZRA, opioid, or gabapentin to DA	Multiagent treatment may avoid use of high doses of a single agent.

APAP = acetaminophen; BZRA = benzodiazepine receptor agonist; DA = dopamine agonist; RLS = restless legs syndrome.

should be tried. If side effects are noted at higher doses of a DA, one might also combine a lower dose of DA with another class of medications. If the RLS is associated with pain, some physicians recommend starting with gabapentin instead of a DA.

Refractory/Severe RLS

Refractory RLS is defined as (1) inadequate initial response despite adequate dose (and timing of dose), (2) response has become inadequate over time, (3) intolerable side effects have occurred, or (4) augmentation is present. The approach to augmentation has already been discussed. Treatment approaches to refractory/severe RLS include (1) switch to another DA, (2) add an opioid, gabapentin, or BZRA, (3) change from a DA to gabapentin, or (4) change to a high-potency opioid. Because of the difficulty in treating severe augmentation, it is best to avoid very high doses of DAs if possible.

CLINICAL REVIEW QUESTIONS

1. A 40-year-old woman has nightly restless legs symptoms that delay her sleep onset. She was started on pramipexole 0.125 mg at bedtime and this was increased to 0.325 mg without much benefit. What do you recommend?

   A. Change to ropinirole.

   B. Increase pramipexole dose to 0.5 mg.

   C. Add tramadol 50 mg.

   D. Administer current dose of pramipexole earlier.

2. A 30-year-old woman has intermittent RLS on long car trips. Although these episodes occur infrequently, they are quite distressing. She has to stop and walk around every 100 miles or the symptoms become intolerable. A recent ferritin level was 100 µg/L. What do you recommend?

   A. Pramipexole 0.125 mg before long car trips.

   B. LD/CD 25/100 mg before long car trips.

   C. Iron supplementation.

   D. Gabapentin 100 mg before long car trips.

3. A 40-year-old man has developed severe RLS symptoms nearly every night. He was started on LD/CD 100/25 mg at bedtime with good initial response. When RLS symptoms returned, the dose was increased to 200/25. After 1 week on this dose, RLS symptoms were noted in both the arms and the legs and the symptoms started at 6 PM rather than 10 PM nightly. What do you recommend?

   A. Increase LD/CD to 300/75 mg.

   B. Take an earlier dose of LD/CD.

   C. Add oxycodone 5 mg nightly at bedtime.

   D. Stop LD/CD and start ropinirole at 0.25 mg.

4. A 25-year-old woman with daily RLS symptoms was started on pramipexole 0.125 mg and this was increased to 0.75 mg over several weeks. The patient feels that her RLS symptoms have improved but continue at a significant level. Her ferritin level is 100 µg/L. What do you recommend?

   A. Increase pramipexole to 1.0 mg.

   B. Switch to ropinirole 0.5 mg.

   C. Add oxycodone 5–10 mg.

   D. Add gabapentin 100 mg.

5. A patient with diabetic neuropathy reports RLS symptoms that are quite painful and distressing. There is a history of alcohol and valium dependence in the past. What do you recommend for initial treatment?

   A. Gabapentin 300 mg in the evening.

   B. Ropinirole 0.25 mg in the evening.

   C. Oxycodone 10 mg in the evening.

   D. Clonazepam 0.25 mg at bedtime.

6. A 50-year-old woman is currently taking pramipexole 1.0 mg and zolpidem 10 mg for severe symptoms of RLS. The symptoms were in fair control but are now present much earlier than when she started treatment. Initially, her symptoms began around 11 PM but now are noted as early as 8 PM. What do you recommend?

   A. Change to pramipexole 0.25 mg at 6 PM and 0.75 mg at 9 PM.

   B. Change from pramipexole to ropinirole.

   C. Add oxycodone 5 mg.

   D. Increase pramipexole dose.

7. A 50-year-old man with a history of snoring undergoes a split-night sleep study. The diagnostic portion shows an apnea-hypopnea index (AHI) of 50/hr. The CPAP titration finds that on CPAP of 10 cm H_2O the AHI is 5/hr. The PLMSI is 50/hr. The patient does not report symptoms of the RLS. The patient's wife does report that he kicks during sleep. What treatment do you recommend?

   A. CPAP of 10 cm H_2O and pramipexole.

   B. CPAP of 10 cm H_2O.

   C. CPAP of 10 cm H_2O and gabapentin.

   D. CPAP and iron supplementation.

8. Which of the following disorders has been associated with PLMS?

   A. Narcolepsy.

   B. RBD

   C. OSA.

   D. All of the above.

9. A 12-year-old boy has difficulty staying awake. He does NOT report an urge to move the legs or unusual sensations. His parents have noted that the patient is a restless sleeper, moves around in bed a lot, and sometimes snores. The patient is "fidgety" in school and has problems concentrating. A PSG is ordered to rule out OSA. The sleep study shows mild snoring, no apneas and hypopneas, and no elevation in end-tidal partial pressure of CO_2. The PLMS index is 15/hr. What is your diagnosis?

   A. RLS.

   B. Snoring.

   C. PLMD.

   D. ADHD.

Answers

1. **D.** Ropinirole and pramipexole should be given 2 hours before bedtime (or evening symptom onset). These medications have a slow onset of action. A higher dose of pramipexole could be needed but the first intervention is to have the patient take the medication earlier.

2. **B.** LD/CD is a useful medication for intermittent RLS owing to the rapid onset of action. However, the duration

of action is short and augmentation frequently occurs with daily use. Iron supplementation is recommended for RLS patients with a ferritin level <45–50 µg/L.

3. **D.** This patient has significant augmentation on LD/CD. This medication should be stopped and the patient changed to a DA. Low iron stores should also be ruled out by a ferritin level in this patient.

4. **C.** The patient is on a fairly high dose of pramipexole for RLS treatment. She is tolerating the medication but significant symptoms persist. It is possible that an increase to 1 mg pramipexole will be effective but could increase the risk of augmentation. However, some would argue that A is also a correct answer. A change to a different DA is another option. The equivalent dose of ropinirole is around twice that of pramipexole. Ropinirole at a dose of 0.5 mg is NOT an equivalent dose compared with pramipexole of 0.75 mg. To avoid the risk of augmentation, most clinicians avoid high doses of DAs. The addition of oxycodone 5 to 10 mg is probably the most effective option. The addition of a BZRA or gabapentin could be tried in this situation. However, 100 mg of gabapentin is unlikely to be effective.

5. **A.** The patient has a history of drug dependence; therefore, benzodiazepines and narcotics should be avoided. Gabapentin is recommended when RLS symptoms are painful. Ropinirole may be effective in this setting but may not improve symptoms of pain. Of note, gabapentin at a dose of 300 mg may not be effective. A dose of 900 to 1500 mg is often needed. Slow upward titration may reduce side effects.

6. **A.** The earlier onset of symptoms is a form of augmentation. Because pramipexole was fairly effective and well tolerated, the first intervention should be use of a split dose with a portion of the medication given earlier in the evening. If this is not effective, either B or C is a reasonable intervention. The patient is already on a high dose of pramipexole; therefore, a further increase in dose in the setting of augmentation is probably not indicated.

7. **B.** The patient has no RLS symptoms. PLMS is frequently associated with OSA and usually does not require treatment. Treatment with CPAP of 10 cm H_2O should be started. If frequent LMs persist and are significantly impairing sleep quality, treatment could then be considered. Iron supplementation should not be started without demonstration of low iron stores.

8. **D.** PLMS have been associated with narcolepsy, the RBD, and OSA.

9. **C.** PLMD. In pediatric patients, PLMD sometimes precedes symptoms of the RLS. A PLMSI of 15/hr might be of no significance in an adult but for a child is significantly elevated. There has been an association between ADHD and RLS/PLMD.

REFERENCES

1. Ondo W: Restless legs syndrome. Neurol Clin 2009;27: 779–799.
2. Trenkwalker C, Hogl B, Winkelmann J: Recent advances in the diagnosis, genetics, and treatment of restless legs syndrome. J Neurol 2009;256:539–543.
3. Coleman RM: Periodic movements in sleep (nocturnal myoclonus) and restless legs syndrome. In Guilleminault C (ed): Sleeping and Waking Disorders: Indications and Techniques. Boston: Butterworths, 1982, pp. 265–295.
4. Earley CJ: Restless legs syndrome. N Engl J Med 2003;348: 2103–2109.
5. Horynak M, Feige B, Riemann B, et al: Periodic leg movements in sleep and periodic limb movement disorder: prevalence, clinical significance, and treatment. Sleep Med Rev 2006; 10:169–177.
6. American Academy of Sleep Medicine: ICSD-2 International Classification of Sleep Disorders, 2nd ed. Diagnostic and Coding Manual. Westchester, IL: American Academy of Sleep Medicine, 2005.
7. Pennestri M, Whittom S, Adam B, et al: PLMS and PLMW in healthy subjects as a function of age: prevalence and interval distribution. Sleep 2006;29:1183–1187.
8. Scofield H, Roth T, Drake C: Periodic limb movements during sleep: population, prevalence, clinical correlates and racial differences. Sleep 2008;3:1221–1227.
9. Claman DM, Redline S, Blackwell T, et al: Prevalence and correlates of periodic limb movements in older women. J Clin Sleep Med 2006;2:438–445.
10. Ancoli-Israel S, Kripke DF, Klauber MR, et al: Periodic leg movements in sleep in community-dwelling elderly. Sleep 1991;14:496–500.
11. Walters AS: Toward a better definition of the restless leg syndrome. The International Restless Leg Syndrome Study Group. Mov Disord 1995;10:634–642.
12. Montplasir J, Boucher S, Poirer G, et al: Clinical, polysomnographic, and genetic characteristics of restless legs syndrome: a study of 133 patients diagnosed with new standard criteria. Mov Disord 1997;12:61–65.
13. Allen RP, Picchietti D, Hening W, et al: Restless legs syndrome: diagnostic criteria, special considerations, and epidemiology. A report from the Restless Legs Syndrome Diagnosis and Epidemiology Workshop at the National Institutes of Health. Sleep Med 2003;4:101–119.
14. Benes H, Walters AS, Allen RP, et al: Definition of restless legs syndrome, how to diagnose it, and how to differentiate it from RLS mimics. Mov Disord 2007;22:S401–S408.
15. Walters AS, Hening W, Rubinstein M, et al: A clinical and polysomnographic comparison of neuroleptic-induced akathisia and the idiopathic restless leg syndrome. Sleep 1991;14: 339–345.
16. Alvarez MV, Driver-Dunckely EE, Caviness JN, et al: Case series of painful legs and moving toes: clinical and electrophysiologic observations. Mov Disord 2008;23:2062–2066.
17. Sun ER, Chen CA, Ho G, et al: Iron and the restless legs syndrome. Sleep 1998;21:381–387.
18. Nofzinger EA, Fasiczka A, Berman S, Thase ME: Bupropion SR reduces periodic limb movements associated with arousal from sleep in depressed patients with period limb movement disorder. J Clin Psychiatry 2000;61:858–862.
19. Yang C, White DP, Winkleman JW: Antidepressants and periodic leg movements of sleep. Biol Psychiatry 2005;58:510–514.
20. Phillips B, Young T, Finn L, et al: Epidemiology of restless leg symptoms in adults. Arch Intern Med 2000;160:2137–2141.
21. Hening WA, Buchfuhrer MJ, Lee HB: Clinical Management of Restless Legs Syndrome. West Islip, NY: Professional Communications, 2008, pp. 53–57.

22. Desautels A, Turecki G, Montplaisir J, et al: Identification of major susceptibility locus for restless legs syndrome on chromosome 12q. Am J Hum Genet 2001;69:1266–1270.

23. Bonati MT, Ferini-Strambi L, Aridon P, et al: Autosomal dominant restless legs syndrome maps on chromosome 14q. Brain 2003;126:1485–1493.

24. Chen S, Ondo WB, Rao S, et al: Genome-wide linkage scan identifies a novel susceptibility locus for RLS on chromosome 9p. Am J Hum Genet 2004;74:876–885.

25. Levchenko A, Provost S, Montplaisir JY, et al: A novel autosomal dominant restless legs syndrome locus maps to chromosome 20p13. Neurology 2006;67:900–901.

26. Levchenko A, Montplaisir JY, Asseline G, et al: Autosomal dominant locus for RLS in French-Canadians on chromosome 16p12.1. Mov Disord 2009;24:40–50.

27. Pichler I, Marroni F, Volpato CG, et al: Linkage analysis identifies a novel locus of restless legs syndrome on chromosome 2q in a South Tyrolean population isolate. Am J Hum Genet 2006;70:716–723.

28. Winklemann J, Shormair B, Lichtner P, et al: Genome wide association study in restless legs syndrome identifies common variants in three genomic regions. Nat Genet 2007;39:1000–1006.

29. Stefannson H, Rye D, Hicks A: A genetic risk factor for periodic limb movements in sleep. N Engl J Med 2007;357:639–647.

30. Winklemann J, Lichtner P, Schormair B, et al: Variants in the neuronal nitric oxide synthetase (nNOS, NOS1) gene are associated with restless legs syndrome. Mov Disord 2007;23:350–358.

31. Paulus W, Dowling P, Rijsman R, et al: Update of the pathophysiology of the restless legs syndrome. Mov Disord 2007;S18:S431–S439.

32. Allen RP, Earley CJ: The role of iron in restless legs syndrome. Mov Disord 2007;22(Suppl 18):S440–S448.

33. Earley C, Connor JR, Beard JL, et al: Ferritin levels in cerebrospinal fluid and restless legs syndrome: effects of different clinical phenotypes. Sleep 2005;28:1069–1075.

34. Earley CJ, Barker PG, Horská A, Allen RP: MRI-determined regional brain iron concentration in early and late onset restless legs syndrome. Sleep Med 2006;7:459–461.

35. Hening W, Walters AS, Allen RP, et al: Impact, diagnosis and management of restless legs syndrome in a primary care population: the REST (RLS Epidemiology, Symptoms, and Treatment) Primary Care Study. Sleep Med 2004;5:237–246.

36. Allen RP, Walters AS, Montplaisir J, et al: Restless legs syndrome prevalence and impact. Arch Intern Med 2005;165:1286–1292.

37. Horynak M, Hundemer HP, Quail D, et al: Relationship of periodic leg movements and severity of RLS syndrome: a study in unmedicated and medicated patients. Clin Neurophysiol 2007;118:1532–1537.

38. International Restless Legs Syndrome Study Group: Validation of the international restless legs syndrome rating scale for the restless legs syndrome. Sleep Med 2003;4:121–122.

39. Hening WA, Allen RP: Restless legs syndrome: the continuing development of diagnostic standards and severity measures. Sleep Med 2003;4:95–97.

40. Picchietti D, Allen RP, Walters AS, et al: Restless legs syndrome: prevalence and impact in children and adolescents—The Peds REST Study. Pediatrics 2007;120:253–266.

41. Picchietti MA, Picchietti DL: Advances in pediatric restless legs syndrome: iron, genetics, diagnosis and treatment. Sleep Med 2010;11:643–651.

42. Simakakjornboon N, Kheirandish-Gozal L, Gozal D: Diagnosis and management of restless legs syndrome in children. Sleep Med Rev 2009;13:149–156.

43. Walters AS, Mandelbaum DE, Lewin DS, et al: Dopaminergic therapy in children with restless legs/periodic limb movements in sleep and ADHD. Dopaminergic Therapy Study Group. Pediatr Neurol 2000;22:182–186.

44. Cortese S, Lecendreux M, Arnulf I, et al: Restless legs syndrome and attention-deficit/hyperactivity disorder: a review of the literature. Sleep 2005;28:1007–1013.

45. The Atlas Task Force of the American Sleep Disorders Association: Recording and scoring leg movements. Sleep 1993;16:749–759.

46. Zucconi M, Ferri R, Allen R, et al: The official World Association of Sleep Medicine (WASM) standards for recording and scoring periodic leg movements in sleep (PLMS) and wakefulness (PLMW) developed in collaboration with a task force from the International Restless Legs Syndrome Study Group (IRLSSG). Sleep Med 2006;7:175–183.

47. Iber C, Ancoli-Israel S, Chesson A, Quan SF, for the American Academy of Sleep Medicine: The AASM Manual for the Scoring of Sleep and Associated Events: Rules, Terminology and Technical Specification, 1st ed. Westchester, IL: American Academy of Sleep Medicine, 2007, pp. 41–42.

48. American Sleep Disorders Association: International Classification of Sleep Disorders, 1st ed. Rochester, MN: American Sleep Disorders Association, 1990.

49. Pollmacher T, Schulz H: Periodic leg movements: their relationship to sleep stages. Sleep 1993;16:572–577.

50. Culpepper WJ, Badia P, Shaffer JI: Time of night patterns in PLMS activity. Sleep 1992;15:306–311.

51. Dickel MJ, Renfrow SD, Moore PT, Berry RB: Rapid eye movement sleep periodic leg movements in patients with spinal cord injury. Sleep 1994;17:733–738.

52. Manconi M, Ferri R, Zucconi M, et al: Time structure analysis of leg movements during sleep in REM sleep behavior disorder. Sleep 2007;30:1779–1785.

53. Fantini ML, Michaud M, Gosseline N, et al: Periodic leg movements in REM sleep behavior disorder and related autonomic and EEG activation. Neurology 2002;59:1889–1894.

54. Michauld M, Poirer G, Lavigne G, Montplasir J: Restless legs syndrome: scoring criteria for leg movements recorded during the suggested immobilization test. Sleep Med 2001;2:317–321.

55. Karadeniz D, Ondze B, Besset A, Billiard M: EEG arousals and awakenings in relations with periodic leg movements during sleep. J Sleep Res 2000;9:273–277.

56. Sforza E, Nicolas A, Lavigne G, et al: EEG and cardiac activation during periodic leg movements in sleep. Neurology 1999;52:786–792.

57. Ali NJ, Davies RJO, Fleetham JA, Stradling JR: Periodic movements of the legs during sleep associated with rises in systemic blood pressure. Sleep 1991;14:163–165.

58. Montplasir J, Boucher S, Grosselin A, et al: Persistence of repetitive EEG arousals (K-alpha complexes) in RLS patients treated with L-dopa. Sleep 1996;19:196–199.

59. Montplasir J, Michaud M, Denesle R, Gosseline A: Periodic leg movements are not more prevalent in insomnia of hypersomnia but are specifically associated with sleep disorders involving a dopaminergic impairment. Sleep Med 2000;1:163–167.

60. Mendelson WB: Are periodic leg movements associated with clinical sleep disturbance? Sleep 1996;19:219–223.

61. Mahowald MW: Periodic limb movements are NOT associated with disturbed sleep. J Clin Sleep Med 2007;3:15–17.

62. Hogl B: Periodic limb movements are associated with disturbed sleep. J Clin Sleep Med 2007;3:12–14.

63. Carrier J, Frenette S, Montplasir J, et al: Effects of periodic leg movements during sleep in middle aged subjects without sleep complaints. Mov Disord 2005;20:1127–1132.

64. Fry JM, DiPhillipo MA, Pressman MR: Periodic leg movements in sleep following treatment of obstructive sleep apnea with nasal continuous positive airway pressure. Chest 1989;96:89–91.

65. Chervin RD: Periodic leg movements and sleepiness in patients evaluated for sleep-disordered breathing. Am J Respir Crit Care Med 2001;164:1454–1458.
66. Exner EN, Collop NA: The association of upper airway resistance with periodic limb movement. Sleep 2000;24:188–192.
67. Baran AS, Allen RC, Douglass AB, et al: Change in periodic limb movement index during treatment of obstructive sleep apnea with continuous positive airway pressure. Sleep 2003; 26:717–720.
68. Hening WA, Allen RP, Earley CJ, et al: An update on the dopaminergic treatment of restless legs syndrome and periodic limb movement disorder. Sleep 2004;27:560–583.
69. Littner MR, Kushida C, Anderson WM, et al: Practice parameters for the dopaminergic treatment of restless legs syndrome and periodic limb movement disorder. Sleep 2004; 27:557–559.
70. Silber MH, Ehrenberg BL, Allen RP, et al: An algorithm for the management of restless legs syndrome. Mayo Clin Proc 2004;79:916–922.
71. Becker PM, Jamieson AO, Brown WD: Dopaminergic agents in restless leg syndrome and periodic leg movements of sleep: response and complications of extended treatment in 49 cases. Sleep 1993;16:713–716.
72. Earley CJ, Allen RP: Pergolide and carbidopa/levodopa periodic leg movements in sleep in a consecutive series of patients. Sleep 1996;19:801–810.
73. Montplaisir J, Nicolas A, Denesle R, et al: Restless leg syndrome improved by pramipexole: a double-blind randomized trial. Neurology 1999;52:938–943.
74. Montplaisir J, Denesle R, Petit D: Pramipexole in the treatment of restless leg syndrome: a follow-up study. Eur J Neurol 2000; 1:27–31.
75. Adler CH, Hauser RA, Sethi K, et al: Ropinirole for restless legs syndrome. Neurology 2004;62:1405–1407.
76. Allen R, Becker PM, Bogan R, et al: Ropinirole decreases periodic leg movements and improves sleep parameters in patients with restless legs syndrome. Sleep 2004;27:907–914.
77. Saletu M, Anderer P, Saletu B, et al: Sleep laboratory studies in periodic limb movement disorder (PLMD) patients as compared to normals and acute effects of ropinirole. Hum Psychopharm 2001;16:177–187.
78. Winklemann JW, Johnson L: Augmentation and tolerance with long-term pramipexole treatment of restless legs syndrome. Sleep Med 2004;5:9–14.
79. Cornelius JR, Tippmann-Peikert M, Slocumb NL, et al: Impulse control disorders with the use of dopaminergic agents in restless legs syndrome: a case-control study. Sleep 2010;33:81–87.
80. Trenkwalder C, Hogl B, Benes H, et al: Augmentation in restless legs syndrome is associated with low ferritin. Sleep Med 2008;9:572–574.
81. Walters AS, Wagner ML, Hening WA, et al: Successful treatment of the idiopathic restless leg syndrome in a randomized double-blind trial of oxycodone versus placebo. Sleep 1993; 16:327–332.
82. Kaplan PW, Allen RP, Bucholz DW, Walters JK: A double-blind, placebo-controlled study of the treatment of periodic limb movements in sleep using carbidopa/levodopa and propoxyphene. Sleep 1993;16:717–723.
83. Happe S, Sauter C, Klosch G, et al: Gabapentin versus ropinirole in the treatment of idiopathic restless legs syndrome. Neuropsychobiology 2003;48:82–86.
84. Garcia-Borreguero D, Larrosa O, de la Llave Y, et al: Treatment of restless legs syndrome with gabapentin. Neurology 2002; 59:1573–1579.
85. Thorp ML, Morris CD, Bagby SP: A crossover study of gabapentin in treatment of restless legs syndrome among hemodialysis patients. Am J Kidney Dis 2001;38:104–108.
86. Kushida CA, Becker PM, Ellengoben AL, et al: Randomized, double-blind, placebo-controlled study of XP135412/GSK1838262 in patients with RLS. Neurology 2009;72: 439–446.
87. Garcia-Borreguero D, Larrosa O, Williams AM, et al: Treatment of restless legs syndrome with pregabalin: a double-blind, placebo-controlled study. Neurology 2010;74:1897–1904.
88. Mitler MM, Browman CP, Menn SJ, et al: Nocturnal myoclonus: treatment efficacy of clonazepam and temazepam. Sleep 1986;9:385–392.
89. Peled R, Lavie P: Double-blind evaluation of clonazepam on periodic leg movements in sleep. J Neurol Neurosurg Psychiatry 1987;50:1679–1681.
90. Bonnet MH, Arand DL: The use of triazolam in older patients with periodic leg movements, fragmented sleep, and daytime sleepiness. J Gerontol 1990;45:M139–M144.
91. Doghramji K, Browman CP, Gaddy JR, et al: Triazolam diminishes daytime sleepiness and sleep fragmentation in patients with periodic leg movements in sleep. J Clin Psychopharmacol 1991;11:284–290.
92. Saletu M, Anderer P, Saletu-Zyhalrz G, et al: Restless legs syndrome (RLS) and periodic limb movement disorder (PLMD): acute placebo-controlled sleep laboratory study with clonazepam. Eur Neuropsychopharmacol 2001;11:153–161.

Chapter 24

Hypersomnias of Central Origin

Chapter Points

- N+C and N–C are two disorders characterized by EDS and symptoms related to the abnormal regulation of wake and sleep. A short REM latency and intrusion of REM sleep features into wake are characteristic of the disorders.
- Cataplexy is characterized by temporary muscle weakness induced by emotional stimuli. The affected individual is conscious and the duration of weakness is usually seconds to minutes. Hearing or telling a joke and laughter are the most common triggers.
- Approximately 60–70% of patients with narcolepsy have cataplexy.
- Cataplexy is the only symptom virtually specific for narcolepsy. Cataplexy in the absence of narcolepsy occurs only in patients with a few rare genetic disorders. Patients with these disorders have abnormal neurological function.
- Approximately 90–95% of patients with N+C have low or absent Hcrt1 in the CSF and absent Hcrt-producing neurons in the lateral hypothalamus.
- Other manifestations of narcolepsy include sleep paralysis, sleep-related hallucination, automatic behavior, disturbed sleep, and the RBD.
- The hallucinations of narcolepsy that occur at nocturnal sleep onset are called **hypnagogic hallucinations** and those on awakening are termed **hypnopompic hallucinations.**
- For N+C, the MSLT is confirmatory. The diagnosis of N–C depends on demonstration of sleep-onset REM periods in the absence of other sleep disorders (such as sleep apnea) that can cause a short REM latency.
- The MSLT criteria for narcolepsy are a mean sleep latency ≤ 8 min and two or more sleep-onset REM periods.
- IH with a long sleep time in contrast to IH without a long sleep time is characterized by a typical sleep duration of longer than 10 hours. The diagnosis depends on exclusion of other disorders that could explain the EDS.
- The MSLT criteria for IH are mean sleep latency <8 minutes and fewer than 2 sleep REM-onset periods.
- Treatments for the EDS of narcolepsy include modafinil (and armodafinil), stimulants (methylphenidate and others), and sodium oxybate.

- Treatments for cataplexy include sodium oxybate (FDA approved) and non–FDA-approved medications including TCAs, SSRIs, and SNRIs. These medications also decrease sleep paralysis and HHs.
- Treatments for the EDS of IH include modafinil (armodafinil) and stimulants.

The hypersomnias of central origin are those conditions in which hypersomnia is due to dysfunction of the central nervous system (CNS). The dysfunction is not due to sleep-related breathing disorders (SRBDs), circadian rhythm sleep disorders, or other causes of disturbed nocturnal sleep. Although the nocturnal sleep in some of these disorders is not normal, the daytime sleepiness is out of proportion to the degree of sleep disturbance. The International Classification of Sleep Disorders, 2nd edition (ICSD-2)[1] lists a number of disorders in the category "Hypersomnias of Central Origin" (Box 24–1). This chapter discusses the disorders with the emphasis on narcolepsy with and without cataplexy.

NARCOLEPSY SYNDROMES

Narcolepsy is a chronic disorder characterized by excessive daytime sleepiness (EDS) and symptoms related to the abnormal regulation of wakefulness and sleep. It is characterized by a short rapid eye movement (REM) latency and intrusion of REM sleep features into the waking state. Approximately 60% to 70% of all patients with narcolepsy have cataplexy.[1-4] Cataplexy consists of temporary muscle weakness following emotional stimuli. Narcolepsy with cataplexy (N+C) and narcolepsy without cataplexy (N–C) are now classified as two distinct disorders but share many of the same features[1-4] (Table 24–1).

As the name implies, definitive *cataplexy* is present in patients with N+C. Following the discovery of hypocretin (Orexin) peptides in 1998,[5,6] it was learned that the majority of patients with N+C have low or undetectable levels of **hypocretin-1 (Hcrt1)** in the cerebrospinal fluid (CSF).[7] However, much more much remains to be determined about the pathophysiology of narcolepsy. In the absence of cataplexy, a diagnosis of N–C depends on demonstration of sleep-onset REM (very short REM latency) and an absence of other disorders to explain this finding.[1-4]

BOX 24-1

Hypersomnias of Central Origin

1. Narcolepsy with cataplexy
2. Narcolepsy without cataplexy
3. Narcolepsy due to medical condition
4. Narcolepsy unspecified
5. Idiopathic hypersomnia with long sleep time
6. Idiopathic hypersomnia without long sleep time
7. Recurrent hypersomnia
8. Behaviorally induced insufficient sleep
9. Hypersomnia due to medical condition
10. Hypersomnia due to drug or substance
11. Hypersomnia not due to substance or known physiologic condition (including hypersomnia due to mental disorder) (nonorganic hypersomnia [NOS])
12. Physiologic (organic) hypersomnia, unspecified

From American Academy of Sleep Medicine: International Classification of Sleep Disorders, 2nd ed. Diagnostic and Coding Manual. Westchester, IL: American Academy of Sleep Medicine, 2005.

History

The key symptoms of narcolepsy were described by Westphal in 1877.[8] The term *narcolepsy,* meaning "to seize with drowsiness," was coined by Gelinau.[8] Aidie termed the loss of muscle tone as "cataplexy" in the early 20th century.[9] Yoss and Daly[10] described the classic tetrad of daytime sleepiness, cataplexy, hypnagogic hallucinations, and sleep paralysis (SP). In 1960, Vogel[11] reported that sleep-onset REM periods were associated with narcolepsy. Initially, the association of narcolepsy with the human leukocyte antigen (HLA) DR2 antigen was described in Japanese patients.[12] Later, the HLA DQB1*0602 was found to be strongly associated with narcolepsy in white and African American populations.[13] In 1998, two groups simultaneously reported the existence of hypocretin (Orexin) peptides present in the lateral and posterior hypothalamus.[5,6] Cleavage of a single precursor protein produces the peptides hypocretin-1 (Orexin A) and hypocretin-2 (Orexin B). In 2000, the association of narcolepsy with cataplexy and low or undetectable levels of CSF Hcrt1 was described.[7]

TABLE 24-1
Features of Narcolepsy

FEATURES OF NARCOLEPSY	COMMENTS	SPECIFIC FOR NARCOLEPSY?
CLASSIC TETRAD SYMPTOMS		
EDS	• Continuous daytime sleepiness, with exacerbations (sleep attacks). • Usually first symptom. • Present in virtually 100% of narcolepsy patients.	No
Cataplexy	• Muscle weakness triggered by emotion. • Most common triggers: hearing or telling a joke. • Onset usually occurs within a few years of the onset of sleepiness. • Duration: Seconds to minutes. • Consciousness preserved at least at beginning of episodes. • Present in 60-70% of patients with narcolepsy.	Yes
Hypnagogic (at sleep onset) or hypnapompic (on awakening) hallucinations	• Vivid dreamlike images that occur at sleep-wake transitions. • Duration: Several minutes. • Can be associated with SP.	No
Sleep paralysis	• A partial or complete paralysis of the skeletal muscles that occurs at sleep onset or sleep offset. • Can be associated with HPH > HH. The patient is awake but can't move. • Can be associated with dyspnea, although the diaphragm is not affected. • Duration: A few seconds to several minutes.	No
OTHER MANIFESTATIONS OF NARCOLEPSY		
Disturbed nocturnal sleep	• Increased stage N1. • Frequent awakenings. • 20-30% have short **nocturnal** REM latency (<15 min). • PLMS is common.	No
Automatic behavior	• Semipurposeful activity with amnesia.	No
REM sleep behavior disorder	• Dream enactment—often violent, REM without atonia.	No

EDS = excessive daytime sleepiness; HH = hypnagogic hallucinations; HPH = hypnopompic hallucinations; PLMS = periodic limb movements during sleep; REM = rapid eye movement; SP = sleep paralysis.

Epidemiology

Narcolepsy is present in about 1/2000 persons. Approximately 60% to 70% of patients with narcolepsy have cataplexy.[14] Men and women are affected equally. The average age of onset in most studies is between 20 and 30 years. However, narcolepsy can begin at any age. Dauvilliers and coworkers[15] found two peaks in the age of onset with one around age 15 and the other around 35 years of age.

Genetics

Familial canine narcolepsy is transmitted as a single autosomal recessive gene (canarc-1) with complete penetrance.[16] This form of narcolepsy is due to an abnormal Hcrt2 receptor. However, the human form of the narcolepsy is not a simple genetic disease. Although the majority of cases of human narcolepsy are sporadic, there have been numerous reports of familial narcolepsy in the literature.[16,17] Studies of families of patients with narcolepsy revealed that the risk of a first-degree relative of a narcoleptic developing N+C is 1% to 2%, a 10 to 40 times higher risk than in the general population.[16] However, studies of identical twins show a high degree of **discordance** for N+C. That is, if one twin has narcolepsy, the other twin will have or develop narcolepsy only about 25% to 31% of the time[16] (Table 24–2). Thus, factors other than genetics are important for the development of human narcolepsy.

HLA Typing

N+C is strongly linked to specific HLAs. Approximately 90% to 95% of patients with N+C have the DQB1*0602 allele regardless of race[16] (see Table 24–2). However, this allele is present in about 12% of Japanese, 25% of whites, and 38% of African Americans *without the syndrome.* The percentage of patients with N–C that are DQB1*0602 positive is lower (40–60%). In general, patients with narcolepsy who are DQB1*602-positive have more severe symptoms.[2]

Importance of Hcrt Neurons

Hcrt neurons located in the lateral or posterior hypothalamus project widely in the CNS (Fig. 24–1A). They augment

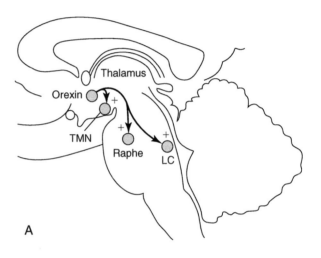

A

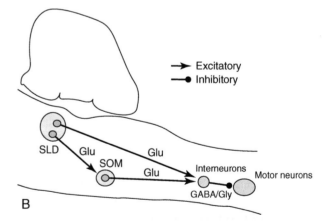

B

FIGURE 24–1 **A,** Orexin (Hypocretin) neurons in the hypothalamus project widely to many brain areas responsible for maintenance of wakefulness including the tuberomammillary nucleus (TMN), dorsal raphe, and locus coeruleus (LC). **B,** Possible pathways mediating atonia of REM sleep. Neurons in the atonia areas of the pons, the sublateral dorsal nucleus (SLD), project directly to interneurons in the spinal cord that inhibit motor neurons. An indirect pathway via the supraolivary medulla (SOM) is also illustrated. Other pathways are also likely important. The atonia neurons are glutaminergic and the inhibitory spinal cord interneurons secrete glycine (Gly) and gamma-aminobutyric acid (GABA). Glu = glucose. *A, Adapted from Scammell TE: The neurobiology, diagnosis, and treatment of narcolepsy. Ann Neurol 2003;53:154–166. B, Vetrivelan R, Fuller PM, Tong Q, Lu J: Medullary circuitry regulating rapid eye movement sleep and motor atonia. J Neurosci 2009;29:9361–9369.*

TABLE 24–2	
Narcolepsy Facts	
INCIDENCE OF NARCOLEPSY	1/2000
FAMILIAL RELATIONSHIP	**RISK FOR DEVELOPING NARCOLEPSY**
Identical twin has narcolepsy with cataplexy.	25–31% of other twin has narcolepsy.
First-degree relative has narcolepsy.	1–2% (10–40 × higher risk).
HLA ANTIGEN PREVALENCE	**HLA DQB1*0602 POSITIVE**
General population.	12–38%.
N+C.	90% (≤10% negative).
N–C.	40–60%.
HYPOCRETIN	**CSF HYPOCRETIN-1**
N+C	Absent or low 90–100%. Normal in up to 10%.
N–C	90% normal levels. 5–10% reduced levels (most + for DQB1*0602).

CSF = cerebrospinal fluid; HLA = human leukocyte antigen; N+C = narcolepsy with cataplexy; N–C = narcolepsy without cataplexy.

the activity of brain areas active during wakefulness (tuber-omammillary nucleus [TMN]—histamine, locus coeruleus—norepinephrine [NE], and dorsal raphe—serotonin).[18-23] Their activity is believed to stabilize the sleep-wake system to prevent abrupt transitions between sleep and wakefulness. Histaminergic neurons are located exclusively in the TMN of the posterior hypothalamus and project to various brain regions associated with regulation of sleep-wake cycles. Activity of these histaminergic neurons is believed to help promote wakefulness. Hcrt neurons project to the TMN and stimulate the TMN neurons via Hcrt2 receptors.

Pathophysiology of Narcolepsy

N+C Group

As noted previously, canine N+C is usually secondary to a defect in the receptor for Hcrt2. Human N+C is associated with absent or very low CSF levels of Hcrt1 (90–100% of patients).[15,24-26] Brains of patients with N+C have reduced staining for Hcrt in the hypothalamus.[27,28] N+C is associated with a loss of approximately 90% of Hcrt neurons. Melanin-concentrating hormone neurons, which are intermixed with Hcrt cells in the normal brain, were not reduced in number, indicating that cell loss is relatively specific for Hcrt neurons. It is believed that hypothalamic Hcrt cells are destroyed before disease onset. Mutations in Hcrt genes do not appear to be the cause of most human narcolepsy.[29] Of note, up to 10% of patients with N+C have normal CSF Hcrt1 levels.[25,26] Thus, other abnormalities of the Hcrt system or other mechanisms must be the cause of the syndrome in these patients. The cause of the loss of Hcrt cells in patients with N+C is unknown. Because of the association of narcolepsy with HLA antigens, an autoimmune mechanism has been hypothesized but has been difficult to document.[30] Elevated anti-streptococcal antibodies were found in one study of patients with recent narcolepsy onset.[31] Another study found that narcolepsy is also associated with a polymorphism in the T-cell receptor alpha gene.[32] Recently, several studies have found that some patients with narcolepsy have elevated levels of antibodies against a protein known as *Tribbles homolog 2 (TRIB2)*.[33-35] In one study, antibodies were found in about 25% of patients with N+C but in only 3.5% in patients with N–C or 4.5% in normal controls.[35] The presence of TRIB2 antibodies was associated with a short duration since disease onset (recent onset of narcolepsy). TRIB2 is produced in Hcrt neurons, providing some of the firmest evidence yet for an autoimmune cause of narcolepsy. However, whether the Tribbles antibodies cause Hcrt damage, occur secondary to damage of the Hcrt neurons, or are simply an associated phenomenon secondary to another cause of Hcrt neuron injury is unknown.[36]

Two investigations have documented low CSF histamine in patients with narcolepsy (with and without cataplexy) and idiopathic hypersomnia (IH).[37,38] As noted previously, histamine secretion is believed important for maintaining wakefulness. It is not clear whether low CSF histamine is a cause or an effect of EDS in these patients. Recall that Hcrt neurons stimulate histaminergic neurons in the TMN. However, CSF histamine was low even in patients **without** Hcrt ligand deficiency (N–C and IH). Therefore, other defects beside Hcrt deficiency must be involved in producing low CSF histamine levels.

N–C Group

The pathophysiology of N–C is not well understood. A small percentage (5–10%) of N–C patients have a reduced CSF Hcrt (most are positive for HLA DQB1*0602). N–C patients negative for the HLA DQB1*0602 almost always have normal CSF Hcrt1 levels.[7,25,26] The etiology of N–C is currently unknown but may represent a dysfunction of the Hcrt system without total loss of Hcrt-producing cells. Thannickal and coworkers[39] examined the brain of one patient with N–C and found a 33% reduction in hypocretin cells (compared to normals) with maximal loss in the posterior hypothalamus. Thus, partial loss of Hcrt neurons and other alterations in the Hcrt system without a reduction in CSF Hcrt could be the etiology of N–C. As noted previously, CSF histamine is low in N–C patients.[37,38] This may be a marker of hypersomnia, or reduced histamine secretion could be part of the pathogenesis of the disorder.

Mechanisms of Cataplexy

The mechanisms inducing cataplexy are still under investigation.[40-42] The atonia of REM sleep is thought to be due to inhibition of the spinal alpha motor neurons of the anterior horn cells by glycine and gamma-aminobutyric acid (GABA) secreted by spinal interneurons (see Fig. 24–1B). The interneurons are activated directly by projections from areas in the pons responsible for atonia or via an intermediate relay area in the ventral medulla. Glutamate is believed to activate the spinal interneurons. The atonia neurons of the pontine reticular formation are located ventral to the locus coeruleus and are often called the *subcoeruleus (SubC)* or *sublaterodorsal nucleus (SLD)*. The neurons are believed to be glutaminergic. During REM sleep, there also appears to be inhibition of pathways normally promoting alpha motor neuron activity.

Cataplexy and the atonia of REM sleep may share some common pathways, but there are important differences. John and colleagues[41] reported that histaminergic neurons in the ventral posterior lateral hypothalamus remain active during cataplexy as opposed to REM sleep (Fig. 24–2). Because histamine is associated with wakefulness, this may at least partially explain why patients remain conscious during cataplexy but not REM sleep. The other important difference between REM-associated atonia and cataplexy is the triggering emotional stimulus for cataplexy. Neural pathways involving the amygdala are thought to be important for the emotional induction of cataplexy.

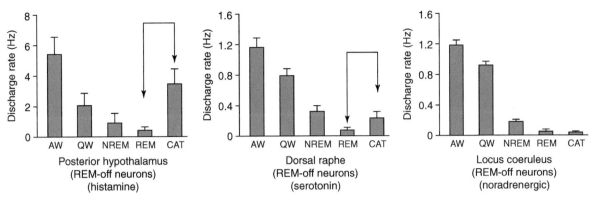

FIGURE 24−2 Posterior hypothalamic (histaminergic) neurons remained active during cataplexy (CAT) whereas dorsal raphe (serotonergic) reduced discharge and locus coeruleus neurons (noradrenergic) nearly ceased discharge. Note the difference between rapid eye movement (REM) and cataplexy for posterior hypothalamic neurons and dorsal raphe neurons. AW = active wake; NREM = non−rapid eye movement; QW = quiet wake. *From John J, Wu MF, Boehmer LN, Siegel JM: Cataplexy-active neurons in the hypothalamus: implications for the role of histamine in sleep and waking behavior. Neuron 2004;42:619−634.*

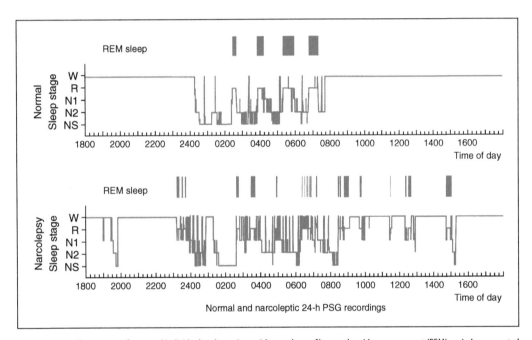

FIGURE 24−3 Hypnogram of a normal individual and a patient with narcolepsy. Sleep and rapid eye movement (REM) periods were noted throughout the day in the patient with narcolepsy. PSG = polysomnography. *From Rogers AE, Aldrich MS, Caruso CC: Patterns of sleep and wakefulness in treated narcolepsy subjects. Sleep 1994;17:590−597.*

Manifestations of Narcolepsy

Similarities and differences between N+C, N−C, and IH are outlined in Table 24-3. IH is discussed in detail in a later section.

Excessive Daytime Sleepiness (N+C and N−C)

The EDS of narcolepsy can occur as discrete "sleep attacks" or as constant sleepiness with intermittent worsening. Unrelenting EDS is usually the *first and most prominent symptom of narcolepsy*.[1−4,43] Sleepiness may occur throughout the day, regardless of the amount or quality of prior nighttime sleep. Sleep episodes may occur at work and social events, while eating, talking, and driving, and in other similarly inappropriate situations. Napping is usually restorative but provides only temporary relief. It has been said that falling asleep while standing or eating is especially suggestive of narcolepsy. Even though patients may sleep at every hour of the day, the total sleep time over a 24-hour period is normal or only slightly increased.[44,45] Rogers and associates[44] performed 24-hour polysomnography (PSG) in a group of narcolepsy patients who were "well controlled." Of 25 subjects with narcolepsy, 10 had no daytime sleep but the other 14 averaged 2.7 naps and 76.2 minutes of sleep during the day (compared with 4.8 min for controls).[44] The two groups did not differ in the total amount of sleep or the total amount of REM sleep in 24 hours. Figure 24−3 compares the 24-hour

TABLE 24-3

Features of Narcolepsy Syndromes versus Idiopathic Hypersomnia

	N+C	N–C	IH
SYMPTOMS			
Daytime sleepiness	Yes	Yes	Yes
Hypnagogic hallucinations (%)	70–86	15–60	40
Sleep paralysis (%)	50–70	25–60	40–50
POLYSOMNOGRAPHY			
Sleep latency	Short	Short	Variable
Nocturnal REM latency < 15 min	33%[†]	24%[†]	Normal REM latency
Disturbed nighttime sleep	Yes	Yes	No
Sleep efficiency (%)*	81	91	93
Stage N1 sleep	Increased	Mildly increased	Normal
24-hr total sleep time	Normal to slight increase	Normal to slight increase	Very increased in patients with IH with long sleep time
MSLT			
Mean sleep latency (min)	2.7[§]	3.5[§]	6.2 ± 3.0[‡]
Sleep-onset REM periods (N)	≥2 (3–3.7 SOREMPs)[§]	≥2 (2–3.3 SOREMPs)[§]	0–1
DQB1*0602 (% positive)	90–100	40–60	52
CSF hypocretin-1	Undetectable in 90–95% ≤10% normal	Normal in 90% Reduced in 5–10%	Normal
Neuropathology	Marked reduction in hypocretin neurons	Unknown	Unknown
Body mass index	Increased in 5–15%	Normal	Normal

*Sleep efficiency = total sleep time/total recording time.
[†]From Aldrich MS, Chervin RD, Malow BA: Value of the multiple sleep latency test (MSLT) for the diagnosis of narcolepsy. Sleep 1997;20:620–629.
[‡]From Arand D, Bonnet M, Hurwitz T, et al: A review by the MSLT and MWT Task Force of the Standards of Practice Committee of the AASM. The clinical use of the MSLT and MWT. Sleep 2005;28:123–147.
[§]From Scammel TE: The neurobiology, diagnosis, and treatment of narcolepsy. Ann Neurol 2003;53:154–166.
CSF = cerebrospinal fluid; IH = idiopathic hypersomnia; MSLT = multiple sleep latency test; N+C = narcolepsy with cataplexy; N–C = narcolepsy without cataplexy; REM = rapid eye movement; SOREMPs = sleep-onset rapid eye movement periods.
Adapted from Scammel TE: The neurobiology, diagnosis, and treatment of narcolepsy. Ann Neurol 2003;53:154–166, with permission.

hypnograms of a patient with narcolepsy and a normal subject. The hypnogram shows sleep episodes scattered throughout the day, and some of the daytime sleep episodes contain REM sleep.

In a study comparing narcoleptics and normal subjects using 24-hour ambulatory monitoring, Broughton and coworkers[45] found no increase in the total amount of sleep in 24 hours. However, narcoleptics had more daytime and less nighttime sleep than normal persons.

Sleep-Related Hallucinations (N+C and N–C)

The sleep-related hallucinations of narcolepsy that occur at nocturnal sleep onset are called **hypnagogic hallucinations (HGHs)** and those on awakening are termed **hypnopompic hallucinations (HPHs)**. The hallucinations are typically bizarre and may be frightening. Patients sometimes have a fair degree of insight that they are hallucinatory in nature, but often consider them no less frightening. The duration is usually less than 10 minutes, and the frequency is quite variable. Visual imagery is the predominant feature for many patients, sometimes with intense colors. A commonly described vision is that of an animal or stranger in the room. Auditory or vestibular hallucinations (sensation of falling) may also occur. The percentage of narcolepsy patients reporting sleep-related hallucinations varies from 20% to 70% depending on whether data are obtained from questionnaire or physician interview.[2-4] A questionnaire study by Aldrich[4] found the proportion of N+C patients reporting sleep-related hallucinations was higher than in the N–C or IH groups. Sleep-related hallucinations (especially HPH) can be associated with SP (discussed in the next section) and can also occur in normal individuals.

Sleep Paralysis (N+C and N–C)

SP is partial or complete paralysis during the onset of sleep or upon awakening. Patients are awake and conscious during the attack. There is no emotional precipitant. The episodes may last longer than a typical cataplectic attack. People who experience SP sometimes experience hallucinations simultaneously. Studies have found that up to 50% to 80% of patients with N+C report SP, with a lower percentage in the N–C group.[4,43]

Adequate ventilation is maintained during SP because diaphragmatic function is spared. However, some patients have a sensation of dyspnea. SP is often very frightening owing to the inability to move, speak, or communicate during the episode. SP is also reported in patients with sleep apnea and occasionally in normal subjects especially after periods of sleep deprivation. **A syndrome of isolated recurrent SP (narcolepsy not present) exists and can be very problematic for affected individuals.**

Disturbed Nocturnal Sleep and Other Symptoms: N+C, N–C

Although HH/HPH, SP, and daytime sleepiness are the classic narcolepsy symptoms, patients often report other associated symptoms that can be significant (see Table 24–1). Narcolepsy patients often experience **disturbed nighttime sleep** with tossing and turning in bed, leg jerks, nightmares, and frequent awakenings. The amount of stage N1 sleep is increased. In general, N+C patients have more disturbed sleep than N–C patients.[1-4] **Automatic behavior** is present in up to 50% of patients. Automatic behavior is defined as performing a seemingly purposeful task with no clear memory of having performed the activity. For example, patients report driving a car and not remembering the trip. They may find themselves doing activities that make no sense like putting salt in iced tea. These episodes typically involve activities that are habitual or not demanding of skill. Inattentiveness related to drowsiness may occur. Aldrich[4] reported that the proportions of patients reporting automatic behavior were similar in groups of N+C and N–C patients. Patients with narcolepsy may also have the **rapid eye movement sleep behavior disorder (RBD).**[46] In this disorder, skeletal muscle atonia is absent during REM sleep and dreams may be acted out. Because the Hcrt system has affects on appetite, it is not surprising that some patients with N+C have an **increased body-mass index.**[4,47] Obstructive sleep apnea (OSA) is also not uncommon.[48] If cataplexy is not present in a patient with OSA, narcolepsy may be suspected only if daytime sleepiness persists after adequate treatment of the sleep apnea. **Periodic leg movements in sleep** (PLMS) are also common in narcolepsy.[49] PLMS may be present during REM sleep, a feature uncommon in most patients with PLMS.

CATAPLEXY: N+C

As the name implies, *cataplexy* is an essential criterion for the diagnosis of N+C. Cataplexy is the only symptom relatively "specific" to narcolepsy.[1-4,50] Isolated cataplexy or cataplexy with sleepiness (secondary narcolepsy) can occur in a few rare neurologic disorders associated with mental retardation and obvious neurologic deficits. These are discussed in a later section. In a patient with daytime sleepiness and a normal neurologic examination, cataplexy is virtually diagnostic of narcolepsy.

Cataplexy is characterized by the sudden, temporary loss of bilateral muscle tone with **preserved consciousness** triggered by strong emotions such as laughter, anger, or surprise.[43,50] After cataplexy episodes, patients have total recall of the entire event. If the episodes last longer than a few minutes, the patient may transition into REM sleep and experience HHs. A systematic survey of symptoms of muscle weakness associated with emotion in a large group of patients with daytime sleepiness found that weakness during joking (telling or hearing a joke), laughter, and anger were the most specific for cataplexy associated with narcolepsy.[43,50] Involvement of the legs also seemed to be more specific for narcolepsy.

When loss of muscle strength during cataplexy is severe, almost all of the voluntary muscles in the body are affected, leading to complete collapse. The muscles of the eyes are not affected during cataplexy; individuals can move their eyes during a cataplectic episode. Diaphragmatic activity is also not impaired. In one study, the legs and knees were most frequently affected during cataplexy.[50] In milder cases of cataplexy, the loss in muscle strength can be quite subtle, involving only a few muscle groups **or occurring unilaterally.** For example, ptosis, difficulty speaking, or partial neck muscle weakness may occur (head nodding). In some patients, partial attacks are more frequent than complete attacks. Loss of muscle function may not be evident, and the patient may experience only a vague feeling of weakness. Patients may fall to the ground, and injuries do occur. However, most people are able to find support at the onset of an attack. The attacks do start abruptly but usually take several seconds to reach their maximum intensity. Episodes of cataplexy usually last from seconds to minutes; rarely does an attack last longer than 2 minutes. Clinical signs during an attack are the loss of muscle tone and loss of deep tendon reflexes including a loss or decrease in the H reflex. During an attack of cataplexy, there are cardiovascular changes consisting of increased blood pressure and decreased heart rate. The phenomenon of virtually continuous attacks of cataplexy (status catapleticus) can occur after sudden withdrawal of medications that suppress cataplexy.

DIAGNOSTIC TESTING FOR NARCOLEPSY

History

Patients with daytime sleepiness are invariably questioned about SP, HH/HPHs, and the severity and nature of the daytime sleepiness. However, none of these historical elements is specific for narcolepsy and they can occur in sleep apnea and other causes of daytime sleepiness including IH[4] (Table 24–4). A history of cataplexy is the most important

TABLE 24-4

Multiple Sleep Latency Test and Narcolepsy Facts

Diagnostic criteria: MSL ≤ 8 min.
≥2 SOREMPs in 5 naps.
MSLs
Narcolepsy 3.1 ± 2.9 min.
Idiopathic hypersomnia 6.2 ± 3.0 min.
Normal 10.5 ± 4.6 min.
30% of the normal population has an MSL <8 min.
REQUIREMENTS FOR VALID MSLT
• Previous PSG excluded causes of abnormal MSLT, TST >360 min.
• Free of drugs that influence sleep for 15 days (at least 5 times the drug half-life).
• Standardized sleep schedule for at least 7 days documented by actigraphy or sleep diary.

MSLs = mean sleep latencies; MSLT = multiple sleep latency test; PSG = polysomnography; SOREMPs = sleep-onset rapid eye movement periods; TST = total sleep time.
Data from references 1, 54, and 55.

TABLE 24-5

Multiple Sleep Latency Test Findings in Patients Evaluated for Daytime Sleepiness

	N+C	N–C*	SRBD
N	106	64	1251
MSL <5 min	87%	81%	39%
MSL <8 min	93%	97%	63%
≥2 SOREMPs	74%	91%	7%
≥2 SOREMPs + MSL <5 min	67%	75%	4%
≥2 SOREMPs + MSL <8 min	71%	91%	6%
SOREMPs on PSG	33%	24%	1%

***Diagnosis made in patients with N–C by repeat MSLT if initial test negative.**
MSL = mean sleep latency; N+C = narcolepsy with cataplexy; N–C = narcolepsy without cataplexy; PSG = polysomnography; SOREMPs = sleep-onset rapid eye movement periods; SRBD = sleep-related breathing disorder.
Adapted from Aldrich MS, Chervin RD, Malow BA: Value of the multiple sleep latency test (MSLT) for the diagnosis of narcolepsy. Sleep 1997;20:620–629.

symptom to elicit. In patients with EDS, unequivocal cataplexy, and a normal neurologic examination, a clinical diagnosis of narcolepsy can be made with some certainty. Even if cataplexy is present, most physicians would still seek objective confirmation with PSG followed by a multiple sleep latency test (MSLT).[1] Daytime naps are often refreshing in patients with narcolepsy. In contrast, naps are not commonly refreshing in patients with IH.

Polysomnography

The nocturnal sleep study is used to rule out other significant sleep disorders (sleep apnea) that might explain daytime sleepiness. Nocturnal PSG often reveals a short sleep latency and impaired sleep quality with increased stage N1 sleep and decreased stage N3 sleep. The total sleep time may be reduced but the amount of REM sleep is usually normal.[51,52] Patients with N+C on average have lower sleep efficiency, lower amounts of stage N3 sleep, more stage N1 sleep, and more awakenings than those with N–C.[2,4] PLMS are common in patients with narcolepsy.[49,52] *Sleep-onset rapid eye movement sleep (SOREM)* is defined as a REM latency less than 15 minutes. Aldrich and colleagues[53] found that 33% of N+C, 24% of N–C, and 1% of SRBD patients had a SOREM on nocturnal PSG. Of interest, the finding of a SOREM period on the nocturnal PSG had a 98.5% specificity and 68% positive predictive value (true positives/total number of positives) for the diagnosis of narcolepsy. Therefore, although a minority of patients with narcolepsy have a nocturnal SOREMP (sleep-onset rapid eye movement period) on a given PSG, the finding is highly suggestive of narcolepsy.

This is especially true if no other factor is present to explain the short REM latency such as depression, OSA, recent withdrawal of REM-suppressing medication, or sleep deprivation.

Multiple Sleep Latency Test

The MSLT is the standard objective test for the assessment of sleepiness and the diagnosis of narcolepsy[53-55] (Table 24–5; see also Table 24–4). Overnight PSG during the patient's habitual sleep period should precede the MSLT. The purpose of the PSG is to exclude other causes of excessive daytime sleepiness such as OSA and periodic limb movement disorder (PLMD). A sleep diary or actigraphy should document a regular and sufficient amount of sleep for at least 7 days before the study. Medications that can alter sleepiness (stimulants) or REM sleep should be withdrawn at least 15 days before testing. REM-suppressing medications can alter the ability to detect REM sleep. However, acute withdrawal of REM-suppressing agents can cause a false-positive test.

The ICSD-2 criteria for the diagnosis of narcolepsy include a mean sleep latency of **8 minutes or less** and two or more SOREMPs during five naps.[1] Aldrich and colleagues[53] found that the MSLT had improved sensitivity when a sleep latency of 8 minutes rather than 5 minutes was used as a criterion for sleep latency in patients with N–C. A meta-analysis found the mean sleep latency for narcolepsy patients to be 3.1 ± 2.9 minutes.[54,55] Up to 30% of the general population have a mean sleep latency less than 8 minutes. However, the finding of two or more SOREMPs is much more specific for narcolepsy. Up to 2% of the normal population will have two SOREMPs, and in other studies, approximately 6% of patients with SRBDs will have a mean sleep latency less than 8 minutes with two SOREMPs on an MSLT.[53,56] A few patients with narcolepsy will occasionally have a mean sleep latency above 10 minutes. However, the mean sleep latency is less than 5 minutes in the vast majority of patients with narcolepsy (Fig. 24-4). The mean sleep latency in patients with SRBDs tends to be higher than in narcolepsy, although overlap does occur.

Unfortunately, the MSLT is not very sensitive or completely specific for the diagnosis of narcolepsy. Aldrich and colleagues[53] reviewed MSLT findings in patients evaluated for daytime sleepiness (see Table 24-5). A diagnosis of narcolepsy in patients without cataplexy required a repeat MSLT in some cases. In patients with N+C, a single MSLT was positive only about 70% of the time. Hence, a negative MSLT does not rule out the diagnosis of narcolepsy. In patients ultimately believed to have only an SRBD, approximately 6% had a positive MSLT[53,56] (see Table 24-5).

It is recommended that sleep apnea be treated adequately before an MSLT is performed to evaluate for narcolepsy. Thus, successful treatment with continuous positive airway pressure (CPAP) should be accomplished for several weeks. Then, the patient should undergo a repeat PSG on CPAP (documenting adequate treatment and sleep) and a subsequent MSLT. If good control of sleep apnea is demonstrated during the night study but the MSLT meets criteria for narcolepsy, one can make a diagnosis of narcolepsy. This assumes adequate adherence to CPAP has been documented. In this setting, most clinicians perform the MSLT with the subjects wearing CPAP.

HLA Typing

Although a high percentage of patients with N+C are positive for the HLA DQB1*602 antigen, this test is not very useful for ruling in narcolepsy (for either N+C or N-C). The HLA DQB1*0602 is found in 12% to 38% of the general population. Therefore, a positive result does not rule in N+C. Conversely, a negative test for presence of DQB1*0602 is not useful because up to 10% of N+C patients and 40% to 60% of N-C patients are negative for the antigen.[1,2,13,57]

CSF Hcrt Levels

Hcrt1 levels of the CSF can be assayed at a few centers. In patients with N+C, over 90% have very low or undetectable Hcrt1 levels. In one study of patients with many neurologic diseases, only patients with N+C and a few patients with Guillain-Barré had undetectable Hcrt levels.[58,59] Patients with a number of neurologic diseases had levels that were lower than normal but still detectable. As noted previously, patients with N-C usually have normal levels of CSF Hcrt1. However, about 10% of N-C patients have low CSF Hcrt1. Most of these N-C patients with low CSF Hcrt1 are positive for the HLA DBQ1*602.[58-60]

Diagnostic Criteria and Important Findings for N+C and N-C Forms of Narcolepsy

Narcolepsy with Cataplexy (N+C) The ICSD-2 diagnostic criteria for N+C[1] are listed in Box 24-2. EDS for at least 3 months

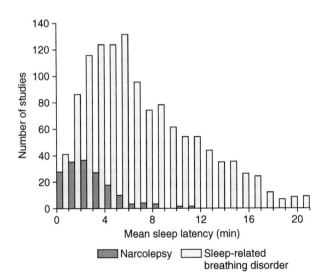

FIGURE 24-4 Distribution of mean sleep latency (MSL) results for groups of patients with narcolepsy and sleep-related breathing disorders. Although considerable overlap is noted, patients with narcolepsy tend to have much lower MSL. *From Aldrich MS, Chervin RD, Malow BA: Value of the multiple sleep latency test (MSLT) for the diagnosis of narcolepsy. Sleep 1997;20:620–629.*

BOX 24-2

Narcolepsy with Cataplexy—Diagnostic Criteria
A. The patient has a complaint of excessive daytime sleepiness occurring almost daily for at least 3 months.
B. A definite history of cataplexy defined as sudden and transient episodes of loss of muscle tone triggered by emotions is present.
Cataplexy = episodes must be triggered by strong emotion—most reliably laughing or joking—and must be bilateral and brief (<2 min). Consciousness must be preserved (at least in the beginning)
Strong evidence = observed cataplexy with loss of DTRs.
C. **The diagnosis of narcolepsy with cataplexy should, whenever possible,** be confirmed by nocturnal PSG followed by an MSLT with a mean sleep latency less than or equal to 8 minutes with two or more SOREMPs observed following sufficient nocturnal sleep (minimum of 6 hr) during the night prior to the test.
Alternatively: CSF hypocretin-1 level <110 pg/mL or less than one third of the mean of normal values.
D. Hypersomnia is not better explained by another sleep disorder, medical or neurologic disorder, medication, or substance use disorder.
CSF = cerebrospinal fluid; DTRs = deep tendon reflexes; MSLT = multiple sleep latency test; PSG = polysomnography; SOREMPs = sleep-onset rapid eye movement periods. From American Academy of Sleep Medicine: International Classification of Sleep Disorders, 2nd ed. Diagnostic and Coding Manual. Westchester, IL: American Academy of Sleep Medicine, 2005.

is required along with cataplexy. When possible, the diagnosis should be confirmed by an MSLT (sleep latency ≤8 min and two or more SOREMPs). A low CSF Hcrt1 level is considered confirmatory even in the absence of an MSLT meeting diagnostic criteria. Other sleep disorders causing the abnormal MSLT should be excluded.

N+C Manifestations Whereas only daytime sleepiness and cataplexy are required to make the diagnosis of N+C, other manifestations such as sleep-related hallucinations, SP, and automatic behavior are often present (see Table 24–1). Only 10% to 15% of patients have the classic symptom tetrad of daytime sleepiness, cataplexy, HGH/HPHs, and SP. Patients with N+C tend to have a higher frequency of SP, HHs, and more severe sleepiness than N–C patients. During PSG, sleep is more disturbed in N+C patients than in N–C patients. On the MSLT, N+C patients tend to have more SOREMPs. Although 90% of N+C patients are positive for DQBQ1*602, this is not useful diagnostically.

Onset of N+C The manifestations of N+C generally begin between the ages of 15 and 30 years.[43] However, this form of narcolepsy can present in the pediatric age group or in patients older than 60 years. EDS alone or in combination with HHs and/or SP is the presenting symptom in approximately 90% of patients.[43] Cataplexy may develop several years after symptoms begin. However, most patients with N+C develop cataplexy within 3 to 5 years of the onset of daytime sleepiness.[14,43] Rarely, cataplexy can precede daytime sleepiness.

Polysomnography Typical findings include a short sleep latency and approximately 20% to 30% have a short **nocturnal** REM latency.[53] Of interest, in one study, the presence of sleep-onset REM during the nocturnal sleep study had a high positive predictive value for the presence of narcolepsy.[53] There tends to be an increase in stage N1 sleep.

Multiple Sleep Latency Test Approximately 70% of patients with N+C will have a MSLT meeting criteria for narcolepsy. The mean sleep latency tends to be slightly less in N+C than in N–C patients and SOREMPs are slightly more frequent than in patients with N–C (see Table 24–3).

Other Studies in N+C
1. Absent to low Hcrt1 in the CSF fluid (90–100%).
2. Absence of Hcrt-staining cells in the hypothalamus.
3. Ninety percent are positive for DQBQ1*602 antigen.

Narcolepsy without Cataplexy (N–C)

The ICSD-2 diagnostic criteria for N–C are listed in Box 24–3. Daytime sleepiness must be present for at least 3 months but typical cataplexy is NOT present. An MSLT shows a mean sleep latency of 8 minutes or less and two or more SOREMPs. The other manifestations of narcolepsy including SP, HHs, and automatic behavior may or may not

---

BOX 24–3

Narcolepsy without Cataplexy—Diagnostic Criteria

A. Complaint of excessive daytime sleepiness almost daily for at least 3 months.
B. Typical cataplexy is not present.
C. Nocturnal PSG followed by MSLT findings:
   - MSL *less than or equal* to 8 min.
   - Two or more SOREMPs (MSLT)
   - Sufficient nocturnal sleep (at least 6 hr).
D. Hypersomnia is not better explained by another sleep disorder, medical or neurologic disorder, medication, or substance use disorder.

MSLT = multiple sleep latency test; PSG = polysomnography; SOREMPs = sleep-onset rapid eye movement periods.
From American Academy of Sleep Medicine: International Classification of Sleep Disorders, 2nd ed. Diagnostic and Coding Manual. Westchester, IL: American Academy of Sleep Medicine, 2005.

---

be present. Compared with patients with N+C, a lower percentage of patients with N–C report SP or HH (see Table 24–3).[2]

Polysomnography (N–C) N–C patients have a short nocturnal sleep latency and 20% to 30% have a short nocturnal REM latency.[53] The amount of stage N1 sleep is increased. N–C patients tend to have less disturbed sleep than N+C patients.

MSLT Findings (N–C) The findings are similar to those of N+C patients. However, there may be a slightly longer mean sleep latency and fewer SOREMPs. Patients with N–C tend to have milder sleepiness and fewer numbers of naps with sleep-onset REM sleep compared with N+C patients. Unfortunately, as discussed previously, an MSLT meeting criteria for the diagnosis of narcolepsy is not completely sensitive or specific. If clinically indicated, repeat testing could be needed. This is in contrast to patients in whom definitive cataplexy is present. A diagnosis of N+C can be made even if the MSLT does not meet criteria if daytime sleepiness and unequivocal cataplexy are present.

TREATMENT OF NARCOLEPSY

The treatment of narcolepsy is usually broken into two components: (1) treatment of EDS and (2) treatment of cataplexy, SP, and HGH/HPHs.[61–64]

Treatment of EDS

The treatment of daytime sleepiness includes conservative measures (adequate sleep time, good sleep hygiene, scheduled daily naps[65]), stimulant medications, alerting medications, and sodium oxybate (Table 24–6). Adequate control of daytime sleepiness can be attained in about 60% to 80% of patients. The stimulant medications used to treat the daytime

TABLE 24–6

Medications Used to Treat Excessive Daytime Sleepiness

MEDICATION (FDA PREGNANCY CATEGORY)	BRAND NAME	DOSE	MAXIMUM DOSE (DAILY)	HALF-LIFE (hr)	SELECTED SIDE EFFECTS
Methylphenidate* (C)	Ritalin	10–30 mg bid or 10–20 mg tid (5, 10, 20 mg tabs)	100 mg	2–4	Nervousness, tremulousness, headache
Methylphenidate SR	Metadate and others Concerta	10–20 mg SR qAM (10, 20 mg tabs) + 10 to 20 mg short-acting in afternoon 18–36 mg SR qAM (18, 27, 36, 54 mg tabs) + 10 to 20 mg short-acting in afternoon			
Dextroamphetamine* (C) Amphetamine/ dextroamphetamine Dextroamphetamine SR Amphetamine/ dextroamphetamine XR	Dexedrine Dextrostat and others Adderall SR Adderall XR	5–60 mg qd 5–30 mg bid (5, 10 mg tabs) (5, 7.5, 12.5, 15 mg tabs) 10 mg SR qAM 5, 10, 15 mg tabs +10 to 20 mg short-acting in afternoon 5, 10, 15, 20, 25, 30 mg capsules	60 mg	10–30	Nervousness, tremulousness, headache
Methamphetamine* (C)	Desoxyn	5 to 60 mg qd (5, 10 mg tabs)	60 mg	12–34	Nervousness, tremulousness, headache
Lisdexamfetamine dimesylate* (C)	Vyvanse	20, 30, 40, 50, 60 mg	70 mg	12–13 (duration of action)	Nervousness, tremulousness, headache
Modafinil† (C)	Provigil	200 or 400 mg qd (100, 200 mg tabs)	400 mg	9–14	Headache, drug interactions, nervousness
Armodafinil† (C)	Nuvigil	150–250 mg daily 150, 250 mg tabs	250 mg	10–14	Headache, drug interactions, nervousness
Sodium oxybate (B)	Xyrem	4.5–9 g/night in 2 divided doses	9 g	1–3	Sedation, enuresis, respiratory suppression
Selegiline (C)	Eldepryl	20–40 mg	40 mg	9–14	Nausea, dizziness, confusion, dry mouth, requires low-tyramine diet, drug interactions

FDA approved for treatment of EDS in narcolepsy: modafinil, armodafinil, dextroamphetamine, methylphenidate, sodium oxybate.

Black box warnings:
Stimulants: Abuse potential.
Sodium oxybate: Abuse potential, should not be used with alcohol or other CNS depressants.
*Schedule II medication (no refills, no telephone prescriptions).
†Schedule IV medication.
CNS = central nervous system; EDS = excessive daytime sleepiness; FDA = U.S. Food and Drug Administration; SR = sustained release.
B and C: *Pregnancy category B:* Animal reproduction studies have failed to demonstrate a risk to the fetus and there are no adequate and well-controlled studies in pregnant women OR Animal studies have shown an adverse effect, but adequate and well-controlled studies in pregnant women have failed to demonstrate a risk to the fetus in any trimester. *Pregnancy category C:* Animal reproduction studies have shown an adverse effect on the fetus and there are no adequate and well-controlled studies in humans, but potential benefits may warrant use of the drug in pregnant women despite potential risks.

sleepiness of narcolepsy include amphetamine (racemic), dextroamphetamine, methamphetamine, and methylphenidate. Dextroamphetamine and methylphenidate are U.S. Food and Drug Administration (FDA) approved for treatment of narcolepsy. A mixture of amphetamine and dextroamphetamine (~25% L-amphetamine and 75% D-amphetamine) is also available (Adderall). Some patients respond best to a mixture, although D-amphetamine may cause less anxiety. Methamphetamine is effective but has a high abuse potential. The FDA does not list narcolepsy as an indication for methamphetamine. The stimulant medications are indirect sympathomimetic stimulants (increase the synaptic availability of dopamine and norepinepherine).

Modafinil and its R enantiomer armodafinil are two alerting medications that are FDA approved for treatment of daytime sleepiness in narcolepsy. There are no studies directly comparing the efficacy of stimulant and alerting medications. However, the relative objective improvement in the sleep latency after medication on the MSLT or maintenance of wakefulness test (MWT) has been compared by computing the pre- and postdrug sleep latency values as a percentage of normal for the test[66] (Fig. 24–5). Because the predrug values differ between the studies, the change from baseline of drug is the main effect of interest. The relative improvements in objective sleepiness are displayed by normalizing the pretreatment (gray bars) and posttreatment (green bars) values of the sleep latency on the MWT or MSLT as a percentage of the published normal values for the MSLT (13.4 min) or the MWT (18.9 min). The largest changes were for methamphetamine and

dextroamphetamine, and the highest postdrug values were for methylphenidate (although baseline values were the highest for this medication). No medication came close to normalizing objective sleepiness.

Stimulant Medications

The stimulant medications increase dopamine transmission by presynaptic mechanisms. The medications inhibit the reuptake of dopamine (DA) and, to a lesser extent, NE and serotonin by the dopamine transporter (DAT).[67-70] The action of amphetamines on DAT causes a reverse efflux of DA through the site as well as blocking reuptake. The amphetamines also inhibit cytoplasmic vesicular storage of DA by the vesicular monoamine transporter (VMAT2). In contrast, methylphenidate has no effect on DA storage. The overall action of the stimulant medications is to increase the synaptic levels of DA.

The peak action of dextroamphetamine, methamphetamine, and methylphenidate is 1 to 3 hours from ingestion, so the medications should be taken at least 1 hour before the time of desired effectiveness. If a sleep attack has begun before medication is taken, a nap may be the best treatment in some patients. Also note that methylphenidate has a much shorter half-life than dextroamphetamine and methamphetamine (see Table 24–6) and must be taken several times a day (bid to tid). Sustained-action forms of the amphetamines and methylphenidate are available. Of note, stimulant medications may have a mild beneficial effect on cataplexy but modafinil has no effect on cataplexy.

The side effects of the stimulant medications include nervousness, headache, loss of appetite, palpitations, irritability, and tremor. All of these medications are schedule II drugs (requiring monthly prescriptions). There are several potential problems with the use of stimulant medications.[66,67] First, tolerance may develop (documented by some but not all studies), requiring escalating doses and leading to ineffectiveness at the highest dose. In some patients, effectiveness can be restored by a "drug holiday"—no medications for several days. Unfortunately, severe sleepiness may occur during that time. Second, the medications can increase blood pressure, although this effect is not usual in normotensive patients.[71] Third, insomnia is a common side effect of stimulants. Thus, they should not be taken near bedtime, especially methamphetamine and dextroamphetamine, both of which have a relatively long half-life. Fourth, attacks of paranoia or hallucinations have been reported with amphetamines, but major psychiatric side effects are rare in the absence of underlying psychiatric disorders.[72] However, use of very high doses of stimulants is associated with an increased risk of adverse outcomes.[72]

Methylphenidate appears to have a lower propensity to produce side effects and is probably the most widely used stimulant medication. However, the relatively short duration of action of methylphenidate is sometimes problematic because patients may experience a sudden decrease in alertness as the medication wears off. One treatment approach is to use sustained-action forms of methylphenidate in the

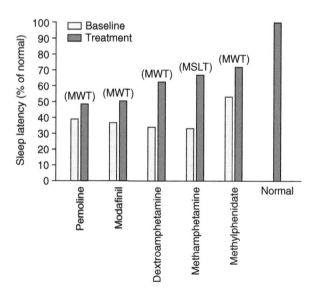

FIGURE 24–5 Comparison of the effects of stimulant medications and modafinil on sleep latency (multiple sleep latency test [MSLT] or maintenance of wakefulness test [MWT]). The pre- and postdrug values were normalized as a percentage of accepted normal values for the tests MSLT (13.4 min) or MWT (18.9 min). The dose of drugs used was 112.5 mg for pemoline, 300 mg for modafinil, 60 mg for dextroamphetamine, 60 mg for methylphenidate, and 40–60 mg for methamphetamine. *From Mitler M, Aldrich MS, Koob GF, et al: ASDA standards of practice: narcolepsy and its treatment with stimulants. Sleep 1994;17:352–371.*

morning with short-acting forms in the afternoon or evening. In some patients, a small dose of short-acting methylphenidate must also be added in the morning to help patients more rapidly achieve alertness for early morning activity. There are individual patients who will tolerate the slower onset of sustained-action medications while they find the shorter-acting medications intolerable (jittery or nervous). The American Academy of Sleep Medicine (AASM) Practice Parameters for Treatment of Narcolepsy and Other Hypersomnias of Central Origin[61] stated "combinations of long- and short-acting stimulants may be indicated and effective for some patients (Option)." Lisdexamfetamine dimesylate (Vyvanse) is a once-daily medication approved for treating attention deficit hyperactivity disorder (ADHD) for ages 6 to 17 and adults. It is a prodrug that is converted to dextroamphetamine in the gastrointestinal tract. This medication has also been used "off label" to treat narcolepsy (see Table 24–6).

Modafinil and Armodafinil

Modafinil and armodafinil (R entaniomer of modafinil) are nonamphetamine wakefulness-promoting medications that are schedule IV medications (refills and telephone orders allowed). They are considered to have less abuse potential than the stimulant medications. Modafinil is considered to be the first-line medication for treatment of EDS associated with narcolepsy.[61,67,73] Randomized, placebo-controlled trials have documented the effectiveness of modafinil in patients with narcolepsy.[73–75]

The elimination half-life of modafinil is 9 to 14 hours, permitting once-daily administration for most patients. Modafinil is usually administered once daily in the morning (200–400 mg). However, some patients taking modafinil in the morning may experience poor control of daytime sleepiness in the afternoon or early evening. They may respond to split dosing (200 mg in AM, 200 mg at 1–2 PM).[76,77] Although the maximum recommended daily dose of modafinil is 400 mg, higher doses have been used. There are some patients in whom adequate control of sleepiness may require a slightly higher dose than 400 mg (400 mg in the AM and 200 mg in the early afternoon).[76,77]

The L enantiomer of modafinil has a shorter half-life (3–4 hr) than the R enantiomer (10–14 hr). Modafinil (racemic, containing both L and R enantiomers) has a similar terminal half-life as armodafinil. Within a few hours after taking modafinil the only enantiomer left in the blood is armodafinil.[78–80] If the same doses of modafinil and armodafinil are given in the morning, the afternoon blood levels of armodafinil are considerably higher. For this reason, a morning dose of armodafinil (150–250 mg) may control afternoon sleepiness better than modafinil. A double-blind study by Harsh and associates[81] documented the efficacy and safety of armodafinil.

There is no evidence that tolerance develops to modafinil or that the drug impairs sleep quality (if taken in the morning). It has a number of advantages including once-daily dosing, low abuse potential, and the fact that it is not a schedule II medication. As noted previously, there are no head-to-head studies comparing effectiveness of modafinil and stimulant medications. However, when compared for the ability to normalize the sleep latency, stimulant medications appear slightly more effective.[66] **Thus, although modafinil is considered the drug of choice for daytime sleepiness in patients with narcolepsy, some patients will respond better to a stimulant.**

The mechanism of action of modafinil is not known,[67,82–84] but the drug likely targets the DA reuptake system. The alerting effect of modafinil is not specific to patients with narcolepsy. Modafinil does not bind the receptors or uptake sites of NE, GABA, adenosine, or benzodiazepines. It does weakly bind to the DAT.[82] Modafinil does enhance the activity of many brain sites associated with wakefulness including the **tuberomammillary nucleus and Hcrt cells** of the perifornical area.[83] However, modafinil does not require the Hcrt system to be effective. Modafinil can reduce the extracellular GABA concentrations.[84] Because GABA is an inhibitory neurotransmitter, this could disinhibit a number of wake-promoting sites such as the tuberomammillary neurons (TMNs). Another possibility is that modafinil may increase dopaminergic signaling. All the brain regions activated by modafinil receive dopaminergic innervation.[85] Wisor and coworkers[70] found that modafinil does not improve wakefulness in mice lacking the DAT. As noted previously, modafinil does bind weakly to the DAT. A study by Gallopin and colleagues[85] found that modafinil blocks reuptake of NE by noradrenergic terminals that interface with sleep-promoting neurons of the ventrolateral preoptic nucleus (VLPO). Higher NE at the VLPO would be wake-promoting because NE inhibits the activity of the VLPO. The mechanism by which modafinil blocks reuptake is unclear because modafinil does not bind to NE receptors. After numerous investigations, the mechanism by which modafinil works is still unknown.[86] In summary, modafinil may promote NE and dopaminergic transmission of wake-promoting centers. Continued research in this area will likely help design more effective treatments for narcolepsy.

The most common side effects of modafinil include headache, nausea, and nervousness. Headache can be minimized by a slow increase in dose. A few cases of severe skin rash (Stevens-Johnson syndrome) have been reported in patients taking modafinil (very low prevalence). Modafinil is metabolized in the liver by the cytochrome P-450 (CYP450) system. Hence, a number of drug interactions are possible. The main interaction of significance is that certain oral contraceptives may be less effective after modafinil is started. Female patients of reproductive age taking oral contraceptives should use additional (or alternative) methods of contraception. Unlike the indirect sympathomimetics, withdrawal of modafinil does not result in a rebound of REM and slow wave sleep. Patients can be switched from stimulants to modafinil without a washout period. However, because stimulant medications have some anticataplectic action, patients changed from methylphenidate to modafinil may require the addition of specific medications for cataplexy.[87]

Sodium Oxybate

Gamma hydroxybutyrate (GHB) is naturally occurring in the CNS and acts as a neurotransmitter at two GHB receptor subtypes. In large doses, the drug acts at GABA-B receptors. It is tasteless and, when given in sufficient doses, can cause rapid sedation and amnesia. This resulted in the compound's use as the "date rape drug." In sufficient doses, respiratory depression and death can occur. Sodium oxybate (SOXB) is the sodium salt of GHB. It is a whitish crystalline powder that is highly soluble in water. SOXB (Xyrem) has been proved to be effective for EDS in narcolepsy as well as for cataplexy.[88-93] Due to the potential for abuse, SOXB is available only from a single central pharmacy.

In many of the studies of SOXB in narcolepsy, patients were allowed to continue on their alerting medication (modafinil) or stimulants. A 4-week study demonstrated a significant reduction in subjective sleepiness (Epworth Sleepiness Scale) at the 9-g dose[88] (Fig. 24–6). A 12-month extension trial showed continued administration of SOXB resulted in progressive improvements in EDS that were maximal after 2 months.[89] A double-blind, placebo-controlled trial found that 9 g of SOXB nightly was associated with a greater than 10-minute median increase in the sleep latency on the MWT.[90] Black and Houghton found that a combination of modafinil and Xyrem was more efficacious than either taken alone in increasing the sleep latency on the MWT (Fig. 24–7).[91]

SOXB is also effective at reducing cataplexy, HH/HPHs, and SP in patients with narcolepsy. This use is discussed in a later section. **It appears that somewhat higher doses of**

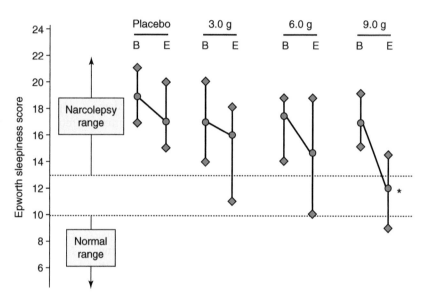

FIGURE 24–6 Effect of sodium oxybate on subjective sleepiness in narcolepsy. Lines are median *(circles)* and 25th and 75th percentile *(diamonds)* values. At 9.0 g, the reduction was significant (*) and the median was just above the normal range. B = baseline; E = end of the study. *From U.S. Xyrem Multicenter Study Group: A randomized, double-blind, placebo-controlled multicenter trial comparing the effects of three doses of orally administered sodium oxybate with placebo for the treatment of narcolepsy. Sleep 2002;25:42–49.*

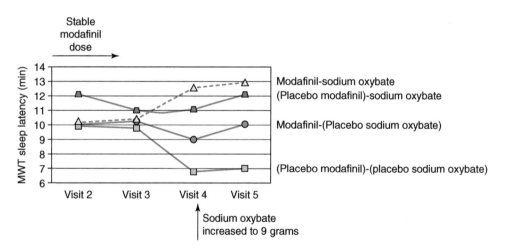

FIGURE 24–7 A combination of modafinil and sodium oxybate may be more effective than sodium oxybate alone in some patients. After visit 3, one group was changed to placebo-modafinil, one group to placebo-sodium oxybate, one group to both placebo-modafinil and placebo-sodium oxybate; one group continued on active medications. Both modafinil and sodium oxybate resulted in a higher sleep latency compared with placebo-placebo. At visit 4, the highest latency was in the group with both active medications. However, there was less benefit from the addition of modafinil at visit 5 after the dose of sodium oxybate was increased to 9 g. MWT = maintenance of wakefulness test. *From Black J, Houghton WC: Sodium oxybate improves excessive daytime sleepiness in narcolepsy. Sleep 2006;29:939–946.*

SOXB may be needed to improve daytime sleepiness as compared with cataplexy.[92,93] The benefits on EDS may take a few months for maximum effect. The FDA approved SOXB for treatment of both daytime sleepiness and cataplexy. SOXB is the only medication FDA approved for cataplexy. The mechanism of action of SOXB with respect to reducing daytime sleepiness is unknown. Studies have shown that the medication reduces nocturnal awakenings and increases stage N3 sleep and consolidates REM periods.[94] Some have hypothesized that sleep consolidation improves daytime sleepiness.

SOXB (Xyrem) is available as a liquid (500 mg/mL) and, because of a short half-life, must be taken at bedtime and repeated 2.5 to 4 hours later. The drug's effect is so rapid that after ingesting each dose of the medication, patients should lie down and remain in bed. SOXB taken on an empty stomach reaches peak concentrations in 0.5 to 1.5 hours and has a half-life of 40 to 60 minutes. Each dose of medication is diluted with 60 mL of water in the child-resistant dosing cups. Both doses should be prepared before going to bed. The dose in the middle of the night should be taken while the patient is sitting in bed. It is very important to note that **food can reduce the bioavailability of SOXB.** SOXB is started at 4.5 g/night taken in divided doses (2.25 g taken at bedtime and repeated 2.5–4 hr [usually ~3 hr] later). The dose is then increased in 1.5-g/night increments each week until a maximum of 9 g/night is reached. One might aim for lower doses in smaller patients. If side effects are intolerable, the dose can be decreased temporarily and then a trial at an increased dose can be tried later. Nausea, dizziness, and enuresis are the most common side effects. SOXB is associated with a high sodium load and this can be a significant concern in patients with congestive heart failure. The simultaneous use of SOXB and alcohol or other CNS depressants is contraindicated.

A study of 4 consecutive nights of SOXB in patients with mild to moderate OSA not on CPAP found no significant worsening in the apnea-hypopnea index (AHI) and mean arterial oxygen saturation (SaO_2).[95] In this study, stage N3 increased but the number of central apneas also increased and a few patients did experience significant oxygen desaturation. Thus, although not an absolute contraindication, SOXB should be used with caution in patients with OSA. If SOXB is used in patients with very severe OSA, adequate treatment of OSA (CPAP) is essential. It may be prudent to perform nocturnal oximetry when SOXB treatment is started or the dose is increased.

Other Interventions for Daytime Sleepiness

Another treatment alternative that can be tried in patients not tolerating stimulants is the irreversible monoamine oxidase (MAO) type B inhibitor selegiline. At doses of 10 to 40 mg/day, this drug has been shown to improve narcoleptic symptoms.[96] Unfortunately, at doses over 20 mg/day, it loses its MAO B inhibitor selectivity and a low-tyramine diet is indicated to avoid the risk of hypertensive reactions. Segeline is metabolized to amphetamine. The drug also has anticataplectic activity in addition to its alerting ability. Patients who experience intolerable side effects with other agents may benefit from this medication as long as they are willing to adhere to a low-tyramine diet.

Improving nocturnal sleep and treatment of concurrent sleep disorders is also important for improving daytime sleepiness. Benzodiazepine receptor agonists may improve sleep quality in some patients. If the restless legs syndrome/PLMS are significantly impairing sleep, specific treatment for these problems may be helpful. The combination of narcolepsy and OSA is commonly encountered. Adequate treatment of OSA with nasal CPAP or other therapies is essential. Good sleep hygiene with a regular sleep schedule and adequate sleep is essential for narcolepsy patients. Some find short scheduled naps to also be beneficial.

Choosing Treatment for Daytime Sleepiness

The AASM has recently published practice parameters regarding the treatment of narcolepsy and central hypersomnias[61] (Table 24-7). For daytime sleepiness, both modafinil and SOXB received Standard recommendations. Due to convenience and tolerability, most physicians would start treatment with modafinil or armodafinil. If modafinil (or armodafinil) is not sufficiently effective, one option is to switch to a stimulant medication. A combination of short-acting and long-acting methylphenidate may be better tolerated in some patients (methylphenidate 20 mg SR qAM and 10–20 mg short-acting in early afternoon). Another option for patients not responding to modafinil is to move directly to SOXB (especially if cataplexy is significant). In some studies, SOXB restored subjective sleepiness to the normal range. However, SOXB is an expensive medication and requires that the patient reliably follow instructions. In any case, if both modafinil and stimulants are not effective, one could prescribe SOXB. Often, modafinil (or stimulant medication) is continued as the dose of SOXB is increased. If treatment of both daytime sleepiness and cataplexy is needed, SOXB would be especially useful. Some patients do not tolerate alternative medications for cataplexy, and in this group, SOXB is also a good option.

Treatment of Cataplexy, HGH/HPHs, and SP

In some patients with N+C, the episodes of cataplexy are so uncommon or mild that treatment is not needed. In others, they constitute an important problem for patients. The medications that are useful for the treatment of cataplexy also suppress the other associated symptoms of narcolepsy including SP and HGH/HPHs (Table 24–8). It should be recalled that these phenomenon can occur in normal individuals and do not require treatment unless recurrent and clinically significant. The classic medications useful in treating cataplexy have a common property of suppressing REM sleep. In the canine form of narcolepsy, drugs increasing NE are the most efficacious.[97]

The tricyclic antidepressants (TCAs) were the first group used to treat cataplexy. The first agent used was imipramine,

TABLE 24–7

American Academy of Sleep Medicine Practice Parameters for Treatment of Narcolepsy and Hypersomnia of Central Origin*

NARCOLEPSY

Daytime sleepiness	Modafinil (Standard)
	Sodium oxybate (Standard)
	Amphetamine (Guideline)
	Methamphetamine (Guideline)
	Dextroamphetamine (Guideline)
	Methylphenidate (Guideline)
	Selegiline (Option)
Cataplexy	Sodium oxybate (Standard)
	Tricyclic antidepressants (Guideline)
	SSRIs (Guideline)
	Venlafaxine (Guideline)
	Selegiline (Option)
Sleep paralysis, hypnagogic hallucinations due to narcolepsy	Sodium oxybate (Option)
	Tricyclic antidepressants (Option)
	SSRIs (Option)
	Venlafaxine (Option)

IDIOPATHIC HYPERSOMNIA

Daytime sleepiness	Modafinil (Option)
	Amphetamine (Option)
	Methamphetamine (Option)
	Dextroamphetamine (Option)
	Methylphenidate (Option)

MEDICAL DISORDERS ASSOCIATED WITH HYPERSOMNIA

Parkinson's disease	Modafinil (Option)
Myotonic dystrophy	Modafinil (Option)
	Methylphenidate (Option)
Multiple sclerosis	Modafinil (Guideline)

RECURRENT HYPERSOMNIA

Episodes (shorter duration, less severe symptoms)	Lithium (Option)
Daytime sleepiness	Modafinil (Option)
	Amphetamine (Option)
	Methamphetamine (Option)
	Dextroamphetamine (Option)
	Methylphenidate (Option)

HYPERSOMNIA DUE TO MEDICAL CONDITION

Daytime sleepiness	Modafinil (Option)
	Amphetamine (Option)
	Methamphetamine (Option)
	Dextroamphetamine (Option)
	Methylphenidate (Option)

*Evidence level: Standard > Guideline > Option.
SSRIs = selective serotonin reuptake inhibitors.
From Morgenthaler TI, Kapur VK, Brown TM, et al: Practice parameters for the treatment of narcolepsy and other hypersomnias of central origin. Sleep 2007;30:1705–1711.

but other TCAs including protriptyline, desipramine, and clomipramine have been used. They are commonly effective in doses less than those used for antidepressant action. Protriptyline, desipramine, and imipramine block reuptake of NE, and clomipramine is a more potent blocker of serotonin reuptake. The major problem with these medications is their anticholinergic side effects. For this reason, these drugs are not the first choice for treatment of cataplexy.

The selective serotonin reuptake inhibitors (SSRIs) such as fluoxetine have also been found useful in treating cataplexy.[98] The SSRIs (fluoxetine) are used in typical antidepressant doses and their effect may be more delayed than that of the TCAs. However, because the SSRIs generally are better tolerated and safer in overdose than TCAs, they are widely used. The selective serotonin and norepinephrine reuptake inhibitors (SNRIs) such as venlafaxine block the reuptake of both serotonin and NE. The extended-release formulation of venlafaxine is preferred because the drug has a short half-life. The SNRIs appear to be particularly useful in treating cataplexy and are generally well tolerated.[67,87] Atomoxetine, an adrenergic reuptake blocker used for ADHD, has also been used as a treatment for cataplexy. Both venlafaxine and atomoxetine can increase blood pressure. Selegiline (Eldepryl) has also been used to treat cataplexy but, due to its side effects and drug interactions, is rarely used.[96]

Although the previous medications were recommended as effective treatments for cataplexy (Guideline) by the recent AASM Practice Parameters for the Treatment of Narcolepsy and Hypersomnia of Central Origin, none of these medications is FDA approved for cataplexy treatment. Abrupt cessation of anticataplectic medications can markedly worsen cataplexy and result in nearly continuous attacks (status cataplecticus). Consistent with the concept that medications that increase NE are effective treatments for cataplexy, there has been a report of exacerbation of cataplexy by the alpha-1 blocker prazosin.[99]

A portion of patients with narcolepsy do not respond well to the traditional medications used to treat cataplexy or are unable to tolerate the side effects. For these patients, SOXB can be an effective option. SOXB is the only FDA-approved treatment for cataplexy and has the additional advantage of treating daytime sleepiness. The method by which the medication decreases cataplexy is unknown. The dosage of SOXB and side effects were previously discussed. The effectiveness of SOXB in decreasing episodes of cataplexy has been documented by placebo-controlled studies.[61,88,92,93] SOXB can improve cataplexy at lower doses (4.5 gm/night)[93] than daytime sleepiness, and the maximum effect takes a few months to be noted (Fig. 24–8).

Future Treatments for Narcolepsy

A number of treatments targeting a proposed autoimmune mechanism have been tried in narcolepsy[3,68,100,101] including steroids, plasma exchange, and immunoglobulins without clear long-term benefit. Another approach would be administration of Hcrt or Hcrt analogues. Central administration

TABLE 24–8

Medications Used for Treatment of Cataplexy, Hypnagogic Hallucinations, and Sleep Paralysis

DRUG (BRAND NAME)	DOSE	MAXIMUM DOSE (DAILY)	HALF-LIFE (hr)	SELECTED SIDE EFFECTS
TRICYCLIC ANTIDEPRESSANTS				
Protriptyline (Vivactil)	5–10 mg bid or tid (5-, 10-, 20-mg tabs)	30 mg	67–89	Dry mouth, urinary hesitancy, constipation
Clomipramine (Anafranil)	Start 50 mg qhs (75–125 mg)	250 mg	32	Dry mouth, sweating, drowsiness
Imipramine (Tofranil)	Start 50 mg qhs (75–125 mg)	300 mg	6–20	Dry mouth, constipation, drowsiness
SSRIS				
Fluoxetine (Prozac)	Start 20 mg qAM (20–60 mg)	80 mg	48–216	Headache, dry mouth, sexual dysfunction
NSRIS				
Venlafaxine (Effexor)	Start 37.5 mg bid (75–100 mg bid)	375 mg	3–7	Nausea, dry mouth, headache, blood pressure elevation, insomnia, nervousness, withdrawal syndrome— wean slowly
	XL form Start 37.5 mg qAM 75–150 mg qAM	225 mg (XL)		
SNRIS				
Atmoxetine (Strattera)	40 mg qAM × 3 days then 40 mg bid or 80 mg qAM (10, 18, 25, 40, 60, 80 mg tabs)	100 mg	5.2	Nausea, dry mouth, headache, blood pressure elevation, insomnia, nervousness
OTHER MEDICATIONS				
Selegiline (Eldepryl)	20–40 mg	40 mg	9–14	Nausea, dizziness, confusion, dry mouth
Sodium oxybate* (Xyrem)	Starting dose 2.25 mg qhs repeated in 2.5–4 hr (see text)	9 g daily in divided doses	0.5–1	Nausea, headache, confusion, enuresis, sleepwalking

*FDA approved for treatment of cataplexy.
FDA = U.S. Food and Drug Administration; NSRIs = nonselective serotonin reuptake inhibitors; SNRIs = selective norepinephrine reuptake inhibitors; SSRIs = selective serotonin reuptake inhibitors.

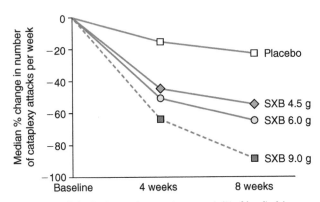

FIGURE 24–8 Reduction in cataplexy attacks per week (% of baseline) in groups treated with 4.5, 6.0, and 9.0 g of sodium oxybate (SXB). There was a significant decrease even with the 4.5-g dose, and the improvement continued from 4 to 8 weeks. Thus, the full benefit of sodium oxybate for treatment of cataplexy may require at least 8 weeks (at least, at 9 g total dose). *From Xyrem International Study Group: Further evidence supporting the use of sodium oxybate for the treatment of cataplexy: a double-blind, placebo-controlled study in 228 patients. Sleep Med 2005;6:415–421.*

of Hcrt1 (more stable that Hcrt2) increases alertness in animals.[101] Development of Hcrt analogues and/or an intranasal approach for administration are being evaluated.[102] Histaminergic compounds are being developed.[68] H3 receptor antagonists bind the H3 receptor (an autoreceptor) blocking the negative feedback of histamine and increasing overall histamine secretion. As mentioned previously, CSF histamine levels are low in narcolepsy and IH.[37,38] As more is learned about the pathophysiology of narcolepsy, improved treatments will undoubtedly be available.

Narcolepsy in Children

The onset of narcolepsy before age 4 is felt to be extremely rare.[1,103] EDS in children may manifest itself as a return to taking daytime naps in a child that previously discontinued napping. In older children, daytime sleepiness may sometimes be manifested as symptoms similar to those of ADHD. Symptoms of cataplexy may be difficult to elicit in children.

Cataplexy can be confused with syncope (except the child is awake) or seizure-like activity. In children with narcolepsy, cataplexy can sometimes be the first symptom and often the first prominent symptom.[104] If cataplexy is the first symptom, an evaluation of narcolepsy due to medical condition (secondary narcolepsy) is indicated (including CNS imaging and genetic testing). In one study, 43% of children had falls as part of their attacks.[104] During cataplexy, knees, head, and jaw were the most often involved. Eyelids, arms, and trunk were less often involved. More rarely, blurred vision, slurred speech, or irregular breathing was noted. A "cataplectic facies" was reported characterized by partially closed eyelids and jaw weakness (open mouth). **In some episodes of childhood cataplexy, a clear-cut emotional trigger may not be noted.** The development of obesity in children associated with the onset of narcolepsy is common (up to 25%) and nocturnal eating syndrome can be present. As discussed in Chapter 14, children tend to have long sleep latencies on the MSLT. For example, the mean sleep latency on the MSLT in one study of normal prepubertal children was 19 ± 16 minutes (in adults, 10.4 ± 4.3).[106] Therefore, use of sleep latency criteria of 8 minutes or less may be problematic. Some clinicians consider a mean sleep latency less than 12 minutes as consistent with daytime sleepiness in children. Conversely, a study by Serra and colleagues[104] found that most of their children diagnosed with N+C had a mean sleep latency of 5.3 minutes with a range of 1 to 13 minutes on the MSLT. A repeat MSLT may be needed because lack of SOREMPs does not rule out the diagnosis. A lumbar puncture for CSF sampling (Hcrt1) could be considered if possible/ambiguous cataplexy is present. The AASM Practice Parameters for Treatment of Narcolepsy and Other Hypersomnias of Central Origin stated that "methylphenidate or modafinil in children 6 to 15 appears to be relatively safe in the treatment of hypersomnias of central origin (Option)."[61] The practice parameters made no recommendation in this age group regarding cataplexy. Fluoxetine, venlafaxine, and SOXB have been used in children.[104,105] A study of Israeli children with narcolepsy reported successful use of modafinil and SOXB for sleepiness.[105]

NARCOLEPSY DUE TO MEDICAL CONDITION

Narcolepsy Due to Medical Condition (NDMC) is a group of disorders also known as **secondary or symptomatic narcolepsy.**[1,107–109] The patient must report or manifest daytime sleepiness. The disorder must be associated with a medical disorder known to cause narcolepsy and the combination of either cataplexy or an MSLT meeting diagnostic criteria for narcolepsy must be present. The ICSD-2 criteria for NDMC are listed in Box 24–4. A low level of CSF Hcrt1 is also acceptable evidence of NDMC.

Medical disorders commonly causing narcolepsy are listed in Box 24–5. Note that if hypersomnia is thought secondary to one of the listed medical conditions but **criteria for narcolepsy are not met,** the diagnosis is "Hypersomnia Due to Medical Condition (HDMC)."

BOX 24–4

Narcolepsy Due to Medical Condition

A. Complaint of daytime sleepiness occurring almost daily for at least 3 months.

B. **One** of the following is observed:

  i. A definite history of cataplexy, defined as sudden and transient episode of loss of muscle tone (muscle weakness) triggered by emotion, is present.

  ii. If cataplexy is not present or is very atypical, PSG monitoring performed over the patient's habitual sleep period followed by an MSLT must demonstrate a mean sleep latency on the MSLT of <8 min with two or more SOREMPs despite sufficient nocturnal sleep prior to the MSLT (minimum of 360 min).

  iii. Hypocretin-1 levels in the CSF <110 pg/mL (or 30% of the normal control values), provided the patient is not comatose.

C. A significant underlying medical or neurologic disorder accounts for the daytime sleepiness.

D. The hypersomnia is not better explained by another sleep disorder, mental disorder, medications use, or substance use disorder.

CSF = cerebrospinal fluid; MSLT = multiple sleep latency test; PSG = polysomnography; SOREMPs = sleep-onset rapid eye movement periods.
From American Academy of Sleep Medicine: International Classification of Sleep Disorders, 2nd ed. Diagnostic and Coding Manual. Westchester, IL: American Academy of Sleep Medicine, 2005.

BOX 24–5

Medical Disorders Causing Narcolepsy Due to Medical Condition

NARCOLEPSY WITH CATAPLEXY
Tumors, sarcoidosis, arteriovenous malformations affecting the hypothalamus
Multiple sclerosis plaques impairing the hypothalamus
Paraneoplastic syndrome anti-Ma2 antibodies
Neimann-Pick type C disease
Possibly Coffin-Lowry syndrome
NARCOLEPSY WITHOUT CATAPLEXY
Head trauma
Myotonic dystrophy
Prader-Willi syndrome (rarely with cataplexy)
Parkinson's disease
Multisystem atrophy

From American Academy of Sleep Medicine: International Classification of Sleep Disorders, 2nd ed. Diagnostic and Coding Manual. Westchester, IL: American Academy of Sleep Medicine, 2005.

Patients with idiopathic narcolepsy usually have a normal neurologic examination and no definite pathology on brain imaging. Patients with NDMC often have specific brain pathology.[107-109] Damage to the hypothalamus due to sarcoidosis, tumors,[110] arteriovenous malformations, or cerebrovascular accidents can cause NDMC. Other reported associations of cerebral disease and narcolepsy include multiple sclerosis and Niemann-Pick disease type C.[111] Daytime sleepiness following closed head injury is a well-known syndrome.[112] However, most patients with daytime sleepiness following head trauma do not have narcolepsy. Postencephalitic narcolepsy was common in the 1920s, but no similar epidemic has been recently described.

Disorders Associated with NDMC, Isolated Cataplexy, or HDMC

Cataplexy can rarely occur with syndromes other than idiopathic narcolepsy. In some cases, a diagnosis of NDMC can be made. In others, it may be difficult to determine whether daytime sleepiness is present (e.g., in the setting of significant mental retardation). The term *isolated cataplexy* implies the presence of cataplexy without daytime sleepiness. Cataplexy has been reported in the **Prader-Willi syndrome (PWS),**[113-116] **Niemann-Pick disease type C,**[111,117,118] **Coffin-Lowry syndrome,**[119,120] **Norrie's disease,**[121,122] **and Moebius syndrome.**[123] These patients have variable mental retardation and/or obvious neurologic deficits in contrast to the patient with "idiopathic" narcolepsy.

Genetic Disorders Causing NDMC or Isolated Cataplexy

Prader-Willi Syndrome **PWS** is a genetic disorder usually associated with a deletion of the long arm of chromosome 15 and is characterized by hyperphagia, obesity, hypogonadotrophic hypogonadism, behavioral disorders, and sleep disorders.[113-116] Abnormal growth hormone secretion results in short stature, reduced muscle mass, and low bone density (scoliosis is common). The characteristic appearance of PWS includes a high narrow forehead, almond-shaped eyes, turned-down lips, a prominent nasal bridge, and small hands and feet. Intelligence is variable but usually ranges from low normal to mild to moderately decreased. **Patients with PWS may have daytime sleepiness from a number of etiologies including sleep apnea, narcolepsy, or the PWS itself.** PWS patients may manifest obstructive apnea, central apnea, hypoventilation, or a mixture of these disorders. EDS is reported commonly in persons with PWS, may begin early in life, and has been correlated with daytime behavioral issues. In fact, EDS has been reported independent of nocturnal sleep problems (sleep apnea), suggesting it is a primary feature of PWS. Some sleepy persons with PWS meet the diagnostic criteria for narcolepsy and PWS is considered a cause of NDMC.[1] Abnormal sleep architecture has been reported in persons with PWS including reduced REM latency and SOREMPs. These findings can be present in PWS patients without significant sleep-related breathing problems. Although PWS is felt to most commonly cause NDMC

without cataplexy, patients with PWS can have cataplexy[114] (accurate history is often difficult to obtain in these patients). Nevsimalova and associates[115] found reduced levels of CSF Hcrt1 levels in four patients with PWS. However, none had cataplexy. Fronczek and coworkers[116] found no difference in the total number of Hcrt-containing neurons in seven PWS patients compared with age-matched controls. If sleepiness is present in PWS but criteria for narcolepsy are not met and sleepiness is NOT felt to be due to sleep apnea, a diagnosis of HDMC is appropriate.

Myotonic Dystrophy

Myotonic dystrophy type 1 (MD1) is an autosomal dominant inherited disorder characterized by myotonia and muscle weakness. The incidence is estimated to be about 1/10,000, so it is a much more rare disorder than narcolepsy. *Myotonia* is defined as **repetitive muscle depolarization resulting in muscle stiffness and impaired relaxation.** The muscles usually involved include facial, masseter, levator palpebra, forearm, hand, pretibial, and sternocleidomastoid. Pharyngeal and laryngeal and muscles of respiration including the diaphragm can be involved. Dysfunction of the hypothalamic region can result in daytime sleepiness or daytime sleepiness with SOREMPs (NDMC).[1,107-109,124] Involvement of upper airway muscles can result in sleep apnea. Some patients have abnormal ventilatory control and hypoventilation. Involvement of the cardiac condition system can occur. There are differences in presentation depending on the age of onset. Congenital MD is apparent at birth and often severe. Juvenile MD is characterized by symptoms that appear between birth and adolescence. Adult-onset MD usually appears in individuals aged 20 to 40 and tends to be slowly progressive. Late-onset MD occurs after age 40 and has mild symptoms.

Daytime sleepiness is a common complaint and can be due to MD (hypersomnia due to medical condition), MD as a cause of secondary narcolepsy (NDMC), or OSA. Thus, several mechanisms can cause daytime sleepiness in patients with MD.

On physical examination, findings include a narrow face, premature frontal balding, distal weakness, and myotonia. MD patients have decreased strength on hand grip but then are slow to relax ("distal myopathy with myotonia"). There is wasting of hand and forearm muscles. PSG can reveal OSA, and PSG + MSLT can meet criteria for narcolepsy or simply document EDS without SOREMPs.

The AASM Practice Parameter on the Treatment of Narcolepsy and Other Hypersomnias of Central Origin[61] stated "methylphenidate and modafinil may be effective treatment for MD" (Option—the lowest recommendation level) (see Table 24-7). Two studies found modafinil to be effective,[124,125] but a more recent small study did not show a benefit.[126]

Rare Genetic Disorders Causing NDMC or Isolated Cataplexy

Niemann-Pick type C disease is a rare autosomal recessive disorder characterized by lysosomal accumulation of unesterfied cholesterol in many tissues as well as lysosomal storage of sphingolipids in the brain and liver. Cataplexy may be seen in up to 10% of children with Niemann-Pick type C disease.[111,117,118] The clinical manifestations and severity are variable. Classic findings include hepatosplenomegaly, vertical supranuclear gaze palsy, ataxia, dystonia, and dementia. In one reported case, the CSF Hcrt was reduced but not into the narcolepsy range.[127]

Coffin-Lowry syndrome is a rare X-linked disorder in which affected males demonstrate severe mental retardation with prominent dysmorphic features usually affecting the face and hands. Typical facial features include a prominent forehead, hypertelorism, a flat nasal bridge, downward-sloping palpebral fissures, and a wide mouth with full lips. Cataplexy has been described in these patients.[119,120]

Norrie's disease is a rare genetic condition that has also been associated with cataplexy. It is an X-linked recessive disorder causing ocular atrophy, mental retardation, deafness, and dysmorphic features.[121,122] Defects in MAO genes occur in some patients.[122]

Moebius syndrome consists of congenital paresis of the seventh cranial nerve, orofacial and limb malformations, and mental retardation. Cataplexy has been reported in children with Moebius syndrome.[123]

IDIOPATHIC HYPERSOMNIA

IH is a poorly understood disorder of unknown etiology characterized by unrefreshing sleep and difficulty awakening.[1,4,53,128,129] In the past, IH was often classified into single and multisymptom forms. However, the ICSD-2 has defined two groups of patients with IH, those with and those without a long sleep time. The diagnosis of IH remains a diagnosis of exclusion of other disorders causing EDS (Box 24–6). There is likely some overlap with patients with N–C. Some patients historically given a diagnosis of IH were later found to have the upper airway resistance syndrome/mild OSA when more sophisticated monitoring techniques such as esophageal pressure monitoring were applied. Atypical depression (hypersomnia instead of insomnia), the insufficient sleep syndrome, medication side effects, narcolepsy (with delayed cataplexy), and medical and neurologic disease must be excluded. The MSLT criteria for IH include a mean sleep latency less than 8 minutes with fewer than two SOREMPs. In IH with long sleep time, an MSLT may not be practical.

IH with Long Sleep Time (IH+LST)

Manifestations Constant and severe daytime sleepiness is reported with prolonged (≤3 hr) but unrefreshing naps and a prolonged nocturnal sleep episode.[1,128] There is great difficulty awakening in the morning or after naps. The major sleep episode is greater than 10 hours (usually 12–14 hr). SP and HHs may be present (see Table 24–3). However, cataplexy is absent.

Autonomic Dysfunction Some patients with IH+LST report symptoms including headaches (often migraine-like in

BOX 24–6

Idiopathic Hypersomnia with Long Sleep Time— Diagnostic Criteria

A. The patient has a complaint of excessive daytime sleepiness occurring almost *daily for at least 3 months.*

B. The patient has prolonged nocturnal sleep time (>10 hr) documented by interview, actigraphy, or sleep logs. Waking up in the morning or at the end of naps is laborious.

C. Nocturnal PSG has excluded other causes of daytime sleepiness.

D. PSG demonstrates a short sleep latency and a major sleep period that is prolonged to more than 10 hours in duration.

E. If an MSLT is performed after the overnight PSG, a mean sleep latency of less than 8 minutes and less than two SOREMPs are demonstrated.
   (Mean sleep latency in idiopathic hypersomnia with long sleep time has been shown to be about 6.2 ± 3.0 min.)

F. Hypersomnia is not better explained by another sleep disorder, medical or neurologic disorder, medication, or substance use disorder.

MSLT = multiple sleep latency test; PSG = polysomnography; SOREMPs = sleep-onset rapid eye movement periods.
From American Academy of Sleep Medicine: International Classification of Sleep Disorders, 2nd ed. Diagnostic and Coding Manual. Westchester, IL: American Academy of Sleep Medicine, 2005.

nature), orthostatic hypotension with symptoms of peripheral vascular dysfunction (Raynaud's phenomenon—vascular constriction on exposure to cold).

Prevalence Unknown; recent studies suggest that there is 1 IH patient for every 10 patients with narcolepsy.

Onset Usually before age 25.

Polysomnography Long sleep time with normal percentages of the sleep stages. In some patients, the amount of stage N3 may be increased. The nocturnal REM latency is normal. Twenty-four-hour PSG demonstrates greater than 10 hours of sleep.

Multiple Sleep Latency Test It may be difficult to awaken a patient to start the MSLT. If performed, an MSLT shows a mean sleep latency (<8 min) and no or one SOREMP. For MSLT to be reliable, it must follow PSG, the patient should be withdrawn from medications affecting REM sleep for 15 days, and regular sleep should occur for at least 7 days before testing. The mean sleep latency for IH was listed as 6.2 ± 3.0 minutes in a recent review of the literature.[55]

CSF Hcrt CSF Hcrt1 levels are normal in patients with IH.[25,26,59] A study also found low CSF histamine[38] in patients with IH. However, this finding was not specific for IH.

Diagnostic Approach CNS imaging is suggested if there is any suspicion of a CNS lesion. The differential diagnosis includes head trauma and sleepiness associated with a psychiatric disorder or structural CNS lesion. A sleep diary or clinical history should eliminate the possibility of the insufficient sleep syndrome.

Treatment Amphetamines, methylphenidate, and modafinil[61,128,130] have all been used with variable success for treatment of daytime sleepiness (see Table 24-7). The AASM Practice Parameters for Treatment of Narcolepsy and Other Hypersomnias of Central Origin state that "modafinil may be effective for treatment of idiopathic hypersomnia (Option)."[61] Amphetamine, methamphetamine, and methylphenidate were also listed as treatments for IH (Option).

IH without Long Sleep Time (IH–LST)
IH without long sleep time (IH–LST) patients have similar symptoms as IH+LST except that the nocturnal sleep time is between 6 and 10 hours. The ICSD-2 criteria are listed in Box 24-7. The disorder has also been called *idiopathic CNS hypersomnia*. Comparison of patients with narcolepsy and IH are also illustrated in Table 24-3.

Manifestations Constant and severe daytime sleepiness is reported with unrefreshing naps and a normal to slightly prolonged nocturnal sleep episode (6–10 hr). Patients may report difficulty awakening in the morning or after naps. SP and HHs may be present. However, cataplexy is absent.

Autonomic Dysfunction Some patients with IH–LST report symptoms including headaches (often migraine in nature), orthostatic hypotension with symptoms of peripheral vascular dysfunction (Raynaud's phenomenon—vascular constriction on exposure to cold).

Prevalence Unknown; recent studies suggest that there is 1 IH patient for every 10 patients with narcolepsy. Males and females are equally affected.

Onset Usually before age 25.

Polysomnography Total sleep time greater than 6 hours but less than 10 hours. Normal distribution of the sleep stages. The sleep efficiency is greater than 85%. The nocturnal REM latency is normal.

Multiple Sleep Latency Test Mean sleep latency (<8 min) and no or one SOREMP.

CSF Hcrt1 Levels CSF Hcrt1 levels are normal in IH patients. One study found CSF histamine to be low.[38]

Diagnostic Approach CNS imaging is suggested if there is any suspicion of a CNS lesion. Psychiatric consultation may also be considered. The differential diagnosis includes head trauma and sleepiness associated with a psychiatric disorder or structural CNS lesion, the chronic fatigue syndrome, behaviorally induced insufficient sleep, and N–C. The PSG should rule out sleep apnea. A sleep diary or clinical history should eliminate the possibility of the insufficient sleep syndrome.

Treatment Same as for IH+LST.

Recurrent Hypersomnia (Including Kleine-Levin Syndrome and Menstrual-Related Hypersomnia)

Kleine-Levin Syndrome
Recurrent episodes of hypersomnia are noted and are clearly associated with behavioral abnormalities.[1,131] These may include binge eating, hypersexuality, abnormal behaviors that exhibit irritability and aggression as well as cognitive abnormalities such as a feel of unreality, confusion, and hallucinations (Box 24–8). Episodes occur 1 to 10 times per year and last a few days to several weeks. Kleine-Levin syndrome (KLS) is rare with just over 200 cases reported. The

BOX 24–7

Idiopathic Hypersomnia without Long Sleep Time—Diagnostic Criteria

A. The patient has a complaint of excessive daytime sleepiness occurring almost daily for at least 3 months.
B. The patient has normal nocturnal sleep (>6 hr but <10 hr), documented by interview, actigraphy, or sleep logs.
C. Nocturnal PSG has excluded other causes of daytime sleepiness.
D. PSG demonstrates a major sleep period that is normal in duration.
E. An MSLT following the overnight PSG demonstrates a mean sleep latency of less than 8 minutes **with fewer** than two SOREMPs.
   (MSL in idiopathic hypersomnia has been shown to be 6.2 + 3.0 min).
F. Hypersomnia is not better explained by another sleep disorder, medical or neurological disorder, medication, or substance use disorder.

MSL = mean sleep latency; MSLT = multiple sleep latency test; PSG = polysomnography; SOREMPs = sleep-onset rapid eye movement periods.

BOX 24–8

Recurrent Hypersomnia (Including Kleine-Levin Syndrome and Menstrual-Related Hypersomnia)

A. The patient experiences recurrent episodes of excessive sleepiness of 2 days to 4 weeks in duration.
B. Episodes recur at least once a year.
C. The patient has normal alertness, cognitive function, and behavior between attacks.
D. Hypersomnia is not better explained by another sleep disorder, medical or neurologic disorder, medication, or substance use disorder.

From American Academy of Sleep Medicine: International Classification of Sleep Disorders, 2nd ed. Diagnostic and Coding Manual. Westchester, IL: American Academy of Sleep Medicine, 2005.

male-to-female ratio is 4/1. In some studies, the frequency of HLA DQB1*602 was increased. Precipitating events including a flulike illness, upper respiratory infection, head trauma, or exposure to anesthesia have been reported. The second decade (adolescence) is the usual time of onset. The disease course usually lasts 1 to several years. Because of the limited number of patients, no large well-controlled study exists. Improvement has been reported with lithium, amantadine, lamotrigine, and valproic acid.[3] The AASM Standard of Practice Paper on Treatment of Narcolepsy and Other Hypersomnias of Central Origin listed lithium as possibly effective.[61] Lithium may reduce the duration of episodes and reduce the undesirable behaviors. Methylphenidate and modafinil could be used for daytime sleepiness.

Menstrual Syndrome

Recurrent episodes of sleepiness associated with the menstrual cycle. The syndrome occurs within the first few months of menarche. Episodes usually last 1 week with resolution at the time of menses. Hormone imbalance is a likely explanation because oral contraceptives result in a prolonged remission.

Other

Recurrent hypersomnia without behavioral abnormalities.

Behaviorally Induced Insufficient Sleep Syndrome

These patients fail to obtain sufficient nocturnal sleep to maintain daytime alertness and mental functioning. The diagnosis depends on patient report or sleep logs but can also be documented by actigraphy. Patients characteristically sleep longer on weekends and vacations. They usually report feeling more refreshed with a longer sleep period. The ICSD-2 criteria for behaviorally induced insufficient sleep syndrome are listed in Box 24–9.

A sleep study is not needed for diagnosis but, if performed owing to suspicion of other disorders, will often show a short sleep latency and high sleep efficiency. There is sometimes evidence of stage N3 or stage R rebound (high amount of those sleep stages).[132] Note that up to 30% of normal populations have a mean sleep latency less than 8 minutes. The complaint of daytime sleepiness and documentation of inadequate sleep are more important than the MSLT finding.

Hypersomnia Due to Medical Condition

In these patients, hypersomnia is due to a medical condition or neurologic disorder. The patients do not meet criteria for narcolepsy due to medical disorder—otherwise that diagnosis would be made. The ICSD-2 criteria for hypersomnia due to medical condition are listed in Box 24–10. Disorders commonly associated with hypersomnia due to medical condition are listed in Box 24–11. Some of these disorders were discussed in previous sections. Note that up to 30% of normal populations have a mean sleep latency less than 8 minutes. A diagnosis of hypersomnia due to medical condition assumes that there is a complaint of daytime sleepiness and that this is not simply the result of a decreased amount of sleep.

BOX 24–9

Behaviorally Induced Insufficient Sleep Syndrome—Diagnostic Criteria

A. The patient has a complaint of excessive sleepiness, or in prepubertal children, a complaint of behavior abnormality suggesting sleepiness. The abnormal sleep pattern is present almost daily for at least 3 months.

B. The patient's habitual sleep episode, established using history, sleep log, or actigraphy is usually shorter than expected for age-adjusted normative data.

C. When the habitual sleep schedule in not maintained (weekends or vacation time), patients will sleep considerably longer than usual.

D. If diagnostic PSG is performed (not required for diagnosis), sleep latency is less than 10 minutes and sleep efficiency greater than 90%. During the MSLT, a short sleep latency *less than 10 minutes* (with or without multiple SOREMPs) may be observed.

E. The hypersomnia is not better explained by another sleep disorder, medical or neurologic disorder, medication, or substance use disorder.

MSLT = multiple sleep latency test; PSG = polysomnography; SOREMPs = sleep-onset rapid eye movement periods.
From American Academy of Sleep Medicine: International Classification of Sleep Disorders, 2nd ed. Diagnostic and Coding Manual. Westchester, IL: American Academy of Sleep Medicine, 2005.

BOX 24–10

Hypersomnia Due to Medical Condition—Diagnostic Criteria

A. The patient has a complaint of excessive daytime sleepiness occurring almost daily for at least 3 months.

B. A significant underlying medical or neurologic disorder accounts for the daytime sleepiness.

C. If an MSLT is performed, the mean sleep latency is less than 8 minutes with no more than one SOREMP after PSG performed during the patient's habitual sleep period, with a minimum total sleep time of 6 hours.

D. The hypersomnia is not better explained by another sleep disorder, medical or neurologic disorder, medication, or substance use disorder.

MSLT = multiple sleep latency test; PSG = polysomnography; SOREMP = sleep-onset rapid eye movement period.
From American Academy of Sleep Medicine: International Classification of Sleep Disorders, 2nd ed. Diagnostic and Coding Manual. Westchester, IL: American Academy of Sleep Medicine, 2005.

Head Trauma Head trauma can be associated with EDS and less commonly a cause of secondary narcolepsy. Part of the hypersomnia could be due to injury to the Hcrt neurons or other wake-promoting systems. Hcrt levels can be reduced after severe head injury. However, true narcolepsy due to head trauma is rare.

Parkinson's Disease Patients with Parkinson's disease may exhibit daytime sleepiness due to medications (sleep attacks with DA agonists in some patients), OSA, and possibly the

BOX 24–11

Disorders Associated with Hypersomnia Due to Medical Condition
A. Posttraumatic hypersomnia. B. Hypersomnia due to Parkinson's disease.
C. Genetic disorders associated with central hypersomnia   Niemann-Pick type C, myotonic dystrophy, Norrie's disease, Prader-Willi syndrome, Moebius syndrome
D. Genetic disorders associated with central hypersomnia and SRBDs   Prader-Willi, myotonic dystrophy
E. Hypersomnia due to endocrine disorder (hypothyroidism) F. Hypersomnia due to central nervous system lesion (infection, tumor) G. Hypersomnia due to toxic metabolic syndrome
SRBDs = sleep-related breathing disorders. From American Academy of Sleep Medicine: International Classification of Sleep Disorders, 2nd ed. Diagnostic and Coding Manual. Westchester, IL: American Academy of Sleep Medicine, 2005.

BOX 24–12

Hypersomnia Due to Drug or Substance
HYPERSOMNIA DUE TO DRUG OR SUBSTANCE (ABUSE)
A. The patient has a complaint of sleepiness or excessive sleep. B. The complaint is believed secondary to current use, recent discontinuation, or prior prolonged use of drugs. C. The hypersomnia is not better explained by another sleep disorder, medical or neurologic disorder, mental disorder, or medication use.
HYPERSOMNIA DUE TO DRUG OR SUBSTANCE (MEDICATIONS)
A. The patient has a complaint of sleepiness or excessive sleep. B. The complaint is believed secondary to current use, recent discontinuation, or prior prolonged use of a prescribed medication. C. The hypersomnia is not better explained by another sleep disorder, medical or neurologic disorder, mental disorder, or substance use disorder.

disease itself.[133] The RBD is very common and may precede Parkinson's disease onset. The Hcrt levels in the CSF are normal but reduced in the lateral ventricles. Recently, one study found a reduction in Hcrt cells in the hypothalamus of patients with Parkinson's disease.[134]

Treatment of Hypersomnia Due to Medical Condition The AASM Practice Parameters for Treatment of Narcolepsy and Hypersomnia of Central Origin (see Table 24–7) stated that modafinil may be effective for treatment of excessive daytime sleepiness in Parkinson's disease (Option), MD (Option), and multiple sclerosis (Guideline).[62] It was also stated that methylphenidate may be indicated for treatment of EDS due to MD (Option). If modafinil is not effective in Parkinson's disease or multiple sclerosis, treatment with methylphenidate could also be tried.

Hypersomnia Due to Drug or Substance

This diagnosis is reserved for patients with excessive sleep or daytime sleepiness believed to be due to substance use (Box 24–12). There is often a historical report of symptoms beginning with the starting of a particular medication. A sleep study is not needed unless there is the suspicion of another sleep disorder. An MSLT may be needed if narcolepsy is suspected. A urine drug screen may help make the diagnosis of substance abuse. The diagnosis is confirmed when symptoms improve after discontinuation of the substance. A list of common medications associated with daytime sleepiness[135] is listed in Box 24–13. One must also remember that medications causing insomnia can indirectly result in daytime sleepiness.

The differential diagnosis of hypersomnia due to drug or medication includes sleep apnea, behaviorally induced

BOX 24–13

Common Medications Associated with Daytime Sleepiness

Benzodiazepines
Hypnotics (especially with long half-life)
Dopamine agonists
Antidepressants
    Sedating (usually > frequent sedation [trazodone, doxepin, mirtazapine])
    Nonsedating (usually <15%)—lower percentage associated with sedation—including citalopram, fluoxetine, paroxetine, sertraline
Narcotics
Antihypertensives: Clonidine, methyldopa
Antihistamines (first generation)
Antiepileptics
    Dilantin, carbamazepine, phenobarbital, lamotrigine, gabapentin, valproic acid, topiramate

insufficient sleep syndrome, or chronic fatigue. Medications can also result in worsening of symptoms of another sleep disorder.

Hypersomnia Not Due to Substance or Known Physiologic Condition

Nonorganic Hypersomnia—Hypersomnia Associated with Mental Disorders

The name of this category is somewhat confusing but most disorders of daytime sleepiness classified here **are associated with mental disorders** (Box 24–14). Women are more commonly affected than men. Sleep is often said to be

BOX 24–14

Hypersomnia Not Due to Substance or Known Physiologic Condition: Nonorganic Hypersomnia—Hypersomnia Associated with Mental Disorders: Diagnostic Criteria and Pathologic Subtypes

DIAGNOSTIC CRITERIA

A. The patient has a complaint of excessive daytime sleepiness or excessive sleep.

B. The complaint is temporally associated with a psychiatric diagnosis.

C. Polysomnography monitoring demonstrates both of the following:
   i. Reduced sleep efficiency and increased frequency and duration of awakenings.
   ii. Variable, often normal, mean sleep latencies on the MSLT.

D. The hypersomnia is not better explained by another sleep disorder, medical or neurologic disorder, mental disorder, or substance use disorder.

PATHOLOGIC SUBTYPES

1. Hypersomnia associated with a major depressive episode.
2. Hypersomnia as a conversion disorder or an undifferentiated somatoform disorder.
3. Hypersomnia associated with seasonal affective disorder.

MSLT = multiple sleep latency test.
From American Academy of Sleep Medicine: International Classification of Sleep Disorders, 2nd ed. Diagnostic and Coding Manual. Westchester, IL: American Academy of Sleep Medicine, 2005.

nonrestorative. The disorder class represents 5% to 7% of patients seen with complaints of EDS.[1,136]

Hypersomnia Associated with a Major Depressive Episode Depression is more often associated with complaints of insomnia. However, hypersomnia is frequently associated with atypical depression (mood reactivity—ability to improve with positive events, overeating) and bipolar type II disorder (major recurrent depression episodes with hypomania episodes). Long hours are spent in bed. However, the sleep latency on MSLT is usually normal.[137]

Hypersomnia Associated with Seasonal Affective Disorder Daytime fatigue, loss of concentration, increased appetite for carbohydrates, and weight gain have been reported with seasonal affective disorder (SAD).

Hypersomnia as a Conversion Disorder or an Undifferentiated Somatoform Disorder Pseudocataplexy and pseudonarcolepsy have been reported.

Physiologic (Organic Hypersomnia), Unspecified

Daily sleepiness for at least 3 months with an MSLT showing sleep latency less than 8 minutes and fewer than two

SOREMPs that do not meet criteria for other disorders are classified here.

CLINICAL REVIEW QUESTIONS

1. A patient is being evaluated for severe daytime sleepiness (Epworth Sleepiness Scale 20/24). He reports sleeping about 7 hours per night. The patient reports neck muscle weakness (head nods) when he hears or tells a joke. He undergoes a PSG followed by an MSLT. The PSG is fairly normal without evidence of sleep apnea. On the MSLT, the mean sleep latency is 4 minutes but only one of five naps has REM sleep. What is the diagnosis?
   A. Narcolepsy without cataplexy.
   B. Idiopathic hypersomnia with long sleep time.
   C. Idiopathic hypersomnia without long sleep time.
   D. Narcolepsy with cataplexy.

2. Which of the following is an effective (and FDA-approved) treatment for both daytime sleepiness and cataplexy?
   A. Sodium oxybate (SOXB).
   B. Fluoxetine.
   C. Modafinil.
   D. Methylphenidate.

3. A patient with daytime sleepiness denies cataplexy. He normally sleeps about 8 hours per night. The nocturnal PSG shows a sleep latency of 5 minutes and a REM latency of 10 minutes. The total sleep time is normal and there is no evidence of sleep apnea, but the periodic limb movement index is 20/hr. The MSLT shows a mean sleep latency of 3 minutes and REM sleep on one of five naps. What is the likely diagnosis?
   A. Narcolepsy without cataplexy.
   B. Idiopathic hypersomnia with long sleep time.
   C. Idiopathic hypersomnia without long sleep time.
   D. PLMD.

4. CSF Hcrt1 is low or undetectable in what percentage of patients with N+C?
   A. 100%.
   B. 90–95%.
   C. 85%.
   D. 70%.

5. A 20-year-old male with N+C is being treated with modafinil 400 mg daily. Daytime sleepiness has improved but is still a problem from 4 to 7 PM. Which of the following would **NOT** be a reasonable intervention?
   A. Change to modafinil 200 mg qAM, 200 mg in early afternoon.
   B. Change to modafinil 300 mg qAM, 100 mg in early afternoon.

C. Change to armodafinil 250 mg qAM.

D. Change to methylphenidate 20–30 mg in the AM.

6. An 18-year-old man is evaluated for three episodes of daytime sleepiness each lasting about 6 weeks that have occurred over the last 8 months. The patient does not have periods of depression. Which of the following is **NOT** true about the patient's disorder?

A. Lithium has been reported to be effective is small case series (delay or preventing recurrences).

B. Hypersexuality can occur during the periods of excessive sleepiness.

C. Reports of derealization and cognitive impairment are common.

D. Increased amount of daily sleep—usually 15 hours or greater.

E. No precipitating event is usually reported.

7. A 40-year-old patient with narcolepsy has disabling daytime sleepiness despite taking modafinil 400 mg daily (Epworth Sleepiness Score 16/24). Cataplexy is not reported. What is the first intervention that you recommend?

A. Increase modafinil to 600 mg daily.

B. Change to methylphenidate 20 mg bid.

C. Begin SOXB.

D. Schedule naps.

8. What duration of nocturnal sleep separates patients with IH+LST from those with IH–LST?

A. Sleep duration >8 hr.

B. Sleep duration >10 hr.

C. Sleep duration >12 hr.

D. Sleep duration >14 hr.

9. Which of the following is **NOT** true about cataplexy?

A. The duration of cataplexy is seconds to several minutes.

B. Laughter or hearing or telling a joke is the most common precipitating event.

C. Consciousness is preserved during episodes of cataplexy.

D. Histamine activity in the tuberomammillary region is lower in cataplexy than in REM sleep.

E. Deep tendon reflexes are absent during an attack of cataplexy.

10. What is the MSLT criterion for diagnosis of narcolepsy?

A. Sleep latency <8 min and two or more SOREMPs.

B. Sleep latency ≤8 min and two or more SOREMPs.

C. Sleep latency <5 min and two or more SOREMPs.

D. Sleep latency ≤5 min and two or more SOREMPs.

11. A patient with Prader-Willi syndrome (PWS) is being evaluated with daytime sleepiness. He denies cataplexy. A PSG shows an AHI of 3/hr. An MSLT shows a sleep latency of 3 minutes and one SOREMP. Which of the following is the most likely diagnosis?

A. Narcolepsy Due to Medical Condition (NDMC).

B. OSA.

C. Hypersomnia Due to Medical Condition.

D. Idiopathic hypersomnia without long sleep time.

12. If one member of a pair of identical twins has narcolepsy, in what percentage of twin pairs is the other twin likely to have or develop narcolepsy?

A. 10%.

B. 30%.

C. 50%.

D. 75%.

13. A patient is diagnosed with narcolepsy. What percentage of his first-degree relatives are likely to have or develop narcolepsy?

A. 1–2%.

B. 5%.

C. 10%.

D. 25%.

14. Which of the following is **NOT** true about modafinil?

A. Headache is the most common side effect.

B. Modafinil can alter the metabolism of oral contraceptives.

C. If modafinil is given in the morning, it can still disturb nocturnal sleep

D. Modafinil is very rarely associated with a life-threatening rash.

Answers

1. **D.** The patient reports cataplexy and daytime sleepiness. In this patient, an MSLT is confirmatory but is not essential for the diagnosis of N+C. Only about 70% of patients with N+C will have an MSLT meeting diagnostic criteria on a given day.

2. **A.** SOXB is effective for the treatment of both daytime sleepiness and cataplexy. Methylphenidate may have a modest anticataplectic effect, but modafinil has no effect on cataplexy. Fluoxetine does not treat daytime sleepiness.

3. **A.** The ICSD-2 diagnostic criteria did not mention the nocturnal REM latency. However, a study by Aldrich and coworkers[53] found that a short nocturnal REM latency had a high specificity for the diagnosis of narcolepsy as well as a moderately high positive predictive

value. PLMS is common in patients with narcolepsy (see Chapter 23).

4. **B.** About 90–95% of patients with N+C have a low or undetectable CSF Hcrt1. However, 5–10% of patients with N+C do not have a reduced CSF Hcrt.

5. **D.** Patients taking modafinil in the morning sometimes have problems with alertness in the late afternoon and early evening. Answers A and B are interventions that might be effective. One might start with A and change to B if reduction in the am modafinil caused worsening of morning sleepiness. Answer C is also reasonable because armodafinil has a longer duration of action and may be more effective than modafinil given as a morning dose. Answer D is unlikely to be effective given the short duration of action of methylphenidate. Sustained-release formulations of methylphenidate might be more useful.

6. **E.** The Kleine-Levin syndrome is characterized by repetitive periods of hypersomnia often associated with hyperphagia and hypersexuality. Over 80% of patients remember an event associated with onset of symptoms. A precipitating event is often identified and has included infection (coldlike symptoms with fever), sleep deprivation, alcohol use, and head trauma.

7. **B.** Modafinil is convenient but not necessarily as effective as stimulant medications. The daytime sleepiness of patients with narcolepsy may respond better to methylphenidate than to modafinil. Although SOXB is also a reasonable option, the patient does not have cataplexy and SOXB is much more expensive than most stimulant medications. Some patients may respond to higher doses of modafinil than 600 mg, but this patient has received little benefit from the medication. Scheduled naps may be helpful but would not be considered as the major therapeutic intervention.

8. **B.** Patients with IH+LST have a nocturnal sleep period >10 hr.

9. **D.** Cataplexy is associated with much **higher** histamine activity in the tuberomammillary area of the ventrolateral hypothalamus during cataplexy than during REM sleep. This is believed to be one of the reasons patients remain conscious during cataplexy.

10. **B.** The MSLT criterion for diagnosis of narcolepsy is a sleep latency ≤8 min and two or more SOREMPs.

11. **C.** PWS can be associated with daytime sleepiness not due to sleep apnea or narcolepsy. The patient does not have cataplexy and does not meet MSLT criteria for narcolepsy. The OSA is too mild to explain the significant daytime sleepiness. The best answer in the case is Hypersomnia Due to a Medical Disorder. If criteria for narcolepsy were present, B would be the correct answer.

12. **B.** 30% of twin pairs are concordant for narcolepsy.

13. **A.** 1–2% of the first-degree relatives are at risk for narcolepsy.

14. **C.** Modafinil does not disturb nocturnal sleep if given in the morning. Women of reproductive age should always be informed that the effectiveness of oral contraceptives may be impaired by modafinil.

REFERENCES

1. American Academy of Sleep Medicine: International Classification of Sleep Disorders, 2nd ed. Diagnostic and Coding Manual. Westchester, IL: American Academy of Sleep Medicine, 2005.
2. Scammell TE: The neurobiology, diagnosis, and treatment of narcolepsy. Ann Neurol 2003;53:154–166.
3. Frenentte E, Kushida CA: Primary hypersomnia of central origin. Semin Neurol 2009;29:354–367.
4. Aldrich MS: The clinical spectrum of narcolepsy and idiopathic hypersomnia. Neurology 1996;46:393–401.
5. De Lecca L, Kilduff TS, Peyron C, et al: The hypocretins: hypothalamic specific peptides with neuroexcitatory activity. Proc Natl Acad Sci U S A 1998;95:322–327.
6. Sakurai T: Orexins and orexin receptors: a family of hypothalamic neuropeptides and G protein–coupled receptors that regulate feeding behavior. Cell 1998;92:573–585.
7. Nishino S, Ripley B, Overeem S, et al: Hypocretin (Orexin) deficiency in human narcolepsy. Lancet 2000;355:39–40.
8. Schenck CH, Bassetti CL, Arnulf I, et al: English translations of the first clinical reports on narcolepsy and cataplexy by Westphal and Gelineau in the late 19th century. J Clin Sleep Med 2007;3:301–311.
9. Adie WJ: Idiopathic narcolepsy: a disease sui generis: with remarks on mechanism of sleep. Brain 1926;49:257–306.
10. Yoss RE, Daly DD: Criteria for the diagnosis of the narcoleptic syndrome. Proc Staff Meet Mayo Clin 1957;32:320–328.
11. Vogel G: Studies in the psychophysiology of dreams, III: the dream of narcolepsy. Arch Gen Psychiatry 1960;3:421–428.
12. Juji T, Sakate M, Honda Y, Doi Y: HLA antigens in Japanese patients with narcolepsy. All patients were DR2 positive. Tissue Antigens 1984;24:316–319.
13. Mignot E, Hayduk R, Black J, et al: HLA DQB1*0602 is associated with cataplexy in 509 narcoleptic patients. Sleep 1997;20:1012–1020.
14. Overeem S, Mignot E, van Dijk JG, Lammers GJ: Narcolepsy: clinical features, new pathophysiologic insights, and future perspectives. J Clin Neurophysiol 2001;18:78–105.
15. Dauvilliers Y, Montplasir J, Molinari N, et al: Age of onset of narcolepsy in two large populations of patients in France and Quebec. Neurology 2001;57:2029–2033.
16. Mignot E: Genetic and familial aspects of narcolepsy. Neurology 1998;50(Suppl 1):S16–S22.
17. Billiard M, Pasquie-Magnetto V, Heckman M, et al: Family studies in narcolepsy. Sleep 1994;17(Suppl):S54–S59.
18. Peyron C, Tighe DK, van den Pol AN, et al: Neurons containing hypocretin (orexin) project to multiple neuronal systems. J Neurosci 1998;18:9996–10015.
19. Erikson KS, Sergeeva O, Brown RE, Haas HL: Orexin/hypocretin-1 excites the histaminergic neurons of the tuberomammillary nucleus. J Neurosci 2001;21:9273–9279.
20. Brown RE, Sergeeva O, Eriksson KS, Haas HL: Orexin A excites serotonergic neurons in the dorsal raphe nucleus of the rat. Neuropharmacology 2001;40:457–459.
21. Hagan J: Orexin A activates locus coeruleus cell firing and increases arousal in the rat. Proc Natl Acad Sci U S A 1999;96:10911–10916.

22. Burlet S, Tyler CJ, Leonard CS: Direct and indirect excitation of laterodorsal tegmental neurons by hypocretin/orexin peptides. Implications for wakefulness and narcolepsy. J Neurosci 2002;22:2862–2872.

23. Korokova T, Sergeeva OA, Eriksson KS, et al: Excitation of ventral tegmental dopaminergic and non-dopaminergic neurons by orexin/hypocretins. J Neurosci 2003;23:7–11.

24. Taheri S, Zeitzer JM, Mignot E: The role of hypocretins (orexins) in sleep regulation and narcolepsy. Annu Rev Neurosci 2002;25:283–313.

25. Ripley BN, Overeem S, Fujiki N, et al: CSF hypocretin/orexin levels in narcolepsy and other neurological conditions. Neurology 2001;57:2253–2258.

26. Mignot E, Lammers GJ, Ripley MS, et al: The role of cerebrospinal fluid hypocretin measurement in the diagnosis of narcolepsy and other hypersomnias. Arch Neurol 2002;59:1553–1562.

27. Thannickal T, Moore RY, Nienbus R, et al: Reduced number of hypocretin neurons in human narcolepsy. Neuron 2000;27:469–474.

28. Thannickal TC, Siegel JM, Nienhuis R, Moore RY: Pattern of hypocretin (orexin) soma and axon loss, and gliosis, in human narcolepsy. Brain Pathol 2003;13:340–351.

29. Hungs M, Lin L, Okun M, et al: Polymorphisms in the vicinity of hypocretin/orexin are not associated with human narcolepsy. Neurology 2001;57:1893–1895.

30. Overeem S, Black JL, Lammers GJ: Narcolepsy: immunological aspects. Sleep Med Rev 2008;12:95–107.

31. Lin A, Nevsimalova S, Piazzi G, et al: Elevated anti-streptococcal antibodies in patients with recent narcolepsy onset. Sleep 2009;32:979–983.

32. Hallmayer J, Faraco J, Lin L, et al: Narcolepsy is strongly associated with the T-cell receptor alpha locus. Nat Genet 2009;41:708–711.

33. Cvetkovic-Lopes V, Bayer L, Dorsaz S, et al: Elevated Tribbles homolog 2–specific antibody levels in narcolepsy patients. J Clin Invest 2010;120:713–719.

34. Toyoda H, Tanaka S, Miyagawa T, et al: Anti-Tribbles homolog 2 autoantibodies in Japanese patients with narcolepsy. Sleep 2010;33:875–878.

35. Kawashima M, Lin L, Tanaka S, et al: Anti-Tribbles homolog 2 (TRIB2) autoantibodies are associated with recent onset in human narcolepsy-cataplexy. Sleep 2010;33:869–874.

36. Lim AS, Scammell TE: The trouble with Tribbles: do antibodies against TRIB2 cause narcolepsy? 1. Sleep 2010;33:857–858.

37. Nishino S, Sakurai E, Nevisimalov S, et al: Decreased CSF histamines in narcolepsy with and without low CSF hypocretin-1 in comparison to healthy controls. Sleep 2009;32:175–180.

38. Kanbayhashi T, Kodama T, Kondo H, et al: CSF histamine contents in narcolepsy, idiopathic hypersomnia and obstructive sleep apnea syndrome. Sleep 2009;32:181–187.

39. Thannickal TC, Nienhuis R, Siegel JM: Localized loss of hypocretin (Orexin) cell in narcolepsy without cataplexy. Sleep 2009;32:993–998.

40. Lai YY, Siegel JM: Medullary regions mediating atonia. J Neurosci 1988;8:4790–4796.

41. John J, Wu MF, Boehmer LN, Siegel JM: Cataplexy-active neurons in the hypothalamus: implications for the role of histamine in sleep and waking behavior. Neuron 2004;42:619–634.

42. Vetrivelan R, Fuller PM, Tong Q, Lu J: Medullary circuitry regulating rapid eye movement sleep and motor atonia. J Neurosci 2009;29:9361–9369.

43. Okun ML, Lin L, Pelin Z, et al: Clinical aspects of narcolepsy-cataplexy across ethnic groups. Sleep 2002;25:27–35.

44. Rogers AE, Aldrich MS, Caruso CC: Patterns of sleep and wakefulness in treated narcolepsy subjects. Sleep 1994;17:590–597.

45. Broughton R, Dunham W, Newman J, et al: Ambulatory 24 hour sleep-wake monitoring in narcolepsy-cataplexy compared to matched controls. Electroencephalogr Clin Neurophysiol 1988;70:473–481.

46. Schenck CH, Mahowald MW: Motor dyscontrol in narcolepsy: rapid-eye-movement (REM) sleep without atonia and REM sleep behavior disorder. Ann Neurol 1992;32:3–10.

47. Schuld A, Hebebrand J, Geller F, et al: Increased body mass index in patients with narcolepsy. Lancet 2000;355:1274–1275.

48. Chokroverty S: Sleep apnea in narcolepsy. Sleep 1986;9:250–253.

49. Dauvilliers Y, Rompre S, Gagnon JF, et al: REM sleep characteristics in narcolepsy and REM sleep behavior disorder. Sleep 2007;30:844–849.

50. Anic-Labat S, Guilleminault C, Kraemer HC, et al: Validation of a cataplexy questionnaire in 983 sleep-disorders patients. Sleep 1999;22:77–87.

51. Mosko SS, Shampain DS, Sassin JF: Nocturnal REM latency and sleep disturbance in narcolepsy. Sleep 1984;7:115–125.

52. Billiard M, Quero-Salva M, De Koninck J, et al: Daytime sleep characteristics and their relationships with night sleep in the narcoleptic patient. Sleep 1986;9:167–174.

53. Aldrich MS, Chervin RD, Malow BA: Value of the multiple sleep latency test (MSLT) for the diagnosis of narcolepsy. Sleep 1997;20:620–629.

54. Littner MR, Kushida C, Wise M, et al: Practice parameters for clinical use of the multiple sleep latency test and the maintenance of wakefulness test. Sleep 2005;28:113–121.

55. Arand D, Bonnet M, Hurwitz T, et al: The clinical use of the MSLT and MWT. Sleep 2005;28:123–144.

56. Chervin RD, Aldrich MS: Sleep onset REM periods during multiple sleep latency tests in patients evaluated for sleep apnea. Am J Respir Crit Care Med 2000;161:426–431.

57. Mignot E, Lin X, Arrigoni J, et al: DBQ1*602 and DQA1*0102 are better markers than DR2 for narcolepsy in Caucasians and Black Americans. Sleep 1994;17(Suppl 8):S60–S67.

58. Mignot E, Chen W, Black J: On the value of measuring CSF hypocretin-1 in diagnosing narcolepsy. Sleep 2003;26:646–649.

59. Nishino S, Kanbayashi T, Fujiki N, et al: CSF hypocretin levels in Guillain-Barré syndrome and other inflammatory neuropathies. Neurology 2003;61:823–825.

60. Krahn LE, Pankratz S, Oliver L, et al: Hypocretin (Orexin) levels in cerebrospinal fluid of patients with narcolepsy: relationship to cataplexy and HLADQB1*0602 status. Sleep 2003;25:733–736.

61. Morgenthaler TI, Kapur VK, Brown TM, et al: Practice parameters for the treatment of narcolepsy and other hypersomnias of central origin. Sleep 2007;30:1705–1711.

62. Littner M, Johnson SF, McCall MV, et al: Standard of Practice Committee of the AASM. Practice Parameters for the treatment of narcolepsy: an update 2000. Sleep 2001;24:451–466.

63. Thorpy M: Therapeutic advances in narcolepsy. Sleep Med 2007;8:427–440.

64. Wise MS, Arand DL, Auger RR, et al: Treatment of narcolepsy and other hypersomnias of central origin. Sleep 2007;30:1712–1727.

65. Mullington J, Broughton R: Scheduled naps in the management of daytime sleepiness in narcolepsy-cataplexy. Sleep 1993:16:444–456.

66. Mitler M, Aldrich MS, Koob GF, et al: ASDA standards of practice: narcolepsy and its treatment with stimulants. Sleep 1994;17:352–371.

67. Mignot E: An update on the pharmacotherapy of excessive daytime sleepiness and cataplexy. Sleep Med Rev 2004;8:333–338.

68. Mignot E, Nishino S: Emerging therapies in narcolepsy-cataplexy. Sleep 2005;28:754–763.

69. Nishino S, Mao J, Sampathkmaran R, et al: Increased dopaminergic transmission mediates the wake-promoting effects of CNS stimulants. Sleep Res Online 1998;1:49–61.

70. Wisor JP, Nishino S, Sora I, et al: Dopaminergic role in stimulant-induced wakefulness. J Neurosci 2001;21:1787–1794.

71. Wallin MT, Mahowald M: Blood pressure effects of long-term stimulant use in disorders of hypersomnolence. J Sleep Res 1998;7:209–215.

72. Auger RR, Goodman SH, Silber MH: Risks of high-dose stimulants in treatment of disorders of excessive somnolence: a case control study. Sleep 2005;28:667–672.

73. Mitler M, Harsch J, Hirshkowitz M, et al: Long-term efficacy and safety of modafinil for the treatment of excessive daytime sleepiness associated with narcolepsy. Sleep 1994;17:352–371.

74. U.S. Modafinil in Narcolepsy Study Group: Randomized trial of modafinil for the treatment of pathological somnolence in narcolepsy. Ann Neurol 1998;43:88–97.

75. U.S. Modafinil in Narcolepsy Study Group: Randomized trial of modafinil as a treatment for the excessive daytime somnolence of narcolepsy. Neurology 2000;53:1166–1175.

76. Schwartz JRL, Feldman NT, Bogan RK: Dose effects of modafinil in sustaining wakefulness in narcolepsy patients with residual evening sleepiness. J Neuropsychiatry Clin Neurosci 2005;7:405–412.

77. Schwartz JRL, Feldman NT, Bogan RK, et al: Dosing regimen effects of modafinil for improving daytime wakefulness in patients with narcolepsy. Clin Neuropharmacol 2003;26:252–257.

78. Darwish M, Kirby M, Hellriegel ET: Comparison of steady-state plasma concentrations of armodafinil and modafinil late in the day following morning administration: post hoc analysis of two randomized, double-blind, placebo-controlled, multiple-dose studies in healthy male subjects. Clin Drug Investig 2009;29:601–612.

79. Darwish M, Kirby M, Hellriegel ET, Robertson P Jr: 1. Armodafinil and modafinil have substantially different pharmacokinetic profiles despite having the same terminal half-lives: analysis of data from three randomized, single-dose, pharmacokinetic studies. Clin Drug Investig 2009;29:613–623.

80. Darwish M, Kirby M, D'Andrea DM, et al: Pharmacokinetics of armodafinil and modafinil after single and multiple doses in patients with excessive sleepiness associated with treated obstructive sleep apnea: a randomized, open-label, crossover study. Clin Ther 2010;32:2074–2087.

81. Harsh JR, Hayduk R, Rosenberg R, et al: The efficacy and safety of armodafinil as treatment for adults with excessive sleepiness associated with narcolepsy. Curr Med Res Opin 2006;22:761–774.

82. Mignot E, Nishino S, Guilleminault C, et al: Modafinil binds to the dopamine uptake carrier site with low affinity. Sleep 1994;17:436–437.

83. Scammell TE, Estabrooke IV, McCarthy MT, et al: Hypothalamic arousal regions are activated during modafinil-induced wakefulness. J Neurosci 2000;20:8620–8628.

84. Ferraro L, Tanganellis S, O'Connor WT, et al: The vigilance promoting drug modafinil decreases GABA release in the medial preoptic area and in the posterior hypothalamus of the awake rat: possible involvement of the serotonergic 5-HT$_3$ receptor. Neurosci Lett 1996;220:5–8.

85. Gallopin T, Luppi PH, Rambert FA, et al: Effect of wake-promoting agent modafinil on sleep-promoting neurons from the ventrolateral preoptic nucleus: an in vitro pharmacologic study. Sleep 2004;27:19–25.

86. Gerrard P, Malcolm R: Mechanisms of modafinil: a review of current research. Neuropsychiatr Dis Treat 2007;3:349–364.

87. Guilleminault C, Aftab FA, Karadeniz D, et al: Problems associated with switch to modafinil—a novel alerting agent in narcolepsy. Eur J Neurol 2000;7:381–384.

88. U.S. Xyrem Multicenter Study Group: A randomized, double-blind, placebo-controlled multicenter trial comparing the effects of three doses of orally administered sodium oxybate with placebo for the treatment of narcolepsy. Sleep 2002;25:42–49.

89. U.S. Xyrem Multicenter Study Group: A 12-month open-label, multi-center extension trial of orally administered sodium oxybate for the treatment of narcolepsy. Sleep 2003;1:31–35.

90. The Xyrem International Study Group: A double-blind, placebo-controlled study demonstrates sodium oxybate is effective for treatment of excessive daytime sleepiness in narcolepsy. J Clin Sleep Med 2005;1:391–397.

91. Black J, Houghton WC: Sodium oxybate improves excessive daytime sleepiness in narcolepsy. Sleep 2006;29:939–946.

92. U.S. Xyrem Multicenter Study Group: Sodium oxybate demonstrates long-term efficacy for the treatment of cataplexy in patients with narcolepsy. Sleep Med 2004;5:119–123.

93. Xyrem International Study Group: Further evidence supporting the use of sodium oxybate for the treatment of cataplexy: a double-blind, placebo-controlled study in 228 patients. Sleep Med 2005;6:415–421.

94. Black J, Pardi D, Hornfledt CS, Inhaber N: The nightly administration of sodium oxybate results in significant reduction in the nocturnal sleep disruption of patients with narcolepsy. Sleep Med 2009;10:829–835.

95. George CFP, Feldman N, Inaber N, et al: A safety trial of sodium oxybate in patients with obstructive sleep apnea. Sleep Med 2010;11:38–42.

96. Mayer G, Ewert-Meier K, Hephata K: Selegeline hydrochloride treatment in narcolepsy: a double-blind, placebo-controlled study. Clin Neuropharmacol 1995;18:306–319.

97. Nishino S, Mignot E: Pharmacological aspects of human and canine narcolepsy. Prog Neurobiol 1997;52:27–78.

98. Frey J, Darbonne C: Fluoxetine suppresses human cataplexy. Neurology 1994;44:707–709.

99. Aldrich M, Rogers AE: Exacerbation of human cataplexy by prazosin. Sleep 1989;12:254–256.

100. Valko PO, Khatami R, Baumann CR, Bassetti CL: No persistent effect of intravenous immunoglobulins in patients with narcolepsy with cataplexy. J Neurol 2008;255:1900–1903.

101. Fujiki N, Yoshida Y, Ripley B, et al: Effects of IV and ICV hypocretin-1 in hypocretin receptor 2 gene mutated narcoleptic dogs and IV hypocretin 1 in a hypocretin-ligand deficient narcoleptic dog. Sleep 2003;26:953–959.

102. Hanson LR, Martinez PM, Taheri S, et al: Intranasal administration of hypocretin 1 bypasses the blood-brain barrier and targets the brain: new strategy for the treatment of narcolepsy. Drug Delivery Technol 2004;4:66–71.

103. Nevsimalova S: Narcolepsy in childhood. Sleep Med Rev 2009;13:169–180.

104. Serra L, Montagna P, Mignot E, et al: Cataplexy features in childhood narcolepsy. Mov Disord 2008;23:858–865.

105. Aran A, Einen M, Lin L, et al: Clinical and therapeutic aspects of childhood narcolepsy-cataplexy: a retrospective study of 51 children. Sleep 2010;33:1457–1464.

106. Carskadon M: The second decade. In Guilleminault C (ed): Sleeping and Waking Disorders: Indications and Techniques. Menlo Park, CA: Addison-Wesley, 1982, pp. 99–125.

107. Malik S, Boeve BF, Krahn LE, et al: Narcolepsy associated with other central nervous system disorders. Neurology 2001;57:539–541.

108. Autret A, Lucas B, Henry-Lebras F, de Toffol B: Symptomatic narcolepsies. Sleep 1996;17:S21–S24.

109. Nishino S, Kanbayashi T: Symptomatic narcolepsy, cataplexy, and hypersomnia, and their implications in the hypothalamic/hypocretin/orexin system. Sleep Med Rev 2005;9:269–310.

110. Aldrich MS, Naylor MW: Narcolepsy associated with lesions of the diencephalon. Neurology 1989;39:1505–1508.

111. Vankova J, Stepanov I, Jech R, et al: Sleep disturbances and hypocretin deficiency in Niemann-Pick disease type C. Sleep 2003;26:427–430.

112. Guilleminault C, Van den Hoed J, Miles L: Posttraumatic excessive daytime sleepiness. Neurology 1983;33:1584–1589.

113. Manni R, Politini L, Nobili L, et al: Hypersomnia in the Prader-Willi syndrome: clinical, electrophysiological features, and underlying factors. Clin Neurophysiol 2001;112:800–805.

114. Tobias ES, Tolmie GJ, Stephenson JBP: Cataplexy in Prader-Willi syndrome. Arch Dis Child 2002;87:170.

115. Nevsimalova S, Vankova J, Stepanova I, et al: Hypocretin deficiency in Prader-Willi syndrome. Eur J Neurol 2005;12:70–72.

116. Fronczek R, Lammers GJ, Balesar R, et al: The number of hypothalamic hypocretin orexin neurons is not affected in PWS. J Clin Endocrinol Metab 2005;90:5466–5470.

117. Kanbayashi T, Abe M, Fujimoto S, et al: Hypocretin deficiency in Niemann-Pick type C with cataplexy. Neuropediatrics 2003;34:52–53.

118. Vanier MT, Suzuki K: Recent advances in elucidating Niemann-Pick C disease. Brain Pathol 1998;8:163–174.

119. Nelson GB, Hahn JS: Stimulus-induced drop episodes in Coffin-Lowry syndrome. Pediatrics 2003;111:197–202.

120. Fryssira H, Kountoupi S, Delaunoy JP, Thomaidis L: A female with Coffin-Lowry syndrome and "cataplexy." Genet Couns 2002;13:405–409.

121. Vossler DG, Wyler AR, Wilkus RJ, et al: Cataplexy and monoamine oxidase deficiency in Norrie disease. Neurology 1996;46:1258–1261.

122. Chen ZY, Denney RM, Breakfield XO: Norrie disease and MAO genes: nearest neighbours. Hum Mol Genet 1995;4:1729–1737.

123. Tyagi A, Harrington H: Cataplexy in association with Moebius syndrome. J Neurol 2003;250:110–111.

124. Talbot K, Stradling J, Crosby J, et al: Reduction in excess daytime sleepiness by modafinil in patients with myotonic dystrophy. Neuromuscul Disord 2003;13:357–364.

125. MacDonald JR, Hill JD, Tarnopolsky MA: Modafinil reduces excessive somnolence and enhances mood in patients with myotonic dystrophy. Neurology 2002;59:1876–1880.

126. Orlikowski D, Chevret S, Quera-Salva MA, et al: Modafinil for the treatment of hypersomnia associated with myotonic muscular dystrophy in adults: a multicenter, prospective, randomized, double-blind, placebo-controlled, 4-week trial. Clin Ther 2009;31:1765–1773.

127. Vankova J, Stepanov I, Jech R, et al: Sleep disturbances and hypocretin deficiency in Niemann-Pick disease type C. Sleep 2003;26:427–430.

128. Bassetti C, Aldrich MS: Idiopathic hypersomnia. Brain 1997;120:1423–1435.

129. Anderson KN, Pilsworth S, Sharples LD, et al: Idiopathic hypersomnia: a study of 77 cases. Sleep 2007;30:1274–1281.

130. Bastujii H, Jouvet M: Successful treatment of idiopathic hypersomnia and narcolepsy with modafinil. Prog Neuropsychopharmacol Biol Psychiatry 1988;12:695–700.

131. Arnulf I, Lin L, Gadoth N, et al: Kleine-Levin syndrome: a systematic study of 108 patients. Ann Neurol 2008:63:482–492.

132. Roehrs T, Zorick F, Sicklesteel J, et al: Excessive daytime sleepiness associated with insufficient sleep. Sleep 1983;6:319–325.

133. Arnulf I, Leu S, Oudiette D: Abnormal sleep and sleepiness in Parkinson's disease. Curr Opin Neurol 2008;21:472–477.

134. Fronczek R, Overeem S, Lee SY, et al: Hypocretin loss in Parkinson's disease. Brain 2007;130:1577–1585.

135. Schweitzer P: Drugs that disturb sleep and wakefulness. In Kryger MH, Roth T, Dement WC (eds): Principles and Practice of Sleep Medicine, 4th ed. Philadelphia: Elsevier Saunders, 2005, pp. 499–518.

136. Plante DT, Winkleman JW: Sleep disturbance in bipolar disorders. Am J Psychiatry 2008;165:830–843.

137. Nofzinger EA, Thase ME, Reynolds CF 3rd, et al: Hypersomnia in bipolar depression: a comparison with narcolepsy using the multiple sleep latency test. Am J Psychiatry 1991;148:1177–1181.

Chapter 25

Insomnia

Chapter Points

- A diagnosis of insomnia requires some type of **daytime impairment** related to nocturnal sleep difficulty.
- **Adjustment insomnia** is characterized by insomnia with a **duration less than 3 months** that is temporally associated with an identifiable stressor and expected to resolve.
- **Psychophysiologic insomnia** must have a **duration of at least 1 month** and is characterized by conditioned sleep-preventing associations—the bedroom is a stimulus for wake not sleep. Patients can often fall asleep better in a novel setting or at home outside the bedroom.
- **Idiopathic insomnia** is present since infancy or childhood, has no identifiable precipitant (insidious onset), and no period of sustained remission.
- **Paradoxical insomnia** is characterized by a **duration of at least 1 month** and complaints of little or no sleep but relatively minor daytime consequences and no or rare naps. The degree of sleep reduction reported far exceeds that noted with objective determinations of sleep (PSG) or estimates of sleep (actigraphy).
- **Inadequate sleep hygiene** is characterized by a **duration of at least 1 month** and improper sleep scheduling, stimulating activities near bedtime, or use of the bed for nonsleep activities.
- **Insomnia Due to Drug or Substance is** characterized by a **duration of at least 1 month** and ongoing dependence and abuse of sleep-disruptive medication or substance with symptoms either during intoxication or withdrawal OR current exposure to medication or substance known to disturb sleep in susceptible individuals. The complaint should be temporally associated with use or withdrawal of the medication or substance.
- **Insomnia Due to Mental Disorder** is characterized by insomnia of a **duration of at least 1 month** that is temporally associated with (or slightly preceding) the onset of the mental disorder, waxes and wanes with the severity of the mental disorder, and is **more prominent than expected for the disorder** such that

the insomnia is causing **marked distress** or is an **independent focus of treatment.**
- **Behavioral Insomnia of Childhood** is divided into **sleep-association type** (requires certain conditions for sleep onset) and **limit-setting type** (refusal to go to sleep).
- The most common cause of insomnia is the presence of a psychiatric disorder.
- The most important characteristic of a BZRA to consider when choosing a medication to treat insomnia is the **duration of action.**
- Hypnotics with a short duration of action are indicated to treat sleep-onset insomnia (e.g., zaleplon, ramelteon).
- BZRAs with intermediate duration of action are indicated to treat sleep-onset or sleep-maintenance insomnia (zolpidem CR, eszopiclone, temazepam). Zolpidem is also effective for sleep-maintenance insomnia in some patients.
- CBT of insomnia (also known as CBTI) is **effective** for both **primary and secondary (co-morbid) insomnia** including insomnia due to medical conditions. **The combination of a hypnotic and CBTI is NOT more effective than CBTI alone for primary insomnia.**
- CBTI is defined as cognitive therapy + stimulus control and/or sleep restriction with or without relaxation therapy.
- Major behavioral techniques with their level of evidence are shown in the following table.

TECHNIQUE	EVIDENCE	BRIEF SUMMARY
Stimulus control	Standard	If not sleepy, get out of bed until sleepy. Have the same wake time every day. Use the bed only for sleep.
Sleep restriction	Standard	Restrict time in bed so sleep ≥ 85% of time in bed.
Relaxation	Guideline	Progressive muscle relaxation. Guided imagery.

TECHNIQUE	EVIDENCE	BRIEF SUMMARY
Biofeedback	Guideline	Reduce somatic tension.
Paradoxical intention	Guideline	Passively remain awake and avoid any effort (intention) to fall asleep.
Sleep hygiene education	No recommendation	Improved sleep scheduling, used bed only for sleep.

- Options for treatment of insomnia in a patient with depression include using (1) a sedating antidepressant at a dose effective for depression, (2) an effective antidepressant + a low dose of a sedating antidepressant, (3) an effective antidepressant + a BZRA. In patients with a history of alcohol or drug dependence, use of a BZRA should be avoided.
- In patients with benign prostatic hypertrophy, medications with anticholinergic side effects should be avoided.

BOX 25–1

Diagnostic Criteria for Insomnia

A. A complaint of difficulty initiating sleep, difficulty maintaining sleep, or waking up too early, or sleep that is chronically nonrestorative or of poor quality. In children, the sleep difficulty is often reported by the caretaker and may consist of observed bedtime resistance or inability to sleep independently.

B. The above sleep difficulty occurs despite **adequate opportunity and circumstances** for sleep.

C. At least one of the following forms of daytime impairment related to the night sleep difficulty is reported by the patient.
   i. Fatigue or malaise.
   ii. Attention, concentration, or memory impairment.
   iii. Social or vocational dysfunction or poor school performance.
   iv. Mood disturbance or irritability.
   v. Daytime sleepiness.
   vi. Motivation, energy, or initiative reduction.
   vii. Proneness to error/accidents at work or while driving.
   viii. Tension, headaches, or gastrointestinal symptoms in response to sleep loss.
   ix. Concerns or worries about sleep.

From American Academy of Sleep Medicine: ICSD-2 International Classification of Sleep Disorders, 2nd ed. Diagnostic and Coding Manual. Westchester, IL: American Academy of Sleep Medicine, 2005.

The International Classification of Sleep Disorders, second edition (ICSD-2)[1] lists diagnostic criteria for insomnia (Box 25–1) that include requirements for an insomnia **sleep complaint, adequate opportunity/sleep**, and some form of **daytime impairment** related to the sleep difficulty. The sleep complaints associated with insomnia include difficulty initiating sleep (**sleep-onset insomnia**), difficulty maintaining sleep (**sleep-maintenance insomnia**), **waking up too early**, or sleep that is chronically **nonrestorative** or poor in quality. A diagnosis of insomnia requires that patients must report at least one of these insomnia complaints. However, it is not uncommon for individual patients to report all of them. There must be adequate opportunity and circumstances for sleep to occur. A diagnosis of insomnia also requires evidence of daytime impairment related to the sleep problem. Patients suffering from insomnia may report a wide variety of complaints (see Box 25–1) including fatigue or malaise, problems with attention or concentration, memory impairment, social or vocational dysfunction, and poor school performance. Other symptoms associated with insomnia include mood disturbance or irritability; daytime sleepiness; reduction in motivation or initiative; proneness to error/accidents at work or while driving; tension headaches or gastrointestinal symptoms in response to sleep loss; and concerns or worries about sleep.[1] In children, the sleep difficulty is often reported by the caretaker and may consist of observed bedtime resistance or inability to sleep independently. Although the minimum duration of insomnia complaints is not specified in the definition of insomnia (see Box 25–1), the diagnostic criteria for several individual insomnia types does specify a minimum duration of 1 month.[1]

PREVALENCE OF INSOMNIA AND RISK FACTORS

It has been estimated that insomnia complaints occur on at least a few nights per year in 33% to 50% of the adult population. Insomnia complaints plus symptoms of impairment due to insomnia occur in 10% to 15% of the population. Specific insomnia disorders occur in 5% to 10%.[2-5] A number of risk factors for the development of insomnia have been identified, including older age, female gender, co-morbid problems (depression and other psychiatric disorders, substance abuse), shift work, unemployment, and lower socioeconomic status. Some studies suggest that single, divorced, and separated patients have greater insomnia rates than married patients. The most common cause of insomnia in patients evaluated by a physician is insomnia due to or associated with depression. Insomnia occurs in the majority of patients (80%) with major depressive or chronic pain disorders. **Persistent insomnia symptoms increase the likelihood of developing a major depression within a 1-year period by a factor of four.**[3] In addition, up to one third of all cases of insomnia are associated with a mental disorder.

INSOMNIA SUBTYPES

The ICSD-2 classification lists a number of distinct sleep disorders associated with insomnia (Box 25–2). The three most common insomnia disorders include adjustment

BOX 25-2

Insomnia Disorders

SUBTYPES OF INSOMNIA DISORDERS

1. Adjustment Insomnia (Acute Insomnia)
2. Psychophysiologic Insomnia (12–15%)
3. Paradoxical Insomnia (<5%)
4. Idiopathic Insomnia (<10%)
5. Insomnia Due to Mental Disorder
6. Inadequate Sleep Hygiene (5–10%)
7. Behavioral Insomnia of Childhood
8. Insomnia Due to Drug or Substance
9. Insomnia Due to Medical Condition
10. Insomnia Not Due to Substance or Known Physiologic Condition, Unspecified
11. Physiologic (Organic) Insomnia, Unspecified

OTHER SLEEP DISORDERS ASSOCIATED WITH INSOMNIA COMPLAINTS

1. Sleep Apnea Syndromes
2. Circadian Rhythm Sleep Disorders
    a. Delayed Sleep Phase Type—sleep-onset insomnia
    b. Advanced Sleep Phase Type—early AM awakening
    c. Irregular Sleep Phase Type—at least 3 sleep episodes per day
    d. Free-Running Type—alternating periods of insomnia and hypersomnia.
3. Restless Legs Syndrome/Periodic Limb Movement Disorders

From American Academy of Sleep Medicine: ICSD-2 International Classification of Sleep Disorders, 2nd ed. Diagnostic and Coding Manual. Westchester, IL: American Academy of Sleep Medicine, 2005.

BOX 25-3

Diagnostic Criteria for Primary Insomnia

A. The predominant complaint is difficulty initiating or maintaining sleep or nonrestorative sleep for at least 1 month.
B. The sleep disorder causes clinically significant **distress** or **impairment** of social, occupation, or other important areas of functioning.
C. The sleep disturbance **does not occur exclusively during the course** of narcolepsy, breathing-related sleep disorder, circadian rhythm sleep disorder, or a parasomnia.
D. The disturbance does not occur exclusively during the course of another **mental disorder** (e.g., Major Depressive Disorder, Generalized Anxiety Disorder, a delirium).
E. The disturbance is not due to the direct physiologic effects of a substance (e.g., a drug of abuse, a medication) or a general medication condition.

From American Psychiatric Association: Diagnostic and Statistical Manual of Mental Disorders. DSM-IV. Washington, DC: American Psychiatric Association, 1994.

include adjustment insomnia, psychophysiologic insomnia, paradoxical insomnia, idiopathic insomnia, and inadequate sleep hygiene. Insomnia associated with a mental disorder is termed *secondary* or *co-morbid insomnia*. The subtypes of insomnia listed in the ICSD-2 classification are each discussed in some detail. However, it is helpful to remember the major characteristics of each type (Table 25–1) when evaluating patients.

EVALUATION OF INSOMNIA COMPLAINTS

Clinical guidelines for the evaluation and management of chronic insomnia in adults have been recently published.[7] This guideline document provides a succinct discussion that is a valuable resource for the clinician. Other, more extensive reviews of evaluation of insomnia and practice parameters for evaluation have also been published.[5,8–10]

A detailed sleep history is the cornerstone of evaluation of insomnia (Box 25–4). First, the nature of the **primary sleep complaint** (problems with sleep onset, sleep maintenance, or quality) should be defined and the **duration of the complaint** determined. The history of the origin of the complaint including age of onset should be explored and particular life events or stressors at the start of the problem should be identified. For example, patients with idiopathic insomnia report problems since childhood or adolescence with an insidious onset. Patients with psychophysiologic insomnia may report that chronic insomnia began after a severe illness. **Presleep conditions** or activities that could affect sleep including the bedroom environment, activities near bedtime, or mental state near bedtime should be explored. The **bedroom environment** should be characterized for factors that might disturb sleep (noise, clock easily seen from the

insomnia, psychophysiologic insomnia, and insomnia due to a mental disorder. A number of other sleep disorders not included in this group can also present with complaints of insomnia (see Box 25–2). The sleep apnea syndromes can be associated with repetitive arousal and sleep-maintenance problems. In patients with **sleep apnea, insomnia symptoms are more likely to be present in women than in men.**[1] The circadian rhythm sleep disorders (CRSDs) can also be associated with insomnia complaints including the **delayed sleep phase syndrome** (sleep-onset insomnia) and the **advanced sleep phase syndrome** (early morning awakening). In the delayed sleep phase type, once the affected individuals are able to fall asleep, they have fairly normal sleep. In the advanced sleep phase syndrome, individuals fall asleep early but then awaken in the early morning hours. In CRSD free-running type, patients may report periods of insomnia alternating with hypersomnia.[1] The **restless legs syndrome/periodic limb movement disorder** can also be associated with symptoms of insomnia or nonrestorative sleep.

Other classifications of insomnia divide disorders into primary and secondary (co-morbid) insomnia. The Diagnostic and Statistical Manual of Mental Disorders, 4th edition (DSM-IV), lists diagnostic criteria for primary insomnia (307.42) (Box 25–3).[6] This type of insomnia would

TABLE 25–1

Major Characteristics of Insomnia Types in International Classification of Sleep Disorders, 2nd Edition

INSOMNIA TYPES	ESSENTIAL FEATURES	CLINICAL CLUES
Adjustment	• Temporally associated with identifiable stressor. • Duration **less than 3 months.** • Expected to resolve.	• Recent psychological, psychosocial, environmental, or physical stressor.
Psychophysiologic	• Duration **at least 1 month.** • Anxiety about sleep. • Heightened arousal when in bed. • Conditioned sleep-preventing associations (bedroom as stimulus for wake not sleep).	• Better sleep in novel environment (away from home) • Can fall asleep outside bedroom or when not trying to sleep
Paradoxical	• Duration **at least 1 month.** • Extreme and physiologically improbable complaints: "I never sleep." • Despite report of little sleep, relatively minor daytime impairment.	• Objective sleep duration much greater than reported. • No or rare naps.
Idiopathic	• Onset in infancy or childhood. • No identifiable precipitant. • No period of sustained remission.	• Lifelong insomnia without remissions. • Insidious onset.
Associated with a mental disorder	• Insomnia present for at least 1 month. • Mental disorder has been diagnosed. • Temporally associated with mental disorder (can precede by a few days of weeks).	• Insomnia waxes and wanes with mental disorder.
Inadequate sleep hygiene	• Improper sleep scheduling. • Use of products that disturb sleep near bedtime. • Stimulating activities near bedtime. • Use of the bed for nonsleep activities.	• Variable bedtime and wake times. • Napping.
Behavioral insomnia of childhood sleep association type	• Falling asleep is an extended process. • Sleep-onset associations demanding. • In absence of associated factors, sleep onset delayed.	• Nighttime awakenings require caregiver for return to sleep.
Behavioral insomnia of childhood limit-setting type	• Difficulty initiating or maintaining sleep • Refusal to go to bed or return to bed after awakening. • Caregiver demonstrates insufficient limit setting to establish appropriate behavior.	• Caregiver demonstrates insufficient limit setting to establish appropriate behavior.

Adapted from Schutte-Rodin S, Broch L, Buysee D, et al: Clinical guideline for the evaluation and management of chronic insomnia in adults. J Clin Sleep Med 2008;4:487–504.

bed, extreme hot or cold temperature). **Activities near bedtime,** including working late on the computer, drinking caffeinated beverages or alcohol in the evening, or exercise near bedtime, may impair the ability to sleep. The **mental status at bedtime** should be explored. Often, patients began worrying about their stresses and problems when retiring for the night. The presence or absence of **nocturnal symptoms** including snoring, gasping during sleep, symptoms of the restless legs syndrome, and body movements should be evaluated.

The **sleep-wake schedule** should be determined by report including variability of bedtime and rise time as well as the frequency and duration of naps. Factors that worsen or improve sleep should be detailed. For example, some patients with psychophysiologic insomnia report sleeping better in a novel environment (**reverse first-night effect**).[11] Patient recall can be supplemented by sleep logs and/or actigraphy

as discussed in a following section. **Daytime function** should be discussed with emphasis on possible consequences of insomnia. Reports of daytime fatigue or impaired cognition and mood are more common than true daytime sleepiness. True daytime sleepiness should trigger suspicion for additional sleep problems such as sleep apnea, narcolepsy, or depression. Daytime activities that may affect sleep such as the amount of caffeine, alcohol, exercise, sunlight exposure, and napping should be detailed. A general medical and psychiatric history is important to identify mental or medical conditions that may affect sleep. **A detailed medication history including over-the-counter medications and substances of abuse is extremely important.**

A physical examination and a general medical history including appropriate laboratory (if not recently performed) should rule out obvious medical causes of insomnia. Examination of the upper airway showing a high Mallampati score

BOX 25–4

Evaluation of Insomnia

1. SLEEP HISTORY

A. Define primary complaint
  - Delayed sleep onset.
  - Sleep maintenance problems.
  - Frequent awakenings/early AM awakening.
  - Nonrestorative sleep.
B. Define time course of complaint—age of onset, precipitating event, or stressor.
C. Presleep conditions (prebedtime activities, bedroom environment, physical and mental status before sleep).
D. Nocturnal symptoms (awakenings, physical or mental symptoms including snoring or body movements).
E. Sleep-wake schedule—by patient report including variability, naps.
F. Daytime function—consequences of insomnia
  - Sleepiness versus fatigue.
  - Impairment of mood, cognitive dysfunction, quality of life.
G. Daytime activities relevant for sleep
  - Sunlight exposure, exercise.
  - Napping.
  - Work schedule and disturbance.
  - Caffeine and alcohol intake.
H. Medical and psychiatric conditions
  - Medications that may affect sleep.
  - Chronic pain.

2. PHYSICAL AND MENTAL STATUS EXAMINATION

3. SUPPORTING INFORMATION

A. Sleep/mood questionnaires
  - Epworth Sleepiness Scale.
  - Dysfunctional Beliefs and Attitudes about Sleep.
  - Pittsburgh Sleep Quality Index.
B. Sleep log for 2 weeks—attention to sleep and wake time variability, general patterns.
C. Actigraphy.

4. SLEEP STUDY—NOT ROUTINELY INDICATED

  - Indicated when concerns that another sleep disorder such as sleep apnea is suspected.

(upper airway narrowing)[12] might trigger suspicions of obstructive sleep apnea.

Questionnaires, Sleep Logs, and Actigraphy

Supporting information from questionnaires (mood, cognition about insomnia), sleep logs, and actigraphy may be helpful in evaluating patients with insomnia (Table 25–2). These may supplement other information obtained from the sleep history. Assessing the patient's attitudes about sleep and the sleep problem is as important as documenting the degree of sleep disturbance. In addition, some patients are hesitant to admit to feelings of depression. Sleep logs and actigraphy provide a more accurate estimate of the patient's sleep quantity than is possible from patient recall.

Questionnaires

A number of questionnaires have been used to evaluate patients with insomnia. The Epworth Sleepiness Scale, as discussed in Chapter 12, is used to assess subjective estimates of propensity to fall asleep in common situations.[13] The Pittsburgh Sleep Quality Index (PSQI) is a 24-item self-report measure of general sleep quality that specifically addresses the preceding 1-month period. The PSQI evaluates seven domains: duration of sleep, sleep disturbance, sleep-onset latency, daytime dysfunction due to sleepiness, sleep efficiency, need for medications to sleep, and overall sleep quality. The PSQI yields a global score and seven component scores (poor sleep: global score > 5).[14,15] The questionnaire has been shown to discriminate healthy patients, patients with depression, and patients with sleep disorders. It was not designed specifically for insomnia but has been used in insomnia assessment and treatment studies. Detailed instructions for use and scoring of the PSQI are available at the University of Pittsburgh Sleep Medicine Institute website: http://www.sleep.pitt.edu/content.asp?id=1484&subid=2316

The Beck Depression Inventory (BDI-I or BDI-II) is a 21-item self-report inventory used to measure manifestations of depression, each item being scored from 0 to 3.[16,17] Higher total scores indicate more severe depressive symptoms. The BDI-II is a revision of the original BDI. The score ranges for the BDI-I are 0 to 9: minimal or no depression;

TABLE 25–2

Questionnaires to Evaluate Patients with Insomnia

Epworth Sleepiness Scale	Propensity to fall asleep in eight situations (0 never, 1 slight, 2 moderate, 3 high chance) with a total score 0 to 24. Normal ≤ 10.
Beck Depression Inventory	BDI-I or BDI-II is a 21-item self-report inventory used to measure depression. BDI-I scores: Minimal or no depression BDI < 10, moderate to severe depression BDI ≥ 19. BDI-II scores: Minimal or no depression BDI < 14, moderate to severe depression BDI ≥ 20.
Pittsburgh Sleep Quality Index	A 24-item self-report measure of sleep qualities (poor sleep: **global score > 5**).
Dysfunctional Beliefs and Attitudes about Sleep Questionnaire	DBAS is a self-rating of 30 statements that is used to assess negative cognitions about sleep. Shorter version of the DBAS-16 also exists (see Appendix 25–1).

BDI = Beck Depression Inventory; DBAS = Dysfunctional Beliefs and Attitudes about Sleep.

10 to 18: mild to moderate depression; 19 to 29: moderate depression; and 30 to 63: severe depression. The score ranges for BDI-II are 0 to 13: minimal or no depression; 14 to 19: mild depression; 20 to 28: moderate depression; and 29 to 63: severe depression. Because primary insomnia and major depression share some daytime symptoms, the usual cutoff scores for the BDI might be less specific for depression in insomnia patients.[18] Indeed, one study evaluating the BDI-II in insomnia patients found that using a cutoff for mild depression of greater than 14 had a high sensitivity (91%) but low specificity (66%) for detecting depression. The authors suggested using a higher cutoff (>17) for mild depression. Using this cutoff the BDI-II had a 79% specificity but an 81% sensitivity for identifying depression.

The Dysfunctional Beliefs and Attitudes about Sleep (DBAS) Questionnaire is a self-rating survey to assess negative cognitions about sleep.[19,20] Reversal of these cognitions is a goal of the cognitive component of CBT (cognitive behavioral therapy). The original DBAS was a 30-item questionnaire in which patients responded using an analog scale (0, strongly disagree; 1, 2, 3. . ., to 10, strongly agree). A shorter version (DBAS-16)[20] has recently been validated and is less time-consuming for patients to complete (Appendix 25–1).

Sleep Logs

Having insomnia patients complete a sleep log (sleep diary) for at least 2 weeks is recommended. Sleep logs are often more accurate than relying on patient recall of their chronic sleep patterns. Sleep logs usually follow a question format (Fig. 25–1) or time plot graphic format (Fig. 25–2). The essential elements include the ability to assess time in bed (TIB), sleep-onset latency (SOL), total sleep time (TST), and the amount of wake after sleep onset (WASO). The TIB is the time period from when the patient gets in bed until the final time the patient leaves the bed in the morning. The WASO includes all wake from sleep onset until the patient leaves the bed in the morning. The patient need report only three of these four parameters because they are related (TIB = SOL + TST + WASO). One can compute a sleep efficiency (= TST × 100/TIB) with normal values exceeding 85%. Sleep logs also typically provide space to record caffeine consumption, bedtime activities, or medications taken for sleep as well as estimates of sleep quality. Sleep logs are very helpful in revealing general patterns of the sleep-wake cycle such as irregular bedtimes and wake times and the amount and frequency of napping. A few characteristic patterns noted in sleep logs are listed in Table 25–3.

SLEEP DIARY										
	Complete before bedtime				Complete in the morning					
Bedtime day Day of week ___ Date ___	Caffeine drinks today (0 if none)	I exercised > 20 minutes	Activity before bed	Sleeping medication? Alcohol? (give times)	I went to bed last night at? PM/AM	I got out of bed this morning at? PM/AM	Last night, I fell asleep in (minutes)	I woke up during the night (how many times?)	Last night, I slept a total of (hours)	When I woke up for the day I felt:
Day 1 Day of week ___ Date ___	___ morning ___ afternoon ___ after supper	___ morning ___ afternoon ___ within 3 hours of bedtime						___ times	___ hours	( ) refreshed ( ) somewhat refreshed ( ) fatigued
Day 2 Day of week ___ Date ___	___ morning ___ afternoon ___ after supper	___ morning ___ afternoon ___ within 3 hours of bedtime						___ times	___ hours	( ) refreshed ( ) somewhat refreshed ( ) fatigued
Day 3 Day of week ___ Date ___	___ morning ___ afternoon ___ after supper	___ morning ___ afternoon ___ within 3 hours of bedtime						___ times	___ hours	( ) refreshed ( ) somewhat refreshed ( ) fatigued
Day 4 Day of week ___ Date ___	___ morning ___ afternoon ___ after supper	___ morning ___ afternoon ___ within 3 hours of bedtime						___ times	___ hours	( ) refreshed ( ) somewhat refreshed ( ) fatigued

FIGURE 25–1 A typical sleep log. From the answers, one can determine the time in bed (TIB), the sleep latency, and the total sleep time. The wake after sleep onset = TIB − sleep latency − total sleep time.

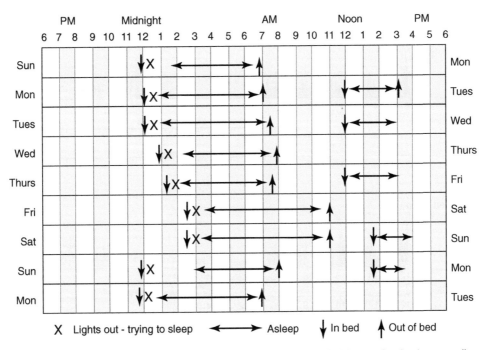

X Lights out - trying to sleep ⟷ Asleep ↓ In bed ↑ Out of bed

FIGURE 25–2 A sleep log (diary) shows inadequate sleep hygiene with **variable bedtimes and wake times** as well as **napping**. Note that on Sunday and Wednesday, the sleep latency was prolonged. Once asleep, the patient had no middle of the night awakenings.

TABLE 25–3	
Some Typical Sleep Log Patterns	
Delayed sleep phase	Late bedtime or long sleep latency, few awakenings, normal sleep duration on weekends or nonwork/nonschool days.
Inadequate sleep hygiene	Irregular wake and rise times, naps.
Psychophysiologic insomnia	Long sleep latency, decreased total sleep time, frequent awakenings. Variability in sleep quality.
Paradoxical insomnia	Nights of minimal or no sleep are reported followed by no or few naps the next day.

Actigraphy

Actigraphy involves use of a portable device (often resembling a watch and typically worn on the wrist) that collects movement information (activity) over an extended period of time (Fig. 25–3). The absence of movement is assumed to be a surrogate of sleep.[21-29] The use of actigraphy is included in the ICSD-2 diagnostic criteria for several CRSDs, paradoxical insomnia, and behaviorally induced insufficient sleep syndrome.[1] Practice parameters for use of actigraphy have been published by the American Academy of Sleep Medicine (AASM).[23,29] Some of the recommendations are listed in Box 25–5. Note that, although actigraphy was said to be indicated for determining the circadian patterns of patients with insomnia, the practice parameters did not state that

BOX 25–5

Selected Recommendations for the Use of Actigraphy According to American Academy of Sleep Medicine Practice Parameters (2007 Update)

1. Actigraphy is a valid method to determine sleep patterns in **normal healthy population** (Standard) and in certain sleep disorders. (Option-Guideline)
2. Actigraphy is indicated to assist in evaluation of patients with suspected **advanced sleep phase syndrome, delayed sleep phase syndrome,** and **shift work disorder** (Guideline); and circadian rhythm disorders, including jet lag, and non–24-hr sleep/wake CRSD. (Option)
3. When PSG is not available, actigraphy is indicated to estimate TST in patients with OSA. (Standard)
4. Actigraphy is indicated as a method to characterize circadian rhythm patterns of sleep disorders in individuals with insomnia including insomnia with depression. (Option)
5. Actigraphy is indicated as a way to determine circadian pattern and estimate average daily sleep time in individuals complaining of hypersomnia. (Option)
6. Actigraphy is useful as an outcome measure in evaluating the response to treatment for circadian rhythm disorders. (Guideline)
7. Actigraphy is useful for evaluation of the response to treatment for patients with insomnia, including insomnia associated with depression. (Guideline)

CRSD = circadian rhythm sleep disorder; OSA = obstructive sleep apnea; PSG = polysomnography; TST = total sleep time.
From Morgenthaler T, Alessi C, Friedman L, et al. Practice parameters for the use of actigraphy in the assessment of sleep and sleep disorders: an update for 2007. Sleep 2007;30:519–529.

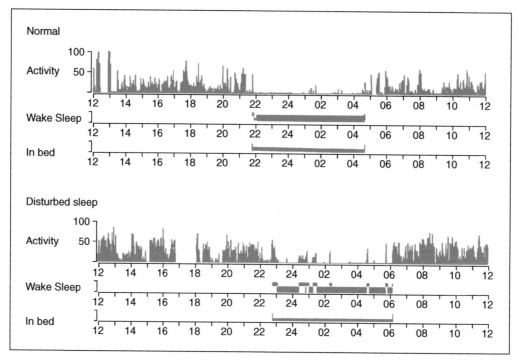

FIGURE 25-3 Examples of actigraphy in a normal subject and a patient with disturbed sleep. **Top,** Normal subject. Measures of activity, actigraphic estimates of wake and sleep, and sleep log reported time in bed are displayed. **Bottom,** A patient with disturbed sleep. Note persistent activity during the sleep period. In the wake sleep data, periods identified as wake (*thin line*) are above periods of sleep (*thicker line*). *Adapted from Córdoba J, Cabrera J, Lataif L, et al: High prevalence of sleep disturbance in cirrhosis. Hepatology 1998;27:339–345.*

actigraphy was indicated as a routine evaluation of patients with insomnia.

Actigraphy does not measure sleep as defined by electro-encephalogram (EEG)/electro-oculogram (EOG)/chin electromyogram (EMG) criteria or the subjective experience of sleep (as measured by sleep logs and questionnaires). Therefore, it is not surprising that estimates of TST, wake time, and the sleep latency from sleep logs and actigraphy may differ from polysomnography (PSG) findings. Algorithms have been developed to estimate TST and WASO from the activity data. Modern actigraphic software allows the clinician to mark periods of possible sleep ("rest periods"). The software then provides automatic estimates of periods of sleep and wake. These can be edited if desired. However, there are limitations to the accuracy of these estimates. Actigraphic estimates of sleep duration, WASO, and sleep latency are more accurate in normal individuals than in patients with insomnia. Periods of low activity in which patients lay quietly in bed but are awake may be scored as sleep by actigraphy software. When performing actigraphy, it is essential to require patients to complete a sleep log (e.g., lights off, lights on, out of bed, actigraph off for shower; TST; sleep latency). This information enables a correct interpretation of acti-graphic tracings. For example, total absence of movement usually indicates that the actigraph has been removed (shower, swimming), but here patient logs are essential to verify device removal. **If the actigraphic estimate of TST far exceeds patient estimates, this would suggest paradoxical insomnia.** Many modern wrist actigraph devices also

provide the capability of recording the amount of ambient light. This is useful in patients with CRSDs in whom light exposure may either exacerbate or improve the underlying disorder. Some actigraphy devices also have event markers that the patient can press when getting in bed, trying to sleep, or after awakening in the morning.

Sleep logs and actigraphy provide complementary information. In a study of patients with insomnia undergoing treatment, Vallières and Morin[24] compared findings from actigraphy and sleep logs with PSG (Fig. 25-4A). Both actigraphy and sleep logs underestimated TST and overestimated wake time. Actigraphy underestimated the sleep latency and sleep logs overestimated the sleep latency. These authors found actigraphy to be more sensitive at detecting treatment effects than sleep logs. In contrast, Sivertsen and coworkers[25] found different results in a group of older adults treated for primary insomnia (expected to have more wake time). Actigraphy slightly overestimated TST and underestimated wake (see Fig. 25-4B). In this study, actigraphy provided a better estimate of TST than of wake time.

Polysomnography

PSG is not indicated for the routine assessment of insomnia.[9,10] However, if there is a suspicion for sleep apnea, periodic limb movement disorder, or a parasomnia, a PSG may be useful. The 2003 AASM practice parameters for the role of PSG in insomnia stated "polysomnography is indicated when the initial diagnosis (insomnia) is uncertain, treatment

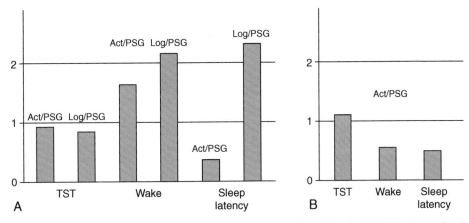

FIGURE 25-4 A, A plot of the ratios of actigraphic (Act)/PSG (polysomnography) and sleep log (Log)/PSG estimates of total sleep time (TST), wake, and sleep latency from the data of a study by Vallèries and Morin in patients with insomnia. Both actigraphy and sleep logs slightly underestimated the total sleep time but overestimated wake time. Sleep logs overestimated sleep latency while actigraphy underestimated sleep latency (laying in bed still but awake). **B,** A plot of data from a study of older insomnias by Sivertsen and coworkers. Actigraphy slightly overestimated TST but underestimated wake and sleep latency. **A,** From Vallières A, Morin CM: Actigraphy in the assessment of insomnia. Sleep 2003;26:902–906. **B,** Sivertsen B, Omvik S, Havik OE, et al: A comparison of actigraphy and polysomnography in older adults treated for chronic primary insomnia. Sleep 2006;29:1353–1358.

fails (either behavioral or pharmacologic), or precipitous arousals occur with violent or injurious behavior (Guideline)."[10] When PSG is performed, typical findings (Box 25–6) in patients with insomnia include a long sleep latency (>30 min), reduced TST, increased WASO, and a reduced sleep efficiency. A long rapid eye movement (REM) latency, high arousal index, increased stage N1, and decreased stage N3 sleep may also be noted. In patients with **paradoxical insomnia, the objective sleep abnormality is much less severe than reported.** It is not unusual for such patients to report little or no sleep following a PSG documenting only mild to moderate decrements in the TST. In some patients with psychophysiologic insomnia, the **"reverse first-night effect"**[11] may be noted. In these patients, the sleep quality in the sleep center is better than that reported at home. It is essential to have all patients complete questionnaires assessing subjective sleep (estimate TST, sleep latency, sleep quality) after PSG.

PHYSIOLOGIC FINDINGS IN PRIMARY INSOMNIA

Some but not all studies have documented increased high-frequency EEG activity, increased whole body and brain metabolic activity, elevated heart rate, and sympathetic nervous system activation (decreased heart rate variability) during both day and night in patients with insomnia. These findings suggest that patients with insomnia are in a state of hyperarousal.[30] Of special interest, functional neuroimaging has found greater global cerebral glucose metabolism during sleep and while awake and a smaller decline in relative metabolism from waking to sleep in wake-promoting regions in patients with insomnia compared with normal controls.[31] In addition, reduced metabolism was found in the prefrontal

BOX 25–6

Typical Polysomnography Findings in Patients with Insomnia

- Increased sleep latency (>30 min)
- Decreased TST
- Decreased sleep efficiency
- Increased stage N1 (%TST)
- Decreased stage N3 (%TST)
- Increased REM latency
- Decreased REM latency (depression)

REM = rapid eye movement; TST = total sleep time.

cortex of patients with primary insomnia while awake. It is not clear whether these findings represent cause or effect. A recent study of magnetic resonance spectroscopy found a global **reduction in gamma-aminobutyric acid (GABA)** in nonmedicated patients with primary insomnia compared with normal controls.[32] This neurotransmitter is generally inhibitory and higher levels would be expected to promote sleep.

INDIVIDUAL INSOMNIA SUBTYPES

Adjustment Insomnia (Acute Insomnia)

Adjustment insomnia, at least in milder forms, is experienced by a large percentage of otherwise normal sleepers at some time in their lives. The 1-year prevalence of adjustment insomnia in adults is 15% to 20%. The problem resolves with time in most cases. **If the insomnia persists beyond 3 months, it is considered a chronic insomnia.** Some cases of psychophysiologic insomnia may have started as adjustment insomnia. Most patients with adjustment insomnia are not evaluated by a sleep specialist. However, they may request hypnotic medication from their primary care physician or self-medicate with over-the-counter sleep aids.

Key Features

Adjustment insomnia is a disorder of less than 3 months' duration that is in response to a definitely identifiable event (Box 25-7). It is expected to resolve but may require treatment if a significant impact on sleep and daytime functioning is noted.

PSG Findings

PSG findings have not been reported.

Differential Diagnosis

Psychophysiologic and paradoxical insomnia typically last longer than 3 months. Insomnia due to medical disorder or medication is temporally associated with starting a medication or the onset of the medical disorder. Insomnia due to mental disorder typically lasts longer than 3 months and waxes and wanes with the mental disorder. Patients with adjustment insomnia can develop a chronic insomnia disorder. Some patients with psychophysiologic insomnia report the onset of their problem after an acute stress. Insomnia due to a mental disorder may develop if the patient with adjustment insomnia develops depression as a result of the acute stressor.

Treatment

Benzodiazepine receptor agonists (BZRAs), ramelteon, anxiolytics, or counseling are used to treat adjustment insomnia (if necessary).

Psychophysiologic Insomnia

Psychophysiologic insomnia is the most common primary insomnia type seen in sleep clinics and it is often called "conditioned or learned insomnia."

BOX 25-7

Adjustment Insomnia—Diagnostic Criteria

A. Patient's symptoms meet criteria for insomnia.
B. The sleep disturbance is temporally associated with an identifiable stressor that is psychological, psychosocial, interpersonal, environmental, or physical in nature.
C. The sleep disturbance is expected to resolve when the acute stressor resolves or when the individual adjusts to the stressor.
D. The sleep disturbance lasts **less than three months.**
E. The sleep disturbance is not better explained by another sleep disorder, medical or neurologic disorder, mental disorder, medication use, or substance abuse.

From American Academy of Sleep Medicine: ICSD-2 International Classification of Sleep Disorders, 2nd ed. Diagnostic and Coding Manual. Westchester, IL: American Academy of Sleep Medicine, 2005.

Key Features

Conditioned sleep difficulty, heightened arousal in bed, and learned sleep-preventing associations are the essential characteristics of this disorder. Mental arousal ("racing mind/thoughts") occurring when trying to go to sleep is a common complaint. The patient becomes conditioned so that the bedroom is a "cue" to develop tension, anxiety, and inability to fall asleep. Some patients sleep better away from home. Patients typically can fall asleep during monotonous activities but not after getting into bed and trying to sleep. For example, a patient may fall asleep while watching television in the living room but become wide awake after entering the bedroom and attempting to sleep. This disorder may start after a precipitating event (death in family, job stress) but then persists owing to perpetuating behaviors even after the precipitating event has resolved. Other patients report a slow onset of symptoms. Patients may report a lifelong pattern of being "light sleepers" or episodically poor sleep (Box 25-8).

Incidence

Psychophysiologic insomnia is present in 1% to 2% of the general population and 12% to 15% of patients seen in sleep centers. This disorder is **more common in women than in men.**

If left untreated, the disorder may persist for decades with periodic worsening.

Objective Findings

Polysomnography Although sleep studies are not indicated for evaluation of most patients with insomnia, typical

---

BOX 25-8

Psychophysiologic Insomnia—Diagnostic Criteria

A. Patient's symptoms meet the criteria for insomnia.
B. Duration of **at least 1 month.**
C. Evidence of **conditioned sleep difficulty** and/or **heightened arousal in bed** as indicated by one or more of the following:
  i. Excessive focus on sleep, anxiety about sleep.
  ii. **Difficulty falling asleep in bed** at desired bedtime or during planned naps BUT no difficulty falling asleep during other monotonous activities when not intending to sleep.
  iii. Ability to sleep **better away from home**.
  iv. **Mental arousal** in bed characterized by either intrusive thoughts or a perceived inability to volitionally cease sleep-preventing mental activity.
  v. **Heightened somatic tension** in bed reflected by a perceived inability to relax the body sufficiently to allow the onset of sleep.
D. The sleep disturbance is not better explained by another sleep disorder, medical or neurologic disorder, mental disorder, medication use, or substance abuse.

From American Academy of Sleep Medicine: ICSD-2 International Classification of Sleep Disorders, 2nd ed. Diagnostic and Coding Manual. Westchester, IL: American Academy of Sleep Medicine, 2005.

findings include a prolonged sleep latency (>30 min), increased WASO, and decreased sleep efficiency. Sometimes, the reverse first-night effect is noted with better sleep in the sleep center than at home. Patients may underestimate their sleep duration but not the "gross underestimation" seen in paradoxical insomnia.

Multiple Sleep Latency Test The sleep latency usually is in the range of 10 to 15 minutes.

Sleep Logs Sleep logs typically show a long sleep latency, reduced TST, increased WASO, and a large number of nocturnal awakenings. Poor sleep quality is often reported. Typically, there is **considerable night-to-night variability** in sleep quality. There may also be evidence of poor sleep hygiene with **prolonged time in bed, napping, and variability in wake times.**

Actigraphy Findings may overestimate or underestimate TST when compared with PSG. Actigraphy typically provides a better estimate of TST than of wake time. Typical actigraphic findings would substantiate patient reports and findings from sleep logs.

Treatment CBT for insomnia and pharmacotherapy are treatment options. These are discussed in a later section of this chapter.

Paradoxical Insomnia (Sleep State Misperception)

Key Features
The severe degree of sleep disturbance reported in patients with paradoxical insomnia (formerly called "sleep state misperception") is out of proportion to the relatively mild daytime impairment **and** the severity of sleep disturbance documented on PSG.

Patients often report little or no sleep on many nights followed by days with relatively minimal dysfunction and no napping. In addition, patients with paradoxical insomnia often report hearing every noise in the house while in the bedroom and/or actively thinking for the entire night. Daytime impairment reported is consistent with other types of insomnia but **is much less severe than expected,** given the severe level of sleep deprivation reported. For example, there are no intrusive sleep episodes or serious mishaps due to loss of alertness, even following nights reportedly without sleep (Box 25–9).

Incidence
Paradoxical insomnia is found in less than 5% of insomnia patients evaluated in sleep clinics.[1]

Objective Findings
Sleep Log Data Sleep log information is usually consistent with the patient's complaints, but **NOT** consistent with objective evidence (from PSG or actigraphic data). There may be nights with little or no sleep reported followed by days with no napping.

BOX 25–9

Paradoxical Insomnia (Sleep State Misperception)—Diagnostic Criteria

A. Symptoms meet criteria for insomnia.
B. Insomnia is present for **at least 1 month.**
C. One or more of the following criteria apply:
   i. Chronic pattern of little or no sleep most nights with rare nights during which relatively normal amount of sleep is obtained.
   ii. Sleep log data during 1 or more weeks of monitoring show an average sleep time well below published age-adjusted normative values, often with no sleep at all indicated for several nights per week: **typically there is an absence of naps following such nights.**
   iii. The patient shows a **consistent mismatch between objective findings** from PSG or actigraphy and **subjective sleep estimates** derived from either sleep report or sleep diary.
D. At least one of the following is observed:
   i. Constant or near-constant awareness of environmental stimuli throughout most nights.
   ii. The patient reports a pattern of **conscious thoughts or rumination** throughout most nights while maintaining a recumbent posture.
E. Daytime impairment reported is consistent with other types of insomnia subtypes, it is much less severe than expected, given the extreme level of sleep deprivation reported; there is no report of intrusive daytime sleep episodes, disorientation, or serious mishaps due to marked loss of alertness or vigilance, even following reportedly sleepless nights.
F. The sleep disturbance is not better explained by another sleep disorder, medical or neurologic disorder, mental disorder, medication use, or substance abuse.

From American Academy of Sleep Medicine: ICSD-2 International Classification of Sleep Disorders, 2nd ed. Diagnostic and Coding Manual. Westchester, IL: American Academy of Sleep Medicine, 2005.

PSG Findings PSG findings indicated lack of significant deficits in TST or an excessively prolonged sleep latency. If abnormalities are noted on the PSG, they are less severe than reported by the patient.

- Reported sleep latency and WASO at least 1.5 times the PSG values.

Multiple Sleep Latency Test The sleep latency in patients with paradoxical insomnia is typically normal or slightly decreased.

Differential Diagnosis
Unlike idiopathic insomnia, paradoxical insomnia does not begin in childhood. In contrast to psychophysiologic insomnia, patients with paradoxical insomnia are more prone to report little or NO sleep on many nights. However, some patients with psychophysiologic insomnia also underestimate their nocturnal sleep. Whereas patients with

paradoxical insomnia often report being aware of the environment for the entire night or ruminating on problems, they tend to have less prominent sleep-preventing associations compared with patients with psychophysiologic insomnia.

Treatment

CBT of insomnia (CBTI), pharmacotherapy, or both are recommended.

Idiopathic Insomnia

Idiopathic insomnia is also called *childhood-onset insomnia*. The patient usually recalls the insidious onset of the insomnia problems in childhood. The history is one of lifelong insomnia problems (Box 25–10).

Key Features

Patients with idiopathic insomnia report this problem since childhood with no periods of significant remission. There is no identifiable cause or precipitating factor. The onset is often insidious.

Epidemiology

Idiopathic insomnia occurs in less than 10% of patients with insomnia. Idiopathic insomnia is a rare disorder occurring in only approximately 0.7% of adolescents.[1]

Objective Findings

Polysomnography PSG findings include a long sleep latency, increased WASO, reduced TST, and low sleep efficiency. These findings are not specific for idiopathic insomnia.

Sleep Log Findings from a sleep log are typically consistent with the patient's complaints.

Differential Diagnosis

Whereas idiopathic insomnia has an insidious onset in childhood, psychophysiologic insomnia starts in adulthood and the time of onset can often be defined. In paradoxical insomnia, a more severe abnormality of sleep is usually reported and the disorder does not start at an early age.

Treatment

CBTI, pharmacotherapy, or both are options. No large studies of treatment outcomes have been published.

Insomnia Due to a Mental Disorder

Insomnia due to mental disorder (IDMD) is the most common form of insomnia seen by sleep physicians (Box 25–11). Many times, patients have **fixated on the insomnia problems while ignoring (denying) or minimizing their other symptoms of depression.**

Key Features

The insomnia is viewed as a consequence of the mental disorder (e.g., depression) and shares the course of the disorder (waxing and waning together). However, insomnia can actually precede the development of depression in some patients. Of note, insomnia complaints are very common in mood disorders and are often considered secondary (co-morbid) to the mood disorder. A separate diagnosis of **insomnia due to mental disorder (IDMD)** is made only if the insomnia is **significant enough to warrant special attention.** Common mental disorders associated with IDMD include major depression, bipolar disorder, and anxiety disorder. In anxiety disorders, prominent sleep-onset insomnia is usually present. **In depressive disorders, especially in older patients, the sleep disturbance is characterized by prominent sleep-maintenance insomnia and early morning awakening. Younger patients with depression may experience more prominent sleep-onset insomnia.**

Epidemiology

IDMD is the **most common cause of insomnia** in patients presenting to sleep disorder centers complaining

---

BOX 25–10

Idiopathic Insomnia—Diagnostic Criteria

A. The patient's symptoms meet criteria for insomnia.
B. The course of the disorder is chronic, as indicated by each of the following:
   a. **Onset during infancy or childhood.**
   b. No identifiable precipitant or cause.
   c. Persistent course with **no periods of sustained remission.**
C. The sleep disturbance is not better explained by another sleep disorder, medical or neurologic disorder, mental disorder, medication use, or substance abuse.

From American Academy of Sleep Medicine: ICSD-2 International Classification of Sleep Disorders, 2nd ed. Diagnostic and Coding Manual. Westchester, IL: American Academy of Sleep Medicine, 2005.

BOX 25–11

Insomnia Due to Mental Disorder— Diagnostic Criteria

A. Patient's symptoms meet criteria for insomnia.
B. The insomnia is present for **at least 1 month.**
C. A mental disorder has been diagnosed by standard criteria (Diagnostic and Statistical Manual of Mental Disorders, 4th edition).
D. Insomnia is temporally associated with the mental disorder; however, in some cases, insomnia may appear a few days or weeks **before the emergence** of the underlying mental disorder.
E. The sleep disturbance is not better explained by another sleep disorder, medical or neurologic disorder, mental disorder, medication use, or substance abuse.

From American Academy of Sleep Medicine: ICSD-2 International Classification of Sleep Disorders, 2nd ed. Diagnostic and Coding Manual. Westchester, IL: American Academy of Sleep Medicine, 2005.

of insomnia. The disorder is **more likely in women than in men.** IDMD occurs in up to 3% of the population.

Objective Findings

Polysomnography PSG if performed shows no specific findings as far as a sleep latency, TST, or WASO. **Patients with depression may have a short REM latency.**

Beck Depression Inventory This inventory reveals an elevated score (BDI-I > 10, BDI-II > 14).

Sleep Logs Sleep logs may show a long sleep latency, decreased TST, early morning awakening, or frequent awakenings. These findings are usually consistent with patient complaints.

Treatment

Treatment of the underlying mental disorder may ultimately improve sleep. However, because the sleep complaints are so prominent, treatment with a hypnotic or the addition of a sedating antidepressant is often needed. **CBT of IDMD is also effective.** Drug treatment of patients with insomnia and mental disorders is discussed in more detail in the "Pharmacologic Treatment of Insomnia" section.

Inadequate Sleep Hygiene

Key Features

This disorder is characterized by behaviors that can potentially disrupt sleep such as exercise or ingestion of caffeine or alcohol near bedtime (Box 25–12). Patients often have irregular bedtimes and wake times and spend too much time in bed. Napping is another behavior that makes nocturnal sleep more difficult. Recommendations for good sleep hygiene are listed in Box 25–13.

Epidemiology

The importance of poor sleep hygiene in the development of insomnia is unknown. Although sleep hygiene education is a part of most treatment programs for insomnia, there is **no evidence for effectiveness of this intervention when used alone.** Insomnia due to inadequate sleep hygiene may develop in adolescence or adulthood. Insomnia due to inadequate sleep hygiene occurs in approximately 5% to 10% of insomnias evaluated in a sleep center. The condition is present in 1% to 2% of adolescents and young adults.

Objective Findings

Sleep Log A typical sleep log of a patient with poor sleep hygiene is shown in Figure 25–2. Findings include variation in wake time, napping, and sleeping much longer on the weekend. Inappropriate use of caffeine and use of over-the-counter medications or alcohol may also be reported on sleep logs.

Long-term Complications Patients with poor sleep hygiene may develop caffeine or alcohol dependence or eventually psychophysiologic insomnia.

BOX 25–12

Inadequate Sleep Hygiene—Diagnostic Criteria

A. Symptoms meet criteria for insomnia.

B. The insomnia is present for **at least 1 month.**

C. Inadequate sleep hygiene practices are evident as indicated by the presence of at least one of the following:

   i. **Improper sleep scheduling** consisting of frequent daytime napping, selecting highly variable bedtimes or rising times, or spending excessive amount of time in bed.

   ii. Routine use of products containing alcohol, nicotine, or caffeine, especially in periods preceding bedtime.

   iii. Engagement in mentally stimulating, physically activating, or emotionally upsetting activities too close to bedtime.

   iv. **Frequent use of the bed for activities other than sleep** (TV watching, reading, studying, snacking, thinking, planning).

   v. Failure to maintain a comfortable sleeping environment.

D. The sleep disturbance is not better explained by another sleep disorder, medical or neurologic disorder, mental disorder, medication use, or substance abuse.

From American Academy of Sleep Medicine: ICSD-2 International Classification of Sleep Disorders, 2nd ed. Diagnostic and Coding Manual. Westchester, IL: American Academy of Sleep Medicine, 2005.

BOX 25–13

Good Sleep Hygiene Practices

- Limit caffeine consumption to before noon.
- No exercise within 2 hours of bedtime.
- Use the bed only for sleep and sex (avoid excessive time in bed).
- Maintain regular waking times.
- Bedroom should be quiet and cool.
- Avoid stimulating activity near bedtime.

Treatment

Education about good sleep hygiene and CBTI, if necessary, are recommended. As noted previously, there is no evidence that education about sleep hygiene alone is effective treatment for the insomnia syndromes. In patients with difficulties entirely due to poor (inadequate) sleep hygiene, one might expect improvement if their sleep habits were improved.

Behavioral Insomnia of Childhood

The behavioral insomnia of childhood (BIOC) including bedtime problems and nighttime awakenings is highly prevalent in young children, occurring in approximately 20% to 30% of infants, toddlers, and preschoolers.[1,33,34] Although BIOC is typically divided into **sleep-onset association type** and **limit-setting type,** there is considerable overlap in most children. If the major emphasis is on **refusal to go to bed** (getting out of bed, verbal protests, crying, and attention-seeking behavior), then limit-setting is the main problem. If sleep either at bedtime or after awakenings **requires certain behaviors** (rocking, feeding, parental presence in the bedroom), then sleep association is the predominant type. Due to variations in culture patterns, what degree of BIOC type behaviors really constitutes a problem is highly variable. In addition, the main complaint is from the caregiver and not the child.

Key Features

The diagnostic criteria for BIOC are listed in Box 25-14.[1] For the **sleep-onset association type,** falling asleep is an extended process that requires special conditions. Sleep onset at night is typically prolonged, problematic, and often demanding for the caregiver. Nighttime awakenings require caregiver interventions for the child to return to sleep. In **limit-setting disorder**, the child has difficulty initiating or maintaining sleep. An essential component is that the caregiver demonstrates insufficient or inappropriate limit-setting to establish appropriate sleeping behavior in the child.

Treatment

Whereas the treatment of adult insomnia is discussed in detail in later sections, a detailed discussion of the treatment of BIOC is presented here due to the unique approaches indicated for this problem (Table 25-4 and Box 25-15).

In 2006, the AASM published practice parameters for treatment of BIOC[33] based on a systematic review.[34] In behavioral therapy, *extinction* means reducing a given behavior's occurrence by withholding or eliminating any reinforcements for that behavior. Several formats are relevant to behavioral insomnia.

Unmodified Extinction The goal of this technique is to reduce undesired behavior (prolonged bedtime protests) by eliminating any reinforcement (parental attention) of the behavior. This involves putting the child to bed and then not responding to any crying or protests. Unmodified extinction has limited parental acceptance.

Modified Extinction In this procedure, reinforcements are not completely eliminated but reduced in "value." For example,

---

BOX 25-14

Behavioral Insomnia of Childhood— Diagnostic Criteria

A. Child's symptoms meet the criteria for insomnia based upon report of the parents or other adult caregivers.

B. Pattern consistent with sleep-onset association or limit-setting type of insomnia described below:

  1. Sleep-onset association type includes **each** of the following:

    i. Falling asleep in an **extended process** that requires **special conditions**.

    ii. Sleep-onset associations are highly problematic or demanding.

    iii. In the absence of the associated condition, sleep onset is significantly delayed or sleep is otherwise disrupted.

    iv. Nighttime awakenings **require caregiver intervention** for the child to return to sleep.

  2. Limit-setting type includes EACH of the following:

    i. Individual has difficulty initiating or maintaining sleep.

    ii. Individual stalls or refuses to go to bed at an appropriate time or refuses to return to bed following a nighttime awakening.

    iii. The caregiver demonstrates insufficient or inappropriate limit setting to establish appropriate sleeping behavior in the child.

From American Academy of Sleep Medicine: ICSD-2 International Classification of Sleep Disorders, 2nd ed. Diagnostic and Coding Manual. Westchester, IL: American Academy of Sleep Medicine, 2005.

BOX 25-15

Recommendations for Behavioral Treatment of Behavioral Insomnia of Childhood

1. **Behavioral interventions** are effective and recommended in the treatment of bedtime problems and night wakings in young children. (Standard)

2. **Unmodified extinction** and **extinction of undesired behavior with parental presence** (modified extinction) are effective and recommend therapies in the treatment of bedtime problems and night wakings.

3. Parental education/prevention is an effective and recommended therapy in treatment of bedtime problems and night wakings. (Standard)

4. Graduated extinction of undesired behavior is an effective and recommended therapy in the treatment of bedtime problems and night wakings. (Guideline)

5. Delayed bedtime with removal from bed (if no sleep) and positive routines is an effective therapy in the treatment of bedtime problems and night wakings. (Guideline)

6. The use of scheduled awakenings is an effective and recommended therapy in the treatment of bedtime problems and night wakings. (Guideline)

7. Insufficient evidence was available to recommend any technique as more effective. (Option)

8. Behavioral interventions are recommended and effective in improving secondary outcomes (child's daytime functioning, parental well-being) in children with bedtime problems and night wakings. (Guideline)

Levels of Evidence: Standard > Guideline > Option.

From Morgenthaler TI, Owens J, Alessi C, et al: Practice parameters for behavioral treatment of bedtime problems and night wakenings in infants and young children. Sleep 2006;29:1277–1281.

TABLE 25-4

Techniques Used for Behavioral Treatment of Insomnia of Childhood

TECHNIQUE	DESCRIPTION	RATIONALE
Unmodified extinction	Involves parents putting the child to bed at a designated bedtime and then ignoring the child until morning (parents continue to monitor for safety issues).	Reduce undesired behaviors (e.g., crying, screaming) by eliminating parental attention (reinforcer).
Graduated extinction	Involves parents ignoring bedtime crying and tantrums for predetermined periods before briefly checking on the child. A progressive (graduated) checking schedule (e.g., 5 min, then 10 min) or fixed checking schedule (e.g., every 5 min) may be used.	Enable a child to develop "self-soothing" skills and be able to fall asleep independently without undesirable sleep associations.
Scheduled awakenings	Involves parents preemptively awakening their child, prior to a typical spontaneous awakening, and providing the "usual" responses (e.g., feeding, rocking, soothing) as if child had awakened spontaneously.	Prevents nightly reinforcement for undesirable behaviors involved with waking.
Positive routines	Parents develop set bedtime routines characterized by enjoyable and quiet activities to establish a behavioral chain leading up to sleep onset.	Removes negative stimuli associated with bedtime.
Delayed (faded) bedtime	Temporarily delaying the bedtime to more closely coincide with the child's natural sleep-onset time, the fading (bedtime) is moved earlier as the child gains success falling asleep quietly.	Reduced arousal at bedtime
Response cost	Response cost involves removing the child from bed for prescribed brief periods of time if the child does not fall asleep within a prescribed time.	A type of stimulus control for child: the bedroom is a place for sleep not crying/attention seeking.
Parental education and prevention	Involves parent education to prevent the occurrence of the development of sleep problems. Behavioral interventions are incorporated into these parent education programs.	Preventing problems before they occur.

Adapted from Mindell JA, Kuhn B, Lewin DS, et al: Behavioral treatment of bedtime problems and night wakings in infants and young children. An American Academy of Sleep Medicine Review. Sleep 2006;29:1263–1276.

extinction with parental presence involves the parent staying in the child's bedroom but not talking with the child, rocking the child, or other behaviors.

Graduated Extinction Parents are instructed to ignore bedtime crying and tantrums for specified periods according to a fixed schedule of progressively longer intervals and to avoid reinforcing protest behavior. For example, suppose a child typically starts crying when placed in the crib. On subsequent nights, bedtime crying is ignored for 10, then 20, then 30, and 60 minutes or more on successive nights.

For these techniques to be effective, parents must be motivated and consistent. It is important that the caregivers choose an approach that they are comfortable with and then apply it every night.

Insomnia Due to Drug or Substance

Insomnia due to drug or substance implies that the insomnia complaints are associated with the use of or withdrawal from a medication or substance. Some patients may often be able to relate the onset of sleep problems with the start of a new medication. In others, the onset is more insidious and may not be noticed.

Key Features

Patients must have ongoing use of a drug or substance associated with symptoms of insomnia. The insomnia can also occur on withdrawal from the agent. In recovering alcoholics, **sleep disturbance may persist for many months after the start of abstinence** (Box 25–16).

Epidemiology

Insomnia complaints due to medications or substances are very common. **Caffeine** is a widely used stimulant that may affect sleep for hours after ingestion. The half-life of caffeine varies from 3 to 7 hours and is longer at higher doses.[35] **Alcohol** may aid sleep onset but tends to cause frequent awakenings in the second part of the night.[36]

Causes

A large number of medications can be associated with insomnia (Table 25–5).[37] Nonsedating antidepressants, anticonvulsants, beta blockers, bronchodilators, and stimulants/alerting agents can all be associated with insomnia. Medications that cause nightmares may also result in insomnia.

Beta Blockers Because beta blockers are frequently used to treat patients with cardiovascular disease, it is important for

BOX 25-16

Insomnia Due to Drug or Substance— Diagnostic Criteria

A. Symptoms meet criteria for insomnia.

B. The insomnia is present for at least 1 month.

C. One of the following applies:

   i. There is current ongoing **dependence on or abuse of a drug or substance** known to have sleep-disruptive properties either during periods of **use or intoxication** or during periods of **withdrawal.**

   ii. The patient has ongoing use of or exposure to a medication, food, or toxin known to have sleep-disruptive properties in susceptible individuals.

   iii. Insomnia is temporally associated with the substance exposure, use, or abuse or acute withdrawal.

D. The sleep disturbance is not better explained by another sleep disorder, medical or neurologic disorder, mental disorder, medication use, or substance abuse.

From American Academy of Sleep Medicine: ICSD-2 International Classification of Sleep Disorders, 2nd ed. Diagnostic and Coding Manual. Westchester, IL: American Academy of Sleep Medicine, 2005.

TABLE 25-5

Medications and Substances Known to Cause Insomnia

ANTICONVULSANTS	STEROIDS
Lamotrigine	Prednisone
ANTIDEPRESSANTS	**DECONGESTANTS**
Bupropion	Phenylpropanolamine
Protriptyline	Pseudoephedrine
Fluoxetine	**BRONCHODILATORS**
Citalopram	
Escitalopram	Theophylline
Venlafaxine	
BETA BLOCKERS	**STIMULANTS/ALERTING AGENTS**
Propanolol	Dextroamphetamine
Pindolol	Methamphetamine
Metoprolol	Modafinil
SUBSTANCES	**IMMUNOSUPPRESSIVE AGENTS**
Caffeine	Interferon
Alcohol: sleep-	Prednisone
maintenance	Mycophenolate
insomnia	**ANTIBIOTICS/ANTIVIRALS**
	Efavirenz (Sustiva)

Adapted from Schweitzer PK: Drugs that disturb sleep and wakefulness. In Kryger MH, Roth T, Dement WC (eds): Principles and Practice of Sleep Medicine, 4th ed. Philadelphia: Elsevier Saunders, 2005, pp. 495–518.

sleep physicians to know that they can cause nightmares and/or sleep disturbance. Beta blockers can reduce nocturnal melatonin secretion. However, the mechanism by which beta blockers disturb sleep is not known. Beta blockers that have high lipid solubility (easily penetrate blood brain barrier—e.g., propanolol) and affect norepinephrine are considered more likely to be associated with nightmares. However, nightmares have also been noted with beta blockers with less lipid solubility. Beta blockers with high lipid solubility include metoprolol, propanolol, and timolol. Atenolol is an example of a beta blocker with lower lipid solubility.

Effects of Alcohol Alcohol is commonly used as a sleep aid and patients often do not connect their sleep problems with **alcohol consumption because most sleep disturbances occur hours after the last drink.**

Patients without Alcoholism Bedtime alcohol may shorten the latency to sleep, at least on the first few nights of consumption. However, bedtime alcohol consumption tends to fragment sleep in the later half of the night. Alcohol also increases the REM latency. Of interest, one study found that late afternoon ("happy hour") **alcohol consumption approximately 6 hours before bedtime increased wakefulness during the second half of sleep.**[36]

Active Alcoholism Sleep disturbances associated with active alcoholism include increased sleep latency, frequent awakening, and decreased subjective sleep quality. Abrupt withdrawal of alcohol can trigger profound insomnia and marked sleep fragmentation. A decrease stage N3 is also typically noted. An increase in REM sleep may also occur with acute withdrawal because alcohol suppresses REM sleep. In some patients during acute alcohol withdrawal, sleep consists of repeated REM episodes interposed on wakefulness.[38]

Abstinent Alcoholic In abstinent alcoholics (recovering alcoholics), sleep disturbance can persist for a long period of time with reduced stage N3 and increased wakefulness (WASO). In one study of patients admitted to alcohol recovery, an increase in REM sleep (REM sleep as % of TST) and an increased REM density (REMs per time in REM sleep) on admission predicted those who relapsed within 3 months.[38] Another study found longer sleep latency, shorter REM latency, and **decreased** stage 4 (stage N3) predicted relapse.[39]

Treatment

The treatment for insomnia due to drug or substance is to withdraw the offending agent. If a withdrawal syndrome is possible, gradual weaning is indicated. If withdrawal of a substance of abuse is planned, this often requires admission to a rehabilitation or mental facility and close medical supervision. If chronic insomnia is present in the recovering alcoholic or patient recovering from other drug addiction, the use of BZRAs is not recommended for treatment. Typically, sedating antidepressants and behavioral treatments are utilized.

BOX 25-17

Insomnia Due to Medical Condition—Diagnostic Criteria

A. Symptoms meet criteria for insomnia.

B. The insomnia is present for **at least 1 month.**

C. The patient has a medical or physiologic condition known to disrupt sleep.

D. Insomnia is clearly associated with the medical condition. The insomnia began near the time of onset of the medical condition and waxes and wanes with fluctuations in the severity of the medical conditions.

E. The sleep disturbance is not better explained by another sleep disorder, medical or neurologic disorder, mental disorder, medication use, or substance abuse.

From American Academy of Sleep Medicine: ICSD-2 International Classification of Sleep Disorders, 2nd ed. Diagnostic and Coding Manual. Westchester, IL: American Academy of Sleep Medicine, 2005.

TABLE 25-6

Stimulus Control Instructions

1. Lie down intending to go to sleep **only when sleepy.**
2. **Do not use the bed for anything except sleep and sex.** Do not use the bed for reading, television watching, eating, or worrying.
3. Do not watch the clock but if you have not fallen asleep in 10 to 15 minutes, get out of bed and go into another room. Stay up as long as you wish or until you feel sleepy and then return to the bedroom.
4. If you cannot fall asleep repeat rule 3 as often as needed.
5. **Get up at the same time every morning** irrespective of how much sleep you got during the night.
   Goal: Help the body acquire a consistent sleep rhythm.
6. **Do not nap during the day.**

From Morgenthaler T, Kramer M, Alessi C, et al: Practice parameters for the psychological and behavioral treatment of insomnia: an update. Sleep 2006;29:1415–1419; and Bootzin RR, Epstein D, Wood JM: Stimulus control instructions. In Hauri P (ed): Case Studies in Insomnia. New York: Plenum, 1991, pp. 19–28.

Insomnia Due to Medical Condition

Many medical disorders can disturb sleep owing to associated pain (rheumatologic disorders), dyspnea or orthopnea (cardiovascular or pulmonary disorders), nocturia (congestive heart failure, diuretic use, benign prostatic hypertrophy, untreated obstructive sleep apnea), and medication side effects. In some patients, improved control of the medical disorder will improve sleep. In others, the sleep disorder will persist, especially if associated with medication side effects (Box 25–17).

Treatment

Behavioral and pharmacologic treatments may be effective if sleep problems persist despite efforts to improve the medical disorder. BZRAs should be used with caution in patients with obstructive sleep apnea and chronic lung disease.

TREATMENT OF INSOMNIA

Cognitive and Behavioral Treatments

Cognitive and behavioral treatments are safe and effective for **sleep-onset and sleep-maintenance insomnia as well as nonrestorative sleep.**[40-46] The efficacy of behavioral treatments is equal to or better than results from pharmacotherapy.[40] Unfortunately, many locales do not have physicians, nurses, or psychologists skilled at this form of treatment. The 2006 update of AASM practice parameters for behavioral treatment of chronic insomnia[44] stated **"psychological and behavioral interventions are effective and recommended in the treatment of chronic primary insomnia, secondary insomnia (due or associated to other medical or psychiatric disorders), insomnia in older adults, and chronic hypnotic users (Standard)."** Levels of evidence for different behavioral techniques are listed in Table 25-6. In 2008, Clinical Guidelines for the Evaluation and Management of Chronic Insomnia in Adults were published.[7]

This document recommended that cognitive and behavioral treatment be utilized as **initial treatment** of insomnia if possible.

Elements of Cognitive and Behavioral Therapy

The AASM practice parameter level of evidence (Standard, Guideline, Option) for the following techniques is listed by the name of the technique.[7,43,44] A combination of techniques is frequently used.

Cognitive Therapy Cognitive therapy is aimed at changing the patient's belief and attitudes about insomnia.[7,44] These dysfunctional cognitions are often identified using questionnaires such as the DBAS (see Appendix 25–1).[19,20] Cognitive therapy uses a psychotherapeutic method to reconstruct cognitive pathways with positive and appropriate concepts about sleep and its effects. Common cognitive distortions that are identified and addressed in the course of treatment include "I can't sleep without medication," "I have a chemical imbalance," "If I can't sleep, I should stay in bed and rest," "My life will be ruined if I can't sleep."[7,20]

Cognitive Behavioral Therapy of Insomnia **(Standard)** Cognitive behavioral therapy (CBT) of insomnia is also sometimes termed *CBTI.* This technique combines cognitive therapy with behavioral techniques. The behavioral component may include **stimulus control therapy and/or sleep restriction therapy with or without use of relaxation therapy.** Sleep hygiene education is often included.

Sleep Hygiene **(No Recommendation)** Up to 30% of patients evaluated for insomnia have inadequate sleep hygiene. Although education about sleep hygiene is always utilized, there is no conclusive evidence that this alone is effective treatment.

Relaxation Therapy (**Standard**) The term *relaxation therapy (RT)* is a generic term that encompasses any number of techniques.[43,44] **Progressive muscle relaxation (PMR)** focuses on somatic arousal and was developed by Edmund Jacobsen. Thus, the technique is often called *Jacobsen PMR*. In this technique, the patient systematically goes through the parts of the body initially tensing muscles, maintaining muscle tension, then relaxing the muscles. The patient is asked to concentrate on the sensations associated with tensing and then relaxation. **Guided imagery relaxation** focuses on cognitive arousal and uses techniques of visualizing a relaxing setting or activity. RT is useful in patients who report or display elevated levels of arousal. The technique can be helpful with **both** sleep-onset and sleep-maintenance insomnia.

Stimulus Control Therapy (**Standard**) This is a specific type of CBT that is based on the idea that arousal occurs as a conditioned response to the stimulus of the sleep (bedroom) environment.[43,45] This technique is among the most effective behavioral treatments. The standard instructions are listed in Table 25–6. The goal of stimulus control therapy (SCT) is to extinguish the negative association between the bed and undesirable outcomes such as wakefulness, frustration, and worry. These associations become conditioned as a result of prolonged efforts to fall asleep and time in bed awake. SCT will replace these negative associations with positive associations between the bed and sleep.

Sleep Restriction Therapy (**Guideline**) Sleep restriction therapy (SRT; Box 25–18) limits the time in bed to the TST as derived from sleep logs.[46] The goal is to improve sleep continuity, enhancing sleep drive with sleep restriction. **Sleep will become more consolidated when long periods in bed and napping are prohibited.** As sleep continuity improves, the time in bed is gradually increased. When using this technique, the patient should be cautioned about sleepiness to prevent accidents or other mishaps.

Paradoxical Intention (**Guideline**) Instructing the patient to passively remain awake and avoid any effort (intention) to fall asleep. The goal is to eliminate performance anxiety.

Biofeedback (**Guideline**) Biofeedback trains the patient to control some physiologic variable through visible or auditory feedback. The goal is to reduce somatic arousal.

Multicomponent Therapy (Without Cognitive Therapy) (**Guideline**) This form of treatment uses multiple behavioral techniques (e.g., SCT, SRT, RT) without cognitive therapy (Table 25–7).

Evidence for Behavioral Treatment

CBTI for periods of 4 to 8 weeks has been proven effective by randomized, controlled trials comparing CBT with standard care or pharmacotherapy. In contrast to pharmacotherapy, the benefits persist when treatment is stopped. Jacobs and colleagues[47] compared CBT, pharmacotherapy (zolpidem 10 mg nightly 28 days then 5 mg nightly for 7 days, then 5 mg every other day for 7 days), combined therapy (zolpidem + CBT), or placebo over 6 weeks of active treatment and another 2 weeks of either drug washout or consolidation of CBT (no treatment sessions). The main

---

BOX 25–18

Sleep Restriction Instructions
1. A sleep log is kept for 1–2 weeks to determine the mean TST.
2. Set bedtime and wakeup time to achieve mean TST with sleep efficiency > 85%.
The minimum TIB is 5 hr.
If TST/TIB = 0.85 then TIB = TST/0.85.
Example: If TST = 310 min, then goal for TIB = 364 (bedtime 11 PM, wake time 5:04 AM.)
3. Adjustments: A. If TST/TIB > 0.85 for 7 days, then add 15–20 min to TIB. B. If TST/TIB < 0.85, decrease TIB every 7 days.

Adapted from Morgenthaler T, Kramer M, Alessi C, et al: Practice parameters for the psychological and behavioral treatment of insomnia: an update. Sleep 2006;29:1415–1419; and Speilman AJ, Saskin P, Thorpy MJ: Treatment of chronic insomnia by restriction of time in bed. Sleep 1987;10:45–56.

TABLE 25–7

Evidence Levels Concerning Behavioral Techniques for Treatment of Insomnia

EFFECTIVE (STANDARD)	EFFECTIVE (GUIDELINE)	NO RECOMMENDATION
Cognitive-behavioral treatment (with or without relaxation therapy)	Paradoxical intention	Improved sleep hygiene
Stimulus control therapy	Biofeedback	
Relaxation therapy	Sleep restriction	
	Multicomponent therapy (combinations of SCT, RT, and SRT without cognitive therapy)	

RT = relaxation therapy; SCT = stimulus control therapy; SRT = sleep restriction therapy.
From Morgenthaler T, Kramer M, Alessi C, et al: Practice parameters for the psychological and behavioral treatment of insomnia: an update. Sleep 2006;29:1415–1419.

outcome was the sleep-onset latency assessed by diary. The greatest improvement was with CBT and there was no advantage to combined treatment. In addition, at follow-up, benefits of CBT were maintained (Fig. 25–5). Edinger and associates[48] compared CBT with RT and quasidesensitization (placebo). The CBT group had a 54% reduction in WASO compared with 16% with relaxation and 12% with placebo. Smith and coworkers[49] compared the effect sizes of CBT and pharmacotherapy with respect to sleep latency, TST, and WASO and found CBT to be equal or better. Figure 25–6 illustrates the time course of improvement in TST with temazepam and CBT from a study by Morin and colleagues.[50] The major point is that, unlike pharmacotherapy, improvement with CBT continues after the active treatment period. **In summary, CBT is effective for measures of sleep-onset insomnia, sleep-maintenance insomnia, and nonrestorative sleep. There is currently no evidence that adding hypnotics (combined treatment) has any advantage.**

CBT in Hypnotic-Dependent Patients and in Co-morbid Insomnia

Although studies to date have not documented an advantage of combining CBT and hypnotics, CBT can be used in patients already on hypnotics with the possible goal of weaning the hypnotics.

Several studies have documented the efficacy of CBT in patients on hypnotics.[51-53] Using structured programs, hypnotic tapering and withdrawal is facilitated by combining the process with CBTI.[51-53] In one study comparing supervised benzodiazepine (BZ) withdrawal, CBT alone, or supervised withdrawal and CBT, all groups significantly reduced BZ use. However, more patients were BZ free in the combined group and both groups with CBT had better improvements in subjective sleep quality.[51] The utility of CBT is not confined to primary insomnia. CBT has also proved effective in secondary (co-morbid) insomnia due to mental or medical disorders.[53] Whereas it is appropriate to optimize treatment of the underlying co-morbid disorder, physicians should remember that CBT as well as hypnotics may improve insomnia complaints.

Pharmacologic Treatment of Insomnia

GABA–BZ–Chloride Ionophore Complex

GABA is the major inhibitory neurotransmitter in the central nervous system. There are two major GABA receptor subtypes $GABA_A$ and $GABA_B$. The $GABA_A$ receptor is associated with a chloride (Cl^-) channel ionophore located in cell membranes. Ionophores are molecular complexes located in cellular lipid membranes that allow transport/passage of compounds across the membrane. The $GABA_A$ receptor is the binding site for several drugs other than GABA including agonists (muscimol, gaboxadol) and antagonists (bicuculline). The $GABA_A$ receptor complex also contains a receptor

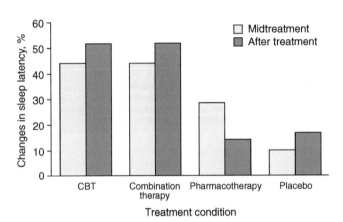

FIGURE 25–5 Percent changes (decreases) in the sleep latency with the four treatment conditions. Combination therapy included a combination of cognitive behavioral therapy (CBT) and pharmacotherapy. CBT was more effective than pharmacotherapy ($P = .03$) and placebo ($P = .02$). Combination therapy was more effective than pharmacotherapy ($P = .02$) or placebo ($P = .001$). Combination therapy and CBT therapy did not differ. *From Jacobs GD, Pace-Schott EF, Stickgold R, Otto MW: Cognitive behavior therapy and pharmacotherapy for insomnia: a randomized controlled trial and direct comparison. Arch Intern Med 2004;164:1888–1896.*

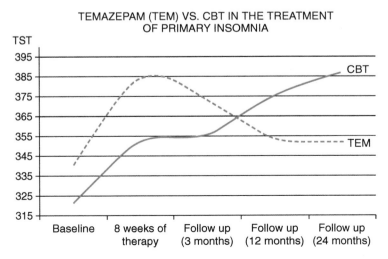

FIGURE 25–6 Total sleep time (TST) in groups treated with temazepam (TEM) and cognitive behavioral treatment (CBT). Note that after 8 weeks of treatment with TEM, the benefits decreased (drug stopped after 8 wk). However, the CBT group continued to show improvement. *From Riemann D, Perlis ML: The treatments of chronic insomnia: a review of benzodiazepine receptor agonists and psychological and behavioral therapies. Sleep Med Rev 2009;13:205–214, data from Morin CM, Colecchi C, Stone J, et al: Behavioral and pharmacological therapies for late life insomnia: a randomized controlled trial. JAMA 1999;281:991–999.*

FIGURE 25-7 **Left,** A schematic representation of the GABA$_A$–benzodiazepine–chloride ionophore complex with five subunits arranged around the chloride pore. **Right,** A view from overhead shows the location of the GABA$_A$ receptors at the junction of the α_1 and β_2 subunits and the benzodiazepine receptor at the junction of the α_1 and γ_2 subunits.

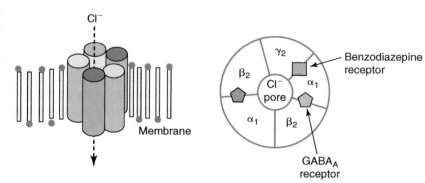

BOX 25-19

GABA$_A$ Receptor and Subunits

GABA$_A$ RECEPTOR COMPLEX

- Five subunits: two alpha, two beta, one gamma subunits
- BZ receptor: between alpha and gamma subunits
- GABA receptor: between alpha and beta subunits
- Barbiturate receptor

SUBUNITS

- Alpha (α_1, α_2, α_3, α_4, α_5, α_6)
- Beta (β_1, β_2, β_3, β_4)
- Gamma (γ_1, γ_2, γ_3)
- Delta (δ)
- Epislon (ε)
- Pi (π)
- Rho (ρ_1, ρ_2, ρ_3)
- Most common GABA$_A$ receptor is (α_1, β_2, γ_2) (understood to mean 2 α_1, 2 β_2, 1 γ_2)

BZ = benzodiazepine; GABA = gamma-aminobutyric acid.

TABLE 25-8

Relative Binding of Benzodiazepine Receptor Subtypes

	ALPHA 1	ALPHA 2	ALPHA 3	ALPHA 5
Zaleplon	17×	2×	2×	1×
Zolpidem	21×	1×	1×	Negligible
Eszopiclone	8×	5×	1×	8×

1× = the lowest affinity of a given drug for any receptor.
Adapted from Nutt DJ, Stahl SM: Searching for perfect sleep: the continuing evolution of GABA$_A$ receptor modulators as hypnotics. J Psychopharmacol 2010;14:1601–1612; Epub 2009;November 26.

for BZs and related compounds, hence, the complex is usually referred to as the **GABA-benzodiazepine-chloride ionophore complex (GBC).**[54-56] When GABA binds the GABA$_A$ receptor on the complex, this allows passage of chloride ions through the membrane, resulting in hyperpolarization and reduced neuronal activity. When BZs and certain nonbenzodiazepine medications bind the BZ receptor on the GBC, the configuration of the GABA receptor changes to **enhance the ability of GABA binding to open the associated chloride channel (increased frequency).** The medications are, therefore, sometimes called *GABA$_A$ receptor modulators.* Medications (including nonbenzodiazepines) that bind the BZ receptor and enhance the ability for GABA to open the chloride channel are called **benzodiazepine receptor agonists (BZRAs).**

The GBC is composed of five protein subunits surrounding the chloride channel (Fig. 25-7). The subunits composing the GBC have different structure and are denoted as alpha, beta, gamma, epsilon, and rho (see Box 25-19).[54,55] The receptor complex is composed of two alpha, two beta, and one gamma subunit. In addition, the alpha, beta, and

gamma subunits have isoforms (e.g., α_1, α_2, α_3, ...). The **GABA binding site** is located between **alpha and beta** subunits and the **BZ receptor site** is located between **alpha and gamma** subunits (see Fig. 25-7). The most common GBC receptor configuration is denoted as α_1, β_2, γ_2 (understood to mean two α_1, two β_2, and one γ_2 subunits) also known as a BZ type 1 receptor. The GBC also has receptors for barbiturates, certain inhaled anesthetics, and alcohol.

GABA$_A$ receptors composed of different alpha subtypes are located in different locations of the central nervous system and mediate different effects (see Box 25-19). GABA$_A$ receptors composed of α_1 subunits mediate sedation (hypnotic effect), amnesia, and anticonvulsant effects. GABA$_A$ receptors associated with α_2 and α_3 subunits mediate anxiolytic and myorelaxant effects.

BZs tend to have high affinity for all these subtypes. The new nonbenzodiazepine BZRAs (zolpidem, zaleplon, eszopiclone), also known as the "Z" hypnotics, have preferential binding to GABA$_A$ receptors containing certain subunits. Zolpidem and zaleplon selectively bind GABA$_A$ receptors containing α1 subunits and are often called *selective BZRAs* (Table 25-8). However, the preferential binding is only relative, and at higher doses, GABA$_A$ receptors containing α_1, α_2, and α_3 are bound. Eszopiclone has receptor binding more like traditional BZs but has many of the same advantages of the other Z hypnotics. Eszopiclone does bind α_1 subunits with higher affinity than α_3 but also binds α_2 subunit receptors with only slightly lower affinity than α_1 subunits.[56] The clinical importance of selective binding for the clinical effects

TABLE 25-9

GABA_A Receptor Alpha Subunits and Associated Actions

	ACTION	PROPORTION OF GABA RECEPTORS	LOCATION
α_1	Sedative, amnestic, anticonvulsant	60%	All brain regions Cortex, hippocampus
α_2	Anxiolytic, myorelaxant	15–20%	Cortex, hippocampus, amygdala, forebrain, hypothalamus
α_3	Anxiolytic, myorelaxant	10–15%	Cerebral cortex, thalamus (reticular nucleus)
α_4, α_6	Insensitive to BZ		Dentate gyrus
α_5	High affinity for BZ Low affinity for zolpidem BZ tolerance		Cerebral cortex, hippocampus

BZ = benzodiazepine; GABA = gamma-aminobutyric acid.

of the Z hypnotics remains uncertain. In addition, the ultimate effect of a BZRA depends not just on receptor affinity but also on the potency of the medication and the achievable drug concentration.

Traditionally, the sedation effects of BZRAs was equated with hypnotic action. However, new information is available from studies in genetically manipulated mice.[55–57] As each of the subunits on the GABA_A receptor is associated with a single gene, genetic manipulation (knock-out, knock-in mice) allows the importance of subunits to be assessed.[56] These studies suggest GABA_A receptors containing α_2 and α_3 subunits, although not associated with sedation, are involved with the control of manifestations of sleep. For example, BZs can induce sleep in α_1 knock-out mice. One study suggests that GABA_A receptors with α_2 subunits were responsible for generating delta waves during non–rapid eye movement (NREM) sleep.[57] GABA_A receptors with α_3 subunits are present in the reticular nucleus of the thalamus—an area responsible for thalamic-cortical oscillations (sleep spindles).[56] In the future, the importance of GABA_A receptors associated with α_2 and α_3 subunits for the control of sleep will be better defined (Table 25–9).

BZRA Effects and Side Effects The BZRAs have a number of important clinical effects including sedation (hypnotic), amnestic, anxiolytic, myorelaxant, and anticonvulsant (Table 25–10). As noted previously, **zolpidem and zaleplon** bind preferentially to BZ receptor-associated α1 subunits and, therefore, have **less anxiolytic and myorelaxant** activity than the classic BZs. However, eszopiclone appears to have more affinity for α_2 units than zolpidem and zaleplon and, therefore, possibly more anxiolytic effects. **All three Z drugs are associated with less reduction in stage N3 than classic BZs (mainly due to less reduction in slow wave amplitude) as well as less rebound insomnia or evidence of tolerance (decreased effect at the same dose).**[58,59] Zaleplon has a very short duration of action (Table 25–11) and may have less residual sedative effects especially after middle of the night dosing.[58–61] Zolpidem has a longer half-life than zaleplon but

TABLE 25-10

Effects of Benzodiazepine Receptor Agonists

ACTIONS

Hypnotic
Amnestic
Anxiolytic
Myorelaxant
Anticonvulsant

SIDE EFFECTS

Sedation
Anterograde amnesia (learning new material)
Ataxia, falls
Sleepwalking, sleep violence, sleep-related eating disorder
Respiratory depression
Tolerance
Dependence, abuse
Rebound insomnia (especially triazolam)

TABLE 25-11

Effects of Benzodiazepine Receptor Agonists on Sleep

- Improved sleep continuity
  - Decreased sleep latency (short- and intermediate-acting BZRAs)
  - Increased total sleep time (intermediate-acting BZRAs)
  - Decreased wake after sleep onset (intermediate-acting BZRAs)

- Decreased stage N3
  - Reduced amplitude of slow waves (less with alpha 1-selective BZRAs)
  - Increased sleep spindles and faster activity

- Decrease in REM sleep: mild, less with alpha 1-selective drugs

BZRAs = benzodiazepine receptor agonists; REM = rapid eye movement.

shorter than eszopiclone. Zolpidem may not increase TST in some patients, and for this reason, zolpidem CR (continuous release) was developed. Zolpidem CR is a coated two-layer tablet with one layer that releases the drug content immediately and another layer that slowly releases additional drug beyond three hours after administration. Zolpidem CR, eszopiclone, and temazepam have intermediate durations of action (Table 25–12) and may be more effective for sleep-maintenance insomnia than medications with a shorter duration of action. However, patients are quite variable in their response to the different hypnotics, and some patients with sleep-maintenance insomnia will respond to generic zolpidem.

The BZRAs have a number of effects on sleep (see Table 25–11). A decrease in sleep latency is common to all medications. Those with an intermediate or longer duration of action also can increase TST and decrease WASO. BZRAs can increase sleep spindle activity and higher EEG frequencies. The BZs reduce stage N3 sleep with no or a mild reduction in REM sleep. The major effect on stage N3 sleep is via a reduction in slow wave amplitude. As mentioned previously, the nonbenzodiazepine BZRAs (Z hypnotics) result in no or minimal decrease in the amount of stage N3 because they do not substantially reduce the amplitude of slow waves. The clinical importance of less reduction in stage N3 sleep is still unclear.

The BZRAs have a number of side effects (see Table 25–10) including anterograde amnesia (decreased ability to learn and retain new information), ataxia (fall risk), as well as residual sedation during the day. Of note, eszopiclone is associated with an unpleasant (often metallic) taste in a significant number of patients (≤25%).[62,63] BZRAs can also be associated with nausea in some patients. They are not recommended for use in nursing women or in pregnant women. In 2007, the U.S. Food and Drug Administration (FDA) required packaging information on the BZRA hypnotics to include a warning regarding several specific potential adverse effects. **The new information states that BZRAs have been associated with sleep behaviors including sleepwalking, eating, driving, and sexual behavior. Patients taking BZRAs should allow for adequate sleep time and NOT take BZRAs in combination with other sedatives, alcohol, or sleep restriction.** Zolpidem is the BZRA most often associated with sleepwalking and the sleep-related eating disorder, but these manifestations can happen with the other BZRAs. Residual sedation is another important side effect of BZRAs. In general, shorter-acting medications are less likely to cause residual sedation.[60,61] Respiratory depression due to the BZRAs hypnotics is uncommon. However, caution is advised with the use of hypnotics in patients with hypoventilation, obstructive sleep apnea, and severe lung disease. Respiratory depression is more likely when BZRAs are combined with other central nervous system depressants such as alcohol or narcotics.

The potential for dependence and abuse resulted in the BZRA hypnotics being classified as Schedule 2 medications. Drugs with high receptor binding affinity such as lorazepam, midazolam, and triazolam cause more side effects with

withdrawal.[58] Triazolam causes rebound insomnia and is no longer recommended as a first-line hypnotic. Significant rebound insomnia has **NOT** been noted in most studies of zaleplon, zolpidem, and eszopiclone.[58,59,62] However, withdrawal side effects and rebound insomnia can potentially occur with all BZRAs and slow withdrawal is recommended if possible.

General Considerations for BZRA Hypnotic Use BZRA hypnotics are well studied and the medications listed in Table 25–12 are FDA approved for treatment of insomnia unless otherwise noted. It is especially important to note the duration of action. The hypnotics are grouped into nonbenzodiazepines and BZs. At this time, the only nonbenzodiazepine available in the United States in generic form is zolpidem. The brand name Z hypnotics are in general quite expensive. Some general considerations for using hypnotics and choosing a specific hypnotic medication are listed in Table 25–13. Ideally, hypnotics should be used on a short term or intermittent basis at the lowest effective dose. A lower dose and more caution is indicated in the elderly or in patients with impaired hepatic function because most BZRAs undergo hepatic metabolism.[7,56] Until 2005, the FDA labeling stated that the hypnotic medications were indicated for short-term use. Since 2005, the duration of action has not been specified. New studies have documented effectiveness of some medications for 6 months or longer[63–66] (Table 25–14). Clinical experience also has noted continued long-term effectiveness (at least by patient report) in a number of BZRA hypnotics. The effect of eszopiclone on sleep latency for a 12-month period (blinded and open-label portions) is illustrated in Figure 25–8.

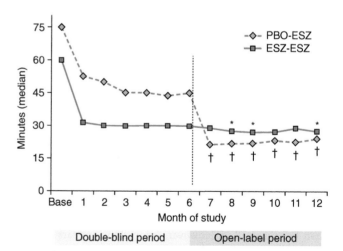

FIGURE 25–8 The continued effect of eszopiclone on sleep latency over a 12-month study. Double-blind and open-label periods are shown. The *squares* (ESZ-ESZ) show patients who used 3 mg of eszopiclone for the entire period. The *diamonds* (PBO-ESZ) show patients originally on placebo but converted to eszopiclone for the last 6 months. Statistical comparisons made against PBO-ESZ and ESZ-ESZ values at 6 months. * = P < .05 ESZ-ESZ during open-label period vs. 6-month ESZ-ESZ value. † = P < .0001 PBO-ESZ group in open-label period vs. 6 month PBO-ESZ value. *From Roth T, Walsh JK, Krystal A, et al: An evaluation of the efficacy and safety of eszopiclone over 12 months in patients with chronic primary insomnia. Sleep Med 2005;6:487–495.*

TABLE 25–12

Commonly Used Benzodiazepine Receptor Agonist and Melatonin Receptor Agonist Hypnotic Medications

BENZODIAZEPINE RECEPTOR AGONISTS USED AS HYPNOTICS (SCHEDULE IV CONTROLLED SUBSTANCES)

NONBENZODIAZEPINES

GENERIC (BRAND NAME)	MEDICATION FORMS	DOSE	ONSET OF ACTION	DURATION OF ACTION	INDICATIONS	SELECTED SIDE EFFECTS AND COMMENTS
Zaleplon (Sonata) Pyrazolopyrimidine	5, 10 mg capsule	10 mg qhs, max 20 mg 5 mg hs in elderly, debilitated, mild to moderate hepatic impairment, or concomitant cimetidine	10–20 min	Short-acting ($T_{1/2}$ = 1 hr)	SOI	Rescue medication if 4 hr left for sleep
Zolpidem generic imidazopyridine	5, 10 mg tablets	10 mg hs, max 10 mg 5 mg in elderly, debilitated, hepatic impairment	10–20 min	Short- to intermediate-acting $T_{1/2}$ 2.5 (1.5–4) hr	SOI, SMI	Generic available in United States Sleep-related eating disorder and sleepwalking reported
Zopidem CR (Ambien CR) imidazopyridine	6.25, 12.5 mg tablets	6.25–12.5 mg qhs 6.25 mg qhs in elderly	10–20 min	Controlled-release, intermediate-acting $T_{1/2}$ 3 hr*	SOI, SMI	Swallow whole not crushed, cut, or chewed
Eszopiclone (Lunesta) Cyclopyrrolones	1, 2, 3 mg tablets	2–3 mg qhs (max 3 mg) 1 mg qhs in elderly and hepatic impairment (max 2 mg)	10–30 min	Intermediate-acting $T_{1/2}$ 6 hr	SOI, SMI	Unpleasant taste common side effect

BENZODIAZEPINES

GENERIC (BRAND NAME)	MEDICATION FORMS	DOSE	ONSET OF ACTION	DURATION OF ACTION	INDICATIONS	SELECTED SIDE EFFECTS AND COMMENTS
Triazolam (Halcion)	0.125 mg 0.25 mg	0.125–0.25 mg qhs 0.125 mg in elderly	10–20 min	Short acting $T_{1/2}$ 2–5 hr	SOI	Rebound insomnia—not a first-line hypnotic
Estazolam (ProSom)	1, 2 mg tablets	1–2 mg hs 0.5 mg in elderly, debilitated	15–30 min	Intermediate-acting $T_{1/2}$ 8–24 hr	SOI, SMI	Residual daytime sleepiness can occur
Temazepam (Restoril)	7.5, 15, 30 mg capsules	15–30 hs 15 mg in elderly, debilitated	45–60 min	Intermediate-acting $T_{1/2}$ 8–20 hr	SOI, SMI	Delayed onset of action
Flurazepam (Dalmane)	15, 30 mg capsule	15–30 mg hs 15 mg hs in elderly, debilitated	15–30 min	Long-acting $T_{1/2}$ 47–100 hr	SMI	Residual daytime sleepiness active metabolites

BENZODIAZEPINES NOT FDA APPROVED AS HYPNOTICS

GENERIC (BRAND NAME)	MEDICATION FORMS	DOSE	ONSET OF ACTION	DURATION OF ACTION	INDICATIONS	SELECTED SIDE EFFECTS AND COMMENTS
Clonazepam (Klonopin)	0.5, 1.0, 2.0 mg	0.25–0.5 mg qhs	Peak levels 1–3 hr	Long-acting $T_{1/2}$ 18–50 hr	SMI	Residual daytime sleepiness Potent BZRA Not FDA approved as hypnotic
Lorazepam (Ativan)	0.5, 1.0 mg	0.5–1.0 mg qhs ≤2–4 mg	Peak levels 1–3 hr	Long-acting $T_{1/2}$ 14 hr		Not FDA approved as hypnotic Wean slowly, can cause withdrawal side effects

MELATONIN RECEPTOR AGONISTS (NOT SCHEDULE IV)

GENERIC (BRAND NAME)	MEDICATION FORMS	DOSE	ONSET OF ACTION	DURATION OF ACTION	INDICATIONS	SELECTED SIDE EFFECTS AND COMMENTS
Ramelteon Rozerem	8 mg tablet	8 mg hs	20–30 min	$T_{1/2}$ 1–2.6 hr Active metabolite MII is 2–5 hours (but 20 X less potent)	SOI	No addiction/dependence potential use with Luvox contraindicated Do not use with hepatic impairment

*Time when drug concentration reaches 50% of maximum = 4.6 hours. Weinling E, McDougall S, Andre F, et al: Pharmacokinetic profile of a new modified release formulation of zolpidem designed to improve sleep maintenance. Funda Clin Pharmacol 2006;20:397–403.

BZRA = benzodiazepine receptor agonist; FDA = U.S. Food and Drug Administration. SMI = sleep-maintenance insomnia; SOI = sleep-onset insomnia.

TABLE 25-13

General Recommendations for Benzodiazepine Receptor Agonist Hypnotic Treatment and Choice of Medication

GENERAL CONSIDERATIONS

1. Use lowest dose for the shortest time possible.
2. Take BZRAs on an empty stomach.
3. BZRAs are not recommended in nursing or pregnant women.
4. Rapid reduction in dose or withdrawal can cause withdrawal symptoms including rebound insomnia.
5. Use with caution in patients with OSA and lung disease (COPD).
6. Do not combine with alcohol; use caution with other sedatives.

CONSIDERATIONS IN CHOICE OF HYPNOTIC

1. Symptom pattern (SOI, SMI, both) and BZRA duration of action.
2. Treatment goals.
3. Past treatment (failures, side effects).
4. Patient preferences.
5. Cost (generic much cheaper).
6. Availability (e.g., covered by health plan).
7. Co-morbid conditions
8. Avoid BZRA if history of medication dependence, alcoholism.
9. Medication interactions
10. Combination of fluvoxamine and ramelteon contraindicated.
11. Side effects (e.g., anticholinergic in patients with benign prostatic hypertrophy).

BZRA = benzodiazepine receptor agonist; COPD = chronic obstructive pulmonary disease; OSA = obstructive sleep apnea; SMI = sleep-maintenance insomnia; SOI = sleep-onset insomnia.

Choice of BZRA Hypnotic Medication The major characteristic of BZRA medications to consider in choosing a hypnotic (see Table 25-13) **is the duration of action.**[7,58] Short-acting medications work for sleep-onset insomnia but may not help with sleep-maintenance insomnia. Triazolam has a short duration of action but is associated with significant rebound insomnia and is no longer considered a first-line agent for insomnia. Zaleplon has a very short duration of action and may be useful as a "rescue medication" for middle of the night dosing (as long as 4-6 hr of potential sleep remain).[60,61] One study of experimental awakening during the middle of the night found morning effects with zolpidem but not with zaleplon.[61] Zolpidem has a short to intermediate action and may work for some but not all patients as treatment of sleep-maintenance insomnia.

Intermediate-acting medications are indicated for sleep-onset and sleep-maintenance insomnia but may cause daytime sedation in some patients. Temazepam, eszopiclone, and zolpidem CR are in this category. Of note, temazepam has a fairly long onset of action in many patients (see Table 25-12) and may not be effective for sleep onset insomnia in some patients. The duration of action of zolpidem CR is 4-6 hours but eszopiclone may be more effective for sleep maintenance insomnia in some patients. On the other hand, zolpidem CR may cause less residual sedation in the morning.

Long-acting medications have an increased risk of daytime sedation and other residual effects. Flurazepam also has active metabolites. It is important to note that sometimes patients who fail to respond to a given BZRA will respond to an alternate BZRA. Lorzepam (Ativan) and clonazepam are two BZ BZRAs that are not FDA approved for primary insomnia. Lorazepam is approved for treatment of anxiety and may work better than approved hypnotics if insomnia is due to anxiety. Although the standard dose for anxiety is 2 to 4 mg, lower doses (0.5-1 mg) may work as a hypnotic. The medication has a relatively long half-life and withdrawal

TABLE 25-14

Studies Documenting Long-term Effectiveness of Benzodiazepine Receptor Agonists

BRZA	STUDY FOCUS	TYPE OF STUDY (LENGTH)	COMMENTS	STUDY
Eszopiclone 3 mg	Adults Chronic insomnia	RCT-DB-PC 6 mo	Efficacy maintained for 6 mo including sleep latency and ability to function during the day	Krystal, 2003[63]
Eszopiclone 3 mg	Adults Chronic insomnia	12 mo total (6-mo open-label extension)	6 mo DB placebo (no benefit) changed to open-label eszopiclone showed benefit over the last 6 mo DB eszopiclone benefits were sustained over 12 mo	Roth, 2005[64]
Eszopiclone 2 mg	Older adults primary and co-morbid insomnia	RCT-DB-PC 12-wk treatment 2-wk withdrawal (SB)	Efficacy maintained No rebound	Ancoli-Israel, 2010[65]
Zolpidem-ER 12.5 mg	Chronic primary insomnia	RCT-DB-PC 24 wk (6 mo)	3-7 nights/wk efficacy maintained Sleep onset and sleep maintenance improved Next day concentration improved Morning sleepiness improved	Krystal, 2008[66]

DB = double-blind; PC = placebo-controlled; RCT = randomized, controlled trial; SB = single-blind.

symptoms may occur after long-term use. Clonazepam is a potent BZRA with a very long half-life and is commonly associated with morning grogginess. However, individual patients may respond well to this medication and not report morning sedation. Starting with the lowest possible dose and having patients plan on a long sleep period is prudent. An occasional rare patient requires up to 2 mg of clonazepam for sleep-maintenance insomnia.

Several studies have compared continuous versus intermittent use of hypnotics and found intermittent hypnotic administration was effective. Walsh and associates[67] compared zolpidem 10 mg (more than 3 but no more than 5 nights per week on as-needed basis) versus placebo and found significant benefits. Hajak and coworkers[68] compared nightly zolpidem, placebo twice weekly, and zolpidem 5 nights per week and found both zolpidem regimens were effective compared with placebo.

Ramelteon (Rozerem)—A Melatonin Receptor Agonist

Ramelteon is the first melatonin receptor agonist approved in the United States for treatment of insomnia.[69-72] It is an MT1/MT2 receptor agonist. The effects at MT1 are thought to inhibit neuronal firing of the suprachiasmatic nucleus (SCN), effectively turning off the alerting signal and allowing sleep to occur. In contrast, MT2 receptor effects are thought to mediate melatonin's phase shifting effects on circadian rhythms. Ramelteon is about 17 times more potent at the MT1/MT2 receptors than melatonin. Studies have shown an absence of next-day residual effects, withdrawal, or rebound effects. The medication lacks abuse potential. Randomized, placebo-controlled studies have demonstrated efficacy of ramelteon with most effects being on sleep latency. The medication has a short half-life. One study by Mayer and colleagues[71] demonstrated that 8 mg of ramelteon 30 minutes before bedtime reduced subjective sleep latency over a 6-month trial. Ramelteon also decreased latency to persistent sleep by PSG over the trial. TST was increased only at week 1. Side effects of ramelteon include headache, nausea, dizziness, somnolence, nightmares, hallucinations, and uncommonly suicidal ideation. Arthralgia and myalgia can also occur. Because ramelteon has no dependence potential, it may be a good choice for patients with alcohol or drug dependency. Ramelteon undergoes hepatic metabolism and should be avoided in patients with severe liver disease. Use of ramelteon is contraindicated in patients taking luvoxamine, because this antidepressant significantly increases the levels of ramelteon in the blood.[7]

Sedating Antidepressants and Antipsychotics

Sedating antidepressants used in doses lower than required for antidepressant effects are widely used as hypnotics (Table 25–15). Until recently, relatively little evidence has

TABLE 25–15

Sedating Antidepressants and Antipsychotics Used "Off-Label" As Hypnotics (Not FDA Approved As Hypnotics Except for Silenor)

NAME GENERIC (BRAND NAME)	DOSE FORMS	HYPNOTIC DOSE	COMMENTS	NOTABLE SIDE EFFECTS
Trazodone	50, 100 mg	25–100 mg qhs	Less anticholinergic side effects than TCAs $T_{1/2}$ 9 (3–14) hr	Priapism Postural hypotension
Mirtazapine (Remeron)	15, 30 mg	7.5–15 mg qhs	$T_{1/2}$ 20–40 hr	Weight gain Higher doses less sedating
TCAs				
Amitryptyline (Elavil)	10, 25, 50 mg	10–25 mg qhs	$T_{1/2}$ 10–26 hr metabolite active (nortriptyline)	Dry mouth, constipation QT prolongation
Doxepin (Sinequan)	10, 25, 50 10 mg/mL	1–10 mg (elixir) 25 mg qhs	$T_{1/2}$ 6–8 hr	Dry mouth, constipation
Doxepin (Silenor)	3, 6 mg	6 mg qhs 3 mg qhs elderly	$T_{1/2}$ 6–8 hr	FDA approved for sleep-maintenance insomnia Cimetidine increases drug levels—max dose of doxepin should not exceed 3 mg if cimetidine co-administered Sertraline can also increase levels of doxepin
SEDATING ANTIPSYCHOTIC MEDICATIONS				
Quetiapine (Seroquel)	25, 50, 100	12.5–50 mg qhs	$T_{1/2}$ 6 hr Intermediate-acting	Weight gain, headache, dizziness Neuroleptic syndrome Tardive dyskinesia Long QT Lens change

FDA = U.S. Food and Drug Administration; TCAs = tricyclic antidepressants.

demonstrated their effectiveness as hypnotics in patients without depression. Trazodone is a sedating antidepressant with minimal anticholinergic activity that is frequently used as a hypnotic. The evidence for its efficacy as a hypnotic in patients without depression is very modest.[73,74] However, some patients seem to benefit from the medication. It is a reasonable hypnotic in co-morbid depression,[75,76] in patients with significant sleep apnea, or in patients with a history of medication dependence. Its main side effects are priapism and postural hypotension. The usual dose is 25 to 100 mg qhs. Mirtazapine (Remeron) is used in low doses as a hypnotic.[77] Of interest, lower doses (7.5 mg and 15 mg) are sometimes more sedating than higher doses. The major side effect is weight gain. Mirtazapine antagonizes alpha 2 receptors and serotonin ($5HT_2$) receptors. Its sedation is believed due to its antihistamine activity. Doxepin (Sinequan, Silenor) and amitriptyline (Elavil) are sedating tricyclic antidepressants that have been used in low doses as hypnotics. They have significant anticholinergic side effects (dry mouth, constipation, urinary retention). It is important to recall that tricyclic antidepressants are very dangerous in overdose. Recently, doxepin has been evaluated with randomized, controlled trials for its utility as a hypnotic in low doses (1, 3, 6 mg). Lower doses avoid significant anticholinergic side effects.[78] In these studies, the major significant effect was a decrease in WASO. The mechanism of hypnotic action of doxepin is antagonism of histamine (H1) receptors. A preparation of doxepin (Silenor) available as 3-mg and 6-mg tablets has recently been approved by the FDA for treatment of sleep-maintenance insomnia. This is the only sedating antidepressant FDA approved for treatment of insomnia. Silenor is fairly expensive. An alternative is to use a low dose of generic doxepin (10 mg or 5 mg using the elixir). Medications with substantial anticholinergic activity can cause urinary retention in patients with benign prostatic hypertrophy. Use of even low-dose doxepin in patients with severe urinary retention should be avoided.

Quetiapine (Seroquel) is a second-generation antipsychotic medication that antagonizes histamine, dopamine D_2, and $5HT_2$ receptors. At low doses, the medication's main effect is as an antihistamine. Quetiapine is indicated for treatment of schizophrenia and bipolar disorder. Side effects include QT prolongation, weight gain, extrapyramidal symptoms, headache, lens changes/cataracts, and decreased white blood cell count. Even at low doses, quetiapine has been associated with significant weight gain. Due to its side effects, this medication is usually not used in patients without significant psychiatric disorders unless other treatments have failed.

Other Medications Used for Insomnia

Other sedating medications have been used for insomnia. Gabapentin (an anticonvulsant structural analog of GABA) is used for chronic pain and the restless legs syndrome. The half-life of gabapentin is approximately 5 to 9 hours, and it is excreted by the kidneys unchanged. Due to the sedative properties of gabapentin, the medication can be used as a hypnotic treatment alternative in patients who do not respond to or tolerate other medications. The usual dose is 300 to 900 mg at bedtime. Side effects include dizziness, ataxia, and less commonly, leukopenia. Gabapentin could potentially be useful in patients with insomnia associated with pain. The use of melatonin has been analyzed with a meta-analysis and appears to have a small effect on sleep latency with little effect on WASO or TST.[79] One problem with both ramelteon and melatonin as hypnotics is that the endogenous melatonin levels are already elevated during the dark hours. The hypnotic dose is 3 to 5 mg. There is some evidence that valerian extracts have some benefit as a hypnotic.[80] Antihistamines (diphenhydramine and doxylamine) are the primary ingredients in over-the-counter sleep aids. There is some limited evidence for their efficacy.[80] The main problem is that they have considerable anticholinergic activity (urinary retention) and can cause daytime sedation.[7]

Pharmacotherapy for Co-morbid Insomnia of Psychiatric Disorders or in Patients with Dependence Issues

Patients with anxiety or major depressive disorders frequently have prominent co-morbid insomnia. In such patients, one might choose to use (1) a sedating antidepressant at antidepressant doses (e.g., mirtazapine 30–45 mg qhs), (2) the combination of an effective nonsedating antidepressant (at antidepressant doses) and a sedating antidepressant at low doses, or (3) the combination of an effective nonsedating antidepressant + BZRA hypnotic. Fava and associates[81] studied a group of patients with both major depressive disorder and insomnia. The combination of fluoxetine (FLX) and placebo was compared with FLX + 3 mg of eszopiclone. Co-administration of eszopiclone resulted in improved subjective sleep latency, WASO, and TST compared with FLX alone. Whereas this result was not unexpected, a surprising finding was that there was also **greater improvement in depression at 4 and 8 weeks with the combination of FLX and eszopiclone.** A similar trial with zolpidem found improvement in sleep but no evidence of greater improvement in depression.[82] It is possible eszopiclone has beneficial antidepressant effects not present with zolpidem. Indeed, eszopiclone does have greater binding affinity for BZ receptors associated with $\alpha 2$ subunits that have an effect on mood. However, a definite benefit of eszopiclone over zolpidem remains to be documented by studies comparing the drugs in a head-to-head comparison in depressed patients. In another study, the use of zolpidem when added to escitalopram (Lexapro) did improve sleep but not anxiety in a group of patients with generalized anxiety disorder.[83] In summary, BZRAs can be used effectively in combination with antidepressants in patients with depression or anxiety associated with prominent insomnia complaints. In patients with a history of past or current **alcohol or BZ dependence,** the use of BZRAs is problematic. For these patients, use of ramelteon (no abuse potential) or a sedating antidepressant may be the best treatment option. However, studies documenting effectiveness of this approach are lacking.

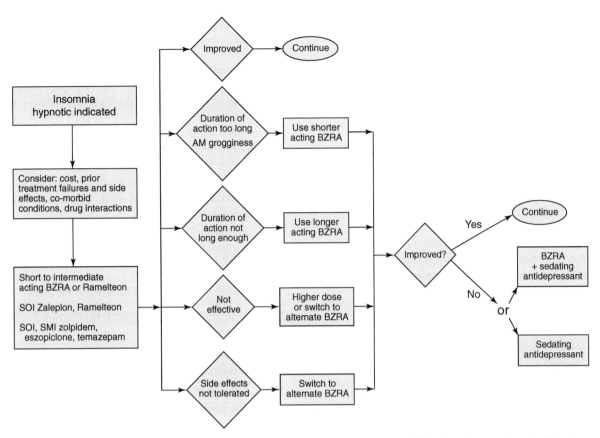

FIGURE 25–9 Clinical pathway for hypnotic treatment of insomnia. BZRA = benzodiazepine receptor agonist; SMI = sleep-maintenance insomnia; SOI = sleep-onset insomnia. *Adapted from Schutte-Rodin S, Broch L, Buysee D, et al: Clinical guideline for the evaluation and management of chronic insomnia in adults. J Clin Sleep Med 2008;4:487–504.*

Pharmacotherapy of Insomnia: Overall Strategy

A general strategy for hypnotic therapy for insomnia[7] is illustrated in Figure 25–9. After considering factors listed in Table 25–13, one could start with ramelteon or zaleplon for sleep-onset insomnia. If sleep-maintenance insomnia is a problem, use of zolpidem, zolpidem CR, eszopiclone, or temazepam could be considered. **In elderly patients or patients with impaired hepatic metabolism, a lower hypnotic dose is prudent.** If the duration of action is not long enough, one can switch to a longer-acting medication. For example, a switch from zolpidem to eszopiclone. If the duration of action is too long (AM sedation), **a switch to a shorter-acting medication or a reduction in dose of the current medication could be tried.** If the medication is not effective, a switch to an alternate BZRA or a change from ramelteon to a BZRA could be considered. Some patients will respond differently to alternate BZRAs. Temazepam may not work well for sleep-onset insomnia in some patients due to its longer onset of action. If anxiety is a major component of insomnia, use of a traditional BZ (e.g., temazepam) or eszopiclone with more anxiolytic activity might be more effective. Recall that zaleplon and zolpidem have little anxiolytic activity. If the current hypnotic medication is not tolerated due to side effects, a switch to an alternate BZRA could also be tried.

If treatment with standard BZRA hypnotics is not successful, one could try a sedating antidepressant. Given the minimal anticholinergic effects associated with trazodone, most physicians would start with this medication when using a sedating antidepressant. However, low-dose doxepin or amitriptyline may be effective in some patients. If sedating antidepressants are not effective (or tolerated at an effective dose), the combination of a BZRA and a sedating antidepressant could be tried (e.g., zolpidem and trazodone).

If patients have a significant pain component to their insomnia, one could try gabapentin for its sedating as well as analgesic effects. If anxiety is a major component of the insomnia or the traditional BZRA hypnotics are not effective, use of lorazepam or clonazepam could be tried. Lastly, one could try a sedating antipsychotic medication in low doses (quetiapine). These drugs have major side effects and are generally to be avoided unless a mental disorder is present or all other options have failed.

CLINICAL REVIEW QUESTIONS

1. A 40-year-old man was prescribed zolpidem for insomnia complaints. His problems with sleep onset have improved but he is still unable to sleep later than 3 to 4 AM. What medication do you prescribe?

A. Zaleplon.

B. Eszopiclone.

C. Flurazepam.

D. Ramelteon.

2. Which of the following behavioral techniques has the least evidence of its efficacy?

A. SCT.

B. RT.

C. SRT.

D. Sleep hygiene education.

E. Multimodality therapy

3. A 60-year-old obese man has a history of alcohol dependence, insomnia, and benign prostatic hypertrophy. What is the most appropriate medication for treatment of his insomnia?

A. Doxepin 25 mg.

B. Amitriptyline 25 mg.

C. Zolpidem 10 mg.

D. Trazodone 50 mg.

E. Diphenhydramine 25 mg.

4. A 30-year-old woman reports problems with insomnia since childhood. There have been no periods of remission. She denies sleeping better in novel environments. During the last few months, her mood and sleep complaints have worsened. What is the most likely diagnosis?

A. Psychophysiologic insomnia.

B. Idiopathic insomnia.

C. Paradoxical insomnia.

D. IDMD.

5. A 30-year-old man complains of episodes of waking up at 3 AM and not being able to return to sleep. These episodes occur about every 2 weeks but are not predictable. What do you prescribe?

A. Zolpidem.

B. Zaleplon.

C. Eszopiclone.

D. Temazepam.

6. A 50-year-old woman is taking a hypnotic for insomnia. Recently, she has been sleepwalking and eating during sleep. Some episodes she can remember but other times she is surprised to find evidence of food consumption when she awakens in the morning. Although the behavior could occur with almost any hypnotic, which of the following BZRAs has been most often associated with the behavior.

A. Zaleplon.

B. Temazepam.

C. Zolpidem.

D. Eszopiclone.

E. Ramelteon.

7. A 45-year-old woman complains of not sleeping at all for 2 to 3 nights each week. Other nights, it takes over an hour to fall asleep and the TST is never over 4 hours. The patient rarely takes naps but feels terrible the next day when she does not sleep the night before. The patient describes laying in bed all night thinking about her work. She kept a sleep log and was studied with actigraphy. One night no sleep was reported but the actigraph estimated about 5 hours of sleep. What is the most likely diagnosis?

A. Idiopathic insomnia.

B. Psychophysiologic insomnia.

C. Paradoxical insomnia.

D. Insomnia associated with a mood disorder.

8. What of the following is NOT true about the $GABA_A$ receptor complex?

A. It contains a chloride ionophore.

B. It is composed of five protein subunits.

C. Binding of a BZRA opens the chloride pore.

D. The complex is usually composed of two alpha, two beta, and one gamma subunits.

9. Which of the following medications is associated with an unpleasant taste?

A. Zolpidem.

B. Eszopiclone.

C. Ramelteon.

D. Trazodone.

10. Which of the following statements about CBTI is not true?

A. It consists of cognitive therapy and one or more of these behavioral treatments (SCT, SRT) with or without RT.

B. It continues to show benefits after the treatment period.

C. It is more effective if combined with hypnotic treatment.

D. It is effective for both primary and secondary insomnia.

11. A 5-year-old boy often awakens during the night and will not return to sleep without at least ½ hour of parental presence and attention. Which diagnosis best describes the problem?

A. Childhood behavioral insomnia—limit-setting type.

B. Childhood behavioral insomnia—sleep-association type.

12. A 50-year-old man with both sleep-onset and sleep-maintenance insomnia is started on 12.5 mg of

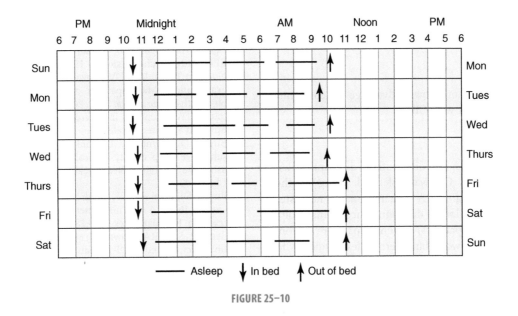

FIGURE 25-10

zolpidem CR. He tolerated the medication and falls asleep quickly but awakens at 4 AM. Which of the following is the most appropriate next step?

A. Eszopiclone.

B. Trazodone.

C. Quetiapine.

D. Ramelteon.

E. Zaleplon.

13. Which of the following is NOT true about adjustment insomnia?

A. Duration must be less than 3 months.

B. It is associated with an identifiable stressor.

C. It is expected to resolve spontaneously in most cases.

D. Duration must be less than 1 month.

14. A patient complains of sleep-onset and sleep-maintenance insomnia. A sleep log is shown in Figure 25–10. Which of the behavioral techniques would be most applicable to this patient?

A. RT.

B. SCT.

C. Sleep hygiene education.

D. SRT.

Answers

1. **B.** A BZRA with a longer duration of action is needed. Zaleplon and ramelteon are short acting. Flurazepam is very long acting and often associated with daytime sedation.

2. **D.** There is no evidence that sleep hygiene education alone is effective treatment for insomnia.

3. **D.** Trazodone. Doxepin (at 25 mg), amitriptyline, and diphenhydramine all have significant anticholinergic activity and could cause urinary retention. Use of zolpidem is relatively contraindicated in a patient with current or prior substance dependence. Trazodone has minimal anticholinergic activity. Recently, low-dose doxepin (1, 3, and 6 mg) has been used and this might be another alternative. In patients with drug dependence, BZRAs should be avoided if possible.

4. **B.** Idiopathic insomnia is characteristically present since childhood without periods of remission. Psychophysiologic and paradoxical insomnia are not present since childhood. IDMD would be a reasonable possibility but the patient had significant insomnia many years before her mood worsened.

5. **B.** Zaleplon is the only medication on the list with a very short half-life. It is most appropriate for "rescue medication" for middle of the night awakening. It should not be used if there are not at least 3 to 4 more hours of possible sleep. If the patient could predict which nights were associated with middle of the night awakening, use of a longer-acting medication at bedtime might also be appropriate.

6. **C.** Zolpidem is the BZRA most associated with sleep-walking, sleep violence, and the sleep-related eating disorder. However, all BZRAs could be associated with these problems.

7. **C.** Paradoxical insomnia is associated with extreme reduction in reported sleep times but relatively little daytime impairment relative to the reported sleep loss. The subjective amount of sleep loss always far exceeds objective determination (PSG or actigraph)

8. **C.** BZRA binding alone is not sufficient to open the pore. Rather, BZRA binding enhances the ability of

GABA binding to open the pore. BZRAs are GABA$_A$ receptor modulators (enhancers).

9. B.

10. C. Studies have not shown advantage to combining hypnotic treatment with CBTI.

11. B.

12. A. Patients may respond differently to different BZRAs. Because zolpidem CR was tolerated, using another intermediate-acting BZRA is a reasonable next step. Eszopiclone (has a longer duration of action than zolpidem CR in some patients) or temazepam are options. Trazodone might work but there is less evidence for efficacy than other BZRAs. The addition of trazodone to zolpidem CR is another option. Quetiapine is an antipsychotic with many side effects. Ramelteon and zaleplon would not be appropriate for sleep-maintenance insomnia.

13. D. The duration must be less than 3 months. Adjustment insomnia is associated with an identifiable stressor and would meet the definition of insomnia only if present for at least 1 month.

14. D. Although all the above behavioral treatments could potentially be helpful, SRT is the one most suggested by the sleep log (see Fig. 25-10). The patient stays in bed almost 12 hours most days. By shortening the time in bed, hopefully the sleep efficiency will increase.

REFERENCES

1. American Academy of Sleep Medicine: ICSD-2 International Classification of Sleep Disorders, 2nd ed. Diagnostic and Coding Manual. Westchester, IL: American Academy of Sleep Medicine, 2005.
2. Ancoli-Israel S, Roth T: Characteristics of insomnia in the United States: results of the 1991 National Sleep Foundation Survey. Sleep 1999;22:S347–S353.
3. Ohayon MM: Epidemiology of insomnia: what we know and what we still need to learn. Sleep Med Rev 2002;6:97–111.
4. Summers MO, Crisostomo MI, Stepanski EJ: Recent developments in the classification, evaluation, and treatment of insomnia. Chest 2006;130:276–286.
5. Mai E, Buysee D: Insomnia, prevalence, impact, pathogenesis, differential diagnosis and evaluation. Sleep Med Clin 2008; 3:167–174.
6. American Psychiatric Association: Diagnostic and Statistical Manual of Mental Disorders, 4th ed. DSM-IV. Washington, DC: American Psychiatric Association, 1994.
7. Schutte-Rodin S, Broch L, Buysee D, et al: Clinical guideline for the evaluation and management of chronic insomnia in adults. J Clin Sleep Med 2008;4:487–504.
8. Sateia MJ, Doghramji K, Hauri P, Morin CM: Evaluation of chronic insomnia. Sleep 2000;23:1–36.
9. Chesson A, Hartse K, McDowell Anderson W, et al: Practice parameters for the evaluation of chronic insomnia. Sleep 2000; 23:1–5.
10. Littner M, Hirshkowitz M, Kramer M, Standards of Practice Committee of the American Academy of Sleep Medicine:

11. Agnew HW, Webb WB, Williams RL: The first night effect: an EEG study. Psychophysiology 1966;2:263–266.
12. Nuckton TJ, Glidden DV, Browner WS, Claman DM: Physical examination: Mallampati as an independent predictor of obstructive sleep apnea. Sleep 2006;29:903–908.
13. Johns MW: Sleepiness in different situations measured by the Epworth Sleepiness Scale. Sleep 1994;17:703–710.
14. Buysee DJ, Reynolds CF, Monk TH, et al: Quantification of subjective sleep quality in healthy elderly men and women using the Pittsburgh Sleep Quality Index (PSQI). Sleep 1991; 14:331–338.
15. Buysse DJ, Reynolds CF, Monk TH, et al: The Pittsburgh Sleep Quality Index: a new instrument for psychiatric practice and research. Psychiatry Res 1989;28:193–213.
16. Beck AT, Steer RA, Brown GK: Manual for the Beck Depression Inventory, 2nd ed. (BDI-II). San Antonio, TX: The Psychological Association, 1996.
17. Beck AT, Ward CH, Mendelson M, et al: An inventory for measuring depression. Arch Gen Psychiatry 1961;4:561–571.
18. Carney CE, Ulmer C, Edinger JD, et al: Assessing depression symptoms in those with insomnia: an examination of the Beck Depression Inventory, 2nd ed (BDI-II). J Psychiatr Res 2009; 43:576–582.
19. Morin CM: Dysfunctional beliefs and attitudes about sleep. Preliminary scale development and description. Behav Ther 1994;Summer:163–164.
20. Morin CM, Vallières A, Ivers H: Dysfunctional beliefs and attitudes about sleep (DBAS): validation of a brief version (DBAS-16). Sleep 2007;30:1547–1554.
21. Hauri PJ, Wisbey J: Wrist actigraphy in insomnia. Sleep 1992;15:293–301.
22. Ancoli-Israel S, Cole R, Alessi C, et al: The role of actigraphy in the study of sleep and circadian rhythms. Sleep 2003; 26:342–392.
23. Littner M, Kushida CA, McDowell Anderson W, et al: Practice parameters for the role of actigraphy in the study of sleep and circadian rhythms: an update for 2002. Sleep 2003; 26:337–341.
24. Vallières A, Morin CM: Actigraphy in the assessment of insomnia. Sleep 2003;26:902–906.
25. Sivertsen B, Omvik S, Havik OE, et al: A comparison of actigraphy and polysomnography in older adults treated for chronic primary insomnia. Sleep 2006;29:1353–1358.
26. Lichstenin KL, Stone KC, Donaldson J, et al: Actigraphy validation with insomnia. Sleep 2006;29:232–239.
27. Kushida C, Chang A, Gadkary C, et al: Comparison of actigraphic, polysomnographic, and subjective assessment of sleep parameters in sleep-disordered patients. Sleep Med 2001;2:389–396.
28. Hedner J, Pillar G, Pittman SD, et al: A novel adaptive wrist actigraphy algorithm for sleep-wake assessment in sleep apnea patients. Sleep 2004;27:1560–1566.
29. Morgenthaler T, Alessi C, Friedman L, et al: Practice parameters for the use of actigraphy in the assessment of sleep and sleep disorders: an update for 2007. Sleep 2007;30:519–529.
30. Bonnet MH, Arand DL: Hyperarousal and insomnia: state of the science. Sleep Med Rev 2010;14:9–15.
31. Nofzinger EA, Buysse DJ, Germain A, et al: Functional neuroimaging evidence for hyperarousal in insomnia. Am J Psychiatry 2004;161:2126–2129.
32. Winkleman JW, Buxton OM, Jensen JE, et al: Reduced brain GABA in primary insomnia: preliminary data from 4T proton magnetic resonance spectroscopy (1H-MRS). Sleep 2008;31: 1499–1506.
33. Morgenthaler TI, Owens J, Alessi C, et al: Practice parameters for behavioral treatment of bedtime problems and night

wakenings in infants and young children. Sleep 2006;29:
1277–1281.

34. Mindell JA, Kuhn B, Lewin DS, et al: Behavioral treatment of
bedtime problems and night wakings in infants and young
children. An American Academy of Sleep Medicine Review.
Sleep 2006;29:1263–1276.

35. Roehrs T, Roth T: Caffeine: sleep and daytime sleepiness. Sleep
Med Rev 2008;12:153–162.

36. Landholt HP, Roth C, Dijik DJ, Borberly AA: Late afternoon
alcohol intake affects nocturnal sleep and the sleep EEG in
middle aged men. J Clin Psychopharmacol 1996;16:428–436.

37. Schweitzer PK: Drugs that disturb sleep and wakefulness. In
Kryger MH, Roth T, Dement WC (eds): Principles and Practice
of Sleep Medicine, 4th ed. Philadelphia: Elsevier Saunders,
2005, pp. 495–518.

38. Gillin JC, Smith TL, Irwoin M, et al: Increased pressure for
rapid eye movement sleep at time of hospital admission
predicts relapse in non-depressed patients with primary alcoholism at 3 month follow-up. Arch Gen Psychiatry 1994;51:
189–197.

39. Brower KJ, Aldrich MS, Hall JM: Polysomnographic and subjective sleep predictors of alcoholic relapse. Alcohol Clin Exp
Res 1998;22:1864–1871.

40. Riemann D, Perlis ML: The treatments of chronic insomnia:
a review of benzodiazepine receptor agonists and psychological and behavioral therapies. Sleep Med Rev 2009;13:
205–214.

41. Morin CM, Hauri PK, Espie CA, et al: Nonpharmacologic
treatment of chronic insomnia. Sleep 1999;22:1134–1156.

42. Chesson AL, McDowell Anderson W, Litter M, et al: Practice
parameters for the nonpharmacologic treatment of chronic
insomnia. Sleep 1999;22:1128–1133.

43. Morin CM, Bootzin RR, Buysee D, et al: Psychological and
behavioral treatment of insomnia: update of recent evidence
(1998–2004). Sleep 2006;29:1398–1414.

44. Morgenthaler T, Kramer M, Alessi C, et al: Practice parameters
for the psychological and behavioral treatment of insomnia: an
update. Sleep 2006;29:1415–1419.

45. Bootzin RR, Epstein D, Wood JM: Stimulus control instructions. In Hauri P (ed): Case Studies in Insomnia. New York:
Plenum, 1991, pp. 19–28.

46. Speilman AJ, Saskin P, Thorpy MJ: Treatment of chronic insomnia by restriction of time in bed. Sleep 1987;10:45–56.

47. Jacobs GD, Pace-Schott EF, Stickgold R, Otto MW: Cognitive
behavior therapy and pharmacotherapy for insomnia: a randomized controlled trial and direct comparison. Arch Intern
Med 2004;164:1888–1896.

48. Edinger JD, Wohlgemuth WK, Radtke RA, et al: Cognitive
behavioral therapy for treatment of chronic primary insomnia.
JAMA 2001;285:1856–1864.

49. Smith MT, Perlis ML, Park A, et al: Comparative meta-analysis
of pharmacotherapy and behavior therapy for persistent
insomnia. Am J Psychiatry 2002;159:5–11.

50. Morin CM, Colecchi C, Stone J, et al: Behavioral and pharmacological therapies for late life insomnia: a randomized controlled trial. JAMA 1999;281:991–999.

51. Morin CM, Bastein C, Guay B, et al: Randomized clinical trial
of supervised tapering and cognitive behavioral therapy to
facilitate benzodiazepine discontinuation in older adults with
chronic insomnia. Am J Psychiatry 2004;161:132–342.

52. Soeffing JP, Lichstein KL, Nau SD, et al: Psychological treatment of insomnia in hypnotic dependent older adults. Sleep
Med 2008;9:165–171.

53. Lichstein KL: Behavioral intervention for special insomnia
populations: hypnotic dependent insomnia and comorbid
insomnia. Sleep Med 2006;7(Suppl 1):S27–S31.

54. Mohler H, Fritschy JM, Rudolph U: A new benzodiazepine
pharmacology. J Pharmacol Exp Ther 2002;300:2–8.

55. Olsen RW, Sieghart W: GABA_A receptors: subtypes provide
diversity of function and pharmacology. Neuropharmacology
2009;56:141–148.

56. Nutt DJ, Stahl SM: Searching for perfect sleep: the continuing
evolution of GABA_A receptor modulators as hypnotics. J Psychopharmacol 2010;24:1601–1612.

57. Kopp C, Rudolph U, Low K, Tobler I: Modulation of rhythmic brain activity by diazepam: GABA_A receptor subtype
and state specificity. Proc Natl Acad Sci U S A 2004;101:
3674–3679.

58. Mitler MM: Non-selective and selective benzodiazepine receptor agonists—where are we today? Sleep 2000;23:S39–S47.

59. Ancoli-Israel S, Walsh JK, Mangano RM, et al: Zaleplon, a
novel nonbenzodiazepine hypnotic, effectively treats insomnia
in elderly patients without causing rebound effects. Prim Care
Companion J Clin Psychiatry 1999;1:114–120.

60. Danjou P, Paty I, Fruncillo R, et al: A comparison of the
residual effects of zaleplon and zolpidem following administration 5 to 2 hours before awakening. Br J Clin Pharmacol 1999;
48:367–374.

61. Zammit GK, Corser B, Doghramji K, et al: Sleep and residual
sedation after administration of zaleplon, zolpidem, and
placebo during experimental middle of the night awakening.
J Clin Sleep Med 2006;4:417–423.

62. Monti JM, Pandi-Perumal SR: Eszopiclone: its use in the
treatment of insomnia. Neuropsychiatr Dis Treat 2007;3:
441–453.

63. Krystal A, Walsh JK, Laska E, et al: Sustained efficacy of eszopiclone over 6 months of nightly treatment: results of a randomized, double-blind, placebo-controlled study in adults with
chronic insomnia. Sleep 2003;26:793–799.

64. Roth T, Walsh JK, Krystal A, et al: An evaluation of the efficacy
and safety of eszopiclone over 12 months in patients with
chronic primary insomnia. Sleep Med 2005;6:487–495.

65. Ancoli-Israel S, Krystal AD, McCall WV, et al: A 12 week,
randomized, double-blind, placebo-controlled study evaluating the effects of eszopiclone 2mg on sleep/wake function in
older adults with primary and comorbid insomnia. Sleep 2010;
33:225–234.

66. Krystal AK, Erman M, Zammit GK, et al: Long-term efficacy
and safety of zolpidem extended-release 12.5mg administered
3 to 7 nights per week for 24 weeks in patients with chronic
primary insomnia: a 6-month, randomized, double-blind,
placebo controlled parallel-group, multi-center study. Sleep
2008;31:79–90.

67. Walsh J, Roth T, Randazzo A, et al: Eight weeks of non-nightly
use of zolpidem for primary insomnia. Sleep 2000;28:1087–
1096.

68. Hajak G, Cluydts R, Declerck A, et al: Continuous versus
non-nightly use of zolpidem in chronic insomnia: results of a
large-double-blind, randomized, outpatient study. Int Clin Psychopharmacol 2002;17:9–17.

69. Roth T, Stubbs C, Walsh JK, et al: Ramelteon (TAK-375), a
selective MT1/MT2-receptor agonist, reduces latency to persistent sleep in a model of transient insomnia related to a novel
sleep environment. Sleep 2005;28:303–307.

70. Erman M, Seiden D, Zammit G, et al: An efficacy, safety, and
dose-response study of ramelteon in patients with chronic
primary insomnia. Sleep Med 2006;7:17–24.

71. Mayer G, Wang-Weigand S, Roth-Schechter B, et al: Efficacy
and safety of 6 month nightly ramelteon administration in
adults with chronic primary insomnia. Sleep 2009;32:351–360.

72. Zammit G, Erman M, Wang-Weigand S, et al: Evaluation of the
efficacy and safety of ramelteon in subjects with chronic insomnia. J Clin Sleep Med 2007;3:495–504.

73. Mendelson W: A review of the evidence for the efficacy and
safety of trazodone in insomnia. J Clin Psychiatry 2005;66:
469–476.

74. Walsh J, Erman M, Erwin CW, et al: Subjective hypnotic efficacy of trazodone and zolpidem in DSMIII-R primary insomnia. Hum Psychopharmacol 1998;13:191–198.

75. Kaynak H, Kaynak D, Gözükirmizi E, et al: The effects of trazodone on sleep in patients treated with stimulant antidepressants. Sleep Med 2004;5:15–20.

76. Nierenberg AA, Adler LA, Peselow E, et al: Trazodone for antidepressant associated insomnia. Am J Psychiatry 1993;151:1069–1072.

77. Winkour A, DeMartins NA, McNally DP, et al: Comparative effects of mirtazapine and fluoxetine on sleep physiology measures in patients with major depression and insomnia. J Clin Psychiatry 2003;64:1224–1229.

78. Roth T, Rogowski R, Hull S, et al: Efficacy and safety of doxepin 1 mg, 3 mg, and 6 mg in adults with primary insomnia. Sleep 2007;30:1555–1561.

79. Brzezinski A, Vangel MG, Wurtman RJ, et al: Effects of exogenous melatonin on sleep. A meta analysis. Sleep Med Rev 2005;9:41–50.

80. Morin CM, Koetter U, Bastien C, et al: Valerian-hops combination and diphenhydramine for treating insomnia: a randomized placebo controlled clinical trial. Sleep 2005;28:1465–1471.

81. Fava M, McCall V, Krystal A, et al: Eszopiclone co-administered with fluoxetine in patients with insomnia coexisting with major depressive disorder. Biol Psychiatry 2006;59:1052–1060.

82. Fava M, Asnis G, Shrivastava R, et al: Zolpidem extended release 12.5 mg co-administered with escitalopram, improves insomnia in patients with comorbid insomnia and major depressive disorder improved insomnia symptoms and next day function in patients with co-morbid disorder. Presented at the American Psychiatric Association 161st Annual Meeting, Washington, DC, 2008.

83. Fava M, Asnis GM, Shrivastava R, et al: Zolpidem extended release improves sleep and next-day symptoms in comorbid insomnia and generalized anxiety disorder. J Clin Psychopharmacol 2009;29:222–230.

Dysfunctional Beliefs and Attitudes about Sleep Worksheet

The DBAS is administered by asking patients to endorse each statement using a Likert scale (0 – 1 – 2 – 3 – 4 – 5 – 6 – 7 – 8 – 9 –10) with 0 = strongly disagree and 10 = strongly agree.

From Morin CM; Vallières A; Ivers H: Dysfunctional Beliefs and Attitudes about Sleep (DBAS): validation of a brief version (DBAS-16). Sleep 2007;30:1547–1554.

DYSFUNCTIONAL BELIEFS AND ATTITUDES ABOUT SLEEP (DBAS)

Name: _____ Date: _____

Several statements reflecting people's beliefs and attitudes about sleep are listed below. Please indicate to what extent you personally agree or disagree with each statement. There is no right or wrong answer. For each statement, circle the number that corresponds to your own **personal belief**. Please respond to all items even though some may not apply directly to your own situation.

Strongly disagree ⟶ Strongly agree

0 1 2 3 4 5 6 ⑦ 8 9 10

1. I need 8 hours of sleep to feel refreshed and function well during the day.

0 1 2 3 4 5 6 7 8 9 10

2. When I don't get proper amount of sleep on a given night, I need to catch up on the next day by napping or on the next night by sleeping longer.

0 1 2 3 4 5 6 7 8 9 10

3. I am concerned that chronic insomnia may have serious consequences on my physical health.

0 1 2 3 4 5 6 7 8 9 10

4. I am worried that I may lose control over my abilities to sleep.

0 1 2 3 4 5 6 7 8 9 10

5. After a poor night's sleep, I know that it will interfere with my daily activities on the next day.

0 1 2 3 4 5 6 7 8 9 10

6. In order to be alert and function well during the day, I believe I would be better off taking a sleeping pill rather than having a poor night's sleep.

0 1 2 3 4 5 6 7 8 9 10

7. When I feel irritable, depressed, or anxious during the day, it is mostly because I did not sleep well the night before.

0 1 2 3 4 5 6 7 8 9 10

8. When I sleep poorly on one night, I know it will disturb my sleep schedule for the whole week.

0 1 2 3 4 5 6 7 8 9 10

9. Without an adequate night's sleep, I can hardly function the next day.

0 1 2 3 4 5 6 7 8 9 10

10. I can't ever predict whether I'll have a good or poor night's sleep.

0 1 2 3 4 5 6 7 8 9 10

11. I have little ability to manage the negative consequences of disturbed sleep.

0 1 2 3 4 5 6 7 8 9 10

12. When I feel tired, have no energy, or just seem not to function well during the day, it is generally because I did not sleep well the night before.

0 1 2 3 4 5 6 7 8 9 10

13. I believe insomnia is essentially the result of a chemical imbalance.

0 1 2 3 4 5 6 7 8 9 10

14. I feel insomnia is ruining my ability to enjoy life and prevents me from doing what I want.

0 1 2 3 4 5 6 7 8 9 10

15. Medication is probably the only solution to sleeplessness.

0 1 2 3 4 5 6 7 8 9 10

16. I avoid or cancel obligations (social, family) after a poor night's sleep.

0 1 2 3 4 5 6 7 8 9 10

Chapter 26

Circadian Rhythm Sleep Disorders

Chapter Points

- In humans, the normal circadian period (tau) is **approximately 24.2 hours** (mean value). Because the period is slightly longer than 24 hours, this requires a slight phase advance daily to maintain entrainment with the light-dark cycle.
- The major circadian pacemaker in humans is the SCN. The SCN is entrained to the light-dark cycle via light stimulation of retinal melanopsin-containing pRGCs. The ganglion cells communicate via the RHT to the SCN. Blue light has the most potent effect.
- The alerting signal from the SCN increases during the day to counter the increasing homeostatic sleep drive (accumulated wake since the last sleep). The alerting signal falls during sleep and the homeostatic sleep drive also falls.
- Melatonin is secreted in darkness by the pineal gland. Light inhibits melatonin secretion by decreasing the activating influences of neurons in the PVH nucleus. The neural pathway from the PVH neurons to the pineal gland is circuitous passing through the spinal cord and superior cervical ganglion (see Fig. 26–2). Melatonin binds to receptors on the SCN and decreases the alerting signal during darkness (promoting sleep).
- The CBTmin occurs about 2 hours before the habitual wake time.
- DLMO is the time that serum melatonin starts to increase above daytime levels under dim light conditions and occurs about 2 to 3 hours before bedtime or 7 hours before CBTmin.
- CBTmin and DLMO can be used as markers of circadian phase. When the circadian rhythm of the body (CBTmin or DLMO) moves to a later clock time, this is said to represent a **phase delay** in circadian rhythms and to an early time **phase advance.**
- Light after the CBTmin induces a phase advance and light before the CBTmin induces a phase delay.
- Melatonin administered before the CBTmin induces a phase advance. Melatonin given after the CBTmin induces a phase delay.

- Bright light "pushes" and melatonin "pulls" on the circadian phase (CBTmin)
- The DSPD is characterized by a delay in sleep period relative to clock time, characterized by late sleep onset and late natural awakening. The DSPD is the most common CRSD seen in sleep clinics and presents as sleep-onset insomnia. If undisturbed by social obligations, patients with DSPD have good sleep maintenance and awaken feeling refreshed.
- Treatments for the DSPD include bright light at or slightly before the natural (unrestricted) wake time (timed to follow CBTmin) or melatonin 5 to 7 hours before habitual sleep-onset time. Both melatonin and light can be used. The patient attempts to go to bed about ½ hour earlier each night and the timing of application of melatonin and light is changed to maintain the initial relationship.
- The ASPD is characterized by an advance in the sleep period relative to clock time characterized by early sleep onset and early awakening. It occurs most commonly in elderly individuals.
- The CRSD-FRT is characterized by a progressive phase delay of 1 to 2 hours per day. It is most common in blind individuals but can occur in sighted individuals and has been described after head trauma.
- The treatment for nonsighted patients with the CRSD-FRT is melatonin given about 1 hour before the desired bedtime. In some studies, a lower dose was more effective than a large dose.
- The ISWR is characterized by at least three different periods of sleep during 24 hours (usually normal total sleep time). This CRSD is most common in elderly patients in nursing homes or institutionalized severely mentally impaired young patients. Treatments include bright light during the day, structured daily activities, and decreased noise and light at night. Melatonin at night is recommended for younger patients with mental retardation but not for elderly nursing home patients.

- Approximately 10% of patients working a night shift have complaints of difficulty staying awake at night or sleeping during the day that are severe enough to be considered an SWD.
- Treatment for night shift workers includes scheduled naps before the shift, bright light during the start of the shift, stimulants (caffeine or modafinil) at the start of the shift, dark glasses on the drive home (if after sunrise), and melatonin or hypnotics before the daytime sleep period. The major sleep period should occur soon after arriving home from work. The sleep environment should be as quiet and dark as possible.
- Jet lag is characterized by a misalignment between endogenous circadian rhythms and local time caused by **rapid travel across at least two time zones.** Eastward travel requires adaptation by a phase advance and adaptation is more difficult than westward travel. Westward travel requires adaptation by a phase delay and adaptation is easier because of the intrinsic tendency for phase delay. Trying to avoid light at times inducing the wrong phase shift and receiving light exposure at correct times inducing the desired phase shift at the new destination are recommended. Melatonin before the desired sleep period or hypnotics may be helpful. Most individuals require about 1 day of adaptation for each time zone crossed.

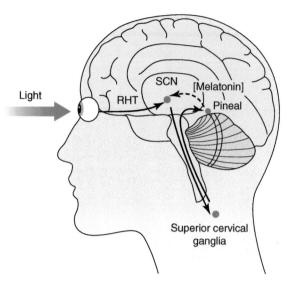

FIGURE 26–1 Light information travels via the retinohypothalamic tract (RHT) to the suprachiasmatic nucleus (SCN). The SCN then signals the pineal via a complex neural pathway passing through the superior cervical ganglion and inhibits melatonin production. In the absence of light (during dark), the inhibition is removed and the pineal secretes melatonin. The melatonin then acts on the SCN to decrease the alerting signal. *From Reid KJ, Zee PC: Circadian rhythm disorders. Semin Neurol 2009;29: 393–405.*

The word *circadian* means "about a day" and describes processes that vary over time with approximately a 24-hour period. In humans, many physiologic processes vary periodically on a nearly 24-hour schedule.[1,2] The major circadian pacemaker in mammals is the suprachiasmatic nucleus (SCN) in the anterior hypothalamus. The nucleus exists as paired structures on each side of the third ventricle above the optic chiasm.[2-4] The SCN contains cells that oscillate independently with a period slightly longer than 24 hours. The SCN controls the rhythms of core body temperature and sleep-wake propensity as well as the secretion of certain hormones (melatonin and cortisol). The period of the rhythm is called *tau* and the **mean value in humans is about 24.2 hours**.[3] Some individuals have a slightly shorter tau and some longer. For humans to maintain synchrony with the light-dark cycle, external stimuli must induce a slight daily advance (shift in circadian rhythms to an earlier clock time) to counteract the intrinsic tendency for phase delay due to a period slightly longer than 24 hours. These external stimuli called *zeitgebers* ("time givers") are said to "entrain" the SCN to the light-dark cycle.

The most potent zeitgeber is non–visual light information. Other zeitgebers include exercise, food, and social activities. The light stimulus reaches the SCN via the retinohypothalamic tract (RHT) (Fig. 26–1). The RHT is a monosynaptic pathway connecting the melanopsin-containing photosensitive retinal ganglion cells (pRGCs) to the SCN.

Nonvisual photoreception also mediates the pupillary light response. Some blind patients continue to be entrained by light due to residual function of the retinal ganglion cells. Whereas the ganglion cells are the major circadian photosensors, the rods and cones also contribute some nonvisual information via communication with the pRGCs.[4,5] The **shorter wavelengths of light (blue)** have the **greatest effect on circadian rhythms**. The primary neurotransmitter of the retinal ganglion cell neurons in the RHT is **glutamate.** However, the neurons also release pituitary adenyl cyclase–activating peptide (PACP) as a co-transmitter that causes similar effects on the SCN neurons. The effects of glutamate are mediated by binding to N-methyl-D-aspartate (NMDA)-type glutamate receptors and the subsequent elevations of intracellular calcium and nitric oxide in the neurons of the SCN. PACP-containing fibers from the retinal ganglion cells also project to the intergeniculate leaflet (IGL), which in turn, project to the SCN. Neurons in the IGL use gamma-aminobutyric acid (GABA) and neuropeptide Y as co-transmitters. Neurons in the IGL may mediate some of the phase-shifting influences of exercise on the SCN. As is discussed later, the intensity, the duration, and the timing of light exposure determine the effect of light on the circadian system.

MELATONIN

The pineal gland secretes a hormone called *melatonin* during the dark cycle.[4-11] In the absence of light, certain dorsal parvocellular neurons in the autonomic subdivision of the paraventricular hypothalamic nucleus (PVH) provide tonic stimulation to the pineal gland via a circuitous pathway[4-7]

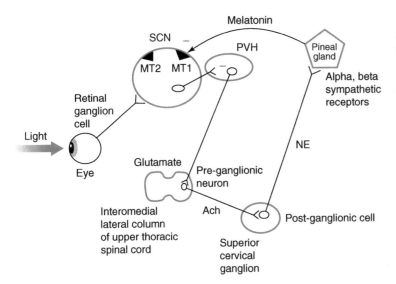

FIGURE 26–2 The suprachiasmatic nucleus (SCN) inhibits melatonin secretion by the pineal via a complicated neural pathway. In the absence of light, dorsal parvocellular neurons in the autonomic subdivision of the paraventricular hypothalamus (PVH) send a tonic signal (glutamate) stimulating preganglionic sympathetic neurons in the thoracic spinal cord that then project to the superior cervical ganglion and stimulate postganglionic neurons. These noradrenergic neurons innervate the pineal gland. Norepinephrine (NE) acting at alpha and beta receptors on the pineal gland results in production and secretion of melatonin. A subset of SCN neurons project directly to the PVH neurons at the origin of the pathway providing stimulation to the pineal gland. When light is present, the SCN inhibits the PVH neurons. In the absence of inhibition (by light), melatonin is produced and secreted by the pineal gland. Ach = acetylcholine; MT = melatonin.

(Fig. 26–2). These PVH glutaminergic neurons project to sympathetic preganglionic neurons in the intermediolateral cell column (IML) of the upper thoracic spinal cord. The preganglionic sympathetic neurons provide a cholinergic projection to postganglionic neurons located in the superior cervical ganglion. The postganglionic neurons are noradrenergic and project to the pineal gland. The release of norepinephrine stimulates the pineal gland via alpha and beta receptors (mainly beta 1). Noradrenergic stimulation on the pineal gland results in increased cyclic adenosine monophosphate (AMP) in the pinealocytes and this induces expression of serotonin N-acetyltransferase (also known as arylalkylamine N-acetyltransferase [AA-NAT]). This enzyme catalyzes the rate-limiting step in the synthesis of melatonin. Therefore, the amount of this enzyme controls the production of melatonin.

In the presence of light, some neurons of the SCN directly inhibit those neurons in the PVH that are responsible for stimulating the pineal gland to secrete melatonin. Thus, light inhibits melatonin secretion and the absence of inhibition (absence of light) allows secretion of melatonin. Melatonin is sometimes called the *dark hormone*. The melatonin secreted by the pineal gland provides inhibitory feedback information to SCN neurons. Therefore, the SCN and pineal gland are mutually inhibitory. Important facts about human circadian rhythms are summarized in Box 26–1.

Melatonin is not essential for circadian rhythms in humans because removal of the pineal gland has minimal effects. In other species such as birds, the pineal gland is essential. The SCN has a high density of two types of melatonin receptors (MT1 and MT2). The MT1 receptor is a G protein–coupled receptor that activates protein kinase C. When melatonin binds the MT1 receptor on SCN neurons, this decreases SCN-alerting signal. The MT2 receptor is a G protein–coupled receptor that inhibits the guanine cyclase pathway and results in a shift in circadian phase. A third type of melatonin receptor (MT3) does not affect the pineal gland. Exogenous melatonin by oral administration can also affect

BOX 26–1

Circadian Physiology—Important Facts

- Circadian ("about a day") denotes processes with approximately a 24-hr period.
- The human period of circadian rhythms (tau) is about 24.2 hr.
- SCN is the major circadian pacemaker in humans.
- SCN function helps maintain alertness by producing an alerting signal during the day and maintaining sleep by a reduced signal at night.
- Usual human alertness:
  - Early afternoon decrease in alertness 2–4 PM.
  - Alertness peaks in the early evening hours.
  - Lowest levels of alertness occur from 4–6 AM.
- Zeitgebers (time givers) entrain the SCN to the physical environment.
- Light (sunlight) is the major zeitgeber.
- Melanopsin-containing retinal ganglion cells are the major circadian photoreceptors and communicate the presence of light to the SCN via the RHT.

RHT = retinohypothalamic tract; SCN = suprachiasmatic nucleus.

the SCN. The half-life of exogenous melatonin is short (30–45 min) unless sustained-release melatonin preparations are used. As might be expected, the effects of exogenous melatonin are largest when no endogenous melatonin is being secreted.[8] Exogenous melatonin can decrease the SCN-alerting signal (hypnotic effects) and cause a phase shift of circadian rhythms (discussed in a later section). Melatonin acting on blood vessels in the skin causes vasodilatation and increased blood flow results in heat loss and lowering of the body temperature.

THE SCN AND SLEEP-WAKE CYCLE

The SCN helps maintain alertness by producing an alerting signal during the day and helps maintains sleep by producing

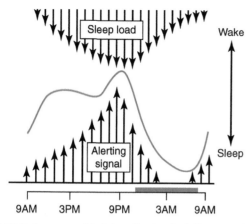

FIGURE 26–3 Opponent model of sleep. The sleep load *(down arrows)* increases proportional to the amount of prior wake and decreases with sleep onset. It is opposed by the alerting signal from the SCN *(up arrows)*. The alerting signal increases to a maximum just before sleep onset to help maintain wakefulness (the forbidden sleep period) but then decreases during the sleep period so that sleep can occur. The *solid line* is the wake-sleep propensity. Note a small dip in the afternoon. *Adapted from Edgar DM, Dement WC, Fuller CA: Effect of SCN lesions on sleep in the squirrel monkey: evidence for opponent processes in sleep-wake regulation. J Neuorsci 1993;13:1065–1079.*

TABLE 26–1		
Sleep-Wake Regulation		
Nighttime sleep	First part of night	• Homeostatic drive is high (from awake all day).
		• Circadian alerting signal is low.
	Second part of night	• Homeostatic drive is lower.
		• Circadian alerting signal is low.
Daytime wakefulness	First part of day	• Homeostatic drive is low (due to prior sleep).
		• Circadian drive is increasing.
	Second part of day	• Homeostatic drive is high and increasing (prior wake).
		• Circadian alerting signal is high (compensation).

BOX 26–2

Markers of Circadian Phase
• CBTmin occurs 2–3 hr before awakening from unconstrained sleep (4–5 AM)
• DLMO occurs ~2–3 hr before typical sleep onset
• CBTmin = DLMO + 7 (i.e., CBTmin occurs about 7 hr later than DLMO)
CBTmin = core body temperature minimum; DLMO = dim light melatonin onset.

a reduced signal at night. The other major influence on sleep propensity is the amount of accumulated wakefulness (time since the last sleep). This **homeostatic process** (sleep load) builds during wakefulness and then falls during sleep. As the pressure for sleep builds, the circadian signal increases to help maintain alertness despite a growing sleep debt but then decreases so that sleep can occur (Fig. 26–3). The two-process model considers the interaction of process S (homeostatic sleep drive) and process C (circadian rhythms, driven in large part by the SCN). The opponent model of sleep[2,9] (SCN-alerting signal vs. sleep load) is illustrated in Figure 26–3. Alertness peaks during the early evening hours. There is a midday decrease in alertness around 2 to 4 PM and the lowest alertness is 4 to 6 AM. The interaction of the opponent processes (homeostatic sleep load and circadian alerting signal) allows humans to be alert during the day and to sleep at night (Table 26–1). The secretion of melatonin at night exerts an inhibitory influence on the SCN that helps maintain sleep by reducing the alerting signal.

The pathways by which the alerting signal of the SCN regulates sleep-wake are complex.[2,5] One of the major pathways is as follows. Neurons in the SCN project to neurons in the ventral subparaventricular zone (vSPZ). This area is immediately dorsal to the SCN. Neurons in the vSPZ then project to the dorsal medial hypothalamus (DMH). Gluta-minergic neurons in the DMH project to the lateral hypo-thalamus neurons producing hypocretin (stabilizing wake-to-sleep transitions). In addition, DMH neurons using GABA as an inhibitory neurotransmitter project to the ven-trolateral preoptic area (VLPO), a sleep-promoting area. These pathways mediate some of the effect of the SCN-alerting signal by inhibiting sleep-promoting areas and stim-ulating areas stabilizing transitions from wake to sleep.

MARKERS OF CIRCADIAN PHASE

The minimum of the core body temperature (CBTmin) and the dim light melatonin onset (DLMO) are two useful markers of the position of an individual's circadian rhythms with respect to the external environment (i.e., time of day) (Box 26–2). The CBTmin occurs about 2 hours before **spontaneous awakening** from nocturnal sleep (4–5 AM in most individuals) (Fig. 26–4).[10–12] The reduction in core body temperature during the sleep period corresponds to the elevation in plasma melatonin. The wakefulness in sleep episode is an estimate of the wake propensity and is maximum in the evening before the sleep period and falls during sleep.

The DLMO occurs about 2 to 3 hours before typical bedtime.[10–15] One can estimate the timing of the **CBTmin** as **DLMO + 7 hours** (see Box 26–2). The DLMO is determined by interval measurement of salivary or plasma melatonin performed in dim light (5 lux; because light inhibits melato-nin secretion) in the evening. A rise in melatonin levels detects the DLMO time (Fig. 26–5). The **melatonin mid-point** can also be used as a circadian marker and occurs about 2 hours before CBTmin. When the circadian rhythm of the body (CBTmin or DLMO) moves to a later clock time, this is said to represent a **phase delay** in circadian rhythms and to an early time **phase advance**. The relationship between the timing of sleep and the circadian phase (as estimated by

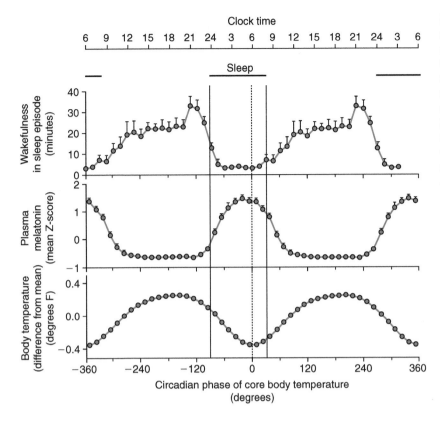

FIGURE 26–4 Schematic representation of the sleep period of a young adult. The minimum of core body temperature (depicted as the *vertical dotted line*) occurs about 2 hours before the end of the sleep period. The core body temperature minimum (CBTmin) also occurs about 1 to 2 hours after the midpoint of melatonin secretion. The amount of wakefulness in sleep (a measure of wake propensity) increases (sleep forbidden zone) just before the sleep period but falls with the onset of melatonin secretion. *From Duffy JF, Dijk DJ, Klerman EB, Czeisler CA: Later endogenous circadian temperature nadir relative to an earlier wake time in older people. Am J Physiol 1998; 275:R1478–R1487.*

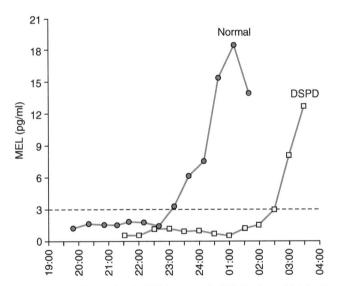

FIGURE 26–5 Salivary melatonin (MEL) for a normal individual and one with delayed sleep phase disorder (DSPD). The dim light melatonin onset (DLMO) is taken as the time at which melatonin reaches 3 pg/mL. This is around 23:00 in the normal individual but is delayed to around 02:30 in the morning in an individual with DSPD. *From Wyatt JK, Stepanski EJ, Kirkby J: Circadian phase in delayed sleep phase syndrome: predictors and temporal stability across multiple assessments. Sleep 2006;29:1075–1080.*

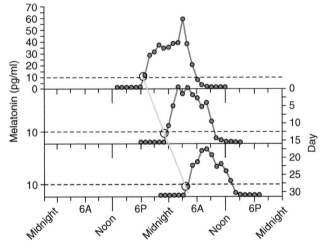

FIGURE 26–6 Melatonin secretion is shown for a patient whose DLMO *(large circles)* occurs progressively later (free-running type of circadian rhythm sleep disorder). *Reproduced from Sack RK, Brandes RW, Kendall AR, Lewy AJ: Entrainment of free-running circadian rhythms by melatonin in blind people. N Engl J Med 2000;343:1070–1077.*

a circadian marker) can be quantified by the time interval (phase angle) between the two rhythms. In Figure 26–6, the progressive delay in the DLMO is evidence of a progressive delay in circadian rhythm in a patient with the circadian rhythm sleep disorder—free-running type (CRSD-FRT), also called the free-running disorder (FRD).[14]

Use of the core body temperature as a marker of circadian rhythms is complicated by the fact that eating, activity, and sleep can affect the timing of CBTmin. In research settings, a constant routine protocol is utilized in which the subject is kept awake at bedrest and fed equally distributed small meals for at least 24 hours. An alternative to the constant routine protocol is to use mathematical adjustments to the temperature rhythm. The DLMO can be affected (masked) by posture and drugs such as beta blockers and caffeine. One can

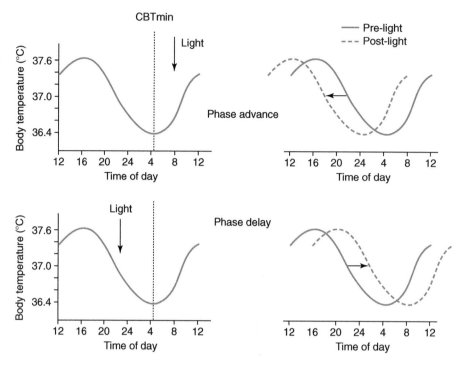

FIGURE 26–7 Phase shifting of the core body temperature minimum (CBTmin) with light. Light after the CBTmin phase advances and light before CBTmin phase delays. *From Berry RB: Sleep Medicine Pearls, 2nd ed. Philadelphia: Hanley & Belfus, 2003, p. 344.*

monitor plasma melatonin (threshold > 10 pg/mL), salivary melatonin (>3 pg/mL), or urinary melatonin metabolite (6-sulfatoxymelatonin [aMT6s]) (see Fig. 26–6).

SHIFTING THE CIRCADIAN RHYTHMS

Phase Shifting by Light

Exposure to light before the CBTmin causes a phase delay and light exposure after the CBTmin causes a phase advance (Fig. 26–7) in circadian rhythm.[15–18] Thus, normal light exposure during the early morning induces a daily phase advance in the circadian rhythms to compensate for the intrinsic tendency to phase delay because tau is slightly longer than 24 hours. The amount of circadian rhythm shifting (also called *phase change)* depends on the timing of light as well as the intensity and duration of light (Box 26–3). In addition, the effect depends on the previous exposure to light.[15–18] For example, a low intensity of light may cause significant shifting of the circadian rhythms in a patient staying in a dark room for several days. Light intensity is measured in lux. Indoor light is typically around 250 lux and outdoor bright light has an intensity over 100,000 lux. For humans exposed to outside light daily (>10,000 lux) for a portion of each day, a relatively high light intensity is needed to shift circadian rhythms. Outside daylight is much more effective at shifting the circadian phase than indoor light. When outdoor light exposure is not practical or possible, light boxes are available (2500 lux) for therapeutic phase shifting by light. One study of subjects kept in a dimly lighted environment found that increasing light intensity above 550 lux added relatively little to the phase shifting ability of light or the ability to suppress melatonin.[19,20] A sigmoid-shaped relationship was noted (Fig. 26–8). However, for

BOX 26–3

Phase Shifting with Light
COMMON LIGHT EXPOSURES
• Bright blue midday sky >100,000 lux
• Sunrise or sunset ~10,000
• Commercial light boxes up to 10,000
• Normal room light ~200
• Moonlight 0.1 lux
PHASE SHIFTING WITH LIGHT
• Short wavelength light (blue ~460 nm)—greatest effect
• Amount of phase shift depends on timing, intensity, and duration of light exposure
• Short pulses of light (intermittent) can also shift circadian rhythms
• Phase advance—light after CBTmin (~3–4 hr after CBTmin greatest effect)
• Phase delay—light before CBTmin (~3–4 hr before CBTmin greatest effect)
• Light in the middle of the day—relatively little effect
CBTmin = core body temperature minimum.

patients chronically exposed to much brighter light, a higher intensity of light would be needed for maximal effect. Natural light is composed of a spectrum from 380 nm (violet) to 760 (red). As noted previously, blue light (460 nm) has greater phase shifting properties than the rest of the visible light spectrum.[20] This may be due to the properties of the mela-nopsin pigment that has maximum absorbance in this range. Recently, light boxes have become available with enriched blue light to minimize the intensity or duration needed for

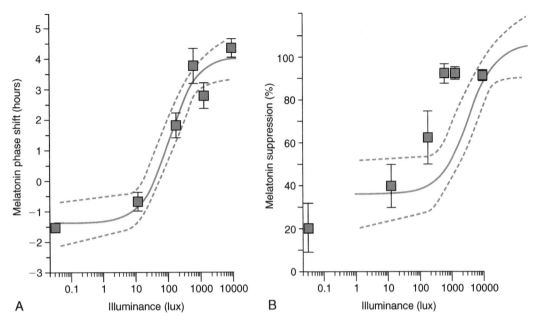

FIGURE 26–8 The amount of phase shifting of melatonin and melatonin suppression against illuminance. The relationship was determined by a subject kept in a controlled environment with dim light except for the light stimulus being tested. *From Zeitzer JM, Dijk DJ, Kronauer RE, et al: Sensitivity of human circadian pacemaker to nocturnal light: melatonin resetting and suppression. J Physiol 2000;526:695–702.*

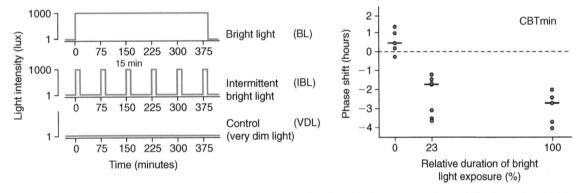

FIGURE 26–9 Intermittent exposure to bright light induces almost as much shift in the core body temperature minimum (CBTmin) as continuous bright light, although the duration of light exposure was about 23% of the time of continuous exposure. 0% light exposure = baseline; 23% light exposure = intermittent light exposure; 100% = continuous light exposure. *Adapted from Gronifer C, Wright KP, Kronauer RE, et al: Efficacy of a single sequence of intermittent bright light pulses for delaying circadian phase in humans. Am J Physiol Endocrinol Metab 2004:287:E174–E181.*

a therapeutic response to light therapy. However, a recent study showed no benefit of light enriched with blue light compared with white light.[21] It is possible that new light boxes with light-emitting diode (LED) emission of monochromatic blue light could be more effective. Intermittent as well as continuous light is also effective at resetting the circadian pacemaker[22,23] (Fig. 26–9). This fact has clinical implications for delivery light treatment when a patient cannot sit in front of a light box for long periods of time.

Phase-Response Curve for Light

The relationship between the timing of light exposure and the amount of phase shift is best presented using a phase response curve (PRC). The curves are constructed by plotting the amount of phase shift versus the timing of the light stimulus (constant stimulus intensity). By convention, the positive vertical axis represents phase advances and the negative axis phase delays. For light, the magnitude of phase shifting depends on the proximity to the CBTmin (Fig. 26–10). In most studies, the maximum phase shift occurs approximately 3 to 4 hours before (phase delay) or after (phase advance) the CBTmin (Fig. 26–11). Light in the middle of the day has minimal phase shifting effects.

Of note, the published PRCs for light vary somewhat depending on the methodology used to determine the PRC. For example, the PRC can be obtained by studying entrained subjects on a constant routine protocol or non-entrained subjects with a free-running routine. Typically, shifts in the DLMO are determined for different timing of light pulses.

PHASE RESPONSE CURVE TO LIGHT

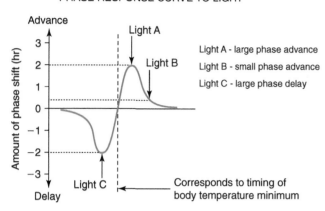

FIGURE 26–10 Schematic of the phase response curve (PRC) for light. The direction of the phase change depends on whether light is applied before or after CBTmin. The maximum phase advance (Light A) occurs about 3 to 4 hours after CBTmin. If light is applied 7 to 8 hours after CBTmin (Light B), the phase advance is much smaller. The maximum phase delay occurs 3 to 4 hours before the CBTmin. At midday to early evening, there is little effect of light on the circadian phase. (See also Fig. 26–11.)

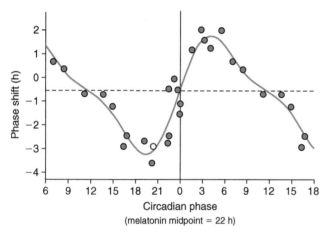

FIGURE 26–11 The PRC to bright light using melatonin midpoints as the circadian phase marker. The determination was made using a constant routine protocol (enforced wakefulness in a semirecumbent position). Phase advances are positive values and phase delays are negative values. They are plotted against the time of the melatonin midpoint (DLMOonset to DLMOoffset). The melatonin midpoint was defined to be 22 hours. The CBTmin is assumed to be 2 hours later (0 hr). The *horizontal dashed line* represents the assumed drift in circadian phase between prestimulus (prelight administration) and poststimulus phase assessments (~3 days). *From Khalsa SBS, Jewett ME, Cajocen C, Czeisler CA: A phase response curve to single bright light pulses in human subjects. J Physiol 2003;549:945–952.*

The phase shifts in circadian rhythms can also be determined by shifts in the CBTmin. However, as noted previously, exercise, food, and other activities can affect CBTmin. Shifts in the DLMO, especially if determined using a constant routine dim light protocol, are felt to more accurately assess the circadian phase than CBTmin.

Figure 26–11 illustrates a PRC for light. This was determined using a constant routine, and shifts in the midpoint

TABLE 26–2		
Phase Shifting with Melatonin and Hypnotic Effects		

- PRC approximately opposite to light PRC (12 hr out of phase).
- Reversal point (phase advance to phase delay) may be slightly before minimum of core body temperature but is always considerably after the DLMO.
- Dose-response curves may vary with dose (0.3 mg vs. 3 mg)
- Note at larger doses, hypnotic effects are noted.
- Exogenous melatonin half-life is about 30 to 45 minutes.
- Given closer to bedtime, melatonin may reduce SCN alerting signal (dampen wake maintenance zone)
- Maximal phase **advance** for different melatonin doses*

Dose	0.3–0.5 mg	3 mg
OPTIMAL TIMING		
Before DLMO	2–3 hr	5 hr
Before habitual sleep onset	4.5–5 hr	7.5 hr
Before CBTmin	9 hr	12 hr

- Maximal phase delay—about 10 hours after DLMO

*From Eastman CI, Burgess HJ: How to travel the world without jet lag. Sleep Med Clin 2009;4:241–255.
CBTmin = core body temperature minimum; DLMO = dim light melatonin onset; PRC = phase response curve; SCN = suprachiasmatic nucleus.

of melatonin secretion (melatonin midpoint) rather than DLMO were measured following a single pulse of light. Again, note that the biggest phase shifts occur when light is administered near the CBTmin.

Phase Shifting by Exogenous Melatonin

Relatively small doses of exogenous melatonin (0.3–0.5 mg) can shift the circadian phase (Table 26–2) if taken at the correct times. As might be expected, the phase shifting effects of exogenous melatonin are minimal during the dark period when the endogenous plasma level of melatonin is high.[24-26] Melatonin in higher doses (3–5 mg) has a direct hypnotic effect[8] as well as a chronobiotic effect. However, the hypnotic effects of melatonin are limited by the drug's short half-life and the fact that if taken at night, the endogenous plasma melatonin is already high.

Melatonin PRC Curve

The PRC curve for melatonin is roughly 12 hours opposite (out of phase) to the light PRC[24-26] (Fig. 26–12). In displays of the melatonin PRC, the timing of melatonin is often expressed relative to DLMO but can also be expressed relative to the estimated CBTmin. Melatonin when given in the early evening before the DLMO results in a phase advance. Melatonin given at the end of the subjective night–early subjective day causes a phase delay (see Fig. 26–12). As expected, the melatonin PRC has flat region (no phase shifting)

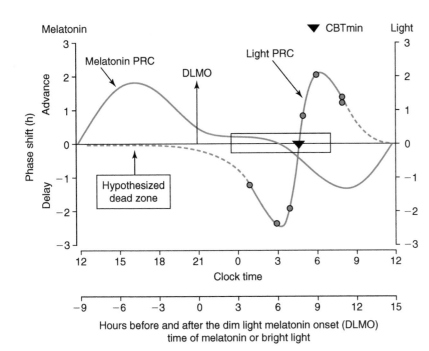

FIGURE 26-12 Phase response curves (PRCs) for light and melatonin (3 mg). The position of DLMO and the core body temperature minimum (CBTmin) are shown. The *rectangle* represents a period of 7.5 hours of sleep. The PRC curves of light and melatonin are approximately out of phase. *From Eastman CI, Burgess HJ: How to travel the world without jet lag. Sleep Med Clin 2009;4:241–255.*

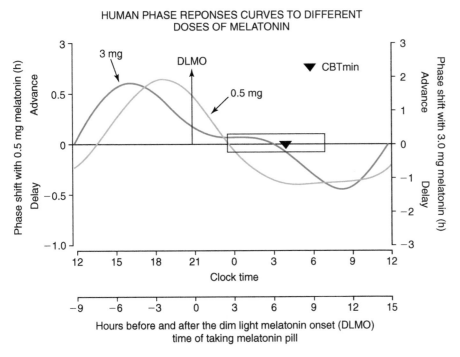

FIGURE 26-13 PRCs for different doses of exogenous melatonin. Note that for the higher dose of melatonin, the maximal effect was noted at an earlier time compared with the DLMO. The *rectangle* illustrates a typical sleep period with core body temperature minimum (CBTmin) shown in the last half of the sleep period. *From Eastman CI, Burgess HJ: How to travel the world without jet lag. Sleep Med Clin 2009;4:241–255.*

between the DLMO and the CBTmin (endogenous melatonin already high). The cross-over point for melatonin (transition from phase advance to phase delay) is during the night but may not precisely coincide with CBTmin. In addition, the shape of the melatonin PRC appears to depend on the dose of melatonin studied and the method of determination of the PRC (Fig. 26-13). Note that the timing of the maximum phase delay induced by melatonin is several hours after the CBTmin. Thus, taking melatonin 1 or 2 hours after spontaneous awakening causes the most phase delay. However, melatonin administration is often not used in the early morning because any hypnotic effects would not be well tolerated outside of a research setting. An exception is when morning sleep is desired by a person working a night shift.

Summary of Effects of Light and Melatonin

A summary of the effects of bright light and melatonin is presented in Figure 26-14 with illustrations of the use of these interventions in two circadian rhythm sleep disorders (CRSDs). Bright light in the evening causes a phase delay and in the early morning a phase advance. Melatonin in the early evening causes a phase advance and in the early morning a phase delay. A simple description of the effects of light and melatonin is that **"bright light pushes and melatonin pulls the circadian rhythms."** In this figure, it is assumed that the CBTmin lies within the initial sleep period of the advanced sleep phase disorder (ASPD) and the delayed sleep phase disorder (DSPD) patients.

GENOMICS OF CRSD

The intrinsic 24-hour rhythm in the SCN neurons is due to the interactions of a number of genes.[27,28] These genes form

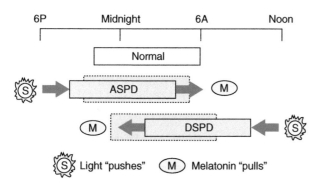

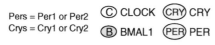

FIGURE 26–14 Summary of effect of light and melatonin on the circadian phase. In patients with the advanced sleep phase disorder (ASPD), melatonin in the late night/early morning phase delays, and in patients with the delayed sleep phase syndrome (DSPD), melatonin in the early evening phase advances. For light, the effects are opposite with early evening light phase delaying and early morning light phase advancing. *Adapted from Barion A, Zee PC: A clinical approach to circadian rhythm sleep disorders. Sleep Med 2007;8:566–577.*

autoregulatory feedback loops on transcription (DNA to mRNA) and translation (mRNA to proteins) that drive the cycling pattern. The feedback is provided by the protein translational products that can either stimulate or repress further gene transcription. A brief description of a few of the many molecular mechanisms responsible for the 24-hour cycle in transcription, translation, and posttranscriptional protein metabolism that drives the rhythmic cycle of the circadian clock genes follows (Fig. 26–15 and Table 26–3). By convention, small letters refer to genes and capital letters refer to protein translational products. For example, transcription and translation of *clock* results in production of the protein **CLOCK.** The human forms of genes are denoted with a preceding h (e.g., *hper2*).

Proteins CLOCK and BMAL1 (synthesized from *clock* and *Bmal1* genes) diffuse into the cytoplasm and associate as heterodimers (CLOCK:BMAL1). These heterodimers then return to the nucleus and bind the Ebox region of genes *Per1, Per2, Cry1,* and *Cry2* and promote transcription of these genes. Ebox is a DNA sequence that usually lies upstream of a gene in a promoter region. The translational products PER and CRY proteins are negative regulators that turn off their own synthesis. The heterodimer PER:CRY and homodimer CRY:CRY diffuse back into the nucleus, inhibiting transcription of the associated genes. That is, PER:CRY and CRY:CRY repress the CLOCK:BMAL1-driven transcription of *Pers* and *Crys.* The synthesis of PER and CRY is under the influence of CLOCK:BMAL1 and can occur only when the level of intranuclear PER and CRY is low enough (after degradation of these proteins). A number of other processes alter these molecular events because PER and CRY can be phosphorylated by several enzymes including casein kinase 1 epsilon (CK1ε), resulting in the ultimate degradation of the

Pers = Per1 or Per2   Ⓒ CLOCK   ⓒⓡⓨ CRY
Crys = Cry1 or Cry2   Ⓑ BMAL1   ⓟⓔⓡ PER

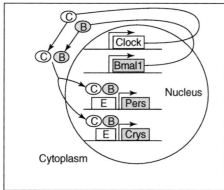

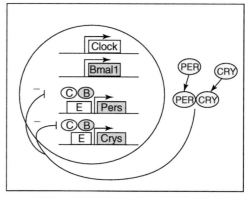

CLOCK: BMAL1 heterodimer binds to Ebox enhancer resulting in increased transcription of Pers and Crys genes

PER and CRY heterodimers and CRY homodimers suppress CLOCK and BMAL1 driven transcription of Pers and Crys

FIGURE 26–15 A schematic of molecular mechanism controlling the circadian clock. Some proteins are inducers of gene transcription, and others inhibit transcription. *Adapted from Vitaterna MH, Pinto LH, Turek FW: Molecular genetic basis for mammalian circadian rhythms. In Kryger MH, Roth T, Dement WC (eds): Principles and Practice of Sleep Medicine, 4th ed. Philadelphia: Elsevier Saunders, 2005, pp. 335–350.*

TABLE 26–3

Circadian Clock Genes

	GENES	PROTEIN
Circadian **L**ocomotor **O**utput **C**ycles **K**aput	*Clock*	CLOCK
Brain and muscle ARNT-like 1	*Bmal1*	BMAL1
Period	*per1, per2, per3*	PER
Timeless	*tim*	TIM
Cryptochrome	*cry1 and 2*	CRY
GENETIC POLYMORPHISMS		
CRSD		
DSPD	*hPer3* and Arylalkylamine *N*-acetyltransferase genes	
ASPD	*hPer2* Phosphorylation site mutation causes reduced degradation of PER (shortening the circadian period)	

ASPD = advanced sleep phase disorder; CRSD = circadian rhythm sleep disorder; DSPD = delayed sleep phase disorder.

BOX 26–5

Circadian Rhythm Sleep Disorders

1. CRSD—Delayed Sleep Phase Type, Delayed Sleep Phase Disorder (DSPD)
2. CRSD—Advanced Sleep Phase Type, Advanced Sleep Phase Disorder (ASPD)
3. CRSD—Irregular Sleep-Wake Type, Irregular Sleep-Wake Rhythm (ISWR)
4. CRSD—Free-Running Type (FRT), Non-entrained Type (non–24-hr Sleep-Wake Syndrome, Free-Running Sleep Disorder)
5. CRSD—Jet Lag Type, Jet Lag Disorder
6. CRSD—Shift-Work Type, Shift-Work Disorder (SWD)
7. CRSD Due to Medical Condition
8. Other CRSD Not Otherwise Specified (NOS)
9. Other, CRSD Due to Drug or Substance

From American Academy of Sleep Medicine: ICSD-2 International Classification of Sleep Disorders, 2nd ed. Diagnostic and Coding Manual. Westchester, IL: American Academy of Sleep Medicine, 2005.

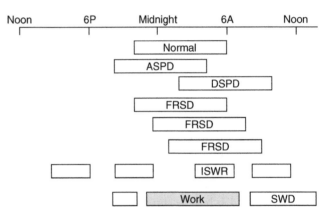

FIGURE 26–16 Schematic diagram of several circadian rhythm sleep disorders. The rectangles represent the timing of sleep. ASPD = advanced sleep phase disorder; DSPD = delayed sleep phase disorder; FRSD = free-running sleep disorder; ISWR = irregular sleep-wake rhythm; SWD = shift-work disorder. *Adapted from Lu BS, Zee PC: Circadian rhythm sleep disorders. Chest 2006;130:1915–1923; and Barion A, Zee PC: A clinical approach to circadian rhythm sleep disorders. Sleep Med 2007;8:566–577.*

BOX 26–4

General Diagnostic Criteria for Circadian Rhythm Sleep Disorder

A. There is a persistent or recurrent pattern of sleep disturbance due primarily to one of the following:
   i. Alterations of the circadian timing system.
   ii. Misalignment between endogenous circadian rhythm and exogenous factors that affects timing or duration of sleep.
B. The circadian-related sleep disruption leads to insomnia, excessive sleepiness, or both.
C. The sleep disturbance is associated with impairment of social, occupational, or other areas of functioning.

From American Academy of Sleep Medicine: ICSD-2 International Classification of Sleep Disorders, 2nd ed. Diagnostic and Coding Manual. Westchester, IL: American Academy of Sleep Medicine, 2005.

protein. The metabolism of PER and CRY influences the stability and rate of entry of protein dimers or heterodimers into the nucleus.

CIRCADIAN RHYTHM SLEEP DISORDERS

The International Classification of Sleep Disorders, second edition (ICSD-2), lists criteria for a CRSD (Box 26–4).[1] There must be alteration of the circadian timing system, usually a **misalignment** between endogenous circadian rhythm and exogenous factors, that affects the timing or duration of sleep. The alteration in circadian timing must lead to a **sleep complaint** (insomnia, excessive sleepiness, or both). Finally,

the change in wake-sleep must be associated with **impairment** including social or occupation functioning. For example, if a person's normal sleep phase is quite delayed but is something that they desire, this would not be a CRSD.[1]

The ICSD-2 lists nine CRSDs (Box 26–5). A large proportion of normal individuals experience problems with sleep or alertness secondary to shift work or jet lag at some point in their lives. The boundary between what constitutes a normal response and what constitutes a disorder is blurry in some disorders such as the shift-work disorder. A schematic of the changes in the habitual sleep period is illustrated in Figure 26–16.

Comprehensive reviews of the existing evidence for evaluation and treatment of these disorders and practice parameters for evaluation and treatment of CRSD were published

BOX 26–6

Morningness-Eveningness Questionnaire, Sleep Logs, and Actigraphy in Circadian Sleep Rhythm Disorder

MEQ

- AASM Practice Parameters: Insufficient evidence to recommend

MEQ SCALE

- Definitely morning type 70–86
- Moderately morning type 59–69
- Moderately evening type 31–41
- Definitely evening type 16–30

SLEEP LOGS

- Indicated in assessment of patients with suspected CRSD (Guideline)

ACTIGRAPHY

- Indicated to assist in evaluation of patients suspected of CRSD (Guideline)
- Useful as an outcome measure in evaluating the response to treatment of CRSD (Guideline)

AASM = American Academy of Sleep Medicine; CRSD = circadian rhythm sleep disorder; MEQ = morningness-eveningness questionnaire.

BOX 26–7

Circadian Rhythm Sleep Disorder—Delayed Sleep Phase Type (Delayed Sleep Phase Disorder)—Diagnostic Criteria

A. Delay in major sleep period in relation to desired sleep time and wakeup time
   a. Chronic or recurrent complaint of inability to fall asleep at a desired conventional clock time.
   b. Inability to awaken at a desired socially accepted time.
B. When allowed to choose preferred schedule, patients have normal sleep quality and duration for age and maintain a delayed but stable phase of entrainment to the 24-hour sleep-wake pattern.
C. Sleep log or actigraphy monitoring (including sleep diary) for at least 7 days demonstrates a stable delay in the timing of the habitual sleep period.

Note: In addition, a delay in the timing of other circadian rhythms, such as the nadir of the core body temperature rhythm, or DLMO, is useful for confirmation of the delayed sleep phase.

D. The sleep disturbance is not better explained by another current sleep disorder, medical or neurologic disorder, mental disorder, medication use, or substance use disorder.

DLMO = dim light melatonin onset.
From American Academy of Sleep Medicine: ICSD-2 International Classification of Sleep Disorders, 2nd ed. Diagnostic and Coding Manual. Westchester, IL: American Academy of Sleep Medicine, 2005.

by the American Academy of Sleep Medicine (AASM) in 2007.[29-31] In evaluating patients for suspected CRSD, the physician utilizes history, a sleep log for at least 7 days, and often actigraphy (Box 26–6). The morningness-eveningness questionnaire (MEQ) is discussed in the following section. The MEQ and markers of circadian phase (DLMO) are used for research studies but the clinical utility for routine evaluation remains to be documented. Polysomnography is not indicated for evaluation of patients with CRSD unless another sleep disorder such as sleep apnea is suspected.

Morningness-Eveningness Questionnaire

The MEQ was developed by Horne and Ostberg in 1976.[32] The MEQ contains 19 questions aimed at determining the natural propensity to perform certain activities during the daily temporal span. Most questions are framed in a preferential manner and require a response to specific times that an individual would prefer to do a certain activity (as opposed to when they actually do it). Each question has answers 0 to 6. The sum ranges from 16 to 86. **Lower values correspond to evening types** (see Box 26–6).

Sleep Logs and Actigraphy

The AASM practice parameters state that sleep logs and actigraphy are indicated for evaluation of patients with suspected or known CRSD[31] (see Box 26–6). Figure 26–16 is a schematic diagram of changes in the sleep period with the different CRSDs compared with normal. In general, sleep logs or actigraphy documents a habitual sleep period compared with normal that is advanced (ASPD), delayed (DSPD), progressively delayed (FRD), irregular (irregular sleep wake rhythm [ISWR]), or with a daytime major sleep episode (shift-work disorder).

Delayed Sleep Phase Disorder

Patients with the DSPD complain of inability to fall asleep at a socially acceptable time—a type of sleep-onset insomnia. If allowed to maintain their own chosen schedule, they would usually sleep for a fairly normal duration and feel rested on arising.[1,16,17,33] However, because of societal pressures, they must awaken earlier than desired and are often sleepy during the day. Therefore, they complain of difficulty waking up and daytime sleepiness (short sleep duration). In contrast to behaviorally induced sleep delay, these patients cannot fall asleep earlier unless very sleep-deprived. Practice parameters for the evaluation and treatment of DSPD have been published (Box 26–7 and Table 26–4).

Epidemiology

The DSPD is the most common CRSD seen in sleep clinics. DSPD is more common in adolescents and young adults with an incidence of 7% to 16% in this population. The incidence in the general population is unknown. Patients with

TABLE 26–4

Recommendations for Evaluation and Treatment of Delayed Sleep Phase Disorder

TOOLS	RECOMMENDATION
EVALUATION	
PSG	Not routinely indicated (S)
MEQ	Insufficient evidence (O)
Circadian phase markers	Insufficient evidence (O)
Actigraphy for diagnosis	Indicated (G)
Actigraphy for response to therapy	Indicated (O)
Sleep log	Indicated (G)
THERAPY	
Planned sleep schedule	Indicated (O)
Timed light exposure	Indicated (G)
Timed melatonin	Indicated (G)
Hypnotics	Not recommended (O)
Stimulants	—
Alerting agents	—

(S) = standard > (G) = guideline > (O) = option; — insufficient evidence; MEQ = morningness-eveningness questionnaire; PSG = polysomnography. From Morgenthaler TI, Lee-Chiong T, Alessi C, et al: Practice parameters for the clinical evaluation and treatment of circadian rhythm sleep disorders. Sleep 2007;30:1445–1459.

DSPD make up about 10% of patients seen in insomnia clinics. The mean age of onset of DSPD is about 20 years.

Pathophysiology

A family history is present in about 40% of patients with DSPD.[1] The DSPD has been associated with **genetic polymorphism in circadian clock gene *hPer3*,**[3,34] **AA-NAT,**[35] **and the *clock* gene.** Another possibility would be an intrinsically long tau. Exposure to bright light in the evening (causing phase delay) or decreased exposure to morning light can exacerbate the problem.

Sleep Logs and Actigraphy

Sleep logs (Fig. 26–17) and actigraphy (Fig. 26–18) typically document a stable delay in the period relative to clock time with a typical sleep-onset time from **1 to 6** AM with wake times in the late morning or early afternoon (10 AM–2 PM). During the work week or school, a forced awakening will cause a short sleep period.

On the weekend or nonschool or nonwork days, longer sleep until late morning/early afternoon is noted. The Horne-Ostberg questionnaire (morning-evening preference) shows a night owl preference (eveningness). The DLMO is delayed in patients with DSPD (see Fig. 26–6). As expected, the CBTmin is also quite delayed. Some studies found the body temperature nadir in DSPD patients to occur earlier during the sleep period than that of normal individuals.[36,37] For example, Watanabe and coworkers[37] found the CBTmin occurred near the middle of the nocturnal sleep period in patients with DSPD in contrast to normal controls in whom

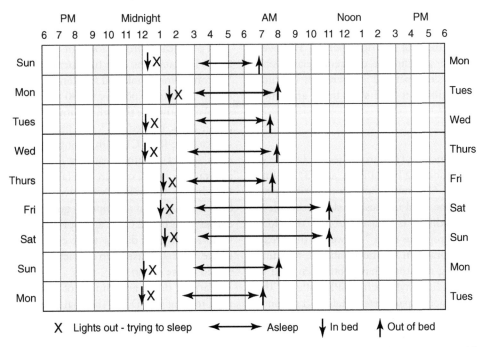

FIGURE 26–17 A sleep log from a patient with DSPD. Note the stable delay in sleep-onset time despite attempts to fall asleep earlier on some nights. On the weekends, sleep continues until the late morning. Note that once the patient is asleep, few awakenings are noted.

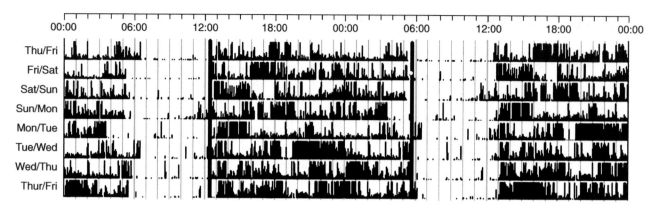

FIGURE 26–18 An actigraph recording of sleep-wake activity, recorded using wrist activity monitoring, from an individual with DSPD. The individual goes to sleep around 5 to 6 AM and wakes between 12 and 1 PM each day. Note that all actigraphy data are double-plotted. A period of 48 consecutive hours is shown on each line. The last 24 hours (second half) of each line is then repeated as the first 24 hours (first half) of the following line (00:00 is midnight). *From Barion A, Zee PC: A clinical approach to circadian rhythm sleep disorders. Sleep Med 2007;8:566–577.*

TABLE 26–5	
Treatment for Delayed Sleep Phase Disorder	
Light therapy	• 2500–10,000 lux 30 min–2 hr. • Timing = at or slightly (1 hr) before spontaneous wake time (ad lib sleep). • Light administered ½–1 hr earlier each day (use alarm if needed). Patient also typically goes to bed earlier. • Restrict light in the evening.
Melatonin	• 0.3–3.0 mg given 5–7 hr before habitual sleep-onset time • 3–5 hr before DLMO. • Large melatonin dose has hypnotic effects.
DLMO = dim light melatonin onset.	

it occurred in the last third of the sleep period. However, other investigators did not find a different relationship between CBTmin and sleep period.[38] Differences in study results may be due to different total sleep times and study designs.

Treatment of DSPD

Treatments for DSPD include (1) chronotherapy (a type of sleep scheduling), (2) morning bright light, and (3) evening melatonin (Table 26–5). Chronotherapy is a prescribed progressive delay in bedtime until the desired sleep schedule is reached.[39] Basically, bedtime is delayed around the clock until it reaches an appropriate time.[39] However, this treatment approach is not practical for most patients. Morning bright light and evening melatonin have both been used to phase advance the circadian rhythms in DSPD patients. The AASM standards of practice parameters state that chronotherapy may be effective (Option) and that morning light exposure and properly timed evening melatonin are indicated to treat DSPD (Guideline)[31] (see Table 26–4). The practice parameters state that the optimal dose and timing of light have not been determined.

In one study, an initial 2-week trial of light therapy at 2500 lux given for 2 hours between 6:00 AM and 9:00 AM in combination with evening light **restriction** demonstrated an advancement of CBTmin of 1.4 hours and an improvement in multiple sleep latencies.[40] A later study reported a 1.5-hour earlier sleep-onset time after 5 days of 3 hours of phototherapy given 1.5 hours after CBTmin.[41]

The optimal timing, dose, and duration of bright light for treatment of DSPD have not been defined but common recommendations are 2500 to 10,000 lux in the morning for 1 to 2 hours. However, a pitfall of this approach is that light may be administered **on the wrong side of the temperature minimum.** For example, if a patient's habitual wake time is 11:00 AM, the CBTmin could be around 8 to 9 AM. Therefore, exposure to bright light at 6 to 8 AM would induce a phase delay in this individual.

A practical approach for light therapy in DSPD (see Table 26–5) is to start the light treatment at 1 or 2 hours before the "unconstrained" habitual awakening time with a light intensity of 2500 to 10,000 lux for 30 minutes to 2 hours (if possible) and advance the light treatment ½ to 1 hour daily (with alarm clock if needed).[42] It is best to estimate the habitual awake time (and CBTmin) using ad lib sleep on the weekends. In fact, starting treatment on the weekends may allow appropriate light exposure at a later clock time than permitted during the school/work week. Once light treatment begins, the patient attempts to go to bed about ½ to 1 hour earlier each night. Once appropriate timing is reached, light treatment 1 to 2 days a week could be used for "maintenance." It is also useful to restrict light in the evening hours (avoid phase delay).

Various doses and timing of melatonin have also been used to treat DSPD.[38,43] The goal is to give melatonin before DLMO to phase advance. Mundey and colleagues[38] used both 0.3 and 3.0 mg of melatonin and found the magnitude of phase advance correlated with the time of administration (earlier better). Of note, in this study, melatonin treatment in DSPD had a greater effect on wake time than sleep-onset time.[38] In another study, 5 mg of melatonin administered 5 hours before the DLMO was effective.[43] However, larger doses of melatonin are more likely to also have a hypnotic effect. **Current reasonable recommendations are to administer 0.3 to 5.0 mg of melatonin 2 to 3 hours before DLMO or 5 to 7 hours before habitual sleep time.** One could make a case for using melatonin 0.3 to 0.5 mg to possibly minimize hypnotic effects if sleepiness at the time of administration is not desirable (see Table 26–5). There is some evidence that use of the combination of light and melatonin may be more effective at inducing a phase advance than either used alone.[44] Side effects of melatonin include headache, dizziness, nausea, and drowsiness. At high doses, melatonin may alter sex hormones.[6] For this reason, some clinicians are hesitant to use the medication long term in adolescents or children.

Advanced Sleep Phase Disorder

The ASPD is thought to be quite rare if diagnostic criteria are strictly followed. Advanced related sleep complaints, particularly early awakening, are more common. Often, patients are able to stay awake but are unable to stay asleep. As a consequence, classic ASPD is fairly rare but early morning awakening is much more common. ASPD is associated with aging, and nonaging ASPD is rare. Early morning awakening can also be noted in depression.

Epidemiology

The prevalence of ASPD is not well documented but believed to be about 1% in middle-aged populations and increases with age. Men and women are equally affected.

Pathophysiology

Familial ASPD has been described with a mutation in the circadian clock gene *hPer2*.[45,46] However, other familial cases do not show this pattern. Causes of ASPD include a short endogenous circadian period or a dominant phase advance region to light. In elderly patients who take early morning walks, this behavior tends to phase advance.

Diagnosis

The ICSD-2 criteria (Box 26–8) require that the sleep period be advanced with respect to the desired sleep time and wakeup times. The use of a sleep log or actigraphy for at **least 7 days** is required to document a stable advance in the normal sleep period. These patients complain of not being able to stay awake in the evening for desired activities and then early morning awakening.[47] The differential diagnosis includes poor sleep hygiene (evening or afternoon naps), caffeine abuse, alcohol, and depression (can cause early morning awakening).

Morningness-Eveningness Questionnaire

Patients with ASPD when completing the MEQ (Horne-Ostberg questionnaire)[32] record answers consistent with "morning type."

BOX 26–8

Circadian Rhythm Sleep Disorder—Advanced Sleep Phase Type (Advanced Sleep Phase Disorder)—Diagnostic Criteria

A. Advance in the major sleep period in relation to desired sleep time and wakeup time
  i. Chronic or recurrent inability to **remain awake** until a desired conventional clock time.
  ii. Inability **to remain asleep** until a desired socially accepted time.
B. When allowed to choose preferred schedule, patients have **normal sleep quality** and **duration** for age and maintain an advanced but **stable phase of entrainment** to the 24-hour sleep-wake pattern.
C. Sleep log or actigraphy monitoring (including sleep diary) for at least 7 days demonstrates a stable **advance** in the timing of the habitual sleep period.

Note: In addition, an advance in the timing of other circadian rhythms, such as the nadir of the core body temperature rhythm, or DLMO, is useful for confirmation of the advanced sleep phase.

D. The sleep disturbance is not better explained by another current sleep disorder, medical or neurologic disorder, mental disorder, medication use, or substance use disorder.

DLMO = dim light melatonin onset.
From American Academy of Sleep Medicine: ICSD-2 International Classification of Sleep Disorders, 2nd ed. Diagnostic and Coding Manual. Westchester, IL: American Academy of Sleep Medicine, 2005.

Sleep Logs and Actigraphy

Patients with ASPD demonstrate a **stable advance in sleep period** with sleep onset 6 PM to 9 PM and awakenings from 2 AM to 5 AM (Fig. 26–19).

Core Body Temperature, Dim Light Melatonin Onset

Circadian phase makers in ASPD patients demonstrate advanced timing (Table 26–6).

Treatment

Chronotherapy (sleep schedule) can be used with a progressive phase advance around the clock until the desired bedtime is reached.[48] For most patients, this is not practical. The most common treatment is bright light in the evening from 7 to 9 PM (Table 26–7 and Boxes 26–9 and 26–10). In one study, 4000 lux was administered for 11 consecutive days then twice weekly for a 3-month period (maintenance).[49] Unfortunately, patients have difficulty complying with this treatment plan. The AASM practice parameters mention evening light as an Option for ASPD (see Table 26–7).[31] Another important form of light therapy is to AVOID early morning light, which tends to cause a phase advance. Although early morning melatonin would be a potential treatment (phase delay), this is not practical and may not be safe if individuals have to function in the morning. Melatonin has sedative

FIGURE 26–19 A typical sleep log for a patient with ASPD. This illustrates an early bedtime and an early rise time. The patient takes naps, which may exacerbate early morning awakening by decreasing sleep load.

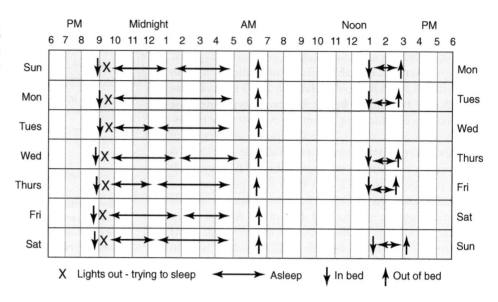

X Lights out - trying to sleep   ←——→ Asleep   ↓ In bed   ↑ Out of bed

TABLE 26–6

Changes in Sleep Pattern in Familial Advanced Sleep Phase Disorder Compared with Controls

	CONTROL	FAMILIAL ASPD	DIFFERENCE (MIN)
Sleep onset	23:10 ± 0:40	19:25 ± 1:44	3:45
Sleep offset	7:44 ± 1:13	04:18 ± 2:00	3:25
DLMO	21:21 ± 0.28	17:31 ± 1:49	3:50
CBTmin	03:35 ± 1:33	23:22 ± 2:55	4:13

ASPD = advanced sleep phase disorder; CBTmin = core body temperature minimum; DLMO = dim light melatonin onset.
Data from Jones C, Campbell S, Zone S, et al: Familial advanced sleep phase syndrome: a short-period circadian rhythm variant in humans. Nat Med 1999;5:1062–1065.
Adapted from Auger RR: Advanced related sleep complaints and advanced sleep phase disorder. Sleep Med Clin 2009;4:219–227.

TABLE 26–7

Recommendations for Evaluation and Treatment of the Advanced Sleep Phase Disorder

TOOLS	RECOMMENDATION
EVALUATION	
PSG	Not routinely indicated (S)
MEQ	Insufficient evidence (O)
Circadian phase markers	Insufficient evidence (O)
Actigraphy for diagnosis	Indicated (G)
Actigraphy for response to therapy	Indicated (O)
Sleep log	Indicated (G)
THERAPY	
Planned sleep schedule	Indicated (O)
Timed light exposure	Indicated (O)
Timed melatonin	Indicated (O)
Hypnotics	—
Stimulants	—
Alerting agents	—

(S) = standard > (G) = guideline > (O) = option; — no recommendation due to lack of evidence; MEQ = morningness-eveningness questionnaire; PSG = polysomnography.
From Morgenthaler TI, Lee-Chiong T, Alessi C, et al: Practice parameters for the clinical evaluation and treatment of circadian rhythm sleep disorders. Sleep 2007;30:1445–1459.

effects especially at higher doses and during periods when the endogenous melatonin is not elevated. However, timed melatonin was listed as indicated (Option) for treatment of ASPD in the AASM practice parameters for CRSD.[31]

CRSD—Irregular Sleep-Wake Type

The CRSD—irregular sleep-wake type (also known as **irregular sleep-wake rhythm [ISWR]**) is characterized by lack of a clearly defined circadian rhythm of sleep and wake behavior. Typically, sleep and wake periods are interspersed throughout the day.[1]

Epidemiology

The prevalence of ISWR is unknown. The disorder occurs most frequently in institutionalized elderly patients with dementia or institutionalized young patients with mental retardation. Precipitating factors include poor sleep hygiene and limited exposure to synchronizing zeitgebers including

outside light, exercise, and social activities. Some patients may have a decrease in the circadian amplitude of the SCN-alerting signal. In others, absence of zeitgebers (decreased light and activity) may be important. Important risk factors for ISWR include age, living in an institutional setting, and dementia or mental retardation (Alzheimer's disease).[50]

BOX 26–9

Treatment of Advanced Sleep Phase Disorder

- Sleep schedule (chronotherapy)—progressive phase advance.
- Light
  - Bright evening light 7–9 PM.
  - Avoid light after temperature minimum (early morning light).
- Melatonin
  - Early AM melatonin potentially effective but sedative effects make this impractical for most patients. Consider a low dose to attempt to minimize sedative effects.

BOX 26–10

Circadian Rhythm Sleep Disorder—Irregular Sleep-Wake Type—Diagnostic Criteria

A. There is a chronic complaint of insomnia, excessive sleepiness, or both.

B. Sleep logs or actigraphy monitoring (including sleep diaries) for at least 7 days demonstrates **multiple irregular sleep bouts (at least three) during a 24-hour period.**

C. Total sleep time per 24 hours is essentially normal for age.

D. The sleep disturbance is not better explained by another current sleep disorder, medical or neurologic disorder, mental disorder, medication use, or substance use disorder.

From American Academy of Sleep Medicine: ICSD-2 International Classification of Sleep Disorders, 2nd ed. Diagnostic and Coding Manual. Westchester, IL: American Academy of Sleep Medicine, 2005.

Etiology

Factors involved in ISWR:

1. Abnormal circadian regulation
   i. Damage or deterioration of the activity of the SCN.
   ii. Diminished response to entraining agents such as light.
2. Behavioral and environmental factors
   i. Decreased exposure to bright light.
   ii. Decreased physical activity and social activities.
   iii. Poor sleep habits.

Sleep Logs and Actigraphy

Monitoring with actigraphy for at least 7 days demonstrates multiple irregular sleep bouts (at least three) during a 24-hour period (Fig. 26–20). The total sleep time is normal for age. The AASM practice parameters for CRSD state that actigraphy is indicated in ISWR for diagnosis and assessing response to treatment.

Diagnosis of ISWR

Diagnosis requires a complaint of daytime sleepiness or insomnia (although the caregiver rather than the patient may complain). Actigraphy or sleep log for at least 7 days

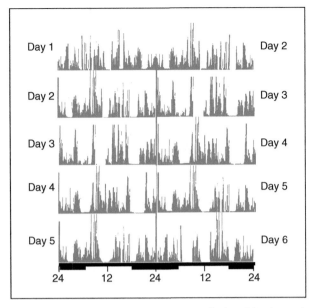

FIGURE 26–20 Actigraphy shows an irregular pattern of wake and sleep in a nursing home patient with dementia. Note that much of the sleep occurred during the day. At least three episodes of sleep were noted during each 24 hours. This is a double plot. Each line is 48 hours. The last 24 hours on one line is repeated as the first 24 hours on the next line.

demonstrates multiple sleep periods (at least three) within 24 hours with approximately a normal total amount of sleep for age. For most patients with ISWR, the sleep log is problematic and this is one setting in which actigraphy is especially helpful. Some actigraph devices also record light exposure, and decreased light exposure may be a predisposing factor for ISWR.

Treatment of ISWR

Treatment of patients with ISWR aims at consolidating both sleep and wake periods. Daytime light has been tried with some benefit.[51] Melatonin has **not** been found to be effective in most studies.[52] A large randomized, controlled trial by Riemersma-ven der Lek and associates[53] compared four conditions (bright light–melatonin, dim light–melatonin, bright light–placebo, and dim light–placebo) in a group of institutionalized elderly patients (87% had dementia). The light conditions included bright (1000 lux) or dim (300 lux) light between 9 AM and 6 PM. The melatonin and placebo conditions included administration of either placebo or 2.5 mg of melatonin in the evening. Light had a modest benefit in improving some cognitive and noncognitive symptoms of dementia. Melatonin (without bright light) decreased the sleep latency and increased total sleep time but impaired mood. Bright light + melatonin did not impair mood but decreased sleep latency and increased total sleep time. Thus, melatonin should probably not be used alone in elderly patients in similar settings. A combination of light and melatonin might be effective. Conversely, melatonin has been shown to be of benefit in some populations of younger developmentally delayed or mentally impaired individuals. A study by Pillar and coworkers[54] found that 4-week treatment with melatonin 3 mg improved sleep duration from 5.9 to 7.3 hours and sleep efficiency from 69.3% to 88% in a group of psychomotor-retarded children.

Interventions to treat ISWR include bright light during the day, structured daytime activities (mixed modality treatment), and decreased noise and nighttime light. Hypnotics have also been used but are associated with side effects (falls or sedation) in the elderly. The AASM practice parameters[31] recommended bright light during the day and mixed-modality therapy (societal activities). Melatonin was recommended only in younger patients with retardation but not for elderly nursing home patients (Option).

CRSD—Free-Running Type (Non–24-Hour Sleep-Wake Syndrome)

The circadian rhythm sleep disorder—free-running type (CRSD-FRT) is characterized by a progressive delay in sleep onset each day (Fig. 26–21, Table 26–8, and Box 26–11). There are periods of time when patients may complain of insomnia, early morning awakening, and daytime sleepiness depending on the relationship of the internal circadian rhythms and external time. These complaints occur when circadian rhythm is out of phase with conventional sleep and wake times. For example, when the CBTmin is during the day, there will be sleepiness during the day and insomnia at night. When the circadian phase is aligned with a normal sleep-wake period, complaints may not be present. **There is a steady drift of the sleep period by 1 to 2 hours each day.**[1,24]

Epidemiology

Up to 50% of totally blind patients have non-entrained circadian rhythms. About 70% have chronic sleep complaints. Rarely, CRSD-FRT occurs in sighted individuals.[55] It has also been described after head trauma.[56] Note that there are some blind patients whose circadian system responds to bright light even though they have no visual perception. Some

TABLE 26–8

Recommendations for Evaluation and Treatment of the Irregular Sleep-Wake Rhythm

TOOLS	RECOMMENDATION
EVALUATION	
PSG	Not routinely indicated (S)
MEQ	Insufficient evidence (O)
Circadian phase markers	Insufficient evidence (O)
Actigraphy for diagnosis	Indicated (O)
Actigraphy for response to therapy	Indicated (O)
Sleep log	Indicated (G)
THERAPY	
Planned sleep schedule	Mixed modality treatment indicated in elderly nursing home patients (G) and in patients with mental retardation (O)
Timed light exposure	Indicated (O)
Timed melatonin	Indicated for certain populations Yes moderate to severe mental retardation (O) Not recommended for elderly/demented NH patients (O)
Hypnotics	—
Stimulants	—
Alerting agents	—

(S) = standard > (G) = guideline > (O) = option; — no recommendation due to lack of evidence; MEQ = morningness-eveningness questionnaire; NH = nursing home; PSG = polysomnography.
From Morgenthaler TI, Lee-Chiong T, Alessi C, et al: Practice parameters for the clinical evaluation and treatment of circadian rhythm sleep disorders. Sleep 2007;30:1445–1459.

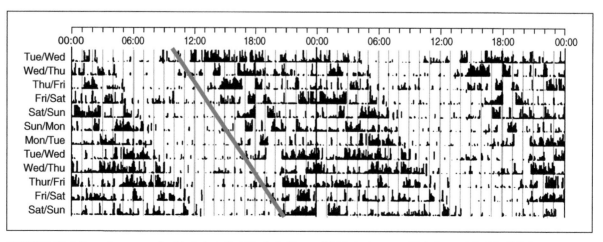

FIGURE 26–21 Actigram shows progressive delay in sleep offset (*blue line*) with a parallel delay in sleep onset. This is characteristic of the CRSD free-running type. *Reproduced with permission from Barion A, Zee PC: A clinical approach to circadian rhythm sleep disorders. Sleep Med 2007;8:566–577.*

BOX 26-11

Circadian Rhythm Sleep Disorder—Free-Running Type (Non–24-Hour Sleep Syndrome)—Diagnostic Criteria

A. There is a complaint of insomnia or excessive daytime sleepiness related to abnormal synchronization between the 24-hour light-dark cycle and the endogenous circadian rhythm of sleep-wake propensity.

B. Sleep log or actigraphy (with sleep diary) for at least 7 days demonstrates a pattern of sleep and wake times that typically delay each day with a period time greater than 24 hours.

Note: Monitoring or sleep logs for greater than 7 days is preferred to document a delay.

C. The sleep disturbance is not better explained by another current sleep disorder, medical or neurologic disorder, mental disorder, medication use, or substance use disorder.

From American Academy of Sleep Medicine: ICSD-2 International Classification of Sleep Disorders, 2nd ed. Diagnostic and Coding Manual. Westchester, IL: American Academy of Sleep Medicine, 2005.

TABLE 26-9

Recommendations for Evaluation and Treatment of Circadian Rhythm Sleep Disorder—Free-Running Type

TOOLS	RECOMMENDATION
EVALUATION	
PSG	Not routinely indicated (S)
MEQ	Insufficient evidence (O)
Circadian phase markers	Insufficient evidence (O)
Actigraphy for diagnosis	Indicated (O)
Actigraphy for response to therapy	Indicated (O)
Sleep log	Indicated (G)
THERAPY	
Planned sleep schedule	Indicated (O)
Timed light exposure	Indicated (O)
Timed melatonin	Indicated sighted (O), indicated unsighted (G)
Hypnotics	—
Stimulants	—
Alerting agents	—

(S) = standard > (G) = guideline > (O) = option; — no recommendation due to lack of evidence; MEQ = morningness-eveningness questionnaire; PSG = polysomnography.
From Morgenthaler TI, Lee-Chiong T, Alessi C, et al: Practice parameters for the clinical evaluation and treatment of circadian rhythm sleep disorders. Sleep 2007;30:1445–1459.

nonvisual function is still present in these patients with ganglion cells and RHT intact.

Pathophysiology

In blind individuals, the absence of non–visual light information to the SCN allows for the intrinsic phase delay to be manifested. The cause of CRSD-FRT in sighted individuals is unknown. They may have a long circadian period (delay is too large to be entrained by ½ hour phase advance from light).

Sleep Logs and Actigraphy

Sleep logs and actigraphy (see Fig. 26–21) demonstrate a progressive phase delay in patients with CRSD-FRT. These demonstrate a progressive phase delay in the sleep period.

CBTmin and DLMO

There is a progressive delay in the CBTmin and the DLMO (see Fig. 26–6).

Treatment of CRSD-FRT

The treatment in blind patients includes melatonin of various doses before desired bedtime (Table 26–9 and Box 26–12). In one study, 10 mg of melatonin was given 1 hour before desired bedtime (Fig. 26–22). A maintenance dose of 0.5 mg of melatonin is used.[57] In a few patients who failed to entrain on 10 mg of melatonin, there was success with a lower dose[58] (see Table 26–9 and Box 26–12). The treatment in sighted patients may include both melatonin and appropriately timed light exposure. Light is timed to oppose the intrinsic progressive phase delay. That is, light should be timed several hours after the CBTmin to induce a phase advance. One might begin treatment during a time when the CBTmin occurs in the early morning (3–5 AM). The goal would be to

BOX 26-12

Treatment in Patients with Circadian Rhythm Sleep Disorder—Free-Running Type

- Blind individuals
  - Melatonin 0.5–10 mg given 1 hour before desired bedtime.
  - Maintenance dose once entrained is 0.5 mg of melatonin.
  - If some light perception, can try AM light.
- Treatment recommendations in sighted individuals are less clear
  - Evening melatonin (phase advance).
  - Maximum daytime sun exposure (bright light after CBTmin to phase advance).
  - Keep regular sleep-wake schedule.

CBTmin = core body temperature minimum.

maintain the CBTmin during the night. A fixed wakeup time with daily light treatment could be used for maintenance.

CRSD–Jet Lag Type

The jet lag type of CRSD is due to a temporary mismatch between internal circadian rhythms (endogenous circadian

FIGURE 26–22 A blind patient with free-running type (tau = 24.3 hr) was treated with 10 mg of melatonin about 1 hour before preferred bedtime. The timing of the DLMO on sequential days is plotted (*circles*). Treatment was started when the DLMO was about 9 PM. Once entrained, the dose was slowly decreased every 2 weeks. Melatonin as low as 0.5 mg maintained entrainment. After treatment stopped, the patient began to free-run again. *Adapted from Lewy AJ, Emens JS, Lefler BJ, et al: Melatonin entrains free-running blind people according to a physiological dose response curve. Chronobiol Int 2005; 22:1093–1106.*

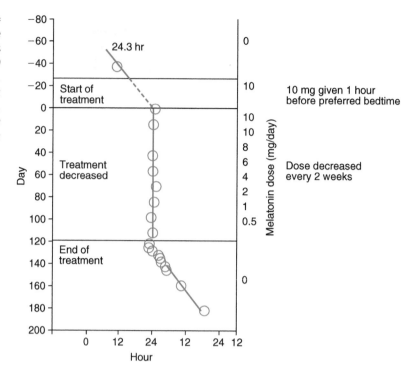

Circadian Rhythm Sleep Disorder—Jet Lag Type—Diagnostic Criteria

A. There is a complaint of insomnia or excessive daytime sleepiness associated with transmeridian jet travel across **at least two time zones.**

B. There is associated impairment of daytime function, general malaise, or somatic symptoms such as gastrointestinal disturbance within 1–2 days after travels.

C. The sleep disturbance is not better explained by another current sleep disorder, medical or neurologic disorder, mental disorder, medication use, or substance use disorder.

From American Academy of Sleep Medicine: ICSD-2 International Classification of Sleep Disorders, 2nd ed. Diagnostic and Coding Manual. Westchester, IL: American Academy of Sleep Medicine, 2005.

clock) and external clock time (sleep-wake pattern) required by rapid change to a new time zone. There must be a **complaint of impairment of sleep and/or daytime function** (Box 26–13).

Epidemiology

The jet lag type of CRSD can occur in all ages but manifestations are worse in the elderly. Jet lag type is a product of our society with approximately one-half million people in the air at any moment worldwide. Aircrews are more vulnerable to jet lag with frequent phase shifting. About one third of travelers do not experience jet lag.

Pathophysiology

Jet lag begins after travel across at least two time zones.[1,59] Desynchrony between body and local time zone is known to cause problems with sleep, alertness, and performance. The degree of dysfunction depends on (1) the number of time zones crossed, (2) the direction of travel (westward travel better tolerated), (3) sleep loss during travel, (4) availability of local time cues (exposure to natural light at destination—depends on weather, business schedule, and other factors), and (5) ability to tolerate circadian misalignment (decreases with age). Westward travel is better tolerated because the body is phase advanced compared with local time. In general, it is easier to adapt (phase delay) because of the intrinsic phase delay (tau >24 hr). In eastward travel, the body is phase delayed. It is more difficult to undergo adaptation to the new time zone with a phase advance. Sleep occurs normally on the rising phase of melatonin rhythm and the falling phase of core temperature rhythm. It is estimated that it takes about 1 day per hour of time zone change to adjust (**maximum adaptation is a phase shift of ½–1 hr/day**, depending on direction of travel). In overnight flights, some degree of sleep loss is inevitable. Flying first class (more room), wearing eye shades or ear plugs, and possibly a hypnotic can minimize sleep loss. If this is not possible, a short nap on arrival at the new destination may help. Drinking adequate fluids and avoiding alcohol may also help. The availability of exposure to natural light in the new destination can be influenced by time of year, weather, and schedule (indoor meetings, societal obligations). The general recommendation is to eat on the destination schedule.

Antidromic Entrainment

Travel over **six time zones** may result in phase shifting in the opposite direction of the direction of travel (i.e., adapting "the wrong way"), so-called **antidromic re-entrainment**. For example, eastern flight requires a phase advance to acclimate to the new time zone. However, after an eastward flight across nine time zones, the traveler's CBTmin normally at 5 AM in the old time zone would occur at 2 PM in the new time zone. Thus, morning light in the new time zone would cause phase delay because light exposure occurs before CBTmin. Of note, some experts recommend that all flights that cross more than 8 to 10 time zones be treated as if they were westward travel (interventions target progressive phase delay).

Symptoms Associated with Jet Lag CRSD

Symptoms associated with jet lag may include (1) daytime tiredness or impaired daytime alertness, (2) inability to get to sleep at night (eastward flight), and (3) early awakening (westward flight). Other symptoms may include disorientation; gastrointestinal problems (poor appetite), inappropriate timing of defecation (gut lag), excessive urination, menstrual abnormalities (flight crew), inappropriate metabolic responses (insulin and other hormones); and heart disease. Symptoms may be worsened by stresses of airplane travel itself or use of caffeine or alcohol.

Treatment of Jet Lag

A number of treatments for jet lag have been recommended depending on the direction of travel (Tables 26–10 to 26–12). Websites are available that allow the traveler to enter current and future locations and a prescription is generated for interventions to minimize jet lag. One difficulty with providing recommendations is in estimating the current CBTmin and also that entrainment in the new destination may depend on societal demands in the new time zone that preclude following the prescription.

General sleep hygiene measures include a dark, quiet sleep environment with earplugs or eye shades if needed. If the plane flight is long, sleeping on the flight during appropriate hours (destination nighttime) may be helpful. In general, daytime naps should be avoided at the destination.

However, napping can improve alertness for special demands (e.g., giving a talk). Napping removes photic stimuli so this can delay adaptation if napping occurs at a time when light exposure would shift circadian rhythms in the correct direction.

Eastward Flights The patient is phase delayed (a phase advance is required) (Fig. 26–23). One method is to phase advance 1 hour per day with bright light in the morning before travel begins (Fig. 26–24).[60,61] At the new destination, morning light should be sought (as long as it is after CBTmin). Evening light should be avoided on arrival at the new destination (to avoid phase delay). Melatonin before CBTmin might be useful if the hypnotic effects would not interfere with wakeful activities. Hypnotics can help with sleep but do not necessarily help with alertness the next day.[62] Even if the individual gets adequate sleep, decreased circadian alertness will occur at time of CBTmin. Stimulants (caffeine) may be

TABLE 26–10	
Jet Lag Facts	
Typical internal clock resetting	92 min/day delay on westward flights. 57 min/day advance on eastward flights.
• Eastern travel	• Difficulty falling asleep—sleep-onset insomnia. • May not notice sleep difficulty the first night in new time zone if sleep deprived (because sleep during flight may have been poor). • Sleep fragmented, decreased REM and stage N3 sleep.
• Western travel	• Less persistent symptoms. • First night: sleep quality good early in sleep period (deprivation). • Increased REM early in sleep period as new bedtime falls nearer to prior REM period. • Early awakenings
REM = rapid eye movement.	

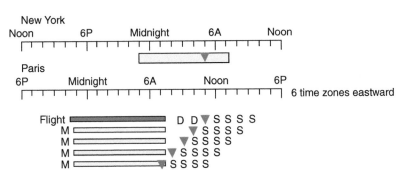

New York: Noon, 6P, Midnight, 6A, Noon
Paris: 6P, Midnight, 6A, Noon, 6P — 6 time zones eastward

Flight D D S S S S / M S S S S (etc.)

D = dark   S = sunlight or bright light   M = melatonin

FIGURE 26–23 Schematic of a flight from New York to Paris (6 time zones eastward). Sleep times are shown as *rectangles* and the CBTmin as *blue triangles*. On arrival, light is avoided (D) before CBTmin to prevent phase delay and sunlight exposure is used after CBTmin to produce a phase advance. Melatonin is taken at bedtime. The circadian phase advances until the CBTmin is within the sleep period *(rectangle)*. However, this process takes several days. For simplicity, timing of melatonin is kept constant.

TABLE 26–11

Recommendations for Jet Lag

	EASTWARD TRAVEL	WESTWARD TRAVEL
	Internal rhythm is phase delayed. Adaptation—phase advance.	Internal rhythm is phase advanced. Adaptation—phase delay.
BEFORE TRAVEL		
Try to reset body clock to minimize necessary change.	Shift sleep 1–2 hr earlier before trip (bright light in AM).	Shift sleep 1–2 hr later before trip (bright light in PM).
DURING TRAVEL		
During flight.	Sleep if possible—especially on long flights—to avoid sleep loss. Sleep during time corresponding to night in the destination if possible. Drink adequate H$_2$O, avoid alcohol.	Sleep if possible—especially on long flights—to avoid sleep loss. Sleep during time corresponding to night in the destination if possible. Drink adequate H$_2$O, avoid alcohol.
ON ARRIVAL		
Anticipated changes in sleep.	Difficulty falling asleep. Difficulty waking up.	Difficulty staying asleep. Early awakening.
Appropriate light exposure.	Seek morning light.	Seek evening light.
If crossing more than eight time zones, avoid light when it may inhibit adaptation.	For the first 2 days after arrival, avoid bright light for the first 2–3 hr after dawn; starting on the third day, seek exposure to bright light in the morning.	For 2–3 days, avoid bright light in the late evening (at dusk); starting on the third day, seek exposure to bright light in the evening.
Melatonin.	Take 0.5–3 mg at local bedtime nightly until you adjust (phase advance).	Take 0.5 mg during the second half of the night (after CBTmin to phase delay).
Hypnotics.	Consider taking at bedtime for a few days.	Consider taking at bedtime for a few days.
Caffeine.	Drink judiciously, avoid after midday.	Drink judiciously, avoid after midday.

CBTmin = core body temperature minimum.
Adapted from Sack RL: Jet lag. N Engl J Med 2010;362:440–447.

FIGURE 26–24 The patient illustrated in Figure 26–23 attempts to reduce the time required for adaptation by use of a preflight phase advance to minimize jet lag on arrival. There are fewer days until the CBTmin *(blue triangles)* is within the desired sleep period *(rectangles).*

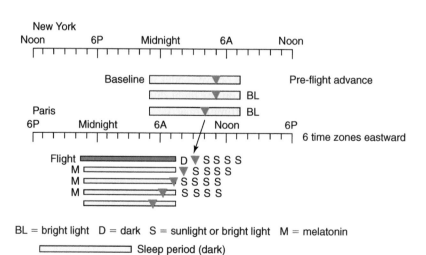

BL = bright light   D = dark   S = sunlight or bright light   M = melatonin

☐ Sleep period (dark)

helpful to maintain alertness during the day in the new locale. A recent study found that 150 mg of armodafinil (R isomer of modafinil) increased wakefulness after eastward travel through six time zones.[63]

Westward Flights The patient is phase advanced relative to local time (a phase delay is required). One could try to phase delay before travel begins (go to bed later, get up later) using evening bright light for 1 to 3 hours. Light should be avoided in the morning in the new destination (if it occurs soon after CBTmin) to prevent phase advance. Exposure to light in the evening (if before CBTmin) may be helpful (phase delay). Melatonin at bedtime in the destination if taken before CBTmin may have hypnotic action but induces phase shift

TABLE 26-12

Recommendations for Evaluation and Treatment of Jet Lag

TOOLS/TREATMENT	RECOMMENDATION
EVALUATION	
PSG	Not routinely indicated (S)
MEQ	Insufficient evidence (O)
Circadian phase markers	Insufficient evidence (O)
Actigraphy for diagnosis	Not routinely indicated (O)
Actigraphy for response to therapy	Not routinely indicated (O)
Sleep log	Indicated (G)
THERAPY	
Planned sleep schedule	Indicated (O)
Timed light exposure	Indicated (O)
Timed melatonin	Indicated (S)
Hypnotics	Indicated (O)
Stimulants	Indicated (O)

(S) = standard > (G) = guideline > (O) = option; MEQ = morningness-eveningness questionnaire; PSG = polysomnography.
From Morgenthaler TI, Lee-Chiong T, Alessi C, et al: Practice parameters for the clinical evaluation and treatment of circadian rhythm sleep disorders. Sleep 2007;30:1445-1459.

BOX 26-14

Circadian Rhythm Sleep Disorder—Shift-Work Type (Shift-Work Disorder)—Diagnostic Criteria

A. There is a complaint of insomnia or excessive daytime sleepiness that is temporally associated with a recurring work schedule that overlaps the usual time for sleep.
B. The symptoms are associated with the shift-work schedule over the course of at least 1 month.
C. Sleep log or actigraphy monitoring (with sleep diaries) for at least 7 days demonstrates disturbed circadian and sleep-time misalignment.
D. The sleep disturbance is not better explained by another current sleep disorder, medical or neurologic disorder, mental disorder, medication use, or substance use disorder.

From American Academy of Sleep Medicine: ICSD-2 International Classification of Sleep Disorders, 2nd ed. Diagnostic and Coding Manual. Westchester, IL: American Academy of Sleep Medicine, 2005.

in the wrong direction (phase advance). If melatonin is used, it is recommended that a small dose (avoid prolonged hypnotic action) be taken during the last half of the night. Taking melatonin on awakening while at the correct time for phase delay may make the individual sleepy (counterproductive). Hypnotics at bedtime can help with sleep but do not necessarily help with alertness the next day. Even if the patients gets adequate sleep, decreased circadian alertness will occur at time of CBTmin. Stimulants (caffeine) may be helpful to maintain alertness during the day in the new locale.

Crossing More than Eight Time Zones Exposure to light at the wrong time should be avoided because this may occur on the wrong side of CBTmin for appropriate adaptation. After eastward flights, avoid very early light (avoid inappropriate phase delay); on westward flights, avoid light at dusk (avoid inappropriate phase advance) for 2 to 3 days.[59] Thereafter, light at the usual times may help with adaptation. Conversely, as noted previously, some physicians recommend attempts at phase delay even if the direction of travel is eastward when more than eight time zones are crossed.

Circadian Rhythm Sleep Disorder—Shift-Work Type

The circadian rhythm sleep disorder—shift work type[1] is characterized by excessive sleepiness or insomnia temporally associated with recurring work schedule that overlaps the usual time for sleep (Box 26-14). The problem must last **at least 1 month.** A sleep log or actigraphy for at least 7 days documents circadian and sleep time misalignment. The boundary between a normal and a pathologic response to circadian stress of unnatural sleep schedule associated with shift work remains unclear. The shift-work disorder is a common problem in industrialized countries due to the need for some occupations and services to continue to function 24 hours per day. The elements of diagnostic evaluation and treatment recommended by the practice parameters of the AASM are listed in Table 26-13.[31]

Epidemiology
Up to 20% of the population in industrialized societies works in an occupation requiring shift work. The total number of night shift workers is 2% to 5% of the population. **About 5% to 10% of shift workers experience such significant insomnia or sleepiness during the shift (or day) to qualify for this disorder.**

Risk Factors
Risk factors include advancing age, possibly women greater than men, morning light exposure (long commute home or morning social obligations, this inhibits adaptive phase resetting). There are also limited data that morning types (MEQ) tend to get shorter daytime sleep after a night shift but further studies are needed.[1]

Pathophysiology
There are a number of exacerbating factors including long shifts (fatigue) and the common practice of resuming normal daytime activities and nighttime sleep on the weekends. The sleepiness at night is often due not only to the **accumulated sleep load** but, more importantly, to **loss of the circadian alerting signal.**

TABLE 26–13

Recommendations for Evaluation and Treatment of Shift-Work Disorder

TOOLS	RECOMMENDATIONS
EVALUATION	
PSG	Not routinely indicated (S)
MEQ	Insufficient evidence (O)
Circadian phase markers	Insufficient evidence (O)
Actigraphy for diagnosis	Indicated (O)
Actigraphy for response to therapy	Indicated (O)
Sleep log	Indicated (G)
THERAPY	
Planned sleep schedule	Indicated (S)
Timed light exposure	Indicated (G)
Timed melatonin	Indicated (G)
Hypnotics	Indicated (G)
Stimulants	Indicated (O) (caffeine)
Alerting agents	Indicated (G)

(S) = standard > (G) = guideline > (O) = option; MEQ = morningness-eveningness questionnaire; PSG = polysomnography.
From Morgenthaler TI, Lee-Chiong T, Alessi C, et al: Practice parameters for the clinical evaluation and treatment of circadian rhythm sleep disorders. Sleep 2007;30:1445–1459.

Sleep Logs and Diaries

Sleep logs and diaries tend to document the altered routine and the effect on sleep.

Circadian Markers

Little CBTmin data are available. Studies of DLMO suggest that night workers are quite variable in their circadian adaptation. Of note, **symptoms do not always correlate with whether or not circadian adaptation has occurred.**

Night Shift Work

The daytime sleep in night shift workers is shorter than normal (5–6 hr). The majority of workers do not have circadian adaptation due to societal obligations. They typically get light after their CBTmin on the drive home and, therefore, phase advance. Bright light during the start of the shift (before CBTmin) and avoiding light in the early morning (preventing phase advance) can potentially **move CBTmin to within the daytime sleep period.**[64] Scheduled naps before or in the early part of the shift may improve alertness.[65,66] Two-hour naps during late afternoon before the evening shift are more effective than 2-hour naps during the shift. In a simulated night shift study over five consecutive nights, Crowley and colleagues[67] studied the effects of different interventions and the effect on shifts in CBTmin and performance (Fig. 26–25). **The groups that shifted the temperature minimum to within the normal sleeping hours had improved nocturnal functioning on the psychomotor vigilance task (PVT).** They used a combination of light during the simulated shift, dark glasses during simulated drive home, and melatonin before sleep. Of interest, the groups with the latest CBTmin at baseline were the ones able to completely entrain to the new schedule.[67,68] Circadian phase

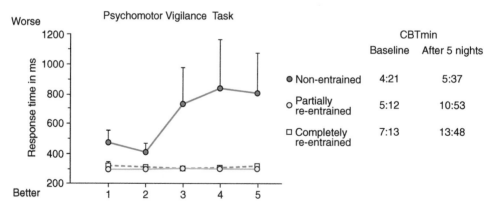

FIGURE 26–25 Change in psychomotor vigilance task (PVT) over five consecutive simulated night shifts in groups non-entrained, partially entrained, and completely re-entrained. The non-entrained group had a worsening in the PVT over five nights (increased response time). The other two groups did not have a deterioration over the five night shifts. The time of core body temperature minimum (CBTmin) is illustrated for each group at baseline and after five nights. The CBTmin shifted to within daytime sleep in the two groups with better function. Subjects were given different combinations of bright light versus dim light during the simulated night shift, dark glasses or normal sunglasses in the morning, and melatonin or placebo before sleep time. *Adapted from Crowley SJ, Tseng CU, Fogg LF, Eastman CI: Complete or partial re-entrainment improves performance, alertness, and mood during shift-work. Sleep 2004;27:1077–1087.*

was measured by DLMO with CBTmin = DLMO + 7 hours. Melatonin given before morning sleep after a night shift resulted in minimal change in total sleep time and added little to circadian shifts induced by interventions with light.[68,69] One study found a significant phase advance with melatonin in the early evening for patients who desire a prolonged sleep period before the night shift.[70]

Sallinen and associates[65] compared four nap strategies (nap duration/timing: 50 min at 1 AM, 50 min at 4 AM, 30 min at 1 AM, 30 min at 4 AM) to the no-nap condition using an experimental night shift protocol. Napping improved reaction time in the second half of the night. The early naps produced increased alertness (assessed by polysomnography sleep latency). In another study, Schweitzer and coworkers[66] showed napping before the night shift, especially when combined with caffeine, improved alertness as assessed with multiple sleep latency test (MSLT) and PVT. The alerting agent modafinil (200 mg given at the start of the night shift) is U.S. Food and Drug Administration (FDA) approved to improve alertness during shift work.[73] However, the medication did not normalize alertness. Recently, armodafinil (the R enantiomer of modafinil) was also demonstrated to be helpful in maintaining alertness during shift work.[72] Hypnotics have also been used in an attempt to improve daytime sleep. Walsh and colleagues[73] found that use of triazolam increased daytime sleep duration by about 50 minutes but did not reduce circadian sleep tendency in the early morning hours.

Rotating Shifts

There is greater sleep loss with rapidly rotating shifts than with slowly rotating shifts (slow = 3-wk periods). Clockwise rotation is better tolerated than counterclockwise due to natural tendency to phase delay.

Complications of Night Shifts

A number of complications of shift work have been proposed including gastrointestinal disturbances (constipation/ diarrhea), obesity, miscarriage, drug dependency, and social and family life disturbances.

Treatment of Shift-Work Disorder

The recommended treatments for shift-work disorder (SWD) are listed in Table 26–13 and Box 26–15. Planned sleep schedule (naps), timed bright light exposure, timed melatonin administration, stimulants (caffeine), and alerting agents (modafinil) were also listed as indicated with various levels of recommendation in the AASM circadian practice parameters.[31] The goals of treatments include interventions to (1) modify circadian rhythms to ameliorate symptoms of circadian rhythm misalignment, (2) decrease sleep load during the night (naps or hypnotics before daytime sleep), or (3) increase alertness (caffeine or modafinil). Stimulants were given the lowest level of recommendation, but evidence for their efficacy is growing. There are actually less convincing data for daytime melatonin than for stimulants. **The rationale behind timed bright light exposure is the supposition that having CBTmin closer to (or within) the daytime**

BOX 26–15

Night Shift Treatment Recommendations

- Bright light for 3–6 hr during the start of shift—phase delay.
- Short scheduled naps (preshift or during shift).
- Avoid bright light on the way home in the AM (use dark goggles if trip home is after sunrise to avoid phase advances).
- Quiet dark sleep environment at home during sleep.
- Melatonin administered in the morning at bedtime (hypnotic and phase delay effects).
- Go to bed as soon as patient reaches home.
- Stimulants/alerting agents at the start of the shift
  - Caffeine (250–400 mg) during first 2 hours of night shift.
  - Modafinil 200 mg (or armodafinil 150 mg) taken 30–60 minutes before start of the night shift (FDA approved for treatment of sleepiness in shift work)
- Hypnotics before daytime sleep—can increase total sleep time but do not help alertness at night.

FDA = U.S. Food and Drug Administration.

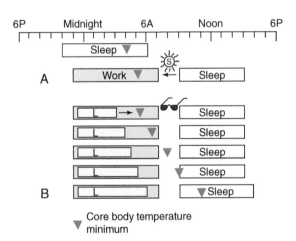

FIGURE 26–26 Interventions for night shift work. **Top line,** A normal sleep period and CBTmin. **A,** Light and activity during the night work shift cause some phase delay. However, light on the commute home opposes this process (causes phase advance). **B,** CBTmin is shifted toward daytime sleep by using bright light (L) during the first part of the work period (shift) and wearing dark goggles on the commute home. Note that the duration of light during the night shift can increase as the CBTmin is progressively delayed.

sleep period will improve sleep quality and amount (Fig. 26–26). Patients should minimize light on the commute home (dark goggles) if possible because this tends to phase advance. In some studies, bright light at the start of the night shift induced a beneficial phase delay.[64,67,68] Bright light also has a direct alerting effect. Melatonin has been used before morning sleep after the night shift both for its soporific effects and for its phase delaying effects (to delay CBTmin into morning sleep time). However, Crowley and colleagues[67,68] found no improvement in morning sleep or phase delay with melatonin given at 8:30 AM (1.8 mg sustained release). The soporific effects of melatonin were also not significant for sleep after night shift work.[69] Another study showed the phase shifting response to melatonin 0.5 mg given at 800 to 1000 hours after the night shift to be variable (compared with placebo), with only a minority of night workers having a phase shifting response.[71] Of note, field studies of actual patients often show much smaller effects of either light or melatonin treatment on shift workers. For example, one study using only 30 minutes of light exposure or 3 mg of melatonin before bedtime showed small effects.[72] In this study, melatonin added 15 to 20 minutes to daytime sleep whereas bright light (short duration) had minimal effects. Napping either before the night shift or during the shift can be helpful.[65,66] Short naps are preferred to decrease sleep inertia. Stimulants at the start of the shift (caffeine, modafinil, or armodafinil) may be helpful but do not completely reverse the fall in alertness that occurs near the CBTmin.[66,73,74] A dark, quiet bedroom or hypnotics may help daytime sleep. As previously noted, whereas use of hypnotics can increase the duration of daytime sleep time, during the day, they have not been shown to improve alertness in the early morning hours during shift work.[75]

CRSD—Due to Medical Condition (Box 26–16)

Disorders Associated with CRSD

1. Dementia—decreased amplitude or absent circadian rhythms.
2. Movement disorders (Parkinson's disease).
3. Blindness.
4. Hepatic encephalopathy.

Treatment

Treatment of underlying medical disorder may or may not improve the CRSD component.

BOX 26–16

Circadian Rhythm Sleep Disorder Due to Medical Condition

A. There is a complaint of insomnia or excessive daytime sleepiness related to alterations of the circadian time-keeping system or misalignment between endogenous circadian rhythm and exogenous factors that affect the timing or duration of sleep.

B. An underlying medical or neurologic disorder predominantly accounts for the circadian sleep disorder.

C. Sleep log or actigraphy monitoring (with sleep diaries) for at least 7 days demonstrates disturbed or low-amplitude circadian rhythmicity.

D. The sleep disturbance is not better explained by another current sleep disorder, medical or neurologic disorder, mental disorder, medication use, or substance use disorder.

From American Academy of Sleep Medicine: ICSD-2 International Classification of Sleep Disorders, 2nd ed. Diagnostic and Coding Manual. Westchester, IL: American Academy of Sleep Medicine, 2005.

CRSD—Not Otherwise Specified

CRSD Due to Drug or Substance

The criteria for CRSD due to drug or substance include disorders that (1) satisfy criteria for a CRSD, (2) are due to a drug or substance, and (3) do not meet criteria for other circadian rhythm disorders.

CLINICAL REVIEW QUESTIONS

1. A 25-year-old man has difficulty falling asleep until 3 AM. On weekends, he sleeps until 10:30 to 11:00 AM. On work days, he uses an alarm clock to wake up at 7:00 AM but has difficulty getting out of bed and is sleepy during the day. What time do you recommend light therapy be initially administered?
   A. 6:00 AM.
   B. 7:00 AM.
   C. 8:00 AM.
   D. 10:00 AM.

2. What is the average circadian period in humans?
   A. 23.8 hr.
   B. 24.0 hr.
   C. 24.2 hr.
   D. 24.6 hr.

3. A graph of core body temperature is shown in Figure 26–27. Bright light at which point (A, B, C, D, or E) results in the maximum phase advance?

4. Which of the following is NOT true about photic input to the SCN?
   A. Photic information travels to the SCN via the RHT.
   B. The major photosensors for entrainment of the SCN are the rods and cones.
   C. Light can entrain some blind individuals.
   D. The SCN pathway mediating inhibition of melatonin travels through the superior cervical ganglion.

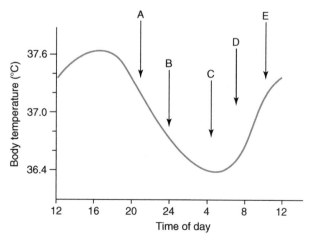

FIGURE 26–27 What should the timing of light be for maximum phase advance (A, B, C, D, E)?

5. Point mutation in which gene has been associated with ASPD?
   A. *Clock*.
   B. Time.
   C. *hPer2*.
   D. Alarm.

6. What intervention would be most helpful in a patient with ASPD?
   A. Evening light.
   B. Morning light.
   C. Evening melatonin.
   D. Morning melatonin.

7. What set of interventions would be most helpful for a night shift worker (Table 26–14)?

8. A blind patient is found to have the non–24-hour circadian rhythm disorder. His desired bedtime is 11 PM. What treatment do you recommend?
   A. Melatonin 5.0 mg at 8 AM.
   B. Melatonin 5.0 mg at 10 PM.
   C. Melatonin 0.5 mg at 7 PM.
   D. Melatonin 0.5 mg at 10 PM.

9. A businessman travels 5 hours eastward. What time should light be avoided in the new time zone?
   A. 6 AM–9 AM.
   B. 11 AM–2 PM.
   C. 2 PM–6 PM.

10. A patient with the DSPD has a habitual sleep time of 3 AM and wake time of 11 AM on the weekends. When should melatonin be administered?
   A. 3 AM.
   B. 2 AM.
   C. 12 midnight.
   D. 9 PM.

11. Which of the following is **not** true about DLMO?
   A. Occurs 2–3 hours before habitual bedtime.
   B. Occurs 1 hour before habitual bedtime.

C. Measured with the subject in dim light.
D. Typical threshold values are 3 pg/mL for salivary and 10 pg/mL for plasma melatonin.

12. A patient with the delayed sleep phase syndrome has a typical wake time on the weekends of 1 PM. He typically has to awaken at 8:30 AM to make a 10:00 AM class. He starts treatment with light by walking to class to get bright light exposure (~9–10 AM). Unfortunately, using this regimen, he is unable to fall asleep any earlier. What do you recommend for initial treatment?
   A. Wear dark glasses on walk to 10 AM class, get bright light exposure after 12 noon.
   B. Wake up at 8 AM, light box for 1 hour, light exposure on walk to 10 AM class.
   C. Wear dark glasses on walk to 10AM class, bright light exposure after 3 PM.
   D. Continue present light exposure, add melatonin 5 hours before habitual sleep time.

Answers

1. **D.** This patient has the DSPD. It is important to use bright light treatment after the CBTmin. The timing of the CBTmin is not known but can be estimated from the spontaneous wake time. In normal subjects, the CBTmin occurs about 2 hours before wake time. It may be somewhat earlier in patients with DSPD. With a normal wake time of 11:00 AM, one could estimate a CBTmin around 9 AM or slightly earlier. Of interest, the patient is exposed to light on his way to work (6–7 AM). This may be on the phase advanced side of his temperature minimum and worsen the problem. He should wear dark glasses on the way to work in the morning.

2. **C.** 24.2 hours.

3. **D.** The maximum phase advance for bright light occurs about 3–4 hours after the CBTmin. C is at the CBTmin, the transition between the phase delay and the phase advance regions. Light at A and B would phase delay. Light at E would have less phase advancing effect.

4. **B.** The major photosensors are the retinal ganglion cells containing melanopsin.

5. **C.** Mutation of *hPer2* gene has been associated with familial ASPD.

6. **A.** Evening light will cause phase delay. Morning melatonin will also cause a phase delay, but the hypnotic effects are undesirable for most patients.

7. **A.** Bright light at the start of the shift, dark glasses on the way home, going to bed on arrival at home, and a nap before the shift are suggested interventions. Light at the end of the shift, on the way home, or during the first hours at home could phase advance. A phase delay so that CBTmin is within the daytime sleep period is desirable.

TABLE 26–14			
Interventions for Night Shift Worker			
A	Bright light start of shift	Dark glasses drive home	Nap before night shift
B	Bright light end of shift	Dark glasses drive home	Nap before night shift
C	Bright light start of shift	Delay bedtime until 11 AM	Nap before night shift
D	Bright light end of shift	Delay bedtime until 11 AM	Nap before night shift

8. D. Melatonin given 1 hour before the desired bedtime is recommended. Although 5 mg may work, some patients will fail to entrain on 5 mg but entrain on a lower dose. However, the AASM practice parameters did not recommend a specific time or dose.

9. A. If the baseline CBTmin is assumed to be 4 AM, this corresponds to 9 AM in the new time zone. The patient must phase advance for adaptation. Light for several hours **before** the CBTmin induces the most significant phase delay. Light exposure should be avoided before 9 AM and pursued from 11 AM to 2 PM to induce the maximum phase advancing effect. Light from 6 to 9 AM may cause phase delay. Light at 2 to 6 PM is so far away from the CBTmin that it has minimal effect.

10. D. Melatonin should be administered 5 to 7 hours before habitual sleep time.

11. B. DLMO occurs about 2 to 3 hours before habitual sleep time.

12. A. The patient's CBTmin is probably around 11 AM (2 hr before typical wake time on weekends). Bright light exposure before 11 AM causes an unwanted phase delay. The best option is to minimize light exposure before 11 AM and then seek bright light exposure for 1–2 hours after 12 noon (after CBTmin for phase advance). Bright light exposure at 3 PM will be less effective than light exposure closer to the CBTmin. Melatonin 5 hours before the habitual bedtime may help, but the most important intervention is use of the correct exposure to light.

REFERENCES

1. American Academy of Sleep Medicine: ICSD-2 International Classification of Sleep Disorders, 2nd ed. Diagnostic and Coding Manual. Westchester, IL: American Academy of Sleep Medicine, 2005.
2. Zee PC, Manthena P: The brain's master circadian clock: implications and opportunities for therapy of sleep disorders. Sleep Med Rev 2007;11:59–70.
3. Czeisler CA, Duffy JF, Shanahan TL, et al: Stability, precision, and nearly 24 hour period of the human circadian pacemaker. Sleep 1999;284:2177–2181.
4. Gooley JJ, Saper CB: Anatomy of the mammalian circadian system. In Kryger MH, Roth T, Dement WC (eds): Principles and Practice of Sleep Medicine. Philadelphia: Elsevier Saunders, 2005, pp. 335–350.
5. Dijk DJ, Archer SN: Light, sleep, and circadian rhythms: together again. PLoS 2009;7:3000145.
6. Brzezinski A: Melatonin in humans. N Engl J Med 1997; 336:186–195.
7. Reid KJ, Zee PC: Circadian rhythm disorders. Semin Neurol 2009;29:393–405.
8. Wyatt JK, Dijk D, Ritz-De Cecco A, et al: Sleep-facilitating effect of exogenous melatonin in healthy young men and women is circadian-phase dependent. Sleep 2006;29:609–618.
9. Edgar DM, Dement WC, Fuller CA: Effect of SCN lesions on sleep in the squirrel monkey: evidence for opponent processes in sleep-wake regulation. J Neuorsci 1993;13:1065–1079.
10. Duffy JF, Dijk DJ, Klerman EB, Czeisler CA: Later endogenous circadian temperature nadir relative to an earlier wake time in older people. Am J Physiol 1998;275:R1478–R1487.
11. Fahey CD, Zee PC: Circadian rhythm sleep disorder and phototherapy. Psychiatr Clin North Am 2006;29:989–1007.
12. Czeisler CA, Buxton OM, Khalsa SBS: The human circadian timing system and sleep-wake regulation. In Kryger MH, Roth T, Dement WC (eds): Principles and Practice of Sleep Medicine, 4th ed. Philadelphia: Elsevier Saunders, 2005, pp. 375–394.
13. Wyatt JK, Stepanski EJ, Kirkby J: Circadian phase in delayed sleep phase syndrome: predictors and temporal stability across multiple assessments. Sleep 2006;29:1075–1080.
14. Sack RK, Brandes RW, Kendall AR, Lewy AJ: Entrainment of free-running circadian rhythms by melatonin in blind people. N Engl J Med 2000;343;1070–1077.
15. Khalsa SBS, Jewett ME, Cajocen C, Czeisler CA: A phase response curve to single bright light pulses in human subjects. J Physiol 2003;549:945–952.
16. Lu BS, Zee PC: Circadian rhythm sleep disorders. Chest 2006;130:1915–1923.
17. Barion A, Zee PC: A clinical approach to circadian rhythm sleep disorders. Sleep Med 2007;8:566–577.
18. Shirani A, St. Louis EK: Illuminating rationale and uses for light therapy. J Clin Sleep Med 2009;5:155–163.
19. Zeitzer JM, Dijk DJ, Kronauer RE, et al: Sensitivity of human circadian pacemaker to nocturnal light: melatonin resetting and suppression. J Physiol 2000;526:695–702.
20. Lockley SW, Brainard GC, Czeisler CA: High sensitivity of the human circadian melatonin rhythm to resetting by short wave length light. J Clin Endocrinol Metab 2003;88:4502–4505.
21. Smith MR, Eastman CR: Phase delaying the human circadian clock with blue-enriched polychromatic light. Chronobiol Int 2009;26:709–725.
22. Rimmer DW, Boivin DB, Shanahan TL, et al: Dynamic resetting of the human circadian pacemaker by intermittent bright light. Am J Physiol Regul Integr Comp Physiol 2000; 279:R1574–R1579.
23. Gronifer C, Wright KP, Kronauer RE, et al: Efficacy of a single sequence of intermittent bright light pulses for delaying circadian phase in humans. Am J Physiol Endocrinol Metab 2004; 287:E174–E181.
24. Lewy AJ, Bauer VK, Ahmed S, et al: The human phase response curve (PRC) to melatonin is about 12 hours out of phase with the PRC to light. Chronobiol Int 1998;15:71–83.
25. Burgess HJ, Revell VL, Eastman CI: A three pulse phase response curve to 3 milligrams of melatonin in humans. J Physiol 2008;586:639–647.
26. Eastman CI, Burgess HJ: How to travel the world without jet lag. Sleep Med Clin 2009;4:241–255.
27. Vitaterna MH, Pinto LH, Turek FW: Molecular genetic basis for mammalian circadian rhythms. In Kryger MH, Roth T, Dement WC (eds): Principles and Practice of Sleep Medicine, 4th ed. Philadelphia: Elsevier Saunders, 2005, pp. 335–350.
28. Piggins HD: Human clock genes. Ann Med 2002;34:394–400.
29. Sack RL, Auckley D, Auger R, et al: Circadian rhythm sleep disorders: part I, basic principles, shift work and jet lag disorders. Sleep 2007;30:1460–1483.
30. Sack RL, Auckley D, Auger R, et al: Circadian rhythm sleep disorders: part II, advanced sleep phase disorder, delayed sleep phase disorder, free-running disorder, and irregular sleep-wake rhythm. Sleep 2007;30:1484–1501.
31. Morgenthaler TI, Lee-Chiong T, Alessi C, et al: Practice parameters for the clinical evaluation and treatment of circadian rhythm sleep disorders. Sleep 2007;30:1445–1459.
32. Horne JA, Ostberg O: A self-assessment questionnaire to determine morningness-eveningness in human circadian rhythms. Int J Chronobiol 1976;4:97–110.

33. Wyatt JK: Delayed sleep phase syndrome: pathophysiology and treatment options. Sleep 2004;27:1195–1203.

34. Archer SN, Robillard DL, Skene DJ, et al: A length polymorphism in the circadian clock gene Per3 is linked to delayed sleep phase syndrome and extreme diurnal preference. Sleep 2003;26:413–415.

35. Hohjoh H, Takasu M, Shishikura K, et al: Significant association of the arylalkylamine N-acetyltransferase (AA-NAT) gene with delayed sleep phase syndrome. Neurogenetics 2003; 4:151–153.

36. Uchiyama M, Okawa M, Shibui K, et al: Altered phase relation between sleep timing and core body temperature in delayed sleep phase syndrome and non-24 hour sleep-wake syndromes in humans. Neurosci Lett 2000;294:101–104.

37. Watanabe T, Kajimura N, Masaaki K, et al: Sleep and circadian rhythm disturbances in patients with delayed sleep phase syndrome. Sleep 2003;26:657–661.

38. Mundey K, Benloucif S, Harsanyhi K, et al: Phase-dependent treatment of delayed sleep phase syndrome with melatonin. Sleep 2005;28:1271–1278.

39. Czeisler CA, Richardson GS, Coleman RM, et al: Chronotherapy: resetting the circadian clocks of patients with delayed sleep phase insomnia. Sleep 1981;4:1–21.

40. Rosenthal NE, Joseph-Vanderpool JR, Levendosky AA, et al: Phase-shifting effects of bright morning light as treatment for delayed sleep phase syndrome. Sleep 1990;13:354–361.

41. Watanabe T, Kajimura N, Kato M, et al: Effects of phototherapy in patients with delayed sleep phase syndrome. Psychiatry Clin Neurosci 1999;53:231–233.

42. Bjorvatn B, Pallesen S: A practical approach to circadian rhythm sleep disorders. Sleep Med Rev 2009;13:47–60.

43. Nagtegall JE, Kerkhof A, Smits MG, et al: Delayed sleep phase syndrome: A placebo controlled cross-over study on the effects of melatonin administered five hours before the individual dim light melatonin onset. J Sleep Res 1998;7:135–143.

44. Revell VL, Burgess HJ, Gazda CJ, et al: Advancing human circadian rhythms with afternoon melatonin and morning intermittent bright light. J Clin Endocrinol Metab 2006;91:54–59.

45. Jones CR, Campbell SS, Zone SE, et al: Familial advanced sleep phase syndrome: a short-period circadian rhythm variant in humans. Nat Med 1999;5:1062–1065.

46. Toh KL, Jones CR, Yan HE, et al: An hPer2 phosphorylation site mutation in familial advanced sleep phase syndrome. Science 2001;291:1040–1043.

47. Auger RR: Advanced related sleep complaints and advanced sleep phase disorder. Sleep Med Clin 2009;4:219–227.

48. Moldofsky H, Musisi S, Phillipson EA: Treatment of a case of advanced sleep phase syndrome by phase advance chronotherapy. Sleep 1986;9:61–65.

49. Lack L, Wright H, Kemp K, et al: The treatment of early morning awakening insomnia with two evenings of bright light. Sleep 2005;28:616–623.

50. Zee PC, Vitiello MV: Circadian rhythm disorder: irregular sleep wake rhythm. Sleep Med Clin 2009;4:213–218.

51. Ancoli-Israel S, Martin JL, Kripke DF, et al: Effect of light treatment on sleep and circadian rhythms in demented nursing home patients. J Am Geriatr Soc 2002;50:282–289.

52. Singer C, Trachtenberg RE, Kaye J, et al: A multicenter, placebo controlled trial of melatonin for sleep disturbance in Alzheimer's disease. Sleep 2003;26:893–901.

53. Riemersma-ven der Lek RF, Swaab DF, Twisk J, et al: Effect of bright light and melatonin on cognitive and noncognitive function in elderly residents of group care facilities. JAMA 2008; 299:2642–2655.

54. Pillar G, Shahar E, Peled N, et al: Melatonin improves sleep wake patterns in psychomotor retarded children. Pediatr Neurol 2000;23:225–228.

55. Hayakawa T, Uchiyama M, Kamei Y, et al: Clinical analysis of sighted patients with non-24 hour sleep-wake syndrome. Sleep 2005;28:945–952.

56. Boivin DB, James FO, Santo BA, et al: Non-24-hour sleep-wake syndrome following a car accident. Neurology 2003;60: 1841–1843.

57. Lewy AJ, Emens JS, Lefler BJ, et al: Melatonin entrains free-running blind people according to a physiological dose response curve. Chronobiol Int 2005;22:1093–1106.

58. Lewy AJ, Bauer VK, Hasler BP, et al: Capturing the circadian rhythms of free-running blind individuals with 0.5 mg of melatonin. Brain Res 2001;918:96–100.

59. Sack RL: Jet lag. N Engl J Med 2010;362:440–447.

60. Eastman CI, Gazda CJ, Burgess HJ, et al: Advancing circadian rhythms before eastward flight: a strategy to prevent or reduce jet lag. Sleep 2005;28:33–44.

61. Revell VL, Eastman CI: How to trick mother nature into letting you fly around or stay up all night. J Biol Rhythm 2005;20:353–365.

62. Jamieson AO, Zammit GK, Rosenberg RS, et al: Zolpidem reduces the sleep disturbance of jet lag. Sleep Med 2001;2: 423–430.

63. Rosenberg RP, Bogan RK, Tiller JM, et al: A phase 3, double-blind, randomized, placebo-controlled study of armodafinil for excessive sleepiness associated with jet lag disorder. Mayo Clin Proc 2010;85:630–638.

64. Boivin DB, James FO: Circadian adaptation to night-shift work by judicious light and dark exposure. J Biol Rhythms 2002; 17:556–567.

65. Sallinen M, Harma M, Akerstedt T, et al: Promoting alertness with a short nap during a night shift. J Sleep Res 1998;7: 240–247.

66. Schweitzer PK, Randazzo AC, Stone K, et al: Laboratory and field studies of naps and caffeine as practical countermeasures for sleep-wake problems associated with night work. Sleep 2006;29:39–50.

67. Crowley SJ, Tseng C, Fogg LF, Eastman CI: Complete or partial re-entrainment improves performance, alertness, and mood during shift-work. Sleep 2004;27:1077–1087.

68. Crowley SJ, Tseng C, Fogg LF, et al: Combinations of bright light, scheduled dark, sunglasses, and melatonin to facilitate circadian entrainment to night shift work. J Biol Rhythms 2003; 18:513–523.

69. Smith MR, Lee C, Crowley SJ, et al: Morning melatonin has limited benefit as a soporific for daytime sleep after night work. Chronobiol Int 2005;22:873–888.

70. Sharkey KM, Eastman CI: Melatonin phase shift human circadian rhythms in a placebo controlled simulated night-work study. Am J Physiol Regul Integr Comp Physiol 2002;282: R454–R463.

71. Sack RL, Lewy AJ: Melatonin as a chronobiotic: treatment of circadian desynchrony in night shift workers and the blind. J Biol Rhythm 1997;12:595–603.

72. Bjorvatn B, Stangenes K, Oyane N, et al: Randomized placebo-controlled field study of the effects of bright light and melatonin in adaptation to shift work. Scand J Work Environ Health 2007;33:204–214.

73. Czeisler CA, Walsh JK, Roth T, et al: Modafinil for excessive sleepiness associated with shift-work sleep disorder. N Engl J Med 2005;353:476–486.

74. Czeisler CA, Walsh JK, Wesnew KA, et al: Armodafinil for treatment of excessive sleepiness associated with shift work disorder: a randomized controlled study. Mayo Clin Proc 2009; 84:958–972.

75. Walsh JK, Sugerman JL, Muehlback MJ, et al: Physiological sleep tendency on a simulated night shift: adaptation and effects of triazolam. Sleep 1988;12:251–264.

Chapter 27

Clinical Electroencephalography and Nocturnal Epilepsy

Chapter Points

- Nocturnal epilepsy can be difficult to differentiate from parasomnias because some patients have seizures only at night, scalp EEG findings may not be visible during seizures, bizarre movements can occur during partial seizures, consciousness can be maintained, and minimal postictal confusion may be present in some cases.
- NFLE manifests as three syndromes: paroxysmal arousals (mimics confusional arousals), nocturnal paroxysmal dystonia (dystonic posturing), and episodic wandering (mimics sleepwalking). The paroxysmal arousals and nocturnal paroxysmal dystonia episodes tend to be brief.
- Factors favoring NFLE over a parasomnia include multiple episodes per night, stereotypical manifestations, onset out of stage N2 versus N3, and certain behaviors (e.g., cycling, fencing, pelvic thrusting) as well as immediate alertness after the episode.
- In roughly 50% of the cases of NFLE, there is no abnormality in the scalp EEG during the seizure (other than artifact due to body movement).
- The partial seizures of TLE are typically complex partial seizures (consciousness is impaired during the seizure). The partial seizures of FLE may be either complex or simple (no impairment of consciousness).
- Seizures from the supplemental motor area may occur with intact responsiveness and no postictal confusion. Classic manifestations of seizures from the supplementary motor area include fencing with head turned away from the outstretched arm, kicking, laughing, or pelvic thrusting. Unlike psychogenic activity, there is an abrupt onset and offset.
- Video PSG is essential for evaluation of patients with possible nocturnal epilepsy. A substantial number of patients with NFLE will not have either ictal or interictal EEG findings and the type of body movements (seminology) can be very helpful in arriving at a correct diagnosis. Using an extended EEG

montage and visualization of waveforms in a 10-second window is recommended.
- The focal seizures of FLE are more likely to occur at night than during the day. The focal seizures of TLE are more likely to occur during the day than during the night. FLE events during the day are more likely to generalize. TLE events during the night are more likely to generalize compared with those occurring during the day.
- Because mastoid electrodes are fairly near the temporal lobes, interictal activity associated with TLE can often be easily seen in standard PSG montages. For example, a left temporal spike may be visible in derivations containing M_1. The spike will be more prominent in C_4-M_1 than in C_3-M_2 even though the spike is on the left.
- Changing to a 10-second window is essential to accurately identify interictal activity because spikes may be difficult to see in the 30-second window. It is useful to examine paroxysmal changes in EEG tracings in a 10-second window to avoid incorrectly assuming that ictal activity is an artifact.

ELECTROENCEPHALOGRAPHIC MONITORING

The international 10-20 system[1,2] for electrode placement for electroencephalographic (EEG) monitoring is illustrated in Figure 27–1. Each electrode is represented by a letter that represents the underlying area or lobe of the brain (F_p = frontopolar; F = frontal; P = parietal; O = occipital; T = temporal) (Fig. 27–2) and numerical subscripts representing position. The odd subscripts are on the left and the even on the right, and the "z" subscripts refer to electrodes in the midline.[1,2] The left and right auricular (earlobe) electrodes are A_1 and A_2. In sleep monitoring, these are actually placed on the mastoids and termed M_1 and M_2.[3] Figure 27–1 illustrates the new electrode nomenclature[1] in which T_7, T_8, P_7, and P_8 have replaced T_3, T_4, T_5, and T_6. In the new nomenclature, all electrodes in a given sagittal plane have the same subscript (F_7, T_7, P_7) and most electrodes in the same coronal plane have the same letter (P_7, P_3, P_z, P_4, P_8). However, many

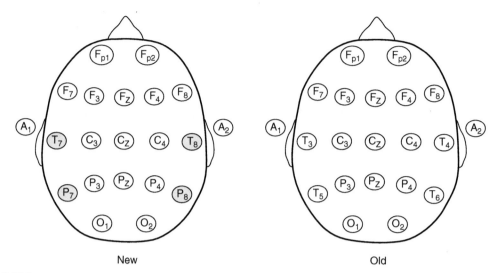

FIGURE 27–1 Electrode nomenclature (new and old terminology). T_3 and T_4 are replaced by T_7 and T_8 and T_5 and T_6 are replaced by P_7 and P_8.

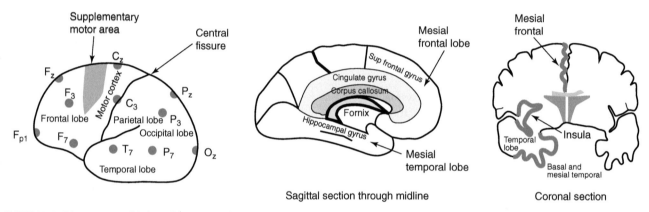

Sagittal section through midline   Coronal section

FIGURE 27–2 Schematic views of the brain illustrate areas of interest for epilepsy and electroencephalography (EEG) monitoring. The central fissure is also known as the Rolandic fissure.

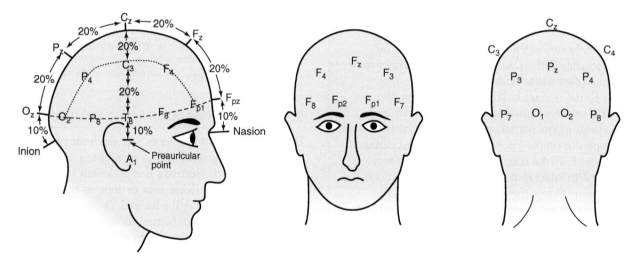

FIGURE 27–3 The 10–20 system of electrode placement. All electrodes are placed either 10% or 20% of the distance between two standard landmarks.

EEG laboratories still use the old electrode nomenclature as does the majority of the published literature on epilepsy. Of note, the *10-20 electrode position*[2] refers to the fact that electrodes are positioned at 10% or 20% of the distance between landmarks such as nasion, inion, or the preauricular points (Fig. 27–3).

BIPOLAR MONITORING AND STANDARD MONTAGES

A **derivation** is the voltage difference between electrodes: for example, F_{p1}-F_3 is the voltage difference between electrodes F_{p1} and F_3. By electroencephalography (EEG) convention, if

F_{p1} is more negative than F_3, the deflection is up.[4,5] A set of derivations is called a **montage.** Montages are designed with a particular purpose in mind. Standard montages for sleep monitoring were illustrated in Chapter 1. Tables 27–1 and 27–2 show standard clinical EEG montages.[6] **Bipolar longitudinal montages** (Fig. 27–4; see also Table 27–1) sequentially compare two adjacent electrodes in chains covering the head in an anteroposterior (AP) direction ("double banana"). In the most frequently used variant (LB-18.1), the chains start at the left temporal area and then progressively move toward the right. Bipolar transverse montages compare two electrodes in chains in the transverse directions (Fig. 27–5; see also Table 27–2). **Referential montages** compare electrodes with the ipsilateral auricular electrodes A_1 and A_2 (see Table 27–2). Different laboratories may display the electrodes in a given montage in different sequences. In modern digital EEG recording, all electrodes are usually recorded against a common reference. Then any two electrodes may be compared by digitally subtracting the signals $(F_7\text{-ref}) - (P_7\text{-ref}) = F_7\text{-}P_7$. Thus, one can change the display montage while recording or later during study review. Digital recording also allows one to visualize multiple time scales. The polysomnography (PSG) window to stage sleep is 30 seconds but the clinical EEG window is 10 seconds. The 10-second time window allows detection of brief, sharply contoured waveforms that may signify seizure activity.

Longitudinal Biopolar

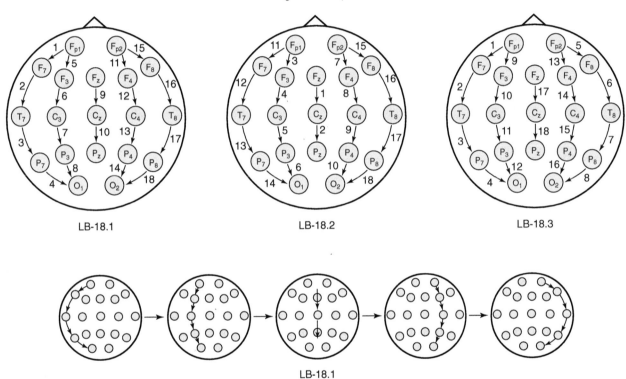

FIGURE 27–4 Longitudinal bipolar montage chains. LB-18.1, LB-18.2, and LB-18.3 are three methods of arranging the derivations for display.

Transverse bipolar

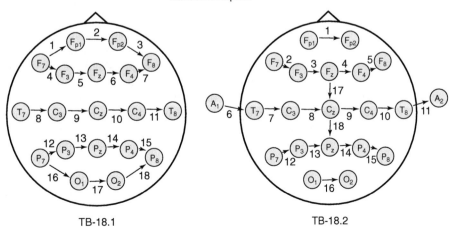

FIGURE 27–5 Transverse bipolar montages.

TABLE 27–1

Longitudinal Bipolar (AP Bipolar) 18-Channel "Double Banana"

LB-18.1		LB-18.2		LB-18.3	
$F_{p1}-F_7$ F_7-T_7 T_7-P_7 P_7-O_1	Left temporal	F_z-C_z C_z-P_z	Vertex	$F_{p1}-F_7$ F_7-T_7 T_7-P_7 P_7-O_1	Left temporal
$F_{p1}-F_3$ F_3-C_3 C_3-P_3 P_3-O_1	Left parasagittal	$F_{p1}-F_3$ F_3-C_3 C_3-P_3 P_3-O_1	Left parasagittal	$F_{p2}-F_8$ F_8-T_8 T_8-P_8 P_8-O_2	Right temporal
F_z-C_z C_z-P_z	Vertex	$F_{p2}-F_4$ F_4-C_4 C_4-P_4 P_4-O_2	Right parasagittal	$F_{p1}-F_3$ F_3-C_3 C_3-P_3 P_3-O_1	Left parasagittal
$F_{p2}-F_4$ F_4-C_4 C_4-P_4 P_4-O_2	Right parasagittal	$F_{p1}-F_7$ F_7-T_7 T_7-P_7 P_7-O_1	Left temporal	$F_{p2}-F_4$ F_4-C_4 C_4-P_4 P_4-O_2	Right parasagittal
$F_{p2}-F_8$ F_8-T_8 T_8-P_8 P_8-O_2	Right temporal	$F_{p2}-F_8$ F_8-T_8 T_8-P_8 P_8-O_2	Right temporal	F_z-C_z C_z-P_z	Vertex

From American Clinical Neurophysiology Society: Guideline 6: a proposal for standard montages to be used in clinical EEG. J Clin Neurophysiol 2006;23:111–117.

If the capacity to add a few electrodes to traditional sleep monitoring exists, one can increase the ability to detect epileptiform activity. For example, one could add two electrodes (T_7, T_8). The derivations F_3-T_7, T_7-O_1, F_4-T_8, and T_8-O_2 would add coverage over much of the frontal and temporal areas. These areas are the predominant foci of seizures occurring mainly during sleep. Other clinicians have utilized the addition of F_z, C_z, F_7, and F_8 to the usual PSG electrodes.[7] The addition of synchronized digital video monitoring to nocturnal EEG or PSG recording greatly enhances the ability of the clinician to diagnose nocturnal events.[8] As is discussed later, many nocturnal seizure disorders are not associated with scalp EEG findings and the patient's actions during the seizure (seminology) may be very helpful in determining whether an episode is likely a parasomnia or nocturnal epilepsy.[8]

WAVEFORM AND SEIZURE TERMINOLOGY

The terminology and identification of epileptic seizures and interictal activity is challenging for physicians without extensive training in EEG (Table 27–3). A **transient** is any isolated wave or complex that stands out compared with background activity. A **spike** is defined as a transient with a pointed peak and a duration of **20 to 70 msec** (Fig. 27–6). On a 30-second page, spikes look like a single vertical line. A **sharp wave** is a transient with a deflection of **70 to 200 msec**.

A **spike and wave complex** is a spike followed by a slow wave (usually wide and often higher amplitude). **Polyspike** complexes often consist of multiple spikes superimposed on

a slow wave. The term **epileptiform activity** literally means "EEG activity resembling that found in patients with epilepsy." This is a somewhat circular definition. **Interictal activity** is defined as abnormal EEG activity that occurs between seizures. Epileptiform activity includes spikes, spike and waves, and polyspike complexes. Abnormal sharp waves are also considered epileptiform or interictal activity. Of course, sharp waves can be normal (e.g., vertex sharp waves). Artifacts can sometimes mimic spikes or spikes and waves. In general, true spike and wave complexes have a "field" (Box 27–1). That is, **true spike and wave activity should be seen in derivations containing several contiguous electrodes.** If a spike and wave is seen only in a single derivation, the activity is usually be an artifact.

Because seizures do not always appear during a given recording (see Box 27–1), the physician reading an EEG or PSG searches for spikes and/or abnormal sharp waves that may represent the interictal footprint of possible seizure activity. However, it should be noted that not all patients with spikes have seizures and not all patients with seizures have detectable interictal activity. Spikes represent abnormal brain activity that is seen as an area of negativity at the scalp. Spikes can be localized (negativity at the scalp over one area of the brain) or appear diffusely. Focal seizures usually, though not invariably, begin at the same location as the interictal spikes. The classic spike is followed by a **slow wave**. Although most common postictally, spike and sharp waves will occur sporadically at any time and may have a slight increase preictally. Using the usual 30-second time window, it may be difficult to appreciate spikes. A switch to a 10-second

TABLE 27–2

Transverse Bipolar and Referential Montages (18 Channels)

TRANSVERSE BIPOLAR		REFERENTIAL		
TB-18.1	TB-18.2	R-18.1	R-18.2	R-18.3
F_7-F_{p1}	F_{p1}-F_{p2}	F_7-A_1	F_z-A_1	F_7-A_1
F_{p1}-F_{p2}		T_7-A_1	P_z-A_2	F_8-A_2
F_{p2}-F_8	F_7-F_3	P_7-A_1		T_7-A_1
	F_3-F_z		F_{p1}-A_1	T_8-A_2
F_7-F_3	F_z-F_4	F_{p1}-A_1	F_{p2}-A_2	P_7-A_1
F_3-F_z	F_4-F_8	F_3-A_1	F_3-A_1	P_8-A_2
F_z-F_4		C_3-A_1	F_4-A_2	
F_4-F_8	A_1-T_7	P_3-A_1	C_3-A_1	F_{p1}-A_1
	T_7-C_3	O_1-A_1	C_4-A_2	F_{p2}-A_2
T_7-C_3	C_3-C_z		P_3-A_1	F_3-A_1
C_3-C_z	C_z-C_4	F_z-A_1	P_4-A_2	F_4-A_2
C_z-C_4	C_4-T_8	P_z-A_1	O_1-A_1	C_3-A_1
C_4-T_8	T_8-A_2		O_2-A_2	C_4-A_2
		F_{p2}-A_2		P_3-A_1
P_7-P_3	P_7-P_3	F_4-A_2	F_7-A_1	P_4-A_2
P_3-P_z	P_3-P_z	C_4-A_2	F_8-A_2	O_1-A_1
P_z-P_4	P_z-P_4	P_4-A_2	T_7-A_1	O_2-A_2
P_4-P_8	P_4-P_8	O_2-A_2	T_8-A_2	
			P_7-A_1	F_z-A_1
P_7-O_1	O_1-O_2	F_8-A_2	P_8-A_2	P_z-A_2
O_1-O_2	F_z-C_z	T_8-A_2		
O_2-P_8	C_z-P_z	P_8-A_2		

From American Clinical Neurophysiology Society: Guideline 6: a proposal for standard montages to be used in clinical EEG. J Clin Neurophysiol 2006;23:111–117.

TABLE 27–3

Waveform Terminology

Spike	Transient with a pointed peak and duration of 20–70 msec
Polyspike	Transient with multiple spikes
Sharp wave	Transient with a pointed peak and duration of 70–200 msec
Interictal discharge	Abnormal (epileptiform) EEG activity that occurs between seizures
Spike and wave	Spike followed by a slow wave
Ictal activity	EEG correlate of a seizure

EEG = electroencephalogram.

BOX 27–1

Useful Facts about Electroencephalography and Epilepsy

INTERICTAL EEG

- A true spike and wave is rarely confined to one derivation—i.e., has a "field" of involvement (especially true if a typical bipolar clinical EEG montage is used).
- A spike confined to one derivation is often an artifact. ECG artifact can mimic spikes.

ICTAL EEG

- Typically, ictal EEG activity "evolves" in
  - Frequency—may increase then exhibit postictal slowing.
  - Field—amount of involved derivations increases.
  - Amplitude—may increase.
- Background rhythms are often suppressed.

EEG AND EPILEPSY

- A single EEG will show epileptiform abnormalities in about 50% of adult patients with epilepsy.
- Diagnostic yield increased to 70% with repeated recordings and/or sleep EEGs.
- A normal EEG does NOT rule out epilepsy.
- An abnormal EEG (epileptiform activity) does NOT rule in epilepsy.

ECG = electrocardiogram; EEG = electroencephalography.

window is indicated to scrutinize any suspicious paroxysmal activity.

PHASE REVERSAL

Localized EEG waveforms (including spikes and sharp waves) will show **phase reversal** if the bipolar chain crosses the area of the localized EEG activity.[4,5] **Phase reversal does not imply an abnormal waveform.** For example, K complexes and vertex sharp waves show phase reversal in montages that cross the location of origin. Phase reversal may help differentiate epileptiform activity such as a spike from artifact. Epileptiform activity is recorded as an electronegative potential. For example, in Figure 27–7A, negative spike activity is seen under electrode T_7. This results in downgoing deflections in F_7-T_7 because T_7 is more negative than F_7. This pattern reverses for T_7-P_7 because now P_7 is more positive than T_7. In this figure, "s" is for spike and "w" is for wave. If the spike focus is located nearly equidistant between two monitoring electrodes (F_8 and T_8) (see Fig. 27–7B), the derivation containing them may show little or no activity (F_8-T_8) and the derivations on either side will show phase reversal ([F_{p2}-F_8] to [T_8-P_8]).

LOCALIZATION IN REFERENTIAL AND PSG MONTAGES

In referential montages, a spike will have greater activity in montages containing electrodes nearer to the location of the

FIGURE 27–6 Sharp waves, spikes, spike and wave, polyspikes, and polyspike and wave. EEG = electroencephalography; PSG = polysomnography.

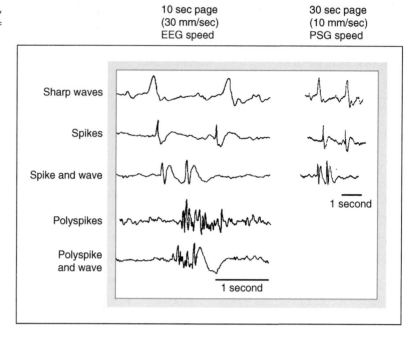

FIGURE 27–7 Examples of phase reversal. **A,** A spike (s; negative) originates at electrode position T_7 and a bipolar chain through the area shows phase reversal. w = wave. **B,** Spike originated in between electrodes. The bipolar pair spanning the location show low amplitude due to cancellation effects but bipolar pairs on either side show phase reversal.

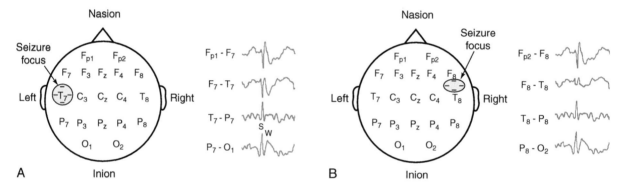

FIGURE 27–8 Difference in localization with a bipolar or a referential montage. In referential montages, the electrode(s) nearest the activity in question has the largest deflection.

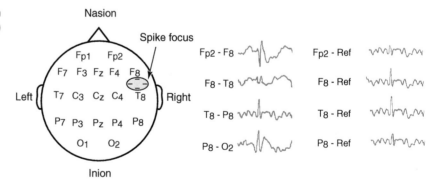

spike. In Figure 27–8, a spike focus is located between F_8 and T_8. On the bipolar montage, this results in the electrical activity being nearly equal in the two electrodes, resulting in minimal activity in F_8-T_8 but a phase reversal in adjacent bipolar pairs. However, in referential recording, the spike results in larger and nearly equal activity in F_8 and T_8 with less activity in adjacent electrodes. In the usual PSG montage,

electrodes are referenced to the opposite mastoid.[3] Therefore, a spike located near F_4 will result in greater deflection in F_4-M_1 compared with C_4-M_1 or O_2-M_1. It is also important to recall that the mastoid electrodes may actually be closer to spikes in the temporal area than the F_4, C_4, and O_2 electrodes. For example, a left temporal focus of activity may be nearer M_1 than F_3, C_3, and O_1. Thus, C_4-M_1 will actually show more activity from a left temporal focus than C_3-M_2 because M_1 is closer to the temporal area than C_3. In the case of a left temporal spike, one would expect to see epileptiform activity in most channels referenced to the left mastoid (M_1).

NORMAL SLEEP WAVEFORMS IN THE 10-SECOND WINDOW

The standard waveforms and eye movements used to stage sleep have a different appearance when viewed in a 10-second window in a standard clinical EEG montage. With digital PSG, one can change the time base (10-second to 30-second window) and vice versa to help with waveform recognition.

Eye Movements and Bell's Phenomenon

Bell's phenomenon describes the reflex upward movement of the front of the eyeball when the eyelids close (or blink). Because the cornea is positive with respect to the retina, this causes a deflection in derivations containing electrodes placed near the eyes (F_{p1}, F_{p2}). Recall that if G_1 becomes positive with respect to G_2, the derivation G_1-G_2 shows a downward deflection. Thus, eyelid closure results in downward deflections in F_{p1}-F_7 and F_{p2}-F_8. This is illustrated in Figures 27–9 to 27–11.

Conjugate vertical eye movements result in characteristic deflections in bipolar derivations. The deflections depend on which electrodes are closer to the eyes. For vertical movements, the F_{p1} and F_{p2} electrodes are more positive (eyes up) or negative (eyes down) compared with adjacent electrodes (see Fig. 27–10). For lateral eye movements, the electrodes F_7 and F_8 become more positive or negative than adjacent electrodes (see Fig. 27–11). Thus, in longitudinal bipolar derivations, vertical eye movements cause in-phase deflections and lateral movements result in out-of-phase deflections.

Posterior Rhythm

The term *alpha rhythm* is used to denote waveforms of 8 to 13 Hz that are prominent in occipital derivations and decrease in amplitude with eye opening. However, the preferred term is **posterior rhythm** or **dominant posterior rhythm (DPR)**. The DPR of infants and children is discussed in Chapter 5. The DPR frequency is slower than 8 Hz in infants and young children. The average frequency of the DPR increases to approximately 8 Hz at 8 years of age in the majority of individuals ("8 Hz by 8 years is OK"). With eyes closed and/or decreased visual attention, the DPR becomes prominent. With drowsiness and transition to stage N1, the occipital derivations show attenuation of the DPR and replacement with theta activity. The effect of eyes open and eyes closed on the DPR in an adult is illustrated in Figure 27–12. As noted previously, eyes closed results in an upward deflection of the eyes (under the eyelids) and a characteristic downward deflection in derivations near the eyes (see Fig. 27–12).

Some familiar waveforms used to stage sleep are displayed in a bipolar montage using a 10-second window in Figure 27–13. Stage R is shown in Figure 27–14. Note the "rapid eye

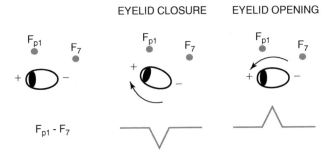

FIGURE 27–9 Bell's phenomenon. With eyelid closure (and blinks), the globe turns upward. This results in characteristic deflections in derivations containing electrodes near the eyes. The cornea is positive with respect to the retina.

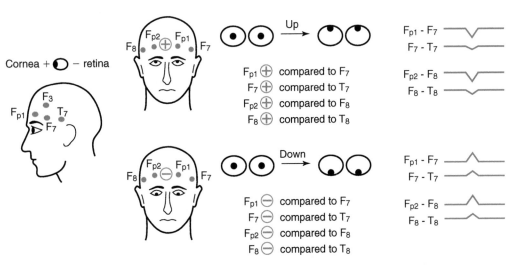

FIGURE 27–10 Effect of vertical eye movements on bipolar derivations containing electrodes near the eyes.

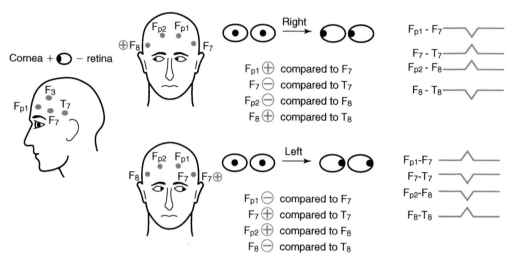

FIGURE 27–11   Effect of lateral eye movements on bipolar derivations containing electrodes near the eyes.

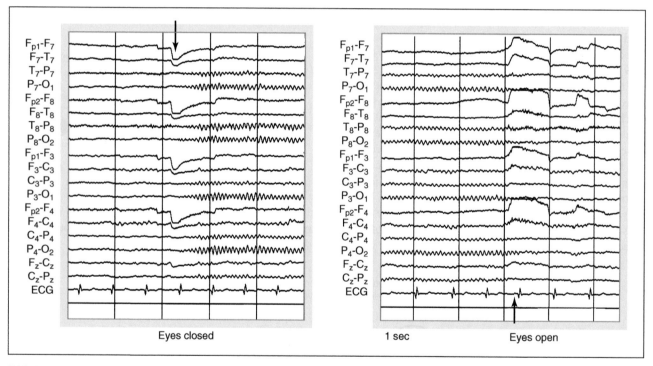

FIGURE 27–12   Effect of eye closure and opening on the alpha rhythm (dominant posterior rhythm). The rhythm is increased with eye closure or visual inattention and attenuated by eye opening and most prominent in derivations containing O_1 and O_2. Recall that with eye closure, the eyes turn upward under the eyelids (Bell's phenomenon). ECG = electrocardiogram.

movements" appear much wider in the 10-second window than in a 30-second time window.

Positive Occipital Sharp Transients of Sleep and Lambda and Mu Rhythms

Positive occipital sharp transients of sleep (POSTS) are sharp waves that can occur normally in non–rapid eye movement (NREM) sleep. They are most prominent in occipital derivations and are positive. Therefore, in O_1-M_2, they would

be downward deflections (O_1 is positive compared with M_2). In Figure 27–15, the POSTS show phase reversal across O_1. The fact that the POSTS are in fact "positive" in the occipital area is documented by the fact that the deflections are up in C_3-O_1 and downward in O_1-M_1.

Lambda waves have similar morphology and location as POSTS but lambda waves are noted during **wakefulness**. Lambda waves are low-voltage triangular waves that appear in the occipital areas. They may be surface positive or negative (POSTS are surface positive) (Fig. 27–16).

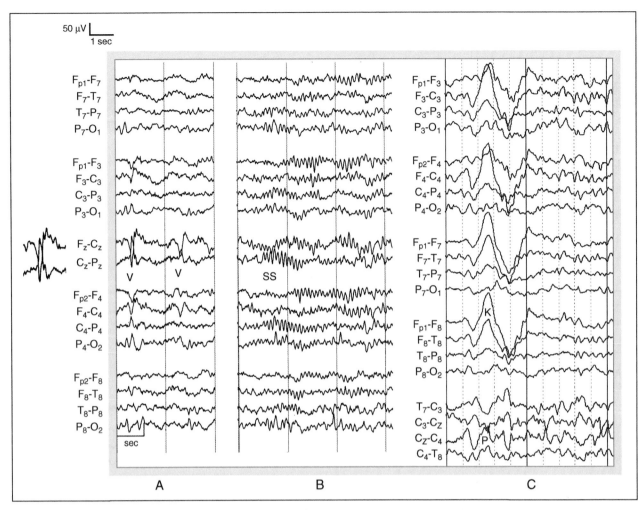

FIGURE 27–13 Waveforms of sleep using a clinical EEG montage (longitudinal bipolar) and a 10-second window. Vertex sharp waves (V; **A**), sleep spindles (SS; **B**), and a K complex (K; **C**) are shown. Note phase reversal across C_z in the vertex sharp waves **(A)** and for K complex in **C** as denoted by P.

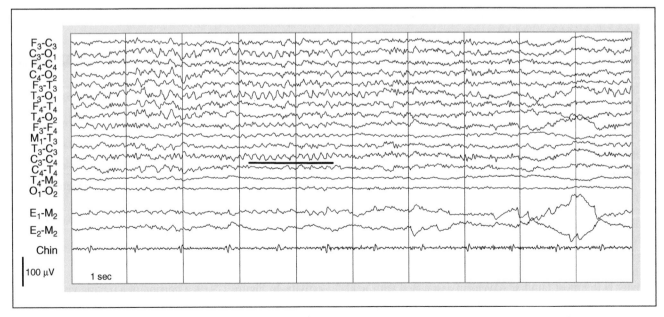

FIGURE 27–14 Stage R using a clinical EEG montage (combination of longitudinal and transverse bipolar) and a 10-second window. The *underlined activity* is a saw-tooth wave (theta activity prominent in central derivations). Note also that alpha activity is common during stage R and usually 1–2 Hz slower. Alpha activity is seen in the occipital derivations at the same time as the saw-tooth waves. However, note that the alpha bursts stop before the saw-tooth activity ends. Note older electrode terminology (T_3, T_4 instead of T_7, T_8).

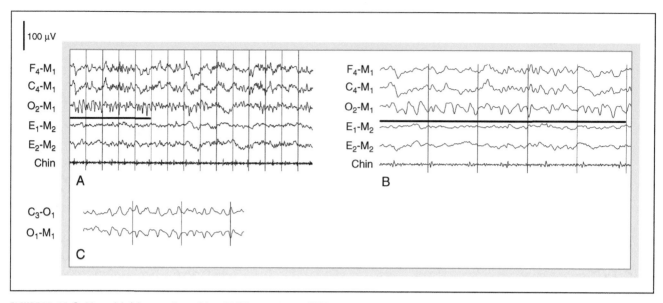

FIGURE 27–15 Positive occipital sharp transients of sleep (POSTS) as seen in typical PSG montage in a 30-second (**A**) and a 10-second window (**B**). **C,** Bipolar derivations containing the occipital electrode show that there is a phase reversal at O_1 and that the waves are positive (downward deflection in O_1-M_1). The vertical lines are 1 second apart.

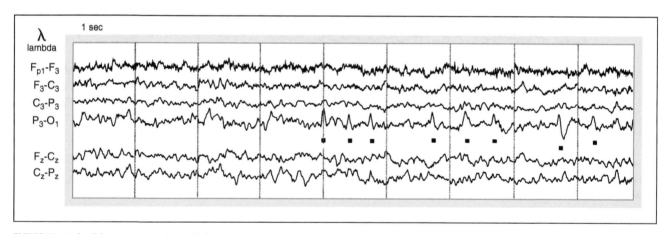

FIGURE 27–16 Lambda waves are noted in the P_3-O_1 derivation and marked by *dots* under the waves. *Adapted from Libenson MH: Practical Approach to Electroencephalography. Philadelphia: Elsevier Saunders, 2010, p. 270.*

Mu rhythm may sometimes be confused with alpha rhythm but differs in a number of features, listed in Table 27–4. Mu rhythm is seen in **central derivations** during wake and has an "archiform" or comblike shape with rounded contour on one side and sharp contour on the other (Fig. 27–17). Mu rhythm is most prominent in **central areas** (rather than occipital) and is reactive to movement of the contralateral hand (rather than opening of the eyes).

ICTAL ACTIVITY

Ictal (seizure) activity may be manifested by rhythmic activity of many types. By definition, to be considered ictal, a given burst of activity must be associated with an abnormality of movement or mentation. Whereas the **spike and wave** activity is the most familiar waveform associated with ictal activity (Fig. 27–18), the pattern of repetitive sharp waves of various frequencies is also common.[4,5] On traditional sleep monitoring montages, ictal activity can even be mistaken for muscle artifact or normal alpha (8–13 Hz) and beta (>13 Hz)

TABLE 27-4		
Mu Rhythm		
	MU	ALPHA
Stage	Wake	Drowsy wake
Frequency (Hz)	8–13	8–13
Location	Central (C_3, C_4)	Occipital
Reactivity, diminished with	Movement of contralateral hand	Opening eyes
Shape	Archiform Comblike	Sinusoidal

activity. In Figure 27–19, a portion of a tracing visualized in a 10-second window shows a spike and wave complex (SW) followed by rhythmic activity of 8 to 9 Hz (R). The rhythmic activity is differentiated from normal alpha rhythm by being more prominent in the eye derivations than in the occipital

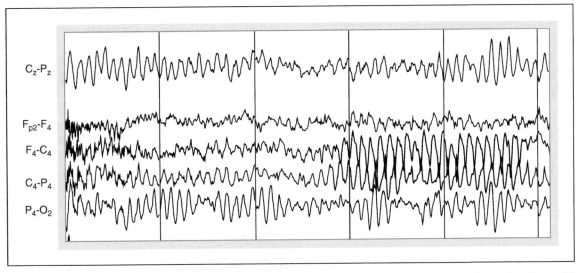

FIGURE 27-17 An example of mu rhythm (archiform "comb" like pattern with phase reversal at C_4). The vertical lines are 1 second apart. *From Libenson MH: Practical Approach to Electroencephalography. Philadelphia: Elsevier Saunders, 2010, p. 272.*

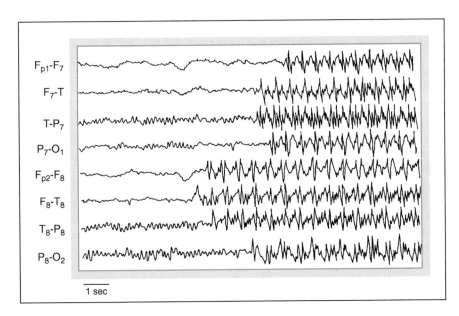

1 sec

FIGURE 27-18 A seizure beginning as focal activity in the right frontal-temporal areas with secondary generalization.

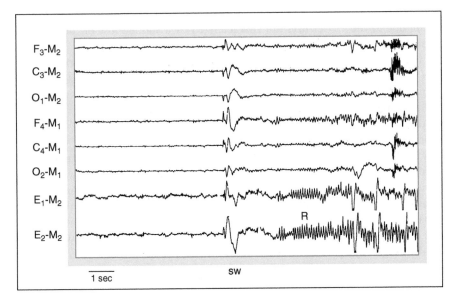

1 sec   sw

FIGURE 27-19 A spike and wave (SW) complex is followed by rhythmic activity (R) in the alpha frequency range that represents ictal activity in a patient with frontal lobe seizure. The origin is the right frontopolar area and the largest amplitude is seen in E_2-M_2 and F_4-M_1.

derivations. This is, in fact, a portion of a frontal seizure manifested by oral automatisms and loss of responsiveness. One might suspect the frontal nature because the activity is higher amplitude in the eye leads (near the frontal lobes). A complete EEG montage documented a right frontal location (note in Fig. 27–19, slightly higher amplitude in E_2-M_1 than in E_1-M_2).

As previously mentioned, ictal activity may not be seen in scalp EEG monitoring. Video recording is absolutely essential because the pattern of movements (seminology) is very important for helping differentiate nonepileptic movements (parasomnias) from epileptic movements. The type of movement and the focal or generalized distribution may help define the type of seizure and/or focus in partial or partial complex seizures. High-resolution magnetic resonance imaging (MRI) or invasive EEG monitoring may also identify the epileptic location in the brain.

Ictal activity can be mistaken for a recording artifact and vice versa. Some useful characteristics of true ictal activity are noted in Box 27–1. True ictal activity evolves (i.e., changes in frequency, amplitude, and distribution) during the episode. There is often EEG slowing after an ictal episode. Synchronized video is very useful to determine whether there are behavioral correlates (e.g., movements) temporally associated with ictal activity.

CLASSIFICATION OF SEIZURES AND TERMINOLOGY

A **seizure** is defined as an episode of disturbance of mental, motor, sensory, or autonomic activity caused by a paroxysmal cerebral neuronal malfunction. **Epilepsy** is defined as a disorder of recurrent seizures. The disorder is called **symptomatic** if there is an identifiable lesion or **idiopathic** if a discrete structural abnormality is not found. The term "idiopathic" is misleading because many seizure disorders classified as idiopathic have a genetic basis and some have a known mechanism.

The most commonly used classification of seizures is based on their manifestations[9] (Box 27–2). Seizure disorders are divided into partial (focal) seizures that are due to the initial involvement of a localized group of neurons limited to one hemisphere. If consciousness is not impaired, the disorder is termed a **simple partial seizure (SPS)**. If consciousness is impaired, the disorder is a **complex partial seizure (CPS)**. An **aura** is an SPS manifested by sensations preceding a seizure and is, in fact, a manifestation of focal epilepsy. **Automatisms** are repetitive movements that may be purposeful but serve no obvious purpose in the actual situation. The **postictal state** is the state following ictal activity often associated with impaired sensorium or confusion. Simple partial seizures may not show an EEG abnormality with scalp EEG recording. Complex partial seizures usually do exhibit some abnormality. Partial seizures may show secondary generalization (see Fig. 27–18), resulting in the ictal activity associated with generalized convulsive seizures.

In Box 27–2, the partial epilepsies are divided into simple partial (consciousness not impaired), complex partial (consciousness impaired), and focal seizures (simple or partial complex) that evolve into generalized seizures. The simple partial seizures are divided into those with (1) motor symptoms, (2) somatosensory symptoms, (3) autonomic symptoms, and (4) psychic symptoms or signs. The complex partial seizures are divided based on whether or not impaired consciousness is apparent at the start of the seizure.

Primary **generalized seizures** are ones in which **initial** manifestations involve both hemispheres usually with loss of consciousness (or impairment), bilateral motor activity, or both. As noted previously, generalized epilepsy is associated with a diffuse origin of the seizure activity and is always associated with impairment (usually loss of consciousness). Generalized epilepsy is divided into **nonconvulsive** (absence or petit mal) epilepsy and **convulsive.**

Nonconvulsive epilepsy is divided into typical (3/sec spike and wave activity) and atypical with slower frequency complexes. Nonconvulsive generalized epilepsy starts in childhood and may resolve by late adolescence to adulthood. Typical absence (petit mal) epilepsy (AE) is associated with impairment of consciousness (staring blankly) without loss of muscle tone or posture. Attacks are triggered by hyperventilation and photic stimuli. Atypical AE is associated with spike and wave complexes of less than 3/sec frequency and may be associated with combinations of impaired consciousness and motor or autonomic changes. Patients with atypical nonconvulsive epilepsy may develop convulsive generalized seizures later in life.

Convulsive generalized epilepsy is divided into **myoclonic, tonic, clonic, tonic-clonic,** and **atonic** seizures. **Myoclonic seizures** are characterized by brief muscle jerking (muscle contraction then relaxation—often involving the shoulder muscles). An example of this type is juvenile myoclonic epilepsy (JME). Tonic seizures are associated with muscle tensing. Clonic seizures manifest with repeated jerking (repeated contraction and relaxation). Generalized tonic-clonic (GTC) seizures (grand mal) are characterized by initial tonic activity followed by clonic activity. Atonic seizures are characterized by a sudden loss of muscle tone (drop attacks).

Unclassified seizures are ones in which the origin (focal or general) has not been determined.

Nocturnal Epilepsy

Seizure disorders are part of the differential diagnosis of "nocturnal spells"—particularly episodes of abnormal motor activity occurring during sleep or soon after awakening. Depending on the type of patients studied, **as many as 10% to 40% of seizures occur exclusively or mainly during sleep.** The lack of daytime seizure activity and the fact that automatisms or episodes of changed sensorium during sleep may not be noted by a bed partner or remembered by the patient make simple partial or partial complex seizures difficult to diagnose. Some seizures such as those associated

BOX 27–2

Classification of Seizures

1. PARTIAL (FOCAL, LOCAL) SEIZURES

A. Simple partial seizzres (consciousness not impaired)
   i. Motor symptoms
      a. Focal motor without march—sustained tonic, intermittent clonic, or a sequence of tonic-clonic movements.
      b. Focal motor with march (Jacksonian)—movements progressively involve adjacent parts of one side of the body.
      c. Versive—turning of head or body, usually in a direction away from the side of the seizure discharge.
      d. Postural—involuntary changes in body posture.
      e. Aphasic—expressive or receptive, global loss of language.
      f. Phonatory (vocalization or arrest of speech).
   ii. Somatosensory or special sensory symptoms
      a. Somatosensory.
      b. Visual—hallucinations.
      c. Auditory—hallucinations of simple or complex sounds.
      d. Olfactory—hallucination of odors, often precedes complex partial seizures.
      e. Gustatory—hallucination of taste.
      f. Vertiginous—transient vertigo.
   iii. Autonomic symptoms or signs: epigastric, pallor, sweating
   iv. Psychic symptoms or signs (usually occur with impairment of consciousness and classified as complex partial)
      a. Dysphasic.
      b. Cognitive.
      c. Dysamnesic (déjà vu).
      d. Affective (fear).
      e. Illusions.
      f. Hallucinations.

B. Complex partial (with impairment of consciousness)
   i. Simple partial onset followed by impairment of consciousness
   ii. Impairment of consciouness at onset
      a. Impairment of consciousness only.
      b. Automatisms.

C. Partial seizures (simple or complex) evolving to generalized seizures.

2. GENERALIZED SEIZURES

A. Nonconvulsive (absence)—petit mal
   i. Typical (3/sec spike and slow wave on EEG)
   ii. Atypical (<3/sec spike and slow wave complexes on EEG)

B. Convulsive
   i. Myoclonic seizures—brief jerks
   ii. Clonic seizures
   iii. Tonic seizures—tensing of muscles
   iv. Tonic-clonic seizures (grand mal)
   v. Atonic ("drop attacks")

3. UNCLASSIFIED SEIZURE

EEG = encephalogram.
Adapted from Commission on Classification and Terminology of the International League Against Epilepsy: Proposal for revised classification of epilepsies and epileptic syndromes. Epilepsia 1981;22:389–399.

with nocturnal frontal lobe epilepsy (NFLE) can occur **without loss of consciousness or postictal confusion** and may be incorrectly assumed to be a parasomnia. The incidence of nocturnal seizures has two peaks—one about 2 hours after bedtime and another between 4 and 5 AM (Table 27–5).[10,11] Daytime seizures are most prevalent in the first hour after awakening. In general, all manifestations of nocturnal seizure disorders are much more common in NREM and rare during rapid eye movement (REM) sleep. Prior sleep deprivation activates seizures; therefore, patients often undergo clinical EEG monitoring in a sleep-deprived state to increase the likelihood of recording seizure activity. Epilepsy syndromes commonly associated with nocturnal seizures are listed in Table 27–6.

Focal Nocturnal Epilepsy—General Characteristics

Focal seizure disorders are often associated with interictal discharges or seizure activity in NREM sleep. The major types of focal nocturnal epilepsy are **frontal lobe epilepsy (FLE) and temporal lobe epilepsy (TLE).** Herman and coworkers[12] studied patients with partial epilepsy undergoing long-term video-EEG monitoring and found that FLE seizures were significantly more common during sleep than wake.[10,11] In contrast, TLE seizures were more common during wake. Figure 27–20 illustrates the percentage of each seizure type that occurs during wake and sleep. Some patients with FLE have seizures only during sleep. TLE is less likely to occur during sleep than during wake. However, because TLE is much more common than FLE, TLE is the most common type of nocturnal seizure. TLE seizures at night are more likely to generalize than TLE seizures during the day. In contrast, FLE seizures during the day are more likely to generalize than those during the night.

Nocturnal simple partial seizures result in focal motor, sensory, autonomic, or psychic manifestations without a change of consciousness. Complex partial seizures usually arise from the mesial or lateral part of the temporal lobe or

TABLE 27-5

Timing of Nocturnal Seizures and Effect of Sleep

Interictal discharges	• NREM > wake > REM
Most frequent timing for nocturnal seizures	• About 2 hours after bedtime • Between 4 and 5 AM
Most frequent time for daytime seizures	• Within 1 hour of awakening
Effect of sleep on seizures	• Incidence of seizures NREM > wake > REM sleep
Factors increasing seizures	• Sleep deprivation • Medications lowering seizure threshold
PARTIAL EPILEPSY	
Interictal activity	• NREM—common • REM—uncommon
Ictal activity	• NREM—common • REM—uncommon
GENERALIZED EPILEPSY	
Interictal activity	• NREM—common • REM—rare
Ictal activity	• NREM—less common • REM—uncommon • After awakening—common

NREM = non–rapid eye movement; REM = rapid eye movement.

TABLE 27-6

Epilepsy Syndromes Associated with Sleep

EPILEPSY SYNDROME	TIME OF ONSET
PARTIAL EPILEPSY	
TLE	Late childhood to early adulthood
FLE (including autosomal dominant FLE)	Late childhood to early adulthood
Secondary generalized partial epilepsy	Late childhood to early adulthood
GENERALIZED EPILEPSY	
Benign centrotemporal epilepsy with centrotemporal spikes	3–13 yr (peak 9–10 yr)
Epilepsy with GTCS on awakening	6–25 yr (peak 11–15 yr)
JME	12–18 yr (peak 14 yr)
Absence epilepsy	3–12 yr (peak 6–7 yr)
Lennox-Gastaut syndrome	1–8 yr (peak 3–5 yr)
Continuous spike and slow wave discharges during sleep	8 mo–11.5 yr

FLE = frontal lobe epilepsy; GTCS = generalized tonic-clonic seizure; JME = juvenile myoclonic epilepsy; TLE = temporal lobe epilepsy.
Adapted from Malow BA: Sleep and epilepsy. Neurol Clin 2005;23:1127.

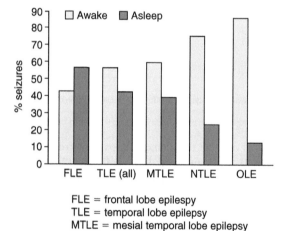

FLE = frontal lobe epilepsy
TLE = temporal lobe epilepsy
MTLE = mesial temporal lobe epilepsy

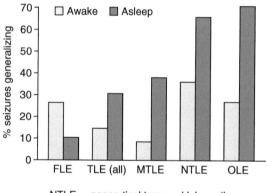

NTLE = neocortical temporal lobe epilepsy
OLE = occipital or parietal lobe epilepsy

FIGURE 27-20 Left, The percentage of different seizure types occurring while awake and asleep. Note that frontal lobe epilepsy (FLE) occurs more often during sleep than awake. Some patients with FLE may have seizures only at night. Temporal lobe epilepsy (TLE) is more likely to occur during awake than sleep. **Right,** The percentage of focal epilepsy that generalized during awake and asleep. TLE occurring during sleep is more likely to generalize. FLE occurring during awake is more likely to generalize. *From Herman ST, Walczak TS, Bazil CW: Distribution of partial seizures during the sleep-wake cycle: differences by seizure onset site. Neurology 2001;56:1456.*

adjacent parts of the frontal lobe. The symptoms consist of changes in the content of consciousness that reduce the patient's ability to interact with the surroundings. They can occur with only a change in consciousness or can include automatisms. For example, lip smacking is a common automatism. Patients with complex partial seizures may have no recollection of the events or only partial memory of the seizure. Patients may remember an aura, a subjective sensation such as a visual or olfactory disturbance that precedes the start of the event.

There have been efforts to identify characteristics allowing differentiation between FLE and TLE. Unfortunately, there is considerable overlap. FLE is more likely to be associated with dystonic posturing (fencing) and TLE more likely to be associated with interictal or ictal activity visualized on the scalp EEG.

TEMPORAL LOBE EPILEPSY

TLE seizures begin focally and usually impair consciousness (complex partial seizures). TLE seizures are more common in NREM sleep but also occur at the transition from NREM to REM sleep. Interictal activity can often be seen even using traditional PSG EEG monitoring because the mastoid electrodes are near the temporal lobes. Very rarely, no abnormal EEG activity may be observed during seizures in some patients with TLE using a full EEG montage of scalp electrodes. TLE seizures may be manifested by lip smacking, staring, episodes of an altered state of consciousness, confused awakenings, and automatic behavior such as sleepwalking or wandering through the house. Of note, partial seizures with complex automatisms including vocalization and violent behavior have been described in a few patients.

TLE can present with seizures that occur only at night. Although FLE seizures are more commonly confined to sleep than TLE seizures, because TLE seizures are much more common, the most common partial seizure disorder occurring only during sleep is TLE. However, as noted previously, for most patients with TLE, seizures are more likely to occur during the day than at night.

Mesial TLE

In adults, hippocampal sclerosis is the most common cause of mesial TLE, whereas in children, cortical dysplasias and low-grade malignancy are most common. Typical mesial TLE consists of complex partial seizures with automatisms. They start as simple partial seizures with sensory symptoms (aura). Typical auras of mesial TLE include epigastric (abdominal) and psychic auras (déjà vu, jamais vu), and fear). Déjà vu ("already seen") is the experience of already experiencing something. Jamais vu ("never seen") is the experience of being unfamiliar with a person or situation that is actually very familiar. The motor manifestations include fine distal automatisms of finger, hands, or orobuccal movements. Interictal EEG shows temporal sharp waves maximal at anterior temporal electrodes. The ictal EEG is often a well-defined theta (5–7 Hz) rhythmic pattern from the temporal region (derivations containing T_7, M_1, T_8, or M_2 depending on the side of the body affected). High-resolution MRI enhances the diagnosis demonstrating atrophy of the hippocampus within the mesial temporal lobe.

Neocortical TLE

Seizures can be simple partial or complex partial depending on the areas of the temporal lobe affected. Interictal EEG shows spikes or sharp waves outside of the anterior temporal area. Ictal EEG can show regional or widespread discharges.

PSG and TLE

The appearance of an interictal spike activity from the temporal lobe in the typical sleep montage can be misleading. The

mastoid electrodes are located fairly close to the temporal lobes. Therefore, derivations containing the mastoid electrode on the same side as the temporal lobe may show prominent activity even if the other part of the derivation is on the other side of the brain. For example, C_4-M_1 might show prominent activity from a left temporal focus despite the fact that C_4 is central in location and on the other side of the brain. Prominent spikes in derivations containing M_1 (near the left temporal lobe) are shown in Figure 27–21. The deflections are downward because M_1 is the second electrode in the derivation. Spikes are surface negative and here M_1 is negative with respect to F_4, C_4, and O_2, resulting in downward deflections.

Ictal activity is shown from the same patient (Fig. 27–22) and consists of repetitive sharp waves most prominent on the left and showing a phase reversal at T_7 localizing the seizure to the left temporal area. At the normal 30-second window, the ictal activity could be mistaken for artifact.

NOCTURNAL FRONTAL LOBE EPILEPSY

NFLE is associated with a wide spectrum of manifestations and is the type of epilepsy most likely mistaken as an NREM or REM parasomnia.[10–14] **In roughly half of the cases of NFLE, there is no abnormality in the scalp EEG during the episodes** and many cases also have no interictal epileptiform activity. In some of the cases with a normal scalp EEG, abnormalities can be demonstrated by invasive EEG monitoring. The NFLE episodes are confined to sleep in most cases, so they are less well observed. Patients often remain conscious with minimal postictal confusion. Nocturnal ambulation such as walking and crying and autonomic activation can mimic sleepwalking and sleep terrors. NFLE exists in familial, sporadic, symptomatic (associated with identifiable structural lesion), and idiopathic forms.

Of focal seizure disorders, approximately 20% have an onset from the frontal lobes. The clinical manifestations of frontal lobe seizures may vary depending on localization of the epileptic focus. Seizures originating from the orbitofrontal areas and the cingulate gyrus (see Fig. 27–2) often resemble those originating from the temporal lobes with staring, nonresponsiveness, and automatisms. Seizure onset in the posterior frontal lobes from the primary motor cortex may have discrete motor manifestation that have a Jacksonian march that begins in the distal muscles of an extremity and moves up the extremity. Patients with a seizure focus located in the midline regions will often have involvement of the supplementary motor cortex eliciting complex motor manifestations such as dystonic posturing, vocalizations, or speech arrest with variable loss of consciousness and minimal postictal confusion. In addition, seizures originating from the cingulate gyrus may also have autonomic features such as tachycardia, tachypnea, pallor, and sweating (see Fig. 27–2). Seizure onset from dorsolateral frontal lobes may be minimal or involve motor manifestations depending on the extent of spread of the seizure activity. As noted previously, patients with FLE seizures frequently do not exhibit interictal EEG activity.

FIGURE 27–21 Spikes (S) are noted in a standard PSG montage in all derivations containing M_1. These spikes are from a left temporal focus (near M_1). ECG = electrocardiogram.

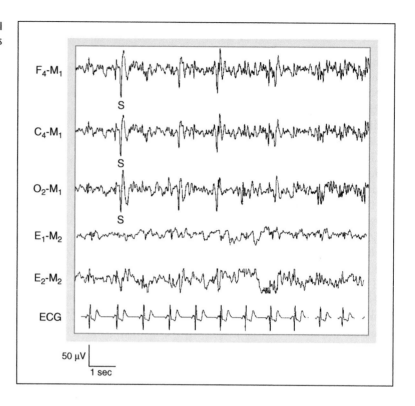

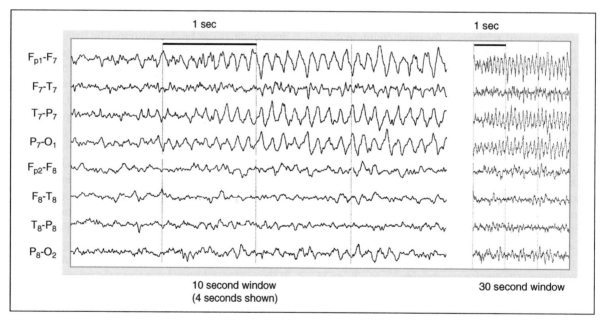

FIGURE 27–22 Bipolar recording from the patient in Figure 27–21 shows ictal activity of approximately 8 Hz in the left frontotemporal derivations. This confirms the suspected left-sided focus noted in Figure 27–21. The low amplitude in F_7-T_7 suggests that the focus is equidistant from both electrodes (see Fig. 27–8).

NFLE Syndromes

Provini and colleagues[13,14] described three general manifestations of NFLE including paroxysmal arousals (PAs), nocturnal paroxysmal dystonia (NPD), and episodic nocturnal wandering (ENW) (Table 27–7). **Paroxysmal arousals** (PAs) typically present during NREM sleep consisting of a stereotypical series of movements lasting 2 to 20 seconds in which the individuals raise their head, sit up, and look around confused with a frightened expression and then scream. Unlike typical sleep terrors, **PAs can occur many times during the night and are very stereotypical.** NPD is characterized by nocturnal coarse movements associated with tonic spasms that often occur multiple times per night. The episodes can be violent or be associated with vocalization. Patients often move the arms and legs with cycling or kicking movements and sometimes adopt a dystonic posture of the limbs. **Episodic nocturnal wanderings (ENWs)** may present

TABLE 27-7

Manifestations of Nocturnal Frontal Lobe Epilepsy

	PA	NPD	ENW
Frequency.	Multiple times per night (mean 2).	Multiple times per night (mean 3).	Multiple times (1–3/night).
Duration of episodes.	Short 20–40 sec.	More prolonged (25–98 sec).	31–180 sec.
	Patients sit up, look around, confused, often with loud scream.	• Arm and leg movements. • Cycling. • Kicking. • Dystonic posture (fencing). • Pelvic thrusting. • Vocalization. • Violence can occur.	• Jump out of bed. • Wander. • Vocalize. • Violent behavior.
Can communicate at end of seizure.	100%.	44% can communicate at end of episode.	100%.
Can communicate during seizure.	12/27.	10/59 during episode.	None.
Stereotypical or varied.	Stereotyped.	Stereotyped.	Stereotyped, agitated somnambulism.
Daytime seizures.	No.	57% (49% secondarily generalized seizures).	13%.
Brain structural abnormality.	0%.	24%.	5%.

NPD = nocturnal paroxysmal dystonia; ENW = episodic nocturnal wandering; PA = paroxysmal arousal.
Adapted from Provini F, Plazzi G, Tinuper P, et al: Nocturnal frontal lobe epilepsy. Brain 1999;122:1017–1031.

with symptoms similar to sleepwalking and sleep terrors. Patients may jump out of bed, wander, vocalize, and show violent behavior during sleep. Classically, treatment with older anticonvulsants (in particular, carbamazepine) or newer anticonvulsants such as levetiracetam at bedtime is generally effective. However, some patients are refractory to antiepileptic medications. It is important to note that a significant proportion of patients with NFLE do have seizures during wakefulness, generalization to tonic-clonic seizures, and a demonstrable brain abnormality.

Familial NFLE

The original description was an autosomal dominant nocturnal frontal lobe epilepsy (ADNFLE) associated with a missense mutation of the neuronal nicotinic acetylcholine receptor (nAChR) alpha 4 subunit. Other mutations of the nAChR gene system have been found and there is genetic heterogeneity in families with ADNFLE. Four known loci are 20q13.2, 15q24, 1q21, and 8p12.3-q12.3. Motor seizures are frequent (nearly every night), often violent, occur in clusters, and are brief (<1 min). The age of onset is variable (2 mo–56 yr). Ninety percent of patients present by age 20 years.

Supplemental Motor Area Epilepsy

Focal seizures arising from the supplementary motor area (SMA), a region anterior to the motor cortex in the midline, is a type of FLE that typically involves unilateral or asymmetrical bilateral tonic posturing and may be associated with facial grimacing, vocalization, or speech arrest (Fig. 27-23). SMA seizures may be preceded by a somatosensory aura.[13-15] Complex automatisms such as kicking, laughing, or pelvic thrusting may be present with **responsiveness often preserved.** A classic manifestation of SMA epilepsy is the "fencing posture" with the head turned toward an outstretched arm (head turns away from side of seizure focus). **Because consciousness is often well preserved and postictal confusion minimal, these episodes are sometimes thought to be psychogenic.** However, unlike psychogenic movements, SMA epilepsy episodes are typically brief and stereotypical.

Parasomnia Versus NFLE

Information contrasting NFLE and NREM parasomnias are listed in Table 27-8. In general, NFLE is associated with greater frequency (episodes per month) and is more likely to consist of multiple episodes in a given night. The manifestations of NREM parasomnias also vary from night to night whereas NFLE seizures have very stereotypical manifestations. They can be bizarre but they always consist of the same activity. EEG is not that helpful in many cases because approximately 40% to 50% of NFLE patients have no interictal or ictal EEG findings (apart from movement and muscle artifact associated with the spells).

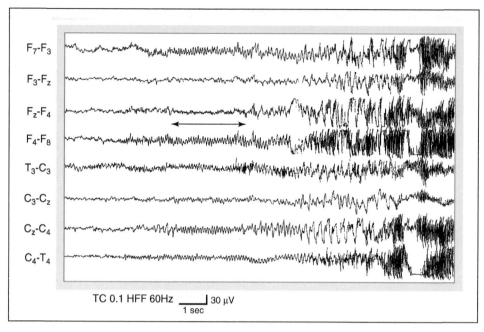

FIGURE 27–23 A nocturnal attack due to frontal lobe epilepsy from the supplemental motor area. Ictal EEG recording of a nocturnal episode of frontal lobe epilepsy. The ictal EEG shows electrodecremental pattern associated with rhythmic low-amplitude 20- to 24-Hz fast activity localized in the right midfrontal region *(horizontal arrow)* that evolved into activity of slower frequency and higher amplitude as the clinical seizure began. HFF = high-frequency filter; TC = time constant. *From Tachiban N, Shinde A, Ikeda A, et al: Supplementary motor area seizure resembling sleep disorder. Sleep 1996;19:813.*

Benign Epilepsy of Childhood with Centrotemporal Spikes

Benign epilepsy of childhood with centrotemporal spikes (BECTS), also known as *rolandic epilepsy,* accounts for 15% to 20% of childhood epilepsy.[10,17] The average age of onset is 6 to 8 years (range 3–13). Seizures occur predominantly during sleep and consist of oropharyngeal signs (hypersalivation and guttural sounds), arrest of speech with clonic jerks, contraction of the mouth, and sometimes clonic jerks of the arms or legs. The onset of seizure activity is about 20 minutes to 3 hours after bedtime. Consciousness is preserved in most cases unless there is secondary generalization. Generalized seizures during sleep may occur. The EEG typically shows centrotemporal or rolandic spikes or sharp waves (Fig. 27–24). In most patients, seizures resolve by adulthood. If treatment is needed, the seizures respond well to medication.

GENERALIZED EPILEPSY SYNDROMES WITH NOCTURNAL SEIZURES

Generalized Epilepsy Syndromes

Primary generalized epilepsies include idiopathic GTC seizures, AE seizures (petit mal), and juvenile myoclonic seizures. GTC seizures consist of a sudden loss of consciousness, a tonic phase of intense muscle contraction, and then a clonic phasic consisting of bilaterally synchronous jerking of the entire body. After the seizure, there is a postictal period of disorientation lasting a variable amount of time.[10,18] AE seizures are manifested as a blank stare during which the patient is unresponsive for 5 to 30 seconds. The characteristic waking EEG pattern is a 3-Hz spike and wave pattern. AE seizures start in childhood and rarely persist into adulthood. The exception is when AE seizures begin after 9 to 10 years of age. JME is a genetically determined condition involving myoclonic jerks in the arms shortly after awakening. Primary generalized seizures are sometimes called **awakening epilepsies** because they commonly occur when the patient is in a drowsy state upon awakening from sleep. Patients with both AE and JME disorders also can have GTC seizures. GTC seizures associated with these disorders usually occur on awakening or shortly thereafter.

Generalized Seizures During or After Sleep

Epilepsy with GTC Seizures on Awakening

In this disorder, GTC seizures occur exclusively or predominantly shortly after awakening (regardless of the time of awakening). Photic stimulation or sleep deprivation can precipitate GTC seizures. Myoclonic or AE seizures may coexist. Complete control is usually possible with antiepileptic medications.

Juvenile Myoclonic Epilepsy

JME is idiopathic (no demonstrable brain lesion) and has a genetic basis with an abnormality on the short arm of chromosome 6.[10,19] Onset is in adolescence, peaking between ages 12 and 18. This is one of the more common forms of generalized epilepsy and consists of a combination of myoclonic

TABLE 27–8

Nocturnal Frontal Lobe Epilepsy Versus Non–Rapid Eye Movement Parasomnias

	NFLE	NREM PARASOMNIA (CONFUSIONAL AROUSALS, SLEEP TERRORS, SLEEPWALKING)
Age at onset (yr ± SD)	14 ± 10 (infancy to adolescence)	<10
Gender	Male/female 7/3	M = F
Ictal EEG	NREM—**sleep stage N2** Normal ictal EEG 44% (higher if only scalp electrodes used) Normal interictal EEG 51%	NREM sleep Stage N3 in children
Movement seminology	Violent, stereotypical	Complex, nonstereotypical
Family history of episodes	39%	62–96%
Episode frequency/ mo	20 ± 11	<1–4
Episode frequency/ night	3 ± 3 (higher with PA, NPD)	1
Episode duration	2 sec–3 min	15 sec–30 min
Clinical course	Increased frequency	Tend to resolve
Triggering factors	None in 78%	Sleep deprivation, alcohol, febrile illness
Autonomic activation	Very common (tachycardia)	Yes in sleep terrors
Episode onset after sleep onset	Any time	First third of night in children
Effect of treatment	Carbamzaepine abolished (20%) or improved episodes (50%)	N/A

EEG = electroencephalogram; N/A = not applicable; NFLE = nocturnal frontal lobe epilepsy; NPD = nocturnal paroxysmal dystonia; NREM = non–rapid eye movement; PA = paroxysmal arousal; SD = standard deviation.
Adapted from Provini F, Plazzi G, Tinuper P, et al: Nocturnal frontal lobe epilepsy. Brain 1999;122:1017–1031.

seizures on awakening, GTC seizures, and AE seizures. The myoclonic seizures occur in clusters on awakening or shortly thereafter. Patients may not seek medical evaluation until after the first associated GTC seizure. The myoclonic seizure may subside during adulthood, but patients often

have persistent GTC seizures requiring lifelong treatment. Antiepileptic medications such as valproate are quite effective but lifelong treatment is usually needed owing to persistence of GTC seizures. The interictal EEG in JME is characterized by diffuse polyspike and slow wave complexes of 4 to 6 Hz, usually maximal at the frontal electrodes. Neurologic examination and brain MRI are usually normal.

Absence Epilepsy

AE is a genetically determined form of generalized epilepsy associated with brief spells, usually lasting less than 10 seconds, characterized by the abrupt cessation of ongoing activity, a blank stare, and abrupt return to awareness with resumption of activity. AE seizures are precipitated by photic stimulation, hyperventilation, and drowsiness.[10] The waking EEG in AE is characterized by diffuse 3/sec spike and wave activity (Fig. 27–25), whereas the sleeping EEG can be associated with polyspike activity. AE responds well to treatment and seizures may decrease as patients age. Unlike complex partial seizures (which can also affect the sensorium), AE is not associated with an aura or postictal confusion.

Lennox-Gastaut Syndrome

This syndrome is associated with generalized tonic, atonic, and atypical AE seizures.[10] There is typically a slow background on interictal EEG with slow (usually 2–2.5 Hz) spike and wave complexes during wake and generalized fast rhythms during sleep (Fig. 27–26). Affected individuals have mental retardation.

ICTAL EFFECTS ON SLEEP

Nocturnal epilepsy can impair sleep quality and result in complaints of daytime sleepiness or insomnia. **Up to 68% of patients with epilepsy complain of daytime sleepiness and 39% complain of insomnia.**[10,11,19,20] Partial and primary generalized seizures can be associated with sleep fragmentation, increased sleep stage shifts, and decreased sleep efficiency. Although antiepileptic drugs (AEDs) can also impair sleep, the sleep of patients with nocturnal epilepsy is usually better on AEDs than without AEDs. That is, seizure control improves sleep quality.

ANTIEPILEPTIC DRUGS—EFFECTS ON SLEEP

The effects of common AEDs[19–21] on sleep are listed in Table 27–9. Published information on this topic is somewhat conflicting and often based on small studies. For most patients, the benefits of seizure control on sleep outweigh side effects of AEDs.

EPILEPSY AND OBSTRUCTIVE SLEEP APNEA

One study in 2003 of unselected adult epilepsy patients found an obstructive sleep apnea (OSA) prevalence of 10.2% (15.4% in men and 5.4% in women).[22] An even

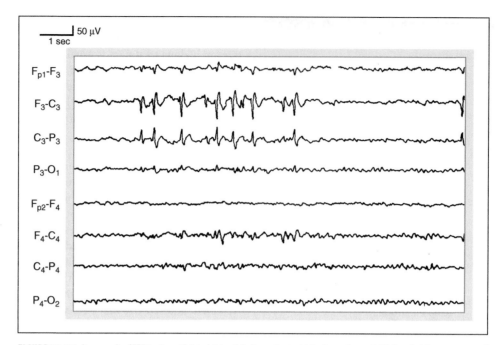

FIGURE 27–24 An example of EEG tracing with interictal activity in a patient with benign epilepsy of childhood with centrotemporal spikes (BECTS). Note the spikes prominent in the frontocentral derivations on the left. There is a phase reversal at C_3. *From Chokroverty S, Quinto C: Sleep and epilepsy. In Chokroverty S (ed): Sleep Disorders Medicine. Boston: Butterworth Heinemann, 1999, p. 711.*

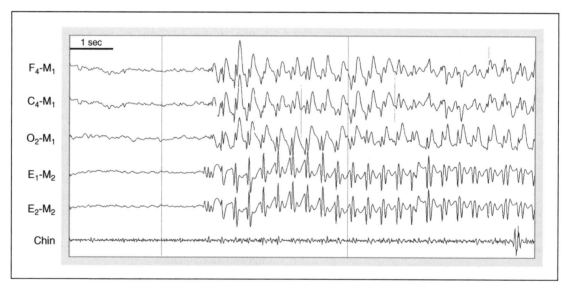

FIGURE 27–25 Three-Hz spike and wave complexes in a patient with absence epilepsy.

higher frequency has been found in patients with refractory epilepsy. **Therefore, a high index of suspicion is indicated when patients with epilepsy report disturbed sleep and snoring.** A randomized, pilot-controlled study of continuous positive airway pressure (CPAP vs. sham) in a group of patients with medically refractory epilepsy and coexistent OSA found a trend for improvement in nocturnal seizures frequency.[23] A 50% or greater reduction in seizure frequency

was noted in 28% of CPAP patients and 15% in the sham group ($P = .40$). Further large studies are needed, but certainly in individual patients, effective treatment of OSA may improve seizure control. The etiology of the benefit of CPAP treatment is not clear. It is known that prior sleep deprivation or disturbance can worsen seizure control. Therefore, improvements in sleep with CPAP treatment may be one mechanism by which seizure control is improved.

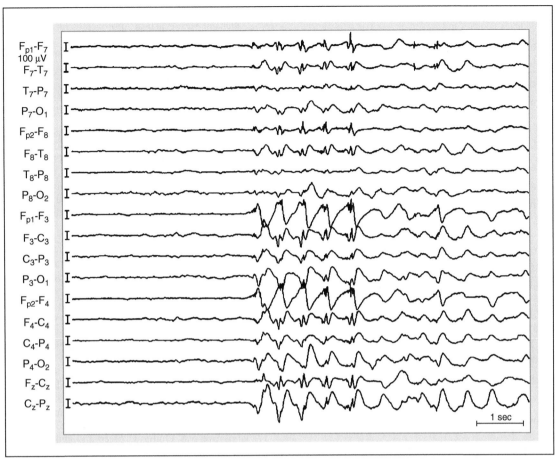

FIGURE 27–26 A tracing from a patient with slow spike and wave activity and the Lennox-Gastaut syndrome. *From Foldvary-Schaefer N, Grigg-Damberger M: Sleep and epilepsy. Sleep Med Clin 2008;3:450.*

TABLE 27–9		
Effects of Common Antiepileptic Drugs on Sleep		
	POSITIVE	**NEGATIVE**
Barbiturates (phenobarbital)	Decreased sleep latency Increased sleep efficiency Increased stage N2	Decreased REM
Carbamazepine	None known	Decreased REM?
Phenytoin	Decreased sleep latency	Increased arousal Increased stage N1 Decreased REM
Valproic acid	None known	Increased stage N1
Gabapentin	Increased stage N3 Decreased arousals	None
Levetiracetam	Increased stage N3	None
REM = rapid eye movement.		

CLINICAL REVIEW QUESTIONS

1. Which of the following characterizes the propensity of nocturnal seizures?
   A. NREM > REM > wake.
   B. Wake > REM > NREM.
   C. NREM > wake > REM.
   D. Wake > NREM > REM.

2. What is the most frequent type of nocturnal partial seizure?
   A. TLE.
   B. NFLE.
   C. AE.
   D. JME.

3. Phase reversal is helpful to:
   A. Identify a transient as epileptiform.
   B. Localize a transient or seizure focus.
   C. A and B.

4. Which of the following statements about POSTS is not true?

    A. They are positive.

    B. They have an occipital location.

    C. They occur during wake.

    D. They are sharp wave.

5. Which of the following is NOT true about mu rhythm?

    A. They are 8 to 13 Hz.

    B. They are most prominent in occipital derivations.

    C. They are attenuated by contralateral arm movement.

    D. They have archiform morphology.

Answers

1. C. NREM > wake > REM. During NREM, seizures out of N2 are more common.

2. A. Although FLE is more likely to occur during the night compared to during the day, NTLE is more common than NFLE as TLE is much more common than FLE. AE is a generalized epilepsy. JME is manifested as myoclonic jerks soon after awakening.

3. B. Phase reversal is helpful for localization but does not imply abnormality.

4. C. POSTS occur during NREM sleep.

5. B. Mu rhythm is more prominent in the central derivations.

REFERENCES

1. American Clinical Neurophysiology Society: Guideline 5: guidelines for standard electrode position nomenclature. J Clin Neurophysiol 2006;23:107–110.
2. International Federation of Societies for Electroencephalography and Clinical Neurophysiology: Ten twenty electrode system. EEG Clin Neurophysiol 1958;10:371–375.
3. Iber C, Ancoli-Israel S, Chesson A, Quan SF, for the American Academy of Sleep Medicine: The AASM Manual for Scoring of Sleep and Associated Events: Rules, Terminology and Technical Specifications, 1st ed. Westchester, IL: American Academy of Sleep Medicine, 2007.
4. Fisch BJ: Spehlman's EEG Primer. New York: Elsevier, 1991.
5. Libenson MH: Practical Approach to Electroencephalography. Philadelphia: Saunders Elsevier, 2010.
6. American Clinical Neurophysiology Society: Guideline 6: a proposal for standard montages to be used in clinical EEG. J Clin Neurophysiol 2006;23:111–117.
7. Foldvary N, Caruso AC, Mascha E, et al: Identifying montages that best detect electrographic seizure activity during polysomnography. Sleep 2000;23:1–9.
8. Foldvary N: Video-encephalography/polysomnography for monitoring nocturnal events. In Lee-Chiong TL, Sateia MJ, Carsakadon MA (eds): Sleep Medicine. Philadelphia: Hanley & Belfus, 2002, pp. 681–688.
9. Commission on Classification and Terminology of the International League Against Epilepsy: Proposal for revised classification of epilepsies and epileptic syndromes. Epilepsia 1989;30:389–399.
10. Malow BA: Sleep and epilepsy. Neurol Clin 2005;23:1127.
11. Bazil CW: Nocturnal seizures. Semin Neurol 2004;24:293–300.
12. Herman ST, Walczak TS, Bazil CW: Distribution of partial seizures during the sleep-wake cycle: differences by seizure onset site. Neurology 2001;56:1453–1459.
13. Provini F, Plazzi G, Montagna P, Lugaresi E: The wide spectrum of nocturnal frontal lobe epilepsy. Sleep Med Rev 2000;4:375–386.
14. Provini F, Plazzi G, Tinuper P, et al: Nocturnal frontal lobe epilepsy. Brain 1999;122:1017–1031.
15. Tachiban N, Shinde A, Ikeda A, et al: Supplementary motor area seizure resembling sleep disorder. Sleep 1996;19:811–816.
16. Derry CP, Harvey AS, Walker MC, et al: NREM arousal parasomnias and their distinction from nocturnal frontal lobe epilepsy: a video EEG analysis. Sleep 2009;32:1637–1644.
17. Chokroverty S, Quinto C: Sleep and epilepsy. In Chokroverty S (ed): Sleep Disorders Medicine. Boston: Butterworth Heinemann, 1999, pp. 697–727.
18. Hrachovy RA, Frost JD: The EEG in selected generalized seizures. J Clin Neurophysiol 2006;23:312–332.
19. Vaughn BV, D'Cruz OF: Sleep and epilepsy. Semin Neurol 2004;24:301–313.
20. Foldvary-Schaefer N, Grigg-Damberger M: Sleep and epilepsy. Sleep Med Clin 2008;3:443–454.
21. Bazil CW: Nocturnal seizures and the effects of anticonvulsants on sleep. Curr Neurol Neurosci Rep 2008;8:149–154.
22. Manni R, Terzaghi M: Comorbidity between epilepsy and sleep disorders. Epilepsy Res 2010;90:171–177.
23. Malow BA, Foldarvy-Schaefer N, Vaught BV, et al: Treating obstructive sleep apnea in adults with epilepsy. Neurology 2008;71:572–577.

Chapter 28

Parasomnias

Chapter Points

- *Parasomnias* are defined as "undesirable physical events or experiences that occur during entry to sleep, within sleep, or during arousals from sleep."
- The indications for evaluation of patients with a suspected parasomnia with PSG include (1) potentially violent or injurious behavior, (2) behavior that is extremely disruptive to household members, (3) the parasomnia results in a complaint of excessive sleepiness, and (4) the parasomnia is associated with medical, psychiatric, or neurologic symptoms or findings.
- If a PSG is indicated for evaluation of a patient for a suspected parasomnia, then use of video PSG (synchronized video and audio) with additional EEG electrodes is recommended.
- The NREM parasomnias include confusional arousals (awakening with confusion), sleepwalking (ambulation during sleep), and sleep terrors (awakening with loud scream and intense fear). In children, NREM parasomnias occur out of stage N3 (first part of the night) but in adults can occur out of stages N1 or N2 during any part of the night. Approximately 60–70% of adults with a NREM parasomnia experienced one or more NREM parasomnias in childhood.
- The REM parasomnias include the RBD, nightmare disorder, and recurrent sleep paralysis.
- Diagnostic criteria for RBD include
  - REM sleep without atonia: the EMG finding of excessive amounts of **sustained or intermittent elevation (transient muscle activity) of submental EMG tone** or excessive phasic submental or (upper or lower) limb EMG twitching.
  - At least one of the following is present:
    - Sleep-related injurious, potentially injurious, or disruptive behavior **by history.**
    - Abnormal REM sleep behavior documented **during PSG monitoring.**
    - Absence of EEG epileptiform activity during REM sleep (unless RBD can be clearly distinguished from any concurrent REM sleep-related seizure disorder).
- The sleep disturbance is not better explained by another sleep disorder, medical or neurologic disorder, mental disorder, or substance use disorder.
- Treatments for RBD include environmental precautions, clonazepam, and/or melatonin (often in high doses).
- The overlap parasomnia consists of manifestations of both an NREM parasomnia and RBD.
- RBD has been associated with narcolepsy, Parkinson's disease, dementia with Lewy bodies, multiple system atrophy, multiple sclerosis, and certain medications. A significant proportion of patients with "idiopathic RBD" later develop Parkinson's disease.
- Nocturnal seizures may mimic parasomnias—especially frontal lobe epilepsy. Features favoring epilepsy over a parasomnia include stereotypical behavior (same manifestations each time) and more than one episode per night.
- The sleep-related eating disorder is manifested by eating and drinking during the main sleep period and is associated with a variable degree of alertness and recall for the eating behavior. The behavior must be associated with one or more of several manifestations including eating peculiar food items, associated with insomnia due to sleep disturbance from the eating episodes, sleep-related injury, dangerous behaviors in pursuit of food, morning anorexia, or adverse consequences of binge eating.
- Catathrenia is characterized by a deep inspiration and long expiratory groan, most commonly during REM sleep.
- *Secondary enuresis* is defined as the onset of enuresis in a patient who has previously been dry for at least 6 months. The diagnosis of OSA should be considered in all children who snore and have secondary enuresis.
- The exploding head syndrome is characterized by a sudden loud imagined noise or sense of violent explosion in the head occurring as the patient is falling asleep on waking during the night. The event is painless but patients usually awaken with fright.

Determining a cause for abnormal movements or behavior during sleep is often a challenging problem for sleep physicians. A **parasomnia** is a motor, verbal, or experiential phenomenon that occurs in association with sleep (at sleep onset, during sleep, or after arousal from sleep) and is often undesirable. The term *parasomnia* comes from a combination of *para* from the Greek prefix meaning "alongside of" with the Latin word *somnus* meaning "sleep." In the usual clinical setting, the term refers to undesirable events. In the International Classification of Sleep Disorders, 2nd edition (ICSD-2),[1] parasomnias are defined as "undesirable physical events or experiences that occur during entry to sleep, within sleep, or during arousals from sleep."

Evaluation of nocturnal "spells or unusual behavior" begins with a detailed history of the nature, age of onset, and time of night of the episodes. Factors (sleep deprivation and medications) that may have affected the behaviors should be explored. A neurologic examination should be performed to rule out associated neurologic disorders. Not all parasomnias require evaluation by polysomnography (PSG). The indications for evaluation with PSG include[2-4]: (1) potentially violent or injurious behavior, (2) the behavior is extremely disruptive to household members, (3) the parasomnia results in a complaint of excessive sleepiness, and (4) the parasomnia is associated with medical, psychiatric, or neurologic symptoms or findings.

Video PSG (usually with synchronized video and audio) is the recommended method of evaluating parasomnias. Today, virtually all digital PSG equipment manufacturers offer synchronized video and audio with their digital PSG recording systems. Additional electroencephalogram (EEG) electrodes are commonly used to monitor patients with a suspected parasomnia to improve the ability to detect interictal or seizure activity. Additional arm electromyogram (EMG) derivations (flexor digitorum) are often performed in addition to right and left tibialis anterior (leg) EMGs to detect transient muscle activity (TMA; phasic muscle activity) during rapid eye movement (REM) sleep. One problem with monitoring parasomnias is that they frequently do not occur every night. Multiple nights of video PSG may be needed.

The ICSD-2 lists a number of parasomnias (Box 28–1).[1] Some parasomnias are associated with non–rapid eye movement (NREM) sleep, some with REM sleep, and some are classified as "other parasomnias" because they can occur during either NREM or REM sleep or during wakefulness soon after arousal from sleep.

NREM PARASOMNIAS

The NREM parasomnias include (1) confusional arousals, (2) sleepwalking, and (3) sleep terrors.[5-8] There is some overlap in these parasomnias and individual patients may manifest behavior consistent with all three types of NREM parasomnias on different nights. Although not listed in the major ICSD-2 diagnostic categories, sleep-related sexual behavior and sleep-related violence are considered variants

---

BOX 28–1

Classification of Parasomnias

A. DISORDERS OF AROUSAL FROM NREM SLEEP

1. Confusional arousals
2. Sleepwalking
3. Sleep terrors

B. DISORDERS USUALLY ASSOCIATED WITH REM SLEEP

1. REM sleep behavior disorder (including parasomnia overlap disorder and status dissociatus)
2. Recurrent isolated sleep paralysis
3. Nightmare disorders

C. OTHER PARASOMNIAS

1. Sleep-related dissociative disorders
2. Sleep enuresis
3. Sleep-related groaning (catathrenia)
4. Exploding head syndrome
5. Sleep-related hallucinations
6. Sleep-related eating disorder
7. Parasomnia, unspecified
8. Parasomnia due to drug or substance
9. Parasomnia due to medical condition

NREM = non–rapid eye movement; REM = rapid eye movement.
From American Academy of Sleep Medicine: ICSD-2 International Classification of Sleep Disorders, 2nd ed. Diagnostic and Coding Manual. Westchester, IL: American Academy of Sleep Medicine, 2005.

---

of the confusional arousal–sleepwalking–sleep terrors spectrum.

Confusional Arousals

Confusional arousals usually occur from stage N3 in the first part of the night but can occur after an arousal from NREM sleep at any hour. In children, confusional arousals usually occur out of stage N3. In adults, confusional arousals may also occur out of stage N1 or stage N2.[1,5] Amnesia for the event is common. Confusional arousal events are brief and, because of amnesia, often go unnoticed unless reported by the bed partner. During awakening, behavior may be inappropriate (especially forced awakening) and even violent. Although behaviors are usually simple (movements in bed, thrashing about, vocalization, or inconsolable crying), they can be more complex. There is frequently an overlap between confusional arousals and sleepwalking. In contrast to sleep terrors, patients with confusional arousals do **NOT** exhibit autonomic hyperactivity or signs of fear or emit a blood-curdling scream.

Prevalence

Confusional arousal episodes are common in children aged younger than 13 years with a prevalence of 17%. In older individuals (>15 yr of age), the prevalence is much lower (3–4%). Men and women are equally affected.

Precipitating and Predisposing Factors

Common factors precipitating confusional arousals include sleep deprivation, bipolar and depressive disorders, obstructive sleep apnea (OSA), and rotating shift/night shift work. There is frequently a family history of similar events in related individuals. In children, the confusional arousals usually resolve after age 5 years.

Variants of Confusional Arousals

The ICSD-2 lists two variants of confusional arousals[1]:

1. Severe morning sleep inertia (sleep drunkenness): This is a variant of confusional arousal in adults and arousal is often out of stage N2 or stage N1 sleep.
2. Sleep-related sexual behaviors: These include masturbation or sexual assault on adults or minors (sleep sex). This entity is described in more detail later in the "Sleepwalking (Somnambulism)" section.

PSG Findings during Confusional Arousals

The EEG during arousal may show persistent delta activity, theta activity, or diffuse poorly reactive alpha activity. Increased chin EMG activity is typical and EMG artifact in the EEG derivations is common (Fig. 28–1). **At event onset, the heart rate increases.**

Diagnosis of Confusional Arousals

The ICSD-2 diagnostic criteria for confusional arousals are listed in Box 28–2. Note that PSG findings are not part of the criteria. Most patients with confusional arousals will not require PSG unless the parasomnia has resulted in injury, the potential for injury, or if treatment is being considered.

Differential Diagnosis of Confusional Arousals

The differential diagnosis of confusional arousals, sleepwalking, and sleep terrors is discussed later in this chapter.

Treatment of Confusional Arousals

Usually, no treatment is needed. There are no controlled studies concerning treatment of confusional arousals. Benzodiazepine receptor agonists (BZRAs) and tricyclic antidepressants (TCAs) have been used.[4-6]

Sleepwalking (Somnambulism)

Sleepwalking is defined as a series of complex behaviors that are initiated during sleep (usually stage N3) and result in ambulation (Boxes 28–3 to 28–5). Activity can vary from simply sitting up in bed to walking. Patients usually are difficult to awaken during these episodes and, if awakened, are confused. Of interest, *the eyes are usually open (wide open and "glassy-eyed") during sleepwalking,*[1,3] but patients may be clumsy in their movements. Talking during sleep (somniloquy) can occur simultaneously. In children, sleepwalking usually occurs during the first third of the night, when stage N3 is present. However, studies in adults have recorded episodes beginning in stage N1 or N2 sleep and frequently in the second half of the night.[5-8] Episodes of sleepwalking in children are rarely violent, and movements often are slow. In

BOX 28–2

Confusional Arousals—Diagnostic Criteria

A. Recurrent mental confusion or confusional behavior occurs during arousal or awakening from nocturnal sleep or a daytime nap.
B. The disturbance is not better explained by another sleep disorder, medical or neurologic disorder, mental disorder, or substance use disorder.

From American Academy of Sleep Medicine: ICSD-2 International Classification of Sleep Disorders, 2nd ed. Diagnostic and Coding Manual. Westchester, IL: American Academy of Sleep Medicine, 2005.

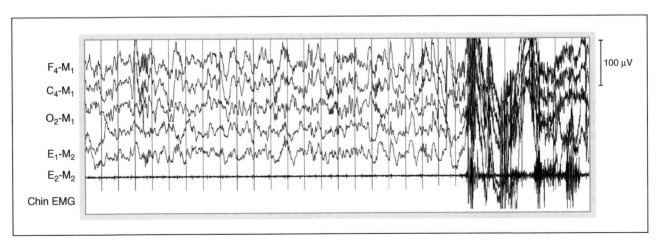

FIGURE 28–1 A 30-second epoch shows a confusional arousal from stage N3 in a 45-year-old adult. There was no evidence of change in airflow before the episode. Note the absence of any change in the electroencephalogram (EEG) or electromyogram (EMG) derivations before the arousal. The patient abruptly sat up and looked around, appearing confused.

BOX 28–3

Sleepwalking (Somnambulism)—Diagnostic Criteria

A. Ambulation occurs during sleep.

B. **Persistence of sleep, an altered state of consciousness, or impaired judgment during ambulation** is demonstrated by at least one of the following:
  i. Difficulty in arousing the person.
  ii. Mental confusion when awakened from an episode.
  iii. Amnesia (complete or partial) for the episode.
  iv. Routine behaviors that occur at inappropriate times.
  v. Inappropriate or nonsensical behaviors.
  vi. Dangerous or potentially dangerous behaviors.

C. The disturbance is not better explained by another sleep disorder, medical or neurologic disorder, mental disorder, or substance use disorder.

From American Academy of Sleep Medicine: ICSD-2 International Classification of Sleep Disorders, 2nd ed. Diagnostic and Coding Manual. Westchester, IL: American Academy of Sleep Medicine, 2005.

BOX 28–4

Predisposing Factors for Sleepwalking and Sleep Terrors

- Genetic
  - Risk of sleepwalking
    - 22% if neither parent affected.
    - 45% if one parent affected by sleepwalking.
    - 60% if both parents have history of sleepwalking.
    - 65% if twin has sleepwalking.
- Sleep deprivation.
- Fever, life stress, novel bedroom.
- Untreated obstructive sleep apnea, or with initial CPAP treatment.
- CNS disease—migraines, head injury, encephalitis.
- Alcohol abuse.
- Medications
  - Zolpidem.
  - Lithium carbonate.
  - Phenothiazines.

CNS = central nervous system; CPAP = continuous positive airway pressure.

BOX 28–5

Sleepwalking Facts

- About 60–70% of adults with sleepwalking had episodes as children.
- Sleepwalking classically occurs during stage N3 in the first part of the night.
- Sleepwalking in some adults can occur in stage N1 or N2 sleep and in the second half of the night.
- The persistence of sleepwalking into adulthood or re-emergence of sleepwalking does NOT always imply underlying psychopathology. However, a significant proportion may have current or past psychopathology.
- Prior sleep deprivation with resulting slow wave sleep rebound (as with nasal CPAP treatment for OSA) can trigger episodes of sleepwalking.
- Treatment of sleepwalking
  - Environmental precautions.
  - Avoid sleep deprivation.
  - Clonazepam and other BZRAs.
  - TCAs.
  - SSRIs.

BZRAs = benzodiazepine receptor agonists; CPAP = continuous positive airway pressure; OSA = obstructive sleep apnea; SSRIs = selective serotonin reuptake inhibitors; TCAs = tricyclic antidepressants.

adults, sleepwalking episodes can be more complex, frenzied, violent, and longer in duration. Episodes of sleepwalking may be terminated by the patient returning to bed or simply lying down and continuing sleep out of bed. Patients are difficult to arouse during sleepwalking episodes. When aroused during sleepwalking, patients are typically very confused. In addition, there is total amnesia for the sleepwalking episodes (see Box 28–4).

Epidemiology and Familial Pattern of Sleepwalking

Sleepwalking can occur as soon as children can walk but peaks between the ages of 4 and 8 occurring in between 10% and 20% of children. **The onset of sleepwalking can also occur in adulthood.** However, **most adult sleepwalkers had episodes during childhood** (60–70% of adults with sleepwalking exhibited this parasomnia during childhood). Sleepwalking usually disappears in adolescence. One study of 100 patients with sleep-related injury found that 33% with sleepwalking had an age of onset after age 16, and 70% had episodes arising from both stages N1 and N2 as well as stage N3. The sleepwalking behaviors were variable in duration and intensity.[6]

Familial, Precipitating, and Predisposing Factors

A number of predisposing and precipitating factors for NREM parasomnias (including sleepwalking) have been identified in children and adults.[1,8,9] There is a definite **familial role in the development of sleepwalking** (see Box 28–4). If one or both parents have a history of sleepwalking, the risk of a child developing sleepwalking episodes is greatly increased. Fever, sleep deprivation, and certain medications (e.g., zolpidem and other BZRAs, phenothiazines, TCAs, lithium) can precipitate the events. Sleepwalking during slow wave sleep rebound has been reported in a patient with OSA treated with nasal continuous positive airway pressure (CPAP).[10] Untreated sleep apnea can also be a predisposing factor, given the frequent arousals associated with respiratory events in this disorder. Effective treatment of sleep apnea can reduce the frequency of sleepwalking in some patients.[11]

The relationship between mental illness and adult NREM parasomnias is a topic of controversy.[6,12] Some have suggested that persistence of sleepwalking into adulthood is a manifestation of underlying psychopathology. However,

Schenck and coworkers[6] found evidence of prior or current psychopathology in only about 48% of adults with sleepwalking/sleep terrors who underwent PSG monitoring for sleep-related injury. Therefore, the adult sleepwalking patients were equally as likely not to have psychopathology as to have this problem. In addition, there was typically no association between sleepwalking/sleep terrors and any concurrent psychopathology with respect to onset, clinical course, or treatment response.[12] However, because mental illness and medication used to treat mental illness can disturb sleep, sleepwalking could well occur or re-emerge in patients with active mental illness.

PSG in Sleepwalking

Although PSG is rarely performed to evaluate cases of sleepwalking, the classic finding is a sudden arousal occurring in stage N3 sleep (Fig. 28–2). During the prolonged arousal, there usually is tachycardia and often persistence of slow wave EEG activity—despite the presence of high-frequency EEG activity and an increase in EMG amplitude. Analysis of a large group of patients with sleepwalking and sleep terrors found that there was no **prearousal buildup of delta activity, increase in heart rate, or prearousal increase in chin EMG.** Postarousal, the EEG showed three patterns: (1) diffuse rhythmic (synchronized) delta activity, (2) diffuse delta and theta activity, and (3) prominent alpha and beta activity.[13] The heart rate is often noted to increase at the onset of the event.

Diagnosis of Sleepwalking

Diagnostic criteria for sleepwalking are listed in Box 28–3 and do not require PSG findings. The ICSD-2 major criteria for a diagnosis of sleepwalking[1] include (A) ambulation during sleep and (B) evidence of persistent sleep, altered consciousness, or **impaired judgment during ambulation.**

Evidence for an altered state of consciousness includes difficulty in arousing the person, mental confusion when awakened from an episode, amnesia (complete or partial) for the episode, and abnormal behaviors. Abnormal behaviors include routine behaviors that occur at inappropriate times, inappropriate or nonsensical behaviors, and dangerous or potentially dangerous behaviors.

Differential Diagnosis of Sleepwalking

The differential diagnosis of sleepwalking is discussed with confusional arousal and sleep terrors in a later section.

Sleep-Related Sexual Behavior and Sleep-Related Violence

The main complications of sleepwalking are social embarrassment and danger of self-injury or injury to others. Violent behavior (self-mutilation or homicide) and sexual assault (sleep sex) have been reported in association with sleepwalking episodes. **Sleep-related sexual behavior or sex-somnia**[14,15] is a parasomnia in which sexual behavior occurs with limited awareness during the act, relative unresponsiveness to the external environment, and amnesia for the event. The behaviors range from sexual vocalizations to intercourse. These actions may include behaviors very atypical for the individual (e.g., anal intercourse). In contrast to typical sleepwalking, these events can exceed 30 minutes.

Sleep-related violence occurs in a state consistent with sleepwalking/sleep terrors and is associated with an emotion of fear or anger. The violent behavior may be directed at individuals in close proximity or those who confront the individual during the parasomnia.[16,17] The patient may either awaken or go back to sleep but typically has amnesia for the event. The violence is often atypical for the individual. Most cases of sleep-related violence occur in middle-aged men with a history of prior sleepwalking.

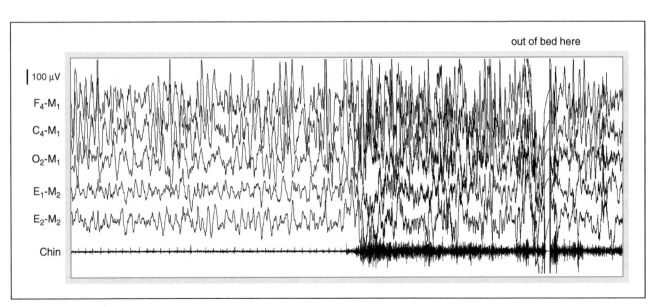

FIGURE 28–2 A 60-second tracing shows an episode of sleepwalking that occurred out of stage N3 in a 5-year-old boy. Note the persistence of slow wave activity during the arousal and subsequent body movements. The patient abruptly aroused, sat up, and left the bed.

Sleep Disorders and the Law

Automatisms are defined as involuntary behavior over which an individual has no control. The behavior may be out of character and the individual may have no recall for the events. The sleep automatisms likely to result in injurious behavior include NREM parasomnias, sleep-related dissociative disorders (SRDDs; discussed in a later section), and sleep-related epilepsy. An important legal question for consideration is **the presence or absence of criminal intent.** When criminal action is taken against the violent sleepwalker, sleep medicine physicians may be called as expert witnesses.[16,17] There are guidelines for expert witness qualifications and testimony.[17] In addition, criteria have been proposed to assist in determination of the putative role of an underlying sleep disorder[17] (Box 28–6).

Treatment of Sleepwalking

The treatment of sleepwalking includes environmental precautions (e.g., closed doors and windows, sleeping on the first level) and avoidance of precipitating causes such as sleep deprivation as well as reassurance. If the episodes are determined to require medication, benzodiazepines, TCAs, or selective serotonin reuptake inhibitors (SSRIs) may be tried. Clonazepam 0.5 to 2.0 mg qhs or temazepam 30 mg qhs are commonly prescribed. Medications should be given early enough before bedtime so that sleepwalking in the first slow wave cycle is prevented. In one study of patients with self-injurious behavior, bedtime clonazepam was successful in controlling sleep terrors/sleepwalking in greater than 80% of cases.[6] However, not all studies have found clonazepam to be this effective. Another study of treatment of patients with sleepwalking found that those with any degree of sleep apnea had fewer sleepwalking episodes if sleep apnea was effectively treated.[11] Conversely, treatment with benzodiazepines was NOT effective in those without sleep-related breathing problems.[11] A recent systematic review of sleepwalking treatments found that no large controlled studies of treatment for sleepwalking have been reported.[18]

Sleep Terrors

Sleep terrors, also called *night terrors* or *pavor nocturnus,* consist of sudden arousal, usually from stage N3 sleep, accompanied by a blood-curdling scream or cry and manifestations of severe fear (behavioral and autonomic) (Boxes 28–7 and 28–8). The affected individual typically is confused, diaphoretic, and tachycardic, and he or she frequently sits up in bed. It is difficult or impossible to communicate with a

---

BOX 28–6

Guidelines for Determination of the Putative Role of a Sleep Disorder in a Violent Act

1. A reason to suspect a sleep disorder exists (history, PSG findings).
2. Duration of episodes is brief (min)—can be much longer.
3. Behavior is abrupt, immediate, impulsive, without apparent motivation, no premeditation.
4. Victim is someone who happened to be present.
5. Immediately upon return of consciousness—horror at event, no attempt to escape or conceal act.
6. Some degree of amnesia for event.
7. In case of sleepwalking, the act must:
   a. Occur upon awakening, usually at least 1 hour after sleep onset.
   b. Occur on attempt to awaken the patient.
   c. Be potentiated by alcohol ingestion, sedative/hypnotic administration, or prior sleep deprivation.

PSG = polysomnography.
Adapted from Mahowald MW, Schenck CH: Parasomnias: sleep walking and the law. Sleep Med Rev 2000;4:321–339.

BOX 28–7

Sleep Terrors—Diagnostic Criteria

A. Sudden episode of terror occurs during sleep, usually initiated by a cry or loud scream that is accompanied by **autonomic nervous system activation** and behavioral manifestations of intense fear.
B. At least one of the following is present:
   i. Difficulty in arousing the person.
   ii. Mental confusion when awakened from episode.
   iii. Amnesia (complete or partial) for the episode.
   iv. Dangerous or potentially dangerous behaviors.
C. The disturbance is not better explained by another sleep disorder, medical or neurologic disorder, mental disorder, medication use, or substance use disorder.

From American Academy of Sleep Medicine: ICSD-2 International Classification of Sleep Disorders, 2nd ed. Diagnostic and Coding Manual. Westchester, IL: American Academy of Sleep Medicine, 2005.

BOX 28–8

Sleep Terror Facts

- In children, sleep terrors occur out of stage N3 in the first part of night.
- In adults, sleep terrors can occur from stage N2 sleep.
- Patients may manifest both sleep terrors and sleepwalking.
- In contrast to confusional arousals, patients with sleep terrors have profound autonomic hyperactivity and manifestations of fear.
- Unlike RBD or nightmares, patients with sleep terrors do not relate dream mentation associated with the event,
- The persistence of sleep terrors into adulthood, re-emergence of sleep terrors in adulthood, or onset of sleep terrors in adulthood is not necessarily evidence that psychopathology is present.
- Sleep terrors have been described in adults during nasal CPAP treatment of OSA.

CPAP = continuous positive airway pressure; OSA = obstructive sleep apnea; RBD = rapid eye movement sleep behavior disorder.

person having a sleep terror, and total amnesia for the event is usual. Patients may sleepwalk during episodes of sleep terrors. Thus, many consider sleepwalking and sleep terrors to be one syndrome with a spectrum of manifestations.

Epidemiology

Sleep terrors typically occur in prepubertal children (≤3%) and subside by adolescence; they are uncommon in adults. Sleep terrors rarely begin in adulthood. As noted previously, one study of patients with sleep terrors/sleepwalking evaluated for sleep-related injury found that 48% had evidence of current or prior psychopathology.[6] However, adults with sleep terrors are just as likely not to have related psychopathology as to have this problem. In addition, sleep terrors/sleepwalking and any concurrent psychopathology are often not closely associated with respect to their onset, clinical course, or treatment response.[12]

Precipitating and Predisposing Factors

Stress, febrile illness, sleep deprivation, and heavy caffeine intake have been identified as inciting agents for sleep terrors. Stressful events and sleep deprivation can sometimes precipitate re-emergence of problems that were present in childhood. Slow wave sleep rebound, such as occurs with nasal CPAP treatment of OSA, has also been associated with episodes of sleep terrors.[19]

PSG Findings Associated with Sleep Terrors

PSG is usually not required to evaluate sleep terrors unless the episodes are frequent, are violent, or have the potential to result in self-injury. When PSG is performed, video PSG is indicated. If seizures are suspected, a complete clinical EEG montage is needed. When a sleep terror is captured, it appears as a sudden arousal from slow wave sleep. The chin EMG amplitude is greatly increased, and alpha waves are present; however, persistent slow wave activity is also noted.

Diagnosis of Sleep Terrors

The ICSD-2 criteria are listed in Box 28-7. The diagnostic criteria include an episode of terror usually **initiated by a loud scream** that is accompanied by **autonomic nervous system activation and behavioral manifestations of intense fear.** In addition, evidence of an altered state of consciousness including difficulty in arousing the person, mental confusion after awakening, and partial or complete amnesia for the event is required.

Treatment of Sleep Terrors

The treatment of sleep terrors is similar to that for confusional arousal and sleepwalking. If the episodes of sleep terrors are infrequent, treatment beyond simple environmental precautions is unnecessary. The medications used for sleepwalking have also been used for sleep terrors. Benzodiazepines, TCAs, and SSRIs have been used with some success. No controlled study has evaluated treatments for sleep terrors.[18] Avoidance of inciting agents is recommended (see Box 28-4).

Differential Diagnosis of NREM Parasomnias

Comparison of characteristics of confusional arousal, sleep terrors, and sleepwalking are listed in Table 28-1. The differential diagnosis of these NREM parasomnias includes the rapid eye movement sleep behavior disorder (RBD), nightmare disorder, nocturnal seizure activity, the posttraumatic stress disorder (PTSD), and nocturnal panic attacks. Nightmare disorders (also called *dream anxiety attacks*) and RBD occur during REM sleep and are more common in the second part of the night. Body movements during RBD can result in patients leaving the bed but rarely the bedroom. RBD usually does not begin until after age 40 and has a strong male predominance. When patients are awakened from RBD episodes they are less confused than in NREM parasomnias. Differentiation of NREM parasomnias from partial complex seizures is difficult without complete EEG monitoring. Seizures tend to be more stereotypical and may occur during the day. Patients with nightmares, the PTSD, and RBD typically can relate complex dream mentation that promoted the event. In sleep-related panic attacks,[20] the patient can awaken from NREM sleep following arousals and develop autonomic activation and fear. However, in contrast to the NREM parasomnias, patients with panic attacks do not have confusion, nonresponsiveness, amnesia, or dramatic motor activity. Panic attacks occur during wakefulness and tend to build in intensity over several minutes.

TABLE 28-1			
Comparison of the Characteristics of Non–Rapid Eye Movement Parasomnias			
	CONFUSIONAL AROUSAL	**SLEEPWALKING**	**SLEEP TERRORS**
Onset	Stage N3 children Stage N2, N3 adults	Same	Same
Autonomic hyperactivity	No	No	Prominent
Loud scream	No	No	Yes
Confusion during episode	Yes	Yes	Yes
Amnesia (partial or complete)	Yes	Yes	Yes

PARASOMNIAS USUALLY ASSOCIATED WITH REM SLEEP (STAGE R)

Parasomnias usually associated with REM sleep (stage R) include RBD, recurrent isolated sleep paralysis, and nightmare disorders (see Box 28–1). RBD has two variants: overlap parasomnia and status dissociatus (SD).

REM Sleep Behavior Disorder (RBD; Including Variants)

RBD is characterized by a loss of the normal muscle atonia associated with REM sleep with dream-enactment behavior (oneirism) that is often violent in nature (Box 28–9).[6,21–24] Dreams are "acted out." Limb and body movements often are violent (e.g., hitting a wall, kicking) and may be associated with emotionally charged utterances. The movements can be related to dream content ("kicking an attacker"), but the patient **may or may not** remember associated dream material when awakened during an episode. Serious injury to the patient or the bed partner can result from these episodes, which typically occur one to four times a week. Because the episodes occur during REM sleep, they are most common during the early morning hours (the second half of the night). There is a strong male predominance and most cases occur after age 50.

Epidemiology of RBD

The median age of onset is about 50 years, and a milder prodrome of sleep talking, simple limb-jerking, or vividly violent dreams may precede the full-blown syndrome. RBD can be idiopathic or associated with a number of neurodegenerative disorders and medications[25–28] (Box 28–10).

BOX 28–9

Rapid Eye Movement Sleep Behavior Disorder—Diagnostic Criteria
A. Presence of REM sleep without atonia: the EMG finding of excessive amounts of **sustained or intermittent elevation of submental EMG tone** or excessive phasic submental or (upper or lower) limb EMG twitching.
B. At least one of the following is present:
i. Sleep-related injurious, potentially injurious, or disruptive behavior **by history.**
ii. Abnormal REM sleep behavior documented **during PSG monitoring.**
C. Absence of EEG epileptiform activity during REM sleep, unless RBD can be clearly distinguished from any concurrent REM sleep-related seizure disorder.
D. The sleep disturbance is not better explained by another sleep disorder, medical or neurologic disorder, mental disorder, or substance use disorder.
EEG = electro-oculogram; EMG = electromyogram; PSG = polysomnography; RBD = rapid eye movement sleep behavior disorder; REM = rapid eye movement. From American Academy of Sleep Medicine: ICSD-2 International Classification of Sleep Disorders, 2nd ed. Diagnostic and Coding Manual. Westchester, IL: American Academy of Sleep Medicine, 2005.

Pathophysiology of RBD

In animal experiments, lesions in areas of the pons (subcoeruleus in cat, sublateral dorsal nucleus in the rat) can result in body movements during REM sleep.[25] As discussed in Chapter 24, descending pathways from atonia regions of the pons result in hyperpolarization and inhibition of spinal motor neurons (mediated by gamma-aminobutyric acid [GABA] and glycine) during REM sleep. Damage to the atonia regions or the descending pathways can result in REM sleep without atonia. However, the precise anatomic changes and pathophysiology associated with REM without atonia in humans remain controversial. Furthermore, REM sleep without atonia is only one of the manifestations of RBD. Areas of the brain such as the limbic system are likely involved in the generation of violent dreams and the associated emotions. Either a disorder or release from inhibition of locomotor pattern generators must also be involved in RBD pathophysiology. The fact that RBD may be a harbinger of future development of disorders such as Parkinson's disease[24,25,27] has led some to hypothesize that dysfunction of areas of the brain such as the striatum may be associated with RBD. One study found reduced striatal dopamine transporters in patients with idiopathic RBD compared with normal controls.[28] Of interest, Parkinson's disease patients had the most severe reduction in striatal dopamine receptors consistent with the idea that RBD may represent an early manifestation of Parkinson's disease in a significant number of patients.

Classifications and Causes of RBD

An acute form of RBD can occur after withdrawal from REM suppressants, such as ethanol. Even after extensive

BOX 28–10

Classification and Causes of Rapid Eye Movement Behavior Disorder
ACUTE RBD
• Alcohol withdrawal
• Substance abuse or withdrawal (barbiturates)
• Medication toxicity (caffeine, MAOIs, TCAs)
CHRONIC RBD
• Idiopathic
• Associated with other sleep disorders
• Narcolepsy
• Associated with alpha synucleopathies
• Parkinson's disease
• Lewy body dementia
• Multiple system atrophy
• Associated or worsened with medications
• SSRIs (fluoxetine, paroxetine)
• Venlafaxine
• Mirtazapine
• TCAs (imipramine)
MAOIs = monoamine oxidase inhibitors; RBD = rapid eye movement sleep behavior disorder; SSRIs = selective serotonin reuptake inhibitors; TCAs = tricyclic antidepressants.

evaluation, about 60% of cases of chronic RBD are idiopathic (see Box 28–10). Causes of chronic RBD include multiple sclerosis, subarachnoid hemorrhage, dementia, ischemic cerebrovascular disease, and brainstem neoplasms.[24–26] RBD can be associated with a number of neurologic disorders including narcolepsy and alpha synucleopathies including Parkinson's disorder, Lewy body dementia, and multiple system atrophy.[24,25] In one study, almost 40% of patients with idiopathic RBD later developed Parkinson's syndrome, although the mean time from onset of RBD to onset of Parkinson's disease was approximately 12 years.[27] There is a strong male predominance in RBD. The acute onset of RBD in a middle-aged woman with other neurologic complaints should raise the possibility of multiple sclerosis. Drug-induced or drug-exacerbated cases of RBD have been reported (see Box 28–10) with the use of monoamine oxidase inhibitors (e.g., phenelzine), TCAs (e.g., imipramine), SSRIs (e.g., fluoxetine), selective serotonin norepinephrine reuptake inhibitors (venlafaxine), and other antidepressants (mirtazapine).[26] **There can also be a sudden exacerbation of RBD when the dose of medications associated with RBD is increased.**

Pseudo-RBD A group of patients with a history of dream-enactment behavior and daytime sleepiness was found to have OSA on PSG but no evidence of REM sleep without atonia.[29] Treatment with CPAP eliminated the behaviors. It is possible that increased pressure for REM sleep (prior REM sleep fragmenation) overwhelms normal REM atonia processes in these cases. **Of note, patients with both true RBD and OSA may also exhibit fewer RBD episodes when adequately treated with CPAP.**

PSG in RBD Video PSG including both leg and arm EMG is recommended. A given PSG study may or may not reveal an episode of abnormal behavior/body movements, because most patients do not have nightly attacks. For this reason, some sleep centers perform multiple sleep studies if the diagnosis remains unclear. However, even if abnormal behavior is not documented by a given PSG, evidence of REM sleep without atonia (tonic or phasic EMG abnormality during REM sleep) is usually present. The American Academy of Sleep Medicine (AASM) scoring manual[30] provides criteria for scoring the EMG activity associated with RBD (Box 28–11). In the chin EMG, sustained muscle activity may be noted. Excessive phasic activity (TMA) may be noted in the chin EMG, limb EMGs (anterior tibial, extensor digitorum), or both (see Chapter 12). TMA in the leg EMG derivations can also be seen without evidence of sustained muscle activity in the chin EMG (Figs. 28–3 and 28–4).

When the chin EMG derivation is abnormal, identification of REM sleep (vs. stage W) may be challenging. Epochs could potentially be scored as stage W (REMs + increased chin EMG). Clues that abnormal REM sleep is present include the presence of saw-tooth waves in the EEG, excessive TMA in the chin and/or limb EMGs, and alterations in airflow associated with bursts of eye movements. The heart rate also may remain constant despite the sudden appearance of increased EMG tone (as opposed to an awakening). TMA

BOX 28–11

Scoring Rules for the Electromyogram Activity Associated with the Rapid Eye Movement Sleep Behavior Disorder

RULES

1. The PSG findings of RBD are characterized by either or both of the following features:
   a. Sustained muscle activity in REM sleep in the **chin EMG.**
   b. Excessive transient muscle activity during REM in the **chin or limb EMG.**

DEFINITIONS

Sustained muscle activity in REM sleep is defined as an epoch of REM sleep with at least 50% of the duration of the epoch having a chin EMG amplitude greater than the minimum amplitude in NREM.

Excessive transient muscle activity in REM sleep: In a 30-second epoch of REM sleep divided into 10 sequential 3-second miniepochs, at least 5 (50%) of the miniepochs contain bursts of transient muscle activity. In RBD, excessive transient muscle activity bursts are 0.1 to 5.0 seconds in duration and at least four times as high in amplitude as the background EMG activity.

EMG = electromyogram; NREM = non–rapid eye movement; PSG = polysomnography; RBD = rapid eye movement sleep behavior disorder; REM = rapid eye movement.
Adapted from Iber C, Ancoli-Israel S, Chesson A, Quan SF for the American Academy of Sleep Medicine: The AASM Manual for the Scoring of Sleep and Associated Events: Rules, Terminology and Technical Specification, 1st ed. Westchester, IL: American Academy of Sleep Medicine, 2007.

can also be mistaken for periodic limb movement in sleep (PLMS) activity. However, TMA usually contains many more brief spikes of activity. Of interest, during RBD body movements, video monitoring of the face will often show **closed eyes but obvious movements of the eyes under the eyelids consistent with REMs.** In contrast, during confusional arousals or sleepwalking, the eyes are typically open with a blank stare and dilated pupils (affected individual is still minimally responsive).

Whereas the AASM scoring manual provides criteria to determine whether a given epoch has sufficient activity in the chin and limb EMGs during REM sleep to be classified as abnormal or excessive (see Box 28–11), the number of such epochs (as a percentage of the total amount of REM sleep) that should be considered to be abnormal was not specified. In fact, it is really not possible to define what is abnormal given the night-to-night variability in manifestations of RBD. Some evidence of REM without atonia can be seen in patients taking SSRIs who have no history of dream enactment. As is discussed in the next section, a diagnosis of RBD requires more than REM sleep without atonia.

Diagnosis of RBD

The ICSD-2 criteria for RBD are listed in Box 28–9. The major points are demonstration of REM sleep without

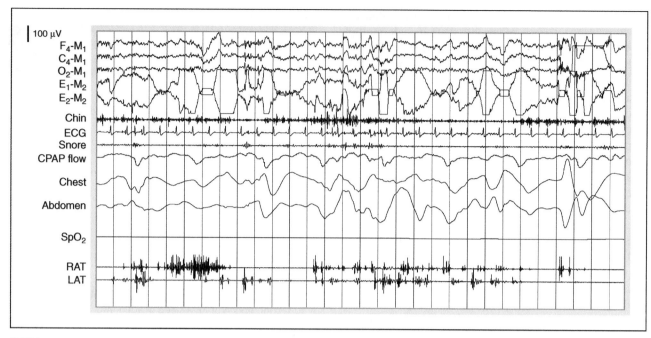

FIGURE 28–3 A 30-second epoch of rapid eye movement (REM) sleep shows both sustained and phasic chin electromyogram (EMG) activity during REM sleep (REM sleep without atonia) and increased transient muscle activity (phasic) in the right anterior tibial (RAT) and left anterior tibial (LAT) EMG derivations. CPAP = continuous positive airway pressure; ECG = electrocardiogram; SpO₂ = pulse oximetry.

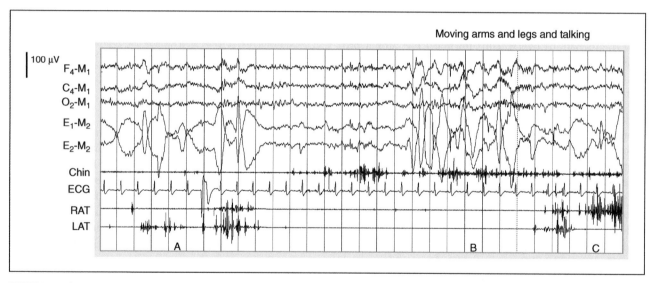

FIGURE 28–4 A 30-second epoch during stage R (REM) sleep. At *A*, the chin EMG is not increased but transient muscle activity is noted in the leg EMG derivations. At *B*, the chin shows sustained and increased phasic EMG activity but there is no increased EMG activity in the legs. At *C*, both chin and leg EMG activity is increased. At *B* and *C*, the patient was moving arms and legs and talking. ECG = electrocardiogram; LAT = left anterior EMG; RAT = right anterior tibial EMG.

atonia (sustained chin EMG activity) or increased TMA during REM sleep (chin, limbs, or both), abnormal dream-enacting behavior documented by history or video PSG, and absence of epileptiform activity during REM sleep (unless RBD can be clearly distinguished from any concurrent REM sleep-related seizure disorder). **Seizure disorders can present with manifestations virtually identical to those of RBD.** Therefore, making a diagnosis of RBD without PSG monitoring is not recommended. Absence of REM without atonia and/or body movements out of NREM sleep would be inconsistent with RBD. Nocturnal epilepsy

occurs most commonly out of NREM sleep but can rarely occur out of REM sleep (NREM > wake > REM). A detailed neurologic evaluation of patients suspected of having RBD is indicated with attention to symptoms and signs of associated neurologic disorders such as Parkinson's disease (see Box 28–10). A magnetic resonance imaging (MRI) study of the brain (to rule out structural causes) and a full clinical EEG (preferably during sleep) are usually performed especially if manifestations are atypical or patients do not respond to therapy. Important facts about RBD are listed in Box 28–12.

BOX 28–12

Rapid Eye Movement Sleep Behavior Disorder Facts

- Male predominance (80–90%)
- Older age (usually presents after 50 yr, but can occur in younger patients)
- Sleep-related injury common
- Dream enactment
- Altered dream process and content—violent and combative
- Tonic and phasic (transient muscle activity) chin EMG activity and phasic limb EMG activity during REM sleep
- Preserved sleep architecture (normal amount of REM sleep, stage N3 can be increased)
- Periodic limb movements during NREM sleep
- Efficacy of clonazepam treatment (>80%)

EMG = electromyogram; NREM = non–rapid eye movement; REM = rapid eye movement.
Adapted from Schenck CH, Mahowald MW: REM sleep behavior disorder: clinical, developmental, and neuroscience perspective 16 years after its formal identification in sleep. Sleep 2002;25:120–138.

BOX 28–13

Treatments for Rapid Eye Movement Sleep Behavior Disorder

- Environmental precautions
- Clonazepam
- Melatonin
- Other less frequently used medications
  - Nonclonazepam BZRAs (temazepam, triazolam, alprazolam)
  - Dopamine agonists (pramipexole)
  - Carbamazepine

BZRAs = benzodiazepine receptor agonists.

Variants of RBD

REM Sleep without Atonia This variant includes findings of REM sleep without atonia without a clinical history of RBD.[31] There can be limb twitching without overt body movements. This is common in patients taking SSRIs. There is some evidence that some of these patients go on to develop RBD.

Parasomnia Overlap Disorder Parasomnia overlap disorder consists of a combination of RBD and NREM parasomnias (sleepwalking, confusional arousals, sleep terrors).[32] Diagnostic criteria for both RBD and one or more of the NREM parasomnias must be met. Most patients with overlap parasomnia had some manifestation of an NREM parasomnia in childhood. Overlap parasomnia can be idiopathic or associated with narcolepsy, multiple sclerosis, brain tumor, and psychiatric disorders. The disorder may respond to treatments used for RBD such as clonazepam.

Status Dissociatus The ICSD-2 states that SD can be considered a subtype of RBD. SD is characterized by state dissociation without identifiable sleep stages but with sleep and dream-related behaviors that resemble RBD.[33] SD represents a breakdown of the typical markers of wake, NREM, and REM sleep. The patient may think she or he is awake but others think she or he is asleep. An underlying medical or neurologic condition, including narcolepsy, Parkinson's disease, dementia with Lewy bodies, and multiple system atrophy, is nearly always present. Of special interest, fatal familial insomnia and advanced human immunodeficiency virus (HIV) can manifest SD.

Useful factors differentiating SD from RBD or the overlap parasomnias are that the sleep stage before SD behavior is not discernible (parasomnia does not occur out of NREM or REM sleep) and the patient when awakened does not realize that he or she has been sleeping. **That is, the behavior occurs out of a state not clearly awake or asleep.**

Differential Diagnosis of RBD

The differential diagnosis of RBD includes sleep-related seizure activity, sleep-related dissociative disorders, PLMS, sleepwalking, sleep terrors, confusional arousals, nocturnal panic attacks, nightmares, and the PTSD. In contrast to RBD, sleepwalking (and variants) classically occurs during slow wave sleep (stage N3) and, hence, is most common in the early portion of the night. Unlike RBD, the majority of adults with sleepwalking had episodes during childhood. When patients are awakened during sleepwalking or sleep terror episodes, they are quite confused and tend to have no memory of dream content. If content is remembered, usually it is not as complex as a typical dream. However, recent studies of sleepwalking and sleep terrors in adults have shown that episodes can begin in stage N2 sleep and during the second part of the night.[6] In addition, the separation between sleepwalking/sleep terrors and RBD is not absolute—some patients have violent behavioral episodes occurring in both NREM and REM sleep (parasomnia overlap disorder). Both nightmares and the PTSD can be associated with violent or terrifying dream content and arousal from sleep.[34] However, complex body movements are uncommon with these disorders. In addition, nocturnal seizure activity usually occurs in NREM sleep, and behaviors typically are more stereotyped and less complex than in RBD. However, cases of a seizure disorder presenting with sleepwalking and/or injurious behavior that mimics RBD have been reported.[6]

Treatment of RBD

There have been no randomized, controlled clinical trials for treatment of RBD. Evidence for treatment comes from case series or anecdotal case reports.[28-31] Treatment options are listed in Box 28–13. A best clinical practice guide to treatment of RBD developed by the Standards of Practice Committee of the American Academy of Sleep Medicine[35] has recently been published following a systematic review of the published literature. Environmental precautions are an essential first step in RBD treatment because, even with effective treatment with medications, breakthrough episodes do occur. Environmental precautions include having the bedmate sleep in a separate room or bed, closed and locked windows and doors, removal of furniture with sharp edges, and use of mattress or pads on the floor near the bed.

The most evidence for effective RBD treatment is for use of clonazepam. Successful treatment of RBD has been achieved with clonazepam 0.5 to 2 mg (≤4 mg) given 30 minutes before bedtime in approximately 80% to 90% of patients. Clonazepam dramatically reduces episode frequency or severity **but usually does not totally eliminate the findings of REM sleep without atonia.** The medication also does not work by decreasing the amount of REM sleep. Clonazepam may modify dream content or inhibit the brainstem locomotor pattern generators. Clonazepam has a half-life of 30 to 40 hours and can cause early morning sedation, confusion, motor incoordination, or memory dysfunction.[35,36] It may also increase risk of falls or worsen OSA. A response hierarchy with increasing doses has been described with the following sequentially decreasing with dose escalation: vigorous violent behavior > complex nonvigorous behavior > simple limb jerking > excessive EMG twitching in stage R. Unfortunately, a significant proportion of RBD patients treated with clonazepam have one or more significant side effects.[36]

Melatonin in doses of 3 to 12 mg has also been found to be effective treatment for RBD either as a sole agent or as an add on to clonazepam.[37] Side effects of melatonin include hallucinations, morning headaches, nightmares, and morning sleepiness. In contrast to clonazepam, some studies suggest that melatonin decreases the number of stage R epochs without atonia.

Successful treatment of RBD has also been reported (case reports with small patient numbers) with pramipexole (total dose 0.75–1.5 mg),[38] paroxetine, acetylcholinesterase inhibitors, BZRAs other than clonazepam (temazepam, triazolam, alprazolam), clozapine, Yi-Gan San (an herbal medication), and carbamazepine.[39] If episodes of what appears to be RBD do NOT respond to clonazepam but DO respond to an antiepileptic medication such as carbamazepine, this is a clue that a seizure disorder rather than RBD may actually be present.

Recurrent Isolated Sleep Paralysis

Recurrent isolated sleep paralysis is characterized by inability to move at sleep onset (hypnagogic) or on awakening (hypnopompic) (Box 28–14).[1] Patients are awake and have full recall for the event. Although diaphragmatic function is not affected, a sensation of dyspnea is common. Episodes can be aborted by the affected individual being touched or spoken to or by making intense efforts to move. The term *isolated* refers to the fact that other sleep disorders such as narcolepsy or idiopathic hypersomnia are not present. The frequency of sleep paralysis episodes is very variable—once per lifetime to several per month. Hallucinatory experiences accompany sleep paralysis in 25% to 75% of individuals.

BOX 28–14

Recurrent Isolated Sleep Paralysis— Diagnostic Criteria

A. The patient complains of inability to move the trunk and all limbs at sleep onset or on awakening from sleep.

B. Each episode lasts seconds to a few minutes.

C. The sleep disturbance is not better explained by another sleep disorder (particularly narcolepsy), a medical or neurologic disorder, mental disorder, medication use, or substance use disorder.

Note: Hallucinatory experiences may be present but are not necessary.

From American Academy of Sleep Medicine: ICSD-2 International Classification of Sleep Disorders, 2nd ed. Diagnostic and Coding Manual. Westchester, IL: American Academy of Sleep Medicine, 2005.

Epidemiology of Sleep Paralysis

Studies of students suggest 15% to 40% experience at least one episode of sleep paralysis. Sleep paralysis is also common in patients with narcolepsy and idiopathic hypersomnia.

Precipitating Events

Sleep disruption, irregular sleep periods, sleep deprivation, and stress are known triggers.[40]

Diagnosis of Recurrent Sleep Paralysis

The ICSD-2 diagnostic criteria are listed in Box 28–14. Note the requirement that the presence of sleep paralysis must not be better explained by another sleep disorder (especially narcolepsy). Sleep paralysis would not be classified as "isolated" if associated with another sleep disorder such as narcolepsy.

Differential Diagnosis of Recurrent Sleep Paralysis

The differential diagnosis of sleep paralysis includes familial periodic paralysis syndromes, atonic seizures, cataplexy, and nocturnal panic attacks. Episodes of familial periodic paralysis (especially hypokalemic period paralysis) last for hours, may be associated with carbohydrate intake, and in the hypokalemic variant, are associated with hypokalemia.[1] In contrast, sleep paralysis is associated with sleep-wake transitions.

Treatment of Sleep Paralysis

In most cases, treatment with medications is not needed. Avoiding sleep deprivation and following a regular sleep pattern may help prevent isolated sleep paralysis: Serotonin reuptake inhibitors (in antidepressant doses) and TCAs (low doses) are usually effective treatment for isolated sleep paralysis. None of these are U.S. Food and Drug Administration (FDA) approved for this indication.

Nightmare Disorder

Nightmare disorder (dream anxiety attacks) are characterized by recurrent nightmares, which are disturbing mental

BOX 28-15

Nightmare Disorder—Diagnostic Criteria

A. Recurrent episodes of awakenings from sleep with recall of intensely disturbing dream mentation, usually involving fear or anxiety, but also anger, sadness, disgust, and other dysphoric emotions.

B. Full alertness or awakening, with little confusion or disorientation; recall of sleep mentation is immediate and clear.

C. At least one of the following associated features is present:
   i. Delayed return to sleep after the episode.
   ii. Occurrence of episodes in the latter half of the habitual sleep period.

From American Academy of Sleep Medicine: ICSD-2 International Classification of Sleep Disorders, 2nd ed. Diagnostic and Coding Manual. Westchester, IL: American Academy of Sleep Medicine, 2005.

BOX 28-16

Medications Commonly Associated with Nightmares

- Beta blockers—propranolol, atenolol
- Cholinergic agonists—donepezil
- Antibiotics—levaquin
- Antiviral agents—amantadine, gancyclovir
- Antiretroviral—efavirenz (Sustiva)
- Dopamine agonists—ropinirole, pramipexole
- Antidepressants—fluoxetine, paroxetine
- Benzodiazepine receptor agonists (zolpidem)
- Melatonin agonist—ramelteon
- Ethanol withdrawal—REM rebound

REM = rapid eye movement.

---

experiences that usually occur during REM sleep and often result in an awakening (Box 28-15). Nightmares can follow acute trauma (acute stress disorder [ASD]) or occur 1 month or more after trauma (PTSD). The dreams of PTSD can occur out of NREM stages N2 or N3, during REM sleep, and at sleep onset. A number of medications can also be associated with nightmares[41] (Box 28-16).

Epidemiology of Nightmare Disorder

Fifty percent to 80% of adults report one or more nightmares.[1] Ten percent to 50% of children age 3 to 5 experience nightmares severe enough to disturb their parents. **Nightmares within 3 months of trauma are present in up to 80% patients with PTSD.**[1]

PSG Recordings in Nightmare Disorder

Few PSG studies of nightmares exist, but typically, accelerated heart rate and respiratory rate precede awakening from REM sleep with report of a nightmare.

Diagnosis of Nightmare Disorder

The ICSD-2 diagnostic criteria for the nightmare disorder are listed in Box 28-15. Note that recurrent episodes

are required. One would probably not classify the rare occurrence of a nightmare as a disorder given the high percentage of normal individuals experiencing an occasional nightmare.

Differential Diagnosis

The differential diagnosis of nightmare disorder includes sleep terrors, RBD, sleep paralysis, SRDDs (to be discussed in a later section), and nocturnal panic attacks. Nocturnal panic attacks occur during or immediately after nocturnal awakenings from NREM sleep. Some patients report that disturbing dreams preceded the attacks but most do not have dream recall.

Treatment of Nightmare Disorder

If a medication is temporally associated with nightmares, a trial of medication discontinuation or change is prudent. Cognitive behavioral treatments have been used to treat nightmares with some success. One behavioral technique called **imagery rehearsal therapy** has proved successful in several studies.[42,43] Patients are asked to rewrite their previous dreams with a positive outcome. In the past, use of medications for nightmares had limited success. Recently, several small studies report success with the alpha 1 blocker **prazosin**. Note that when prazosin is started, the drug should be initiated with a dose of 1 mg at bedtime to avoid severe first-dose hypotension (often orthostatic hypotension). The drug can then be titrated upward slowly over several nights. A parallel placebo-controlled study in traumatic nightmares in PTSD associated with combat showed improvements in sleep and reduction in nightmares. A relatively high dose (mean 13 mg) was reached over a protracted period of upward titration.[44] Another study using a crossover design and a dose of 2 to 6 mg at bedtime also found benefit in civilian trauma PTSD.[45] One study also reported success in reducing disturbing nightmares using topiramate in PTSD patients.[46] However, neither prazosin or topiramate are FDA approved for treatment of nightmares in PTSD. Prazosin must be used with caution to avoid hypotension.

OTHER PARASOMNIAS

Sleep-Related Dissociative Disorders

The ICSD-2[1] states "sleep-related dissociative disorders (SRDD) emerge throughout the sleep period **during well-established EEG wakefulness**, either at transition from wakefulness to sleep or within several minutes after awakening from stage N1, N2, or R" (Box 28-17). An important distinction from other parasomnias is that whereas typical parasomnias tend to emerge almost simultaneously with arousal, the SRDDs emerge from **well-established wakefulness.**

The Diagnostic and Statistical Manual of Mental Disorders, 4th edition (DSM-IV), states that "a dissociative disorder is characterized by a disruption in the usually integrated functions of consciousness, memory, identity, or perception of the environment."[47] An SRDD would include dissociative

BOX 28–17

Sleep-Related Dissociative Disorders—Diagnostic Criteria

A. A dissociative disorder must fulfill Diagnostic and Statistical Manual of Mental Disorders, 4th ed. (DSM-IV), criteria and **emerges in close association with the main sleep period.**

B. One of the following is present:

   i. PSG demonstrates a dissociative episode or episodes that emerge during sustained EEG wakefulness, either in the transition from wakefulness to sleep or after an awakening from NREM or REM sleep.

   ii. In the absence of a PSG-recorded episode of dissociation, the history provided by observers is compelling for a sleep-related dissociative disorder, particularly if the sleep-related behaviors are similar to observed daytime dissociative behaviors.

C. The sleep disturbance is not better explained by another sleep disorder, a medical or neurologic disorder, mental disorder, medication use, or substance use disorder.

EEG = electroencephalogram; NREM = non–rapid eye movement; PSG = polysomnography; REM = rapid eye movement.
From American Academy of Sleep Medicine: ICSD-2 International Classification of Sleep Disorders, 2nd ed. Diagnostic and Coding Manual. Westchester, IL: American Academy of Sleep Medicine, 2005.

BOX 28–18

Sleep-Related Dissociative Disorders Facts

• SRDDs occur out of established wakefulness.
• Most patients have daytime DD.
• There is a female predominance.
• Most patients have a history of physical or sexual trauma/abuse.

DD = dissociative disorder; SRDD = sleep-related dissociative disorder.

BOX 28–19

Sleep Enuresis—Diagnostic Criteria

PRIMARY SLEEP ENURESIS

A. The patient is older than 5 years.
B. The patient exhibits recurrent involuntary voiding during sleep, occurring at least twice a week.
C. The patient has never been consistently dry during sleep.

SECONDARY SLEEP ENURESIS

A. The patient is older than 5 years.
B. The patient exhibits recurrent involuntary voiding during sleep, occurring at least twice a week.
C. The patient has been **previously consistently dry during sleep for at least 6 months.**

From American Academy of Sleep Medicine: ICSD-2 International Classification of Sleep Disorders, 2nd ed. Diagnostic and Coding Manual. Westchester, IL: American Academy of Sleep Medicine, 2005.

behavior that occurred out of wakefulness during the sleep period in which there was an impairment of identity, memory, or state of consciousness.

Types of Dissociative Disorders Associated with Sleep

There are five diagnostic categories of DDs in DSM-IV[47] including (1) dissociative identity disorder (formerly multiple personality disorder), (2) dissociative fugue, (3) dissociative amnesia, (4) depersonalization disorder, and (5) dissociative disorder not otherwise specified (DD NOS). Of these, three are considered SRDD: dissociative identity disorder, dissociative fugue, and DD NOS. Most but not all patients with SRDD have both daytime DD episodes as well as previous episodes of SRDD.[1,48]

Dissociative Identity Disorder In dissociative identity disorder, a person displays multiple identities and personalities each with its own pattern of perceiving and integrating with the environment. A minimum of two personalities is required.

Dissociative Fugue State The dissociative fugue state is characterized by reversible amnesia for personal identity and memories usually lasting hours to days. A dissociative fugue state usually involves unplanned travel or wandering and is sometimes associated with establishment of a new identity. After the episode, prior memories return but there is amnesia for the fugue episode.

Dissociative Disorder Not Otherwise Specified The classification DD NOS is used for a DD that does not fit the criteria for a specific DD.

Epidemiology **SRDD are more common in females.**[1] In patients with SRDD, the age of onset is usually from childhood to middle adulthood. In one study of 100 consecutive patients referred to a sleep disorders clinic, 7% were diagnosed with SRDDs.[6] **The majority of patients with SRDDs have a history of physical or sexual trauma/abuse.**

Diagnosis of SRDD The ICSD-2 diagnostic criteria are listed in Box 28–17 and important facts are displayed in Box 28–18.

Treatment of SRDDs The treatment of SRDD involves the treatment of the underling DD. Psychotherapy is the main treatment for DD with the goal of encouraging communication of conflicts and increased insight. The overall goal is to help the individual come to terms with the stress or trauma that triggered the DD.

Sleep Enuresis

Sleep enuresis is characterized by involuntary voiding during sleep. Sleep enuresis is divided into **primary sleep enuresis** and **secondary sleep enuresis** (Box 28–19).[49] In primary enuresis, the patient **has never been consistently dry after age 5 years.** In secondary enuresis, the patient was *previously*

BOX 28-20

Causes of Secondary Enuresis

1. Inability to concentrate urine (DI, nephrogenic DI, sickle cell anemia).
2. Increased urine production (caffeine, medications).
3. Urinary tract pathology—UTI, malformations of urinary tract.
4. Chronic constipation and encopresis (bulging colon constricts bladder capacity).
5. Neurologic disorders: seizures, neurogenic bladder.
6. OSA.
7. Psychosocial stress: parental divorce, neglect, physical or sexual abuse.

DI = diabetes insipidus; OSA = obstructive sleep apnea; UTI = urinary tract infection.

BOX 28-21

Treatments for Sleep-Related Enuresis

- Behavioral treatments (frequent daytime voiding, fluid restriction at night).
- Alarm treatments (wet bed triggers alarm).
- Evaluation for sleep apnea and genitourinary pathology if indicated.
- Drug therapy: vasopressin, anticholinergics (oxybutynin), tricyclic antidepressants.

consistently dry. The classification is useful because each group has characteristic causes.

Primary Enuresis

The patient either fails to arouse from sleep when the bladder is full or fails to inhibit a bladder contraction. These are both acquired skills and are developed at different ages in different individuals. A limit of age 5 years is somewhat arbitrary. The spontaneous "cure" rate for enuresis after age 5 is approximately 15%/year. Some children with primary enuresis have absence of the nocturnal secretion of vasopressin (antidiuretic hormone). In primary enuresis, the ratio of **males to females is 3:2. Hereditary factors** are important in primary enuresis. The risk of sleep-related enuresis is 77% if both parents had enuresis and 44% when one parent had enuresis.

Secondary Enuresis

Secondary enuresis has a number of causes (Box 28-20). Evaluation commonly involves history (for snoring and signs of sleep apnea) and a urinalysis (looking for infection, diabetes, and other evidence of renal disease). Ultrasonography of the pelvis is recommended, especially in children with daytime symptoms. Nocturia or frequent urination suggests small bladder capacity. Daytime incontinence or failure to respond to treatment is an indication for referral to a specialist. Physical examination should check for neurologic impairment and stigmata of spinal cord abnormality. The anal wink should also be assessed. Palpation of the abdomen may show retained stool, which can compress the bladder and reduce capacity.

PSG in Evaluation of Enuresis

A sleep study is indicated if OSA or nocturnal seizures are suspected. Untreated OSA in children can worsen or cause enuresis.[49-51] Therefore, **sleep apnea should be considered in all children being evaluated for enuresis,** especially secondary enuresis. Episodes of **enuresis can occur in all sleep stages,** during nocturnal wakefulness, and in association with transient arousals.

Treatments for Enuresis

Treatments for enuresis are listed in Box 28-21. These include behavioral techniques to encourage regular voiding during the day, alarm treatments (alarm sounds when bedwetting is detected), evaluation for genitourinary malformations, and drug therapy (e.g., vasopressin, anticholinergics, TCAs).[49] The medications that are used are treatments and not cures. Relapse will occur if medication is suddenly discontinued. Oral vasopressins (fast-melting formulations 120–360 µg before bedtime) reduce urine volume. The nasal spray formulations have a longer duration of action and are no longer recommended (more risk for hyponatremia). With vasopressin, the major concern is hyponatremia, which can be avoided by fluid restriction after dinner. The anticholinergic oxybutynin, tablets or syrup, before bedtime relaxes the bladder. A combination of vasopressin and oxybutynin has also been used. TCAs (imipramine 25–50 mg before bedtime) are effective but the mechanism is unclear. Because of substantial side effects, TCAs are third-line treatment.

Sleep-Related Groaning—Catathrenia

Sleep-related groaning (catathrenia) is a chronic (often nightly) disorder characterized by expiratory groaning, **most often out of REM sleep** (especially in the REM episodes in the second part of the night). Catathrenia can also occur in NREM sleep. It may be associated with bradypneic episodes (slow respiratory rate) with **long exhalations.** Typically, a large inspiration is followed by a protracted expiration during which a monotonous vocalization ("mournful moaning or groaning") is produced (Fig. 28-5). The catathrenia events tend to occur in clusters and are often associated with bradycardia. Patients are usually unaware of the groaning. The disorder is thought to be benign and its main complication is disturbance of the bed partner.[52-55]

Epidemiology

Catathrenia is very rare, with onset usually in adolescence or early adulthood (mean age 19 yr with a range of 5–36 yr).[1] The prevalence of catathrenia is **greater in men than in women.**

Polysomnography

Catathrenia events usually occur in the second part of the night and may occur in clusters resembling a run of central

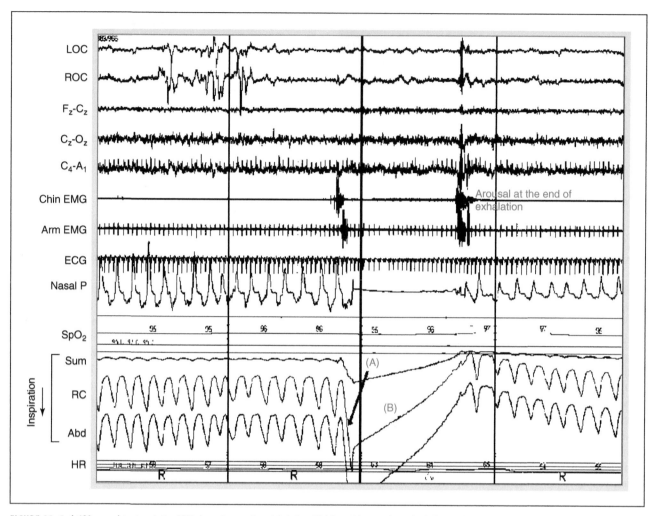

FIGURE 28–5 A 120-second tracing during REM sleep shows a deep inhalation *(A)* followed by a prolonged exhalation *(B)* associated with monotonous sound generation (groaning). Note that in the Sum, rib cage (RC), and abdominal (Abd) tracings, the direction of inspiration is downward and exhalation upward. The absence of nasal pressure excursions is due to exhalation through the mouth during groaning. ECG = electrocardiogram; EMG = electromyogram; HR = heart rate; LOC = left outer canthus; Nasal P = nasal pressure; ROC = right outer canthus; SpO_2 = pulse oximetry. *Reproduced from Ramar K, Olson EJ, Morgenthaler TI: Catathrenia. Sleep Med 2008;9:457–459.*

apneas. An EEG arousal with or without body movement often marks the end of the event.

Diagnosis of Catathrenia

The ICSD-2 criteria for catatherenia are listed in Box 28–22. Diagnosis can be based on **history or PSG.** Clusters of catathrenia events can be confused with central apneas. However, in central apneas, an exhalation precedes the long **inspiratory** pause. In contrast, in catathrenia, a deep inspiration precedes the long **expiratory** pause (see Fig. 28–5). Mild bradycardia during the exhalation is common.

Differential Diagnosis of Catathrenia

The differential diagnosis of catathrenia includes stridor, sleep-related laryngospasm, and sleep talking. Stridor can be inspiratory or expiratory, occurs with every breath, and does not have a prolonged expiratory phase. **Sleep-related laryngospasm** is associated with a sense of suffocation. Sleep talking consists of words rather than groans.

BOX 28–22

Sleep-Related Groaning (Catathrenia)— Diagnostic Criteria
A. History of regularly occurring groaning (or related monotonous vocalization) occurring during sleep.
OR
B. PSG with respiratory sound monitoring reveals characteristic respiratory dysrhythmia predominantly or exclusively during REM sleep.
PSG = polysomnography; REM = rapid eye movement. From American Academy of Sleep Medicine: ICSD-2 International Classification of Sleep Disorders, 2nd ed. Diagnostic and Coding Manual. Westchester, IL: American Academy of Sleep Medicine, 2005.

Treatment of Catathrenia

Not all cases require treatment. Multiple medications have been tried without success. There are two case reports of a benefit from CPAP treatment,[56,57] whereas another study did not find a benefit from CPAP.[54]

Exploding Head Syndrome

The exploding head syndrome (EHS) is characterized by a sudden loud imagined noise or sense of violent explosion in the head occurring as the patient is falling asleep or upon wakening during the night.[1,58] The event can be described as a painless loud bang, a clash of cymbals, or a bomb exploding.

Epidemiology

The median age of onset is 58 years, but it can occur at any age.[1]

Diagnosis

The ICSD-2 diagnostic criteria for the exploding head syndrome are listed in Box 28–23. Note that **pain is absent and the patient typically arouses with a sense of fright.**

Demographics

The prevalence is not known; however, the EHS is **more common in women than in men.** Onset at all ages has been reported.

Polysomnography

Limited data suggest the exploding head events **occur during drowsiness** while the subject is still awake.

Differential Diagnosis of Sleep-Related Headaches

A number of sleep-related headaches exist.[1,59–61] For detailed information on diagnostic criteria for different headache syndromes, the reader can review the International Classification of Headache Disorders, 2nd edition,[61] published by the International Headache Society:

1. Idiopathic stabbing headache (icepick headache)—sudden jabbing pain on the side of head.

BOX 28–23

Exploding Head Syndrome—Diagnostic Criteria
A. The patient complains of a sudden loud noise or sense of explosion in the head either at the **wake-sleep transition** or upon **waking during the night.**
B. The experience is **NOT** associated with significant **pain** complaints.
C. The patient rouses immediately after the event, usually with a sense of fright.
Note: In a minority of cases, a flash of light or myoclonic jerk may accompany the event.
From American Academy of Sleep Medicine: ICSD-2 International Classification of Sleep Disorders, 2nd ed. Diagnostic and Coding Manual. Westchester, IL: American Academy of Sleep Medicine, 2005.

2. Thunderclap headache—a severe headache associated with subarachnoid hemorrhage or other causes. It usually does not occur at sleep onset.
3. Sleep-related migraines—unilateral throbbing often associated with photophobia and nausea.
4. Cluster headaches—unilateral headaches with retroperi-orbital pain lasting 15 minutes to 3 hours. The clusters of headaches last 1 week to 1 year separated by pain-free periods.
5. Nocturnal paroxysmal hemicrania—unilateral headache on one side of the face near the eye, often with swollen eyelid and nasal congestion. It responds to indomethacin. The headaches may occur multiple times during the day.
6. Simple partial seizures—usually not at sleep onset.
7. Sleep starts (hypnic jerks)—motor phenomenon with sudden myoclonic jerks.
8. Hypnic headaches—a rare disorder during which the headache awakens the patient with two of the following characteristics: (1) occurs more than 15 times monthly, (2) lasts longer than 15 minutes after awakening, and (3) occurs after age 50.[60,61] In addition, there should be no autonomic symptoms and no more than one of the following: nausea, photophobia, and phonophobia. Hypnic headaches commonly awaken patients 4 to 6 hours after sleep onset.

Treatment of Exploding Head Syndrome

Only a few case reports of treatment of the exploding head syndrome have been published. Flunarizine (a calcium channel blocker not available in the United States),[62] nifedipine,[63] and clomipramine[58] have been effective in individual cases.

Sleep-Related Hallucinations

Sleep-related hallucinations (SRHs) include **hypnagogic hallucinations** (HGHs) at sleep onset, **hypnopompic hallucinations** (HPHs) on awakening from sleep, and **complex nocturnal visual hallucinations** (CNVHs).[1] SRHs are primarily visual hallucinatory experiences that occur at sleep onset or on awakening. However, they may include auditory, tactile, or kinetic phenomena (sensation of motion or falling). SRHs may be difficult to differentiate from sleep-onset or sleep-termination dreaming.

CNVHs are a variant of SRHs in which hallucinations occur **after full awakening from sleep** (in wakefulness after arousal from sleep).[1,64] Usually, the affected individual does **NOT remember a specific dream.** The hallucinations are complex vivid visual images (multicolor), usually of people or animals, that are relatively immobile and may be distorted. Although patients realize that they are awake, the hallucinations can be very frightening. CNVHs can occur in patients taking beta blocker medication and those with neurologic degenerative disorders such as Lewy body dementia. However, CNVHs can occur in neurologically intact individuals. Of interest, in one description of CNVHs, many of the patients also had other parasomnias.[64]

Epidemiology

HGH events have a prevalence of 25% to 35% and HPH events have a prevalence of 7% to 13%. Both HGHs and HPHs are more common in younger patients. SRHs can occur in association with sleep paralysis.

Factors Precipitating SRH

Precipitating factors include current drug use, mood disorder, anxiety, and past alcohol use.

Associations with SRHs

1. HGHs and HPHs are common, can occur in normal subjects, and are common in patients with narcolepsy or idiopathic hypersomnia.
2. CNVHs are rare and can occur in idiopathic form. There may be an association with a neurologic disorder: narcolepsy, Parkinson's disease, dementia with Lewy bodies, visual loss (Charles Bonnet hallucinations), midbrain and diencephalic pathology (peduncular hallucinosis), and the use of beta blocker medications.

PSG in SRHs

Little PSG data are available, but HGHs likely represent sleep-onset REM periods **whereas HPHs occur at arousal out of REM sleep.** CNVH events have also occurred out of NREM sleep.

Diagnosis of SRHs

The ICSD-2 diagnostic criteria for SRHs are listed in Box 28–24.

Treatment

No significant information on treatment of CNVHs exists. If due to beta blocker medications, these should be withdrawn. One approach could be REM suppressants such as SSRIs or TCAs. These medications are effective in HPHs or HGHs in patients with narcolepsy.

BOX 28–24

Sleep Related Hallucinations—Diagnostic Criteria

A. The patient experiences hallucinations just prior to sleep onset (hypnagogic) or on awakening during the night or in the morning (hypnopompic).
B. Hallucinations are primarily visual.
C. The disturbance is not better explained by another sleep disorder, medical or neurologic disorder, mental disorder, medication use, or substance use disorder.

Note: Hypnogogic or hypnopompic hallucinations may be difficult to differentiate from sleep-onset or sleep-termination dreaming. Complex nocturnal visual hallucinations may clearly occur in wakefulness following arousal from sleep.

From American Academy of Sleep Medicine: ICSD-2 International Classification of Sleep Disorders, 2nd ed. Diagnostic and Coding Manual. Westchester, IL: American Academy of Sleep Medicine, 2005.

Sleep-Related Eating Disorders

Sleep-related eating disorders (SREDs) are manifested by eating and drinking during the main sleep period (Boxes 28–25 and 28–26). The behavior must be associated with one or more of several manifestations including eating peculiar food items, associated with insomnia due to sleep disturbance from the eating episodes, sleep-related injury, dangerous behaviors in pursuit of food, morning anorexia, or adverse consequences of binge eating. In the past, SRED was differentiated from nocturnal eating syndrome (NES) by the level of alertness during the episodes and the degree of recall.[1,4,65-67] However, there is considerable overlap between SRED and NES. In the current ICSD-2 diagnostic criteria for SRED, altered awareness and lack of recall are NOT required.[1]

In SRED, **the degree of alertness and recall for the eating behavior are variable.** Some patients cannot be brought to full consciousness during the eating events and

BOX 28–25

Sleep-Related Eating Disorder— Diagnostic Criteria

A. Recurrent episodes of involuntary eating and drinking occur **during the main sleep period.**
B. One or more of the following must be present with the **recurrent episodes of involuntatry eating** and drinking:
   i. Consumption of **peculiar forms or combinations** of food or inedible or toxic substance.
   ii. **Insomnia** related to sleep disruption from repeated episodes of eating, with a complaint of **nonrestorative sleep, daytime fatigue, or somnolence.**
   iii. **Sleep-related injury.**
   iv. **Dangerous behaviors** performed while in the pursuit of food or while cooking food.
   v. Morning anorexia.
   vi. Adverse health consequence for current binge of high-calorie foods.
C. The disturbance is not better explained by another sleep disorder, medical or neurologic disorder, mental disorder, medication use, or substance use disorder.

From American Academy of Sleep Medicine: ICSD-2 International Classification of Sleep Disorders, 2nd ed. Diagnostic and Coding Manual. Westchester, IL: American Academy of Sleep Medicine, 2005.

BOX 28–26

Sleep-Related Eating Disorder Facts

- Strong female predominance
- Variable awareness/alertness during episodes
- Eating unusual foods (e.g., raw, frozen, toxic)
- Variable recall (partial amnesia)
- Co-morbid with other sleep disorders and eating disorders
- Topiramate, pramipexole, and sertraline are possible treatments

have no recall of the event. Others are relatively alert during the episode and have considerable recall of the event the next morning. The amount of alertness can even vary between episodes on a given night. **A sensation of hunger is usually missing** and patients may eat in an "out of control" manner.[1] Patients often eat peculiar, nonedible, or even dangerous substances. These may include frozen food, coffee grounds, and cat food. Of interest, alcoholic beverages are rarely consumed. High-calorie foods are often chosen. There may be **multiple episodes of eating during a single night.**

Demographics

SRED is much more common in females than in males. Females make up 66% to 83% of affected individuals in most series. The prevalence is higher in patients with other eating disorders. Typical age of onset of SRED is 20 to 30 years.

Pathophysiology

The cause of SRED is unknown but **more than 50% of patients have another parasomnia** and the strong female predominance is typical of eating disorders.

Causes of SRED and Association with Other Sleep Disorders

The causes and associations of SRED are listed in Box 28–27. An idiopathic form does exist when no obvious cause or association is identified. SRED is most commonly associated with sleepwalking but can occur with PLMD, restless leg syndrome, OSA, and circadian rhythm disorders (irregular sleep phase). Medication-induced SRED has been reported with BZRAs,[66,67] including zolpidem and triazolam, and psychotropic medications (lithium). **Zolpidem is by far the medication most commonly associated with the SRED.** Zolpidem-associated SRED is especially common if patients take higher than the recommended dose (e.g., zolpidem 20 mg). Patients also report triggering of episodes by stress,

BOX 28–27

Causes of Sleep-Related Eating Disorder

1. Idiopathic—less common than #2
2. Associated with another sleep disorder
   a. Sleepwalking—most common association
   b. Obstructive sleep apnea
   c. PLMD, RLS
   d. Circadian rhythm sleep disorders (esp. irregular sleep-wake type)
3. Associated with medication
   a. BZRAs: zolpidem, triazolam
   b. Psychotropic medications (lithium, olanzapine, risperidone)
   c. Anticholinergic medications

BZRAs = benzodiazepine receptor agonists; PLMD = periodic limb movement disorder; RLS = restless legs syndrome.

cigarette smoking cessation, and cessation of alcohol or other drugs of abuse.[1,66]

PSG in SRED

PSG may show multiple arousals from stage N3 with behavior typical of confusional arousal (with or without attempted eating behavior). Sometimes, OSA or PLMS is also noted.

SRED Complications

Complications include weight gain or injury due to preparation of food (cooking—e.g., burns, opening cans, cutting food with a knife).

Diagnosis

The ICSD-2 diagnostic criteria are listed in Box 28–25. Observations by a significant other, finding evidence of nocturnal eating behavior (e.g., open food packages, dirty plates), videotaping, and self-report (in patients with some recall) have been used to make a diagnosis.

Differential Diagnosis

Other possible etiologies of this behavior include NES, recurrent hypersomnia (Kleine-Levin syndrome—hyperphagia, hypersomnia). Whereas NES is said to be characterized by full alertness (Table 28–2), there is considerable overlap between SRED and NES. Some clinicians consider them to be two eating disorders at the opposite ends of the spectrum of awareness.

Treatment

If SRED is medication associated (zolpidem), the medication should be withdrawn. Patients may not have the behavior with another medication in the same class (e.g., switch from zolpidem to eszopiclone). Sometimes, medication-induced SRED will continue, at least temporarily, even with discontinuation of the offending medication. **Topiramate appears to be the best-documented treatment**, although sertraline, carbidopa/levodopa, and pramipexole have been used successfully.[68-72] In one study, the mean dose of topiramate was 218 mg, although patients may note an improvement at a 100-mg dose.[70] The side effects of topiramate include weight loss, paresthesias, renal calculi, cognitive dysfunction, and orthostasis. In one series, up to 41% of patients discontinued the medication because of side effects. If SRED is associated with sleepwalking, clonazepam has sometimes been effective.

Parasomnia, Unspecified

This diagnosis is used on a temporary basis when the parasomnia is believed to be secondary to a psychiatric diagnosis but before this diagnosis can be made with certainty.

Parasomnia Due to Drug or Substance

This category can be used when a temporal association between starting a medication and the onset of a parasomnia can be documented.

TABLE 28–2

Traditional Characteristics of Sleep-Related Eating Disorder and Nocturnal Eating Syndrome

	SLEEP-RELATED EATING DISORDER	NOCTURNAL EATING SYNDROME
State of consciousness	Partial to full arousal state	Fully awake during compulsive eating.
Timing of onset	Onset out of sleep period	**Eating between evening meal and onset of nocturnal sleep** or Eating **during complete awakenings** from sleep.
Food	Unusual foods or toxic substances Preference for high-caloric foods Foods NOT typically preferred during daytime (e.g., raw food, cat food, frozen food)	Absence of bizarre or atypical foods.
Recall	Partial or complete amnesia	Complete recall.
State in AM	Morning anorexia and abdominal distention	Morning anorexia can occur, bulimia can occur.
Associated disorders	Associated with sleepwalking OSA, PLMS	Associated with eating and psychiatric disorders.
Gender	Female 60–80%	Female < 60%.

Note that in the ICSD-2 diagnostic criteria, there is no requirement for amnesia or an impaired state of consciousness for diagnosis of the sleep-related eating disorder. ICSD-2 = International Classification of Sleep Disorders, 2nd ed.; OSA = obstructive sleep apnea; PLMS = periodic limb movement during sleep.

Parasomnia Due to Medical Condition

The parasomnia emerges as a manifestation of an underlying neurologic or medical disorder. RBD is often associated with Parkinson's disease, Lewy body with dementia, and multiple system atrophy. An entity known as agrypnia excitia is characterized by generalized motor overactivity, impaired ability to initiate and maintain sleep ("wakeful dreaming"), loss of stage N3 sleep, and autonomic sympathetic activation. Agrypnia excitia can be found associated with delirium tremens and fatal familial insomnia.[1]

OTHER NOCTURNAL BEHAVIORS IN THE DIFFERENTIAL DIAGNOSIS OF PARASOMNIA

The ICSD-2 classifies a number of nocturnal behaviors under other categories including sleep-related movement disorders (bruxism and rhythmic movement disorder) and "Isolated Symptoms and Apparently Normal Variants and Unresolved Issues" (sleep talking, hypnic jerks, propiospinal myoclonus, hypnagogic foot tremor, and alternating leg movement activity). Hypnagogic foot tremor, alternating leg movement activity, and the rhythmic movement disorder are discussed in Chapter 12.

Sleep Talking (Somniloquy)

Sleep talking is usually reported by the bed partner or someone asleep near the affected individual.[1] Although few sleep recordings have been performed, sleep talking can arise **from NREM or REM sleep.** Vocalizations have been described associated with sleepwalking, RBD, PTSD, SRED,

BOX 28–28

Hypnic Jerks—Diagnostic Criteria

A. Patient complains of sudden brief jerks at sleep onset, mainly affecting the legs or arms.

B. The jerks are associated with at least one of the following:
   i. A subjective feeling of falling.
   ii. A sensory flash.
   iii. A hypnagogic dream.

C. The disorder is not better explained by another sleep disorder, medical, or neurologic disorder, mental disorder, medication use, or substance use disorder

From American Academy of Sleep Medicine: ICSD-2 International Classification of Sleep Disorders, 2nd ed. Diagnostic and Coding Manual. Westchester, IL: American Academy of Sleep Medicine, 2005.

on arousal from OSA, and with nocturnal seizures. Sleep talking has few consequences unless it disturbs the sleep of others or the content of the talking contains material upsetting to the listener (calling out the name of an ex-wife while the current wife is present).

Hypnic Jerks

Hypnic jerks (sleep starts) are brief total body jerks that occur at sleep onset.[1] These are entirely normal. They may be associated with a sense of falling. The jerks may affect the body asymmetrically. There is usually a single jerk at the start of the sleep episode at transitions from wakefulness to sleep. Multiple jerks may sometimes occur (Box 28–28).

Propiospinal Myoclonus

Propriospinal myoclonus at sleep onset (Box 28–29) consists of sudden muscular jerks that occur in transition from wakefulness to light sleep. Jerks involve the abdominal and trunk muscles with spread to involve limbs and neck muscles.[73]

Differential Diagnosis of Nocturnal Behavior

Table 28–3 lists notable behavior often seen during the sleep period. The categories include normal phenomena (including those with no known clinical significance), sleep-related movement disorders, parasomnias, psychiatric disorders, and nocturnal seizure disorders.

THE DIFFERENTIAL DIAGNOSIS OF PARASOMNIAS

In one study of 100 adults referred for evaluation of sleep-related injury,[6] 54 had sleep terrors/sleepwalking, 36 had the RBD, 7 had SRDD, 2 had nocturnal seizures, and 1 had sleep apnea. Table 28–3 presents disorders classified as parasomnias and other disorders. Some comparisons between the disorders are presented in Table 28–4. Nocturnal epilepsy is discussed in Chapter 27 and psychiatric disorders in Chapter 29. Many prior classifications of nocturnal "spells" included the disorders **nocturnal paroxysmal dystonia** (NPD) and **nocturnal wandering.** These are now believed to be manifestations of nocturnal frontal lobe epilepsy. Whereas sleep-related epilepsy is covered in detail in Chapter 27, frontal lobe epilepsy is briefly discussed here because these patients typically have seizures confined to the night and typical manifestations mimic parasomnias.

Nocturnal frontal lobe epilepsy can present as paroxysmal arousals, NPD, and episodic nocturnal wandering (ENW).[74]

BOX 28–29

Propiospinal Myoclonus at Sleep Onset— Diagnostic Criteria

A. The patient complains of sudden jerks, mainly of the abdomen, trunk, and neck.

B. The jerks arise upon relaxed wakefulness and drowsiness and disappear on mental activation and at sleep onset.

C. The disorder is not better explained by another sleep disorder, medical, or neurologic disorder, mental disorder, medication use, or substance use disorder.

From American Academy of Sleep Medicine: ICSD-2 International Classification of Sleep Disorders, 2nd ed. Diagnostic and Coding Manual. Westchester, IL: American Academy of Sleep Medicine, 2005.

TABLE 28–3

Differential Diagnosis of Unusual Behavior Associated with Sleep

GROUP	DIAGNOSIS	USUAL SLEEP STAGE
"Normal sleep phenomenon" Apparently normal variants	Sleep starts (hypnic jerks)	Sleep onset
	Nightmares (REM anxiety attacks)	REM >> NREM
	Hypnogogic foot tremor	Wake or arousal from NREM
	Alternating leg movement activity	Wake or arousal from NREM
	Sleep talking (somniloquy)	NREM and REM
Sleep-related movement disorders	Periodic limb movements in sleep	NREM > REM
	Bruxism	Any sleep stage, N2 most common
	Rhythmic movement disorder	Stage W, NREM, REM
Parasomnias	Confusional arousal	NREM
	Sleepwalking (somnambulism)	NREM
	Sleep terrors	NREM
	REM sleep behavior disorder	REM
	Recurrent sleep paralysis	REM-wake transition
	Nightmare disorders	REM >> NREM
	Overlap parasomnia	NREM and REM
	Sleep-related dissociative disorder	Occurs from established wake
	Enuresis	NREM and REM
	Catathrenia (sleep-related groaning)	REM >> NREM
Psychiatric disorders	Panic attacks	From wake after arousal from NREM
	Posttraumatic stress disorder	REM and NREM
Seizure disorders	Nocturnal seizures	NREM > Wake > REM

NREM = non–rapid eye movement; REM = rapid eye movement.

TABLE 28-4

Common Features Associated with Nocturnal Events

	NREM PARASOMNIA CONFUSIONAL AROUSALS, SLEEPWALKING, SLEEP TERRORS	REM BEHAVIOR DISORDER	NIGHTMARES	SEIZURE
Time of night	Children—early Adults—early or late	Late	Late > early	Any
Sleep stage at start	Children—Stage N3 Adults—Stages N2, N3	REM	REM	NREM > Wake > REM
Screams	Yes in sleep terrors No in confusional arousals, sleepwalking	Can occur, talking, yelling more common	Rare, talking more common	Rare
Autonomic activation	Extreme in sleep terrors	Mild	Mild	Mild
Walking	Yes—sleepwalking No—confusional arousals, sleep terrors	Rare	No	Can occur Walking (nocturnal wandering) Stereotypical behavior
Confusion after episode on awakening	Usual	No	Rare	Usual
Age	Child—common Adult—less common	Adult > 50 yr Male	Any age	Adult
Episodes also in wake	No	No	No	Usual
CNS lesion	No	Can occur	No	Common

CNS = central nervous system; NREM = non–rapid eye movement; REM = rapid eye movement.

Paroxysmal arousals typically present during NREM sleep consisting of a stereotypical series of movements lasting 2 to 20 seconds in which the individuals raise their head, sit up, and look around confused with a frightened expression then scream. NPD is characterized by nocturnal coarse movements associated with tonic spasms that often occur multiple times per night. The episodes can be violent or be associated with vocalization. Patients often move the arms and legs with cycling or kicking movements and sometimes adopt a dystonic posture of the limbs. ENWs may present with symptoms similar to sleepwalking and sleep terrors. Patients may jump out of bed, wander, vocalize, and show violent behavior during sleep. Treatment with older anticonvulsants such as carbamazepine or newer anticonvulsants such as levetiracetam at bedtime is effective.

Among psychiatric disorders, **panic attacks** can present as nocturnal spells. Panic attacks occur **from wakefulness after arousal from sleep.**[20] The individual is alert and the severity builds with intense fear, tachycardia, dyspnea, chest pain, or flushing. Whereas nocturnal panic attacks usually occur in patients with known daytime attacks, a few patients may have panic attacks only at night. PTSD patients also may complain of terrifying dreams and may awaken with episodes similar to sleep terrors.[34] They are usually not confused on awakening and may have vivid dream recall.

CLINICAL REVIEW QUESTIONS

1. Which of the following is NOT true about sleepwalking in adults?

   A. Approximately 60% to 70% have a history of sleepwalking in childhood.

   B. It can be precipitated by sleep deprivation.

   C. Approximately 50% of patients with adult-onset sleepwalking have psychopathology.

   D. It always occurs out of stage N3.

2. Which of the following disorders is NOT commonly associated with RBD?

   A. Narcolepsy.

   B. Parkinson's disease.

   C. Dementia with Lewy bodies.

   D. Alzheimer's disease.

   E. Multiple system atrophy.

3. Which of the following medications are associated with RBD?

   A. Fluoxetine.

   B. Venlafaxine.

   C. Mirtazapine.

D. TCAs.

E. All of the above.

4. Which of the following is true about RBD?

   A. It typically occurs in the first half of the night.

   B. Women > men.

   C. It responds to clonazepam in approximately 80% of patients.

   D. It responds to 0.3 to 0.5 mg of melatonin.

   E. Dream recall is always present.

5. What characteristic(s) are true about nocturnal panic attacks?

   A. They are associated with autonomic hyperactivity, tachycardia.

   B. The patient is alert during a panic attack.

   C. The patient has amnesia for the event.

   D. B and C.

   E. A and B.

6. Which of the following factors favor nocturnal epilepsy over a parasomnia?

   A. Confusion following the event.

   B. Stereotypical behavior.

   C. Several episodes per night.

   D. Amnesia for the event.

   E. B and C.

   F. A and B.

7. Which of the following is true concerning the SRED?

   A. Patients are not alert during events.

   B. Amnesia for SRED events is always present.

   C. Prevalence of SRED: men > women.

   D. Zolpidem is the medication most often associated with SRED.

   E. Normal foods are eaten.

8. Which of the following characterize events associated with the exploding head syndrome?

   A. They are painless.

   B. Men > women.

   C. They occur out of NREM sleep.

   D. They are not associated with fright.

9. In which of the following situations would a diagnosis of RBD be indicated?

   A. REM sleep without atonia, history of dream enactment.

   B. REM without atonia, body movements on video PSG during REM sleep.

   C. REM without atonia, no body movements during PSG, no history of dream-enacting behavior.

   D. No evidence of REM with atonia, violent movements out of REM sleep.

E. A and B.

F. C and D.

10. Which of the following patterns is NOT considered compatible with RBD?

    A. Chin EMG—sustained tonic activity during REM sleep.

    B. Chin EMG—TMA (phasic) during REM sleep.

    C. Leg EMG—sustained tonic activity.

    D. Leg EMG—TMA (phasic).

    E. Chin EMG—sustained tonic activity and TMA during REM sleep.

11. Which of the following describes catathrenia?

    A. Deep inspiration, prolonged expiratory groan, slow breathing rate.

    B. Long inspiratory groan, slow breathing rate.

    C. NREM > REM sleep.

    D. Women > men.

    E. Patient complains of disturbed sleep.

12. A child was previously dry until age 8 when he began to have frequent nocturnal enuretic episodes. He also was noted to snore loudly and to have difficulty concentrating in classes. Which of the following are true?

    A. The patient has secondary enuresis.

    B. One of his parents likely had enuresis.

    C. OSA should be considered.

    D. A and B.

    E. A and C.

Answers

1. D. Sleepwalking in adults can occur out of stages N1 and N2 as well as N3.

2. D. Although RBD can occur with patients with Alzheimer's disease, it is not typical of that disorder.

3. E. All of the above.

4. C. RBD responds to clonazepam in about 80% of cases, although many patients experience side effects. Melatonin, often in doses up to 12 mg may also be effective. RBD is typically a disorder of men older than 50 years of age. Because this parasomnia occurs out of REM sleep, the usual timing is the second part of the night.

5. E. Unlike NREM parasomnias, during panic attacks, patients are alert and do not have amnesia for the event. Panic attacks may occur out of NREM sleep and be associated with autonomic hyperactivity and intense fear.

6. E. Stereotypical behaviors (same manifestations with every episode) and several episodes per night are more

common with nocturnal epilepsy. Confusion after the event and amnesia can occur with both NREM parasomnias and many types of nocturnal seizures.

7. **D.** Zolpidem is the medication most often associated with SRED. Alertness during event and recall of the event are highly variable. **SRED is much more common in women than in men.** Although normal foods (especially those high in carbohydrates) may be eaten, frozen foods and nonfoods are also sometimes consumed.

8. **A.** Exploding head episodes are painless. They may be associated with a noise. Episodes occur during drowsiness rather than after arousal from sleep. More women than men have the syndrome.

9. **E.** A diagnosis of RBD requires PSG evidence of REM sleep without atonia and either body movements during REM sleep noted on a PSG or a history of dream enactment. A PSG showing evidence of REM sleep without atonia without other findings does not meet diagnostic criteria. This pattern can simply mean that the patient is taking an SSRI or similar medication. In pseudo-RBD (severe untreated OSA), body movements can be noted during REM sleep with **NO** evidence of REM sleep without atonia.[29]

10. **C.** Sustained leg EMG activity is not considered evidence of REM sleep without atonia.

11. **A.** Catathrenia is much more common in REM than in NREM and is characterized by a prolonged expiratory groan/moan often with a slow breathing rate. Catathrenia is more common in men than in women. This parasomnia is believed to have no direct consequences for the patient but can significantly disturb the sleep of the bed partner.

12. **E.** Because the patient was previously dry, he has secondary enuresis. Heritable factors are associated with primary enuresis. Enuresis can be a manifestation of OSA.

REFERENCES

1. American Academy of Sleep Medicine: ICSD-2 International Classification of Sleep Disorders, 2nd ed. Diagnostic and Coding Manual. Westchester, IL: American Academy of Sleep Medicine, 2005.
2. Mahowald MW, Ettinger MG: Things that go bump in the night—parasomnias revisited. J Clin Neurophysiol 1990;7: 119–143.
3. Bornermann MA, Mahowald MW, Schenck CH: Parasomnias: clinical features and forensic implications. Chest 2006;130: 605–610.
4. Plante DT, Winkelmann JW: Parasomnias: psychiatric considerations. Sleep Med Clin 2008;3:217–229.
5. Mahowald MW, Bornemann MA: NREM sleep-arousal parasomnias. In Kryger MH, Roth T, Dement WH (eds): Principles and Practice of Sleep Medicine. Philadelphia: Elsevier Saunders, 2005, pp. 889–896.
6. Schenck CH, Milner DM, Hurwitz TD, et al: A polysomnographic and clinical report of sleep related injury in 100 adult patients. Am J Psychiatry 1989;146:1166–1172.
7. Crisp AH: The sleepwalking/night terrors syndrome in adults. Postgrad Med J 1996;72:599–604.
8. Pressman MR: Factors that predispose, prime and precipitate NREM parasomnias in adults: clinical and forensic implications. Sleep Med Rev 2007;11:5–30.
9. Hublin C, Krapio J, Partinen M, et al: Prevalence and genetics of sleep walking: a population-based twin study. Neurology 1997;48:177–181.
10. Millman RP, Kipp GJ, Carskadon MA: Sleepwalking precipitated by treatment of sleep apnea with nasal CPAP. Chest 1991;99;750–751.
11. Guilleminault C, Kirisogluc C, Bao G, et al: Adult chronic sleepwalking and its treatment based on polysomnography. Brain 2005;128:1062–1069.
12. Schenck CH, Mahowald MW: On the reported association of psychopathology with sleep terrors in adults. Sleep 2000; 23:1–2.
13. Schenck C, Pareja JA, Patterson AL, Mahowald MW: Analysis of polysomnographic events surrounding 252 slow wave sleep arousals in thirty-eight adults with injurious sleep walking and sleep terrors. J Clin Neurophysiol 1998;15:159–166.
14. Shapiro CM, Trajanovic NN, Fedoroff JP: Sex-somnia. A new parasomnia? Can J Psychiatry 2003;48:311–317.
15. Schenck CH, Arnulf I, Mahowald MW: Sleep and sex: what can go wrong? A review of the literature on sexual related disorders and abnormal sexual behaviors and experiences. Sleep 2007; 30:683–702.
16. Cartwright R: Sleep walking violence: a sleep disorder, a legal dilemma, and a psychological challenge. Am J Psychiatry 2004; 161:1149–1158.
17. Mahowald MW, Schenck CH: Parasomnias: sleep walking and the law. Sleep Med Rev 2000;4:321–339.
18. Harris M, Grunstein RR: Treatments for somnambulism in adults: assessing the evidence. Sleep Med Rev 2009;13: 295–297.
19. Pressman MR, Meyer TJ, Kendrick-Mohamed J, et al: Night terrors in adults precipitated by sleep apnea. Sleep 1995;18: 773–775.
20. Craske MG, Tsao JCI: Assessment and treatment of nocturnal panic attacks. Sleep Med Rev 2005;9:173–184.
21. Schenck CH, Bundlie SR, Patterson AL, et al: Rapid eye movement sleep behavior disorder: a treatable parasomnia affecting older males. JAMA 1987;257:1786–1789.
22. Mahowald MW, Schneck CH: REM sleep parasomnias. In Kryger MH, Roth T, Dement WH (eds): Principles and Practice of Sleep Medicine. Philadelphia: Elsevier Saunders, 2005, pp. 897–914.
23. Olson EJ, Boeve BF, Silber MH: Rapid eye movement sleep behavior disorder: demographic, clinical, and sleep laboratory findings in 93 cases. Brain 2000;123:331–339.
24. Schenck CH, Mahowald MW: REM sleep behavior disorder: clinical, developmental, and neuroscience perspective 16 years after its formal identification in sleep. Sleep 2002;25:120–138.
25. Boeve BF, Silber MH, Saper CB, et al: Pathophysiology of REM sleep behavior disorder and relevance to neurodegenerative disease. Brain 2007;130:2770–2788.
26. Hoque R, Chesson AL: Pharmacologically induced/exacerbated restless legs syndrome/periodic limb movements of sleep, and REM behavior disorder/REM sleep without atonia: literature review, qualitative scoring, and comparative analysis. J Clin Sleep Med 2010;15:79–83.
27. Schenck CH, Bundlie SR, Mahowald MW: Delayed emergence of a parkinsonian disorder in 38% of 29 older men initially diagnosed with idiopathic rapid eye movement sleep disorder. Neurology 1996;46:388–393.

28. Eisensehr I, Linke R, Noachtar S, et al: Reduced striatal dopamine transporters in idiopathic rapid eye movement sleep behavior disorder. Comparison with Parkinson's disease and controls. Brain 2000;123:1155–1160.

29. Iranzo A, Santamaria J: Severe obstructive sleep apnea/hypopnea mimicking REM sleep behavior disorder. Sleep 2005;28:203–206.

30. Iber C, Ancoli-Israel S, Chesson A, Quan SF, for the American Academy of Sleep Medicine: The AASM Manual for the Scoring of Sleep and Associated Events: Rules, Terminology and Technical Specification, 1st ed. Westchester, IL: American Academy of Sleep Medicine, 2007.

31. Winklemann JW, James L: Serotonergic antidepressants are associated with REM sleep without atonia. Sleep 2004;27:317–321.

32. Schenck CH, Boyd JL, Mahowald MW: A parasomnia overlap disorder involving sleep walking, sleep terrors, and REM sleep behavior disorder in 33 polysomnographically confirmed cases. Sleep 1997;20:972–981.

33. Mahowald MW, Schenck CH: Status dissociatus—a perspective on states of being. Sleep 1991;14:69–79.

34. Husain AM, Miller PP, Carwile ST: REM sleep behavior disorder: potential relationship to post-traumatic stress disorder. J Clin Neurophysiol 2001;18:148–157.

35. Aurora RN, Zak RS, Maganti RK, et al: Best practice guidelines for the treatment of REM sleep behavior disorder (RBD). J Clin Sleep Med 2010;6:85–95.

36. Anderson KN, Shneerson JM: Drug treatment of REM sleep behavior disorder: the use of drug therapies other than clonazepam. J Clin Sleep Med 2009;5:235–239.

37. Boeve BF, Silber MH, Ferman TJ: Melatonin for treatment of REM sleep behavior disorder in neurological disorders: results in 14 patients. Sleep Med 2003;4:281–284.

38. Schmidt MH, Koshal VB, Schmidt HS: Use of pramipexole in REM sleep behavior disorder: results from a case series. Sleep Med 2006;7:418–423.

39. Bamford CR: Carbamazepine in REM sleep behavior disorder. Sleep 1993;16:33–34.

40. Tackuchi T, Fukuda K, Sasaki Y, et al: Factors related to the occurrence of isolated sleep paralysis elicited during a multiphasic sleep-wake schedule. Sleep 2002;25:89–96.

41. Pagel JF, Helfter P: Drug-induced nightmares—an etiology-based review. Hum Psychopharmacol Clin Exp 2003;18:59–67.

42. Lancee J, Spoormaker MI, Krakow B, Van den Bout J: A systematic review of cognitive-behavioral treatment for nightmares: toward a well-established treatment. J Clin Exp Med 2008;4:475–480.

43. Krakow B, Hollifield M, Johnston L, et al: Imagery rehearsal therapy for chronic nightmares in sexual assault survivors with post-traumatic stress disorder. JAMA 2001;286:537–545.

44. Raskind MA, Peskind ER, Hoff DJ, et al: A parallel group placebo-controlled study of prazosin for trauma nightmares and sleep disturbance in combat veterans with post-traumatic stress disorder. Biol Psychiatry 2007;61:928–934.

45. Taylor FB, Martin P, Thompson C, et al: Prazosin effects on objective sleep measures and clinical symptoms in civilian trauma PTSD: a placebo-controlled study. Biol Psychiatry 2008;63:629–632.

46. Berlant JL: Prospective open-label study of add-on and monotherapy topiramate in civilians with chronic nonhallucinatory posttraumatic stress disorder. BMC Psychiatry 2004;4:24.

47. American Psychiatric Association: Diagnostic and Statistical Manual of Mental Disorders, 4th ed. Washington, DC: American Psychiatric Association, 1994.

48. Agargun M, Kara H, Ozer O, et al: Characteristics of patients with nocturnal dissociative disorders. Sleep Hypnosis 2001;3:131–134.

49. Robson WLM: Evaluation and management of enuresis. N Engl J Med 2009;360:1429–1436.

50. Brooks LJ, Topol HI: Enuresis in children with sleep apnea. J Pediatr 2003;142:515–518.

51. Barone JG, Hanson C, DaJusta DG, et al: Nocturnal enuresis and overweight are associated with obstructive sleep apnea. Pediatrics 2009;124:e53–e59.

52. Vetrugno R, Provini F, Plazzi G, et al: Catathrenia (nocturnal groaning): a new type of parasomnia. Neurology 2001;56:681–683.

53. Siddiqui F, Walters AS, Chokroverty S: Catathrenia: a rare parasomnia which may mimic central sleep apnea on polysomnogram. Sleep Med 2008;9:460–461.

54. Pevernagie DA, Boon PA, Mariman AN, et al: Vocalization during episodes of prolonged expiration: a parasomnia related to REM sleep. Sleep Med 2001;2:19–30.

55. Ramar K, Olson EJ, Morgenthaler TI: Catathrenia. Sleep Med 2008;9:457–459.

56. Iriarte J, Alegre M, Urrestarazu E, et al: Continuous positive airway pressure as treatment for catathrenia (nocturnal groaning). Neurology 2006;66:609–610.

57. Songu M, Yilmaz H, Uucetruk AV, et al: Effect of CPAP therapy on catathrenia and OSA: a case report and review of the literature. Sleep Breath 2008;12:401–405.

58. Sachs C, Svanborg E: The exploding head syndrome: polysomnographic recordings and therapeutic suggestions. Sleep 1991;14:263–266.

59. Evers S, Goadsby PJ: Hypnic headache. Neurology 2003;60;905–909.

60. Alberti A: Headache and sleep. Sleep Med Rev 2006;10:431–437.

61. International Classification of Headache Disorders, 2nd ed. (ICHD-II): International Headache Society. Cephalagia 2004;24(Suppl 1):46–54.

62. Chakraverty A: Exploding head syndrome: a report of two new cases. Cephalgia 2007;28:399–400.

63. Jacome DE: Exploding head syndrome and idiopathic stabbing headache relieved by nifedipine. Cephalagia 2001;21:617–618.

64. Silber MH, Hansen MR, Girish M: Complex nocturnal visual hallucinations. Sleep Med 2005;6:363–366.

65. Schenck CH, Hurwitz TD, Bundlie SR, Mahowald MW: Sleep-related eating disorders: polysomnographic correlates of a heterogeneous syndrome distinct from daytime eating disorders. Sleep 1991;14:419–431.

66. Howell MJ, Schenck CH, Crow SJ: A review of nighttime eating disorders. Sleep Med Rev 2009;13:23–34.

67. Morgenthaler TI, Silber MH: Amnestic sleep-related eating disorder associated with zolpidem. Sleep Med 2002;3:323–327.

68. Howell MJ, Schenck CH: Treatment of nocturnal eating disorders. Curr Treatment Options Neurol 2009;11:333–339.

69. Winkelmann JW: Treatment of nocturnal eating syndrome and sleep-related eating disorder with topirmate. Sleep Med 2003;4:243–246.

70. Winkelmann JW: Efficacy and tolerability of open-label topiramate in the treatment of sleep-related eating disorder: a retrospective case series. J Clin Psychiatry 2006;67:1729–1734.

71. Provini F, Albani R, Vetrugno R, et al: A pilot double-blind placebo-controlled trial of low-dose pramipexole in sleep-related eating disorder. Eur J Neurol 2005;12:432–436.

72. O'Reardon JP, Allison KC, Martino NS, et al: A randomized, placebo-controlled trial of sertraline in the treatment of night eating syndrome. Am J Psychiatry 2006;163:893–898.

73. Verrugno R, Provini F, Meletti S, et al: Propiospinal myoclonus at the sleep-wake transition: a new type of parasomnia. Sleep 2001;24:835–843.

74. Provini F, Plazzi G, Montagna P, Lugaresi E: The wide spectrum of nocturnal frontal lobe epilepsy. Sleep Med Rev 2000;4;375–386.

Chapter 29

Psychiatry and Sleep

Chapter Points

- A significant proportion of patients with a sleep complaint have a psychiatric illness and a significant number of patients with a psychiatric illness have a sleep complaint.
- Insomnia or hypersomnia nearly every day is one of the nine major criteria for diagnosis of an MDE.
- During an MDE, approximately 80% of patients complain of symptoms of insomnia (frequent awakenings, early morning awakening) and 20% complain of hypersomnia.
- PSG during a depressive episode shows a long sleep latency, reduced sleep efficiency, reduced stage N3, a short REM latency, a longer first REM period, and a higher REM density early in the night. Early morning awakening may also be present.
- Insomnia can precede an MDE and is often the last symptom of depression to resolve. Some but not all studies suggest that the persistence of sleep complaints is a risk factor for relapse of depression.
- During MEs, the patient reports a decreased need for sleep (feeling rested on a few hours of sleep). Sleep loss can precipitate an ME.
- Hypomanic episodes have characteristics similar to those of MEs except for the following three conditions: severe impairment is not present, hospitalization is not necessary, and there are no psychotic features. If any of the three are present, the episode is considered an ME.
- A summary of duration criteria for the mood episodes:
  - MDE: 2 weeks.
  - ME: 1 week.
  - Mixed episode: 1 week.
  - Hypomanic episode: 4 days.
- Bipolar disorder I requires:
  - A current (or recent) hypomanic, ME, mixed episode, or MDE.
  - If the current episode is hypomanic or an MDE, there must be history of a prior mixed episode or ME.
- Note that, unlike diagnostic criteria for bipolar disorder II, the presence of at least one MDE is not required.

- Bipolar disorder II consists of at least one hypomanic episode, one or more depressive episodes, and no history of current (or prior) MEs or mixed episodes.
- Relapse rates for bipolar disorder patients are very high, even on maintenance therapy. Bipolar disorder is a significant risk factor for suicide.
- Most patients with nocturnal panic attacks have similar episodes during the day. However, panic attacks can occur mainly at night and must be differentiated from NREM parasomnias such as sleep terrors.
- The treatment of panic disorder includes behavioral psychotherapy/relaxation techniques, an SSRI (e.g., paroxetine or sertraline), and an antianxiety medication such as alprazolam or clonazepam. The SSRI is typically started in a low dose in combination with an antianxiety medication to prevent initial worsening of symptoms. The antianxiety medication can later be tapered in many cases.
- Disturbing nightmares are a significant problem impairing sleep in PTSD. Imagery rehearsal therapy and prazosin are two relatively new treatment options.

Psychiatric disorders are among the most common health problems, with over 15% to 20% of Americans being treated for a significant psychiatric illness in any given year.[1] Almost one third of individuals with significant complaints of insomnia or hypersomnia show evidence of psychiatric disorders.[2-5] Psychiatric disorders account for the largest diagnostic category for patients with sleep complaints. Conversely, sleep complaints are part of the diagnostic criteria for many psychiatric disorders and are a source of considerable morbidity. The psychiatric disorders commonly affecting sleep (or vice versa) are listed in Box 29-1.

MOOD DISORDERS

Mood disorders are the most common category of psychiatric disorders followed by anxiety disorders. The mood disorders include major depressive disorder (MDD) and the bipolar disorders. The mood disorders are defined on the basis of the occurrence of mood episodes. Several types of

BOX 29–1

Psychiatric Disorders Commonly Affecting Sleep
MOOD DISORDERS
• Major depressive disorder
• Bipolar disorder I
• Bipolar disorder II
ANXIETY DISORDERS
• Panic disorder
• Posttraumatic stress disorder
• Generalized anxiety disorder

mood episodes (major depressive, manic, hypomanic, and mixed) are defined later. When mood episodes occur in a temporal pattern together with other diagnostic features, they define the characteristics of the mood disorder. Note that all mood episodes with the exception of hypomania have "**impairment**" as a criterion.

Depression Questionnaires and Severity Rating Scales

A number of depression scales are available for use by the sleep clinician in helping evaluate patients for possible depression or measuring improvement with treatment. The Beck Depression Inventory was mentioned in Chapter 25 on insomnia.[6] The Hamilton Depression Scale (HAMD) is a 17, 21, or 24 question instrument that is widely used for research.[7] The Montgomery-Åsberg Depression Rating Scale (MADRS) is a 10-item diagnostic questionnaire used to measure the severity of depressive episodes in patients.[8] It was developed to be sensitive to the changes brought on by antidepressants and other forms of treatment. The Patient Health Questionnaire (PHQ-9) is a short 9-question instrument (Appendix 29–1)[9] that the patient can quickly fill out and is easy to use. The PHQ-9 has been validated and may be used to screen patients with sleep disorders for depression.

Mood Episodes

Major Depressive Episode

A major depressive episode (MDE; Box 29–2) is defined by **five** (or more) of the following **nine symptoms** having been present during the **same 2-week period** and representing a **change from previous functioning;** at least one of the symptoms is either (1) depressed mood or (2) loss of interest or pleasure (Diagnostic and Statistical Manual of Mental Disorders, 4th edition [DSM-IV]).[2]

1. Depressed mood.*
2. Markedly diminished interest or pleasure.*

---

*Essential symptoms.

BOX 29–2

Major Depressive Episode

A. **Five (or more)** of the following **nine symptoms** have been present during the **same 2-week period** and represent a change from previous functioning; at least one of the symptoms is either (1) depressed mood or (2) loss of interest or pleasure.

1. **Depressed mood,** present most of the day, nearly every day, as indicated by either subjective report (e.g., feels sad or empty) or observation made by others (e.g., appears tearful). *Note:* In children and adolescents can be irritable mood.
2. **Markedly diminished interest or pleasure** in all, or almost all, activities most of the day, nearly every day (as indicated by either subjective report or observation made by others).
3. Significant **weight loss** when not dieting or **weight gain** (e.g., change of > 5% of body weight in a month), or **decrease or increase in appetite** nearly every day.
4. **Insomnia or hypersomnia** nearly every day.
5. **Psychomotor agitation or retardation** present nearly every day (observable by others, not merely subjective feelings of restlessness or being slowed down).
6. **Fatigue or loss of energy** nearly every day.
7. **Feelings of worthlessness or excessive or inappropriate guilt** (which may be delusional) nearly every day.
8. Diminished ability to **think or concentrate,** or indecisiveness nearly every day.*
9. **Recurrent thoughts of death** (not just fear of dying), recurrent suicidal ideation without a specific plan, or a suicide attempt or specific plan for committing suicide.

B. Symptoms do not meet criteria for a mixed episode.

C. Symptoms cause clinically significant distress or **impairment** in social, occupational, or other important areas of functioning.

D. Symptoms are not due to the direct physiologic effects of a substance (e.g., drug of abuse, a medication, or other treatment) or general medical condition (e.g., hypothyroidism).

E. Symptoms are not better accounted for by bereavement (i.e., after the loss of a loved one), the symptoms persist for longer than 2 months or are characterized by marked functional impairment, morbid preoccupation with worthlessness, suicidal ideation, psychotic symptoms, or psychomotor retardations.

*Either by subjective report or observed by others.
Adapted from American Psychiatric Association: Diagnostic and Statistical Manual of Mental Disorders, 4th ed. Washington, DC: American Psychiatric Association, 2000.

3. Significant weight loss, when not dieting, or weight gain, or decrease or increase in appetite.
4. Insomnia or hypersomnia nearly every day.
5. Psychomotor agitation or retardation nearly every day (observable by others, not merely subjective feelings or restlessness or being slowed down).

BOX 29–3

Subtypes of Depressive Episodes

MELANCHOLIC (RETARDED) SUBTYPE	ATYPICAL (ANXIOUS) SUBTYPE
• Minimal mood reactivity 　• Look depressed or flat during interview • Insomnia • Loss of appetite and weight loss • Severe anhedonia 　• Inability to find pleasure in anything • Diurnal variability 　• Worse in morning • More common in older age groups 　• Particularly in elderly and medically ill	• *Mood reactivity* must be present 　• Can feel much better or even normal in social situations • Do not always "look depressed" during interview • At least two of four additional symptoms: 　• Hypersomnia 　• Hyperphagia/weight gain 　• Rejection sensitivity—fear of negative social evaluation 　• Laden fatigue • More likely in younger age groups • In one study, 60% of adults with atypical subtype had bipolar II disorder

BOX 29–4

Sleep and Major Depressive Episodes

- Symptoms
  - 80% of depressive episodes are associated with insomnia
    - Early AM awakening.
    - Frequent awakening.
- 15–20% hypersomnia.
- PSG findings
  - Prolonged sleep latency.
  - Increased wake, early AM awakening, frequent awakenings.
  - Decreased stage N3, decreased N3 in the early part of the night.
  - REM abnormalities.
    - Short REM latency.
    - Increased REM density.
    - Increased REM early in the night.
    - Increased REM (%TST).
- MSLT—does NOT demonstrate severe sleepiness.
- Sleep abnormalities may persist after remission.
- Persistent abnormalities may be associated with risk of recurrence.

MSLT = multiple sleep latency test; PSG = polysomnography; REM = rapid eye movement; TST = total sleep time.

6. Fatigue or loss of energy.
7. Feelings of worthlessness or excessive or inappropriate guilt (which may be delusional) nearly every day (not merely self-reproach or guilt about being sick).
8. Diminished ability to think or concentrate or indecisiveness nearly every day.[†]
9. Recurrent thoughts of death (not just fear of dying), recurrent suicidal ideation without a specific plan, or a suicide attempt or specific plan for committing suicide.

In order to meet criteria for an MDE, symptoms must not meet criteria for a mixed episode, must cause significant distress or impairment, and are not a result of another process or medication/substance. In addition, the symptoms are not explained by bereavement. An MDE can occur in either bipolar disorders or unipolar depression (MDD). A useful mnemonic for symptoms of depression = depressed mood + SIGECAPS = **S**leep, **I**nterest, **G**uilt, **E**nergy, **C**oncentration, **A**ppetite, **P**leasure, and **S**uicidality.

MDEs are sometimes divided into melancholic and atypical subtypes (Box 29–3). The **melancholic** subtype is associated with **insomnia** whereas **hypersomnia** is characteristic of the **atypical** subtype. The melancholic subtype usually has worse symptoms in the morning. An atypical depressive episode is also characterized by mood reactivity (ability for mood to temporarily improve in response to a positive or stimulating situation), increased appetite and weight, laden fatigue (a sense of heaviness or being weighed down), and rejection sensitivity (fear of social rejection). Unipolar depressive episodes are more often of the melancholic type

and the atypical subtype is more characteristic of bipolar depressive episodes.

Impact of MDE on Sleep The impact of an MDE on sleep is summarized in Box 29–4. A sleep complaint (insomnia or hypersomnia) is one of the primary diagnostic criteria for an MDE. Nearly 80% of depressive episodes are associated with insomnia.[3,4] The insomnia complaints include early morning awakening and frequent awakenings. However, up to 15% to 20% of patients complain of hypersomnia during an MDE. The polysomnography (PSG) findings in patients during an MDE[4,5] include **a prolonged sleep latency, increased wake after sleep onset, decreased stage N3, and rapid eye movement (REM; stage R) abnormalities. The stage R abnormalities include a short REM latency, an increased length of the first REM episode, and an increased REM density in the early part of the night.** Recall that the REM density (number of REMs per time) is typically low during the first REM episodes. Symptoms of insomnia or PSG abnormalities may persist after remission of depression.[5,10–14] Rush and coworkers[10] found a short REM latency (<65 min) in 11/13 patients during active depression, and in those 11 patients, a short REM latency persisted in 8 after clinical remission. Dombrovski and colleagues[14] found that anxiety and possibly residual sleep disturbance predicted early recurrence. However, Yang and associates[15] did not find that persistent sleep disturbance predicted recurrence. Even if patients with an MDE complain of hypersomnia, the multiple sleep latency test (MSLT) does not usually reveal severe sleepiness.[3,4,16]

[†]Either by subjective report or observed by others.

Manic Episode

Manic episodes (MEs) are distinct periods of abnormally and persistently elevated, expansive, or irritable mood, lasting **at least 1 week** (or any duration if hospitalization is necessary) (Box 29–5). If the **mood is irritable, four** of the following are needed, otherwise **three** of the following[2]:

1. Inflated self-esteem or grandiosity.
2. Decreased need for sleep (e.g., feels rested after 3 hr of sleep).
3. More talkative than usual or pressure to keep talking.
4. Flight of ideas or subjective experience that thoughts are racing.
5. Distractability (i.e., attention too easily drawn to unimportant or irrelevant external stimuli).
6. Increase in goal-directed activity (either socially, at work or school, or sexually) or psychomotor agitation.

7. Excessive involvement in pleasurable activities that have a high potential for painful consequences (e.g., engaging in unrestrained buying sprees, sexual indiscretions, or foolish business investments).

In MEs, the symptoms do not meet criteria for a mixed episode (defined later). The disturbance is sufficiently **severe to cause marked impairment** in occupational function or in usual social activities or relationships with others or to **necessitate hospitalization to prevent harm to self or others,** or there are **psychotic features.** Note that the symptoms noted previously are essentially the same for hypomania episodes (discussed in a later section), **BUT** in **hypomania, there is NO** marked impairment, need for hospitalization, or psychotic features.

Impact of Mania on Sleep MEs are associated with marked insomnia, but the patient awakens refreshed after a few hours of sleep. PSG findings include reduced stage N3, a short REM latency, and an increased REM density.[11,17–19] **Of note, sleep loss can trigger MEs**[20,21] (Box 29–6).

Mixed Episode

In mixed episodes, criteria are met both for an ME and for an MDE (except for duration) **nearly every day during at least a 1-week period.**[2] The disturbance is sufficiently **severe to cause marked impairment** in occupational function or in usual social activities or relationships with others or to **necessitate hospitalization** to prevent harm to self or others, or there **are psychotic features.** Symptoms are not due to the direct physiologic effects of a substance (e.g., drug of abuse, a medication, or other treatment) or general medical condition (e.g., hypothyroidism). The mixed episode combines symptoms of both mania and depression. The patient may be effusive and grandiose one moment and crying the next (Box 29–7).

Hypomanic Episode

A hypomanic episode is a distinct period of persistently elevated, expansive, or irritable mood, lasting throughout at

---

BOX 29–5

Manic Episode

A. Distinct period of abnormally and persistently elevated, expansive, or irritable mood, lasting **at least 1 week** (or any duration if hospitalization is necessary).

B. During the period of mood disturbance, **three (or more)** of the following symptoms have persisted (**four if the mood is only irritable**) and have been present to a significant degree:
1. **Inflated self-esteem or grandiosity.**
2. **Decreased need for sleep** (e.g., feels rested after 3 hr of sleep).
3. More talkative than usual or **pressure to keep talking.**
4. **Flight of ideas** or subjective experience that thoughts are racing.
5. **Distractability** (i.e., attention too easily drawn to unimportant or irrelevant external stimuli).
6. Increase in **goal-directed activity** (either socially, at work or school, or sexually) or **psychomotor agitation.**
7. **Excessive involvement in pleasurable activities** that have a high potential for painful consequences (e.g., engaging in unrestrained buying sprees, sexual indiscretions, or foolish business investments).

C. Symptoms do not meet criteria for mixed episode.

D. Mood disturbance is sufficiently **severe to cause marked impairment** in occupational function or in usual social activities or relationships with others or to **necessitate hospitalization to prevent harm to self or others**, or there are **psychotic features.**

Manic episodes cause marked impairment or have psychotic features (in contrast, hypomania mood disturbance does NOT cause marked impairment, does NOT necessitate hospitalization, and has NO psychotic features).

Adapted from American Psychiatric Association: Diagnostic and Statistical Manual of Mental Disorders, 4th ed. Washington, DC: American Psychiatric Association, 2000.

BOX 29–6

Manic/Hypomanic Episodes and Sleep

MANIC EPISODES

- Marked insomnia.
- Refreshed with only a few hours of sleep.
- PSG findings
  - Reduced stage N3.
  - Short REM latency.
  - Increased REM density.
- Sleep loss can trigger mania.

HYPOMANIC EPISODES

- Report of decreased sleep need.

PSG = polysomnography; REM = rapid eye movement.

BOX 29–7

Mixed Episode

A. Criteria are met both for a manic episode and for a major depressive episode (except for duration) **nearly every day during at least a 1-week period.**

B. Mood disturbance is **sufficiently severe to cause marked impairment** in occupational function or in usual social activities or relationships with others or to **necessitate hospitalization** to prevent harm to self or others, or there **are psychotic features.**

C. Symptoms are not due to the direct physiologic effects of a substance (e.g., drug of abuse, a medication, or other treatment) or general medical condition (e.g., hypothyroidism).

Adapted from American Psychiatric Association: Diagnostic and Statistical Manual of Mental Disorders, 4th ed. Washington, DC: American Psychiatric Association, 2000.

BOX 29–8

Hypomanic Episode

A. A distinct period of persistently elevated, expansive, or irritable mood, lasting throughout at least **4 days,** that is clearly different for the usual nondepressed mood.

B. During the period of mood disturbance, three (or more) of the following symptoms have persisted (four if the mood is only irritable) and have been present to a significant degree:

   i. Inflated self-esteem or grandiosity.

   ii. Decreased need for sleep (rested on 3 hours of sleep).

   iii. More talkative than usual or pressure to keep talking.

   iv. Flight of ideas or subjective experience that thoughts are racing.

   v. Distractability.

   vi. Increase in goal-directed activity or psychomotor agitation.

   vii. Excessive involvement in pleasurable activities that have a high potential for painful consequences (e.g., buying sprees, sexual indiscretions, or foolish business investments).

C. The episode is associated with an unequivocal change in functioning that is uncharacteristic of the person when not symptomatic.

D. The disturbance in mood and the change in functioning are observable by others.

E. The episode is **NOT SEVERE** enough to cause **marked impairment** in social or occupational function, or to **necessitate hospitalization**, and there are **NO psychotic features.**

F. The symptoms are not due to the direct physiologic effects of a substance (e.g., a drug of abuse, a medication, or other treatment) or a general medical condition (e.g., hypothyroidism).

Adapted from American Psychiatric Association: Diagnostic and Statistical Manual of Mental Disorders, 4th ed. Washington, DC: American Psychiatric Association, 2000.

least 4 days, that is clearly different from the usual nondepressed mood (Box 29–8).[2] During the period of mood disturbance, three (or more) of the following symptoms have persisted (four if the mood is only irritable) and have been present to a significant degree:

1. Inflated self-esteem or grandiosity.
2. Decreased need for sleep (**rested on 3 hr of sleep).**
3. More talkative than usual or pressure to keep talking.
4. Flight of ideas or subjective experience that thoughts are racing.
5. Distractability.
6. Increase in goal-directed activity or psychomotor agitation.
7. Excessive involvement in pleasurable activities that have a high potential for painful consequences (e.g., buying sprees, sexual indiscretions, or foolish business investments).

Episodes of hypomania are associated with an unequivocal change in functioning that is uncharacteristic of the person when she or he is not symptomatic. Of note, the disturbance in mood and the change in functioning are observable by others. Although all the previous statements are similar to those of MEs, the following differentiate hypomania from mania. The hypomania episode is **NOT SEVERE** enough to cause **marked impairment** in social or occupational function, or to **necessitate hospitalization,** and there are **NO psychotic features** (no delusions or hallucinations are present). **Note that a diagnosis of a hypomanic episode requires a minimum duration of 4 days whereas the minimum duration of symptoms for diagnosis of an ME is 1 week** (see Box 29–8).

Impact of Hypomania on Sleep Complaint of insomnia (mainly short sleep duration) or decreased need for sleep. In general, patients with hypomania report similar sleep symptoms as mania, but they are not as severe and do not cause the patient significant distress. In fact, patients may enjoy more energy and a lower sleep requirement.

Summary of Minimum Episode Durations
MDE: 2 weeks.
ME: 1 week.
Mixed episode: 1 week.
Hypomanic episode: 4 days.

Mood Disorders

The major mood disorders are listed in Box 29–9. This is not a complete list. For additional disorders refer to the DSM-IV.[2] These mood disorders are diagnosed based on occurrence of mood episodes (Fig. 29–1).

Major Depressive Disorder
The MDDs include (1) MDD—single episode or (2) MDD—recurrent (Box 29–10).[2] To be considered separate episodes, the depressive episodes must be separated by at least **2**

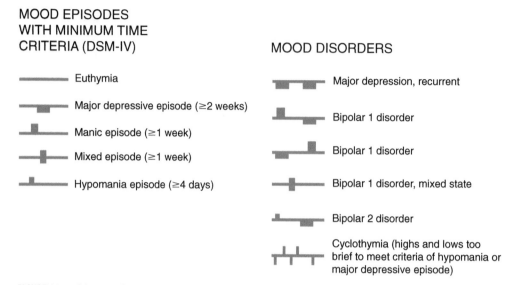

FIGURE 29-1 Schematic of episodes (showing minimum durations) and examples of mood disorders (elevations about and below baseline represent elevated or depressed mood). *Adapted from Priviter MR, Lness JM: Psychiatry Mentor, 2nd ed. Philadelphia: FA Davis, 2008, p. 121.*

BOX 29-9

Mood Disorders

   I. Major depressive disorder (no hypomania, mixed, manic episodes)
      1. Major depressive disorder, single episode
      2. Major depressive disorder, recurrent
  II. Dysthmic disorder
 III. Bipolar disorder I (at least one manic or mixed episode)
  IV. Bipolar disorder II (at least one hypomanic episode, one or more MDEs, and no manic or mixed episodes)
   V. Cyclothymic disorder

BOX 29-10

Major Depressive Disorder

1. Major depressive disorder, single episode
   A. Presence of a single major depressive episode.
   B. There has NEVER been a manic, mixed, or hypomanic episode.
2. Major depressive disorder, recurrent
   A. Presence of two or more depressive episodes—to be considered separate episodes, there must be an **interval of at least 2 consecutive months** in which criteria for major depressive episodes are NOT met.
   B. There has NEVER been a manic, mixed, or hypomanic episode.

Adapted from American Psychiatric Association: Diagnostic and Statistical Manual of Mental Disorders, 4th ed. Washington, DC: American Psychiatric Association, 2000.

---

consecutive months in which diagnostic criteria for MDE are not met. In MDD, there is NO history of a manic, mixed, or hypomanic episode. MDD is sometimes called "unipolar depression."

Sleep and MDD At least 60% to 80% of patients with an MDD report at least one of the following sleep complaints: difficulty falling asleep (38%), frequent awakenings (39%), or early morning awakening (41%) (Box 29-11).[3,13] Subjective complaints of insomnia may improve but are not necessarily normalized with remission from major depression.[12-15] Insomnia is often the last symptom to improve in patients treated for MDD. In addition, **insomnia is the most common residual complaint in patients who have recovered from depression.** Some studies have suggested that the persistence of sleep disturbance during remission from depression is predictive of a relapse.[13,14] However, a recent double-blind withdrawal of fluoxetine (FLX) after successful treatment[15] was unable to show a predictive value of residual sleep disturbance for the risk of recurrence of depression. Patients having a response to FLX during an open-label study received placebo or FLX during withdrawal. Sleep components of the

---

BOX 29-11

Sleep in Major Depressive Episode

- Insomnia in 65%—frequently sleep-maintenance insomnia, early AM awakening.
- Insomnia may precede the depressive episode.
- Insomnia is the most common residual symptom after remission.
- Residual insomnia may be predictive of recurrence of depression. However, a recent study did not replicate this finding.

HAMD were used to determine whether residual sleep complaints correlated with an increased chance of relapse. No sleep complaint was associated with higher rate of relapse of depression.

Depression and insomnia appear to have a reciprocal relationship **because insomnia frequently precedes the** onset of depression and has been found to be strongly predictive of future depressive episodes. Individuals with **persistent insomnia have been found to be 4 to 10 times more likely to subsequently develop depression** than those with short-term insomnia or no insomnia.[22] Patients with depression and persistent insomnia are 1.8 to 3.5 times more likely to remain depressed, compared with patients with no insomnia.[23]

Of interest, sleep deprivation or restriction has been found to have an acute antidepressant effect on patients with unipolar depression.[24,25] With recovery sleep, 50% to 80% of patients have a relapse. As noted previously, sleep loss can also precipitate mania in some patients.

Differential Diagnosis of Sleep Disturbance in MDE Differential diagnosis: If insomnia complaints are prominent, psychophysiologic insomnia or inadequate sleep hygiene should be considered. If hypersomnia complaints are prominent, then one should consider obstructive sleep apnea (OSA), narcolepsy, or insufficient sleep.

Treatment of Depression A detailed discussion of the treatment of depression is beyond the scope of this chapter. Psychotherapy and medications are often used alone or in combination. Many antidepressants are available.[26–33] Often, the choice is based on side effects and which symptoms are most prominent (anxiety, fatigue). Individual patients may respond to a different medication if treatment with an initial antidepressant is not successful. It is important to get a good drug history. If a patient previously responded to a medication, he or she is likely to have a good response again (Table 29–1). The older **tricyclic antidepressants** (TCAs) block the reuptake of serotonin and norepinephrine and are effective treatment for depression. However, the TCAs are not selective in the blockade of receptors and are associated with prominent anticholinergic side effects (constipation, dry mouth). They are also lethal in overdose. The selective serotonin reuptake inhibitors (SSRIs) are safer in overdose and in general have fewer side effects than TCAs. They vary in a number of properties. For example, the half-life of FLX is very long. The SSRIs can cause either daytime sedation or insomnia. If they cause insomnia, they should be given in the morning. If they cause sedation, they should be given at bedtime. SSRIs can also have prominent sexual side effects or result in weight gain in some patients. There is some evidence that escitalopram (Lexapro) is the most effective (or at least as effective)[29,30] for unipolar depression as other commonly used antidepressants and is well tolerated. Escitalopram also has fewer drug interactions than many other antidepressants. Some studies suggest that citalopram (racemic) is less effective than escitalopram. If escitalopram cannot be used due to financial issues, sertraline is a good alternative.

Bupropion is a unique medication with serotonin and dopamine uptake blocking effects. It has fewer sexual side effects than SSRIs and weight gain is less of a problem. It must be taken two or three times a day unless used in the extended-release form (Wellbutrin XL). It should not be used in patients with a seizure disorder. Venlafaxine (Effexor)

TABLE 29–1
Depression Treatment Strategy

UNIPOLAR DEPRESSION—GENERAL APPROACH

- Escitalopram (Lexapro)
  - Highest response rate in some meta-analyses.
  - Favorable side effect profile.
- Wellbutrin XL (bupropion, generics require multiple doses, possibly less effective)
  - Some clinicians feel less effective for depression but may be better tolerated than SSRIs.
  - Best side effect profile.
  - No weight gain.
  - Minimal sexual side effects.
- Sertraline (Zoloft)
  - Possibly most effective generic SSRI, well tolerated.
- Other SSRIs
  - Fluoxetine (long half-life, can be used for SNRI withdrawal side).
  - Citalopram (Celexa).
  - Paroxetine (Paxil) if anxiety a major component, sedating.

PROMINENT MELANCHOLIC MANIFESTATIONS

- Tricyclic antidepressants classic treatment
  - Affects both NE and 5HT.
  - More side effects, lethal in overdose.
- Good initial antidepressant choices
  - Wellbutrin XL (bupropion).
  - Venlafaxine (Effexor) (prominent withdrawal side effects).
  - Mirtazapine (Remeron) (helps with sleep).
- Augmentation strategies based on primary residual symptoms
  - Treat insomnia (see Table 29–3), anxiety, appetite.
  - Treat anergy/cognitive deficits
  - Stimulant, modafinil, armodafinil*

PROMINENT ATYPICAL FEATURES

- Monoamine oxidase inhibitor classic treatment
  - All three monoamines—5HTP, DA, and NE.
  - Rarely used due to required dietary restrictions, cannot be used with SSRIs (serotonin syndrome).
- Start with SSRI (tricyclics less effective).
- Augmentation usually necessary
  - Aripiprazole, Wellbutrin XL.
  - Stimulant, modafinil*, armodafinil*.

*Not FDA approved for treatment of depression.
DA = dopamine agonist; 5HT = serotonin; 5HTP = 5-hydroxy-L-tryptophan; NE = norepinephrine; SNRI = selective norepinephrine reuptake inhibitor; SSRI = selective serotonin reuptake inhibitor.

and desvenlafaxine (Pristiq) block reuptake of serotonin at lower doses and serotonin and norepinephrine at higher doses (selective norepinephrine reuptake inhibitors [SNRIs]). They are very effective antidepressants but can increase anxiety and cause a severe withdrawal syndrome if not tapered. Venlafaxine and desvenlafaxine can also increase blood pressure. Duloxetine (Cymbalta) blocks uptake of serotonin and norepinephrine (SNRI) and is used both as an antidepressant and to treat chronic pain (U.S. Food and Drug Administration [FDA] approved for treatment of fibromyalgia). **Mirtazapine (Remeron)** is a unique medication that

TABLE 29–2

Factors to Consider in Choosing an Antidepressant

- Previous medication history
  - Use a medication with a previous good response (unless side effects)
  - Avoid a medication if previous negative response or negative response to two or more in subclass
- Choose best fit for depression subtype
- Ability to treat co-morbid psychiatric or medical disorder
- Patient preference
  - Side effect profile
  - Cost issues

blocks histamine, central alpha 2 receptors, and $5HT_2$ and $5HT_3$ serotonin receptors. In low doses (7.5–15 mg), mirtazapine is more sedating compared with higher doses. The typical effective antidepressant dose is 30 to 45 mg. Mirtazapine, like bupropion, is less likely to cause sexual side effects but can cause significant weight gain. Mirtazapine may help patients with anxiety. Blockade of $5HT_2$ receptors may improve sleep quality.

An approach for choosing an antidepressant for treatment of depression is listed in Table 29–2. If the patient has prominent melancholic or atypical features, one might consider different medications. If the patient does not respond to an effective dose of the initial medication, either trial of another medication or the addition of another agent (augmentation) could be considered. Note that the serotonin syndrome (agitation, tachycardia, hyperthermia) can rarely occur when two medications blocking serotonin re-uptake are used together. The syndrome is most common with use of an SSRI + MAOI (contraindicated). Do not start an SSRI until a MAOI has been stopped for 21 days. Do not start a MAOI unless an SSRI has been stopped for up to five weeks (depending on SSRI half-life).

A detailed discussion of the use of second-generation antipsychotics (SGAs)[34-36] (e.g., quetiapine, aripiprazole) or alerting agents (modafinil)[37] for augmentation of treatment of depression is beyond the scope of this chapter. However, the reader should be aware that such medications are being used for this purpose. **Aripiprazole** (Abilify) is FDA approved for adjunctive therapy of major depression. This medication tends to cause less metabolic side effects (weight gain) than other SGAs. **Quetiapine** (Seroquel) is approved as both an adjunctive and a single agent treatment for depression.[35,36]

Effects of Antidepressants on Sleep A discussion of the effects of antidepressants on sleep (Table 29–3) is complicated by the fact that the results can vary depending on whether normal or depressed individuals are studied. The acute and chronic effects may also vary.[27,28] The literature is somewhat conflicting on the effects of a few medications. In general, antidepressants increase the REM latency and decrease the amount of REM sleep. Bupropion is one of the few medications that can actually increase the amount of REM sleep, although it increases the REM latency (at least in depressed patients). Nefazodone is a sedating antidepressant that also

tends to increase REM sleep.[38] It can cause severe hepatotoxicity and is rarely used today. Mirtazapine also has been reported to be associated with no or only mild reduction in the amount of REM sleep. The monoamine oxidase inhibitors (MAOIs) are less commonly used but are the most powerful suppressors of REM sleep. In general, sedating antidepressants have a beneficial effect on sleep efficiency whereas nonsedating antidepressants tend to decrease sleep efficiency. Of note, **if patients respond to an antidepressant, their subjective estimate of their sleep quality may improve even if objective sleep quality by PSG does not.** A study comparing fluoxetine and nefazodone showed subjective improvements in sleep quality with both medications but only patients on the sedating nefazodone had objective improvements in sleep.[38]

Pharmacotherapy for Co-morbid Insomnia of Psychiatric Disorders Patients with an MDD frequently have prominent co-morbid insomnia. In such patients, one might choose to use (1) a sedating antidepressant at antidepressant doses (e.g., mirtazapine 30–45 mg qhs), (2) the combination of an effective nonsedating antidepressant (at antidepressant doses) and a sedating antidepressant at low doses, (3) the combination of an effective nonsedating antidepressant and a benzodiazepine receptor agonist [BZRA] hypnotic), or (4) the combination of an antidepressant and a sedating atypical antipsychotic (quetiapine). Sedating antidepressants and antipsychotics commonly used for their hypnotic effect are listed in Table 29–4. For information on BZRA hypnotics, see Chapter 25.

Several sedating antidepressants are used in lower than antidepressant doses for their sedating properties. Doxepin is a sedating antidepressant but has anticholinergic side effects. It has been used in low doses (25 mg) as a hypnotic. It has recently been approved by the FDA for sleep maintenance in very low doses (3, 6 mg Silenor). Silenor is much more expensive than generic doxepin. Trazodone is used in low doses (50 mg) as a hypnotic but rarely in higher doses as an antidepressant. Trazodone can be used in combination with an SSRI to reduce antidepressant-associated insomnia.[39] Trazodone can rarely cause priapism but has minimal anticholinergic side effects compared with sedating TCAs. Because of the lack of anticholinergic side effects and availability of generic medication, trazodone is widely used as a hypnotic. As discussed in Chapter 25, the evidence for its hypnotic efficacy in patients who are not depressed is limited.

The utility of using the combination of an antidepressant and a BZRA has recently been studied using placebo-controlled trials. Fava and coworkers[40] studied a group of patients with both MDD and insomnia. The combination of FLX and placebo was compared with FLX + 3 mg of eszopiclone. Co-administration of eszopiclone resulted in improved subjective sleep latency, wake after sleep onset (WASO), and total sleep time compared with FLX alone. Although this result was not unexpected, a surprising finding was that there was also greater improvement in depression at 8 weeks with the combination of FLX and eszopiclone (Fig. 29–2). A

TABLE 29-3
Effects of Antidepressants on Sleep

	CONTINUITY	STAGE N3	REM	REM LATENCY	SEDATION
TCAs					
Amitriptyline	↑↑↑	↑	↓↓↓	↑	++++
Doxepin	↑↑↑	↑↑↑	↓↓	↑	++++
Imipramine	↑↔	↑	↓↓	↑	++
Nortriptyline	↑	↑	↓↓	↑	++
Desipramine	↔	↑	↓↓	↑	+
Clomipramine	↑↔	↑	↓↓↓↓	↑	↔
MAOIs					
Phenelzine	↓	↔	↓↓↓↓	↑↑↑↑	↔
SSRIs					
Fluoxetine	↓	↓	↓	↑	±
Paroxetine	↓↓	↓	↓↓	↑	+
Sertraline	↔	↔↓	↓	↑	+
Citalopram	↔	↓	↓	↑	+
Escitalopram	↔	↓	↓	↑	+
SNRIs					
Venlafaxine	↓	↔↓	↓↓	↑↑	++
Desvenlafaxine	Same				
Duloxetine	Same				
ATYPICAL					
Bupropion	↓↔	↔	↔↑	↔	↔
Trazodone	↑	↔↑	↓	↑	++++
Mirtazapine	↑	↔↑	↔↓	↔	3+ (low doses)

Up arrows = increased; down arrows = decreased; horizontal arrows = no or minimal change; plus signs (1–4) = increasing amount of sedation; MAOIs = monoamine oxidase inhibitors; REM = rapid eye movement; SNRIs = selective norepinephrine reuptake inhibitors; SSRIs = selective serotonin reuptake inhibitors; TCAs = tricyclic antidepressants.

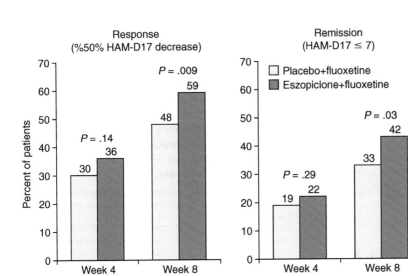

FIGURE 29-2 Eszopiclone + fluoxetine resulted in a significantly greater improvement in the Hamilton Depression Scale (HAM) at 8 weeks as determined by both relapse and remission compared with placebo + fluoxetine. *From Fava M, McCall V, Krystal A, et al: Eszopiclone co-administered with fluoxetine in patients with insomnia coexisting with major depressive disorder. Biol Psychiatry 2006;59:1052–1060.*

TABLE 29–4

Antidepressants and Atypical Antipsychotics Used for Sleep

NAME GENERIC (BRAND NAME)	DOSE FORMS	HYPNOTIC DOSE	COMMENTS	NOTABLE SIDE EFFECTS
Trazodone	50, 100 mg	25–100 mg qhs	Less anticholinergic side effects than TCAs $T_{1/2}$ 9 (3–14) hr	Priapism (1/8000 males) Postural hypotension
Mirtazapine (Remeron)	15, 30 mg	7.5–15 mg qhs	$T_{1/2}$ 20–40 hr	Weight gain Higher doses possibly less sedating
TCAs				
Amitryptyline (Elavil)	10, 25, 50 mg	10–25 mg qhs	$T_{1/2}$ 10–26 hr metabolite active (nortriptyline)	Dry mouth, constipation QT prolongation
Doxepin (Sinequan)	10, 25, 50 10 mg/mL	1–10 mg (elixir) 25 mg qhs	$T_{1/2}$ 6–8 hr	Dry mouth, constipation
Doxepin (Silenor)	3, 6 mg	6 mg qhs 3 mg qhs elderly	$T_{1/2}$ 6–8 hr	FDA approved for sleep-maintenance insomnia Cimetidine increases drug levels—max dose of doxepin should not exceed 3 mg Sertraline can also increase levels of doxepin
SEDATING ANTIPSYCHOTIC MEDICATIONS				
Quetiapine (Seroquel)	25, 50, 100 mg	12.5–50 mg qhs	$T_{1/2}$ 6 hr Intermediate acting	Headache, dizziness Neuroleptic syndrome Tardive dyskinesia Long QT Lens change

FDA = U.S. Food and Drug Administration; TCAs = tricyclic antidepressants.

similar trial with zolpidem found improvement in sleep but no evidence of greater improvement in depression.[41]

In patients with a history of past or current alcohol or benzodiazepine dependence, the use of BZRAs is problematic. For these patients, use of ramelteon (a melatonin receptor agonist with no abuse potential) or a sedating antidepressant may be the best treatment option. Ramelteon is approved only for sleep-onset insomnia and is not useful to improve sleep maintenance. It should NOT be used with the SSRI luvoxamine, which causes increased melatonin levels.

Quetiapine (Seroquel) is an SGA medication that antagonizes histamine, dopamine D_2, and serotonin $5HT_2$ receptors. At low doses, the medication's main effect is as an antihistamine. Therefore, it can be used in low doses as a hypnotic. Quetiapine is indicated for treatment of schizophrenia and bipolar disorder. As noted previously, quetiapine has been used as a second medication (augmentation) in treatment-resistant depression[35] or as a single antidepressant medication.[36] Side effects of quetiapine include QT prolongation, weight gain, extrapyramidal symptoms, headache, lens changes/cataracts, and decreased white blood cell count. Even at low doses, quetiapine has been associated with significant weight gain.

Dysthymic Disorder

Dysthymic disorder (Box 29–12) is manifested by a depressed mood for most of the day, for more days than

BOX 29–12

Dysthmic Disorder

A. Depressed mood for most of the day, for more days than not, as indicated either by subjective account or observation by others, **for at least 2 years.**

B. Presence while depressed of two or more of the following:
   i. Poor appetite or overeating.
   ii. Insomnia or hypersomnia.
   iii. Low energy or fatigue.
   iv. Low self-esteem.
   v. Poor concentration or difficulty making decision.
   vi. Feelings of hopelessness.

C. During the 2-year period of the disturbance, the person has never been **without** the symptoms in criterion A or B for more than 2 months at a time.

D. No major depressive episodes have been present the first 2 years of the disturbance.

E. There has never been a **manic episode, mixed episode, or hypomanic episode** and criteria have never been met for **cyclothymic disorder.**

Adapted from American Psychiatric Association: Diagnostic and Statistical Manual of Mental Disorders, 4th ed. Washington, DC: American Psychiatric Association, 2000.

not for at least 2 years. During depressed mood and two or more of the following are present[2]:

1. Poor appetite or overeating.
2. Insomnia or hypersomnia.
3. Low energy or fatigue.
4. Low self-esteem.
5. Poor concentration or difficulty making decisions.
6. Feelings of hopelessness.

The diagnosis of dysthymic disorder is NOT made if there has been an MDE during the 2-year period qualifying for dysthymic disorder. In addition, an ME, a hypomanic episode, or a mixed episode cannot have occurred previously.

Cyclothymic Disorder The diagnostic criteria for cyclothymic disorder (Box 29–13) require that the patient have numerous periods of both hypomania and depressive symptoms for 2 years that do not meet criteria for MDEs.[2] The periods of depressive or hypomanic symptoms can disturb sleep.

Bipolar Disorders

The bipolar disorders include bipolar I (BP-I) and bipolar II (BP-II)[2] (Box 29–14). The major difference between these disorders is that the "up" period in BP-II is hypomania and the patient has never had an ME or mixed episode. A BP-I patient can have hypomania or most recently be depressed **BUT** the diagnosis of BP-I requires **a current or previous mixed episode or ME.** The difference between mania and

hypomania is one of degree of severity. Patients with mania are severely impaired and are often hospitalized. Their actions often cause financial or physical harm to themselves or others.

In summary:
1. BP-I diagnosis requires:
   A. A current (or recent) hypomanic episode, ME, mixed episode, or MDE.
   B. If the current episode is hypomanic or an MDE, there must be history of a prior mixed episode or ME.
   Note that, unlike diagnostic criteria for BP-II, the presence of at least one MDE is not required.
2. BP-II diagnosis requires at least one hypomanic episode, one or more depressive episodes, and no history of current (or prior) MEs or mixed episodes.

Bipolar Depression

The depression of BP disorders is problematic for several reasons. First, treatment of depression in BP-I patients can send the patient into mania unless they are on a mood stabilizer. Second, there is a great risk of suicide during the depressive phase—a lifetime risk of suicide attempts up to 25%! Third, only a few medications are actually FDA approved for bipolar depression. Some bipolar patients present with complaints of depression and may be misdiagnosed as MDD (unipolar depression) rather than bipolar depression. It is important to question patients carefully about prior symptoms consistent with mania or hypomania. There are no pathognomonic characteristics of BP-I depression compared with unipolar depression. Table 29–5 present characteristics that are more probable in each category.[42]

Sleep in Bipolar Disorder

In BP-I, there is usually severe insomnia and a reduced need for sleep during MEs or hypomanic episodes. BP-II patients

---

BOX 29–13

Diagnostic Criteria for Cyclothymic Disorder

A. For at least 2 years, the presence of numerous periods with hypomanic symptoms and numerous periods of depressive symptoms that do not meet criteria for major depressive episodes. For children and adolescents, the duration must be at least 1 year.

B. During the above 2-year period, the person has not been without the symptoms of criterion A for more than 2 months at a time.

C. No major depressive episode, manic episode, or mixed episode has been present during the first 2 years of the disturbance.

D. The symptoms in criterion A are not better accounted for by schizoaffective disorder and are not superimposed on schizophreniform disorder, delusional disorder, or psychotic disorder not otherwise classified.

E. Symptoms are not due to physical effects of a substance or a general medical condition.

F. The symptoms cause clinical significant disorder or impairment in social, occupation, or other important areas.

Adapted from American Psychiatric Association: Diagnostic and Statistical Manual of Mental Disorders, 4th ed. Washington, DC: American Psychiatric Association, 2000.

BOX 29–14

Bipolar Disorders

BIPOLAR I DISORDER (AT LEAST ONE MANIC OR MIXED EPISODE)

A. Currently (or recently) hypomanic, manic, mixed, or major depressive episode.

B. If current episode is hypomanic or major depressive episode, there has previously been at least one manic or mixed episode.

BIPOLAR II DISORDER (AT LEAST ONE HYPOMANIC EPISODE, NO MANIC, NO MIXED)

A. Presence (or history) of one or more major depressive episodes.

B. Presence (or history) of at least one hypomanic episode.

C. There has never been a manic or mixed episode.

Adapted from American Psychiatric Association: Diagnostic and Statistical Manual of Mental Disorders, 4th ed. Washington, DC: American Psychiatric Association, 2000.

TABLE 29–5

Manifestations of Patients with Bipolar and Unipolar Depression

BIPOLAR I DEPRESSION MORE LIKELY	UNIPOLAR DEPRESSION MORE LIKELY
Hypersomnia	Prominent insomnia
Hyperphagia	Reduced appetite, weight
Psychomotor retardation	loss
Earlier age of onset of	Normal activity levels
first episode	Later age of onset of first
Psychotic features	episode
(pathologic guilt)	Somatic complaints
Lability of mood	No family history of bipolar
Family history of bipolar	
disorder	

From Mitchell PB, Goodwin GM, Johnson GF, Hirschfeld RMA: Diagnostic guidelines for bipolar depression: a probabilistic approach. Bipolar Disord 2008;10:144–152.

BOX 29–15

Bipolar Disorder I—Treatment Phases and Goals

- Mania/mixed
  - Rapid onset of action
  - Relief of symptoms
  - No depression induction
  - Typical treatments: divalproex, SGA, or a combination
- Bipolar depression
  - Relief of symptoms
  - No mania induction
  - Typical treatments: antimanic medication (lithium or divalproex) + lamotrigine, quetiapine XR, or a combination of olanzapine and fluoxetine
- Maintenance
  - Prevention of relapse into mania or depression
  - Reduction of co-morbid anxiety
  - Typical treatments: lithium, divalproex, lithium + lamotrigine; aripiprazole or ziprasidone frequently added in patients with frequent relapse

SGA = second-generation antipsychotic (aripiprazole, olanzapine, quetiapine).

do not have full-blown mania; they are less likely to present with episodes of severely short sleep duration. However, insomnia can still be a significant problem. **During bipolar depression, hypersomnia complaints are often more prominent than insomnia complaints.** However, insomnia can also be a significant problem in these patients as well. Adequate treatment of the mania and depression in patients with bipolar disorders is essential to improve sleep in these patients. Specific treatments for insomnia in bipolar patients would include use of BZRA hypnotics, ramelteon, lorazepam, clonazepam, and sedating SGAs (Seroquel). One would not use sedating antidepressants (at least at an antidepressant dose) in BP-I patients to avoid the precipitation of mania.

Genetics in Mood Disorders

Genetic factors account for 33% of the risk of major depression and more than 85% of the risk of bipolar disorder.[43]

Treatment of Bipolar Disorders

The treatment of bipolar disorders is complex.[44,45] A brief overview follows. Most sleep physicians who are not psychiatrists will probably not be the primary physician treating a patient for bipolar disorder. However, an understanding of the approach is important. A well-known treatment algorithm, the Texas Implementation of Medical Algorithm (TIMA) for bipolar disorder, may be found at http://www.dshs.state.tx.us/mhprograms/pdf/TIMABDalgos2005.pdf

Other treatment guidelines are available.[46,47] The treatment of bipolar disorders is usually grouped into three treatment phases: acute bipolar mania/mixed, bipolar depression, and bipolar maintenance (Box 29–15). The medications FDA approved for the different treatment phases are listed in Table 29–6. The major medication groups used include mood stabilizers and atypical antipsychotics. Antidepressants can be used for BP-I depression but usually only after several other medications have failed and always in combination with an antimanic medication (mood stabilizer). In

BP-II patients who have not displayed a manic episode over many years of depressive episodes, some clinicians will use an antidepressant without a mood stabilizer.

Acute Mania The newer atypical antipsychotic drugs such as risperidone (Risperdal), quetiapine (Seroquel), aripiprazole (Abilify), ziprasidone (Geodon), and olanzapine (Zyprexa) are often used in acutely manic patients because these medications have a rapid onset of psychomotor inhibition, which may be life-saving in the case of a violent or psychotic patient. These medications are approved for use in acute mania, alone or in combination with lithium or divalproex. The approved mood stabilizers for mania include lithium, divalproex (Depakote), and carbamazepine (Tegretol). Divalproex (Depakote) is an enteric-coated formulation of sodium valproate and valproic acid in a 1:1 molar ratio. Valproic acid (Depakene) and injectable sodium valproate (Depacon) are other available formulations. Divalproex is available in a long-acting preparation (Depakote ER), allowing once-daily dosing. The combination of an atypical antipsychotic and a mood stabilizer is also often used for severe mania. Lithium must be titrated up slowly and is not the drug of choice for acute severe mania. Antimania effects occur after 1 to 3 weeks of lithium at therapeutic doses. If lithium is used for acute mania, it usually requires the addition of another medication. Lithium side effects are experienced by up to 30% of patients taking this medication and include tremor, nausea, weight gain, fatigue, and mild cognitive impairment. A number of medications have important drug interactions with lithium. For example, diuretics and nonsteroidal anti-inflammatory drugs (NSAIDs) can reduce renal clearance (increase lithium levels). Divalproex is probably the mood stabilizer of choice for acute mania in this situation because it can be titrated up fairly rapidly

TABLE 29–6

U.S. Food and Drug Administration–Approved Medications for Bipolar Disorder

GENERIC	TRADE	MANIA	MIXED	MAINTENANCE	DEPRESSION
Valproic acid/valproate	Depakote	X	X	NFA	NFA
Carbamazepam ER	Equetro	X	X		
Lamotrigine	Lamictal			X (BP-I)	NFA
Lithium		X	X	X	NFA
Aripiprazole	Abilify	X	X	X	
Ziprasidone	Geodon	X	X	X	
Risperidone	Risperdal	X	X		
Quetiapine XR	Seroquel	X†	X	X*	X (BP-I and BP-II)
Olanzapine	Zyprexia	X	X	X	
Olanzapine + fluoxetine	Symbyax				X (BP-I)

*Approved for maintenance as adjunctive treatment with lithium or divalproex.
†Approved for combination with lithium or valproic acid.
BP-I, BP-II = bipolar I and II; FDA = U.S. Food and Drug Administration; NFA = not FDA approved for this indication but often used.

(20–30 mg/kg/day on a tid schedule). In less urgent cases, the medication is started at 250 mg with a meal on day 1, then increased to 250 mg tid for 3 to 6 days. Mania typically begins improving 1 to 4 days after drug levels exceed 50 μg/mL. Side effects of divalproex include nausea, vomiting, dyspepsia, and diarrhea. When titrated up rapidly, divalproex can also cause sedation. Rare but very severe side effects include hepatoxicity, leukopenia, thrombocytopenia, and pancreatitis. Drug levels can be obtained before the morning dose with a therapeutic range of 50 to 125 μg/mL (commonly felt > 75 needed for mania). Both lithium and divalproex have been associated with an increased risk of birth defects. Of note, **lithium increases stage N3 sleep and decreases REM sleep.**

Mixed Episode The treatment of a mixed episode is similar to the treatment of mania.

Maintenance Treatment The goal of maintenance treatment is to prevent relapse of mania and depressive episodes. **The cumulative rate of relapse after an episode of mania in the absence of maintenance treatment is 50% at 12 months and nearly 90% at 60 months.** Lithium and lamotrigene are the two mood stabilizers that are FDA approved for maintenance treatment. Divalproex is not FDA approved for maintenance treatment but is also widely used for this application. Lithium has the advantage of also preventing bipolar depression and reducing suicide risk. It appears to have an advantage over divalproex in these respects. Lamotrigine (Lamictal) may be used as a mood stabilizer for maintenance. Lamotrigine also has antidepressant effects and, therefore, is useful for maintenance. This medication requires a slow upward titration (over 6 wk) to avoid a significant skin rash. It can be associated with the Stevens-Johnson syndrome. Lamotrigine is NOT approved for acute mania. Aripiprazole (Abilify) and

ziprasidone (Geodone) are the only antipsychotic medications currently approved for maintenance. Aripiprazole is a partial dopamine D_2 agonist and serotonin $5HT_{1A}$ agonist as well as an antagonist at $5HT_{2A}$ receptors. Ziprasidone antagonizes dopamine D_2 receptors and serotonin $5HT_2$ receptors. Of note, even with maintenance treatment relapse of mania or depression may occur in up to 30 to 40% of BP-I patients in the first year and up to 75% over five years.

Bipolar Depression Treatment of bipolar depression is often challenging.[47] Few medications are actually FDA approved for treatment of bipolar depression. Quetiapine XR or a combination of olanzapine and FLX (Symbyax) are the only medications FDA approved for bipolar depression. One problem with the olanzapine/FLX combination is that FLX has a very long half-life. If mania occurs, the residual effects can be problematic.

Studies have NOT documented an advantage of the addition of a standard antidepressant to a mood stabilizer in treatment of bipolar depression.[48] The addition of an antidepressant can worsen anxiety, increase mood instability, or trigger a switch to mania. However, individual patients may benefit from the long-term combination of a mood stabilizer and an antidepressant. If an antidepressant is used, the activating ones like venlafaxine or duloxetine are more likely to cause switches (mania). Bupropion or a nonfluoxetine SSRI are used by many clinicians.

Although not FDA approved for bipolar depression, most treatment algorithms (Fig. 29–3) use a mood stabilizer (lithium or divalproex) as the initial step. Lithium is generally more effective for bipolar depression than divalproex. Many clinicians would next add lamotrigine, which has antidepressant activity. If this was not successful, quetiapine or the olanzapine/FLX combination could be added. If this does not work, antidepressants are then often added.

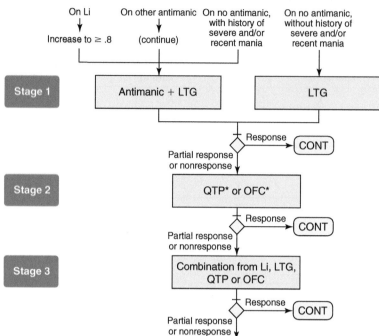

ALGORITHM FOR THE TREATMENT OF
BIPOLAR DISORDER I—CURRENTLY DEPRESSED

Antimanic = Li, valproex
Li = lithium
LTG = lamotrigine
QTP = quetiapine
OFC = olanzapine + fluoxetine combination
CONT = continue

FIGURE 29–3 The first three stages of a five-stage algorithm for treatment of bipolar depression (Bipolar Disorder I—Currently Depressed). Stage 1 consists of an antimanic medication (lithium or divalproex) and lamotrigine. Stage 2 consists of either quetiapine or the olanzapine + fluoxetine combination used alone. *There is overlap with the medications in Stage 1. The stage 1 medications are gradually withdrawn. QTP or OFC used alone after taper of stage 1 medications (if taper possible). Stage 3 means a combination of a medication used in stage 2 and one or more medications used in stage 1. For example: Lithium + lamotrigine + quetiapine. *From Texas Implementation of Medication Algorithm for Bipolar Disorders. Austin: Texas Department of State Health Services, 2005.*

TABLE 29–7
Anxiety Disorders

- Panic disorder with agoraphobia
- Panic disorder without agoraphobia
- Agoraphobia without panic disorder
- Specific phobia
- Obsessive compulsive disorder
- Posttraumatic stress disorder
- Acute stress disorder
- Generalized anxiety disorder
- Anxiety disorder due to a general medical condition
- Substance-induced anxiety disorder
- Anxiety disorder—NOS
- Social phobia

NOS = not otherwise specified.
Adapted from American Psychiatric Association: Diagnostic and Statistical Manual of Mental Disorders, 4th ed. Washington, DC: American Psychiatric Association, 2000.

ANXIETY DISORDERS

Table 29–7 is a list of anxiety disorders.

Panic Disorder

Panic Attack

A panic attack (Box 29–16) is characterized[2] by a discrete period of intense fear or discomfort in which four (or more) of the following symptoms developed abruptly and reached a peak within 10 minutes: palpitation, pounding heart, or accelerated heart rate; sweating; trembling or shaking; sensation of shortness of breath or smothering; feeling of choking, chest pain or distress; nausea or abdominal discomfort; feeling dizzy, unsteady, lightheaded, or faint; derealization (feelings of unreality) or depersonalization (being detached from oneself); fear of losing control or going crazy; fear of dying; paresthesias (numbness or tingling sensation); and chills or hot flashes. **Panic attacks can occur at night (nocturnal panic). Patients usually (but not always) have a history of panic attacks during the day** (see Box 29–16).

Panic Disorder

Panic disorder is characterized by patients who have recurrent panic attacks, OR if only one panic attack has occurred, the attack has been followed by 1 month (or more) of the following: persistent concern about having additional attacks, worry about the implications of the attack or its consequences, or a significant change in behavior related to the attacks (Box 29–17). The attacks are not due to a substance, medication, or general medication condition.[2,49] Note that the DSM-IV has classifications of panic disorder with or without agoraphobia, as well as agoraphobia. Agoraphobia is fear of being in a place that is unfamiliar or for which there is no easy escape or which they have no familiarity. The fear could be having a panic attack and not being able to escape and being embarrassed. Agoraphobia without panic attack is a separate disorder. Patients with this disorder have agoraphobia, but it is not tied to apprehension about a panic attack but to apprehension about being in a strange place or being out in the open or near crowds (social anxiety) (Boxes 29–17 and 29–18).

BOX 29–16

Criteria for Panic Attack

A. A discrete period of intense fear or discomfort in which four (or more) of the following symptoms developed abruptly and reached a peak within 10 minutes:
   i. Palpitation, pounding heart, or accelerated heart rate
   ii. Sweating
   iii. Trembling or shaking
   iv. Sensation of shortness of breath or smothering
   v. Feeling of choking
   vi. Chest pain or distress
   vii. Nausea or abdominal discomfort
   viii. Feeling dizzy, unsteady, lightheaded, or faint
   ix. Derealization (feelings of unreality) or depersonalization (being detached from oneself)
   x. Fear of losing control or going crazy
   xi. Fear of dying
   xii. Paresthesias (numbness of tingling sensation)
   xiii. Chills or hot flashes

Adapted from American Psychiatric Association: Diagnostic and Statistical Manual of Mental Disorders, 4th ed. Washington, DC: American Psychiatric Association, 2000.

BOX 29–17

Criteria for Diagnosis of Panic Disorder

A. Both (i) and (ii) are present
   i. Recurrent unexpected panic attacks.
   ii. At least one of the attacks has been followed by 1 month (or more) of the following:
      a. Persistent concern about having additional attacks.
      b. Worry about the implications of the attack or its consequences (e.g., losing control, having a heart attack, "going crazy").
      c. A significant change in behavior related to the attacks.
B. The panic attacks are not due to the direct physiologic effects of a substance (e.g., a drug of abuse, medication) or a general medical condition (e.g., hyperthyroidism).
C. The panic attacks are not better accounted for by another mental disorder (e.g., social phobia, specific phobias, obsessive-compulsive disorder, PSTD, or separation anxiety disorder).

PTSD = posttraumatic stress disorder.
Adapted from American Psychiatric Association: Diagnostic and Statistical Manual of Mental Disorders, 4th ed. Washington, DC: American Psychiatric Association, 2000.

Sleep and Panic Disorder A nocturnal panic attack is in the differential diagnosis of parasomnias including night terrors. The majority of patients with panic **disorder** have at least one nocturnal panic attack. About one third of patients with panic disorder have recurrent nocturnal panic attacks. Of those panic disorder patients with nocturnal panic attacks, up to two thirds report insomnia often associated with fear of returning to sleep.[49] The symptom of dyspnea appears to be more common in nocturnal panic attacks. The attacks occur from non–rapid eye movement (NREM) sleep, commonly at the transition from stage N2 to stage N3 sleep. In most patients, sleep architecture is normal (normal REM latency and sleep efficiency). However, some patients may develop sleep phobia—and this can be associated with findings consistent with insomnia (Box 29–19).

Differential Diagnosis of Panic Attack The differential diagnosis of panic attacks includes night terrors, nightmares, posttraumatic stress disorder (PTSD), and REM behavior disorder.

BOX 29–18

Sleep and Panic Disorder

- Most patients with nocturnal panic attacks also have daytime panic attacks.
- Majority of patients with panic disorder have at least one nocturnal panic attack.
- One third or more of patients have recurrent nocturnal panic attacks.
- Usually during NREM sleep at transition to stage N3.
- Two thirds of patients with panic disorder report sleep-onset and sleep-maintenance insomnia (fear of returning to sleep).
- In contrast to a NREM parasomnia, the patient is awake.
- In contrast to nightmares, there is no dream recall.
- If SSRIs are started, they should be started at low doses to avoid exacerbation of nocturnal panic.

NREM = non–rapid eye movement; SSRIs = selective serotonin reuptake inhibitors.

BOX 29–19

Differential Diagnosis of Nocturnal Panic Attacks

1. Medical disorder (hyperthyroidism, pheochromocytoma)
2. Paroxysmal nocturnal dyspnea (CHF)
3. Arousal from OSA
4. Arousal for GERD
5. Nocturnal laryngospasm
6. NREM parasomnia—night terrors
7. PTSD
8. RBD

CHF = congestive heart failure; GERD = gastroesophageal reflux disease; NREM = non–rapid eye movement; OSA = obstructive sleep apnea; PTSD = posttraumatic stress disorder; RBD = rapid eye movement sleep behavior disorder.

Night terrors usually begin in childhood and during the episodes the individual is not well aware of his or her surroundings and does not remember the episodes in the morning. In panic attacks, the patient is awake and aware of his or her surroundings. In nightmares, the patient usually is aware of a frightening dream. In contrast, patients with panic attacks remember the episode, but typically do not report a terrifying dream. In nocturnal laryngospasm, the patient wakes up choking with near-total cessation for airflow from 5 to 43 seconds with stridor.

Treatment of Panic Disorder The treatment of panic attacks includes behavioral psychotherapy or relaxation techniques and pharmacotherapy.[49,50] Although benzodiazepines (e.g., alprazolam, clonazepam) were the classic treatments for panic disorder, the long-term treatment of the panic disorder is an antidepressant. Both SSRIs (e.g., paroxetine, sertraline) and TCAs (e.g., imipramine) must be started at very low doses or the panic attack initially may be exacerbated. For example, paroxetine is started at 10 mg daily or imipramine at 10 to 25 mg daily. The doses are slowly increased to 20 to 40 mg for paroxetine or 100 to 200 mg for imipramine, as tolerated. Because improvements may take 4 to 6 weeks or longer, many physicians add benzodiazepines during the early course of therapy. Alprazolam (Xanax) has a short half-life and many psychiatrists prefer to use clonazepam, which has a long duration of action. This is especially true for patients requiring antianxiety treatment during the day. Unfortunately, clonazepam (long duration of action) can be quite sedating in some patients. Alprazolam is available in an extended action preparation (Xanax XR), which prevents the need for repeated dosing.

Generalized Anxiety Disorder

Generalized anxiety disorder (GAD) is characterized by excessive anxiety and worry (apprehensive expectation), occurring more days than not for a period of at least 6 months, about a number of events or activities (Box 29–20). The individual finds it difficult to control the worry. The anxiety and worry are with three (or more) of the following six symptoms (with at least one symptom present for more days than not for the past 6 mo)[2,51]: (1) restlessness or feeling keyed up or on edge, (2) being easily fatigued, (3) difficulty concentrating or mind going blank, (4) irritability, (5) muscle tension, or (6) sleep disturbance (difficulty falling or staying asleep or restless unsatisfying sleep).

Sleep in GAD

Chronic subjective sleep disturbance is common among people with GAD. Few PSG results are available but usually describe increased sleep latency and reduced sleep efficiency and total sleep time, as well as sleep continuity disturbance and reduced slow wave sleep. Fava and coworkers[52] compared the combination of extended-release zolpidem and escitalopram versus placebo and escitalopram in a group of patients with insomnia and co-morbid GAD. The group with

---

BOX 29–20

Generalized Affective Disorder— Diagnostic Criteria

A. Excessive anxiety and worry (apprehensive expectation), occurring more days than not for at least 6 months, about a number of events or activities (such as work or school performance).

B. The person finds it difficult to control the worry.

C. The anxiety and worry are associated with three (or more) of the following six symptoms (with at least one symptom present for more days than not for the past 6 months):

   i. Restlessness or feeling keyed up or on edge.

   ii. Being easily fatigued.

   iii. Difficulty concentrating or mind going blank.

   iv. Irritability.

   v. Muscle tension.

   vi. Sleep disturbance (difficulty falling or staying asleep or restless unsatisfying sleep).

D. The focus of anxiety and worry is NOT confined to features of an axis I disorder (i.e., another major psychiatric disorder: e.g., worry about having a panic attack, being embarrassed in public with social phobia, being contaminated in obsessive compulsive disorder).

Adapted from American Psychiatric Association: Diagnostic and Statistical Manual of Mental Disorders, 4th ed. Washington, DC: American Psychiatric Association, 2000.

---

the addition of zolpidem had improved insomnia (subjective total sleep time) and next day symptoms (but not anxiety symptoms). Note that zolpidem is a BZRA hypnotic without antianxiety activity. Medications such as clonazepam and lorazepam could be used for sleep in GAD patients for both their hypnotic and their antianxiety effects. Alprazolam is another alternative, although it may have less hypnotic activity because it tends to be less sedating. Note that clonazepam, lorazepam, and alprazolam are not FDA approved for use as hypnotics.

Differential Diagnosis of Sleep Problems with GAD In psychophysiologic insomnia, patients are anxious about their sleep but not to the degree as in GAD, and in psychophysiologic insomnia, the anxiety is focused on sleep. Other anxiety disorders such as phobia, or anxiety about medical conditions, or substance use anxiety should be considered.

Treatment of GAD Treatment includes psychotherapy, benzodiazepines (alprazolam [Xanax], lorazepam [Ativan], diazepam [Valium], clonazepam [Klonopin]), and SSRI/SNRIs. The medications with demonstrated effectiveness include citalopram (Celexa), escitalopram (Lexapro), paroxetine (Paxil), and sertraline (Zoloft).[51,53] Some patients may feel more anxious when starting an SSRI, and benzodiazepines can be used during the first 4 to 6 weeks of treatment. A discontinuation syndrome has been described with alprazolam after only 6 to 8 weeks of treatment. In general, all benzodiazepines should be weaned rather than abruptly discontinued.

Posttraumatic Stress Disorder

PTSD[2] is a disorder of symptoms (Box 29–21) that occur after exposure to an extremely traumatic stressor involving (1) direct personal experience of an event that involves actual or threatened death, serious injury, or other threat to one's physical integrity; (2) witnessing an event that involves death, injury, or a threat to the physical integrity of another person; or (3) learning about unexpected or violent death, serious harm, or threat of death or injury experienced by a family member or other close associate. The person's response to the event must involve intense fear, helplessness, or horror. The characteristic symptoms resulting from the exposure to the extreme trauma include persistent re-experiencing of the traumatic event, persistent avoidance of stimuli associated with the trauma and numbing of general responsiveness, and persistent symptoms of increased arousal.

Associated Features

Recurrent distressing dreams (i.e., nightmares) of the traumatic event are one of the diagnostic features of PTSD. For many patients with PTSD, the associated nightmares represent one of the most frequently occurring and problematic aspects of the disorder. Persistent nightmares may also be one of the most enduring symptoms in PTSD (see "Treatment of Nightmares in PTSD"). High percentages of patients (70–90%) describe subjective sleep disturbance. However, PSG studies of patients with PTSD have yielded variable and inconclusive findings[54–56] in regard to abnormalities in REM sleep, and controlled studies have not found consistent abnormalities with sleep architecture. Increased rates of sleep-related breathing disturbance have been reported in trauma victims.

Symptoms of PTSD can begin immediately after the event or have a delayed onset (up to years later). Patients with PTSD also report a heightened startle response. Given a common exposure to a traumatic event, **PTSD appears to occur more frequently in women than in men.** Patients with PTSD also may have depression and may abuse ethanol or other substances.

BOX 29–21

Posttraumatic Stress Disorder—Diagnostic Criteria

A. The person has been exposed to a traumatic event in which both of the following were present:
   i. The person experienced, witnessed, or was confronted with an event or events that involved actual or threatened death or serious injury, or a threat to the physical integrity of self or others.
   ii. The person's response involved intense fear, helplessness, or horror.
   Note: In children, this may be expressed instead by disorganized or agitated behavior.
B. The traumatic event is persistently re-experienced in one (or more) of the following ways:
   i. Recurrent and intrusive distressing recollections of the event, including images, thoughts, or perceptions.
   Note: In young children, repetitive play may occur in which themes or aspects of the trauma are expressed.
   ii. Recurrent distressing dreams of the event.
   Note: In children, there may be frightening dreams without recognizable content.
   iii. Acting or feeling as if the traumatic event were recurring (includes a sense of reliving the experience, illusions, hallucinations, and dissociative flashback episodes, including those that occur on awakening or when intoxicated).
   Note: In young children, trauma-specific reenactment may occur.
   iv. Intense psychological distress at exposure to internal or external cues that symbolize or resemble an aspect of the traumatic event.

   v. Physiologic reactivity on exposure to internal or external cues that symbolize or resemble an aspect of the traumatic event.
C. Persistent avoidance of stimuli associated with the trauma and numbing of general responsiveness (not present before the trauma), as indicated by three (or more) of the following:
   i. Efforts to avoid thoughts, feelings, or conversation associated with the trauma.
   ii. Efforts to avoid activities, places, or people that arouse recollection of the trauma.
   iii. Inability to recall important aspects of the trauma.
   iv. Markedly diminished interest or participation in significant activities.
   v. Feeling of detachment or estrangement from others.
   vi. Restrict range of affect (e.g., inability to have loving feelings).
   vii. Sense of foreshortened future (e.g., does not expect to have a career, marriage, children, or a normal lifespan).
D. Persistent symptoms of increased arousal (not present before the trauma) as indicated by two or more of the following:
   i. Difficulty falling or staying asleep.
   ii. Irritability or outbursts of anger.
   iii. Difficulty concentrating.
   iv. Hypervigilance.
   v. Excessive startle response.
E. Duration of the disturbance (symptoms in criteria B, C, and D) is more than 1 month.

Adapted from American Psychiatric Association: Diagnostic and Statistical Manual of Mental Disorders, 4th ed. Washington, DC: American Psychiatric Association, 2000.

Differential Diagnosis of Nocturnal Event Due to PTSD

The differential of awakening with anxiety includes sleep panic disorder, REM sleep behavior disorder, and night terrors. Unlike patients with panic attacks during sleep, patients with PTSD can recount a dream of a specific traumatic event. In contrast to night terrors, patients become alert quickly after awakening. Sleep studies in patients with PTSD have produced conflicting results. The duration of REM latency and the amount of REM sleep have varied among studies. This may be a reflection of the fact that some patients with PTSD are also suffering from depression. Several studies have found an increase in REM density in patients with PTSD (as in depression), an increase in body movements during sleep, and the presence of periodic limb movements in sleep (PLMS).[54,56] Some patients may have REM sleep without atonia, but some are already on SSRIs that can cause this finding.

Treatment of PTSD—General Considerations

The treatment of PTSD includes counseling and medication. Although many patients with PTSD have anxiety, benzodiazepines have not been effective, and withdrawal of these medications may produce a flair of symptoms.[57] **Sertraline and paroxetine are the only antidepressants FDA approved for treatment of PTSD.** However, other SSRIs may also be effective. Sertraline was shown to be effective in a double-blind, placebo-controlled study.[58] Open-label trials of paroxetine[59] and escitalopram[60] in PTSD have also been published.

Treatment of Nightmares in PTSD

As noted previously, recurrent disturbing nightmares may be an important problem in PTSD and do not always respond to general PTSD treatments. Cognitive behavioral treatments have been used to treat nightmares with some success. One behavior technique called **imagery rehearsal therapy** has proved successful in several studies.[61] Patients are asked to rewrite their previous dreams with a positive outcome. In the past, use of medications for nightmares had limited success. Recently, several small studies report success with the alpha 1 blocker **prazosin**.[62,63] Note that when prazosin is started, the drug should be initiated with a dose of 1 mg at bedtime to avoid severe first-dose hypotension (often orthostatic hypotension). The drug can then be titrated upward slowly over several nights. A parallel placebo-controlled study in trauma nightmares in PTSD due to combat showed improvements in sleep and reduction in nightmares with prazosin. A relatively high dose (mean 13 mg) was reached over a protracted period of upward titration.[62] Another study using a cross-over design and a dose of 2 to 6 mg at bedtime also found benefit in civilian trauma PTSD.[63] One study also reported success in reducing disturbing nightmares using topiramate in PTSD patients.[64] However, neither prazosin nor topiramate is FDA approved for treatment of nightmares in PTSD.

CLINICAL REVIEW QUESTIONS

1. Which of the following is true about MDEs?
   A. Insomnia complaints in 80% of patients.
   B. Hypersomnia complaints in about 50% of patients.
   C. Hypersomnia complaints in 60% of patients.
   D. Insomnia complaints in 40% of patients.

2. Which of the following is a common PSG finding during MDE?
   A. Short sleep latency.
   B. Short REM latency.
   C. Increased total sleep time.
   D. Increased REM sleep in the last part of the night.
   E. Decreased REM density.

3. The most common misdiagnosis in bipolar depression is:
   A. Anxiety disorder.
   B. Substance abuse.
   C. Personality disorder.
   D. Unipolar depression.

4. Treatment of bipolar depression in BP-I patients with antidepressants may lead to:
   A. Anxiety.
   B. Greater mood instability.
   C. Mania induction.
   D. B and C.
   E. A, B, and C.

5. The family of a 50-year-old man reports a recent change in his behavior. He has been sleeping 5 hours per night but seems well rested. The patient "never stops talking" and switches from one topic to another. He starts many new projects that he never completes. The patient has continued to work and manage his home responsibilities. He had an episode of depression about a year ago. What is the best description of the behavior?
   A. BP-I.
   B. BP-II
   C. MDD.
   D. Cyclothymic in up phase.

6. Which of the following would be more typical for bipolar depression than for unipolar depression?
   A. Loss of appetite.
   B. Hypersomnia.
   C. Normal activity.
   D. No family history of bipolar disorder.

7. During a PSG, a patient suddenly arouses from stage N2 and sits up in bed and appears awake. He does not return to sleep and develops tachycardia. He signals for the technologist, who comes to evaluate him. The patient is trembling and sweaty but completely alert and responsive. He

reports feeling that he is about to die. What is the most likely diagnosis?

A. Confusional arousal.

B. Nocturnal frontal lobe epilepsy.

C. Panic attack.

D. Sleep terror.

Answers

1. A. MDE is characterized by complaints of insomnia in a majority of patients.

2. B. PSG in MDE shows short REM latency, long sleep latency, decreased total sleep time, more REM sleep in the first part of the night.

3. D. Unipolar depression is often diagnosed because a history for prior mania or hypomania was not sought by the treating clinician.

4. E. Treatment with antidepressant (especially without a mood stabilizer) can cause mania, mood instability, and anxiety.

5. B. The patient is able to work and is not disabled, but there has been a significant acute change in his behavior. There is a history of previous depression. The best diagnosis based on current knowledge is BP-II based on the current hypomanic episode.

6. B. Hypersomnia can occur with unipolar MDD but is more typical of bipolar depression.

7. C. Panic attack. Panic attacks occur during established wake (including after arousal from sleep) with manifestations of pounding heart, diaphoresis and often chest pain or choking.

REFERENCES

1. Kessler RC, Demler O, Frank RG, et al: Prevalence and treatment of mental disorders, 1990 to 2003. N Engl J Med 2005; 352:2515–2523.
2. American Psychiatric Association: Diagnostic and Statistical Manual of Mental Disorders, 4th ed. Washington, DC: American Psychiatric Association, 2000.
3. Peterson MJ, Benca RM: Sleep in mood disorders. Psychiatr Clin North Am 2006;29:1009–1032.
4. Benca RM, Obermeyer WH, Thisted RA, et al: Sleep and psychiatric disorders: a meta-analysis. Arch Gen Psychiatry 1992; 49:651–668.
5. Kupfer DJ: Sleep research in depressive illness: clinical implications—a tasting menu. Biol Psychiatry 1995;38: 391–403.
6. Beck AT, Steer RA, Brown GK: Manual for the Beck Depression Inventory, 2nd ed (BDI-II). San Antonio, TX: The Psychological Association, 1996.
7. Hamilton M: A rating scale for depression. J Neurol Neurosurg Psychiatry 1960;23:56–62.
8. Montgomery SA, Åsberg M: A new depression scale designed to be sensitive to change. Br J Psychiatry 1979;134:382–389.
9. Kroenke K, Spitzer RL, Williams JBW: The PHQ-9. Validity of a brief depression severity measure. J Gen Intern Med 2001; 16:606–613.
10. Rush AJ, Erman MK, Giles DE, et al: Polysomnographic findings in recently drug-free and clinically remitted depressed patients. Arch Gen Psychiatry 1986;43:878–884.
11. Hudson JI, Lipinski JF, Keck PE Jr, et al: Polysomnographic characteristics of young manic patients. Comparison with unipolar depressed patients and normal control subjects. Arch Gen Psychiatry 1992;49:378–383.
12. Reynolds CF 3rd, Frank E, Houck PR, et al: Which elderly patients with remitted depression remain well with continued interpersonal psychotherapy after discontinuation of antidepressant medication? Am J Psychiatry 1997;154:958–962.
13. Nierenberg AA, Keefe BR, Leslie VC, et al: Residual symptoms in depressed patients who respond acutely to fluoxetine. J Clin Psychiatry 1999;60:221–225.
14. Dombrovski AY, Mulsant BH, Houck PR, et al: Residual symptoms and recurrence during maintenance treatment of late life depression. J Affect Disord 2007;103:77–82.
15. Yang H, Sinicropi-Yao L, Chuzi S, et al: Residual sleep disturbance and risk of relapse during the continuation/maintenance phase treatment of major depressive disorder with the selective serotonin reuptake inhibitor fluoxetine. Ann Gen Psychiatry 2010;9:10.
16. Nofzinger EA, Thase ME, Reynolds CF 3rd, et al: Hypersomnia in bipolar depression: a comparison with narcolepsy using the multiple sleep latency test. Am J Psychiatry 1991;148: 1177–1181.
17. Hudson JI, Lipinski JF, Frankenburg FR, et al: Electroencephalographic sleep in mania. Arch Gen Psychiatry 1988;45: 267–273.
18. Bauer M, Grof P, Rasgon N, et al: Temporal relation between sleep and mood in patients with bipolar disorder. Bipolar Disord 2006;8:160–167.
19. Leibenluft E, Albert PS, Rosenthal NE, et al: Relationship between sleep and mood in patients with rapid-cycling bipolar disorder. Psychiatry Res 1996;63:161–168.
20. Wehr TA: Sleep loss: a preventable cause of mania and other excited states. J Clin Psychiatry 1989;50(Suppl):8–16.
21. Wehr TA: Sleep loss as a possible mediator of diverse causes of mania. Br J Psychiatry 1991;159:576–578.
22. Taylor DJ, Lichstein KL, Durrence HH, et al: Epidemiology of insomnia, depression, and anxiety. Sleep 2005;28:1457–1464.
23. Pigeon WR, Hegel M, Unützer J, et al: Is insomnia a perpetuating factor for late-life depression in the IMPACT cohort? Sleep 2008;31:481–488.
24. Vogel GW, Vogel F, McAbee RS, Thurmond AJ: Improvement of depression by REM sleep deprivation. New findings and a theory. Arch Gen Psychiatry 1980;37:247–253.
25. Giedke H, Schwärzler F: Therapeutic use of sleep deprivation in depression. Sleep Med Rev 2002;6:361–377.
26. Kent JM: SNaRIs, NaSSAs, and NaRIs: new agents for the treatment of depression. Lancet 2000;355:911–918.
27. Mayers AG, Baldwin DS: Antidepressants and their effect on sleep. Hum Psychopharmacol 2005;20:533–559.
28. Winokur A, Gary KA, Rodner S, et al: Depression, sleep physiology, and antidepressant drugs. Depress Anxiety 2001; 14:19–28.
29. Ali MK, Lam RW: Comparative efficacy of escitalopram in the treatment of major depressive disorder. Neuropsychiatr Dis Treat 2011;7:39–49.
30. Garnock-Jones KP, McCormack PL: Escitalopram: a review of its use in the management of major depressive disorder in adults. CNS Drugs 2010;24:769–796.
31. Gaynes BN, Rush AJ, Trivedi MH, et al: The STAR*D study: treating depression in the real world. Cleve Clin J Med 2008; 75:57–66.

32. Gursky JT, Krahn LE: The effects of antidepressants on sleep: a review. Harvard Rev Psychiatry 2000;8:298–306.

33. Dubovsky SL, Dubovsky AN: Psychopharmacology for neurologists. Semin Neurol 2009;29:200–219.

34. Chen J, Gao K, Kemp DE: Second-generation antipsychotics in major depressive disorder: update and clinical perspective. Curr Opin Psychiatry 2011;24:10–17.

35. Anderson IM, Sarsfield A, Haddad PM: Efficacy, safety and tolerability of quetiapine augmentation in treatment resistant depression: an open-label, pilot study. J Affect Disord 2009; 117:116–119.

36. Bortnick B, El-Khalili N, Banov M, et al: Efficacy and tolerability of extended release quetiapine fumarate (quetiapine XR) monotherapy in major depressive disorder: a placebo-controlled, randomized study. J Affect Disord 2011;128:83–94.

37. Abolfazli R, Hosseini M, Ghanizadeh A, et al: Double-blind randomized parallel-group clinical trial of efficacy of the combination fluoxetine plus modafinil versus fluoxetine plus placebo in the treatment of major depression. Depress Anxiety 2011;28:297–302.

38. Gillin JC, Rapaport M, Erman MK, et al: A comparison of nefazodone and fluoxetine on mood and on objective, subjective, and clinician-rated measures of sleep in depressed patients. J Clin Psychiatry 1997;58:186–192.

39. Nierenberg AA, Adler LA, Peselow E, et al: Trazodone for antidepressant-associated insomnia. Am J Psychiatry 1994; 151:1069.

40. Fava M, McCall V, Krystal A, et al: Eszopiclone co-administered with fluoxetine in patients with insomnia coexisting with major depressive disorder. Biol Psychiatry 2006;59:1052–1060.

41. Fava M, Asnis GM, Shrivastava RK, et al: Improved insomnia symptoms and sleep-related next-day functioning in patients with comorbid major depressive disorder and insomnia following concomitant zolpidem extended-release 12.5 mg and escitalopram treatment: a randomized controlled trial. J Clin Psychiatry Epub ahead of print 2010;December 28.

42. Mitchell PB, Goodwin GM, Johnson GF, Hirschfeld RMA: Diagnostic guidelines for bipolar depression: a probabilistic approach. Bipolar Disord 2008;10:144–152.

43. McGuffin P, Rijsdijk F, Andrew M, et al: The heritability of bipolar affective disorder and the genetic relationship to unipolar depression. Arch Gen Psychiatry 2003;60:497–502.

44. Suppes T, Dennehy EB, Hirschfeld RM, et al, Texas Consensus Conference Panel on Medication Treatment of Bipolar Disorder: The Texas implementation of medication algorithms: update to the algorithms for treatment of bipolar I disorder. J Clin Psychiatry 2005;66:870–886.

45. Fountoulakis KN: An update of evidence-based treatment of bipolar depression: where do we stand? Curr Opin Psychiatry 2010;23:19–24.

46. Hilty DM, Leamon MH, Lim RF, et al: Diagnosis and treatment of bipolar disorder in the primary care setting: a concise review. Prim Psychiatry 2006;13:77–85.

47. Nivoli AM, Colom F, Murru A, et al: New treatment guidelines for acute bipolar depression: a systematic review. J Affect Disord 2011;129:14–26; Epub 2010;June 8.

48. Sachs GS, Nierenberg AA, Calabrese JR, et al: Effectiveness of adjunctive antidepressant treatment for bipolar depression. N Engl J Med 2007;356:1711–1722.

49. Mellman TA, Ude TW: Patients with frequent sleep panic: clinical findings and response to medication treatment. J Clin Psychiatry 1990;51:513–516.

50. Moroze G, Rosenbaum JF: Efficacy, safety, and gradual discontinuation of clonazepam in panic disorder: a placebo-controlled, multicenter study using optimized doses. J Clin Psychiatry 1999;60:604–612.

51. Fricchione G: Generalized anxiety disorders. N Engl J Med 2004;351:675–682.

52. Fava M, Asnis GM, Shrivastava R, et al: Zolpidem extended-release improves sleep and next-day symptoms in comorbid insomnia and generalized anxiety disorder. J Clin Psychopharmacol 2009;29:222–230.

53. Stein DJ: Algorithms for primary care: an evidence-based approach to the pharmacotherapy of depression and anxiety disorders. Prim Psychiatry 2004;11:55–78.

54. Ross RJ, Ball WA, Dinges DR, et al: Rapid eye movement sleep disturbance in posttraumatic stress disorder. Biol Psychiatry 1994;35:195–202.

55. Mellman TA, Nolan B, Hedding J, et al: A polysomnographic comparison of veterans with combat-related PTSD, depressed men, and non-ill controls. Sleep 1997;20:46–51.

56. Brown TM, Boudewyns PA: Periodic limb movements of sleep in combat veterans with posttraumatic stress disorder. J Trauma Stress 1996;9:129–136.

57. Davis LL, English BA, Ambrose SM, et al: Pharmacotherapy for post-traumatic stress disorder: a comprehensive review. Expert Opin Pharmacother 2001;2:1583–1595.

58. Davidson JR, Rothbaum BO, van der Kolk BA, et al: Multicenter, double-blind comparison of sertraline and placebo in the treatment of posttraumatic stress disorder. Arch Gen Psychiatry 2001;58:485–492.

59. Kim Y, Asukai N, Konishi T, et al: Clinical evaluation of paroxetine in post-traumatic stress disorder (PTSD): 52-week, non-comparative open-label study for clinical use experience. Psychiatry Clin Neurosci 2008;62:646–652.

60. Robert S, Hamner MB, Ulmer HG, et al: Open-label trial of escitalopram in the treatment of posttraumatic stress disorder. J Clin Psychiatry 2006;67:1522–1526.

61. Krakow B, Hollifield M, Johnston L, et al: Imagery rehearsal therapy for chronic nightmares in sexual assault survivors with post traumatic stress disorder. JAMA 2001;286:537–545.

62. Raskind MA, Peskind ER, Hoff DJ, et al: A parallel group placebo-controlled study of prazosin for trauma nightmares and sleep disturbance in combat veterans with post-traumatic stress disorder. Biol Psychiatry 2007;61:928–934.

63. Taylor FB, Martin P, Thompson C, et al: Prazosin effects on objective sleep measures and clinical symptoms in civilian trauma PTSD: a placebo-controlled study. Biol Psychiatry 2008;63:629–632.

64. Berlant JL: Prospective open-label study of add-on and monotherapy topiramate in civilians with chronic nonhallucinatory posttraumatic stress disorder. BMC Psychiatry 2004;4:24.

Patient Health Questionnaire (PHQ-9)

Over the last 2 weeks, how often have you been bothered by any of the following problems? Put an X in the box that indicates your answer.	NOT AT ALL	SEVERAL DAYS	MORE THAN HALF THE DAYS	NEARLY EVERY DAY
1. Little interest or pleasure in doing things.	0	1	2	3
2. Feeling down, depressed, or hopeless.	0	1	2	3
3. Trouble falling or staying asleep or sleeping too much.	0	1	2	3
4. Feeling tired or having little energy.	0	1	2	3
5. Poor appetite or overeating.	0	1	2	3
6. Feeling bad about yourself or that you are a failure or have let yourself or your family down.	0	1	2	3
7. Trouble concentrating on things, such as reading the newspaper or watching television.	0	1	2	3
8. Moving or speaking so slowly that other people could have noticed. Or the opposite—being so fidgety or restless that you have been moving around a lot more than usual.	0	1	2	3
9. Thoughts that you would be better off dead or of hurting yourself in some way.	0	1	2	3
10. If you checked off any problems, how difficult have these problems made it for you to do your work, take care of things at home, or get along with other people?	Not at all	Somewhat difficult	Very difficult	Extremely difficult

1–4 minimal depression, 5–9 mild depression, 10–14 moderate depression, 15–19 moderately severe depression, 20–27 severe depression.

PHQ-9 is adapted from PrimeMD today, developed by Dr. RL Spitzer, JBW Williams, K Kroenke, and colleagues, with an education grant from Pfizer, Inc. Use of the PHQ-9 may only be made in accordance with the terms of use available at http://www.pfizer.com
Copyright © 1999 Pfizer, Inc.

Chapter 30

Sleep and Nonrespiratory Physiology—Impact on Selected Medical Disorders

Chapter Points

- The secretion of GH and PRL by the pituitary is controlled mainly by the timing of sleep. GH secretion in men is tightly tied to the first cycle of stage N3 sleep. PRL secretion is increased during sleep (inhibited by wakefulness).
- The secretion of ACTH, cortisol, and TSH are mainly controlled by circadian timing (time of day) influences with weaker sleep-related effects. The secretion of ACTH and cortisol peaks soon after awakening. TSH secretion is under circadian control (peaks during the night). Sleep inhibits TSH secretion.
- Ghrelin is a hormone secreted by the stomach that stimulates the appetite and is increased by sleep loss. Leptin is a hormone secreted by adipose tissue that increases satiety. Leptin is decreased by sleep loss. Studies suggest that individuals with decreased total sleep time have an increased risk of developing obesity.
- The normal defense mechanisms to minimize the detrimental effects of GER are not present during sleep. Saliva secretion virtually stops and reflex swallowing to clear refluxed material is not present. This results in a prolonged ACT. The absence of symptoms does not eliminate the presence of GER. Esophageal pH monitoring often shows significant GER episodes in asymptomatic patients.
- Nocturnal GER is common in patients with OSA and is improved with CPAP treatment.
- Alpha-delta sleep (alpha anomaly) is not specific to fibromyalgia. Alpha anomaly may be seen in psychiatric disorders, in many chronic pain syndromes, and in normal individuals.
- Sleep in patients with the FS is abnormal and studies have shown decreased total sleep time, increased arousals, and decreased stage N3 and REM sleep. At least in some patients, a poor night of sleep is associated with worse daytime symptoms.

This chapter reviews aspects of endocrine, gastrointestinal, rheumatologic, and renal physiology and related medical disorders relevant to sleep medicine. It is not a comprehensive review of any area.

ENDOCRINE PHYSIOLOGY AND SLEEP

The timing of the secretion of important hormones with respect to sleep and circadian control is briefly reviewed. The secretion of some hormones is tied to sleep, whereas others are under circadian control. A common strategy to determine whether sleep or circadian influence predominates is to move the timing of sleep and determine what happens to the pattern of hormone secretion.

GROWTH HORMONE

Growth hormone (GH) is secreted by somatotroph cells of the anterior pituitary under hypothalamic control. GH secretion is increased by **GHRH** (growth hormone–releasing hormone) and decreased by **somatostatin,** both secreted by the hypothalamus. GH secretion is also increased by acylated ghrelin (ghrelin is secreted by the stomach). The most reliable burst of GH secretion is associated with the first slow wave sleep **(stage N3)** cycle (any time of the day).[1,2] This is associated with increased GHRH and decreased somatostatin.

In healthy adults, the 24-hour profile of plasma GH consists of stable low levels abruptly interrupted by bursts of secretion (Box 30–1 and Fig. 30–1). The most reproducible GH pulse occurs shortly after sleep onset. In men, the sleep-onset GH pulse is the largest and often the only secretory pulse over the 24-hour day. In women, daytime GH pulses are more frequent and the sleep-onset pulse does not account for the majority of the 24-hour secretory output (Fig. 30–2). The amount of GH released is proportional to slow wave activity. Figure 30–1 shows a large burst of GH secretion after sleep onset. During the next nighttime period, the subject is awake and there is only a slight increase in GH secretion. The subject is allowed to sleep at 11 AM,

FIGURE 30–1 Mean 24-hour profile of plasma growth hormone (GH) during a 53-hour period including 8 hours of nocturnal sleep *(dark blue bar)*, 28 hours of continuous wakefulness (nocturnal hours: *white bar)*, and 8 hours of daytime sleep *(light blue bar)*. Subjects were young healthy men. The *shaded area* corresponds to normal 24-hour conditions. The *vertical bar* at each time point represents the standard error of the mean (SEM). The temporal organization of GH secretion is mainly regulated by the **homeostatic control of sleep** such that shifted sleep is associated with a shift in the secretion of GH. *Adapted from Van Cauter E, Spiegel K: Circadian and sleep control of hormones. In Turek FW, Zee PC (eds): Regulation of Sleep and Circadian Rhythms. New York: Marcel Dekker, 1999, p. 399, with permission.*

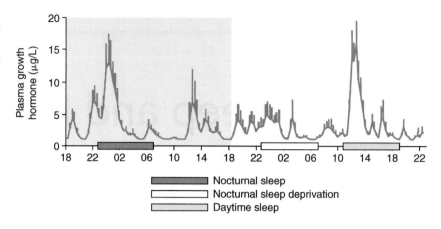

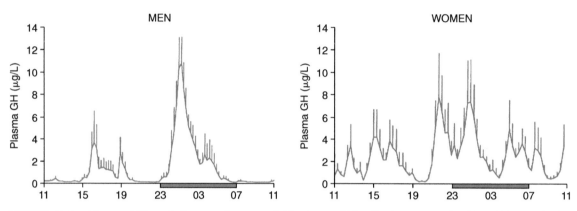

FIGURE 30–2 Growth hormone (GH) secretion in a group of young men **(left)** and women **(right).** The plots are mean values. The *dark blue bar* is the sleep period. Men have most of their GH secretion during sleep, but in women, bursts during the day are more common. *From Van Cauter E, Plat L, Copinschi G: Interrelations between sleep and the somatotropic axis. Sleep 1998;21:553–566.*

BOX 30–1

Growth Hormone and Sleep
• Men—sleep-onset GH pulse is generally the largest, and often the only, secretory pulse observed over the 24-hour span. • Women—daytime GH pulses are more frequent, and the sleep-associated pulse, although still present, in the vast majority of individual profiles does not account for the majority of the 24-hour secretory output. • GH secretion is tied to **sleep onset** (start of stage N3 sleep) rather than time of day. • Amount of GH secretion correlates with duration of stage N3 episodes.
GH = growth hormone.

and sleep onset is followed by a large burst in GH secretion.

Etiology of Sleep-Related GH Burst

The sleep-related burst of GH secretion is due to increased GHRH activity during stage N3 and decreased somatostatin. There is a circadian (time of day) peak in GH at the time of

normal sleep (slight increase in GH secretion occurs at night even when individuals are awake) likely due to a decrease in somatostatin. Of interest, ghrelin is also highest at night (peaks during first part of the night) and could contribute to the weak circadian component to control of GH release. An acyl chain (octanoate residue) is added to ghrelin by the enzyme ghrelin-O-acyltransferase before it can bind GH secretagogue receptors. It is not known whether acetylated ghrelin increases at night.

GHRH and GH—Effects on Sleep

Injections of GHRH stimulate stage N3 and slow wave activity (electroencephalogram [EEG] spectral power in the delta range). In contrast, injections of GH appear to enhance rapid eye movement (REM) sleep, particularly in rodents.[3] Somatostatin injections impair sleep quality in older, but not in young, adult humans.[4]

Changes in GH Secretion with Age

The nocturnal increase in GH decreases with age in parallel with the amount of stage N3 (formerly termed stages 3 + 4; Fig. 30–3).[5]

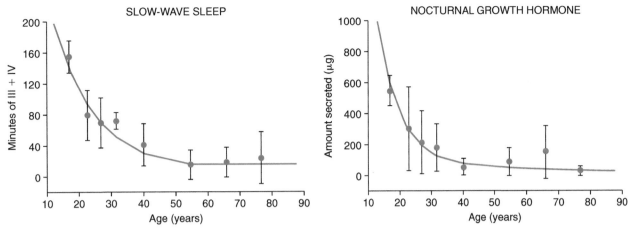

FIGURE 30–3 Patterns of the amount of slow wave sleep (stage N3, formerly stages III + IV) and nocturnal GH secretion throughout aging, obtained in 102 healthy nonobese men, ages 18 to 83 years, who were grouped according to age bracket (mean ± SEM for each age bracket). GH decreases with age in parallel to the amount of slow wave sleep. *Data from Van Cauter E, Plat L, Copinschi G: Interrelations between sleep and the somatotropic axis. Sleep 1998;21:553–566.*

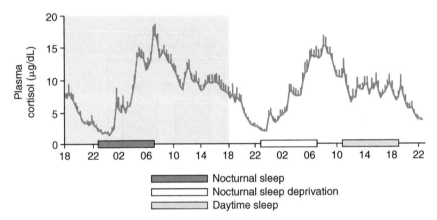

FIGURE 30–4 Mean 24-hour profile of plasma cortisol during a 53-hour period including 8 hours of nocturnal sleep *(dark blue bar)*, 28 hours of continuous wakefulness (nocturnal hours: *white bar*), and 8 hours of daytime sleep *(light blue bar)*. Subjects were young healthy men. The *shaded area* corresponds to normal 24-hour conditions. The *vertical bar* at each time point represents the SEM. The plasma cortisol remains largely synchronized to clock time even when sleep is shifted, indicating a predominant role of circadian rhythmicity in the control of hypothalamus-pituitary-adrenal axis activity. *Adapted from Van Cauter E, Spiegel K: Circadian and sleep control of hormones. In Turek FW, Zee PC (eds): Regulation of Sleep and Circadian Rhythms. New York: Marcel Dekker, 1999, p. 399, with permission.*

SLEEP AND THE CORTICOTROPIC AXIS

The adrenals secrete cortisol under the control of pituitary adrenocorticotropic hormone (ACTH). There is strong **circadian control of ACTH** secretion (and cortisol). The plasma levels of cortisol and ACTH peak in the early morning and decline during the day (Box 30–2 and Fig. 30–4). The nadir of cortisol and ACTH levels is during the first part of sleep. The levels start to climb a few hours before waking. During shifted sleep, the cortisol rhythm remains tied to clock time. There is a weak sleep-related component. The presence of **sleep causes inhibition** and maintains low levels early in the sleep period (Fig. 30–5). Awakening at the end of sleep is associated with a burst of cortisol secretion.

Sleep Deprivation and Sleep Loss

Sleep deprivation induces a 15% decrease in **amplitude** of the 24-hour cortisol rhythm (i.e., peak to trough of excursion is smaller). In the absence of sleep, the nadir in the early part of the sleep period is not as low and the peak following in the morning is not as high (absence of stimulating effects of awakening). However, sleep fragmentation causes a burst of cortisol and higher morning levels. The night of sleep

BOX 30–2

Adrenocorticotropic Hormone (ACTH) and Cortisol

- Under circadian control (peak around 7 AM).
- Nadir shortly after the typical time of sleep onset (does not depend on sleep).
- Peak levels in the early morning then decline over the day.
- The overall shape of the corticotropic profile is not markedly affected by the absence of sleep or by sleep at an unusual time of day.
- During sleep deprivation, the nocturnal cortisol is higher (amplitude of oscillation reduced—i.e., early night not as low, early AM not as high).

deprivation induces less recovery (less impact on morning stimulation by ACTH). Older adults tend to have higher evening cortisol levels (Fig. 30–6; see also Box 30–2).

SLEEP AND THE THYROID AXIS

TSH (secreted by the pituitary) stimulates the thyroid gland to secrete the hormones thyroxine (T_4) and triiodothyronine

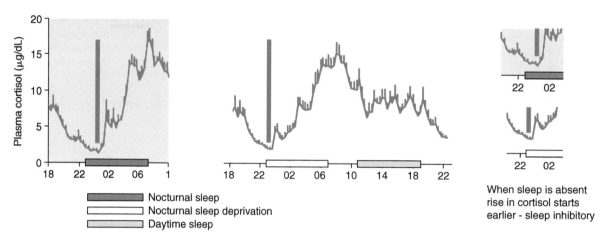

Nocturnal sleep
Nocturnal sleep deprivation
Daytime sleep

When sleep is absent rise in cortisol starts earlier - sleep inhibitory

FIGURE 30-5 When sleep is present, it is inhibitory on cortisol secretion. When sleep is absent, the start of the rise in cortisol is earlier. The *vertical bar* shows the time of onset in the upswing in cortisol secretion. An enlargement of the areas is shown to the **right.** *Adapted from Van Cauter E, Spiegel K: Circadian and sleep control of hormones. In Turek FW, Zee PC (eds): Regulation of Sleep and Circadian Rhythms. New York: Marcel Dekker, 1999, p. 399.*

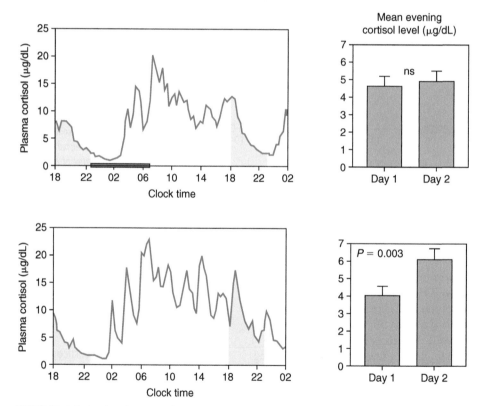

FIGURE 30-6 During sleep deprivation, the nocturnal cortisol is greater. Mean profiles of plasma cortisol for two groups of healthy young subjects during a 32-hour period with normal sleep **(upper panel)** and sleep deprivation **(lower panel).** The *dark bar* represents the sleep period. The *shaded areas* represent cortisol secretion between 18:00 and 23:00 on Day 1 and Day 2 (before and after the night shown). The mean of these areas determines the mean evening cortisol level **(bar graphs).** In the **top panel,** the mean of the two *shaded areas* is virtually identical **(bar graph to the right of the upper panel).** In the **bottom panel,** sleep deprivation results in an increase in the mean evening cortisol level **(bar graph to the right of the bottom panel).** Thus, sleep deprivation results in a higher nocturnal cortisol and higher late evening cortisol levels. *From Van Cauter E: Endocrine physiology. In Kryger MH, Roth T, Dement WC (eds): Principles and Practice of Sleep Medicine. Philadelphia: Elsevier, 2005, p. 270.*

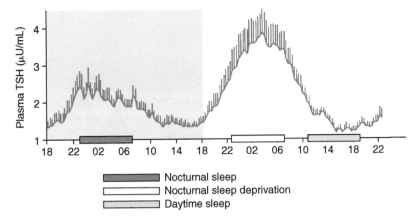

FIGURE 30–7 Mean 24-hour profiles of levels of plasma thyroid-stimulating hormone (TSH) during a 53-hour period including 8 hours of nocturnal sleep *(dark blue bar)*, 28 hours of continuous wake *(white bar)*, and 8 hours of daytime sleep *(light blue bar)*. Subjects were young healthy men. The *shaded area* corresponds to normal 24-hour conditions. The *vertical bar* at each time point represents the SEM. The nocturnal elevation of plasma TSH remains synchronized to clock time even when sleep is shifted. The effect of nocturnal sleep is an inhibition of TSH secretion that is relieved by sleep deprivation, resulting in an augmentation of the nocturnal TSH rise. The inhibitory effects of sleep on TSH secretion depend on the time of day. Daytime sleep does not significantly alter (inhibit) TSH levels, which are already low at that time of day because of circadian influences. *Adapted from Van Cauter E, Spiegel K: Circadian and sleep control of hormones. In Turek FW, Zee PC (eds): Regulation of Sleep and Circadian Rhythms. New York: Marcel Dekker, 1999, p. 399, with permission.*

(T_3). TSH production is controlled by **thyrotropin-releasing hormone** (TRH), which is manufactured in the hypothalamus and transported to the anterior pituitary gland where it stimulates TSH production and release. **Somatostatin** is also produced by the hypothalamus and has an opposite effect on the pituitary production of TSH, decreasing or inhibiting its release.

The level of thyroid hormones (T_3 and T_4) in the blood has an effect on the pituitary release of TSH. When the levels of T_3 and T_4 are low, the production of TSH is increased, and conversely, when levels of T_3 and T_4 are high, TSH production is decreased. This effect creates a regulatory negative feedback loop.

TSH Secretion

Daytime levels of plasma TSH are low and relatively stable. There is a rapid elevation of TSH starting in the early evening and culminating in a **nocturnal maximum** occurring around the end of the first third of the sleep period (Box 30–3 and Fig. 30–7). The latter part of the sleep period is associated with a progressive decline in TSH. Because the start of the nocturnal rise in TSH occurs **well before sleep onset,** it likely reflects a **circadian effect. Sleep exerts an inhibitory influence on TSH secretion,**[1,2] and sleep deprivation relieves this inhibition, resulting in higher TSH during the night. The inhibition of TSH by sleep is greatest during stage N3 sleep and the inhibition is greater on recovery sleep from prior sleep deprivation (more stage N3, higher delta power).

The suppression of TSH by sleep depends on the time of day. When sleep occurs during daytime hours, TSH secretion is not suppressed significantly below normal daytime levels. Thus, the inhibitory effect of sleep on TSH secretion

BOX 30–3

Thyroid-Stimulating Hormone (TSH) and the Thyroid Axis

- Circadian control (higher at night).
- Peak in midsleep period (middle of the night).
- Stable level during the day.
- Sleep inhibitory at night (higher if no sleep).

appears to be operative when the nighttime elevation has taken place, indicating an interaction of the effects of circadian time and the effects of sleep. Awakenings interrupting nocturnal sleep appear to relieve the inhibition of TSH and are consistently associated with a short-term TSH elevation.

Thyroid Hormone Levels

Circadian and sleep-related variations in thyroid hormones have been difficult to demonstrate. Thyroid hormones are bound to serum proteins, and thus, peripheral concentrations are affected by diurnal variations in hemodilution caused by postural changes. However, under conditions of sleep deprivation, the increased amplitude of the TSH rhythm may result in a detectable increase in plasma T_3 levels, paralleling the nocturnal TSH rise.

SLEEP AND PROLACTIN SECRETION

Pituitary prolactin (PRL) secretion is regulated by neuroendocrine neurons in the hypothalamus, the most important ones being the neurosecretory tuberoinfundibulum (TIDA)

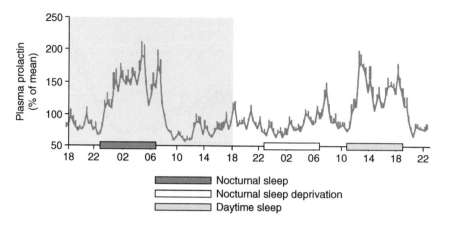

FIGURE 30-8 Mean 24-hour profile of plasma prolactin (PRL) during a 53-hour period including 8 hours of nocturnal sleep (*dark blue bar*), 28 hours of continuous wakefulness (nocturnal hours: *white bar*), and 8 hours of daytime sleep (*light blue bar*). Subjects were young healthy men. The *shaded area* corresponds to normal 24-hour conditions. The *vertical bar* at each time point represents the SEM. The temporal pattern of PRL secretion is mainly regulated by sleep so that shifted sleep is associated with a shift in the secretion of PRL. *Adapted from Van Cauter E, Spiegel K: Circadian and sleep control of hormones. In Van Cauter E, Spiegel K (eds): Circadian and Sleep Control of Hormones. In Turek FW, Zee PC (eds): Regulation of Sleep and Circadian Rhythms. New York: Marcel Dekker, 1999, p. 399.*

BOX 30-4

Sleep and Prolactin

- PRL—timing of secretion is primarily sleep related (sleep stimulatory).
- PRL secretion has a possible role in circadian control of REM sleep and in the amount of stage N3 sleep.

PRL = prolactin; REM = rapid eye movement.

TABLE 30-1

Summary of Major Control of Major Hormones

HORMONE	PRIMARY	SECONDARY
GH	Sleep (stimulatory, onset stage N3)	Weak circadian effect (increased GH secretion at night)—low somatostatin?
ACTH, cortisol	Circadian (peaks around 7 AM)	Sleep inhibitory
TSH	Circadian (peaks around 2 AM)	Sleep inhibitory
Prolactin	Sleep (stimulatory)	Circadian effect—sleep is more stimulatory when it occurs at night

ACTH = adrenocorticotropic hormone; GH = growth hormone; TSH—thyroid-stimulating hormone.

neurons of the arcuate nucleus, which secrete **dopamine** to act on the dopamine-2 receptors of lactotrophs, **causing inhibition** of PRL secretion. **Thyrotropin-releasing factor** (TRH) has a **stimulatory** effect on PRL release. Vasoactive intestinal peptide (VIP) secretion by the hypothalamus also stimulates PRL release.

PRL levels show a bimodal pattern. They are minimal around noon, **increase somewhat during the afternoon,** and then **increase shortly before sleep onset** (Fig. 30–8). **Decreased dopaminergic inhibition of PRL during sleep is likely to be the primary mechanism underlying nocturnal PRL elevation.** In adults of both sexes, the nocturnal maximum corresponds to an average increase of more than 200% above the minimum level. Morning awakenings and awakenings interrupting sleep are consistently associated with a rapid inhibition of PRL secretion. Studies of the PRL profiles during daytime naps or after shifts of the sleep period have consistently demonstrated that **sleep onset, irrespective of the time of day, has a stimulatory effect on PRL release**[1,2] (Box 30–4). Note that the stimulatory effect of sleep on PRL secretion is greatest at night.

Evidence for the Role of PRL in Regulation of Sleep

Several studies have examined the possible relationship between pulsatile PRL release during sleep and the alternation of REM and non–rapid eye movement (NREM) stages. Using power spectral analysis of the EEG, a close temporal association between increased PRL secretion and delta wave activity is apparent. Awakenings inhibit nocturnal PRL release. **Thus, fragmented sleep generally is associated with lower nocturnal PRL levels.** The primary effect of

prolactin secretion may be stimulation of REM sleep. However, this has been demonstrated only in rodents. The effect may be observed 1 to 2 hours after treatment. The stimulatory effect of PRL on REM sleep depends on time of day (observed only during light—the inactive period in rodents).

There is also some evidence for an involvement of PRL in stage N3 regulation. Stage N3 sleep is enhanced in patients with hyperprolactinemia and in women who breast-feed and have high PRL levels compared with women who bottle-feed their infants.[6,7]

Summary of Control of Hormone Secretion

A summary of the control of secretion of GH, cortisol, TSH, and PRL is listed in Table 30–1. The table highlights that the secretion of some hormones is tied to sleep and others to circadian control. There may be a weaker secondary effect of sleep on hormone secretion primarily under circadian control and a weaker circadian effect on hormone secretion primarily under sleep control. A mnemonic for remembering the major control mechanisms: **GPS – ATC = Growth** hormone and **P**rolactin under **S**leep-wake control and

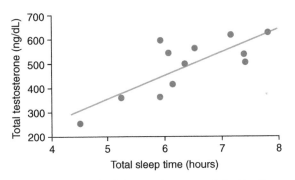

FIGURE 30–9 Morning levels of plasma total testosterone in healthy older men in relation to the amount of their nocturnal total sleep measured by polysomnography. A superimposed *best-fit line* illustrates the unadjusted bivariate correlation of these variables. Total sleep time is highly correlated with the total testosterone the following morning. *From Penev PD: Association between sleep and morning testosterone levels in older men. Sleep 2007;30:428, with permission.*

ACTH (cortisol) and TSH primarily under Circadian control.

SLEEP AND THE GONADAL AXIS

The 24-hour patterns of gonadotropin release and gonadal steroid levels vary according to the stage of life and are gender dependent.[8,9] In prepubertal children, luteinizing hormone (LH) and follicle-stimulating hormone (FSH) are secreted in pulses of low amplitude, and a sleep onset–augmentation effect is present in the majority of both girls and boys. As the child approaches puberty, the amplitude of the nocturnal pulses increases and the diurnal rhythm becomes more evident. A large nocturnal increase in gonadotropins is one of the hallmarks of puberty. In pubertal boys, the nocturnal rise of testosterone parallels the elevation of gonadotropins, whereas in pubertal girls, higher concentrations of estradiol occur during the daytime instead of the nighttime.[9] It has been proposed that the lack of parallelism between the diurnal variation of gonadotropins and estradiol reflects a 6- to 10-hour delay between gonadotropin stimulation and the ovarian response related to the time required for aromatization of estradiol.

In young adult men, the day-night variation of plasma LH levels is dampened or even undetectable,[10] whereas a marked diurnal rhythm in circulating testosterone levels persists with minimal levels in the late evening, and a clear nocturnal elevation results in maximal levels in the early morning.[11] Sleep fragmentation in normal men decreases the nocturnal rise in testosterone if REM sleep does not occur. The sleep related rise in testosterone appears to be linked to the first REM period.[11,12]

In elderly men, the morning level of testosterone depends on the amount of sleep. Higher levels correlate with more sleep. A recent study has indicated that the **amount of nighttime sleep is a strong predictor of morning testosterone levels** in healthy older men[13] (Fig. 30–9).

In adult women, diurnal and pulsatile LH variations are markedly modulated by the menstrual cycle. In postmenopausal women, gonadotropin levels are elevated, and show no consistent circadian patten.

LEPTIN AND GHRELIN

Appetite is regulated by the interaction between metabolic and hormonal signals and neural mechanisms.[14] The arcuate nucleus of the hypothalamus has two opposing sets of neuronal circuitry, appetite-simulating and appetite-inhibiting, and several peripheral hormonal signals have been identified that affect these neuronal regions.[15] The peripheral signals included leptin and ghrelin (Box 30–5). **Leptin** is primarily secreted by adipose tissue and appears to promote satiety.[15] **Ghrelin** is a peptide released primarily from the stomach.[16] Studies in humans also indicate that ghrelin increases appetite and food intake. Plasma ghrelin levels are rapidly suppressed by food intake and then rebound after 1.5 to 2 hours, paralleling the resurgence in hunger. Thus, leptin and ghrelin exert opposing effects on appetite. Animal studies suggest that leptin and ghrelin also have opposing effects on energy expenditure (leptin increasing energy expenditure), but the picture is less clear in humans. Under normal conditions, the 24-hour profile of human plasma leptin levels shows a marked nocturnal rise. When leptin levels were studied with continuous enteral nutrition, leptin levels still rose at night.[17] Ghrelin levels typically rise during the first half of the night, then decrease in the second half even in the fasting condition.[18] A mnemonic for the effect of **Gh**relin is "**G**otta **H**ave **F**ood."

There have been several studies of the effect of sleep loss on ghrelin and leptin levels. The results have varied between studies. However, in general, **sleep loss leads to increased ghrelin and decreased leptin.**[14] This would tend to increase food intake and perhaps decrease energy utilization. Some of the variable findings from studies may been due to the fact

---

BOX 30–5

Sleep Loss, Leptin, Ghrelin

SLEEP LOSS IS ASSOCIATED WITH:

- Impaired glucose metabolism.
- Lower leptin levels.
- Higher ghrelin levels.
- Increased risk of obesity (chronic short sleep duration).

LEPTIN

- Secreted by adipose tissue.
- Promotes satiety.
- Leptin levels rise at night.

GHRELIN (PEPTIDE)

- Secreted by the stomach.
- Increases appetite.
- Intake of food suppresses ghrelin secretion.
- Levels increase in the first part of the night then fall in the second part.

that nocturnal sleep times were not very reduced or that variable degrees of obesity were present in the populations studied.

OBESITY AND SLEEP DURATION

Numerous cross-sectional population studies have tried to determine whether obesity is associated with sleep loss.[14] Two longitudinal studies are mentioned. Analysis of data from the first National Health and Nutrition Examination Survey (NHANES I) indicated that subjects between the ages of 32 and 49 years with self-reported sleep durations at baseline of less than 7 hours had higher average body mass indices (BMIs) and were more likely to be obese than subjects with sleep durations of 7 hours.[19] A second longitudinal study analyzed the association between sleep and BMI over a 13-year period and reported that the odds ratio for sleep duration predicting obesity was 0.50, which means that every extra hour increase of sleep duration was associated with a 50% reduction in risk of obesity.[20] In humans, part of the tendency for weight gain after sleep loss is that sleep loss may reduce energy expenditure. In rodents, leptin increases energy expenditure and ghrelin decreases expenditure. In rodents, sleep loss experiments involve constant movement or other activity and rodents do not gain weight even with increased food intake. The importance of leptin and ghrelin on energy expenditure in humans remains to be documented.

SLEEP AND GLUCOSE TOLERANCE

Sleep has important effects on glucose metabolism, suggesting that sleep disturbances may adversely affect glucose tolerance. In a study by Scheen and coworkers,[21] subjects received a constant glucose infusion during (1) nocturnal sleep, (2) nocturnal sleep deprivation, and (3) daytime recovery sleep. The investigators analyzed plasma glucose levels, insulin secretion rates (ISRs), and plasma GH and cortisol levels. Plasma glucose and ISR markedly increased during early nocturnal sleep and returned to presleep levels during late sleep. These changes in glucose and ISR appeared to reflect the predominance of slow wave activity (stage N3) in early sleep and of REM and wake stages in late sleep. Major differences in glucose and ISR profiles were observed during sleep deprivation as glucose and ISR remained essentially stable during the first part of the night and then decreased significantly, despite the persistence of bedrest and constant glucose infusion.

During daytime recovery sleep, slow wave activity (stage N3) was increased, glucose levels peaked earlier during nocturnal sleep, and the decreases of glucose and ISR in late sleep were reduced by one half. Thus, sleep has important effects on brain and tissue glucose utilization, suggesting that sleep disturbances may adversely affect glucose tolerance. Spiegel and colleagues[22] studied 11 healthy volunteers using a protocol of experimental sleep restriction (4 hr/night × 6 nights) followed by a recovery period (12 hr/night × 6

nights). The study found decreased glucose tolerance in the sleep-debt condition compared with the fully rested condition. Evening cortisol concentrations were raised and activity of the sympathetic nervous system was increased in the sleep-debt condition.

Gottlieb and associates[23] analyzed a subsample of the population from the Sleep Heart Health Study (1486 subjects; 722 men and 764 women).

The usual sleep time was obtained by self-report. Statistical adjustments made for numerous covariates including age, gender, race, apnea-hypopnea index (AHI), and waist girth. Lower sleep time was associated with impaired glucose tolerance and diabetes mellitus based on serum glucose measurements (fasting and 2-hr).

Chapter 17 discusses the evidence that OSA is associated with impaired glucose tolerance and an increased risk of developing diabetes. The major confounder is the presence of obesity. A cross-sectional analysis of the Sleep Heart Health data[24] was performed (2588 participants aged 52–96 yr; 46% men) on individuals without known diabetes. Sleep-disordered breathing (SDB) was defined as a respiratory disturbance index of 10 events/hr or greater. **Impaired fasting glucose** (IFG), **impaired glucose tolerance** (IGT), occult diabetes, and body weight were classified according to recent accepted guidelines. Participants with and without SDB were compared on prevalence and odds ratios for measures of **impaired glucose metabolism** (IGM) after adjusting for age, sex, race, BMI, and waist circumference. SDB was observed in 209 non-overweight and 1036 overweight/obese participants. SDB groups had significantly higher adjusted prevalence and adjusted odds ratios of IFG, IFG plus IGT, and occult diabetes. The adjusted odds ratio for all subjects was 1.3 for IFG, 1.2 for IGT, 1.4 for IFG plus IGT, and 1.7 for occult diabetes. SDB was associated with occult diabetes, IFG, and IFG plus IGT after adjusting for age, sex, race, BMI, and waist circumference. The magnitude of these associations was similar in non-overweight and overweight participants. The consistency of associations across all measures of IGM and body habitus groups and the significant association between SDB and IFG plus IGT (a risk factor for rapid progression to diabetes, cardiovascular disease, and mortality) suggest the importance of SDB as a risk factor for clinically important levels of metabolic dysfunction. Chapter 17 discusses some studies showing that continuous positive airway pressure (CPAP) may improve glucose control in some patients with both obstructive sleep apnea (OSA) and diabetes. At least in some studies, CPAP treatment has more significant effects in patients who are not obese.

SLEEP AND GASTROINTESTINAL PHYSIOLOGY AND DISORDERS

Gastric and Intestinal Function

There is a peak in acid secretion occurring between 10 PM and 2 AM. Basal waking acid secretion is minimal unless stimulated by food. The peak in acid secretion is under

BOX 30–6

Important Facts about Gastroesophageal Reflux

GER AND SLEEP

- 45–50% of patients with GER have nocturnal symptoms
  - Prolonged sleep latency.
  - Frequent awakenings.
- Fewer but longer GER episodes at night.
- GER is common in OSA patients (50–75%).

GER AND PULMONARY COMPLICATIONS

- Exacerbation of nocturnal asthma.
- Nocturnal pulmonary aspiration.
- Increased incidence of GERD in pulmonary fibrosis.
- Sleep-related laryngospasm (possible role for GER).

GER AND GASTROINTESTINAL COMPLICATIONS

- Erosive esophagitis.
- Increased risk for Barrett's esophagus?
- Increased risk esophageal carcinoma?
- Nocturnal GER.
  - May increase risk of GER complications.
  - Can cause significant sleep disturbance.

NOCTURNAL MECHANISMS WORSENING DAMAGE FROM GER

- Saliva production virtually stops during sleep.
- Swallowing occurs only after arousal from sleep.
- Prolonged ACT.
- Transient LES relaxation after arousal from sleep or during wake.
- Most sleep-related reflux occurs during or following arousal from stage N2 sleep.

ACT = acid contact time; GER = gastroesophageal reflux; GERD = gastroesophageal reflux disease; LES = lower esophageal sphincter; NREM = non–rapid eye movement; OSA = obstructive sleep apnea.

BOX 30–7

pH Monitoring Definitions

pH PROBE POSITION

- pH probe placed 5 cm H_2O above LES (GE junction about 42 cm H_2O from nares).
- LES pressure determined manometrically (pressure transducers).
- LES position determined by pH measurement.
  - Probe is inserted until pH drops to 1.5–2.5, is slowly withdrawn until pH = 4, and then slowly withdrawn to 5–7 cm H_2O above this point.

DEFINITIONS

- Reflux episodes—pH drops below 4.
- Clearance defined as when PH returns to 4.
- Clearance interval—time from initial pH drop below 4 until return to above 4.
- Acid contact time—time below pH of 4.
  - Expresses as % of time in 24 hours.
  - Normally 4–6%.

GE = gastroesophageal; LES = lower esophageal sphincter.

esophagus to pH 5.5 to 6.5 (normal esophageal pH) (Boxes 30–6 and 30–7).

Nocturnal Gastroesophageal Reflux

Gastroesophageal reflux (GER) during sleep is common, with up to 10% of the population reporting symptoms of nocturnal reflux in survey studies.[26,27] In a Gallup poll of heartburn patients, 79% reported nighttime heartburn, of which 75% noted that heartburn negatively affected their sleep. Despite medical therapy for GER, only 49% had adequate control of their nocturnal symptoms.[27,28] Nocturnal GER is potentially more injurious than diurnal GER because **acid clearance mechanisms are impaired during sleep**. When episodes of GER occur during sleep, acid contact time (ACT) is prolonged. During sleep salivary flow virtually stops and the frequency of swallowing is very decreased (e.g., 6/hr). The clearance of refluxed material occurs only after arousal from sleep. Most nocturnal GER episodes occur during prolonged wake or after arousal from stage N2 sleep.

Freidin and coworkers[28] compared normal subjects and patients with reflux esophagitis with nocturnal monitoring of pH, esophageal manometry, and sleep stage. The LES pressures were similar in normal subjects and patients. Both groups had similar LES pressure during both wakefulness and sleep. The patients had many more reflux episodes. However, most nocturnal reflux episodes occurred during wake periods and some occurred after brief arousals from sleep. Transient lower esophageal sphincter relaxations (TLESRs) accounted for most of these episodes. Symptomatic reflux (especially at night) is believed to be a possible risk factor for the development of esophageal adenocarcinoma[29] and Barrett's esophagus[30] (a precursor of adenocarcinoma). However, not all studies have found a higher

circadian control and is not definitely altered by sleep or sleep stage.[25] There is delayed gastric emptying during sleep. Intestinal and colonic activity are generally decreased during sleep. Rectal motor activity increases during sleep but propulsion is retrograde. This and the fact that anal sphincter tone (while reduced) remains higher than rectal tone prevent anal leakage during sleep.

Gastroesophageal Reflux and Sleep

Normal Gastroesophageal Physiology

The lower esophageal sphincter (LES) prevents reflux of stomach contents into the esophagus. In the upright position, postprandial gastric distention causes brief relaxation of the LES with transient reflux that is quickly cleared. A number of factors assist in clearance or neutralization of stomach contents: (1) volume clearance—two or three swallows induce clearance of reflux material, and (2) acid neutralization—saliva itself buffers the acidity of refluxed material. These mechanisms quickly return the distal

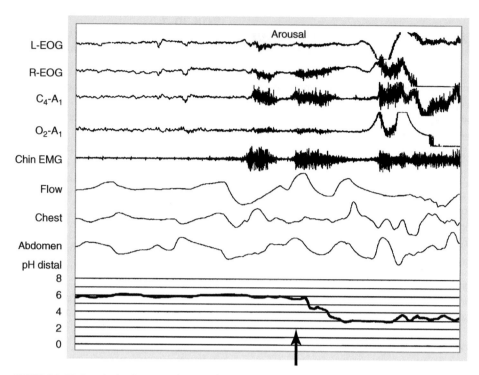

FIGURE 30–10 An episode of gastroesophageal reflux (GER) follows an arousal. Note that the pH drops below 4. EMG = electromyogram; EOG = electro-oculogram. *From Berry RB, Harding SM: Sleep and medical disorders. Med Clin North Am 2004;88:679–703.*

incidence of complaints of nocturnal reflux in patients with Barrett's esophagus.[31] Symptoms of nocturnal GER include multiple awakenings, substernal burning or chest discomfort, indigestion, and heartburn. Other symptoms include a sour or bitter taste in the mouth, regurgitation, coughing, and choking.

pH Monitoring

Esophageal pH testing (see Box 30–7) is used to diagnose GER and has a sensitivity and specificity of approximately 90%.[32] It can be performed as an ambulatory study or integrated with polysomnography (sleep monitoring) for temporal correlation of sleep-related events such as arousals. Esophageal pH testing is performed by placing a pH probe in the distal esophagus (5 cm above the LES). Many laboratories utilize dual pH probes, in which a proximal pH probe is also placed at the upper esophageal sphincter or in the pharynx. A GER episode is defined by the presence of material that has a pH less than 4. Figure 30–10 shows a GER event after an arousal from sleep. **ACT, defined as the time with a pH less than 4**, is often computed as absolute time or as a percentage of monitoring time or sleep time. A normal ACT is often assumed to be less than 4%. **GER episodes should be suspected on routine polysomnography if there is an arousal followed by a prolonged period of increased chin electromyogram (manifestation of swallowing)** (see Fig. 30–10).

Nocturnal Asthma and GER

Recently, there has been considerable interest in the relationship between nocturnal GER and asthma. Some

experimental evidence suggests that GER can worsen airway function with or without aspiration into the lungs. Jack and colleagues[33] monitored both tracheal and esophageal pH in four nocturnal asthmatics with GER. There were 37 episodes of esophageal reflux of which 5 episodes were associated with a fall in tracheal pH. Tracheal acid episodes were associated with prolonged reflux episodes, nocturnal awakenings, and bronchospasm during the night. Aspiration, however, may not be required to trigger changes in bronchial tone. Afferent vagal fibers are present in the lower esophagus and could trigger changes in bronchial tone when stimulated by gastric contents. Cuttitta and associates[34] evaluated spontaneous reflux episodes and airway patency during the night in seven asthmatics with GER. Multiple stepwise linear regression analysis revealed that the most important predictor of change in lower respiratory resistance was the **duration of esophageal acid exposure.** Both long and short GER episodes (those < 5 min and those > 5 min) were associated with higher respiratory resistance compared with baseline. These data collectively suggest that esophageal acid is able to elicit nocturnal bronchoconstriction. Given these findings, an important question is whether or not treatment of nocturnal GER can improve asthma. Some uncontrolled studies have shown a benefit in asthma with aggressive treatment of GER.[35] A large parallel-group, randomized, double-blind study of esomperazole for treatment of poorly controlled asthma (patient did **not** complain of GER) found no difference in episodes of asthma excerbations.[36] GER was found in 40% of patients using pH monitoring (asymptomatic). No subgroup of patients could be identified in which treatment of GER improved asthma. The investigators concluded that GER (in patients asymptomatic with respect to GER) is unlikely to be a major factor in uncontrolled asthma. However, this group of patients did not have GER symptoms. Treatment of patients with asthma and symptomatic GER could be considered (for GER alone) but may also help asthma in individual patients.

GER and OSA

Given the negative intrathoracic pressure during obstructive apnea and the frequent arousals from sleep, one would suspect that nocturnal GER is common in patients with OSA. Green and coworkers[37] prospectively examined 331 OSA patients. Significant nighttime GER was found in 62% of subjects before OSA treatment. Patients compliant with CPAP had a 48% improvement in their nocturnal GER symptoms. There was no change in nighttime reflux symptoms if patients did not use CPAP. Furthermore, there was a strong correlation between higher levels of CPAP and improvement in nocturnal GER symptom scores (higher pressure levels associated with more improvement). This study shows that nocturnal reflux is common in OSA patients and that nasal CPAP decreases the frequency of nocturnal GER symptoms. Of note, the fact that nocturnal GER is common in OSA patients and that CPAP reduces GER does not necessarily prove that OSA causes GER. In some studies, episodes of GER were not correlated with apneic events.[38] CPAP by increasing the pressure gradient between the thorax and the stomach may also reduce GER independent of the effects of CPAP on OSA. Tawk and colleagues[39] studied a group of OSA patients (AHI > 20/hr) and a 24-hour ACT of at least 6%. They performed 24-hour pH monitoring before and after 1 week of CPAP. The final monitoring was performed with the subjects wearing CPAP at night. The ACT fell as did the number of reflux episodes (Fig. 30–11). Eighty-one percent of subjects had ACT reduced to normal range (<4%).

Sleep-Related Laryngospasm

GER may also have a role in sleep-related laryngospasm (SRL). Episodes of SRL consist of the patient abruptly awakening with an intense feeling of suffocation often accompanied with stridor and choking sensations.[40] Other features include intense anxiety, rapid heart rate, sensation of impending death, and residual hoarseness. The differential diagnosis for SRL includes OSA, epilepsy, sleep choking syndrome, sleep terrors, vocal cord dysfunction, and other upper airway pathologies. Thurnheer and associates[41] noted that 9 of 10 patients with SRL had GER documented by esophageal pH testing. Six patients responded to antireflux therapy, showing that GER may be associated with SRL.

Treatment of Nocturnal GER

Patients should not eat for at least 2 hours before bedtime and avoid foods that promote GER, including high-fat foods, caffeine, chocolate, mint, alcohol, tomato products, citrus,

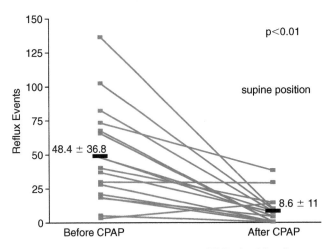

FIGURE 30–11 Continuous positive airway pressure (CPAP) reduced the reflux events in the supine position in patients with obstructive sleep apnea (OSA) and GER. *From Tawk M, Goodrich S, Kinasewitz G, Orr W: The effect of 1 week of continuous positive airway pressure treatment in obstructive sleep apnea patients with concomitant gastroesophageal reflux. Chest 2006;130:1003–1008.*

and sodas. Medications that promote reflux should be avoided, including calcium channel blockers, theophylline, prostaglandins, and bisphosphonates. Smoking significantly decreases LES pressure, so all patients should be encouraged to stop smoking. Patients should lose weight if they are obese and sleep in loose-fitting clothing. Positional therapy can also be used. Sleeping with the head of the bed elevated 6 inches with a full-length wedge or placing blocks under the head of the bed may be useful. **The right lateral decubitus position worsens GER, whereas the left lateral decubitus posture seems to be the best sleep position for sleep-related GER.**[42]

Medications to treat sleep-related GER include antacids for acute symptom control, H_2 receptor antagonists, proton pump inhibitors, and prokinetic agents.[43] H_2 receptor antagonists provide heartburn relief in 60% of patients and can be given before sleep onset. Proton pump inhibitors provide superior gastric acid suppression. One study found that 40 mg of omeprazole with dinner, or omeprazole, 20 mg, before breakfast and with dinner, resulted in better gastric acid suppression than giving 40 mg before breakfast only.[44] **Of note, proton pump inhibitors should be given before the evening meal rather than before bedtime to treat nocturnal GER.** Some data suggest there may be nocturnal acid breakthrough despite proton pump inhibitor therapy.[45] Whether nocturnal gastric acid breakthrough is clinically important in GER is not known. Metoclopramide is the only prokinetic agent available in the United States and has a high prevalence (20–50%) of central nervous system side effects. Prokinetic agents can be used concomitantly with gastric acid–suppressive agents. Antireflux surgery, primarily fundoplication (both open and laparoscopic methods), is successful in 80% to 90% of patients. Long-term results, however, show that many surgically treated patients use antireflux medications regularly.[46]

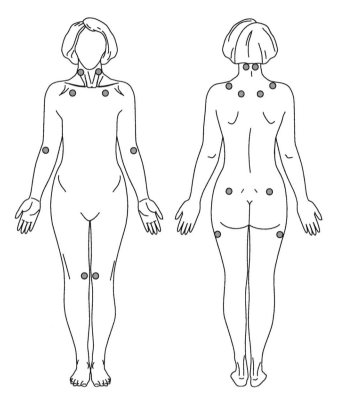

FIGURE 30–12 Location of tender points used to diagnose fibromyalgia. *From Wolfe F, Smythe HA, Yunus MB, et al: The American College of Rheumatology 1990 criteria for the classification of fibromyalgia: report of the multi-center criteria committee. Arthritis Rheum 1990;33:160–172.*

SLEEP AND RHEUMATOLOGY

Fibromyalgia Syndrome

Manifestations of Fibromyalgia

Fibromyalgia syndrome (FS) is defined by the American College of Rheumatology as the presence of widespread musculoskeletal pain for at least 3 months, which is bilateral above and below the waist, including axial pain and the presence of 11 of 18 tender points[47] (Fig. 30–12). FS should be considered a syndrome rather than a disease process. Fibromyalgia affects about 3% of the population aged 30 to 50 years and **70% to 90% of patients are women.**[48] Depression is common in the disorder. The pathophysiology of FS is very complex.[49–52] A possible mechanism is thought to be central sensitization of nociceptive neurons in the dorsal horn of the spinal cord with activation of N-methyl-D-aspartate receptors. This central sensitization results in generalized heightened pain sensitivity caused by pathologic nociceptive processing within the central nervous system. There is a threefold increase in substance P and a decrease in serotonin levels in the cerebrospinal fluid.[52]

Sleep in FS

Sleep complaints are common and include nonrestorative sleep, fragmented sleep, and insomnia. Poor sleep seems to worsen pain symptoms in 67% of the patients.[48] Sleep studies in FS patients have shown decreased total sleep time, decreased stage N3 and REM sleep, and increased arousals.[48] An interesting EEG pattern (alpha sleep or alpha-NREM anomaly) was first described in FS patients by Roizenberg and coworkers[53] and Branco and colleagues.[54] This is characterized by prominent alpha activity (8–13 Hz) persisting into NREM sleep (alpha intrusion). Alpha activity is normally present during relaxed wake and after brief awakenings (arousals) but is normally virtually absent during stages N2 and N3 except as associated with arousals. Alpha intrusion into stage N3 (slow wave or delta sleep) is called **alpha-delta sleep.** Since that time, it has been recognized that the alpha-NREM sleep anomaly is not specific for FS and is not present in all patients with FS. **Other groups in which the alpha-NREM sleep anomaly can be found include patients with chronic pain syndromes, depression, and diverse causes of nonrestorative sleep.** Indeed, alpha sleep has been seen in up to 15% of normal subjects.[55] In a variant of alpha sleep (phasic alpha activity), alpha intrusion is seen mainly during stage N3 rather than being present diffusely in NREM sleep. In one study, phasic alpha activity seemed to be present in FS patients with prominent sleep disturbance, subjective feeling of superficial sleep, and more pain and stiffness.[53] Chapter 4 contains sleep tracings illustrating the alpha anomaly.

Treatment of FS

Treatments for FS include antidepressants, anticonvulsants (to treat pain), hypnotics, muscle relaxers, cognitive therapy, exercise, biofeedback, and hypnosis.[56,57] Patients should incorporate good sleep hygiene habits. Furthermore, screening for primary sleep disorders is also indicated. Of note, FS patients have a higher prevalence of restless legs syndrome than controls.[58] Some FS patients have clinical improvement with low doses of antidepressants, whereas others require the

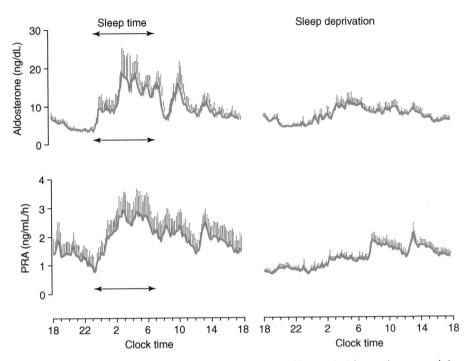

FIGURE 30–13 Mean 24-hour profiles of plasma renin activity (PRA) and aldosterone in eight normal young men during normal nocturnal sleep and acute sleep deprivation. The *vertical bar* at each time point represents the SEM. Sleep deprivation blunts the nocturnal increase in PRA and aldosterone. *From Charloux A, Gronfier C, Chapotot F, et al: Sleep deprivation blunts the nighttime increase in aldosterone release in humans. J Sleep Res 2001;10:29, with permission.*

usual doses needed for an antidepressant effect. Traditionally, low doses of tricyclic antidepressants (both serotonin and norepinephrine reuptake inhibitors) such as amitryptiline 25 to 50 mg qhs were used for FS.[59] The selective serotonin reuptake inhibitors (SSRIs) have not been very effective as treatment for FS unless depression was present. Two medications selectively blocking reuptake of both serotonin and norepinephrine (SNRIs) are U.S. Food and Drug Administration (FDA) approved for treatment of FS. These medications are duloxetine (Cymbalta) and milnacipran (Savella)[57] (Table 30–2). Venlafaxine (Effexor, also an SNRI) has also been used but is not FDA approved for FS. The SNRIs appear to work in both depressed and nondepressed patients with FS.[60–63] **Pregabalin (Lyrica)** is an anticonvulsant that has also been FDA approved for FS. Gabapentin is another anticonvulsant that has been used for chronic pain syndromes including FS (not FDA approved for FS). Both pregabalin and gabapentin have been shown to have benefit in FS patients.[64,65] Muscle relaxants such as cyclobenzaprine have also been used.[66] Studies have shown benefit from treatment of FS with sodium oxybate.[67,68]

Sodium oxybate is believed to work in FS by improving sleep quality. Sodium oxybate is currently FDA approved for treatment of narcolepsy (cataplexy and daytime sleepiness). An application was made to the FDA for an indication for the use of sodium oxybate as a treatment for FS. However, this application was rejected in part because the large FS population and the potential for abuse of medication ("date rape drug").

SLEEP AND RENAL

Renin-Aldosterone and Sleep

Water and sodium homeostasis depends on coordination of a number of factors including several hormones. Arginine vasopressin (AVP) is secreted by the posterior pituitary and is also known as antidiuretic hormone (ADH). AVP is secreted in bursts but is independent of sleep stage. AVP results in reabsorption of water from the collecting duct of the kidney. Renin is secreted by the juxtaglomerular cells of the kidney and aldosterone secreted by the adrenal cortex. Renin hydrolyzes angiotensinogen (produced by the liver) to produce angiotensin I. Angiotensin I is metabolized by lung endothelial cells containing angiotensin-converting enzyme (ACE) to angiotensin II. Angiotensin II is a potent vasoconstrictor and also stimulates the adrenal to produce aldosterone. Aldosterone causes absorption of sodium and water and excretion of potassium. Atrial natriuretic peptide (ANP) is secreted by the atrial myocytes in response to stretch and other influences. ANP causes an increase in the renal excretion of sodium and is a mechanism to respond to fluid overload. ANP is elevated in untreated sleep apnea (negative intrathoracic pressure swings stretch the atria), resulting in nocturia. Patients with untreated OSA have nocturnal natriuresis. Urine volume and electrolyte secretion is normally lower at night. In particular, REM sleep is associated with decreased urine flow and increased osmolality.

Plasma renin activity (PRA) and aldosterone levels are elevated during sleep.[69–72] This effect is mainly **related to**

sleep rather than circadian factors. The usual nocturnal rise in PRA and aldosterone is blunted by sleep deprivation[71] (Fig. 30–13). PRA increases during NREM sleep and decreases during REM sleep. REM sleep is associated with increased sympathetic tone, which increases renin. This seems inconsistent with lower renin during REM sleep. However, the dip in renin during REM sleep may occur from lower blood pressure and sympathetic tone during NREM sleep. Renin activity is already sharply decreasing before REM sleep occurs. At the transition from REM sleep to NREM sleep, renin levels are already rising.

CLINICAL REVIEW QUESTIONS

1. Secretion of GH is most closely tied to which of the following?
   A. First period of stage N3.
   B. First REM period.
   C. Time of day (circadian).
   D. Time of awakening.

2. Which of the following about PRL secretion is true?
   A. It is predominantly under circadian control.
   B. It is inhibited by sleep.
   C. It is stimulated by sleep.
   D. It is increased by dopaminergic signaling from the hypothalamus.
   E. It is inhibited by TRH.

3. Which of the following is true about cortisol secretion?
   A. It is closely tied to timing of sleep.
   B. Nocturnal levels are increased by sleep deprivation.
   C. Lowest levels are in the morning.
   D. Lowest levels are in the evening.

4. Which of the following is true about TSH secretion?
   A. It is stimulated by sleep.
   B. It is inhibited by sleep.
   C. TSH stimulation is under circadian control.
   D. A and B.
   E. B and C.

5. Which of the following are NOT true about leptin and ghrelin?
   A. Ghrelin stimulates the appetite.
   B. Leptin stimulates the appetite.
   C. Eating reduces ghrelin secretion.
   D. Ghrelin levels are higher at night.
   E. Sleep loss decreases leptin and increases ghrelin.

6. A GER episode is defined by a pH less than which number?
   A. pH < 3.
   B. pH < 4.
   C. pH < 5.
   D. pH < 6.

7. Which of the following states are true concerning nocturnal GER?
   A. It typically occurs during sleep.
   B. It occurs during wake or after arousals.
   C. Acid clearance at night is normal.
   D. Acid clearance at night is abnormal.
   E. B and D.

Answers

1. **A.** GH secretion is linked to the first period of stage N3.

2. **C.** Sleep stimulates PRL secretion. Dopamine inhibits PRL secretion and TRH increases it.

3. **B.** Cortisol secretion is under circadian control. Highest cortisol levels are around 7 AM. The lowest levels are during the first part of the sleep period. Sleep deprivation increases nocturnal levels.

4. **E.** TSH secretion is under circadian control but is inhibited by sleep.

5. **B.** Leptin induces satiety. The other statements are true.

6. **B.** pH < 4.

7. **E.** Nocturnal GER occurs after arousals. Acid clearance is reduced because saliva secretion stops during sleep and swallowing does not occur.

REFERENCES

1. Van Cauter E, Spiegel K: Circadian and sleep control of hormones. In Turek FW, Zee PC (eds): Regulation of Sleep and Circadian Rhythms. New York: Marcel Dekker, 1999, p. 399.
2. Pannain S, Van Cauter E: Modulation of endocrine function by sleep-wake homeostasis and circadian rhythmicity. Sleep Med Clin 2007;2:147–159.
3. Mendelson WB, Slater S, Gold P, Gillin JC: The effect of growth hormone administration on human sleep: a dose-response study. Biol Psychiatry 1980;15:613–618.
4. Beranek L, Obál FJ, Taishi P, et al: Changes in rat sleep after single and repeated injections of the long-acting somatostatin analog octreotide. Am J Physiol 1997;273:R1484–R1491.
5. Van Cauter E, Plat L, Copinschi G: Interrelations between sleep and the somatotropic axis. Sleep 1998;21:553–566.
6. Frieboes RM, Murck H, Stalla GK, et al: Enhanced slow-wave sleep in patients with hyperprolactinemia. J Clin Endocrinol Metab 1998;83:2706–2710.
7. Blyton DM, Sullivan CE, Edwards N: Lactation is associated with an increase in slow-wave sleep in women. J Sleep Res 2002;11:297–303.
8. Van Cauter E, Copinschi G: Endocrine and other biological rhythms. In DeGroot LJ, Jameson JL (eds): Endocrinology, Vol. 1. Philadelphia: Elsevier Saunders, 2006, pp. 341–372.
9. Goji K: Twenty-four-hour concentration profiles of gonadotropin and estradiol (E2) in prepubertal and early pubertal

girls: the diurnal rise of E2 is opposite the nocturnal rise of gonadotropin. J Clin Endocrinol Metab 1993;77:1629–1635.

10. Fehm HL, Clausing J, Kern W, et al: Sleep-associated augmentation and synchronization of luteinizing hormone pulses in adult men. Neuroendocrinology 1991;54:192–195.

11. Luboshitzky R, Zabari Z, Shen-Orr Z, et al: Disruption of the nocturnal testosterone rhythm by sleep fragmentation in normal men. J Clin Endocrinol Metab 2001;86:1134–1139.

12. Luboshitzky R, Herer P, Levi M, et al: Relationship between rapid eye movement sleep and testosterone secretion in normal men. J Androl 1999;20:731–737.

13. Penev P: Association between sleep and morning testosterone levels in older men. Sleep 2007;30:427–432.

14. Knutson KL, Spiegel K, Penev P, Van Cauter E: The metabolic consequences of sleep deprivation. Sleep Med Rev 2007;11:163–178.

15. Gale SM, Castracane VD, Mantzoros CS: Energy homeostasis, obesity and eating disorders: recent advances in endocrinology. J Nutr 2004;134:295–298.

16. van der Lely A, Tschop M, Heiman M, Ghigo E: Biological, physiological, pathophysiological, and pharmacological aspects of ghrelin. Endocr Rev 2004;25:426–457.

17. Simon C, Gronfier C, Schlienger JL, Brandenberger G: Circadian and ultradian variations of leptin in normal man under continuous enteral nutrition: relationship to sleep and body temperature. J Clin Endocrinol Metab 1998;83:1893–1899.

18. Dzaja A, Dalal MA, Himmerich H, et al: Sleep enhances nocturnal plasma ghrelin levels in healthy subjects. Am J Physiol Endocrinol Metab 2004;286:E963–E967.

19. Gangwisch JE, Malaspina D, Boden-Albala B, Heymsfield SB: Inadequate sleep as a risk factor for obesity: analyses of the NHANES I. Sleep 2005;28:1289–1296.

20. Hasler G, Buysse D, Klaghofer R, et al: The association between short sleep duration and obesity in young adults: a 13-year prospective study. Sleep 2004;27:661–666.

21. Scheen AJ, Byrne MM, Plat L, et al: Relationships between sleep quality and glucose regulation in normal humans. Am J Physiol 1996;271:E261–E270.

22. Spiegel K, Leproult R, Van Cauter E: Impact of sleep debt on metabolic and endocrine function. Lancet 1999;354:1435–1439.

23. Gottlieb DJ, Punjabi NM, Newman AB, et al: Association of sleep time with diabetes mellitus and impaired glucose tolerance. Arch Intern Med 2005;165:863–867.

24. Seicean S, Kirchner HL, Gottlieb DJ, et al: Sleep-disordered breathing and impaired glucose metabolism in normal-weight and overweight/obese individuals: the Sleep Heart Health Study. Diabetes Care 2008;31:1001–1006.

25. Orr WC: Gastrointestinal physiology. In Kryger M, Roth T, Dement WC (eds): Principles and Practice of Sleep Medicine. Philadelphia: Elsevier, 2005, pp. 283–291.

26. Farup C, Kleinman L, Sloan S, et al: The impact of nocturnal symptoms associated with gastroesophageal reflux disease on health-related quality of life. Arch Intern Med 2001;161:45–70.

27. Shaker R, Castell DO, Schoenfeld PS, Spechler SJ: Nighttime heartburn is an underappreciated clinical problem that impacts sleep and daytime function: the results of a Gallup Survey conducted on behalf of the American Gastroenterological Association. Am J Gastroenterol 2003;98:1487–1493.

28. Freidin N, Fisher MJ, Taylor W, et al: Sleep and nocturnal acid reflux in normal subjects and patients with reflux oesophagitis. Gut 1991;32:1275–1279.

29. Lagergren J, Bergstrom R, Lindgren A, Nuyren O: Symptomatic gastroesophageal reflux as a risk factor or esophageal adenocarcinoma. N Engl J Med 1999;340:825–831.

30. Gerson LB, Edson R, Lavori PW, Triadafilopoulos G: Use of a simple symptom questionnaire to predict Barrett's esophagus in patients with symptoms of gastroesophageal reflux. Am J Gastroenterol 2001;96:2005–2012.

31. Eloubeidi MA, Provenzale D: Clinical and demographic predictors of Barrett's esophagus among patients with gastroesophageal reflux disease: a multivariable analysis in veterans. J Clin Gastroenterol 2001;33:306–309.

32. Kahrilas PJ, Quigley EMM: Clinical esophageal pH recording: a technical review for practice guideline development. Gastroenterology 1996;110:1982–1996.

33. Jack CIA, Calverley PMA, Donnelly RJ, et al: Simultaneous tracheal and oesophageal pH measurement in asthmatic patients with gastro-oesophageal reflux. Thorax 1995;50:201–204.

34. Cuttitta G, Cibella F, Visconti A, et al: Spontaneous gastroesophageal reflux and airway patency during the night in adult asthmatics. Am J Respir Crit Care Med 2000;161:177–181.

35. Harding SM, Richter JE, Guzzo MR, et al: Asthma and gastroesophageal reflux: acid suppressive therapy improves asthma outcomes. Am J Med 1996:100:395–405.

36. ALA Asthma Clinical Research Centers: Efficacy of esomeprazole for treatment of poorly controlled asthma. N Engl J Med 2009;360:1487–1499.

37. Green BT, Broughton WA, O'Connor JB: Marked improvement in nocturnal gastroesophageal reflux in a large cohort of patients with obstructive sleep apnea. Arch Intern Med 2003;163:41–45.

38. Graf KI, Karaus M, Heinemann S, et al: Gastroesophageal reflux in patients with sleep apnea syndrome. Z Gastroenterol 1995;33:689–693.

39. Tawk M, Goodrich S, Kinasewitz G, Orr W: The effect of 1 week of continuous positive airway pressure treatment in obstructive sleep apnea patients with concomitant gastroesophageal reflux. Chest 2006;130:1003–1008.

40. American Academy of Sleep Medicine: International Classification of Sleep Disorders, 2nd ed. Westchester, IL: American Academy of Sleep Medicine, 2005.

41. Thurnheer R, Henz S, Knoblauch A: Sleep-related laryngospasm. Eur Respir J 1997;10:2084–2086.

42. Khoury RM, Camacho-Lobato L, Katz PO, et al: Influence of spontaneous sleep positions on nighttime recumbent reflux in patients with gastroesophageal reflux disease. Am J Gastroenterol 1999;94:2069–2073.

43. Berry RB, Harding SM: Sleep and medical disorders. Med Clin North Am 2004;88:679–703.

44. Kuo B, Castell DO: Optimal dosing of omeprazole 40 mg daily: effects on gastric and esophageal pH and serum gastrin in healthy controls. Am J Gastroenterol 1996;91:1532–1538.

45. Peghini PL, Katz PO, Bracy NA, et al: Nocturnal recovery of gastric acid secretion with twice-daily dosing of proton pump inhibitors. Am J Gastroenterol 1998;93:763–767.

46. Spechler SJ, Lee E, Ahnen D, et al: Long-term outcome of medical and surgical therapies for gastroesophageal reflux disease: follow-up of a randomized controlled trial. JAMA 2001;285:2331–2338.

47. Wolfe F, Smythe HA, Yunus MB, et al: The American College of Rheumatology 1990 criteria for the classification of fibromyalgia: report of the multi-center criteria committee. Arthritis Rheum 1990;33:160–172.

48. Harding SM: Sleep in fibromyalgia patients: subjective and objective findings. Am J Med Sci 1998;315:367–376.

49. Okifugi A, Turk DC: Stress and psychophysiological dysregulation in patients with fibromyalgia syndrome. Appl Psychophysiol Biofeedback 2002;27:129–141.

50. Neeck G: Pathogenic mechanisms of fibromyalgia. Ageing Res Rev 2002;1:243–255.

51. Pillemer SR, Bradley LA, Crofford LJ, et al: The neuroscience and endocrinology of fibromyalgia. Arthritis Rheum 1997;40:1928–1939.

52. Staud R, Spaeth M: Psychophysical and neurochemical abnormalities of pain processing in fibromyalgia. CNS Spectr 2008;13(3 Suppl 5):12–17.

53. Roizenblatt S, Moldofsky H, Benedito-Silva AA, Tufik S: Alpha sleep characteristics in fibromyalgia. Arthritis Rheum 2001;44:222–230.

54. Branco J, Atalaia A, Paiva T: Sleep cycles and alpha-delta sleep in fibromyalgia syndrome. J Rheumatol 1994;21:1113–1117.

55. Mahowald ML, Mahowald MW: Nighttime sleep and daytime functioning (sleepiness and fatigue) in less well-defined chronic rheumatic diseases with particular reference to the "alpha-delta NREM sleep anomaly." Sleep Med 2000;1:195–207.

56. Dussias P, Kalali AH, Staud R: Treatment of fibromyalgia. Psychiatry (Edgemont) 2010;7:15–18.

57. Staud R: Pharmacological treatment of fibromyalgia syndrome. Drugs 2010;70:1–14.

58. Yunus MB, Aldag J: Restless legs syndrome and leg cramps in fibromyalgia syndrome: a controlled study. BMJ 1996;312:1339.

59. Goldenberg D, Mayskiy M, Mossey C, et al: A randomized, double-blind crossover trial of fluoxetine and amitriptyline in the treatment of fibromyalgia. Arthritis Rheum 1996;39:1852–1859.

60. Mease PJ, Clauw DJ, Gendreau RM, et al: The efficacy and safety of milnacipran for treatment of fibromyalgia: a randomized, double-blind, placebo-controlled trial. J Rheumatol 2009;36:398–409.

61. Choy EHS, Mease PJ, Kajdasz DK, et al: Safety and tolerability of duloxetine in the treatment of patients with fibromyalgia: pooled analysis of data from five clinical trials. Clin Rheumatol 2009;28:1035–1044.

62. Iyengar S, Webster AA, Hemrick-Luecke SK, et al: Efficacy of duloxetine, a potent and balanced serotonin-norepinephrine reuptake inhibitor in persistent pain models in rats. J Pharmacol Exp Ther 2004;311:576–584.

63. Arnold LM, Rosen A, Pritchett YL, et al: A randomized, double-blind, placebo-controlled trial of duloxetine in the treatment of women with fibromyalgia with or without major depressive disorder. Pain 2005;119:5–15.

64. Hauser W, Bernardy K, Uceyler N, et al: Treatment of fibromyalgia syndrome with gabapentin and pregabalin: a meta-analysis of randomized controlled trials. Pain 2009;145:69–81.

65. Arnold LM, Goldenberg DL, Stanford SB, et al: Gabapentin in the treatment of fibromyalgia: a randomized, double-blind, placebo-controlled, multicenter trial. Arthritis Rheum 2007;56:1336–1344.

66. Tofferi JK, Jackson JL, O'Malley PG: Treatment of fibromyalgia with cyclobenzaprine: a meta-analysis. Arthritis Rheum 2004;51:9–13.

67. Scharf MB, Baumann M, Berkowitz DV: The effects of sodium oxybate on clinical symptoms and sleep patterns in patients with fibromyalgia. J Rheumatol 2003;30:1070–1074.

68. Moldofsky H, Inhaber NH, Guinta DR, Alvarez-Horine SB: Effects of sodium oxybate on sleep physiology and sleep/wake-related symptoms in patients with fibromyalgia syndrome: a double-blind, randomized, placebo-controlled study. J Rheumatol 2010;37:2156–2166; Epub 2010;August 3.

69. Brandenberger G, Krauth MO, Ehrhart J, et al: Modulation of episodic renin release during sleep in humans. Hypertension 1990;15:370–375.

70. Luthringer R, Brandenberger G, Schaltenbrand N, et al: Slow wave electroencephalographic activity parallels renin oscillations during sleep in humans. Electroencephalogr Clin Neurophysiol 1995;95:318–322.

71. Charloux A, Gronfier C, Lonsdorfer-Wolf E, et al: Aldosterone release during the sleep wake cycle in humans. Am J Physiol 1999;276:E43–E49.

72. Charloux A, Gronfier C, Chapotot F, et al: Sleep deprivation blunts the night time increase in aldosterone release in humans. J Sleep Res 2001;10:27–33.

Chapter 31

Sleep and Neurologic Disorders

Chapter Points

- AD is the most common cause of dementia and can be associated with the irregular sleep-wake rhythm disorder and sundowning. In early AD, there is a decrease in stage N3. In late AD, there is a decrease in REM sleep and an increase in the REM latency.
- OSA is common in AD patients and, if successfully treated with CPAP, can improve sleep quality and mood as well as slow the rate of cognitive decline.
- Donepezil (Aricept), a cholinesterase inhibitor, is used in AD to improve cognition but is often associated with insomnia. Morning dosing is suggested to minimize sleep disturbance. Some studies have suggested that evening doses of rivastigmine and galantamine can improve sleep quality. Cholinesterase inhibitors and cholinergic medications in general tend to increase REM sleep. Rivastigmine has been reported to cause RBD in AD patients.
- PSP is characterized by vertical gaze palsy and prominent sleep-maintenance insomnia (worse than in AD) and nocturia. PSP patients have a large reduction in the amount of REM sleep. PSG will often show absence of vertical eye movements during REM sleep. RBD occurs in approximately 13% to 30% of PSP patients.
- The sleep of patients with PD is impaired by rigidity, tremor (tends to resolve with sleep onset), dyskinesias, OSA, RBD, and nocturnal hallucinations. Patients with PD can manifest excessive daytime sleepiness even if OSA is not present. Modafinil may be helpful, although the published evidence is conflicting.
- PD+ disorders are manifested by parkinsonism (bradykinesia and rigidity), no or decreased response to levodopa, sensitivity to dopamine blockers, and a more rapid course than PD. PD+ disorders include PSP, DLBD, and MSA.
- Patients with DLBD have prominent dementia much earlier in the disease course compared with PD. The patients frequently have visual hallucinations and are exquisitely sensitive to dopamine blockers (can

develop severe rigidity). The RBD is common in patients with DLBD.
- MSA patients have various amounts of striatonigral degeneration (rigidity and bradykinesia), olivopontocerebellar degeneration (cerebellar dysfunction, ataxia, falls), and autonomic dysfunction (erectile dysfunction, orthostatic hypotension, bladder dysfunction). The RBD is very common in MSA patients.
- Stridor (especially during sleep) is a well-known manifestation of MSA and denotes a poor prognosis.
- FFI is a familial autosomal dominant prion disease with progressive insomnia and dementia. PET shows a characteristic absent or very low activity of the thalamus.
- There is a high prevalence of sleep apnea in patients who have had a recent stroke. OSA is the most common form of sleep apnea but central sleep apnea (including CSB) can occur. If OSA is present, this is associated with a worse prognosis but CPAP treatment can improve outcomes.

SLEEP AND NEURODEGENERATIVE DISORDERS

Sleep complaints are very common in patients with neurodegenerative disorders (Box 31–1). Some basic knowledge about these disorders is essential for the sleep clinician. The major neurodegenerative disorders are discussed briefly with an emphasis on the effects on sleep.

Synucleopathies

The synucleopathies are chronic and progressive disorders associated with a decline in cognitive, behavioral, and autonomic functions.[1,2] The two major categories are taupathies and alpha synucleopathies (Table 31–1). The taupathies are disorders associated with intracellular disposition of abnormally phosphorylated tau (a microtubule-associated protein) usually expressed as neurofibrillary tangles, neurophil threads, and abnormal tau filaments (Pick bodies). Tau

BOX 31–1

Sleep Disorders in Neurodegenerative Disorders
• Insomnia—sleep onset, sleep maintenance, fragmented sleep
• Hypersomnia
• Sleep apnea syndromes
• Hypersomnia due to the neurologic disorder
• Excessive nocturnal motor activity (including RBD)
• Circadian rhythm disorders
• Sundowning
RBD = rapid eye movement sleep behavior disorder.

TABLE 31–1

Neurodegenerative Disorders

TAUPATHIES	ALPHA SYNUCLEOPATHIES
• Alzheimer's disease (AD)	• Parkinson's disease (PD)
• Progressive supranuclear palsy (PSP)	• Diffuse Lewy body dementia (DLBD)
• Corticobasal degeneration (CBD)	• Multiple system atrophy (MSA)
• Frontotemporal dementia (FTD)	
• Pick's disease	

proteins are involved in maintaining the cell shape and serve as tracks for axonal transport. The taupathy disorders include Alzheimer's disease (AD), progressive supranuclear palsy (PSP), corticobasal degeneration (CBD), frontotemporal dementia (FTD), and Pick's disease. Alpha synuclein is a protein that helps in the transportation of dopamine-laden vesicles from the cell body to the synapses. The alpha synucleopathies include Parkinson's disease (PD), diffuse Lewy body dementia (DLBD), and multiple system atrophy (MSA).

Dementias

Dementia is defined as a clinical syndrome characterized by acquired loss of cognitive and emotional abilities severe enough to interfere with daily functioning.[1,2] In evaluating any patients with dementia, it is important to rule out treatable causes including medication side effects, hypothyroidism, vitamin B_{12} deficiency, depression, and occult obstructive sleep apnea (OSA). Pseudodementia of the elderly is due to depression and can be associated with a short rapid eye movement (REM) latency and high REM density. In contrast, patients with AD tend to have a low REM density, long REM latency, and a reduction in the amount of REM sleep. AD is by far the most common cause of dementia with DLBD the next most common (Box 31–2).

Alzheimer's Disease

AD is the most common cause of dementia (>60% of dementias). The diagnosis is one of exclusion. The hallmark is a

BOX 31–2

Major Dementias
• Alzheimer's disease (60–80%)
• Diffuse Lewy body dementia (20%)
• Others (vascular, metabolic)

gradual onset of short-term memory problems. The APO4E genotype is a risk factor for AD. Sleep disturbance worsens in parallel with cognitive dysfunction. Patients with AD suffer from *sundowning* (Box 31–3), which is defined as nocturnal exacerbation of disruptive behavior or agitation in older patients. This is likely the most common cause of institutionalization in patients with AD. Some of the key points concerning AD are listed in Box 31–4.

Etiology of Sleep Disturbances in AD A number of factors may contribute to sleep disturbance in AD. Degeneration of neurons in a number of areas including the optic nerve, retinal ganglion cells, and suprachiasmatic nucleus may contribute to circadian rhythm disturbances in AD.[3–5] These patients may manifest the irregular sleep-wake rhythm disorder. Institutional factors can worsen circadian rhythm disorders by decreasing normal zeitgebers (light and activity) and disturbing nocturnal sleep (noise). Poor sleep hygiene including daytime sleeping and decreased physical activity may impair sleep-wake rhythms.

Sleep Disturbances in AD A number of sleep disturbances are present in AD and vary with the course of the illness (Table 31–2). Early in the illness, there is disruption of sleep-wake rhythms, nocturnal awakenings, and decreased stage N3 sleep. Late in the disease course, there is a reduction in REM sleep and increased REM latency as well as **excessive daytime sleepiness.** Whereas both OSA and medications can contribute to daytime sleepiness in AD patients, sleepiness can occur simply as a manifestation of AD. The disruption of the sleep-wake rhythms manifests itself with large amounts of daytime sleep and often an irregular sleep-wake rhythm disorder. As noted previously, there is degeneration of both the suprachiasmatic nucleus (SCN) neurons and the pineal neurons. Recently, a decrease in melatonin MT1 receptors in the SCN has been demonstrated.[5] This could be one reason for the poor response to melatonin in AD. A large multicenter trial of melatonin did not show an improvement in elderly patients in group facilities.[6] A recent study in AD found that combined bright light and melatonin decreased aggressive behavior and modestly improved sleep efficiency and decreased nocturnal restlessness.[7]

OSA in AD OSA is common among patients with AD, and several studies have suggested that continuous positive airway pressure (CPAP) treatment of AD patients with OSA can slow the deterioration of cognition and improve sleep and mood.[8]

BOX 31–3

Sundowning

Definition: Nocturnal exacerbation of disruptive behavior or agitation in older patients

Factors

- Early bedtime
- Use of sedatives
- Advanced cognitive impairment
- Associated medical conditions

BOX 31–4

Alzheimer's Disease

- Most common cause of dementia (60% of cases of dementia)
- Progressive intellectual deterioration in middle to late adult life
- RBD much **less** common than in other causes of dementia
- Sundowning common
- Treatment is with cholinergic medications

RBD = rapid eye movement sleep behavior disorder.

TABLE 31–2

Sleep Disturbance in Alzheimer's Disease

EARLY AD	LATE AD
Disruption of sleep-wake rhythms	Reduction in REM
Increased nocturnal awakenings	Increased REM latency
Decreased stage N3	EDS and daytime napping—not associated with OSA or medications

AD = Alzheimer's disease; EDS = excessive daytime sleepiness; OSA = obstructive sleep apnea; REM = rapid eye movement.

Treatment of AD Patients with AD have reduced cerebral production of choline acetyl transferease, which leads to a decrease in acetylcholine synthesis and impaired cortical cholinergic function. Cholinergic medications (cholinesterase inhibitors) are used to treat AD and are beneficial.[9] However, cholinergic medications can cause sleep disturbance. The cholinergic medications used to treat AD include donepezil (Aricept), rivastigmine (Excelone), and galantamine (Razadyne, formerly Reminyl). The dosage of the medications is listed in Appendix 31–1. The cholinesterase inhibitors tend to increase REM sleep.

Memantine (Namenda), an *N*-methyl-D-aspartate (NMDA) receptor antagonist, is approved for treatment of moderate to severe AD. It is thought to prevent excitotoxicity from excessive glutamate actions at NMDA receptors that can cause neuronal dysfunction. Memantine's side effects

BOX 31–5

Sleep Disturbance in Progressive Supranuclear Palsy

- Sleep disturbance present in most patients (>50%)
  - Insomnia is the most common sleep disorder (more severe than in AD or PD).
  - RBD occurs (13–30%)—tends to **start concomitantly or soon after onset of** PSP (unlike RBD in PD, which starts BEFORE manifestations of motor and cognitive dysfunction).
- Factors leading to insomnia
  - Immobility in bed.
  - Difficulty with transfer.
  - Frequent nocturia.

AD = Alzheimer's disease; PD = Parkinson's disease; PSP = progressive supranuclear palsy; RBD = rapid eye movement sleep behavior disorder.

include hallucinations and dizziness (most common side effect). Treatment with memantine can be combined with a cholinesterase inhibitor. Some studies have shown a benefit from combined treatment.

Medication-Induced Insomnia in AD Donepezil (Aricept) up to 10 mg has been associated with incident insomnia up to 18%. Morning dosing of donepezil is recommended to minimize insomnia. Whereas donepezil is a once-a-day medication, rivastigmine is bid to tid and must be titrated up slowly. Rivastigmine and galantamine have more gastrointestinal side effects than donepezil. The sleep of some AD patients may improve with evening doses of galantamine or rivastigmine.[10,11] Stahl and coworkers[10] reviewed the results of double-blind studies of galantamine and found no higher incidence of sleep side effects than with placebo. Rivastigmine improved sleep complaints in some studies.[11,12] Whereas cholinesterase inhibitors have been reported to improve rapid eye movement sleep behavior disorder (RBD) in idiopathic RBD patients, rivastigmine has been reported to cause RBD in patients with AD.[13]

Progressive Supranuclear Palsy

PSP is characterized by supranuclear extraocular gaze palsy. Manifestations include a pseudobulbar palsy (upper neuron lesion to corticobulbar tract with dysarthria and choking), akinetic rigidity, ataxic gait and falling, limb and axial rigidity, and frontal lobe type dementia. There is a lack of response to dopaminergic medications.[1,2]

Sleep disturbance will be present in most patients (Box 31–5). Insomnia is the most common complaint (worse than in AD or PD). Patients have **an absence or a drastic reduction in REM sleep. Nocturia is a common problem.** One study comparing patients with AD and PSP found unsuspected OSA in approximately 50% of both groups.[14,15] A high and nearly equal percentage of both groups had REM sleep without atonia. However, clinical RBD was less common in PSP than in PD (7/20 vs. 13/20). If RBD is present in PSG, it presents concomitantly with other findings. In contrast, RBD can occur many years before the onset of PD.

Physical Examination Impaired voluntary vertical gaze especially in downward direction is an early finding.

Epidemiology in PSP Patients with PSP have a mean age of 63 and the mean survival from symptoms is 9 years.

Histology Tau-positive neurofibrillary tangles are present in multiple subcortical nuclei including the locus coeruleus. There is relative preservation of the hippocampus and cortex.

Sleep in PSP PSP patients have severe sleep-maintenance insomnia (worse than PD). Sleep complaints in PSP include an increased sleep latency, increased arousals, increased awakening frequency, decreased REM sleep, and increased REM latency.[14,15]

Polysomnography in PSP Polysomnography (PSG) reveals absence of vertical eye movements during REM sleep. Horizontal movements are present but are slower.

Corticobasal Degeneration

CBD is a neurodegenerative disorder characterized by progressive asymmetrical rigidity, apraxia, and other findings reflecting cortical and basal ganglia dysfunction.[1,2] Tau-positive astrocytic threads and oligodendral coiled bodies are noted. **Apraxia** is characterized by loss of the ability to execute or carry out learned purposeful movements, despite having the desire and the physical ability to perform the movements. It is a **disorder of motor planning,** which may be acquired or developmental but may not be caused by incoordination.

Frontotemporal Dementia

FTD is a type of cortical dementia resembling AD.[1,2] It is characterized by insidious onset, early loss of insight, social decline, emotional blunting, relative preservation of perception and memory, perseverance, and echolalia. Computed tomography (CT) or magnetic resonance imaging (MRI) shows frontal or anterior temporal atrophy.

Parkinsonism Syndromes (PD, PD+)

The term *parkinsonism* is used to refer to a group of manifestations including tremor, rigidity, bradykinesia, and postural instability. Parkinsonism is found in both PD and Parkinson Plus (PD+) disorders (Box 31–6).[16,17] The PD+ disorders include those characterized by parkinsonism and other manifestations. The PD+ disorders include PSP, DLBD, and MSA. Of note, the brains of PD patients do have Lewy bodies (LBs), but in DLBD, the distribution of LBs is more dense and more diverse. DLBD patients have more prominent dementia than noted in patients with PD. The dementia

---

BOX 31–6

Disorders Associated with Parkinsonism

Parkinsonism = tremor, rigidity, bradykinesia, and postural instability

Disorders with parkinsonism

- PD—also known as idiopathic parkinsonism
- PD+—disorders **with parkinsonism** + other manifestations
  - PSP
  - CBD
  - DLBD
  - MSA
- Medication side effects (dopamine blockers)
- Wilson's disease (hereditary copper accumulation)—presents in younger patients with parkinsonism features, diagnosis by slit lamp examination showing Kayser-Fleischer rings

CBD = corticobasal degeneration; DLBD = diffuse Lewy body dementia; MSA = multiple system atrophy; PD = Parkinson's disease; PSP = progressive supranuclear palsy.

---

of DLBD also present much earlier in the course of the disease than the dementia associated with PD. However, there is overlap between PD and DLBD. The PD+ disorders tend to progress more quickly than PD. The typically anti-Parkinson's medications are either less effective or completely ineffective in PD+ disorders. **PD+ patients are also very sensitive to dopamine blockers.**

Differential Diagnosis of Parkinsonism
1. Essential tremor—responds to beta blocker, worse on intention, improved with alcohol.
2. Wilson's disease—a disorder of hereditary copper accumulation. The typical presentation is a young person who has parkinsonian features. Diagnosis is by performing a slit lamp examination for Kayser-Fleischer rings.

Parkinson's Disease

PD is also called *primary parkinsonism* or *idiopathic PD*. The term *idiopathic* means "no secondary systemic cause." The etiology of PD is partially understood and, in this sense, is not truly idiopathic. PD is a chronic neurodegenerative disorder associated with a loss of dopaminergic neurons (substantia nigra and other sites). It is characterized by bradykinesia (slowing of physical movement), akinesia (loss of physical movement), rigidity, resting tremor, postural instability, and a good response to levodopa (LD; Box 31–7).[16,17] The disorder often starts unilaterally. Movements are slow and reduced facial expressiveness is noted (masklike facies) with infrequent blinking and a monotonous voice. Gait is slow and shuffling with small steps. The tremor in PD is a resting tremor—maximal when limb is at rest and disappearing with voluntary movement and sleep. Secondary symptoms may include cognitive dysfunction and subtle language problems.

BOX 31-7

Parkinson's Disease Manifestations

- Resting tremor (pill rolling).
- Gabellar reflex (sensitive but not specific)—breakdown of frontal lobe inhibition.
- Masklike facies.
- Small handwriting (micrographia).
- Walking without arm swinging.
- Flexed forward posture when walking with small shuffling steps.
- RBD in 20–30%—often precedes PD manifestations—sometimes by 10 years.
- Insomnia in 50%.
- OSA.

OSA = obstructive sleep apnea; PD = Parkinson's disease; RBD = rapid eye movement sleep behavior disorder.

Nonmotor manifestations of PD include sleep disorders, dementia, orthostatic hypotension, oily skin, and seborrheic dermatitis. The sleep disorders in PD can occur secondary to medication side effects but are also a primary manifestation of PD. PD patients have a sixfold increased risk of dementia. Physical findings in PD include resting pill rolling tremor, gabellar tap (tap of forehead elicits continued blinking [a frontal lob sign]), and cogwheel rigidity (joint stiffness and increased muscle tone). Imaging of the central nervous system (MRI, CT scan) is typically normal. The neuropathology of PD includes the presence of LBs. A major component of LB is alpha synuclein. Secondary parkinsonism can occur secondary to drugs such as dopamine blockers (phenothiazines and butyrophenones) or head trauma.

Differential Diagnosis of PD

1. Essential tremor—Responds to beta blocker, worse on intention, improved with alcohol.
2. PD+ disorders—If cognitive dysfunction occurs early in the disease course of a patient with parkinsonism, DLBD would be suspected. If **early postural instability + supranuclear gaze palsy** is prominent early, the PSP should be suspected. If autonomic dysfunction is prominent early (erectile dysfunction or syncope), MSA should be suspected.
3. CBD—If CT or MRI shows prominent asymmetry with patchy changes and cortical deficits (apraxia) are prominent, CBD should be suspected.

Treatment of PD A detailed discussion of the treatment of PD is beyond the scope of this chapter. A very comprehensive and useful discussion of PD is recommended.[18] A number of different medications have been used to treat PD (Table 31-3). The usual treatment of PD is with levodopa/carbidopa (LD/CD). CD prevents peripheral metabolism of LD to dopamine, thus reducing side effects and allowing for more LD to reach the central nervous system. Patients may respond to LD/CD but have a number of reported problems. "On times" refers to periods of time when symptoms go away or improve markedly. "Off times" refers to periods of time when symptoms return. "Wearing off time" refers to times when symptoms are under less control. **Dyskinesias,** manifested by sudden jerky or uncontrolled movements of the limbs and neck, are side effects of LD/CD treatment. **Dystonias** consisting of abnormal posture or cramps of the extremities or trunk can occur.

Dopamine agonists (DAs) are less likely to cause dyskinesia but have some dose-dependent side effects of their own. In low doses, DAs tend to cause sleepiness or promote sleep. Ropinirole or pramipexole have dopamine D_2/D_3 receptor activity and can stimulate autoreceptors to decrease dopamine release. In high doses, DAs can cause insomnia, frequent awakenings, and a reduction in the amount of stage N3. Another serious side effect of DA treatment of PD patients is the often unpredictable sudden onset of severe daytime sleepiness.

Catechol-O-methyl transferase (COMT) inhibitors have also been used as adjunctive medications in PD. This enzyme is involved in degrading neurotransmitters including dopamine. The COMT inhibitors available include entacapone (Comtan) and tolcapone (Tasmar). Entacapone is only peripherally active, whereas tolcapone is active in both the peripheral and the central nervous system. Tolcapone can be hepatotoxic, whereas entacapone is not. These medications can permit LD to last longer or maintain higher levels of effectiveness.

Anticholinergic agents are typically used in younger patients without cognitive impairment in whom tremor is the major feature. The concept behind the use of these agents is that PD has upset the cholinergic-dopaminergic balance in the basal ganglia due to loss of dopaminergic neurons. Anticholinergic drugs restore the balance. The anticholinergic drugs do not work for other PD manifestations. LD can also help tremor. The two anticholinergic drugs most commonly used include **trihexyphenidyl (Artane)** and **benzotropine (Cogentin)**. Trihexyphenidyl is started at 0.5 to 1 mg bid and gradually increased to 2 mg tid as tolerated. Benzotropine is used in doses of 0.5 to 2 mg bid. Side effects of these medications including memory impairment and hallucinations limit their use. The anticholinergic side effects include dry mouth, constipation, and urinary retention. Of note, LD improves tremor as well as rigidity and can be used to treat tremor in patients not tolerating anticholinergic medications.

Amantadine is an antiviral agent that can improve rigidity, akinesia, or tremor in approximately two thirds of patients. The mechanism of action is unknown. The usual dose of amantadine is 100 to 200 mg one to three times daily. The dose should be lower in patients with renal failure. The starting dose of amantadine is 100 mg daily with slow increases as tolerated. Side effects include confusion, hallucinations, insomnia, and nightmares.

Selegiline (Deprenyl, Eldepryl), a selective monoamine oxidase B (MAO-B) inhibitor, is approved for use in PD patients as an adjunct to LD because it modestly increases the percent of "on" time in advanced PD patients. When used

TABLE 31–3

Medications Used to Treat Parkinson's Disease

Dopamine precursor LD/CD 10/100, 25/100, 25/100	• Very effective for akinetic symptoms or tremor. Start ½ of 25/100 tid, titrate up to 25/100 tid.
SR LD/CD (25/100, 50/200 ER)	• Poorly and slowly absorbed, 30% higher dose needed for same effect. • Very low dose of SR can cause nausea owing to inadequate CD.
DAs Ropinirole (Requip) Pramipexole (Mirapex)	• Less likely than LD to cause dyskinesias. • Can cause sudden episodes of severe sleepiness. • Dopamine dysregulation syndrome. • Some recommend using DAs in younger patients as "neuroprotective."
COMT Inhibitors Tolcapone (Tasmar) Entacapone (Comtan)	• These medications prolong the effect of LD and can allow a reduction in dose. COMT inhibition reduces the peripheral methylation of LD or dopamine, which increases the plasma half-life of LD; thus, prolongs action of LD. • Entacapone—peripheral inhibition of COMT. • Tolcapone—peripheral and central inhibition of COMT. • Tolcapone—deaths from hepatotoxicity.
Amantadine	• Antiviral. • May improve rigidity, akinesia, and tremor. • Monotherapy or combined with LD.
Trihexyphenidyl (Artane) Benzotropine (Cogentin)	• For younger patients with predominant tremor. • Side effects include cognitive impairment and typical anticholinergic side effects (dry mouth, urinary retention, constipation).
MAOI (segiline)	• MAO-B inhibitor • Modest benefit; can be used with LD to reduce motor fluctuations.

CD = carbidopa; COMT = catechol-*O*-methyl transferase; DAs = dopamine agonists; ER = extended-release; LD = levodopa; MAO = monoamine oxidase; MAOI = monoamine oxidase inhibitor; SR = sustained release.

alone at 5 mg bid, it is well tolerated. When used with LD, it can increase dopaminergic side effects. Some clinicians use selegiline at a lower dose in combination with LD to decrease motor fluctuations. Other clinicians use selegiline as a putative neuroprotective therapy.

There is controversy about which dopaminergic medication is most appropriate for initiation of treatment of PD. The most common approach is to start with LD/CD if symptoms are significant. LD/CD is particularly effective for rigidity. However, patients taking LD/CD can develop dyskinesias. This tends to happen if patients have been on the medication for years or if high doses are used. If a patient on LD/CD develops dyskinesias, she or he can be switched to a DA. Conversely, some clinics recommend starting a DA as initial dopaminergic treatment. It is possible that DAs have a neuroprotective effect not present with LD/CD.

Sleep-Related Manifestations of PD Patients with PD have a number of sleep-related manifestations and disturbances (Table 31–4).[19,20] Treating the nocturnal manifestations of PD can be challenging.

SLEEP DISTURBANCE DUE TO MOTOR MANIFESTATIONS Patients with PD have motor symptoms including tremor that are worse during wakefulness (Fig. 31–1) and usually decrease or are abolished with sleep. The tremor often stops with the onset of alpha activity during drowsiness even before the onset of stage N1 or N2. Tremor is rare during stage N3. However, in some patients, motor manifestations persist during sleep. Examples of motor findings associated with sleep include repeated eye blinking at onset of sleep, blepharospasm at the onset of REM sleep, and prolonged tonic contractions of limb extensor or flexor muscles during non–rapid eye movement (NREM) sleep. Because of rigidity, patients with PD have difficulty changing body position during the night. Early morning akinesia and painful off dystonia can be problematic. LD/CD has a short duration of action. The DAs have a longer duration of action and may be useful in patients with motor manifestations during sleep.

DAYTIME SLEEPINESS IN PD Excessive daytime sleepiness (EDS) not due to OSA or medications is a well-known phenomenon in PD. Sleep attacks were once thought due to side effects from DAs. Most recent studies suggest medications used to treat PD may worsen EDS but that the underlying disease process is the most common cause of EDS in PD. Studies have reported 50% loss of hypocretin neurons in patients with PD.[21] Treatment of EDS not due to OSA in PD patients includes modafinil, bupropion, and traditional stimulants. Fatigue can also be a major complaint. The American Academy of Sleep Medicine (AASM) practice parameters for treatment of central hypersomnia[22] state that modafinil may

TABLE 31–4
Sleep Disturbance in Parkinson's Disease

PATHOPHYSIOLOGY	MANIFESTATION	TREATMENT
Changes in cholinergic and monoaminergic systems	Impaired wake-sleep control Decreased REM sleep	Cautious use of sedating antidepressants and hypnotics
Bradykinesia and rigidity	Decreased body shifts during sleep → discomfort and increased awakenings Impaired ability to use the bathroom	Sustained-release LD/CD or DAs
Tremor	Arousals Insomnia	Sustained release CD/LD or DAs
Drug-induced dyskinesia	Jerks, arousals	Decrease evening LD/CD or DAs
Abnormal motor control of respiratory and upper airway muscles	OSA (BMI often normal)	CPAP
RBD	• Disturbed REM sleep • Injury to self or bed partner • RBD • May precede other findings by years • Prevalence 15–30%	• Clonazepam • Melatonin • ?Dopamine agonists
PLMS, RLS	Arousals, difficult sleep onset	Dopamine agonists
Depression and anxiety	Insomnia Difficulty with sleep onset Early AM awakening	Cautious use of hypnotics and antidepressants
Dementia	Nocturnal confusional episodes	Quetiapine Aricept

BMI = body mass index; CD = carbidopa; CPAP = continuous positive airway pressure; DAs = dopamine agonists; LD = levodopa; OSA = obstructive sleep apnea; PLMS = periodic limb movements during sleep; RBD = rapid eye movement sleep behavior disorder; REM = rapid eye movement; RLS = restless legs syndrome.
Adapted from Comella CL: Sleep disorders in Parkinson's disease. Curr Treat Options Neurol 2008;10:215–221.

be an effective treatment of daytime sleepiness in PD. However, the evidence from studies of the effects of modafinil in PD is somewhat conflicting. A study by Ondo and colleagues[23] found no significant improvement in the Epworth Sleepiness Scale (ESS; subjective sleepiness). A study by Hogl and associates[24] found an improvement in the ESS but no increase in the sleep latency on the maintenance of wakefulness test (MWT). An uncontrolled study by Nieves and Lang[25] found improvement in the ESS with modafinil in PD patients. Another study investigated whether modafinil would improve fatigue in PD. Using a double-blind, placebo-controlled design, Lou and coworkers[26] noted no improvement in fatigue symptoms, no improvement in ESS, and some improvement in finger tapping. In summary, even though the evidence is less than totally convincing, a trial of modafinil is indicated if daytime sleepiness is a significant problem for a patient with PD. Of course, the possibility of OSA should be eliminated. As noted previously, treatment with DAs can be associated with sudden attacks of severe daytime sleepiness. One case report found that the addition of modafinil to DA therapy reduced the severity of this DA side effect.[27]

NOCTURNAL BEHAVIOR: RBD, NOCTURNAL HALLUCINATIONS, NOCTURNAL PSYCHOSIS **RBD** occurs in 20% to 40% of patients with PD. It

can be the earliest manifestation, occurring many years before other PD symptoms and signs. In general, treatment options for RBD in PD are similar to those for idiopathic RBD. DAs have been reported to be effective treatment of RBD in some patients.

Nocturnal hallucinations can occur in PD and disturb sleep. A recent study compared sleep between groups of PD patients with and without visual hallucinations. Whereas both groups slept poorly, the group with visual hallucinations had much poorer sleep.[28]

Drug-induced psychosis is a major problem in PD. It can occur in up to 22% and is a major cause of placing patients in a chronic care facility. Treatments have included reducing the dose of anti-Parkinson's medication, adding a neuroleptic drug, or discontinuing PD treatment for a period of time. Low-dose clozapine was found effective even if anti-Parkinson's medications were still taken and did not worsen tremor. In this study, doses of 6.25 to 50 mg were used (far lower than the 300–900 mg used for schizophrenia). The drug can cause leukopenia.[29] Quetiapine has also been effective for drug-induced psychosis but can cause problems with glucose control and oversedation.[30]

Dementia in PD A study found modest benefit from donepezil and the drug did not cause worsening of PD.[31] Another study

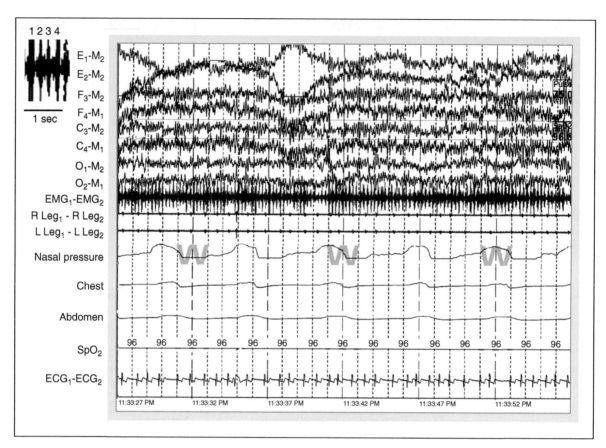

FIGURE 31–1 A 30-second tracing during wakefulness in a patient with Parkinson's disease shows a classic 4-Hz tremor noted in the chin electromyogram (EMG). RLeg$_1$-RLeg$_2$ and LLeg$_1$-LLeg$_2$ are the right and left anterior tibial EMG derivations. ECG = electrocardiogram; SpO$_2$ = pulse oximetry.

has reported some benefit from memantine in patients with PD with dementia or DLBD.[32]

Diffuse Lewy Body Dementia

DLBD is also known as dementia with Lewy bodies (DLB), Lewy body dementia, or diffuse Lewy body disease. DLBD is a type of dementia characterized anatomically by the presence of Lewy bodies, clumps of alpha synuclein and ubiquitine proteins in neurons. In this disorder, loss of cholinergic neurons results in cognitive dysfunction and loss of dopamine neurons results in parkinsonism (Box 31–8). If dementia occurs **more than 1 year after** other symptoms in PD, the disorder is called *PD with dementia*. If dementia occurs within the first year of parkinsonism, the diagnosis is DLBD. **DLBD tends to progress much more rapidly than PD.**

Manifestations of DLBD The major manifestations of DLBD[33] include (1) fluctuating cognition with great variation in attention and alertness from day to day and hour to hour, (2) recurrent visual hallucination (75% of patients with DLBD), (3) motor features of parkinsonism (tremor less common in DLBD than in PD), (4) RBD (50–75%), and (5) problems with orthostasis, including repeated falls, syncope (fainting),

and transient loss of consciousness. **The RBD can have an onset years before the other manifestations of DLBD (similar to PD).**

VISUAL HALLUCINATIONS The most common reported hallucination is of people or animals. The patient may misinterpret what he or she sees. For example, the patient may open a drawer full of socks but see snakes.

SENSITIVITY TO DA BLOCKERS An important characteristic of DLBD is exquisite sensitivity to dopamine blockers. When given dopamine blockers, patients with DLBD can develop life-threatening rigidity or malignant neuroleptic syndrome. Anticholinergic drugs such as benadryl or hytrin can worsen dementia.

DEMENTIA VARIANT A variant of DLB and RBD but without parkinsonism or hallucinations has been reported. This disorder may be a variant of DLBD.[34]

Multiple System Atrophy

MSA is a neurodegenerative disorder characterized by a combination of parkinsonism, dysautonomia, cerebellar dysfunction, and features of pyramidal tract dysfunction (Box

31–9).[35] Some patients have more prominent dysfunction in one category. MSA is sometimes divided into three separate conditions (Table 31–5). These include (1) striatonigral degeneration, (2) olivopontocerebellar degeneration, and (3) progressive autonomic failure (Shy-Drager syndrome). A recent consensus conference[35] recommended new MSA terminology and the term *Shy-Drager* was not used in this classification, although it is widely used in the literature.

Symptoms

1. Autonomic dysfunction (erectile dysfunction, bladder control—urgency, incomplete emptying, constipation, abnormal breathing during sleep, orthostatic hypotension).
2. Parkinsonism = rigidity ± tremor, bradykinesia, and postural instability. The tremor of MSA is irregular and usually not a pill rolling tremor as seen in PD.
3. Gait ataxia (poor coordination/unsteady walking) may be a presenting symptom. Ataxia of speech (cerebellar dysarthria) is also common and manifested by slow and slurred speech and sudden uncontrolled alterations in loudness of voice.

Epidemiology of MSA The typical age of onset of MSA is 50 to 60 years. The disease course is fairly rapid with onset to death in about 9 years. The disorder progresses more rapidly than PD.

Diagnosis The second consensus conference on MSA defined two categories of MSA based on the predominant symptoms at the time of evaluation[35]:

1. MSA-P—MSA with predominant parkinsonism (also called *striatonigral degeneration, parkinsonian variant*).
2. MSA-C—MSA with predominant cerebellar features. MSA in which cerebellar features predominate is also called *sporadic olivopontocerebellar atrophy*.

Pathology of MSA The pathology of MSA involves alpha synuclein oligodendral inclusions in the brainstem, cerebellum, and spinal cord. Glial cytoplasmic inclusions (Papp-Lantos bodies) appear in the brain centers involved with control of movement, balance, and autonomic control centers.

Vocal Cord Palsy and Stridor in MSA Stridor may occur in up to 30% of patients with MSA. It can be much worse during

---

BOX 31–8

Diffuse Lewy Body Dementia

- Fluctuating cognition and alertness.
- Visual hallucinations in 70%.
- Orthostasis and frequent falls.
- Motor manifestations of parkinsonism (rigidity, tremor less common than in PD).
- Onset of dementia within 1 year of symptoms of parkinsonism.
- RBD is very common (50–80%).
- Life-threatening rigidity with dopamine blockers.

PD = Parkinson's disease; RBD = rapid eye movement sleep behavior disorder.

BOX 31–9

Manifestations of Multiple System Atrophy

- Age of onset 50–60 years.
- Onset to death in 9 years.
- Not seen: hallucinations and dementia.
- Orthostatic hypotension a major problem.
- Variants
  - Striatonigral degeneration—rigidity, bradykinesis.
  - Olivopontocerebellar atrophy—prominent ataxia, postural instability.
  - Shy-Drager—autonomic dysfunction.
- Stridor—poor prognostic sign, normal awake laryngeal examination does not exclude.
- Sleep disorders very common (>70%).
- RBD very common (80–95% of patients).
- OSA.

OSA = obstructive sleep apnea; RBD = rapid eye movement sleep behavior disorder.

TABLE 31–5

Classifications of Multiple System Atrophy

	CHARACTERISTICS	1996 CONSESNUS CONFERENCE	2007 CONSENSUS CONFERENCE
Striatonigral degeneration	Predominantly Parkinson's type symptoms	MSA-P	MSA-P
Sporadic OPCA	Progressive ataxia of gait, limbs, and speech (cerebellar dysarthria)	MSA-C	MSA-C
Shy-Drager syndrome	Characterized by parkinsonism + pronounced failure of the autonomic nervous system	MSA-A	No longer used

MSA = multiple system atrophy; OPCA = sporadic olivopontocerebellar atrophy.
From Gillman S, Wenning P, Low PA, et al: Second consensus statement of the diagnosis of multiple system atrophy. Neurology 2008;71:670–676.

sleep. **A normal laryngeal examination during wakefulness does not rule out the problem.**[36] The presence of stridor is associated with a poor prognosis (compared with MSA patients without stridor) and has traditionally been managed by tracheostomy. Recently, CPAP has been used to assist with stridor at night.[36,37] Patients with MSA often have OSA as well as worsening stridor during sleep. The etiology of stridor is controversial but is likely due to overactivity of the vocal cord adductors (close vocal cords) and underactivity of vocal cord abductors (posterior cricoarytenoid muscles [PCAs]). A neuropathy of the recurrent laryngeal nerves that innervate the PCA muscles may be involved. The syndrome of stridor in many patients is a dystonia rather than vocal cord paralysis. In others, there is complete vocal cord immobility. Sudden death has been reported in MSA patients with stridor even though treated with tracheostomy or CPAP.[37,38]

Central Apnea and Cheyne-Stokes Breathing Central apnea, nocturnal hypoventilation, and Cheyne-Stokes breathing (CSB) have been reported in MSA, especially in patients with prominent autonomic features.[39]

Treatment of MSA The treatment of MSA is mostly supportive. There is usually no or only a short initial response to LD. Patients with stridor can be treated with CPAP or tracheostomy (although sudden death can still occur at night).

Other Neurodegenerative Disorders

Fatal Familial Insomnia
Fatal familial insomnia (FFI) is a familial autosomal dominant prion disorder associated with the D178N mutation and methionine-methionine genotype at codon 129 in the prion protein gene on chromosome 20.[40,41] Of note, the D178N mutation and valine-valine genotype at codon 129 are associated with familial Creutzfeldt-Jakob disease (CJD).

Topography of Degeneration
Methionine-methionine genotype at codon 129 produces dorsomedial and anteroventral thalamic dysfunction, whereas the valine-valine genotype of CJD is associated with more general cortical involvement.

FFI Manifestations
FFI manifestations include insomnia, dementia, ataxia, dysarthria, dysautonomia, hallucinations, and hypersomnolence. The duration from onset to death varies from a few months to 4 years.

Diagnosis
The International Classification of Sleep Disorders, 2nd edition (ICSD-2), diagnostic criteria for FFI are listed in Box 31–10. The PSG in FFI reveals severe disruption of the sleep-wake cycle, loss of sleep spindles, reduction in stage N3 and stage R, as well as reduced sleep efficiency. REM sleep without atonia can occur.

Positron Emission Tomography Scan
Positron emission tomography (PET) reveals nearly absent or very low activity of the thalamus.

Summary
FFI should be considered in any patient with prominent sleep-wake disturbance and dementia. Treatment is supportive.

Sleep Disturbances in Stroke

Important points concerning stroke and sleep are listed in Box 31–11. SDB occurs in 50% to 70% of stroke patients (defined by apnea-hypopnea index [AHI] > 10/hr).[42–46] Central sleep apnea including CSB can be noted, especially soon after stroke, but tends to decrease with time. CSB in some chronic stroke patients is associated with heart failure.[45,46] Other patients with stroke and central sleep apnea have occult heart failure.[47] OSA is the most common

---

BOX 31–10

Fatal Familial Insomnia—Diagnostic Criteria
A. Complaint of insomnia is initially present and becomes progressively more severe.
B. Progressive autonomic hyperactivity with pyrexia, hypersalivation, hyperhydrosis, cardiac and respiratory dysfunction, tremor-like muscle activity.

C. Polysomnographic monitoring demonstrates
    i. Loss of sleep spindles.
    ii. Loss of slow wave sleep.
    iii. Dissociated REM sleep.

D. The disorder is not better explained by another sleep disorder, medical or neurologic disorder, mental disorder, medication use, or substance use disorder.
OR
E. A missense GAC to AAC mutation at codon 17 of the *PRNP* gene (d178N) co-segregating with the methionine polymorphism at codon 129 of the *PRNP* on the mutated allele is found (this mutation is absent in sporadic fatal familial insomnia).

REM = rapid eye movement.
Adapted from International Classification of Sleep Disorders, 2nd ed. Westchester, IL: American Academy of Sleep Medicine, 2005.

BOX 31–11

Stroke and Sleep Apnea
• OSA > CSA are common in patients after CVA. • If OSA is present, adequate treatment may improve outcome. • CPAP treatment is often challenging, especially in nonsleepy patients. • Incidence of stroke increased in men with mild to moderate OSA.

CSA = central sleep apnea; CVA = cerebrovascular accident; OSA = obstructive sleep apnea.

disorder following a cerebrovascular accident (CVA). OSA also tends to improve with time, but a substantial number of patients still have OSA at 2 to 3 months after stroke. However, the presence of sleep apnea following a CVA raises questions about the temporal relationship with stroke. Does brain damage from CVA cause sleep apnea or did sleep apnea precede the stroke? If so, is the presence of sleep apnea an independent risk factor for the development of a CVA? The Sleep Heart Health Study did show an increased risk of having a CVA (prevalence) if OSA is present.[48] In a recently published study, Redline and colleagues[49] evaluated the Sleep Heart Health data and found an increased risk for **incident** ischemic stroke in **men** with mild to moderate OSA. In this study, data were adjusted for a number of confounders that complicate the analysis including obesity. If there is a causal role for OSA in stroke, what are the mechanisms? OSA could predispose a patient to atherosclerosis, hypertension, and early morning hemoconcentration. These factors would increase the risk of stroke. During sleep apnea, there are increases in intracranial pressure (ICP)[50] and decreases in cerebral blood flow.[51] There is an increase in ICP with each apneic event and the rise tends to be correlated with the length of apnea. The increase in ICP is thought secondary to increases in central venous pressure, systemic pressure, and cerebral vasodilatation from rises in arterial partial pressure of carbon dioxide ($PaCO_2$) during events. Because cerebral perfusion is proportional to the mean arterial pressure (MAP)—ICP, increases in ICP may reduce perfusion pressure even if MAP also rises. Studies of cerebral blood flow velocity using Doppler monitoring have shown that flow velocity increases in early apnea, then has approximately a 25% fall below baseline at end apnea.[51]

There is some evidence that the presence of OSA in patients who have suffered a CVA is a poor prognostic sign regardless of whether OSA precedes or follows the CVA. Good and associates[52] found that the Barthel index (a multifaced scale measuring mobility and activities of daily living that is used to assess patients after stroke) was significantly lower in patients with OSA and CVA compared with those with no evidence of OSA after CVA. The presence of OSA was determined at discharge and the Barthel index was lower at 3 and 12 months in the OSA-CVA group. Martinez-Garcia and coworkers[53] found that CPAP treatment reduced mortality in patients found to have OSA following an ischemic stroke. This study suggests that physicians need to be more aggressive about ruling out OSA in patients with a recent CVA. Unfortunately, CPAP adherence following CVA is often very suboptimal.

After stroke, other sleep-wake disorders may impair recovery. Insomnia can occur but treatment should be cautious unless sleep apnea is excluded. Daytime sleepiness can occur even if sleep apnea is not present. Poststroke hypersomnia can be found after subcortical (caudate-putamen), thalamomesencephalic, medial pontomedullary, and cortical strokes. In one study, up to 12% of patients developed new-onset restless legs syndrome after stroke.[54] Pontine-tegmental strokes can lead to RBD.

CLINICAL REVIEW QUESTIONS

1. In which of the following dementias is RBD relatively uncommon?
   A. PSP.
   B. AD.
   C. PD.
   D. MSA.
   E. DLBD.

2. What neurodegenerative disorder is not an alpha synucleinopathy?
   A. PSP.
   B. MSA.
   C. PD.
   D. DLBD.

3. Which of these neurodegenerative disorders is frequently associated with stridor?
   A. PD.
   B. AD.
   C. PSP.
   D. DLBD.
   E. MSA.

4. In which of the following disorders is sundowning a prominent feature?
   A. AD.
   B. PD.
   C. PSP.
   D. MSA.

5. Which of the following is NOT a PD+ disorder?
   A. PSP.
   B. AD.
   C. MSA.
   D. DLB.

6. Which of the following is true about PD+ disorders compared with PD?
   A. There is a good response to LD.
   B. They have a slower downhill course than PD.
   C. They are very sensitive to dopamine blockers.
   D. Dementia is less common early.

7. Which of the following is true about patients with DLBD?
   A. Dopamine blockers can cause life-threatening rigidity.
   B. Dementia starts about 2 years after rigidity and loss of balance.
   C. Visual hallucinations occur in 5%.
   D. They respond well to LD.

Answers

1. **B.** RBD is uncommon in AD. RBD is very common in PD, DLB, and MSA and tends to precede other neurologic manifestations. RBD occurs in about 13% of PSP patients and tends to start concomitantly with other manifestations.

2. **A.** PSP is a tau disorder.

3. **E.** MSA is associated with stridor.

4. **A.** Sundowning is common in AD.

5. **B.** AD is not a PD+ disorder.

6. **C.** PD+ patients are very sensitive to dopamine blockers. They have a more rapid course than those with PD, they have minimal response to LD, and dementia can be prominent early (DLBD).

7. **A.** Dopamine blockers can cause life-threatening rigidity. Visual hallucinations are very common—up to 70%.

REFERENCES

1. Chokroverty S: Sleep and neurodegenerative diseases. Semin Neurol 2009;29:446–468.
2. Avidan AY: Sleep and neurological problems in the elderly. Sleep Med Clin 2006;1:273–292.
3. Hofman MA, Swaab DF: Living by the clock: the circadian pacemaker in older people. Ageing Res Rev 2006;5:33–51.
4. Wu Y, Swaab DF: Disturbance and strategies for reactivation of the circadian rhythm system in aging and Alzheimer's disease. Sleep Med 2007;8:623–636.
5. Zee PC, Vitiello MV: Circadian rhythm sleep disorder: irregular sleep-wake rhythm type. Sleep Med Clin 2009;4:213–218.
6. Singer C, Tractenberg RE, Kaye J, et al: A multicenter, placebo-controlled trial of melatonin of sleep disturbance in Alzheimer's disease. Sleep 2003;26:893–901.
7. Riemersma-van der Lek RF, Swaab DF, Twisk J: Effect of bright light and melatonin on cognitive and noncognitive function in elderly residents of group care facilities. JAMA 2008;299: 2647–2655.
8. Cooke JR, Ayalon L, Palmer BW, et al: Sustained use of CPAP slows deterioration of cognition, sleep, and mood in patients with Alzheimer's disease and obstructive sleep apnea: a preliminary study. J Clin Sleep Med 2009;5:305–309.
9. Birks J: Cholinesterase inhibitors for Alzheimer's disease. Cochrane Database Syst Rev 2006;1:CD005593.
10. Stahl SM, Markowitz JS, Papadopoulos G, Sadik K: Examination of nighttime sleep-related problems during double-blind, placebo-controlled trials of galantamine in patients with Alzheimer's disease. Curr Med Res Opin 2004;20: 517–524.
11. Gauthier S, Juby A, Dalziel W, et al, EXPLORE Investigators: Effects of rivastigmine on common symptomatology of Alzheimer's disease (EXPLORE). Curr Med Res Opin 2010;26: 1149–1160.
12. Grossberg G, Irwin P, Satlin A, et al: Rivastigmine in Alzheimer's disease: efficacy over two years. Am J Geriatr Psychiatry 2004;12:420–431.
13. Yeh SB, Yeh PY, Schenck CH: Rivastigmine-induced REM sleep behavior disorder (RBD) in a 88-year-old man with Alzheimer's disease. J Clin Sleep Med 2010;15:192–195.
14. Sixel-Döring F, Schweitzer M, Mollenhauer B, Trenkwalder C: Polysomnographic findings, video-based sleep analysis and sleep perception in progressive supranuclear palsy. Sleep Med 2009;10:407–415.
15. Arnulf I, Merino-Andreu M, Bloch F, et al: REM sleep behavior disorder and REM sleep without atonia in patients with progressive supranuclear palsy. Sleep 2005;28:349–354.
16. Jankovic J: "Parkinson's disease": Clinical features and diagnosis. J Neurol Neurosurg Psychiatry 2008;79:368–376.
17. Reichmann H: Clinical criteria for the diagnosis of Parkinson's disease. Neurodegener Dis 2010;7:284–290.
18. Olanow CW, Watts RL, Koller WC: An algorithm for the management of Parkinson's disease (2001): treatment guidelines. Neurology 2001;56:1–88.
19. Comella CL: Sleep disorders in Parkinson's disease. Curr Treat Options Neurol 2008;10:215–221.
20. Manni R, Terzaghi M, Repetto A, et al: Complex paroxysmal nocturnal behaviors in Parkinson's disease. Mov Disord 2010;25:985–990.
21. Thannickal TC, Lai YY, Siegel JM: Hypocretin (orexin) cell loss in Parkinson's disease. Brain 2007;130:1586–1595.
22. Morgenthaler TI, Kapur VK, Brown TM, et al, Standards of Practice Committee of the AASM: Practice parameters for the treatment of narcolepsy and other hypersomnias of central origin. Sleep 2007;30:1705–1711.
23. Ondo WG, Fayle F, Atassi F, Jankovic J: Modafinil for daytime somnolence in Parkinson's disease: double-blind, placebo-controlled parallel trial. J Neurol Neurosurg Psychiatry 2005;76: 1636–1639.
24. Hogl B, Saletu M, Brandauer E, et al: Modafinil for the treatment of daytime sleepiness in Parkinson's disease: a double-blind, randomized, crossover, placebo-controlled polygraphic trial. Sleep 2002;25:905–909.
25. Nieves AV, Lang AE: Treatment of excessive daytime sleepiness in patients with Parkinson's disease with modafinil. Clin Neuropharmacol 2002;25:111–114.
26. Lou JS, Dimitrov DM, Park BS, et al: Using modafinil to treat fatigue in Parkinson disease: a double-blind, placebo-controlled pilot study. Clin Neuropharmacol 2009;32:305–310.
27. Hauser RA, Walha MN, Anderson WM: Modafinil treatment of pramipexole associated somnolence. Mov Disord 2000; 15:1269–1271.
28. Barnes J, Connelly V, Wiggs L, et al: Sleep patterns in Parkinson's disease patients with visual hallucinations. Int J Neurosci 2010;120:564–569.
29. Parkinson Study Group: Low-dose clozapine for the treatment of drug induced psychosis in Parkinson's disease. N Engl J Med 1999;340:757–763.
30. Juri C, Chana P, Tapia J, et al: Quetiapine for insomnia in Parkinson disease: results from an open label trial. Clin Neuropharmacol 2005;28:185–187.
31. Trieschmann MM, Reichwein S, Simuni T: Donepezil for dementia in Parkinson's disease: a randomised, double-blind, placebo-controlled, crossover study. J Neurol Neurosurg Psychiatry 2005;76:934–939.
32. Emre M, Tsolaki M, Bonuccelli U, et al, on behalf of the 11018 Study Investigators: Memantine for patients with Parkinson's disease dementia or dementia with Lewy bodies: a randomised, double-blind, placebo-controlled trial. Lancet Neurol 2010; 9:969–977; Epub 2010;August 20.
33. McKeith JG, Galasko D, Kosaka K, et al: Consensus guideline for the clinical and pathological diagnosis of dementia with Lewy bodies: report of Consortium on DLB International Workshop. Neurology 1996;47:1113–1124.
34. Ferman T, Boeve B, Smith G, et al: Dementia with Lewy bodies may present as dementia with REM sleep behavior disorder without parkinsonism or hallucinations. J Int Neuropsychol Soc 2002;8:907–914.

35. Gillman S, Wenning P, Low PA, et al: Second consensus statement of the diagnosis of multiple system atrophy. Neurology 2008;71:670–676.

36. Iranzo A: Management of sleep-disordered breathing in multiple system atrophy. Sleep Med 2005;6:297–300.

37. Kuźniar TJ, Morgenthaler TI, Prakash UBS, et al: Effects of continuous positive airway pressure on stridor in multiple system atrophy—sleep laryngoscopy. J Clin Sleep Med 2009; 5:65–67.

38. Silber MH, Levine S: Stridor and death in multiple system atrophy. Mov Disord 2000;15;699–714.

39. Sadaoka T, Kakitsub N, Fujiwara Y, et al: Sleep-related breathing disorders in patients with multiple system atrophy and vocal fold palsy. Sleep 1996;19:479–484.

40. Lugaresi E, Tobler I, Montagna P, et al: Fatal familial insomnia and dysautonomia with selective degeneration of thalamic nuclei. N Engl J Med 1986;315:997–1003.

41. Montagna P, Gambetti P, Cortelli P, Lugaresi E: Familial and sporadic fatal insomnia. Lancet Neurol 2003;2:167–176.

42. Hermann DM, Bassetti CL: Sleep-related breathing and sleep wake disturbances in ischemic stroke. Neurology 2009;73: 1313–1322.

43. Turkington P, Bamfor J, Wanklyn P, et al: Prevalence and predictors of upper airway obstruction in the first 24 hours after acute stroke. Stroke 2002;33:2037–2041.

44. Para O, Arboix A, Bechichi S, et al: Time course of sleep-related breathing disorders in first-ever stroke or transient ischemic attack. Am J Respir Crit Care Med 2000;161:375–380.

45. Siccoli MM, Valko PO, Hermann DM, Bassetti CL: Central periodic breathing during sleep in 74 patients with acute ischemic stroke—neurogenic and cardiogenic factors. J Neurol 2008;255:1687–1692.

46. Hermann DM, Siccoli M, Kirov P, et al: Central periodic breathing during sleep in ischemic stroke. Stroke 2007;38: 1082–1084.

47. Nopmaneejumruslers C, Kaneko Y, Hajek V, et al: Cheyne-Stokes respiration in stroke: relationship to hypocapnia and occult cardiac dysfunction. Am J Respir Crit Care Med 2005;171:1048–1052.

48. Shahar E, Whitney CW, Redline S, et al: Sleep-disordered breathing and cardiovascular disease: cross-sectional results of the Sleep Heart Health Study. Am J Respir Crit Care Med 2001;163:19–25.

49. Redline S, Yenokyan G, Gottlieb DJ, et al: Obstructive sleep apnea-hypopnea and incident stroke: the Sleep Heart Health study. Am J Respir Crit Care Med 2010;182:269–277.

50. Sugita Y, Susami I, Yoshio T, et al: Marked episodic elevation of cerebral spinal fluid pressure during nocturnal sleep in patients with sleep apnea hypersomnia syndrome. Electroencephalogr Clin Neurophysiol 1985;60:214–219.

51. Balfors EM: Impairment of cerebral perfusion during obstructive sleep apneas. Am J Respir Crit Care Med 1994;150: 1587–1591.

52. Good DC, Henkle JQ, Gelber D, et al: Sleep disordered breathing and poor functional outcome after stroke. Stroke 1996; 27:252–259.

53. Martinez-Garcia MA, Soler-Cataluna JJ, Ejarque-Martinez L, et al: Continuous positive airway pressure treatment reduces mortality in patients with ischemic stroke and obstructive sleep apnea: a five-year follow-up. Am J Respir Crit Care Med 2008;180:36–41.

54. Lee SJ, Kim JS, Song IU, et al: Post-stroke restless legs syndrome and lesion location. Anatomical considerations. Mov Disord 2008;24:77–84.

Medications Used to Treat Alzheimer's Disease

	STARTING DOSE	MAINTENANCE DOSE	COMMENTS
Cholinesterase Inhibitors			
Donepezil	5 mg po qd Increase after 4–6 wk	10 mg qd	Given in AM
Rivastigmine			
Patch	4.6 mg/24 hr	Increase to 9.5 mg/24 hr after 4 wk	Rash, fewer side effects than pill
Pill	1.5 mg bid	Increase in 1.5-mg increments bid every 2–4 wk until 6 mg bid	Give with meals
Galantamine			Give with meals
Immediate release	4 mg bid	Increase in 4-mg increments monthly until 12 mg bid	
Extended release	8 mg qd	Increase in 8-mg increments monthly until 24 mg daily	
Neuroprotective			

Memantine (Namendia) an NMDA receptor antagonist.
Can cause hallucinations and dizziness (most common side effect).
Can be used with cholinesterase inhibitors.

NMDA = *N*-methyl-D-aspartate.

Glossary

A

AASM American Academy of Sleep Medicine.

AASM scoring manual The AASM Manual for the Scoring of Sleep and Associated Events. Iber C, Ancoli-Israel S, Chesson AL, Quan SF. Westchester, IL, American Academy of Sleep Medicine, 2007.

Adaptive servoventilation A mode of positive airway pressure that varies pressure support (IPAP-EPAP) to stabilize ventilation (or flow). ASV is used for Cheyne-Stokes breathing or complex sleep apnea.

Advanced sleep phase syndrome (ASPS) Characterized by early sleep onset and early wake time relative to societal (clock) norms in the external world.

Alpha activity EEG activity of 8–13 Hz (see Alpha rhythm).

Alpha-delta sleep Prominent alpha activity occurring during stage N3 sleep.

Alpha rhythm 8- to 13-Hz activity recorded over the occipital region during eye closure and attenuated with eye opening.

Alpha sleep Prominent alpha activity occurring during NREM sleep.

Apnea Absence of air flow (≥90% reduction) at the nose and mouth for 10 seconds or longer (using oronasal thermal sensor or CPAP flow).

Apnea-hypopnea index (AHI) The number of apneas and hypopneas per hour of sleep.

Arousal In NREM sleep, an arousal is an abrupt shift in EEG frequency including alpha, theta, and/or frequencies greater than 16 Hz (but not spindles) that lasts at least 3 seconds with at least 10 seconds of stable sleep preceding the change. Scoring of an arousal during REM sleep requires a concurrent increase in the submental EMG that lasts at least 1 second.

ASDA American Sleep Disorders Association, now called the American Academy of Sleep Medicine.

AutoCPAP (APAP) Autoadjusting or autotitrating CPAP units that deliver the lowest required pressure at any time needed to maintain upper airway patency.

Automatisms Involuntary or unconscious movements often described as purposeless. They may mimic purposeful behaviors but are of no benefit.

B

Beta activity EEG activity greater than 13 Hz.

Bilevel positive airway pressure (BPAP) Method of ventilation allowing separately adjustable pressure levels in inspiration (inspiratory positive airway pressure [IPAP]) and expiration (expiratory positive airway pressure [EPAP]).

Biocalibration Recording of voluntary maneuvers during wakefulness at the beginning of polysomnography to determine if the EEG, EOG, chin and leg EMG, ECG, airflow, respiratory effort, and oximetry signals are adequate. Electrodes of sensors are replaced or repositioned if necessary. Biocalibrations are useful to determine if alpha rhythm is produced with eye closure and to note the appearance of eyes open wakefulness.

Bruxism Clinching or grinding of the teeth (see Chapter 12 for scoring rules).

C

C₃, C₄ Central EEG electrode on the right (left) side of the head.

Capnogram Tracing of exhaled PCO_2 versus time. The plateau of the deflection from each exhalation is the end-tidal PCO_2 (an estimate of the arterial PCO_2).

Cataplexy Sudden loss of muscle tone (especially antigravity muscles) at moments of high emotion (e.g., surprise, laughter, fear) with preservation of consciousness, characteristic of narcolepsy.

Central apnea Apnea associated with an absence of respiratory effort.

Cheyne-Stokes breathing Crescendo-decrescendo pattern of breathing with central apneas or hypopneas at the nadir.

Chronic obstructive pulmonary disease (COPD) Chronic bronchitis, emphysema, or a mixture.

Circadian rhythm sleep disorder (CRSD) Pattern of sleep disturbance due to alterations of the circadian timing system or misalignment between endogenous circadian rhythm and exogenous factors (clock time, societal demands) that affects timing or duration of sleep.

Confusional arousals A parasomnia characterized by confusion after a spontaneous or forced arousal from sleep. Confusional arousals tend to occur out of stage N3 sleep. In contrast to sleep terrors, there is no autonomic hyperactivity, signs of fear, or blood-curdling scream.

Continuous positive airway pressure (CPAP) Maintenance of positive airway pressure during inspiration and expiration.

Core body temperature minimum (CBTmin) Minimum core body temperature occurs about 2 hours before habitual wake time, a marker of circadian phase.

CPAP flow The flow signal from the positive airway pressure device utilized in polysomnography (also known as PAP flow).

D

Delayed sleep phase syndrome (DSPS) Characterized by delayed sleep onset and final wake-time relative to societal (clock) norms in the external world.

Delta activity EEG activity at less than 4 Hz. In human sleep staging, slow wave activity (SWA) is defined as a frequency 0.5 to 2 Hz with greater than 75 μV peak-to-peak amplitude (See Slow wave activity).

Derivation A set of two electrodes and the voltage difference between them (e.g., C_4-M_1).

Desaturation Fall in arterial oxygen saturation from baseline, usually a 4% or greater decrease.

Dim light melatonin onset (DLMO) The time that serum melatonin starts to increase above daytime levels under dim light conditions. The DLMO occurs about 2 to 3 hours before habitual bedtime or 7 hours before CBTmin and is a marker of circadian timing (see Chapter 26).

Diurnal Pertaining to daytime.

E

E₁, E₂ Left and right electrode positions to recorded eye movements. The recommended derivations are E_1-M_2 and E_2-M_2. E_1 is 1 cm below the left outer canthus and E_2 is 1 cm above the right outer canthus (see Chapter 1).

Early morning awakening Final awakening earlier than expected; characteristic of depression, sleep-maintenance insomnia, or the advanced sleep phase syndrome.

Electroencephalogram (EEG) Recording of brain electrical activity.

Electromyogram (EMG) Recording of the electrical activity of a muscle. In routine sleep monitoring, surface electrodes monitor EMG activity in the chin area (three electrodes) and the right and left anterior tibialis muscle (see Chapters 1 and 7).

Electro-oculogram (EOG) Recording of the electrical activity generated during eye movements. In some texts the term is spelled without a hyphen (electrooculogram).

EPAP Expiratory positive airway pressure.

Epoch A period of time usually corresponding to 30 seconds (one page of recording at a paper speed of 10 mm/sec).

Epworth Sleepiness Scale (ESS) A score from 0 to 24 of the propensity to fall asleep in eight normal situations (see Chapter 14). Normal is 10 or less, and 24 is the maximal ESS score (the most sleepy).

F

F₃, F₄ Frontal electrodes over the right and left frontocentral portions of the brain.

FEV₁/FVC Ratio of the forced expiratory volume in 1 second to the forced vital capacity. Reduced in obstructive airway disease. In this text, normal is ≥0.70 and 90% of predicted.

Forced expiratory volume in 1 second (FEV₁) The volume of air in liters exhaled in the first 1 second of a maximal forced vital capacity maneuver. In this text, normal is assumed to be 80% to 120% of predicted.

Forced vital capacity (FVC) Volume of air in liters exhaled from maximal inhalation (total lung capacity) to residual volume (maximal exhalation) during a forced maneuver. In this text, normal is assumed to be 80% to 120% of predicted.

H

Hypnagogic An event occurring on transition from wake to sleep.

Hypnagogic hallucination Vivid imagery at sleep onset; a feature of narcolepsy in which REM periods occur at sleep onset (see Chapter 24).

Hypnic jerk (sleep start) Brief total body jerk at sleep onset.

Hypnogram A graphical overview of the cyclic nature of sleep (see Chapter 6).

Hypnopompic An event occurring on transition from sleep to wakefulness.

Hypnopompic hallucination Vivid imagery at the transition from sleep to wake (see Chapter 24).

Hypocretins Two peptides, Hcrt 1 and Hcrt 2 (also known as orexins A and B), that are secreted by lateral posterior hypothalamic neurons. Hypocretins project to many brain areas involved with the control of sleep and wake. CSF hypocretin 1 is absent or very low in 90% to 95% of patients with narcolepsy + cataplexy (see Chapters 7 and 24).

Hypopnea Reduction in air flow for 10 seconds or longer. Definitions vary (see Chapter 9).

I

ICSD-1, ICSD-2 International Classification of Sleep Disorders, 1st and 2nd editions.

Interictal Refers to transient focal or generalized discharges between seizure events.

K

K complex A well-delineated large-amplitude biphasic complex consisting of a negative sharp wave (upward deflection) followed by a positive component (downward) standing out from the background EEG, with a total duration of 0.5 seconds or longer, usually maximal in the frontal derivations.

K complex with arousal An arousal is associated with a K complex when it commences no more than 1 second after termination of the K complex.

L

Laser-assisted uvuloplasty (LAUP) Palatoplasty performed with a laser.

Left outer canthus (LOC) Outer corner of the left eye (formerly left eye electrode placed slightly lateral and below the LOC).

Low-amplitude mixed frequency activity (LAMF) Low amplitude, predominantly 4 to 7 Hz activity.

Low chin EMG tone (REM level) Baseline chin EMG activity in the chin derivation no higher than in any other sleep stage and usually the lowest level of the entire recording (see Chapter 3).

M

M_1, M_2 Left and right mastoid electrodes (formerly A_1 and A_2). Frontal, central, occipital, E_1, and E_2 electrodes are referred to the mastoid electrodes (see Chapter 1).

Maintenance of wakefulness test (MWT) Test to determine the ability to stay awake (see Chapter 14).

Major body movement (MBM) Movement and muscle artifact obscuring the EEG for more than half of the epoch to the extent that the sleep stage cannot be determined (see Chapter 3 for scoring rules for epochs with a MBM).

Mean sleep latency (MSL) The mean of sleep latencies recorded during naps over the course of a multiple sleep latency test or a maintenance of wakefulness test.

Mixed apnea Apnea composed of an initial central part followed by an obstructive component.

Montage The particular arrangement of a number of derivations that are displayed simultaneously in a polysomnogram.

Movement arousal Defined in the R&K scoring manual as an increase in the chin EMG accompanied by a change in pattern on any additional channel. For EEG channels, qualifying changes include a decrease in amplitude, paroxysmal high-voltage activity, or an increase in alpha activity. Not used in the AASM scoring manual.

Movement time (MT) The total duration of epochs in which the sleep stage is indeterminant owing to movement artifact in the EEG. Not used in the AASM scoring manual (see Major body movement).

Multiple sleep latency test (MSLT) Test to determine the mean sleep latency during daytime naps as an objective measure of daytime sleepiness and the presence of REM sleep without 15 minutes of sleep onset (sleep-onset REM periods). A diagnosis of narcolepsy requires 2 or more SOREMPs (see Chapter 14).

N

Nasal pressure Used to detect airflow = $K \times flow^2$, where K is a constant (see Chapter 7).

Non–rapid eye movement (NREM) sleep Sleep stages N1, N2, N3.

O

O_1, O_2 Occipital EEG electrode on the left and right side of the head.

Obesity-hypoventilation syndrome (OHS) Daytime hypoventilation (hypercapnia) not secondary to lung disease in an obese patient, usually accompanied by severe obstructive sleep apnea.

Obstructive apnea Apnea with persistent respiratory effort.

Obstructive sleep apnea syndrome (OSAS) Syndrome characterized by obstructive and mixed apnea and hypopneas. In adults, the diagnostic criteria include an AHI of 5/hr or greater with symptoms or 15/hr with or without symptoms.

Overlap syndrome Obstructive sleep apnea plus chronic obstructive pulmonary disease (OSA + COPD).

P

Paradoxical insomnia The patient shows a **consistent mismatch between objective findings** from PSG or actigraphy and **subjective sleep estimates** derived from either sleep report or sleep diary (see Chapter 25).

Parasomnia A condition associated with or occurring from sleep. Disorders of arousal or partial arousal. Examples include sleepwalking, night terrors, and REM sleep behavior disorder (see Chapter 28).

Periodic limb (leg) movement–arousal index (PLM-arousal index) Number of PLMs associated with arousal per hour of sleep.

Periodic limb movement disorder (PLMD) A disorder of sleep disturbance resulting in a sleep complaint (insomnia or, less often, excessive daytime sleepiness) secondary to PLMS when other causes have been ruled out. A diagnosis of RLS excludes a diagnosis of PLMD. A diagnosis of PLMD requires a PLMS index greater than 5/hr in children or 15/hr in adults. However, the normal range of the PLMS index is not well defined and can be higher than 15/hr in normal elderly individuals (see Chapter 23).

Periodic limb (leg) movement in sleep (PLMS) Leg movements characterized by foot flexion, big toe extension, and partial flexion at hip and knee. To be considered part of a PLMS series (e.g., a PLM separately by ≥5 and ≤90 seconds from onset to onset of consecutive movements), a leg movement must be 0.5 to 10 seconds in duration and must occur in a group (sequence) of four or more movements (see Chapters 12 and 23).

Periodic limb (leg) movement in sleep index (PLMS index or PLMSI) Number of movements per hour of sleep.

Phase response curve (PRC) A curve characterizing the magnitude and direction of the shift of the internal clock (circadian rhythm) induced by light (or exogenous melatonin) as a function of the timing of light relative to the baseline circadian rhythm (relative to the nadir in body temperature).

Phasic REM sleep REM sleep in which rapid eye movements are present.

Polysomnography The detailed monitoring of sleep.

Popping artifact High-voltage artifact caused by temporary disconnection of electrodes from the skin (see Chapter 4).

Psychophysiologic insomnia Conditioned sleep difficulty falling asleep in bed at the desired time (the bedroom is a stimulus for arousal), heightened arousal and difficulty relaxing in bed, excessive focus on sleep, and ability to sleep better away from home.

R

R&K The sleep staging criteria of Rechtschaffen and Kales, published in A Manual of Standardized Terminology Techniques and Scoring System for Sleep Stages of Human Sleep. Los Angeles: UCLA, Brain Information Service/Brain Research Institute, 1968.

Rapid eye movement density Number of eye movements per time in REM sleep. Normally highest during the last REM peiods of the night.

Rapid eye movement sleep Stage R (see Chapters 3 and 5 for scoring rules).

Rapid eye movement sleep behavior disorder (RBD) A parasomnia occurring from REM sleep associated with REM without atonia and dream enactment often with body movements and violent behavior (see Chapter 28).

Rapid eye movements (REMs) Conjugate, irregular, sharply peaked eye movements with an initial deflection lasting less than 500 msec. REMs can be seen during eyes open wake or stage R.

Recording time; time in bed (TIB) Total time of sleep monitoring from lights out to lights on.

REM latency Time from sleep onset to the start of stage R.

Respiratory arousal index (RAI) Arousals secondary to an apnea or hypopnea, and in some sleep laboratoies, respiratory effort–related arousals.

Respiratory disturbance index (RDI) Definitions vary, RDI = AHI, RDI = AHI + RERA index, RDI = apneas + hypopneas/monitoring time (Centers for Medicare and Medicaid Services definition used for home sleep testing). The RDI was not defined in the AASM scoring manual OR in the ICSD-2.

Respiratory effort–related arousal (RERA) An event characterized by an arousal following a period of increased respiratory effort lasting 10 seconds or longer that does not qualify as an obstructive apnea or hypopnea. Increased respiratory effort is detected by increased esophageal pressure deflections or flattening of the nasal pressure signal (see Chapter 8).

Respiratory inductance plethysmography (RIP) A method of detecting chest and abdominal movement secondary to changes in the inductance (a component of impedance) of bands around those regions. Used to detect respiratory effort (see Chapters 7 and 8).

Restless legs syndrome (RLS) Syndrome marked by URGE: urge to move legs, rest makes symptoms worse, gets better with movement (partial temporary improvement), and worse in the evening. The urge to move is often associated with uncomfortable sensation in the legs that can be temporarily relieved by movement.

Right outer canthus (ROC) Right outer corner of the eye. The ROC electrode is placed lateral to the ROC and slightly above the eye. The ROC terminology and electrode placement has been replaced by the E_2 electrode (AASM scoring manual).

S

Saw-tooth waves Trains of sharply contoured or triangular, often serrated, 2- to 6-Hz waves maximal over the central regions, characteristically seen during stage R, often before a burst of eye movements.

Sharp wave Duration 70 to 200 msec.

Sleep architecture The relative amounts of the different sleep stages composing sleep and timing of sleep cycles (see Chapter 6).

Sleep efficiency Usually defined as total sleep time × 100/time in bed.

Sleep hygiene Conditions and practices that promote continuous and effective sleep.

Sleep latency Time from lights out (statistic of monitoring period) to the first epoch of any stage of sleep.

Sleep-maintenance insomnia Difficulty maintaining sleep; frequent awakenings.

Sleep-onset insomnia Difficulty falling asleep (usually sleep latency > 30 min).

Sleep paralysis Inability to move while still awake at sleep onset (hypnagogic) or at the end of a sleep period (hypnopompic). Sleep paralysis can occur in normal individuals but is one of the symptoms of narcolepsy. Episodes of sleep paralysis may be associated with hallucinations.

Sleep period time (SPT) Time from sleep onset until the final awakening. Not used in the AASM scoring manual.

Sleep spindle EEG activity of 11 to 16 Hz (most commonly 12–14 Hz) with a duration of 0.5 second or greater, usually maximal in central derivations, characteristic of stage N2 (can also occur in stage N3) (see Chapters 1 and 3).

Sleep stages Stage N1 (formerly stage 1), stage N2 (formerly stage 2), stage N3 (formerly stage 3 + stage 4), and stage R (formerly stage REM) (see Chapters 3 and 5 for scoring criteria).

Sleep starts (hypnic jerk) Brief whole body jerk at sleep onset.

Sleep state misperception (see Paradoxical insomnia).

Sleep terrors A parasomnia characterized by sudden awakening from NREM sleep (usually stage N3 in children, but any stage of NREM sleep in adults) with a cry or scream, confusion, and autonomic hyperactivity.

Sleepwalking (somnambulism) Characterized by a partial awakening from NREM sleep (classically from stage N3 in children, but also N1 and N2 in adults) with complex movements including walking.

Slow rolling eye movement or slow eye movements (SEMs) Smooth, undulating eye movements occurring during drowsy wakefulness and stage N1 sleep.

Slow wave activity (SWA) Waves of frequency 0.5 to 2 Hz with a peak-to-peak amplitude greater than 75 µV. The amount of SWA determines whether stage N2 or N3 is present. Score stage N3 when SWA is 20% or higher.

Slow waves (delta waves) EEG waves with a frequency of 1 to 4 Hz (see Slow wave activity).

SOREMPs Sleep-onset rapid eye movement periods. Stage R begins 15 minutes or less (clock time) after sleep onset.

Spike An EEG transient with a pointed peak and a duration of 20 to 70 msec.

Suprachiasmatic nucleus (SCN) Major circadian pacemaker in humans (see Chapter 27).

Sweat artifact Slow undulations in EEG and EOG tracings secondary to sweat (see Chapter 4).

T

Ten-twenty system An international standard for the placement of EEG electrodes in which spacing of electrodes is 10% or 20% of the distance between landmarks on the head (see Chapters 1 and 27).

Theta activity EEG activity at 4 to 7 Hz.

Three-minute rule An R&K scoring rule for determining how long stage N2 could continue without a sleep spindle or K complex. Not used in the AASM scoring manual.

Time in bed (TIB) Recording time – total monitoring time, from lights out to lights on.

Tonic REM sleep REM sleep in which rapid eye movements are absent.

Total sleep time (TST) Total minutes of stages N1, N2, N3, and R.

Transient muscle activity (TMA) Short irregular bursts of EMG activity usually with a duration less than 0.25 seconds superimposed on low EMG tone during stage R. The activity may be seen in the chin or anterior tibial EMG derivations. Formerly called phasic activity.

U

Upper airway resistance syndrome (UARS) Syndrome characterized by daytime sleepiness secondary to frequent arousals related to increased respiratory effort during periods of high upper airway resistance (narrowing) without an abnormal amount of frank apnea or hypopnea. Most authorities believe it is simply a mild form of OSA.

Uvulopalatopharyngoplasty (UPPP) An upper airway surgery for sleep apnea and snoring. The uvula, a portion of the soft palate, and excess pharyngeal tissues are removed.

V

Vertex sharp wave A negative sharp wave (upward deflection) with highest amplitude in derivations containing electrodes near the vertex (e.g., C_z) characteristic of stage N1 (typically near transition to stage N2). According to the AASM scoring manual, vertex sharp waves have a duration less than 500 msec (usually sharp waves are defined as <200 msec).

W

Wake after sleep onset (WASO) Wake after sleep onset during the time in bed (wake from sleep onset to lights on).

Note: Page numbers followed by f refer to figures; page numbers followed by t refer to tables; page numbers followed by b refer to boxes.

Printed and bound by CPI Group (UK) Ltd, Croydon, CR0 4YY

03/10/2024

01040303-0008